Textbook of

Clinical

Biochemistry

Textbook of
Clinical
Biochemistry

Ramnik Sood MD (Pathology), Gold Medalist

Consultant Pathologis⁻/Molecular Pathologist
Speciality Diagnostic Labs, Goa, India

Specialist A, Consultant
Laboratory Medicine/Histopathology/Cytopathology
United Arab Emirates

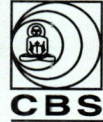

CBS

CBS Publishers & Distributors Pvt Ltd

New Delhi • Bengaluru • Chennai • Kochi • Kolkata • Mumbai

Bhopal • Bhubaneswar • Hyderabad • Jharkhand • Nagpur • Patna • Pune • Uttarakhand • Dhaka (Bangladesh)

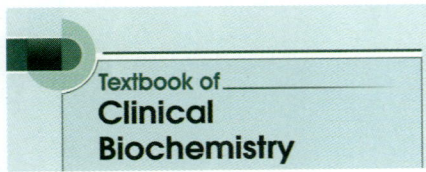

Textbook of
**Clinical
Biochemistry**

ISBN: 978-93-87964-26-6

First Edition: 2019

Published by Satish Kumar Jain and produced by Varun Jain for

CBS Publishers & Distributors Pvt Ltd
4819/XI Prahlad Street, 24 Ansari Road, Daryaganj, New Delhi 110 002, India.
Ph: 23289259, 23266861, 23266867   Fax: 011-23243014   Website: www.cbspd.com
e-mail: delhi@cbspd.com; cbspubs@airtelmail.in.

Corporate Office: 204 FIE, Industrial Area, Patparganj, Delhi 110 092
Ph: 4934 4934   Fax: 4934 4935   e-mail: publishing@cbspd.com; publicity@cbspd.com

Branches

- **Bengaluru:** Seema House 2975, 17th Cross, K.R. Road,
  Banasankari 2nd Stage, Bengaluru 560 070, Karnataka
  Ph: +91-80-26771678/79   Fax: +91-80-26771680   e-mail: bangalore@cbspd.com
- **Chennai:** 7, Subbaraya Street, Shenoy Nagar, Chennai 600 030, Tamil Nadu
  Ph: +91-44-26680620, 26681266   Fax: +91-44-42032115   e-mail: chennai@cbspd.com
- **Kochi:** 42/1325, 1326, Power House Road, Opp KSEB Power House,
  Ernakulam 682 018, Kochi, Kerala
  Ph: +91-484-4059061-65   Fax: +91-484-4059065   e-mail: kochi@cbspd.com
- **Kolkata:** 6/B, Ground Floor, Rameswar Shaw Road, Kolkata-700 014, West Bengal
  Ph: +91-33-22891126, 22891127, 22891128   e-mail: kolkata@cbspd.com
- **Mumbai:** 83-C, Dr E Moses Road, Worli, Mumbai-400018, Maharashtra
  Ph: +91-22-24902340/41   Fax: +91-22-24902342   e-mail: mumbai@cbspd.com

Representatives

• **Bhopal**	0-8319310552	• **Bhubaneswar**	0-9911037372	• **Hyderabad**	0-9885175004
• **Jharkhand**	0-9811541605	• **Nagpur**	0-9021734563	• **Patna**	0-9334159340
• **Pune**	0-9623451994	• **Uttarakhand**	0-9716462459	• **Dhaka (Bangladesh)**	01912-003485

Printed at: Goyal Offset Printers, GT Karnal Road, Industrial Area, Delhi, India *to*

*All avid readers hungry for
more and more knowledge about less and less*

Ramnik Sood

Foreword

Laboratory medicine is fundamental to practice multidisciplinary healthcare. An efficient laboratory, providing accurate and precise results of measured analytes with a meaningful interpretation in a reasonable turnaround time is a vital to patient centered approach.

One of the most dominant components of laboratory medicine is clinical biochemistry. Earliest to arrive it still continues to be at the forefront of advances in the field of laboratory medicine. The new age clinical chemistry using high throughput machines backed by powerful computational techniques have transformed the practice of biochemistry bringing in revolutionary changes to patient care. Nucleic acid chemistry and field of molecular medicine are a gift of basic and advanced clinical biochemistry. The expanding horizon of clinical chemistry necessitates a fresh look at theory, practice, and interpretation of results in the light of clinical details. The current project is an effort to create a learning experience that amalgamates analytic principles, techniques, and the correlation of results with disease states.

One should not be surprised to learn that the delivery of healthcare has been undergoing major transformation for several decades. The laboratory medicine has been transformed in innumerable ways as well. These changes have impacted the laboratory professionals in a very positive manner. Today, the students' greatest asset is their mental skills and their ability to acquire and apply knowledge. The laboratory professionals are now considered knowledge workers, and a student's ability to successfully become such knowledge workers depends on their instruction and exposure to quality education.

There are increased emphasis on improving the quality of patient care, individual patient outcomes, financial responsibility, and total quality management. Now, more than ever, clinical laboratorians need to be concerned with disease correlations, interpretations, problem solving, quality assurances, and cost-effectiveness. They need to know not only how of tests but also more importantly what, why, and when. This book shall help you develop that faculty.

It is a privilege and an honor to have been invited to take part in such a quality endeavor as this exceptional textbook. I find it truly a useful asset not only to medical laboratory scientists but also to medical and paramedical healthcare workers undergoing training. In addition, it will serve as a reference book in any medical laboratory and resource material for training instructors as well.

I wish the author and the publisher a great success.

Dr Anurag Mehta
MD (Pathology), Gold Medalist
Former Professor and Head
Department of Pathology/Laboratory Medicine Armed
Forces Medical College, Pune, India

Currently Director
Laboratory and Transfusion Services Molecular
Diagnostics, Research and Bio-repository
Rajiv Gandhi Cancer Institute and Research Center
Delhi, India

Preface

Clinical biochemistry (also known as medical biochemistry or chemical pathology) is the laboratory service absolutely essential for medical practice or branch of laboratory medicine in which chemical and biochemical methods are applied to the study of disease. The results of the biochemical investigations carried out in a clinical biochemistry laboratory will help the clinicians to determine the diseases (diagnosis) and for follow-up of the treatment/recovery from the illness (prognosis).

Biochemical investigations are used extensively in medicine, both in relation to diseases that have an obvious metabolic basis (e.g. diabetes mellitus, hypothyroidism) and those in which biochemical changes are a consequence of the disease (e.g. kidney failure, malabsorption). The principal uses of biochemical investigations are for diagnosis, prognosis, monitoring, and screening.

Understanding these principles are a necessary requirement of the knowledge worker in the laboratory medicine. This significant professional role provides effective laboratory services that will improve medical-decision making and thus patient safety while reducing medical errors.

I sincerely hope that clinical biochemistry specialist and educators find this book to be a worthy and useful tool to support their professional activities.

I am thankful to Mr YN Arjuna Senior Vice President—Publishing, editiorial and Publicity, Mrs Ritu Chawla AGM—Production, Mr Parmod Kumar, Mrs Baljeet Kaur, and all publishing team of CBS Publishers & Distributors, New Delhi, for their excellent inputs in shaping the book to its present form.

I welcome comments, suggestions, and corrections from the readers.

Ramnik Sood
MD (Pathology), Gold Medalist

Contents

Biochemical Investigations in Clinical Medicine

INTRODUCTION

Clinical pathology (also known as **clinical chemistry** or **chemical biochemistry)** is a laboratory service absolutely essential for medical practice or branch of laboratory medicine in which chemical and biochemical methods are applied to the study of disease. The results of the biochemical investigations carried out in a clinical chemistry laboratory will help the clinicians to determine the diseases (diagnosis) and for follow-up of the treatment/recovery from the illness (prognosis).

A central function of the **clinical pathology** or **chemical pathology** laboratory is to provide biochemical information for the management of patients. Such information will be of value only if it is accurate and relevant, and if its significance is appreciated by the clinician so that it can be used appropriately to guide clinical decision-making. This chapter examines how biochemical data are acquired and how they should be used.

Biochemical investigations are used extensively in medicine, both in relation to diseases that have an obvious metabolic basis (e.g. diabetes mellitus, hypothyroidism) and those in which biochemical changes are a consequence of the disease (e.g. kidney failure, malabsorption). The principal uses of biochemical investigations are for diagnosis, prognosis, monitoring, and screening (Fig. 1.1).

DIAGNOSIS

1. **Clinical diagnosis** based on signs, symptoms, and laboratory findings during life.
2. **Differential diagnosis** the determination of which one of several diseases may be producing the symptoms.
3. **Medical diagnosis** based on information from sources, such as findings from a physical examination,

interview with the patient or family or both, medical history of the patient and family, and clinical findings as reported by laboratory tests and radiologic studies.

4. **Physical diagnosis** based on information obtained by inspection, palpation, percussion, and auscultation.
5. **Diagnosis-related groups** (DRG) a system of classification or grouping of patients according to medical diagnosis for purposes of paying hospitalization costs.

Frequently, a confident diagnosis can be made on the basis of the history combined with the findings on examination. Failing this, it is usually possible to formulate a differential diagnosis, in effect a short list of possible diagnoses. Biochemical and other investigations can then be used to distinguish between them.

Investigations may be selected to help either confirm or refute a diagnosis, and it is important that the clinician appreciates how useful the chosen investigations are for these purposes. Making a diagnosis, even if incomplete, such as a diagnosis of hypoglycemia without knowing its cause, may allow treatment to be initiated.

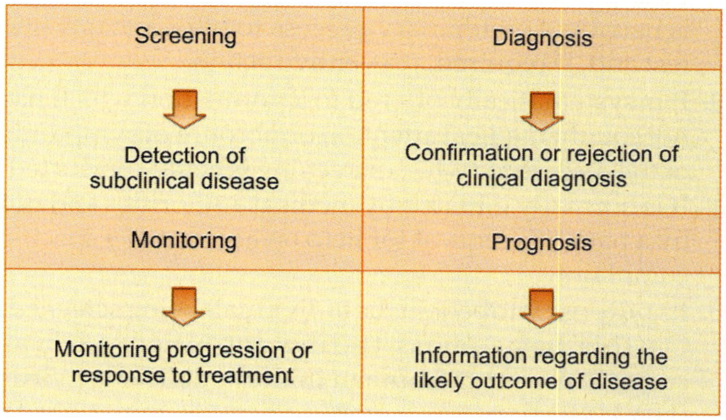

Screening	Diagnosis
⬇	⬇
Detection of subclinical disease	Confirmation or rejection of clinical diagnosis
Monitoring	Prognosis
⬇	⬇
Monitoring progression or response to treatment	Information regarding the likely outcome of disease

Fig. 1.1: The principal functions of biochemical tests

PROGNOSIS

A forecast of the probable course and outcome of an attack of disease and the prospects of recovery as indicated by the nature of the disease and the symptoms of the case. For example, serial measurements of plasma creatinine concentration in progressive kidney disease are used to indicate when dialysis may be required. Investigations can also indicate the risk of developing a particular condition. For example, the risk of coronary artery disease increases with increasing plasma cholesterol concentration. However, such risks are calculated from epidemiological data and cannot give a precise prediction for a particular individual.

MONITORING

A major use of biochemical investigations is to follow the course of an illness and to monitor the effects of treatment. To do this, there must be a suitable analyte, for instance glycated hemoglobin in patients with diabetes mellitus. Biochemical investigations can also be used to detect complications of treatment, such as hypokalemia during treatment with diuretics, and are extensively used to screen for possible drug toxicity, particularly in trials, but also in some cases when a drug is in established use.

SCREENING

Screening is a strategy used in a population to identify an unrecognized disease in individuals without signs or symptoms, *to identify individuals at sufficient risk of a specific disorder to benefit from further investigation or direct preventive action, among persons who have not sought medical attention on account of symptoms of that disorder*. There is no universally accepted definition of medical screening a general agreement that the activity contains three elements:

1. It is a process of selection with the purpose of identifying those individuals who are at a sufficiently high risk of a specific disorder to warrant further investigation or sometimes direct preventive action. It is usually a preliminary process to offer a diagnostic test and, if required, preventive action.
2. It is systematically offered to a population which has not sought medical attention on account of symptoms of the disease for which screening is being conducted. It is normally initiated by medical authorities and not by a patient's request for help on account of a specific complaint.
3. Its purpose is to benefit the individuals being screened. On this basis, mass testing activities, such as surveillance for the human immunodeficiency virus (HIV) infection or pre-employment examinations to test fitness for work, would not be classified as medical screening. The best-known example is the mass screening of all newborn babies for phenylketonuria (PKU), congenital hypothyroidism and some other conditions, i.e. carried out in many countries.

SPECIMEN COLLECTION

The Test Request

The specimen for analysis must be collected and transported to the laboratory according to a specified procedure if the data are to be of clinical value. This procedure begins with the clinician making a test request, either on paper, or increasingly, electronically. The completed request should include:

1. Patient's name, sex and date of birth, hospital or other identification number/ward/clinic/address
2. Name of requesting doctor (telephone/pager number for urgent requests)
3. Clinical diagnosis/problem
4. Test(s) requested
5. Type of specimen
6. Date and time of sampling
7. Relevant treatment (e.g. drugs)

The provision of sufficient information reliably to identify the patient is self-evidently essential, but the omission of any of the above may either cause delay in analysis and reporting or make it impossible to interpret the results. Many laboratories publish a minimum data set without which they will refuse to analyze samples.

Relevant clinical information and details of treatment, especially with drugs, are necessary to allow laboratory staff to assess the results in their clinical context. Drugs may interfere with the analytical methods *in vitro* or may cause changes *in vivo* that suggest a pathological process; for instance, some psychotropic drugs increase plasma prolactin concentration.

All laboratories should publish user guides, which should provide information including the test repertoire, specimen requirements, turnaround time, protocols for dynamic function testing and local or national guidelines for the investigation or monitoring of particular conditions, together with contact details for making enquiries to the laboratory.

THE PATIENT

Some analytes are affected by variables such as posture, time of day, etc., and it may be necessary to standardize the conditions, under which the specimen is obtained. Factors of importance in this respect are listed in Table 1.1.

Table 1.1	Examples of important factors that influence biochemical variables	
Factor	**Example of variable affected**	
Age	Alkaline phosphatase, urate	
Sex	Gonadal steroids, creatinine	
Ethnicity	Creatine kinase	
Pregnancy	Urea, iron	
Posture	Proteins	
Exercise	Creatine kinase, growth hormone	
Stress	Prolactin	
Nutritional status	Glucose, triglyceride, amino acids	
Time	Cortisol	
Drugs	Triglycerides, γ-glutamyl transferase	
Artificial light exposure	Bilirubin	

Even when standardized conditions are used for sampling, the results of repeated quantitative tests (e.g. daily measurements of fasting blood glucose concentration) will themselves show a Gaussian distribution, clustering about the 'usual' value for the individual. Typically, the scatter, which can be assessed by determining the standard deviation (SD), is less for analytes subject to strict regulation (e.g. fasting blood glucose and plasma calcium concentrations) than for others (e.g. plasma enzyme activities). This **biological variation** can be expressed as the coefficient of variation (CV) for repeated tests, where $CV = SD \times 100 / mean$ value.

THE SPECIMEN

Proper specimen collection and handling are vital for assuring accurate results. Improper technique in obtaining and preserving specimens may yield false or invalid values. Most biochemical analyses are made on serum or plasma, but occasionally whole blood is required (e.g. for blood gases), and analyses of urine, cerebrospinal fluid (CSF), pleural fluid, etc., can also be valuable. For most analyses on serum or plasma either fluid is acceptable, but in some instances it is of critical importance which of these is used; for example, serum is required for protein electrophoresis and plasma for measurement of renin activity. **Hemolysis** must be avoided when blood is drawn and, if the patient is receiving intravenous (IV) therapy, blood must be drawn from a remote site (e.g. the opposite arm) to avoid contamination. Hemolysis causes increase in plasma potassium and phosphate concentrations and aspartate aminotransferase activity, owing to leakage from red cells. If hemolysis is a consequence of a delay in centrifugation to separate blood cells from plasma, glucose concentration can fall. Other analytes may also be affected by hemolysis, depending on the analytical method used. The laboratory should always draw attention to potentially spurious results. It should be noted that leakage from cells *in vitro* can cause increase in plasma potassium and phosphate concentrations even in the absence of obvious hemolysis, particularly in patients with high white blood cell or platelet counts.

Collecting a blood specimen into the **wrong container** can lead to (usually obviously) erroneous results. Citrate and ethylenediaminetetraacetic acid (EDTA) which are used as anticoagulants in containers used for some hematological tests, combine with calcium and cause low measured concentrations in the plasma; so does oxalate (the anticoagulant in containers for blood glucose measurement, which also contain fluoride to inhibit glycolysis), and it is clearly inappropriate to collect blood for lithium measurement into a container with lithium heparin as an anticoagulant. Laboratory user guides should provide clear guidance on the types of specimen, and where appropriate, the sampling conditions, for all laboratory tests. This should include guidance on the sequence in which individual specimen tubes are filled to avoid any possibility of contamination. For example, blood should be collected into 'plain tubes' (not containing an anticoagulant or other additive) before being collected into a tube containing, e.g. EDTA.

All specimens must be correctly labelled and transported to the laboratory without any delay. There should be a written protocol for discarding incorrectly collected or labelled specimens. For tests on serum or plasma, the fluid is then separated from blood cells by centrifugation and then analysed. When analysis is delayed, or when specimens are sent to distant laboratories for analysis, degradation of labile analytes must be prevented by refrigerating or freezing the serum or plasma.

Equal care is needed with the collection and transportation of other specimens, such as urine and cerebrospinal fluid (CSF). All specimens should be considered as potentially hazardous and handled accordingly. However, special precautions are necessary for obtaining and handling specimens from patients infected (thought to be infected) with high-risk pathogens. It is important to remember that carriers may be asymptomatic. Infection may be acquired by spillage of blood and other body fluids onto recently broken skin, by accidental scratches, puncture wounds from needles, instruments or possibly by splashing into the eye, nostrils, and lips of susceptible persons.

UNACCEPTABLE SPECIMENS
Unlabeled or Mislabeled Specimen

Chemical pathology laboratory requires the users and clients to place at least two patient identifiers on every specimen's label. The most common and appropriate patient identifiers are: Name, Birth date, Assigned Patient ID Number and Assigned Specimen ID Number. The patient's floor, clinic, hospital or provider, or the specimen's collection date is not a valid identifier.

The identifiers used must appear on both the specimen and on the requisition forms. The laboratory cannot accept responsibility for identification of unlabeled/mislabeled specimens. If a specimen is unlabeled or mislabeled:

1. The ordering location will be notified.
2. The requested lab work will be cancelled, except in rare cases, where recollection of the specimen would place the patient in danger, and the specimen is reasonably identifiable. In those rare instances, the originating person(s) must receive authorization from the chief medical office, chief nursing officer, or state nurse. If authorization is given, the originating person must then identify the specimen(s) and sign the original requisition indicating acceptance of responsibility for the identification of the specimen. In this rare event, the specimen will be processed and the laboratory will complete an 'unusual incident report' documenting the event.

Discrepancy between Specimen Label and Requisition Form

A requisition form must accompany specimen(s) sent to the laboratory. The patient's name and hospital number on the requisition form must match name and number mentioned on specimen container.

When a discrepancy exists, specimens are unacceptable and the policy that is followed is the same as that described above for unlabeled/mislabeled specimens.

Specimen Condition

All specimens sent to the laboratory must be collected according to the department specifications.

1. Examples of sample collection errors include:
   - Improper patient preparation
   - Improper specimen handling in transport to the lab
   - Incorrect specimen container type
   - Incorrect preservative used in specimen collection
   - Insufficient quantity of specimen
   - Hemolysis
   - Contaminated or damaged specimen
   - Needle left on syringe
2. If a specimen is judged to be unacceptable for testing, the ordering location will be notified, no specimen should be discarded without notifying the ordering location.

Urgent Requests

All requests for urgent biochemical tests must be clearly marked to avoid unnecessary delays (Table 1.2). Although laboratories should endeavor to generate results as quickly as possible, some requests will be urgent in that their results may have an immediate bearing on the management of the patient. Examples include the measurement of serum paracetamol concentration in a patient who has taken a drug overdose, measurement of serum troponin concentration in a patient with chest pain, and measurement of serum potassium concentration in a patient with acute kidney injury (renal failure). Special provision must be made for such samples to be 'fast-tracked' through the analytical process, albeit in full accordance with procedures to ensure quality, and the results reported to the requesting clinician as soon as they have been validated.

Repeat Requesting

The appropriate use of laboratory tests is necessary for optimal patient care. Increased laboratory use is appropriate if it allows accurate diagnoses to be made, ideal treatment to be identified and monitored, accurate prognoses to be established, and patients' hospital stays to be shortened. Serial analyses will be required, and the question arises how frequently these should be performed. This will depend on both physiological and pathological factors. For example, in patients being treated with thyroxine for hypothyroidism, it can take several weeks for the plasma concentration of thyroid stimulating hormone (TSH) to stabilize at a new value after a change in the dose of thyroxine: repeating thyroid function tests in a patient whose dose of thyroxine has been changed at an interval of <1 month may therefore provide misleading information, and could prompt a doctor who is not cognizant with the rate of response to make a further change of dose prematurely. In contrast, plasma glucose and potassium concentrations can change

Table 1.2	Definitions and guidelines for ordering laboratory testing
STAT	To be requested when medically indicated and specifically ordered as such by a physician, i.e. an unstable patient in a life-threatening situation.
ASAP	To be requested when a degree of medical urgency exists, but the patient is stable.
TIMED	To be requested for determination of medication levels, the results are usually available the same day.
TODAY	To be requested when results are needed the same day, but there is no medical emergency.
ROUTINE	To be scheduled or obtained when practical, the results are usually available the next day.

very rapidly in patients being treated for diabetic ketoacidosis, and it may be appropriate to make measurements as frequently as every 1–2 hours, at least initially. Laboratory user guides may include guidance on repeat testing, based on locally or nationally agreed protocols.

SAMPLE ANALYSIS AND REPORTING OF RESULTS

Analysis

The ideal analytical method is **accurate, precise, sensitive** and **specific.** It gives a correct result (accurate, Fig. 1.2) that is the same if repeated (precision, Fig. 1.2). It measures low concentrations of the analyte (sensitive) and is not subject to interference by other substances (specific). In addition, it should preferably be cheap, simple and quick to perform. In practice, no test is ideal, but the pathologist must ensure that the results are sufficiently reliable to be clinically useful. Laboratory staff makes considerable efforts to achieve this, and analytical methods are subject to rigorous quality control and quality assurance procedures.

Nevertheless, there will always be a potential for some degree of imprecision or **analytical variation** in a result. The extent of this can be assessed by making repeated analyses (using exactly the same method) on the same sample (cf. biological variation, above). The results will cluster about a mean for which the SD can be calculated. The imprecision of the analysis can be expressed as the CV, where $CV = SD \times 100 / \text{mean result}$. As will be discussed later in this chapter, an understanding of the concepts of both analytical and biological variation is essential to the informed interpretation of laboratory data.

It is important to appreciate that results obtained using different methods may not be interchangeable. When a comparison between two results is being made for clinical purposes, the same analytical method should be used on both occasions.

It is often appropriate to perform a group of related tests on a specimen. For example, plasma calcium and phosphate concentrations and alkaline phosphatase activity all provide information that may be useful in the diagnosis of bone disease; several liver 'function' tests may usefully be grouped together. Such groupings are sometimes referred to as 'biochemical profiles'. Many currently available analyzers can perform numerous assays simultaneously on a single specimen. However, it may be tempting to perform all the assays on every specimen, this approach generates an enormous amount of information, some of which may be unwanted, ignored, or misinterpreted (e.g. an elevated creatine kinase (CK) activity in someone who has recently undertaken severe exercise being construed as evidence of myocardial damage). Worst of all, it may actually divert the clinician's attention from important results. Discrete analysis, i.e. performing only the necessary tests required to answer the clinical question (e.g. 'is this patient's jaundice cholestatic or due to hepatocellular disease?'), is to be preferred.

Reporting Results

Once analysis has been completed and the necessary quality control checks made and found to be satisfactory, a report can be issued. Cumulative reports, which show previous as well as current results, allow trends in data to be picked out at a glance. It may be appropriate to add a comment to a report to assist the clinician with its

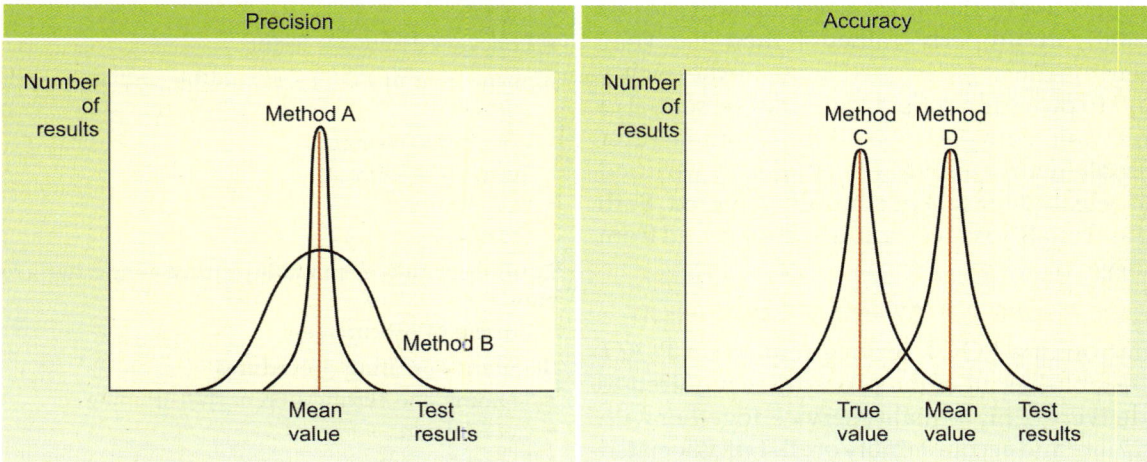

Fig. 1.2: Precision and accuracy of biochemical tests. Both the graphs show the distribution of results for repeated analysis of the same sample by different methods. Precision—the mean value is the same in each case, but the scatter about the mean is less in method A than in method B. Method A is, therefore, more precise. Accuracy—both are equally precise, but in method D, the mean value differs from the true value. The mean for method C is equal to the true value. Both the methods are equally precise, but method C is more accurate

interpretation. Results that indicate a need for rapid clinical intervention should be communicated to the requesting clinician as a matter of urgency.

Point-of-Care Testing

It is defined as 'testing at or near the site of patient care whenever the medical care is needed, since not all analyses need to be performed in a central laboratory'. The purpose of point-of-care testing (POCT) is to provide immediate information to physicians about the patient's condition, so that this information can be integrated into appropriate treatment decisions that improve patient outcomes, i.e. reduce patient's criticality, morbidity, and mortality. Reagent sticks for testing urine at the bedside or in the clinic have long been available. Various substances, including glucose, protein, bilirubin, ketones, and nitrites (indicative of urinary tract infection), can be tested for using such sticks.

The testing of blood for analytes, such as glucose, hydrogen ion and blood gases at point of care has also been available for some time. Indeed, the availability of easily used instruments to measure glucose allows patients with diabetes to monitor their blood glucose concentrations at home. In recent years, manufacturers have developed instruments that can perform a wide range of tests suitable for use at the point of care. Such instruments allow the more rapid provision of analytical results for patients in whom they are required urgently (e.g. in intensive therapy units), but may also be used for convenience. It is clearly desirable that such instruments should be capable of providing results that are as robust with regard to accuracy and precision as those provided by the main laboratory. These instruments are designed to be very simple to operate, but it is nevertheless essential that individuals using them, who will usually not be laboratory staff, are properly trained in their use. They should adhere to protocols designed to ensure the quality of results and to provide a robust audit trail, essential to be able to follow up with patients should a manufacturer convey a problem after a lot has been quality certified initially and released for sale or clinically released. Both the training and quality issues should be supervised from the laboratory.

POINT-OF-CARE TESTING POLICY AND ACCOUNTABILITY

Implementation of a POCT service requires a POCT policy that establishes all of the procedures required to ensure the delivery of high-quality service, together with the responsibility and accountability of all staff associated with the POCT. This may be (1) part of the organization's total quality management system, (2) part of its clinical governance policy, and (3) required for accreditation purposes. The elements of a POCT policy are shown in Table 1.3.

Sources of Error

Traditionally, chemical pathology laboratory practice can be divided into three phases (pre-analytical, analytical, and post-analytical). All the three phases of the total testing process can be targeted individually for improving quality; errors can be minimized by scrupulous adherence to robust, agreed protocols at every stage of the testing process; this means a lot more than ensuring that the analysis is performed correctly. Errors can occur at various stages in the process. It is published that most errors occur in the pre- and post-analytical phases in the field of laboratory medicine (Table 1.4).

Pre-analytical Errors

The pre-analytical phase of the total laboratory testing process is where the majority of laboratory errors occur. Pre-analytical errors can occur at the time of patient assessment, test order entry, request completion, patient identification, specimen collection, specimen transport, or specimen receipt in the laboratory. Some of the other common sources of pre-analytical errors are the

Table 1.3	Elements of a point-of-care testing (POCT) policy

Catalog information-review time
- Approved by
- Original distribution
- Related policies
- Further information
- Policy replaces

Introduction—background
- Definition
- Accreditation of services
- Audit of services

Laboratory services in the organization-location
- Logistics
- Policy on diagnostic testing

Management of POCT—committee and accountability
- Officers
- Committee members
- Terms of reference
- Responsibilities
- Meetings

Equipment and consumable procurement-criteria for procurement
- Process of procurement

Standard operating procedures
- Training and certification of staff-training
- Certification
- Recertification

Quality control and quality assurance procedures
- Documentation and review

Health and safety procedures

Bibliography

Table 1.4	Types and rates of errors in the three stages of the laboratory testing process	
Phase of total testing process	**Type of error**	**Rates**
Pre-analytical	Inappropriate test request Order entry errors Misidentification of patient Inappropriate container Inadequate sample collection and transport Inadequate sample/anticoagulant volume ratio Insufficient sample volume Sorting and routing errors Labeling errors	46–68.2%
Analytical	Equipment malfunction Sample mix-ups/interference Undetected failure in quality control Procedure not followed	7–13%
Post-analytical	Failure in reporting Erroneous validation of analytical data Improper data entry	8.5–47%

following—ordering tests on the wrong patient, ordering the wrong test, misidentifying the patient, choosing the inappropriate collection container, or labeling containers improperly.

A comprehensive plan to prevent pre-analytical errors has five interrelated steps:
1. Developing clear written procedures.
2. Enhancing health care professional training.
3. Automating functions, both for support operations and for executive operations.
4. Monitoring quality indicators.
5. Improving communication among health care professionals and fostering interdepartmental cooperation.

Types and Rates of Errors in the Three Stages of the Laboratory Testing Process

Written procedures must clearly explain how to identify a patient, collect and label a specimen, and subsequently transport the specimen, and prepare it for analysis. Those individuals performing the pre-analytical procedures must understand not only what the procedures are, but also why they are important to follow. They need to know not only what happens if the correct steps are not followed, but also what errors can occur and what effect they can have on the sample and ultimately the patient. There must be ongoing training for these employees and competencies must be assessed annually.

Modern robotic technologies and information systems can also help reduce pre-analytical errors. Computerized order entry simplifies test ordering and eliminates a second person from transcribing the orders. Automated phlebotomy tray preparation provides a complete set of labeled blood tubes and labels for hand labeling in a single tray for each patient. Pre-analytical robotic workstations

automate some of the steps and reduce the number of manual steps involving more people. Barcodes also simplify specimen routing and tracking.

Recent advances in laboratory technology have made available, new and more reliable means for the automated detection of the serum indices, including the hemolysis index. Visual detection of hemolysis must be abandoned due to low sensitivity and low reproducibility. Laboratory personnel must ask for new samples when hemolysis is detected. If a new sample cannot be obtained, it is the responsibility of the laboratory specialist to communicate the problem to the clinician. The data obtained from the serum indices can be used to monitor the quality of the collection process.

Analytical Errors

Focusing first on the analytical phase of laboratory testing, the analytical phase begins when the patient specimen is prepared in the laboratory for testing, and it ends when the test result is interpreted and verified by the technologist in the laboratory. Not processing a specimen properly prior to analysis or substances interfering with assay performance can affect test results in the analytical phase. Establishing and verifying test method performance specifications as to test accuracy, precision, sensitivity, specificity, and linearity are other areas where errors can occur in the analytical phase of laboratory testing.

The laboratory has spent decades improving analytical quality by establishing internal quality controls (IQC) and external quality assessment (EQA). The role of EQA and proficiency testing (PT) is to provide reliable information allowing laboratories to assess and monitor the quality status of internal procedures and processes, the suitability of the diagnostic systems, the accountability and competence of the staff, along with the definition of measurement uncertainty in laboratory results. The responsibility of laboratory professionals is to appropriately analyze EQA/PT samples and reports, detect trends or bias that may not be apparent in single results, investigate root causes producing unacceptable performances, apply and monitor opportune actions for removing the underlying cause(s), verify the effectiveness, and above all, determine whether the problem affected clinical decision-making.

Post-analytical Errors

Post-analytical quality, the ultimate check on the consistency of pre- and intra-analytical quality, can be considered as the overall quality. It ties together not only the quality of the question to be answered, the analytical quality achieved and the usefulness of the answer obtained, but also the context of the patient and the perceived abilities of the physician to interpret and utilize laboratory information. Similar to the pre-analytical step, the post-analytical phase can be subdivided into one phase performed within the laboratory and another (post-post-analytical phase) in which the clinicians receive, interpret and react to laboratory results.

Post-analytical Procedures Performed within the Laboratory

The post-analytical procedures performed within the laboratory include verifying laboratory results, feeding them into the laboratory information system, and communicating them to the clinicians in a number of ways (in particular, by producing a report and making any necessary oral communications regarding 'alert' or panic results). In this step, the most common mistakes, accounting for 18.5–47% of total laboratory errors, are wrong validation, results that are delayed, not reported or reported to the wrong providers, and incorrect results reported because of post-analytical data entry errors and transcription errors.

Manual test validation is a time-consuming process with large inter-individual variation; moreover, it slows down the response of the laboratory to the clinic, thus causing delay in the diagnostic and therapeutic process. This validation process can be automated; some automated validation systems with satisfactory sensitivity and specificity have been developed and introduced into clinical laboratories. As yet, however, it has not been proven that validation systems allow clinical laboratories to reduce errors, thus improving patient safety and outcomes. This is owing to difficulties in performing longitudinal studies with a design that allows the identification of real errors and a comparison with historical error rates. However, validation systems

may be considered valid 'preventive action'. Another well-recognized source of post-analytical problems is inter-laboratory variability and inaccuracy of reference intervals. Reference intervals for healthy subjects and diseased populations are important benchmarks for the clinical interpretation of laboratory test values. The use of different, sometimes erroneous, reference intervals may markedly affect the clinical interpretation of laboratory data, leading to errors in clinical decision-making. The production and release of the laboratory report is the crucial step in post-analytical procedures, as its format, content, and communication significantly affect the interpretation and utilization of laboratory data by clinicians. The importance of information technology in improving reliability and security of result reporting is widely recognized.

Requirements for information technology in laboratory medicine now go well beyond the provision of purely analytical data and include fundamental aspects of data communication, namely the notification of results that fall within established critical or alert intervals. In particular, the possible role of interpretative comments in improving patient outcomes has generated a lot of interest. Guidelines for the provision of interpretative comments have been released and schemes for assessing the quality of comments have been initiated. The results obtained indicate that interpretation provided by laboratory professionals with inadequate expertise can be dangerous, and highlight the need for improvement in the standard of interpretation currently provided.

Post-analytical Procedures Performed Outside the Laboratory

In the post-analytical phase performed outside laboratory control (post-post-analytical phase), the clinician receives, reads and interprets the results, and makes a decision on the basis of information from the laboratory and other sources. There is evidence that laboratory information is only partially utilized; a recent report demonstrates that 45% of the results for urgent laboratory tests requested by the emergency department of one hospital were never accessed, or were accessed far too late. In addition, numerous errors can occur at this stage, as admitted by some clinicians on completing questionnaires, but problems can be generated at the laboratory-clinician interface. In fact, results released by the laboratory may not contain all the information needed by the clinician; the laboratory report may even contain information that the clinician considers superfluous or irrelevant. It has also been underlined that the introduction of new and complex tests, including genetic testing, may increase the complexity of medical management, and this, in turn, may influence the interpretation and clinical applicability of new and promising laboratory tests.

Monitoring Errors

The success of any efforts made to reduce errors must be monitored in order to assess the efficacy of the measures taken. Quality indicators must be used for assessment. In the testing process areas involving non-laboratory personnel, interdepartmental communication, and cooperation are crucial to avoid errors. Therefore, the entire health care system must be involved in improving the total testing process. There must be adequate and effective training of personnel throughout the institution to be competent in following processes and procedures.

Incident Reporting in Laboratory Diagnostics

While major efforts have been made to monitor the pre-analytical phase and provide reliable solutions, it is surprising that concrete formal programs of incident reporting have not been so pervasive in laboratory diagnostics. The major focus in health care is placed on incident reporting for several medical conditions with lesser effort devoted to translating this noteworthy practice into laboratory diagnostics. If, in fact, laboratory errors are being under reported, then current statistics reveal only a small portion of the medical errors actually taking place. There is an urgent need to establish a reliable policy of error recording, possibly through informatics aids, and settle universally agreed 'laboratory sentinel events' throughout the total testing process, which would allow gaining important information about serious incidents and holding both providers and stakeholders accountable for patient safety. Some of these sentinel events have already been identified, including inappropriate test requests and patient misidentification (pre-analytical phase), use of wrong assays, severe analytical errors, tests performed on unsuitable samples, release of lab results in spite of poor quality controls (analytical phase), and failure to alert critical values and wrong report destination (post-analytical phase).

Development and widespread implementation of a total quality management (TQM) system is the most effective strategy to minimize uncertainty in laboratory diagnostics. Pragmatically, this can be achieved using three complementary actions, i.e. preventing adverse events (error prevention), making them visible (error detection), and mitigating their adverse consequences when they occur (error management).

Other methodologies can also be used to prevent errors. Failure mode and effect analysis (FMEA) has been a broadly cited reliable approach to risk management. It is a systematic process for identifying potential process failures before they occur, with the aim to eliminate them or minimize the relative risk.

Interpretation of Results

When the result of a biochemical test is obtained, the clinician should ask the following questions:

- Is the result the correct one for the patient?
- Does the result fit with the clinical findings? Remember to treat the patient and not the 'laboratory numbers'.
- Is the result normal?
- If the result is abnormal, is the abnormality of diagnostic significance or is it a nonspecific finding?
- If it is one of a series of results, has there been a change and, if so, is this change clinically significant?

Is the Result Normal?

For the majority of tests, the individual's results for any constituent are distributed around this mean in a 'normal' (Gaussian) statistical theory predicts that approximately 95% of the values in the population will lie within the range given by the mean ±2 SDs (Fig. 1.3); of the remaining 5%, half of the values will be higher and half will be lower than the limits of this range; such results are not necessarily abnormal for that individual. All that can be said with certainty is that the probability that a result is abnormal increases the further it is from the mean or median until, eventually, this probability approaches 100%. Furthermore, a normal result does not necessarily exclude the disease that is being sought; a test result within the population reference range may be abnormal for that individual.

Very few biochemical tests clearly separate a 'normal' population from an 'abnormal' population. For most there is a range of values in which 'normal' and 'abnormal'

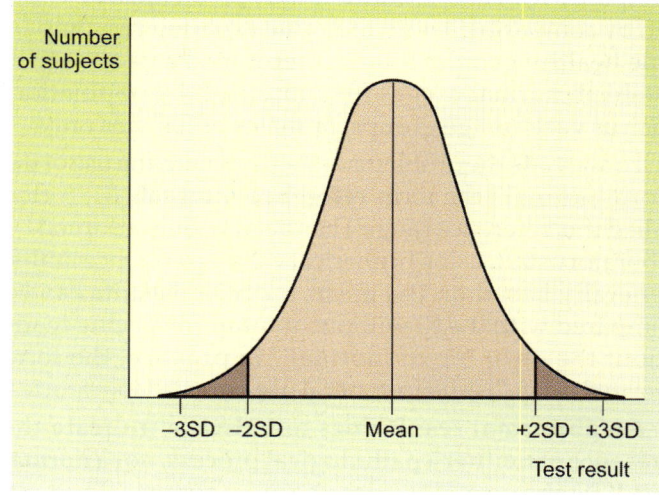

Fig. 1.3: Gaussian distribution

overlap, the extent of the overlap differing for individual tests. There are 5% chances, that one result will fall outside the reference range.

When establishing the range of values for a particular variable in healthy people, it is conventional to first examine a representative sample of sufficient size to determine whether or not the values fall in a Gaussian distribution. The range (mean ±2 SDs) can then be calculated; this, in statistical terms, is the 'normal range'. Several important points arise from this:

1. Although it is assumed that the population is healthy, values from 5% of individuals by definition lie outside the normal range. This suggests that, if the measurements were to be made in a group of comparable individuals, 1 in 20 would have a value outside this range.
2. The specialized statistical use of the word 'normal', does not equate with what is generally meant by the word, i.e. 'habitual' or 'usually encountered'.
3. The statistical 'normal' may not be related to another common use of the word, which is to imply freedom from risk. For example, there is an association between increased risk of coronary heart disease and plasma cholesterol concentrations even within the normal range as derived from measurements on apparently healthy men.

Thus, the normal range for an analyte, defined and calculated as described, has severe limitations. It only identifies the range of values that can be expected to occur most often in individuals who are comparable with those in the population for whom the range was derived. It is not necessarily normal in terms of being 'ideal', nor is it associated with no risk of having or developing disease. Furthermore, by definition it will exclude values from some healthy individuals. In all cases, like must be compared with like. An individual's result must be assessed by comparing it with the value expected for comparable healthy people. It may, therefore, be necessary to establish normal ranges for subsets of the population, such as various age groups, or males or females only.

To alleviate the problems associated with the use of the word 'normal', the term **reference interval** (RI) (often called the 'reference range') has been widely adopted by laboratory staff, using numerical values (reference limits) generally based on the mean ± 2 SDs. Results can be compared with the RI without assumptions being made about the meaning of 'normal'. In practice, the term 'normal range' is still in general use outside laboratories.

An abnormal result does not always indicate the presence of neither a pathological process, nor a normal result its absence. However, the more abnormal a result, i.e. the greater its difference from the limits of the reference interval, the greater is the probability that it is related to a pathological process.

In practice, there is rarely an absolute demarcation between normal values and those seen in disease: equivocal results must be investigated further. If an important decision in the management of a patient is to be based upon a single result, it is vital that the cut-off point, or 'decision level', is chosen to ensure that the test functions efficiently. In screening for PKU, e.g. the blood concentration of phenylalanine selected to indicate a positive result must include all infants with the condition; in other words, there must be no false negatives. Because there is some overlap in the values seen in the presence and absence of PKU, this inevitably means that some normal children will test positive (false positives) and will be subjected to further investigation. Generally, it is unusual to have to determine a patient's management on the basis of one result alone.

It has been explained that 5% of healthy people will, by definition, have a value for a given variable that is outside the reference interval. If a second and independent variable is measured, the probability that this result will be 'abnormal' is also 0.05 (5%). However, the abnormal results may not arise in the same individuals and the overall probability of an abnormal result from at least one test will be >5%. It follows that the more tests that are performed on an individual, the greater the probability that the result of one of them will be abnormal; for 10 independent variables, the probability is 0.4; in other words, at least one abnormal result would be expected in 40% of healthy people. For 20 variables, the probability is 0.64.

Although biochemical parameters are frequently to some extent, interdependent (e.g. albumin and total protein), the use of multichannel analyzers to produce biochemical profiles inevitably risks generating a number of spuriously abnormal results. Before any decision can be made on the basis of such results, some information is required about the probability that they are indicative of a pathological process.

Is the Abnormality of Diagnostic Significance?

If the result of a previous test is available, the clinician will be able to compare the results and decide whether any difference between them is significant. This will depend on the precision of the assay itself (a measure of its reproducibility) and the natural biological variation.

The probability that the difference between two results is **analytically significant** at a level of $p = <0.05$ is 2.8 times the analytical SD. Thus, for plasma calcium concentration, with an analytical SD of 0.04 mmol/L, an apparent increase in calcium concentration from

2.54 mmol/L to 2.62 mmol/L ($2 \times$ SD) is within the limits of expected analytical variation, whereas an increase from 2.54 to 2.70 ($4 \times$ SD) is not. However, to decide whether an analytical change is **clinically significant** it is necessary to consider the extent of natural **biological variation**. The effects of analytical and biological variation can be assessed by calculating the overall standard deviation of the test, given by:

$$SD = \sqrt{SD_A^2 + SD_B^2}$$

in the above equation, SD_A and SD_B are the SDs for the analytical and biological variation respectively. If the difference between two test results exceeds 2.8 times the SD of the test, the difference can be regarded as of potential clinical significance—the probability of this difference being a result of analytical and biological variation is <0.05. It should be appreciated, however, that setting the level of significance at a probability of <0.05 is arbitrary (albeit conventional). It does not mean that a difference of less than that equating to this probability cannot be of significance, nor that a greater difference necessarily is significant. If undertaking a major intervention depends on a result, it may be desirable only to make this decision if the probability that the change is not the result of innate variation is considerably greater.

Is this Change Clinically Significant?

If the result is consistent with clinical findings, it is evidence in favor of the clinical diagnosis. If it is not consistent, the explanation must be sought. There may have been a mistake in the collection, labelling or analysis of the sample, or in the reporting of the result. In practice, it may be simplest to request a further sample and to repeat the test. If the result is confirmed, the utility of the test in the clinical context should be considered and the clinical diagnosis itself may have to be reviewed.

The Clinical Utility of Laboratory Investigations

In using the result of a test, it is important to know how reliable the test is and how suitable it is for its intended purpose. Thus, the laboratory personnel must ensure, as far as is practicable, that the data are accurate and precise, and the clinician should appreciate how useful the test is in the context in which it is used. Various properties of a test can be calculated to provide this information.

Specificity and Sensitivity

The specificity is an ability of a measurement to correctly identify those who do not have the condition in question. The word 'specificity' refers to how narrowly a test is targeted; does it only identify people with that particular type of disease (is it specific to that condition?), i.e. 'true

negative' (TN). Sensitivity is the ability of a measurement or screening test to identify those who have a condition, i.e. 'true positive' (TP). A specificity of 90% implies that 10% of disease-free people would be classified as having the disease on the basis of the test result; they would have a 'false positive' (FP) result. A sensitivity of 90% implies that only 90% of people known to have the disease would be diagnosed as having it on the basis of that test alone; 10% would be 'false negatives' (FN).

Specificity and sensitivity are calculated as follows:

$$Specificity = \frac{TN}{All\ without\ disease\ [FP + TN]} \times 100$$

$$Sensitivity = \frac{TP}{All\ with\ disease\ [TP + FN]} \times 100$$

An ideal diagnostic test would be 100% sensitive, giving positive results in all subjects with a particular disease, and also 100% specific, giving negative results in all subjects free of the disease. Because the ranges of results in quantitative tests that can occur in health and in disease almost always show some overlap, individual tests do not achieve such high standards. Factors that increase the specificity of a test tend to decrease the sensitivity, and vice versa. To take an extreme example, if it were decided to diagnose hyperthyroidism only if the plasma free thyroxine concentration were at least 32 pmol/L (the upper limit of the reference range is 26 pmol/L), the test would have effectively 100% specificity; positive results (>32 pmol/L) would only be seen in thyrotoxicosis (an exception is a very rare condition in which patients are resistant to thyroid hormones). On the other hand, the test would have a low sensitivity in that many patients with mild hyperthyroidism would be misdiagnosed. If a concentration of 20 pmol/L were used, the test would be very sensitive (all those with hyperthyroidism would be correctly assigned) but have low specificity, because many normal people would also be diagnosed as having the condition. These concepts are illustrated in Fig. 1.4.

Whether it is desirable to maximize specificity or sensitivity depends on the nature of the condition that the test is used to diagnose and the consequences of making an incorrect diagnosis. For example, sensitivity is paramount in a screening test for a harmful condition, but the inevitable false positive results mean that all positive results will have to be investigated further. However, in selecting patients for a trial of a new treatment, a highly specific test is more appropriate to ensure that the treatment is being given only to patients who have a particular condition. In some cases, this decision may not be straightforward. For example, in the context of chest pain and suspected acute myocardial infarction, where the possible options are to identify all those who have had a myocardial infarction ('rule in') or to identify all those who have definitely not ('rule out'). The preferred option should depend on the relative outcomes of treatment and non-treatment for patients in the two groups.

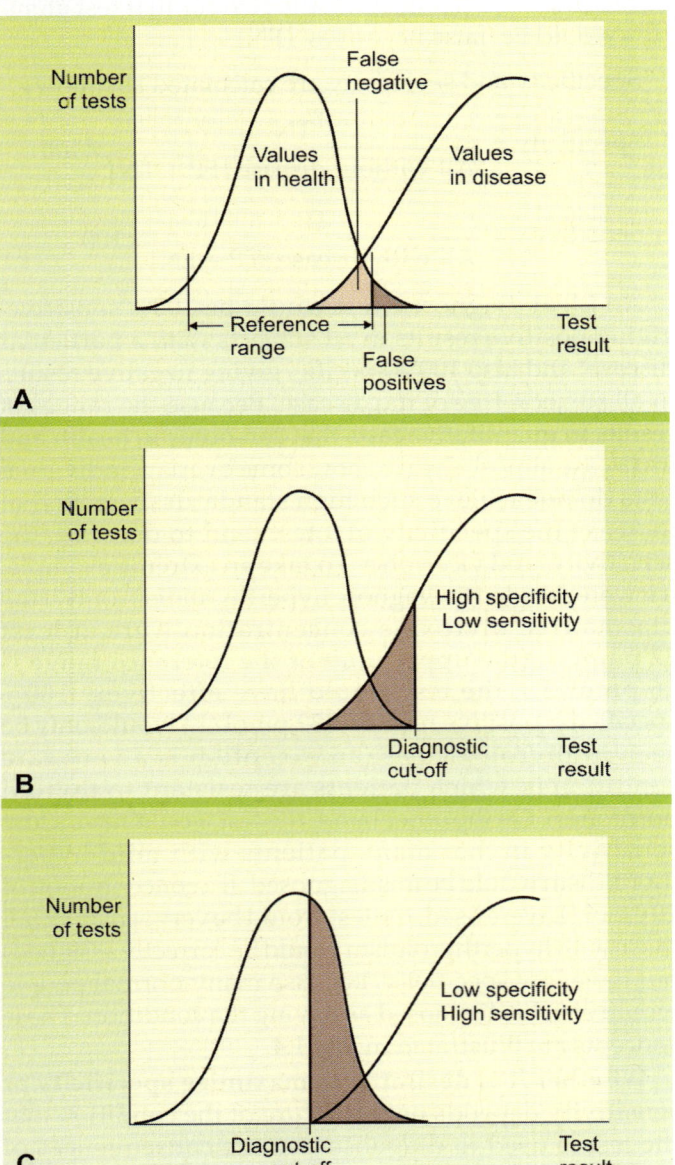

Fig. 1.4: Because the range of values for a test results in health and disease overlap (A), some patients with disease will have results within the reference range (false negatives), while some individuals free of disease will have results outside this range (false positives). If the diagnostic cut-off value for a test is set too high (B), there will be no false positives, but many false negatives; specificity is increased but sensitivity decreases. If the diagnostic cut-off value is set too low (C), the number of false positives, and sensitivity, increases, at the expense of a decrease in specificity

One way of comparing the sensitivity and specificity of different tests is to construct **receiver operating characteristic curves** (ROC curves). Each test is performed in each of a series of appropriate individuals. The specificity and sensitivity are calculated using different cut-off values to determine whether a given result is positive or negative (Fig. 1.5). The curves can then be assessed to determine which test performs the best in the specific circumstances for which it is required.

Accuracy and Precision

Statistical measurements of accuracy and precision reveal a lab test's basic reliability. These terms, which describe sources of variability, are not interchangeable. A test method can be precise (reliable reproducibility) without being accurate (measuring what it is supposed to measure and its true value) or vice versa.

The word 'precision' refers to be precise when repeated analyses on the same sample give similar results. When a test method is precise, the amount of random variation is small. The test method can be trusted because results are reliably reproduced time after time. The word 'accuracy' refers to be accurate when the test value approaches the absolute 'true' value of the substance (analyte) being measured. Results from every test performed are compared to known 'control specimens' that have undergone multiple evaluations and compared to the 'gold' standard for that assay, thus analyzed to the best testing standards available.

Although a test that is 100% accurate and 100% precise is ideal, in practice, test methodology, instrumentation, and laboratory operations all contribute to small, but

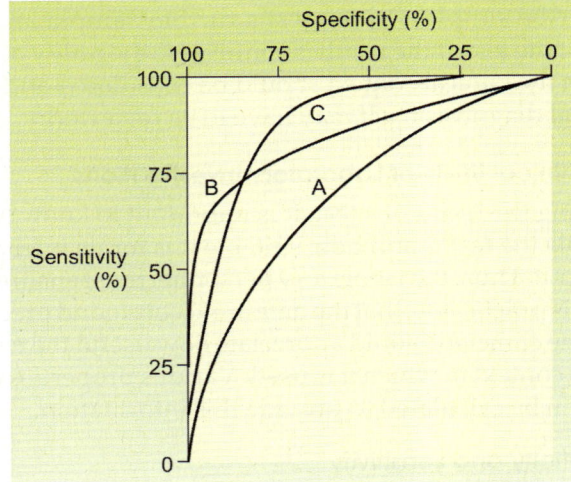

Fig. 1.5: Receiver operating characteristic (ROC) curves for three hypothetical tests, A, B, and C. Examination of the curves shows that test A performs less well in terms of both sensitivity and specificity than tests B and C. Test B has better specificity than C, but C has better sensitivity

measurable variations in results. The small amount of variability that typically occurs does not usually detract from the test's value and statistically is insignificant. The level of precision and accuracy that can be obtained is specific to each test method, but is constantly monitored for reliability through comprehensive quality control and quality assurance procedures. Therefore, when your blood is tested more than once by the same laboratory, your test results should not change much unless your condition has changed. There may be some differences between laboratories in precision and accuracy due to different analytical instrumentation or methodologies, however, the test results are reported with standardized reference intervals specific for that laboratory. This helps your health care provider to correctly interpret the information and its relevance to that reference interval.

Efficiency

The efficiency of a test is the number of correct results divided by the total number of tests. Thus, efficiency is given by:

$$\text{Efficiency} = \frac{TP + TN}{\text{Total number of tests}} \times 100$$

When sensitivity and specificity are equally important, the test with the greatest efficiency should be used.

Predictive Values

Even a highly specific and sensitive test may not necessarily perform well in a clinical context. This is because the ability of a test to diagnose disease depends on the prevalence of the condition in the population being studied (prevalence is the number of people with the condition in relation to the population). This ability is given by the 'predictive value' (PV). PV_{+ve}, **the PV for a positive result, is the percentage of all positive results that are true positives,** that is:

$$PV_{+ve} = \frac{TP}{TP + FP} \times 100$$

If a condition has a low prevalence and the test is <100% specific, many false positives will result and the PV will be low.

A high predictive value for a positive test is important if the appropriate management of a patient with a true positive result would be potentially dangerous if applied to someone with a false positive result. However, when a test is used for **screening,** (i.e. the detection of a condition in asymptomatic individuals), the appropriate management is to perform further (diagnostic) tests, and although these may cause inconvenience for subjects with false positive results, they are unlikely to be harmful.

In order not to miss cases, a screening test should have a very high PV_{-ve}, **the PV for a negative result; this is the percentage of all negative results that are true negatives,** that is:

$$PV_{-ve} = \frac{TN}{TN + FN} \times 100$$

This conclusion follows directly from the fact that the test must be highly sensitive.

For clarity, this discussion has centered on the use of single tests for diagnostic purposes, but in practice, the clinician will combine clinical information and, often, the results of several investigations to make a diagnosis. If the tests are used rationally, the PV of positive results will be higher; as the tests will be used only in patients who have other features suggesting a particular diagnosis (the prevalence of the disease in question would be higher in a group of such people than in the general population). For example, although Cushing's disease is rare, making the PV of a positive test for the condition in the general population low, in practice one would only investigate patients suspected on clinical grounds of having the condition and in whom the prevalence will therefore be higher. This may be self-evident, but doctors frequently order tests on flimsy clinical grounds and fail to appreciate how unhelpful, or even misleading, the results may be.

Likelihood Ratios

Likelihood ratios (LRs) express the odds that a given finding (e.g. a particular result) would occur in a person with, as opposed to without, a particular condition. As such, LRs directly link the pre-test and post-test probability of a disease in a specific patient. Simplified, LRs tells us how many times more likely particular test result is in 5 subjects with the disease than in those without disease. When probabilities are equal, such test is of no value and its LRs = 1.

Likelihood ratio for positive test results (LR_{+ve}) tells us how much more likely the positive test result is to occur in subjects with the disease compared to those without the disease. LR_{+ve} is usually higher than 1 because it is more likely that the positive test result will occur in subjects with the disease than in subject without the disease.

LR_{+ve} can be simply calculated according to the following formula:

$$LR_{+ve} = \text{Sensitivity} / (1 - \text{Specificity})$$

LR_{+ve} is the best indicator for ruling-in diagnosis. The higher the LR_{+ve} the test is more indicative of a disease. Good diagnostic tests have $LR_{+ve} >10$ and their positive result has a significant contribution to the diagnosis.

Likelihood ratio for negative test result (LR_{-ve}) represents the ratio of the probability that a negative result will occur in subjects with the disease to the probability that the same result will occur in subjects without the disease. Therefore, LR tells us how much less likely the negative test result is to occur in a patient than in a subject without disease. LR_{-ve} is usually less than 1 because it is less likely that negative test result occurs in subjects with than in subjects without disease. LR_{-ve} is calculated according to the following formula:

$$LR_{-ve} = (1 - Sensitivity)/Specificity$$

LR_{-ve} is a good indicator for ruling-out the diagnosis. Good diagnostic tests have $LR_{-ve} < 0.1$. The lower the LR_{-ve} the more significant contribution of the test is in ruling-out, i.e. in lowering the posterior probability of the subject having the disease.

Since both specificity and sensitivity are used to calculate the likelihood ratio, it is clear that neither LR_{+ve} nor LR_{-ve} depend on the disease prevalence in examined groups. Consequently, the likelihood ratios from one study are applicable to some other clinical setting, as long as the definition of the disease is not changed. If the way of defining the disease varies, none of the calculated measures will apply in some other clinical context.

Evidence-based Clinical Biochemistry

An approach to summarizing the results of **sensitivity** and **specificity** analyses for various cutting points on diagnostic or **screening tests** that also takes account of the prevalence of the condition in the population under study. The likelihood ratio expresses how much the estimated odds of the patient having the disease increase following a positive test score, or decrease following a negative test score. Such an approach is advocated as a part of the practice of evidence-based medicine. The **likelihood ratio** is the probability that a given test result would occur in a person with the target disorder divided by the probability, that the same result would occur in a person without the disorder.

An LR_{+ve} ratio indicates how much more likely a person with the disease is to have a positive test result than a person without the disease.

$$LR_{+ve} = Sensitivity/(1 - Specificity)$$

An LR_{-ve} ratio indicates how much more likely a person without the disease is to have a negative test result, compared to a person with the disease.

$$LR_{-ve} = (1 - Sensitivity)/Specificity$$

Clinical Audit

Clinical audit is a systematic review and evaluation of current practice against research based standards with a view to improve clinical care for patients. It involves identifying an area of practice, setting standards or guidelines (e.g. a protocol for investigation of patients suspected of having a particular condition), implementing changes designed to achieve these and then examining compliance with them and the effects on patient care. The cycle is completed by review of the standards in the light of this analysis and their modification as required. It should be followed by re-audit after an appropriate interval. Whether undertaken in the context of formal audit or not, ongoing liaison between the providers and users of laboratory services is essential to ensure that the service meets the latter's needs. It also provides a forum for laboratory staff to educate users about changes in practice designed to improve the service.

The term 'audit' is also applied to procedures used by some laboratory accreditation bodies to examine the internal functioning of laboratories. It is beyond the scope of this book to describe such procedures.

Critical Values

Represent values which require immediate notification and clinical intervention to avoid or attenuate patient morbidity and mortality.

Establishing a Critical Values List

Although there are many regulations specifying that laboratories must define and communicate critical values, it may seem surprising that regulations do not state which laboratory tests require critical value limits and notification. Indeed, individual clinical laboratories face unique challenges that reflect institutional organization, clinical demand, patient population, instrumentation, and staffing. Such variations have hindered the development of universal standards for critical value reporting across laboratories.

The idea of a universal critical value list is appealing to many laboratorians and clinicians. For example, many clinicians would likely consider a sodium (Na^+) level of (160 mmol/L) a 'critical' value regardless of which laboratory performs the test. Indeed, the practice of assigning the laboratory director responsibility for creating and refining the critical value list has led to similar overall inclusion of tests between laboratories without there being a universal mandate or requirement. As an example, virtually all laboratories include Na^+ on their critical value list precisely because it is important for patient care. Furthermore, not communicating a critically elevated Na^+ level could have medicolegal ramifications if an adverse clinical outcome occurred. Defining (and then mandating) a universal set of thresholds for tests, however, would be a daunting task given the scarcity of outcomes-based data on critical value thresholds. Inherent variability in assay-specific reference intervals between institutions is also a complicating factor. An individual laboratory director can account for this variability by defining critical ranges consistent with his or her own assays and instrumentation.

How should a laboratory determine which tests to include on a critical value list? Moreover, how should the critical high and low thresholds be established? While ultimately, this determination is the responsibility of the laboratory director, it should be made in communication with the clinicians who use laboratory services, as well as with a medical review board of the institution, if applicable. This task may include meeting with relevant physicians, medical and surgical section chiefs, hospital administrators, and/or nurse managers to discuss critical value policies and to determine, if there are any tests that should be included (or omitted) and whether any thresholds should be adjusted according to clinical needs.

Not every laboratory test should have critical values associated with it. Critical value lists are, by nature, limited to not hinder the clinical effectiveness of notification (Table 1.5). Critical lists that are too inclusive (or that have critical value thresholds that require excessive notification) place an unnecessary burden on laboratory staff. Such lists annoy clinicians, foster a negative attitude toward important laboratory services, and most important, provide uncertain additional benefit

to patient care. At the other extreme, lists that are too exclusive (or with thresholds that are too high or low) might not prevent adverse clinical outcomes, as a delay in the recognition of life-threatening laboratory results by clinicians can be disastrous. A balance must be achieved.

Critical Values Reporting and Communication

Phone Call System

The notification given is reported in a register (a quality document) together with the date, the time of the call, the patient's identification, bar code, location, test result, the physician communicating the critical value, and the recipient of the information.

Computerized Notification System: Alerting System and SMS

The instrument, middle ware, or laboratory information system (LIS) will notify the laboratory staff (usually the performing technologist) of the critical value. Laboratory policies must clearly indicate whether the assay should be verified and/or repeated before reporting and, if so, within what time frame.

Laboratory procedures must indicate 'by whom and to whom' critical results are reported, as well as the acceptable length of time between the availability and reporting of critical results. Documentation is required including date, time, responsible laboratory individual and the person whom notified.

Table 1.5	Critical laboratory values		
Test	**Unit (SI)**	**Low threshold**	**High threshold**
Clinical chemistry (adult)			
CO$_2$ (bicarbonate)	mmol/L	10	40
Calcium	mmol/L	1.5	3.25
Calcium, ionized	mmol/L	0.75	1.63
Glucose	mmol/L	2.2	27.8
Magnesium	mmol/L	0.50	2.5
Phosphorus	mmol/L	0.32	3.2
Potassium (plasma)	mmol/L	2.5	6.2
Sodium	mmol/L	115	160
Glucose tolerance	mmol/L	3.3	27.8
CSF glucose	mmol/L	1.1	
CSF protein	g/L		3.0
Free T$_4$	pmol/L		45.0
TSH	mIU/L		100
Clinical chemistry (pediatric)			
Ammonia	imol/L		150
Total bilirubin (newborn <30 days)	imol/L		306
Glucose (newborn <30 days)	mmol/L	1.7	11.1
Glucose (1 month to 1 year)	mmol/L	1.7	16.7
Potassium (newborn <10 days)	**(mmol/L)**	**2.0 (2.0)**	**7.0 (7.0)**
Sodium (newborn <10 days)	**(mmol/L)**	**125 (125)**	**160 (160)**

The critical values notifications should be made by one of the team members involved in performing the procedure using a call center for critical value notifications. Several hospitals have implemented the use of automated notification systems for critical value reporting by transmitting the critical values from the LIS to a hospital clinical information system trigger the generation of text messages directed to the responsible clinician's mobile phone and computer. If the clinician does not confirm receipt in the clinical information system within 60 minutes, results are communicated by telephone. This approach improved the speed of communication and another automated paging system was developed for critical value notification. In that program, critical values transmitted from the LIS, generate a page containing the patient name, medical record number, collection time, critical result, and reference range. The clinician must confirm receipt of the critical value by dialing a phone number listed in the message. If the clinician does not respond within 10 minutes (or rejects the notification), the call is escalated to a trained group of operators which proceed with telephone notification. Implementation of that system increased documentation of critical value receipt by physicians and decreased the median time for notification.

It should be emphasized that automated solutions should allow for an *escalation policy* to ensure communication of critical results, when clinicians do not acknowledge receipt.

Laboratory contact information should also be available so that clinicians with additional questions can ask a laboratory professional or medical director as appropriate. Patient privacy requirements should also be considered with automation.

To whom should critical values be reported?

Notification should be done to a physician or the individual or entity requesting the test and the individual responsible for using the test results.

Types of Specimens

Types of biological specimens that are analyzed in clinical laboratories include (1) whole blood, (2) serum, (3) plasma, (4) urine, (5) feces, (6) saliva, (7) spinal, synovial, amniotic, pleural, pericardial, and ascitic fluids, and (8) various types of solid tissues.

Plasma and Serum

Plasma, the liquid component of blood, comprises 55% of the total blood volume. It can separate by artificially spinning or centrifuging the blood at high rotations of 3000 rpm or higher (Fig. 1.6). The blood cells and platelets that make up about 45% of the blood are

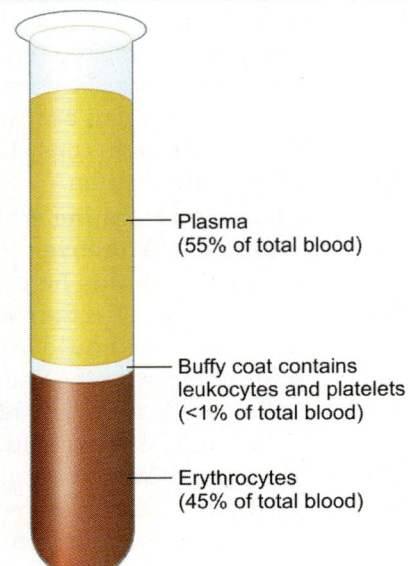

Plasma
(55% of total blood)

Buffy coat contains
leukocytes and platelets
(<1% of total blood)

Erythrocytes
(45% of total blood)

Fig. 1.6: Blood sample after centrifugation—the liquid components of blood called plasma (yellow section), can be separated from the erythrocytes (red section) and platelets (white section) by using a centrifuging or spinning the blood

separated by centrifugal forces to the bottom of a specimen tube, leaving the plasma as the upper layer. Plasma consists of 90% water along with various substances required for maintaining the body's pH, osmotic load, and for protecting the body. The plasma also contains the coagulation factors and antibodies.

Serum, the plasma component of blood which lacks coagulation factors, is similar to interstitial fluid in which the correct composition of key ions acting as electrolytes is essential for normal functioning of muscles and nerves. Other components in the serum include proteins, which assist with maintaining pH and osmotic balance while giving viscosity to the blood; antibodies, or specialized proteins that are important for defense against viruses and bacteria; lipids, including cholesterol, which are transported in the serum; and various other substances including nutrients, hormones, metabolic waste, and external substances, such as drugs, viruses, and bacteria.

Human serum albumin, the most abundant protein in human blood plasma, is synthesized in the liver. Albumin, which constitutes about one-half of the blood serum protein, transports hormones and fatty acids, buffers pH, and maintains osmotic pressures. Immunoglobulin, a protein antibody produced in the mucosal lining, plays an important role in antibody-mediated immunity.

Handling of Specimens for Analysis

Steps that are important for obtaining a valid specimen for analysis include (1) identification, (2) preservation, (3) separation and storage, and (4) transport.

Identification of Specimens

Proper identification of the specimen must be maintained at each step of the testing process. The minimum information on a label should include a patient's name, location, identifying number, and the date and time of collection. All labels should conform to the laboratory's stated requirements to facilitate proper processing of specimens. No specific labeling should be attached to specimens from patients with infectious diseases to suggest that these specimens should be handled with special care. All specimens should be treated as if they are potentially infectious.

In practice, every specimen container must be adequately labeled even if the specimen must be placed in ice, or if the container is so small that a label cannot be placed along the tube, as might happen with a capillary blood tube. Direct labeling of a capillary blood tube by folding the label like a flag around the tube is preferred. For small volumes of urine submitted in a screw-cap urine cup and any specimen submitted in a screw-cap test tube or cup, the label should be placed on the cup or tube directly, not on the cap.

Preservation of Specimens

The practitioner must ensure that specimens are collected into the correct container and are properly labeled; in addition, specimens must be properly treated both during transport to the laboratory and from the time the serum, plasma, or cells have been separated until analysis. For some tests, specimens must be kept at 4°C from the time the blood is drawn until the specimens are analyzed, or until the serum or plasma is separated from the cells. Examples are specimens for ammonia and blood gas determinations, such as PCO_2, PO_2, and blood pH. Transfer of these specimens to the laboratory must be done by placing the specimen container in ice water. Specimens for acid phosphatase, lactate, and pyruvate, and certain hormone tests (e.g. gastrin and renin activity) should be treated the same way. A notable decrease in pyruvate and increase in lactate concentration occurs within a few minutes at ambient temperature.

For all test constituents that are thermally labile, serum and plasma should be separated from cells in a refrigerated centrifuge. Specimens for bilirubin or carotene and for some drugs, such as methotrexate, must be protected from both daylight and fluorescent light to prevent photo-degradation.

Hemolysis may occur in pneumatic tube systems unless the tubes are completely filled and movement of the blood tubes inside the specimen carrier is prevented. The pneumatic tube system should be designed to eliminate sharp curves and sudden stops of specimen carriers, because these factors are responsible for much of the hemolysis that may occur. With many systems, however, the plasma hemoglobin concentration may be increased, and the serum activity of red cell enzymes, such as lactate dehydrogenase, may also be increased. Nonetheless, the amount of hemolysis is usually so small that it can be ignored. In special cases, such as a patient's undergoing chemotherapy whose cells are fragile, samples should be centrifuged before they are placed in the pneumatic tube system or identified as 'messenger delivery only'.

For specimens that are collected in a remote facility within frequent transportation by courier to a central laboratory, proper specimen processing must be done in the remote facility so that appropriately separated and preserved plasma or serum is delivered to the laboratory. This necessitates that there mote facility has ready access to all commonly used preservatives and wet ice.

Separation and Storage of Specimens

Plasma or serum should be separated from cells as soon as possible and certainly within 2 hours. Premature separation of serum, however, may permit continued formation of fibrin, which can clog sampling devices in testing equipment. If it is impossible to centrifuge a blood specimen within 2 hours, the specimen should be held at room temperature rather than at 4°C to decrease hemolysis. For most plasma samples used for molecular diagnostics, the plasma should be removed from the primary tube promptly after centrifugation and held at −20°C in a freezer capable of maintaining this temperature.

Frostfree freezers should be avoided because they have a wide temperature swing during the freeze-thaw cycle. Note, however, that 4°C or −20°C is not the optimum storage temperature for all tests; some lactate dehydrogenase isoenzymes, for instance, are more stable at room temperature than at 4°C. Although changes in concentration of test constituents have been observed when serum or plasma is stored in a gel separator tube in a refrigerator for 24 hours, these changes do not appear to be large enough to be of clinical significance.

Specimen tubes should be centrifuged with stoppers in place. Closure reduces evaporation, which occurs rapidly in a warm centrifuge with the air currents set up by centrifugation. Stoppers also prevent aerosolization of infectious particles. Specimen tubes containing volatiles, such as ethanol, *must* be stoppered while they are spun. Centrifuging specimens with the stopper in place maintains anaerobic conditions, which are important in the measurement of carbondioxide and ionized calcium. Removal of the stopper before centrifugation allows loss of carbon dioxide and an increase in blood pH. Control of pH is especially important for the enzymatic measurement of acid phosphatase, which is labile under alkaline conditions engendered by CO_2 loss.

Transport of Specimens

Although the remaining discussion uses the specific example of referral laboratory testing by another laboratory, many of the issues discussed, such as regulations related to shipping, are also relevant to a laboratory that receives specimens from outlying clinics via a (laboratory-owned and/or operated) courier service. This may involve validating specific transport/storage conditions that are in conflict with existing clinical and laboratory standards institute (CLSI) recommendations. Before a referral laboratory is used for any tests, the quality of its work should be verified by the referring laboratory.

Guidelines for selection and evaluation of a referral laboratory have been published. For laboratories accredited by the College of American Pathologists (CAP), it is a requirement that the referring laboratory validate that the referral laboratory is clinical laboratory improvement amendments (CLIA) certified by obtaining a copy of the CLIA certificate before specimens are shipped. For molecular diagnostic testing, this is of particular importance, because often the latest genetic test being requested by a physician has not yet been moved from research interest status to patient care status and may not be available in a CLIA-certified laboratory.

Specimen type and quantity and specimen handling requirements of the referral laboratory must be observed, and in laboratories operating under CLIA regulations, test results reported by a referral laboratory must be identified as such when they are filed in a patient's chart. The director of a referring laboratory has the responsibility to ensure that specimens will be adequately transported to the referral laboratory.

Also, the director should determine the benefits of different services and should keep in mind that the fastest service is usually the most expensive. The director should also know that specimens should not be sent to a referral laboratory at the end of the days, because more delays in transit occur during weekends than during the working days, and deterioration of specimens is more likely. It should be assumed that transport from a referring laboratory to a referral laboratory may take as long as 72 hours.

Under optimal conditions, a referring laboratory should retain enough specimen for retesting should an unanticipated problem arise during shipment. The tube used for holding a specimen (primary container) should be so constructed that the contents do not escape if the container is exposed to atmosphere (50 kPa) may be encountered during air transport, together with vibration, and specimens should be protected from these adverse conditions by a suitable container.

Variability in temperature is a significant factor causing instability of test constituents. Polypropylene and polyethylene containers are usually suitable for specimen transport. Glass should be avoided. Polystyrene is unsuitable because it may crack when frozen. Containers must be leakproof and should have a teflon-lined screw cap that does not loosen under the variety of temperatures to which the container may be exposed. The materials of both stopper and container must be inert and must not have any effect on the concentration of the analyte.

The shipping or secondary container used to hold one or more specimen tubes or bottles must be constructed to prevent the tubes from banging against each other. Corrugated, fiberboard, or Styrofoam® boxes designed to fit around a single specimen tube are commonly used.

A padded shipping envelope provides adequate protection for shipping single specimens. When specimens are shipped as drops of blood on filter paper (e.g. for neonatal screening), the paper should be enclosed in a paper envelope to ensure that the sample remains dry. The initial paper envelope can be placed in a shipping envelope and transported to the testing facility; rapid shipping is rarely required for dried blood on paper.

For transport of frozen or refrigerated specimens, a Styrofoam® container should be used. The container walls should be 1 inch (2.5 cm) thick to provide effective insulation. The container should be vented to prevent buildup of carbondioxide under pressure and a possible explosion. Solid carbondioxide (dry ice) is the most convenient refrigerant material for keeping specimens frozen, and temperatures as low as $-70°C$ can be achieved. The amount of dry ice required in a container depends on the size of the container, the efficiency of its insulation, and the length of time for which the specimens must be kept frozen. One piece of solid dry ice (about 3 inches × 4 inches × 1 inch) in a container with 1-inch Styrofoam® walls and a volume of 125 cubic inches (2000 cm^3) will maintain a single specimen frozen for 48 hours.

Various laws and regulations apply to the shipment of biological specimens. Although they theoretically apply only to etiologic agents (known infectious agents), all specimens should be transported as if the same regulations applied. Airlines have rigid regulations covering the transport of specimens. Airlines deem dry ice a hazardous material, therefore, the transport of most clinical laboratory specimens is affected by the regulations, and those who package the specimens should be trained in the appropriate regulations, such as those put forth by the United States Air International Transport Association (IATA).

The various modes of transport of specimens influence the shipping time and cost, and each laboratory will need to make its own assessment as to adequate service. The objective is to ensure that the properly collected, processed, and identified specimen arrives at the testing facility in time and under the correct storage conditions so that the analytical phase can then proceed.

BIBLIOGRAPHY

1. Altman DE, Clancy C, Blendon RJ. Improving patient safety. Five years after the IOM report. N Engl J Med. 2004; 351: 2041–2.

2. Astion ML, Shojana KG, Hamil TR, et al. Classifying laboratory incident reports to identify problems that jeopardize patient safety. Am J Clin Pathol. 2003; 120: 18–26.

3. Auchinleck GF, Lines RB, Godolphin WJ. Cost-effectiveness and benefits of automation and robotics. In: Kost GJ, editor. Clinical automation, robotics and optimization. New York: John Wiley & Sons, 1996.

4. Belk WP, Sunderman FW. A survey of the accuracy of chemical analyses in clinical laboratories. Am J Clin Pathol. 1947;17:853–61.

5. Biosca C, Ricós C, Jiménez CV, et al. Are equally spaced collections necessary to assess biological variation? Evidence from renal transplant recipients. Clin Chim Acta. 2000; 301:79–85.

6. Biosca C, Ricós C, Jiménez CV, et al. Model for establishing biological variation in non-healthy: renal post transplantation. Clin Chem. 1997; 43:2206–8.

7. Biosca C, Ricós C, Lauzurica R, et al. Reference change value concept combining two delta values to predict crises in renal post-transplantation. Clin Chem. 2001; 47:2146–8.

8. Bjerner J, Nustad K, Norum LF, et al. Immunometric assay interference: incidence and prevention. Clin Chem. 2002; 48: 613–21.

9. Bonini P, Plebani M, Ceriotti F, et al. Errors in laboratory medicine. Clin Chem. 2002; 48:691–8.

10. Boone DJ. Is it safe to have a laboratory test? Accred Qual Assur. 2004; 10:5–9.

11. Busch MP, Kleinman SH, Nemo GJ. Current and emerging infectious risks of blood transfusions. J Am Med Assoc. 2003; 289:959–62.

12. Coffin CM, Spilker K, Lowichik A, et al. Critical values in pediatric surgical pathology: definition, implementation, and reporting in a children's hospital. Am J Clin Pathol. 2007; 128: 1035–1040.

13. College of American Pathologists. Laboratory accreditation checklist. http://www.cap.org/apps/cap.portal. Accessed January 18; 2009.

14. Corberand JX, Rogari E, Laharrague P, et al. Computer-assisted validation system applied to hematology: Valab-haemato. Ann Biol Clin (Paris). 1994; 52:447–50.

15. Cotlove E, Harri EK, Wiliams GZ. Biological and analytical components of variation in long term studies of serum constituents in normal subjects. III. Physiological and medical implications. Clin Chem. 1970; 16:1028–32.

16. Dale JC, Howanitz PJ. Patient satisfaction in phlebotomy: a College of American Pathologists Q-Probes study. Lab Med. 1996; 27:188–92.

17. Dighe AS, Rao A, Coakley AB, et al. Analysis of laboratory critical value reporting at a large academic medical center. Am J Clin Pathol. 2006; 125:758–64.

18. Dighe AS, Soderberg BL, Laposata M. Narrative interpretations for clinical laboratory evaluations, Am J Clin Pathol. 2001; 116 (Suppl 1): S123–8.

19. Fihn SD, McDonell M, Martin D, et al. Risk factors for complications of chronic anticoagulation: a multicenter study. Warfarin Optimized Outpatient Follow-up Study Group. Ann Intern Med. 1993; 118:511–20.

20. Forsman RW. Why is the laboratory an afterthought form an aged care organizations? Clin Chem. 1996; 42: 813–6.

21. Fraser CG, Cummings ST, Wilkinson SP, et al. Biological variation of 26 clinical chemistry analytes in elderly people. Clin Chem. 1989; 35:783–6.

22. Fraser CG, Harris EK. Generation and application of data on biological variation in clinical chemistry. Crit Rev Clin Lab Sci. 1989; 27,5:409–37.

23. Fraser CG, Hyltoft Petersen P, Libeer JC, et al. Proposals for setting generally applicable quality goals solely based on biology. Ann Clin Biochem. 1997; 34:8–12.

24. Fraser CG. BV in clinical chemistry. An update: collated data 1988-1991. Arch Pathol Lab Med. 1992; 116:916–23.

25. Fraser CG. Changes in serial results. In: Biological variation: from principles to practice. Washington: AACC Press. 2001; 67–90.

26. Fraser CG. The application of theoretical goals based on BV data in proficiency testing. Arch Pathol Lab Med. 1988; 112:404–15.

27. Fraser FG. The nature of BV. In: Fraser CG. Biological variation: from principles to practice. Washington: AACC Press Washington. 2001;1–28.

28. Fuentes-Arderiu X, Castineiras-Lacambra MJ, Panadero-Garcia MT. Evaluation of the VALAB expert system. Eur J Clin Chem Clin Biochem. 1997; 35:711–4.

29. Goldschmidt HM, Lent RW. Gross errors and work flow analysis in the clinical laboratory. Klin Biochem Metab. 1995;3:131–40.

30. Goldschmidt HM. Postanalytical factors and their influence on analytical quality specifications. Scand J Clin Lab Invest. 1999;59:551–4.

31. Gowans EMS, Hyltoft Petersen P, Blaabjerg O, et al. Analytical goals for the acceptance of common reference intervals for laboratories throughout a geographical area. Scan J Clin Lab Invest. 1988; 48:757–64.

32. Grasbeck R. The evolution of the reference value concept. Clin Chem Lab Med. 2004; 42:692–7.

33. Hanna D, Griswold P, Leape LL, et al. Communicating critical test results: safe practice recommendations. Jt Comm J Qual Patient Saf. 2005; 31:68–80.

34. Harris EK. Statistical principles underlying analytic goal-setting in clinical chemistry. Am J Clin Pathol. 1979;72: 374–82.

35. Haverstick DM. Critical value called, read-back obtained [editorial]. Am J Clin Pathol. 2004;121:790–791.

36. Henny J, Petersen HP. Reference values: from philosophy to a tool for laboratory medicine. Clin Chem Lab Med. 2004; 42:686–91.

37. Holman JW, Mifflin TE, Felder RA, et al. Evaluation of an automated preanalytical robotic work station at two academic health centers. Clin Chem. 2002; 48:540–8.

38. Howanitz JH, Howanitz PJ. Evaluation of total serum calcium critical values. Arch Pathol Lab Med. 2006;130: 828–30.

39. Howanitz PJ, Cembrowski GS. Post analytical quality improvement: a College of American Pathologists Q-Probes study of elevated calcium results in 525 institutions. Arch Pathol Lab Med. 2000; 124:504–10.

40. Howanitz PJ, Renner SW, Walsh MK. Continuous wristband monitoring over 2 years decreases identification errors: a College of American Pathologists Q-Tracks study. Arch Pathol Lab Med. 2002; 126:809–15.

41. Howanitz PJ, Steindel SJ, Heard NV. Laboratory critical values policies and procedures: a College of American Pathologists Q-Probes study in 623 institutions. Arch Pathol Lab Med. 2002; 126:663–69.

42. Howanitz PJ, Steindel SJ. Digoxin therapeutic drug monitoring practices: a College of American Pathologists Q-Probes study of 666 institutions and 18,679 toxic levels. Arch Pathol Lab Med. 1993; 117:573–7.

43. Howanitz PJ. Errors in laboratory medicine. Practical lessons to improve patient safety. Arch Pathol Lab Med. 2005; 129:1252–61.

44. International Organization for Standardization. ISO 15189: 2007: Medical laboratories: particular requirements for quality and competence. Geneva, Switzerland: International Organization for Standardization.

45. Ismail AA, Barth JH. Wrong biochemical results. Br Med J. 2001; 323:705–6.

46. Ismail AA, Walker PL, Barth JH, et al. Wrong biochemistry results: two case reports and observational study in 5310 patients on potentially misleading thyroid-stimulating hormone and gonadotropin immunoassay results. Clin Chem. 2002; 48:2023–9.

47. Jenkins JJ, Mac Crawford J, Bissell MG. Studying critical values: adverse event identification following a critical laboratory values study at the Ohio State University Medical Center. Am J Clin Pathol. 2007;128:604–9.

48. Jones BA, Calam RR, Howanitz PJ. Chemistry specimen acceptability: a College of American Pathologists Q-Probes study of 453 laboratories. Arch Pathol Lab Med. 1997;121: 19–26.

49. Jones R, O'Connor J. Information management and informatics: need for a modern pathology service. Ann Clin Biochem. 2004; 41:183–91.

50. Kalra J. Medical errors: impact on clinical laboratories and other critical areas. Clin Biochem. 2004; 37:1052–62.

51. Kazmierczak SC, Catrou PG. Analytical interference. More than just a laboratory problem. Am J Clin Pathol. 2000; 113:9–11.

52. Kenny D, Fraser CG, Hyltoft Petersen P, et al. Consensus agreement. In: Hyltoft Petersen P, Fraser CG, Kallner A, et al. Strategies to set global analytical quality specifications in laboratory medicine. Scan J Clin Lab Invest 1999; 59(7):585.

53. Khoury M, Burnett L, McKay MA. Error rate in Australian chemical pathology laboratories. Med J Aust. 1996;165: 128–30.

54. Kilpatrick ES, Holding S. Use of computer terminals onwards to access emergency test results: a retrospective-study. Br Med J. 2001; 322:1101–3.

55. Kim EK, Sikaris KA, Gill J, et al. Quality assessment of interpretative commenting in clinical chemistry. Clin Chem. 2004; 50:632–7.

56. Klee GG, Schryver PG, Kisabeth RM. Analytical bias specifications based on the analysis of effects on performance of medical guidelines. Scand J Clin Lab Invest. 1999; 59: 509–12.

57. Klee GG. Clinical interpretation of reference intervals and reference limits. A plea for assay harmonization. Clin Chem Lab Med. 2004; 42:752–7.

58. Kratz A, Soderberg BL, Szczepiorkowski ZM, et al. The generation of narrative interpretations in laboratory medicine. Am J Clin Pathol. 2001; 116(Suppl 1):S133–40.

59. Kricka LJ. Interferences in immunoassays—still a threat. Clin Chem. 2000; 46:1037–8.

60. Landefeld CS, Beyth RJ. Anticoagulant-related bleeding: clinical epidemiology, prediction, and prevention. Am J Med. 1993; 95:315–328.

61. Laposata M. Patient-specific narrative interpretations of complex clinical laboratory evaluations: who is competent to provide them? Clin Chem. 2004; 50:471–2.

62. Laposata ME, Laposata M, Van Cott EM, et al. Physician survey of a laboratory medicine interpretive service and evaluation of the influence of interpretations on laboratory test ordering. Arch Pathol Lab Med. 2004; 128:1424–7.

63. Lapworth R, Teal TK. Laboratory blunders revisited. Ann Clin Biochem. 1994; 31:78–84.

64. Leape LL, Berwick DM. Five years after To Err Is Human. J Am Med Assoc. 2005; 293:2384–90.

65. Levine MN, Hirsh J, Landefeld S, et al. Hemorrhagic complications of anticoagulant treatment. Chest. 1992; 102(Suppl 4):352–363.

66. Lippi G, Brocco G, Franchini M, et al. Comparison of serum creatinine, uric acid, albumin and glucose in male professional endurance athletes compared with healthy controls. Clin Chem Lab Med. 2004; 42:644–7.

67. Lippi G, Brocco G, Salvagno GL, et al. High-workload endurance training may increase the serum ischemia modified albumin concentrations. Clin Chem Lab Med. 2005; 43:741–4.

68. Lippi G, Franchini M, Guidi G. Haematocrit measurement and antidoping policies. Clin Lab Haematol. 2002; 24:65–6.

69. Lippi G, Salvagno GL, Montagnana M, et al. Influence of short-term venous stasis on clinical chemistry testing. Clin Chem Lab Med. 2005; 43: 869–75.

70. Lundberg GD. When to panic over abnormal values. MLO Med Lab Obs. 1972; 4:47–54.

71. Makuch R, Simon R. Sample size requirements for evaluating a conservative therapy. Cancer Treat Rep. 1978; 62:1037–40.

72. Marchand M, Guibourdenche J, Saada J, et al. Real time validation of paediatric biochemical reports using the Valab-Biochem system. Ann Clin Biochem. 1997; 34:389–95.

73. Marks V. False-positive immunoassay results: a multicenter survey of erroneous immunoassay results from assays of 74 analytes in 10 donors from 66 laboratories in seven countries. Clin Chem. 2002; 48: 2008–16.

74. Oberholzer M, Östreicher M, Christen H, et al. Methods in qualitative image analysis. Histochem Cell Biol. 1996; 105:333–55.

75. Oosterhuis WP, Ulenkate HJ, Goldsmidt HM. Evaluation of Lab Respond, a new automated validation system for clinical laboratory test results. Clin Chem. 2000; 46 1811–7.

76. Plebani M, Bonini P. Interdepartmental cooperation may help avoid errors in medical laboratories. Br Med J. 2002; 324: 423–4.

77. Plebani M, Carraro P. Mistakes in a stat laboratory: types and frequency. Clin Chem. 1997; 43:1348–51.

78. Plebani M. Charting the course of medical laboratories in a changing environment. Clin Chim Acta. 2002; 319:87–100.

79. Porth AJ. Plamix. Einintegratives Verfahrenzur Plausibilität-skontrolle. Mitt Dtsch Ges Klin Chem. 1995; 26:91–5.

80. Renner SW, Howanitz PJ, Bachner P. Wristband identi-fication errors reporting in 712 hospitals: a College of American Pathologists Q-Probe study of quality issues in transfusion practice. Arch Pathol Lab Med. 1993; 117:573–7.

81. Ricós C, Álvarez V, Garía-Lario JV, et al. Current databases on BV: pros, cons and progress. In: Hyltoft Petersen P, Fraser CG, Kallner A, Kenny D. Scan J Clin Lab Invest. 1999; 59,7:491–500.

82. Ricós C, Arbós MA. Quality goals for hormone testing. Ann Clin Biochem. 1990; 1–21.

83. Ricós C, Cava F, García-Lario JV, et al. The reference change value: a proposal to interpret laboratory reports in serial testing based on biological variation. Scand J Clin Lab Invest. 2004; 64:175–84.

84. Romero A, Munoz M, Ramos JR, et al. Identification of preanalytical mistakes in the stat section of the clinical laboratory. Clin Chem Lab Med. 2005; 43:974–5.

85. Schifman RB, Meier FA. Viral hepatitis serology test utili-zation. Q-Probes 93-01. Northfield, IL: College of American Pathologists, 1993.

86. Schifman RB, Steindel SJ, Howanitz PJ. Quality of telephone support by clinical laboratories: a College of American Pathologists Q-Probes study involving 459 institutions. Am J Clin Pathol. 1996; 105:517A–518A.

87. Sebastián MA, Lirón FJ, Fuentes X. Intra and inter-individual biological variability data bank. Eur J Clin Chem Clin Biochem. 1997; 35:845–52.

88. Solomon DH, Hashimoto H, Daltroy L, et al. Techniques to improve physicians' use of diagnostic tests: anew conceptual framework. J Am Med Assoc. 1998;280 2020–7.

89. Stankovic AK. The laboratory is a key partner in assuring patient safety. Clin Lab Med. 2004; 24:1023–35.

90. Steindel SJ, Howanitz PJ, Renner SW. Reasons for proficiency testing failures in clinical chemistry and blood gas analysis. Arch Pathol Lab Med. 1996; 120:1094–101.

91. Steindel SJ, Tetrault G. Quality control practices for calcium, cholesterol, digoxin and haemoglobin: a College of American Pathologists Q-Probes study in 505 hospital laboratories. Arch Pathol Lab Med. 1998; 122:401–8.

92. Stroobants AK, Goldschmidt HM, Plebani M. Error budget calculations in laboratory medicine: linking the concepts of biological variation and allowable medical errors. Clin Chim Acta. 2003; 333:169–76.

93. The Royal College of Pathologists. Guidelines for the provision of interpretative comments on biochemical reports. Bull R Coll Pathol. 1998; 104:25–8.

94. Tietz textbook of clinical chemistry 3rd edition, Philadelphia, WB Saunders company, 1995.

95. Tietz textbook of clinical chemistry and molecular biology 5th edition, Philadelphia, WB Saunders Company, 2012.

96. Ulenkate HJLM, Oosterhuis WP, Goldschmidt HMJ. Design of 'RESPOND': an automated validation system for clinical laboratory test results [Abstract]. Ned Tijdschr Klin Chem. 1997; 22:153–4.

97. Ulenkate HJLM, Oosterhuis WP, Osmanovic N, Goldschmidt HMJ. Selfreporting validation software (VALAB and Lab Respond) compared with clinical chemists [Abstract]. Clin Chem Lab Med. 1999; 37:S250.

98. Valdiguié PM, Rogari E, Corberand JX, et al. The performance of the knowledge-based system VALAB revisited: an evaluation after five years. Eur J Clin Chem Clin Biochem. 1996;34:371–6.

99. Valdiguie PM, Rogari E, Philippe H. VALAB: expert system for validation of biochemical data. Clin Chem. 1992; 38: 83–7.

100. Valenstein P, Meier F. Outpatient order accuracy. A College of American Pathologists Q-Probes study of requisition order entry accuracy in 660 institutions. Arch Pathol Lab Med. 1999; 123:1145–50.

101. Valenstein PN, Howanitz PJ. Ordering accuracy: a College of American Pathologists Q-Probes study of 577 institutions. Arch Pathol Lab Med. 1995; 119:117–22.

102. van der Meer FJ, Rosendaal FR, Vandenbroucke JP, et al. Bleeding complications in oral anticoagulant therapy: an analysis of risk factors. Arch Intern Med. 1993; 153: 1557–62.

103. Vasikaran SD, Penberthy L, Gill J, et al. Review of a pilot quality-assessment program for interpretative comments Ann Clin Biochem. 2002; 39:250–60.

104. Westgard JO. Six Sigma quality design and control. Madison, WI: Westgard QC. Inc. 2001.

105. William Marshall, MártaLapsley, Stephen K Bangert. Elsevier.com: Clin Chem, 7th edition ISBN-9780723437031, 2012.

106. Witte DL, VanNess SA, Angstadt DS, et al. Errors, mistakes, blunders, outliers, or unacceptable results: how many? Clin Chem. 1997; 43:1352–6.

107. Witte DL, VanNess SA, Angstadt DS, et al. Errors, mistakes, blunders, outliers, or unacceptable results: how many? Clin Chem. 1997; 43:1352–6.

108. Young DS. Conveying the importance of the preanalytical phase. Clin Chem Lab Med. 2003; 41:884–7.

109. Zardo L, Secchiero S, Sciacovelli L, et al. Reference intervals: are inter laboratory differences appropriate? Clin Chem Lab Med. 1999; 37:1131–3.

2

The Body Buffer Systems and Blood Gases

INTRODUCTION

Acid-base homeostasis is the part of human homeostasis concerning the proper balance between acids and bases, also called body pH. The body's acid-base homeostasis is normally tightly regulated, keeping the arterial blood pH between 7.35 and 7.45. The human body has one of the most complicated and effective buffer systems which are responsible for maintaining human life.

The pH is the measurement used to determine acidity or alkalinity of arterial blood. It is inversely proportional to the number of hydrogen ions (H^+) in the blood. The pH of a solution is measured on a scale from 1 (very acidic) to 14 (very alkalotic). A liquid with a pH of 7, such as water is neutral (neither acidic nor alkalotic). The further away from 7 in either direction indicates the strength of the acid or base. An acid can donate the hydrogen ion (H^+) and the base is a substance which can accept the ion.

The body is in a state of constant change. Thus, the pH is constantly changing within a narrow range of values. This of course is called the homeostatic process. Body waste products are constantly being produced and affecting the pH of the blood. In order for normal metabolism to take place, the body must maintain the narrow range at all times. When the pH is below 7.35, the blood is said to be acidic. Changes in body system functions that occur in an acidic state include a decrease in the force of cardiac contractions, a decrease in the vascular response to catecholamines, and a diminished response to the effects and actions of certain medications. When the pH is above 7.45, the blood is said to be alkalotic.

An alkalotic state interferes with tissue oxygenation and normal neurological and muscular functioning. Significant changes in the blood pH above 7.8 or below 6.8 will interfere with cellular functioning, and if uncorrected, will lead to death (Fig. 2.1).

Three different buffer systems exist in blood; the bicarbonate buffer and the phosphate buffer are composed of 'simple' chemicals. In addition, the carbonyl groups (–COOH) and the amide group (–NH₂) present on proteins allow some of these to act as buffers. Several buffering agents that reversibly bind hydrogen ions and impede any change in pH exist. Extracellular buffers include bicarbonate and ammonia, whereas proteins and phosphate act as intracellular buffers (Table 2.1).

The main buffer that neutralizes hydrogen ions released from cells is the bicarbonate buffer. Another

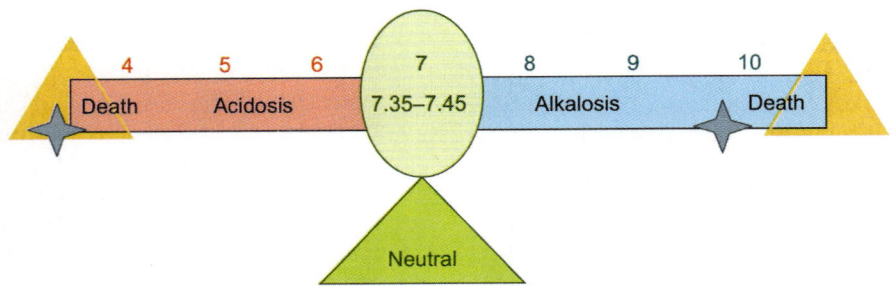

Fig. 2.1: Normal pH of human arterial blood has a pH between 7.35 and 7.45

Table 2.1	Body buffer systems	
Site	**Buffer system**	**Comment**
ISF	Bicarbonate	For metabolic acids
	Phosphate	Not important because concentration too low
	Protein	Not important because concentration too low
Blood	Bicarbonate	Important for metabolic acids
	Hemoglobin	Important for carbon dioxide
	Plasma protein	Minor buffer
	Phosphate	Concentration too low
ICF	Proteins	Important buffer
	Phosphates	Important buffer
Urine	Phosphate	Responsible for most of 'titratable acidity'
	Ammonia	Important—formation of NH_4^+
Bone	Calcium carbonate	In prolonged metabolic acidosis

ICF, intracellular fluid; ISF, interstitial fluid

important buffer is hemoglobin, which contributes to buffering of hydrogen ion generated from the carbonic anhydrase reaction. Hydrogen ion is neutralized by intracellular buffers, mainly proteins and phosphates.

The bicarbonate buffering system is especially a key, as carbon dioxide (CO_2) can be shifted through carbonic acid (H_2CO_3) to hydrogen ions (H^+) and bicarbonate ions (HCO_3^-):

$$H_2O + CO_2 \leftrightarrow H_2CO_3 \leftrightarrow H^+ + HCO_3^-$$

Acid-base imbalances that overcome the buffer system can be compensated in the short term by changing the rate of ventilation. This alters the concentration of carbon dioxide in the blood, shifting the above reaction according to Le Chatelier's principle, which in turn alters the pH.

The kidneys are slower to compensate, but renal physiology has several powerful mechanisms to control pH by the excretion of excess acid or base. In response to acidosis, tubular cells reabsorb more bicarbonate from the tubular fluid, collecting duct cells secrete more hydrogen and generate more bicarbonate, and ammoniagenesis leads to increased formation of the NH_3 buffer. In response to alkalosis, the kidneys may excrete more bicarbonate by decreasing hydrogen ion secretion from the tubular epithelial cells, and lowering rates of glutamine metabolism and ammonium excretion.

ACID-BASE HOMEOSTASIS

Acid-base homeostasis is one of the homeostatic mechanisms required to maintain health. It refers to the equilibrium between acids and bases; it is also referred to as body pH. An acid is a substance capable of giving up a hydrogen ion during a chemical exchange, and a base is a substance that can accept it. The positively charged hydrogen ion (H^+) is the active constituent of all acids.

Most of the body's metabolic processes produce acids as their end products, but a somewhat alkaline body fluid is required as a medium for vital cellular activities. Therefore, chemical exchanges of hydrogen ions must take place continuously in order to maintain a state of equilibrium. An optimal pH (hydrogen ion concentration) between 7.35 and 7.45 must be maintained; otherwise, the enzyme systems and other biochemical and metabolic activities will not function normally.

The body's response to a change in acid-base homeostasis has three components (Fig. 2.2):

1. **The chemical buffer systems (immediate response):** Buffering is a rapid physicochemical phenomenon. The body has a large buffer capacity. The buffering of fixed acids by bicarbonate changes the $[HCO_3^-]$ numerator in the ratio (in the Henderson-Hasselbalch equation).

   $$pH = pK'a + \log_{10}([HCO_3^-]/0.03 \times pCO_2)$$

2. **The respiratory regulation (alteration in ventilation):** Adjustment of the denominator pCO_2 (in the Henderson-Hasselbalch equation) by alterations in ventilation is relatively rapid (minutes to hours).

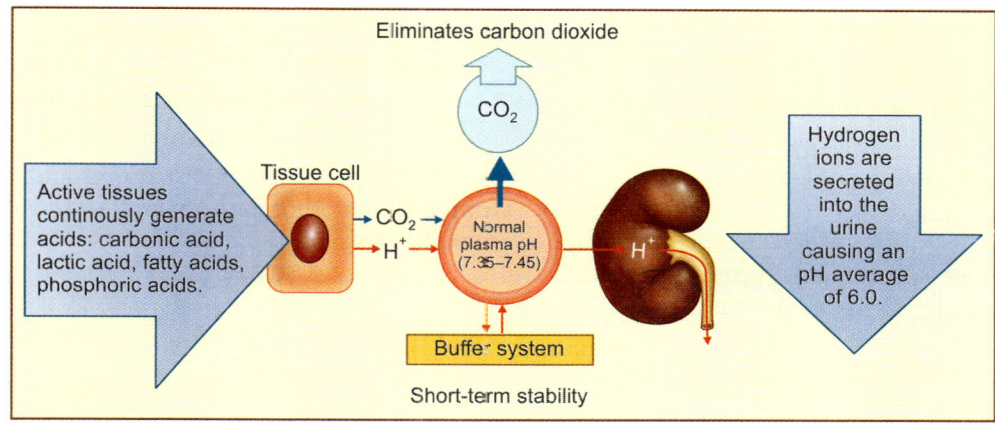

Fig. 2.2: The body response to a change in acid-base homeostasis has three components

An increased CO_2 excretion due to hyperventilation will result in one of the three acid-base outcomes:
- Correction of a respiratory acidosis
- Production of a respiratory alkalosis
- Compensation for a metabolic acidosis

Which of these three circumstances is present cannot be deduced merely from the observation of the presence of hyperventilation in a patient.

This respiratory response is particularly useful physiologically because of its effect on intracellular pH as well as extracellular pH. Carbon dioxide crosses cell membranes easily so changes in pCO_2 affect intracellular pH rapidly and in a predictable direction.

The system has to be able to respond quickly and to have a high capacity because of the huge amounts of respiratory acid to be excreted.

3. **Renal regulation and role of the kidneys (alteration in bicarbonate excretion):** This much slower process (several days to reach maximum capacity) involves adjustment of bicarbonate excretion by the kidney. This system is responsible for the excretion of the fixed acids and for compensatory changes in plasma $[HCO_3^-]$ in the presence of respiratory acid-base disorders.

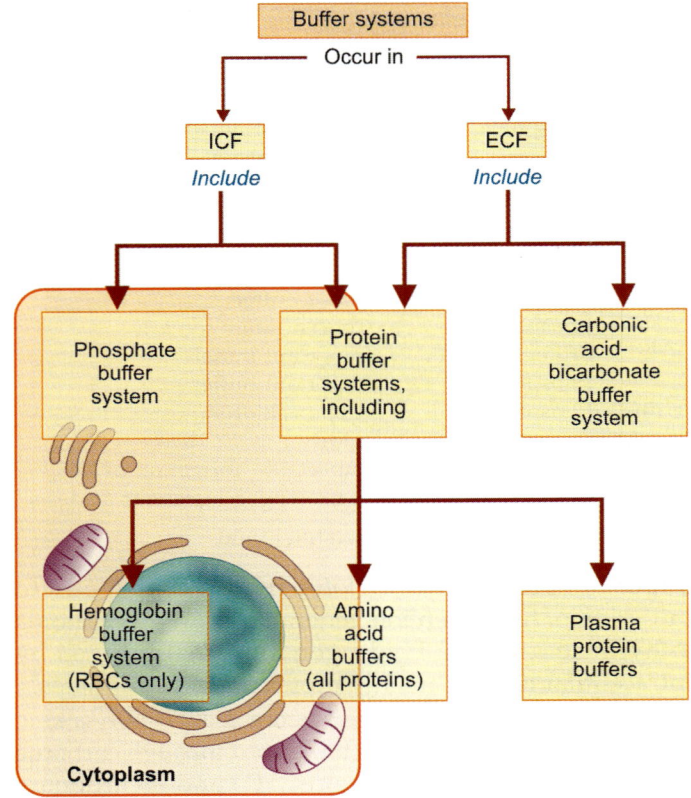

Fig. 2.3: The three main buffer systems in the body

CHEMICAL BUFFER SYSTEMS

Various buffer systems exist in body fluids to correct both excess acidity and alkalinity. The main buffer systems involved in the maintenance of body pH are (Fig. 2.3)
- Carbonic acid-bicarbonate buffer system
- Phosphate buffer
- Protein buffer

In extracellular fluid (ECF), the carbonic acid-bicarbonate buffer system is quantitatively the most important for buffering metabolic acids. Its effectiveness is greatly increased by ventilatory changes which attempt to maintain a constant pCO_2 and by renal mechanisms, which result in changes in plasma bicarbonate.

In blood, hemoglobin is the most important buffer for CO_2 because of its high concentration and its large number of histidine residues.

Carbonic Acid-Bicarbonate Buffer System

The main buffer system in the ECF is the carbonic acid-bicarbonate buffer system. This is responsible for about 80% of extracellular buffering. It is the most important ECF buffer for metabolic acids, but it cannot buffer respiratory acid-base disorders. The components are

easily measured and are related to each other by the Henderson-Hasselbalch equation.

$$pH = pK'a + \log_{10} ([HCO_3^-]/0.03 \times pCO_2)$$

The pK'a value is dependent on the temperature, $[H^+]$ and the ionic concentration of the solution. It has a value of 6.099 at a temperature of 37°C and a plasma pH of 7.4. At a temperature of 30°C and pH of 7.0, it has a value of 6.148. For practical purposes, a value of 6.1 is generally assumed and corrections for temperature, pH of plasma and ionic strength are not used except in precise experimental work.

The pK'a is derived from the Ka value of the following reaction:

$$H_2O + CO_2 \leftrightarrow H_2CO_3 \leftrightarrow H^+ + HCO_3^-$$

(where CO_2 refers to dissolved CO_2)

The concentration of carbonic acid is very low compared to the other components so the above equation is usually simplified to:

$$H_2O + CO_2 \leftrightarrow H^+ + HCO_3^-$$

By the law of mass action:

$$Ka = [H^+] \cdot [HCO_3^-]/[CO_2] \cdot [H_2O]$$

The concentration of H_2O is so large compared to the other components, the small loss of water due to this reaction changes its concentration by only an extremely small amount. This means that $[H_2O]$ is effectively constant. This allows further simplification as the two constants (Ka and $[H_2O]$) can be combined into a new constant K'a.

$$K'a = Ka \times [H_2O] = [H^+] \cdot [HCO_3^-]/[CO_2]$$

The excretion of CO_2 via the lungs is particularly important because of the rapidity of the response. The adjustment of pCO_2 by change in alveolar ventilation has been referred to as physiological buffering.

The bicarbonate buffer system is an effective buffer system despite having a low pKa because the body also controls pCO_2.

The glomerular filtrate contains the same concentration of bicarbonate ions as the plasma. At normal rates of glomerular filtration, approximately 4300 mmol/24 h of bicarbonate is filtered by the renal glomeruli. If this bicarbonate were not reabsorbed, copious amounts would be excreted in the urine, depleting the body's buffering capacity and causing an acidosis. In health, at normal plasma bicarbonate concentrations, virtually all the filtered bicarbonate is reabsorbed.

The luminal surface of renal tubular cells is impermeable to bicarbonate and, therefore, direct reabsorption cannot occur. Within the renal tubular cells, carbonic acid is formed from carbon dioxide and water (Fig. 2.4). This otherwise rather slow reaction is catalyzed in the kidneys by the enzyme carbonate dehydratase (carbonic anhydrase). The carbonic acid thus formed dissociates into hydrogen and bicarbonate ions. The bicarbonate ions pass across the basolateral borders of the cells into the interstitial fluid. The hydrogen ions are secreted across the luminal membrane in exchange for sodium ions, which accompany bicarbonate into the interstitial fluid (Fig. 2.4). The formation of bicarbonate and hydrogen ions is promoted by their continuous removal and by the presence of carbonate dehydratase.

In the tubular fluid, hydrogen ions combine with bicarbonate to form carbonic acid, most of which dissociates into carbon dioxide and water. Some of the carbon dioxide diffuses back into the renal tubular cells (and is converted via carbonic acid into bicarbonate and hydrogen ions), while the remainder is excreted in the urine. This whole process, which takes place primarily in the proximal convoluted tubules, effectively results in the reabsorption of filtered bicarbonate.

Although hydrogen ions are secreted into the tubular fluid during bicarbonate reabsorption, this does not represent net acid excretion. The formation of these hydrogen ions merely provides the means for the reabsorption of bicarbonate. Net acid excretion depends on the same reactions occurring in the renal tubular cells, but in addition, requires the presence of a suitable buffer system in the urine. This is because the minimum urinary pH that can be generated, 4.6, is equivalent to a hydrogen ion concentration of approximately 25 μmol/L. Given a normal urine volume of 1.5 L/24 h, free hydrogen ion excretion can account for less than a thousandth of the total amount that has to be excreted.

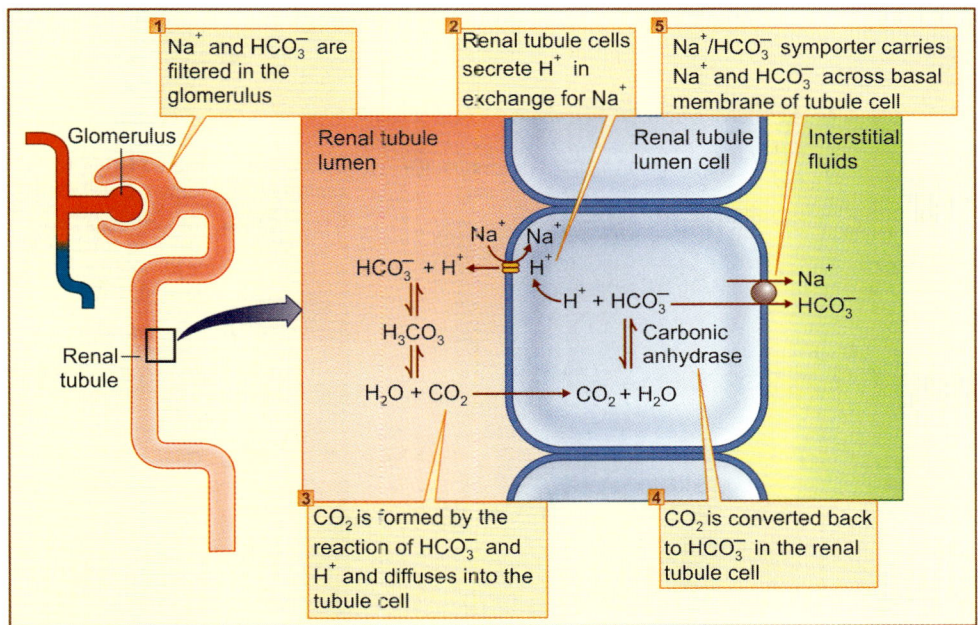

Fig. 2.4: Hydrogen and bicarbonate ions are generated in renal tubular cells and the hydrogen ions are secreted in exchange for sodium into the tubular lumen where they combine with filtered bicarbonate to form carbon dioxide and water. Bicarbonate ions diffuse with sodium from the tubular cells into the interstitial fluid and thence into the plasma

PHOSPHATE BUFFERS

The phosphate buffer system is not an important blood buffer, as its concentration is too low. It presents in the glomerular filtrate, approximately 80% being in the form of the divalent anion HPO_4^{2-}, this combines with hydrogen ions and is converted to $H_2PO_4^-$:

$$HPO_4^{2-} + H^+ \leftrightarrow H_2PO_4^-$$

At the minimum urinary pH, virtually all the phosphate is in the $H_2PO_4^-$ form. About 30–40 mmol of hydrogen ions are normally excreted in this way every 24 hours.

Ammonia

Ammonia produced by the deamination of glutamine in renal tubular cells, is also an important urinary buffer. The enzyme that catalyzes this reaction, i.e. glutaminase, is induced in states of chronic acidosis, allowing increased ammonia production and hence increased hydrogen ion excretion via ammonium ions. Ammonia can readily diffuse across cell membranes, but ammonium ions, formed when ammonia buffers hydrogen ions cannot. Passive reabsorption of ammonium ions is therefore prevented.

$$NH_3 + H^+ \leftrightarrow NH_4^+$$

At normal intracellular hydrogen ion concentrations, most ammonia is present as ammonium ions. Diffusion of ammonia out of the cell disturbs the equilibrium, causing more ammonia to be formed. The simultaneous production of hydrogen ions would seem to negate the process. However, these ions are used up in gluconeogenesis, when they combine with glutamate formed by the deamination of glutamine. There may also be some shift of hepatic urea synthesis to glutamine synthesis. Urinary hydrogen ion excretion is summarized in (Fig. 2.5). Acidification of the urine takes place primarily in the distal parts of the distal convoluted tubules and in the collecting ducts, where an ATP-dependent H^+-pump in the α-intercalated cells secretes hydrogen ions in exchange for potassium ions. In addition, sodium reabsorption by the principal cells creates an electrochemical gradient that engenders the secretion of potassium and hydrogen ions. Aldosterone facilitates hydrogen ion secretion directly by stimulating the H^+-pump and indirectly through enhancing sodium reabsorption.

It will be apparent that hydrogen and bicarbonate ions are generated in equimolar amounts in renal tubular cells. This is essential for the reabsorption of filtered bicarbonate, but also means that, when a hydrogen ion is excreted in the urine, a bicarbonate ion is produced and retained. This process effectively regenerates the bicarbonate ions consumed when hydrogen ions are buffered.

There is considerable secretion of both acid (by the stomach) and bicarbonate (by the pancreas and small intestine) into the gut, but these processes are normally in homeostasis and in health doing not contribute to net hydrogen ion excretion.

Hemoglobin is an important blood buffer particularly for buffering CO_2.

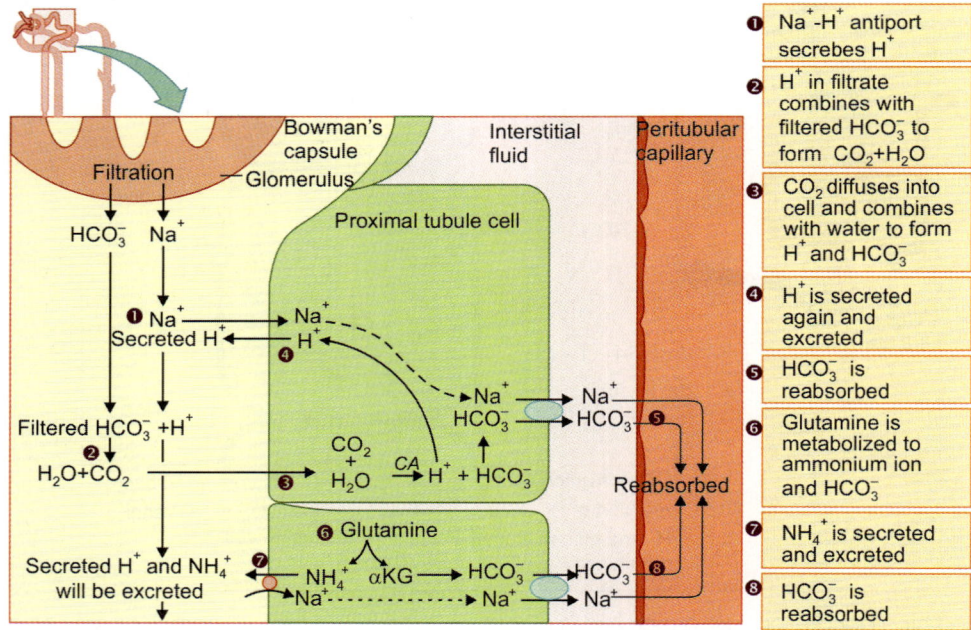

Fig. 2.5: The hydrogen ions are excreted in the urine buffered by phosphate and ammonia, while the bicarbonate enters the ECF, replacing that which was consumed in buffering

Protein buffers in blood include hemoglobin (150 g/L) and plasma proteins (70 g/L). Buffering is by the imidazole group of the histidine residues which has a pKa of about 6.8. This is suitable for effective buffering at physiological pH. Hemoglobin is quantitatively about 6 times more important than the plasma proteins as it is present in about twice the concentration and contains about 3 times the number of histidine residues per molecule. For example, if blood pH changed from 7.5 to 6.5, hemoglobin would buffer 27.5 mmol/L of H^+ and total plasma protein buffering would account for only 4.2 mmol/L of H^+.

Deoxyhemoglobin is a more effective buffer than oxyhemoglobin and this change in buffer capacity contributes about 30% of the Haldane effect. The main factor accounting for the Haldane effect in CO_2 transport is the much greater ability of deoxyhemoglobin to form carbamino compounds.

In red blood cells, metabolism is anerobic and little carbon dioxide is produced. Carbon dioxide thus diffuses into red cells down a concentration gradient and carbonic acid is formed, facilitated by carbonate dehydratase (Fig. 2.6). Hemoglobin buffers the hydrogen ions formed when the carbonic acid dissociates is a more powerful buffer when in the deoxygenated state and the proportion in this state increases during the passage of blood through capillary beds, as oxygen is lost to the tissues.

The overall effect of this process is that carbon dioxide is converted to bicarbonate in red blood cells. This bicarbonate diffuses out of the red cells because a concentration gradient develops; electrochemical neutrality is maintained by inward diffusion of chloride ions (the chloride shift). In the lungs, the reverse process occurs; the oxygenation reduces its buffering capacity,

liberating hydrogen ions; these combine with bicarbonate to form carbon dioxide, which diffuses into the alveoli to be excreted in the expired air while bicarbonate diffuses into the cells from the plasma.

Most of the carbon dioxide in the blood is present in the form of bicarbonate. Dissolved carbon dioxide, carbonic acid and carbamino compounds (compounds of carbon dioxide and protein) account for less than 2.0 mmol/L in a total carbon dioxide concentration of approximately 26 mmol/L. The terms 'bicarbonate' and 'total carbon dioxide' are frequently used synonymously. They are not strictly the same, but may be considered to be so for most practical clinical purposes. It is technically difficult to measure bicarbonate concentration alone; most analytical techniques for bicarbonate, actually measure total carbon dioxide.

ROLE OF BONE BUFFERING

The carbonate and phosphate salts in bone act as a long-term supply of buffer especially during prolonged metabolic acidosis.

Bone consists of matrix within which specialised cells are dispersed. The matrix is composed of organic (collagen and other proteins in ground substance) and inorganic [hydroxyapatite crystals, general formula $Ca_{10}(PO_4)_6(OH)_2$] components. The hydroxyapatite crystals make up two-thirds of the total bone volume, but they are extremely small and consequently have a huge total surface area. The crystals contain a large amount of carbonate (CO_3^{2-}) as this anion can be substituted for both phosphate and hydroxyl ions in the apatite crystals. Bone is the main CO_2 reservoir in the body and contains carbonate and bicarbonate equivalent to 5 moles of CO_2 out of a total body CO_2 store of 6 moles.

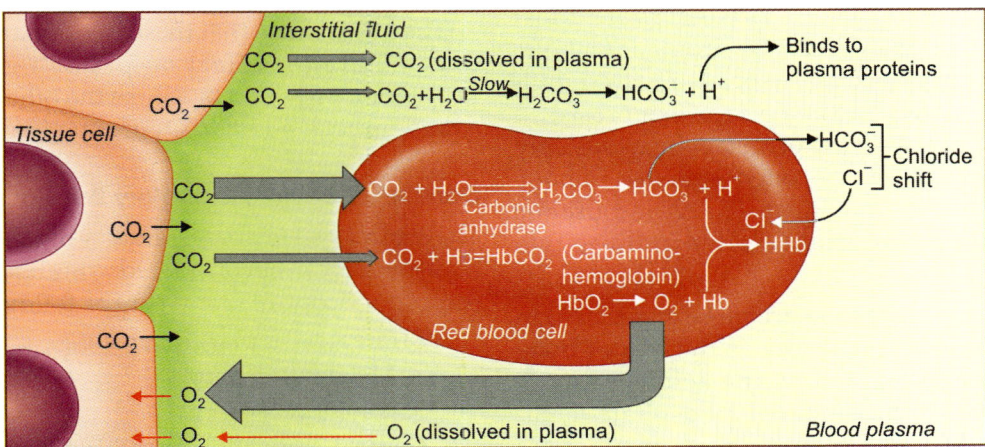

Fig. 2.6: Transport of carbon dioxide in the blood. In capillary beds, carbon dioxide diffuses into red blood cells and combines with water to form carbonic acid; the reaction is catalyzed by carbonate dehydratase. The carbonic acid dissociates to form hydrogen ions, which are buffered by hemoglobin, and bicarbonate, which diffuses out of the cell; chloride diffuses in to maintain electrochemical neutrality. In the alveoli, the process reverses; carbon dioxide is produced from bicarbonate and is excreted in the expired air

CO_2 in bone is in two forms—bicarbonate (HCO_3^-) and carbonate (CO_3^{2-}). The bicarbonate makes up a readily exchangeable pool, because it is present in the bone water which makes up the 'hydration shell' around each of the hydroxyapatite crystals. The carbonate is present in the crystals and its release requires dissolution of the crystals. This is a much slower process, but the amounts of buffer involved are much larger.

How Does Bone Act as a Buffer?

Two processes are involved:
- Ionic exchange
- Dissolution of bone crystal

Bone can take up H^+ in exchange for Ca^{2+}, Na^+, and K^+ (ionic exchange) or release of HCO^{3-}, CO_3^-, or HPO_4^{2-}. In acute metabolic acidosis uptake of H^+ by bone in exchange for Na^+ and K^+ is involved in buffering as this can occur rapidly without any bone breakdown. A part of the so called 'intracellular buffering' of acute metabolic disorders may represent some of this acute buffering by bone. In chronic metabolic acidosis, the main buffering mechanism by far is release of calcium carbonate from bone. The mechanism by which this dissolution of bone crystal occurs involves two processes:
- Direct physicochemical breakdown of crystals in response to [H^+]
- Osteoclastic reabsorption of bone.

The involvement of these processes in buffering is independent of parathyroid hormone. Intracellular acidosis in osteoclasts results in a decrease in intracellular Ca^{2+} and this stimulates these cells.

Bone is probably involved in providing some buffering for all acid-base disturbances. Little experimental evidence is available for respiratory disorders. Most research has been concerned with chronic metabolic acidosis, as these conditions are associated with significant loss of bone mineral (osteomalacia, osteoporosis). In terms of duration only two types of metabolic acidosis are long-lasting enough to be associated with loss of bone mineral, i.e. renal tubular acidosis (RTA) and uremic acidosis. Bone is an important buffer in these two conditions.

In uremia, additional factors are more significant in causing the renal osteodystrophy as the loss of bone mineral cannot be explained by the acidosis alone. Changes in vitamin D metabolism, phosphate metabolism and secondary hyperparathyroidism are more important than the acidosis in causing loss of bone mineral in uremic patients. The loss of bone mineral due to these other factors releases substantial amounts of buffer.

RESPIRATORY REGULATION

'Respiratory regulation' refers to changes in pH due to pCO_2 changes from alterations in ventilation. This change in ventilation can occur rapidly with significant effects on pH. Carbon dioxide is lipid soluble and crosses cell membranes rapidly, so changes in pCO_2 result in rapid changes in [H^+] in all body fluid compartments.

A quantitative appreciation of respiratory regulation requires knowledge of two relationships which provide the connection between alveolar ventilation and pH via pCO_2. These two relationships are:
- First equation—alveolar ventilation (V_A) and pCO_2.
- Second equation—pCO_2 and pH.

1. **First equation (alveolar ventilation—arterial pCO_2 relationship):**
   Relationship: Changes in alveolar ventilation are inversely related to changes in arterial pCO_2 (and directly proportional to total body CO_2 production).
   pCO_2 is proportional to [V_{CO_2}/V_A]
   where:
   - pCO_2 = Arterial partial pressure of CO_2
   - V_{CO_2} = Carbon dioxide production by the body
   - V_A = Alveolar ventilation
   Alternatively, this formula can be expressed as:
   $$pCO_2 = 0.863 \times [V_{CO_2}/V_A]$$
   (If V_{CO_2} has units of mL/min at STP and V_A has units of L/min at 37°C and at atmospheric pressure).

2. **Second equation (Henderson-Hasselbalch equation):**
   Relationship: These changes in arterial pCO_2 cause changes in pH (as defined in the Henderson-Hasselbalch equation).

The key point is that these two equations can be used to calculate the effect on pH of a given change in ventilation provided of course the other variables in the equations (e.g. body's CO_2 production) are known.

Control System for Respiratory Regulation

The control system for respiratory regulation of acid-base homeostasis can be considered using basic elements of the respiratory control system are as follows:

1. **Strategically placed sensors:**
   - Mechanoreceptors
   - Chemoreceptors
2. **Central controller:** Breathing is mainly controlled at the level of brainstem. The normal automatic and periodic nature of breathing is triggered and controlled by the respiratory centers located in the pons and medulla. These centers are not located in

a special nucleus or a group of nuclei, but they are rather poor defined collection of neurons.
- Medullary respiratory centre
- Apneustic centre
- Pneumotaxic centre

3. **Respiratory muscles:** Diaphragm, intercostal muscles, and the other accessory respiratory muscles work in coordination for normal breathing under central controller. There is evidence suggesting that in premature newborn babies this coordination is not mature enough and this could be responsible for the sudden infant death syndrome.

Renal Regulation and Role of the Kidneys

The discussion above has described the mechanisms involved in renal acid excretion and mentioned some factors which regulate acid excretion.

The main factors which regulate renal bicarbonate reabsorption and acid excretion are as follows:

1. **Extracellular volume:** Volume depletion is associated with Na^+ retention and this also enhances HCO_3^- reabsorption. Conversely, ECF volume expansion results in renal Na^+ excretion and secondary decrease in HCO_3^- reabsorption.

2. **Arterial pCO_2:** An increase in arterial pCO_2 results in increased renal H^+ secretion and increased bicarbonate reabsorption. The converse also applies Hypercapnia results in an intracellular acidosis and this result in enhanced H^+ secretion. The cellular processes involved have not been clearly delineated This renal bicarbonate retention is the renal compensation for a chronic respiratory acidosis.

3. **Potassium and chloride deficiency:** Potassium has a role in bicarbonate reabsorption. Low intracellular K^+ levels result in increased HCO_3^- reabsorption in the kidney. Chloride deficiency is extremely important in the maintenance of a metabolic alkalosis because it prevents excretion of the excess HCO_3^- (i.e. now the bicarbonate instead of chloride is reabsorbed with Na^+ to maintain electroneutrality).

4. **Aldosterone and cortisol (hydrocortisone):** Aldosterone at normal levels has no role in renal regulation of acid-base homeostasis. Aldosterone depletion or excess does have indirect effects. High aldosterone levels result in increased Na^+ reabsorption and increased urinary excretion of H^+ and K^+ resulting in a metabolic alkalosis. Conversely, it might be thought that hypoaldosteronism would be associated with a metabolic acidosis, but this is very uncommon, but may occur if there is coexistent significant interstitial renal disease.

5. **Phosphate excretion:** Phosphate is the main component of titratable acidity. The amount of phosphate present in the distal tubule does not vary greatly. Consequently, changes in phosphate excretion do not have a significant regulatory role in response to an acid load.

6. **Reduction in glomerular filtration rate:** It has recently been established that a reduction in glomerular filtration rate (GFR) is a very important mechanism responsible for the maintenance of a metabolic alkalosis. The filtered load of bicarbonate is reduced proportionately with a reduction in GFR.

7. **Ammonium:** The kidney responds to an acid load by increasing tubular production and urinary excretion of NH_4^+. The mechanism involves an acidosis-stimulated enhancement of glutamine utilization by the kidney resulting in increased production of NH_4^+ and HCO_3^- by the tubule cells. This is very important in increasing renal acid excretion during a chronic metabolic acidosis. There is a lag period; the increase in ammonium excretion takes several days to reach its maximum following an acute acid load. Ammonium excretion can increase up to about 300 mmol/day in a chronic metabolic acidosis so this is important in renal acid-base regulation in this situation. Ammonium excretion increases with decrease in urine pH and this relationship is markedly enhanced with acidosis.

As pH falls, the three factors involved in increased H^+ excretion are:

1. **Increased ammonium excretion** increases steadily with decrease in urine pH and this effect is augmented in acidosis. This is the main regulatory factor because it can be increased significantly.

2. **Increased titratable acidity (TA)**
   - Increased buffering by phosphate (but negligible further effect on H^+ excretion if pH <5.5 as too far from pKa so minimal amounts of HPO_4^{2-} remaining)
   - Increased buffering by other organic acids (if present) may be important at lower pH values as their pKa is lower (e.g. creatinine, keto-anions)

3. **Bicarbonate:** Reabsorption is complete at low urinary pH so none is lost in the urine (such loss would antagonize the effects of an increased TA or ammonium excretion on acid excretion).

ACID-BASE DISORDERS

Pathophysiologic disturbances that tend to increase or decrease hydrogen ion concentration called acidosis and alkalosis respectively. Four components can be identified in the pathophysiology of hydrogen ion disorders (acid-base disorders):

1. Generation
2. Buffering
3. Compensation
4. Correction

Primary disturbances in pCO_2 cause the respiratory acid-base disorders, whereas primary alterations in bicarbonate are responsible for the metabolic disturbances (Fig. 2.7). Each primary disturbance elicits a compensatory response, which is usually incomplete, but returns the pH toward normal.

Classification of the Acid-base Disorders

Acid-base disorders are classified as either respiratory or metabolic according to whether or not there is a primary change in pCO_2. The term acidosis signifies a tendency for the [H$^+$] to be above normal, and alkalosis for it to be below normal.

Primary mixed acid-base disorders, i.e. disorders of combined respiratory and metabolic origin, are common. However, the secondary, or compensatory, responses to a primary disorder of hydrogen ion homoeostasis may produce changes in the measured indices indistinguishable from those seen in primary mixed disorders.

RESPIRATORY ACIDOSIS

A respiratory acidosis is a primary acid-base disorder in which arterial pCO_2 rises to a level higher than expected. At onset, the acidosis is designated as an 'acute respiratory acidosis'. The body's initial compensatory response is limited during this phase. As the body's renal compensatory response increases over the next few days, the pH returns towards the normal value and the condition is now a 'chronic respiratory acidosis'.

The differentiation between acute and chronic is determined by time, but occurs because of the renal compensatory response.

The arterial pCO_2 is normally maintained at a level of about 40 mmHg by a balance between production of CO_2 by the body and its removal by alveolar ventilation. If the inspired gas contains no CO_2, then this relationship can be expressed by:

$$pCO_2 \text{ is proportional to } V_{CO_2}/V_A$$

where:

V_{CO_2} is CO_2 production by the body
V_A is alveolar ventilation

An increase in arterial pCO_2 can occur by one of three possible mechanisms:

- Presence of excess CO_2 in the inspired gas
- Decreased alveolar ventilation
- Increased production of CO_2 by the body

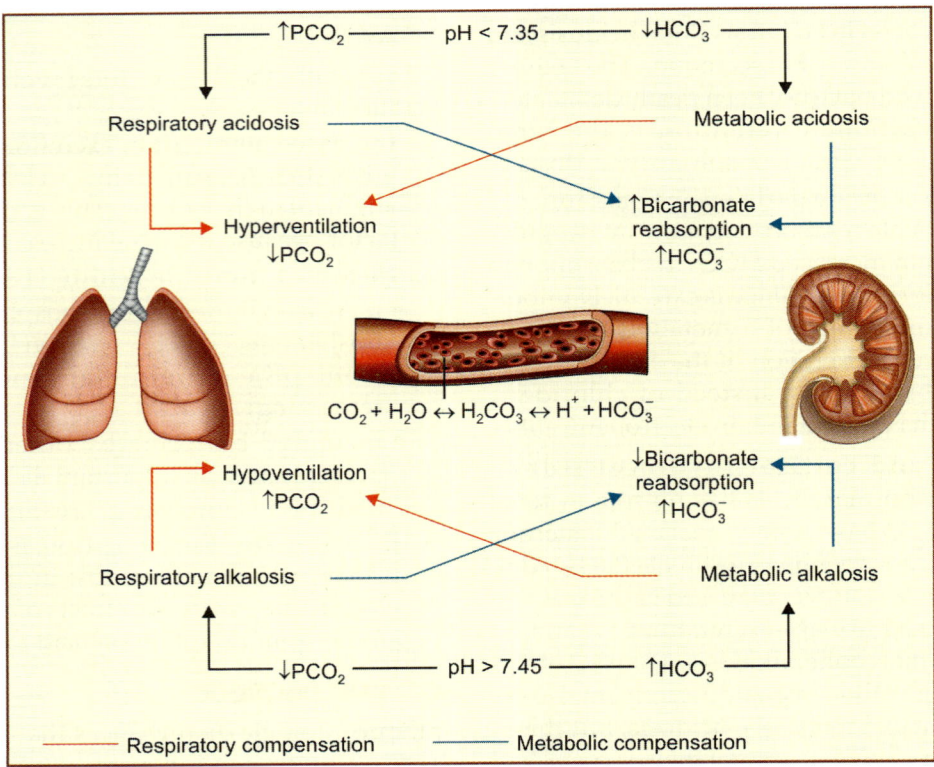

Fig. 2.7: Respiratory and metabolic acidosis and alkalosis

CO2 gas can be added to the inspired gas or it may be present because of rebreathing. Anesthetists are familiar with both these mechanisms. In these situations, hypercapnia can be induced even in the presence of normal alveolar ventilation and normal carbon dioxide production by the body.

An adult at rest produces about 200 mL of CO_2 per minute—this is excreted via the lungs and the arterial pCO_2 remains constant. An increased production of CO_2 would lead to a respiratory acidosis if ventilation remained constant. The system controlling arterial pCO_2 is very efficient, (i.e. rapid and effective) and any increase in pCO_2 very promptly results in a large increase in ventilation. The result is that increased CO_2 production almost never results in respiratory acidosis. It is only in situations where ventilation is fixed that increased production will cause respiratory acidosis. Examples of this would be a ventilated patient who develops acute malignant hyperthermia; the arterial pCO_2 will rise unless the alveolar ventilation is substantially increased.

Etiology

Most cases of respiratory acidosis are due to decreased alveolar ventilation that it may impair oxygen uptake. The defect leading to this can occur at any level in the respiratory control mechanism. This provides a convenient way to classify causes (Table 2.2).

The degree of arterial hypoxemia will be related to the amount of hypoventilation. Increasing the percent of oxygen in the inspired gas can completely correct the hypoxemia if hypoventilation is the only factor involved. If pulmonary disease leading to shunt or ventilation-perfusion mismatch is present, then the hypoxemia will not be so easily corrected. The following list classifies causes by the mechanism or site causing the respiratory acidosis.

In clinically practice, nearly all cases are due to inadequate alveolar ventilation. This is a very important point. Nevertheless, the rare causes should be considered especially in anesthetic and intensive care practice, where patients are often intubated and connected to circuits. Particular issues here include:

- Malignant hyperthermia (MH) is an extremely rare, but potentially fatal condition which occurs almost exclusively in anesthetized patients exposed to certain drugs.
- Various circuit misconnections and malfunctions, or soda lime exhaustion, can result in significant rebreathing of expired carbon dioxide.
- Patients who are paralyzed and on controlled ventilation, cannot increase their alveolar ventilation to excrete any increased amounts of CO_2 produced by the body (e.g. in hypercatabolic states such as sepsis or MH).

Table 2.2	Causes of respiratory acidosis (classified by mechanism)

A: Inadequate alveolar ventilation

Central respiratory depression and other CNS problems
- Drug depression of resp. center (e.g. by opiates, sedatives, and anesthetics)
- CNS trauma, infarct, haemorrhage or tumor
- Hypoventilation of obesity (e.g. Pickwickian syndrome)
- Cervical cord trauma or lesions (at or above C4 level)
- High central neural blockade
- Poliomyelitis
- Tetanus
- Cardiac arrest with cerebral hypoxia

Nerve or Muscle disorders
- Guillain-Barre syndrome
- Myasthenia gravis
- Muscle relaxant drugs
- Toxins, e.g. organophosphates, snake venom
- Various myopathies

Lung or chest wall defects
- Acute respiratory failure in chronic obstructive airways disease
- Chest trauma—flail chest, contusion, and hemothorax
- Pneumothorax
- Diaphragmatic paralysis or splinting
- Pulmonary oedema
- Adult respiratory distress syndrome
- Restrictive lung disease
- Aspiration

Airway disorders
- Upper airway obstruction
- Laryngospasm
- Bronchospasm/Asthma

External factors
- Inadequate mechanical ventilation

B: Overproduction of carbon dioxide

Hypercatabolic disorders
- Malignant hyperthermia

C: Increased intake of carbon dioxide

Rebreathing of CO_2-containing expired gas
Addition of CO_2 to inspired gas
Insufflation of CO_2 into body cavity (e.g. for laparoscopic surgery)

- Exogenous carbon dioxide is introduced into the body in certain procedures (e.g. laparoscopy) and this increases the amount of carbon dioxide to be excreted by the lungs.
- Adding CO_2 to the inspired gas as a respiratory stimulant has resulted in adverse outcomes in the past (this practice is now abandoned in modern anesthetic practice).

Symptoms and Signs

Symptoms and signs depend on the rate and degree of pCO_2 increase. CO_2 rapidly diffuses across the blood-brain barrier. Symptoms and signs are a result of high CNS CO_2 concentrations (low CNS pH) and any accompanying hypoxemia.

Acute (or acutely worsening chronic) respiratory acidosis causes headache, confusion, anxiety, drowsiness, and stupor (CO_2 narcosis). Slowly developing, stable respiratory acidosis (as in chronic obstructive pulmonary disease) may be well tolerated, but patients may have memory loss, sleep disturbances, excessive daytime sleepiness, and personality changes. Signs include gait disturbance, tremor, blunted deep tendon reflexes, myoclonic jerks, asterix is, and papilledema.

Maintenance

A rise in arterial pCO_2 is a potent stimulus to ventilation, so a respiratory acidosis will rapidly correct unless some abnormal factor is maintaining the hypoventilation.

This feedback mechanism is responsible for the normal tight control of arterial pCO_2. The factor causing the disorder is also the factor maintaining it. The prevailing arterial pCO_2 represents the balance between the effects of the primary cause and the respiratory stimulation due to the increased pCO_2.

Other than by ventilatory assistance, the pCO_2 will return to normal only by correction of the cause of the decreased alveolar ventilation.

An extremely high arterial pCO_2 has direct Anesthetic effects and this will lead to a worsening of the situation either by central depression of ventilation or as a result of loss of airway patency or protection.

Metabolic Effects

1. **Depression of intracellular metabolism:** As CO_2 rapidly and easily crosses lipid barriers, a respiratory acidosis has rapid and generally depressing effects on intracellular metabolism.

   Hypercapnia will rapidly cause an intracellular acidosis in all cells in the body. The clinical picture will be affected by the arterial hypoxemia that is usually present. The effects described below are the metabolic effects of hypercapnia rather than respiratory acidosis. Patients with respiratory acidosis can be hypocapnic if a severe metabolic acidosis is also present.

2. **Importance of cerebral effects:** The cerebral effects of hypercapnia are usually the most important. These effects are:
   - Increased cerebral blood flow
   - Increased intracranial pressure
   - Potent stimulation of ventilation

This can result in dyspnea, disorientation, acute confusion, headache, mental obtundation or even focal neurologic signs. Patients with marked elevations of arterial pCO_2 may be comatose, but several factors contribute to this:
- Anesthetic effects of very high arterial pCO_2 (i.e. >100 mmHg)
- Arterial hypoxemia
- Increased intracranial pressure

As a practical clinical example, the rise in intracranial pressure due to hypercapnia may be particularly marked in patients with intracranial pathology (e.g. tumor, head injury) as the usual compensatory mechanism of CSF translocation may be readily exhausted. Any associated hypoxemia will contribute to an adverse outcome.

3. **Effects on cardiovascular system:** The effects on the cardiovascular system are a balance between the direct and indirect effects. Typically, the patient is warm, flushed, sweaty, tachycardic and has a bouncing pulse.

   The clinical picture may be modified by effects of hypoxemia, other illnesses, and the patient's medication. Arrhythmias may be present particularly if significant hypoxemia is present or sympathomimetic have been used.

   Acutely, the acidosis will cause a right shift of the oxygen dissociation curve. If the acidosis persists, a decrease in red cell 2, 3 diphosphoglycerate (DPG) occurs which shifts the curve back to the left.

Compensation

1. **The compensatory response is a rise in the bicarbonate level:** This rise has an immediate component (due to a resetting of the physicochemical equilibrium point) which raises the bicarbonate slightly.

   Next is a slower component where a further rise in plasma bicarbonate due to enhanced renal retention of bicarbonate. The additional effect on plasma bicarbonate of the renal retention is what converts an 'acute' respiratory acidosis into a 'chronic' respiratory acidosis.

   As can be seen by inspection of the Henderson-Hasselbalch equation (below), an increased $[HCO_3^-]$, will counteract the effect (on the pH) of an increased pCO_2, because it returns the value of the $[HCO_3^-]/0.03\ pCO_2$ ratios towards normal.

$$pH = pK'a + \log_{10}([HCO_3^-]/0.03 \times pCO_2)$$

2. **Buffering in acute respiratory acidosis:** The compensatory response to an acute respiratory acidosis is limited to buffering. By the law of mass

action, the increased arterial pCO_2 causes a shift to the right in the following reaction:

$$CO_2 + H_2O \leftrightarrow H_2CO_3 \leftrightarrow H^+ + HCO_3^-$$

In the blood, this reaction occurs rapidly inside red blood cells because of the presence of carbonic anhydrase. The hydrogen ion produced is buffered by intracellular proteins and by phosphates. Consequently, in the red cell, the buffering is mostly by hemoglobin. This buffering by removal of hydrogen ion pulls the reaction to the right resulting in an increased bicarbonate production. The bicarbonate exchanges for chloride ion across the erythrocyte membrane and the plasma bicarbonate level rises. In an acute acidosis, there is insufficient time for the kidneys to respond to the increased arterial pCO_2, so this is the only cause of the increased plasma bicarbonate in this early phase. The increase in bicarbonate only partially returns the extracellular pH towards normal.

Empirically, the $[HCO_3^-]$ rises by 1 mmol/L for every 10 mmHg increase in pCO_2 above its reference value of 40 mmHg. For example, if arterial pCO_2 has risen acutely from 40 mmHg to 60 mmHg (due to decreased alveolar ventilation) then this acute rise of two tens, (i.e. 60–40 = 20 mmHg rise) results in a rise of plasma bicarbonate by 2 from its reference value of 24 mmol/L up to 26 mmol/L. Consequently, we would predict that if this acute respiratory acidosis was the only base disorder present, then plasma bicarbonate would be 26 mmol/L.

Though very important for carriage of carbon dioxide in the blood, the bicarbonate system is not responsible for any buffering of a respiratory acid-base disorder. This is because a system cannot buffer itself. If HCO_3^- were to react with H^+ produced from the dissociation of H_2CO_3, this would just produce H_2CO_3 again-reversing the reaction is not 'buffering'.

Ninety-nine percent of the buffering of an acute respiratory acidosis occurs intracellularly. Proteins (especially hemoglobin in red cells) and phosphates are the most important buffers involved. These take up the H^+ produced from the dissociation of H_2CO_3. This intracellular buffering results in a further increase in intracellular $[HCO_3^-]$, because it pulls the CO_2 hydration reaction to the right. The HCO_3^- that leaves the cell causes the rise in extra-cellular HCO_3. The amount of buffering is limited by the concentration of protein as that is low relative to the amount of carbon dioxide requiring buffering.

3. **Chronic respiratory acidosis (renal bicarbonate retention):** With continuation of the acidosis, the kidneys respond by retaining bicarbonate. If the respiratory acidosis persists then the plasma bicarbonate rises to an even higher level because of renal retention of bicarbonate.

Thus, in a chronic respiratory acidosis there are two factors present which elevate the plasma bicarbonate:

- *Firstly:* The acute physicochemical change and consequent buffering especially by intracellular protein (immediate onset, as occurs with an acute respiratory acidosis.)
- *Secondly:* The renal retention of bicarbonate, as renal function is altered by the elevated arterial pCO_2 and additional bicarbonate is added to the blood passing through the kidney.

4. **Maximal compensation versus full compensation:** The increase in plasma $[HCO_3^-]$ results in an increase in amount of bicarbonate filtered in the kidney and this amount increases as plasma bicarbonate continues to increase. Eventually, a new steady state is reached which is referred to as 'maximal compensation'.

This level of compensation has long been believed to be less than that required to return the plasma pH to normal. That is the actual compensation (maximal compensation) is less than 'full compensation'. If the pH was found to actually be within the normal range, the interpretation of this was that there was a coexisting metabolic alkalosis (e.g. due to the use of diuretics or corticosteroids) or there had been transient hyperventilation from the stress of arterial puncture.

Correction

Restoration of adequate alveolar ventilation: The pCO_2 rapidly returns to normal with restoration of adequate alveolar ventilation. Treatment usually needs to be directed to correction of the primary cause if this is possible. In severe cases, intubation and mechanical ventilation will be necessary to restore alveolar ventilation.

If a chronically elevated arterial pCO_2 is returned to normal relatively quickly (as can happen if the patient is intubated and ventilated), then the patient is in the situation of having elevated bicarbonate (due renal compensation) without there being the physiological need for it anymore. The elevated bicarbonate is typically slow to fall as return to normal requires renal excretion of the excess bicarbonate. The kidney normally has a large capacity to excrete bicarbonate but several factors, particularly chloride depletion, impair this. Consequently, the bicarbonate level can remain persistently elevated; this state is referred to as 'posthypercapnic alkalosis.

The general factors causing maintenance of high bicarbonate levels in this situation are the same as those involved in maintenance of a metabolic alkalosis. These factors are chloride depletion, potassium depletion, ECF volume depletion, and reduction of GFR.

Assessment

The arterial pCO_2 value is used to quantify the magnitude of the alteration in alveolar ventilation (assuming CO_2 production is constant and inspired pCO_2 is negligible). The arterial pCO_2 alone is not satisfactory for assessing the magnitude of a respiratory acidosis in some cases. In particular, coexisting metabolic acid-base disorders cause compensatory changes in pCO_2 and these must be accounted for.

The best available quantitative index of the magnitude of a respiratory acidosis is the difference between the 'actual' pCO_2 and the 'expected' pCO_2.

- Actual pCO_2—the measured value obtained from arterial blood gas analysis.
- Expected pCO_2—the value of pCO_2 that we calculate would be present taking into account the presence of any metabolic acid-base disorder. If there is no metabolic acid-base disorder then a pCO_2 of 40 mmHg is taken as the reference point, i.e. we would use 40 mmHg as the expected pCO_2.

The reason we have to allow for a metabolic acid-base disorder is that the pCO_2 value changes from 40 mmHg due solely to the body's compensatory ventilatory response to a metabolic acidosis or alkalosis so just using a value of 40 mmHg as normal would be wrong and lead us to incorrect conclusions.

With an acute metabolic acidosis, the body responds by increasing alveolar ventilation. This response is compensatory because hyperventilation results in a decrease in arterial pCO_2 which tends to return the arterial pH towards 7.4 partially correcting the acute deviation of plasma pH from normal. The value of pCO_2 at maximal compensation can be predicted using a simple bedside 'rule of thumb' and this calculated value is the 'expected' pCO_2 which we use to compare with the 'actual' (measured) pCO_2 value.

Prevention

1. Inadequate alveolar ventilation is the underlying problem in nearly all patients so any patient who could have impaired ventilation is at risk of developing respiratory acidosis. So recognise these at-risk situations.
2. Inadequate ventilation will also necessarily affect arterial oxygenation so steps to avoid, recognise and/or treat arterial hypoxemia are very important.

The simple measure of providing supplemental oxygen by face mask to patients can often correct or prevent hypoxemia.

Some particular medical situations where prevention can be utilised are:

- Better airway care and attention to safe positioning of cerebrally obtunded patients (i.e. prevent airway obstruction).
- Increased care in the use of drugs (such as CNS sedatives or opiate drugs) which can depress ventilation.
- Increased attention to the care of patients at risk of aspiration (e.g. unconscious patients).
- Ensuring adequate reversal of neuromuscular relaxants.

METABOLIC ACIDOSIS

The primary abnormality in metabolic acidosis is either increased production or decreased excretion of hydrogen ions other than from carbon dioxide. In some cases, both may contribute. Loss of bicarbonate from the body can also, indirectly, cause an acidosis. Excess hydrogen ions are buffered by bicarbonate as in the following reaction:

$$H^+ + HCO_3^- \leftrightarrow H_2CO_3$$

and other buffers. The carbonic acid, thus, formed dissociates as in the following reaction:

$$CO_2 + H_2O \leftrightarrow H_2CO_3$$

and the carbon dioxide is lost in the expired air. This buffering limits the potential rise in hydrogen ion concentration, but at the expense of a reduction in bicarbonate concentration, which is a constant feature of metabolic acidosis.

Etiology

1. **Classification by pathophysiological mechanism:** A decrease in plasma bicarbonate can be caused by two mechanisms:
   - A gain of strong acid
   - A loss of base

   All causes of a metabolic acidosis must work by these mechanisms. The gain of strong acid may be endogenous, (i.e. ketoacids from lipid metabolism) or exogenous (NH_4Cl infusion). Bicarbonate loss may occur via the bowel (diarrhea, small bowel fistulas) or via the kidneys (carbonic anhydrase inhibitors and renal tubular acidosis).

2. **Classification by anion gap:** An alternative to the above is to classify the causes of metabolic acidosis into two groups depending on whether the anion gap is elevated or normal. These two groups are referred to as (Table 2.3):
   - 'High anion gap metabolic acidosis (HAGMA)'
   - 'Normal anion gap metabolic acidosis'

This is the most clinically useful way to classify metabolic acidosis and it is used extensively when assessing metabolic acidosis. The further subdivisions within this classification are outlined in the Table 2.3.

High Anion Gap Acidosis

Ketoacidosis

Ketoacidosis is a high anion gap metabolic acidosis due to an excessive blood concentration of ketone bodies (keto-anions). Ketone bodies (acetoacetate, beta-hydroxybutyrate, and acetone) are released into the blood from the liver when hepatic lipid metabolism has changed to a state of increased ketogenesis, a relative or absolute insulin deficiency is present in all cases.

The main ketone bodies are acetoacetate and beta-hydroxybutyrate and the ratio between these two acid anions depends on the prevailing redox state, (i.e. as assessed by the $NADH/NAD^+$ ratio).

Diabetic Ketoacidosis

An absolute or relative lack of insulin leads to diabetic metabolic decompensation with hyperglycemia and ketoacidosis. A precipitating factor (i.e. infection and stress) which causes an excess of stress hormones (which antagonize the actions of insulin) may be present.

Starvation Ketoacidosis

When hepatic glycogen stores are exhausted (i.e. after 12–24 hours of total fasting), the liver produces ketones to provide an energy substrate for peripheral tissues. Ketoacidosis can appear after an overnight fast, but it typically requires 3–14 days of starvation to reach maximal severity. Typical keto-anion levels are only 1–2 mmol/L and this will not much alter the anion gap. The acidosis even with quite prolonged fasting is only ever of mild to moderate severity with keto-anion levels up to a maximum of 3–5 mmol/L and plasma pH down to 7.3. This is probably due to the insulin level, which though lower, is still enough to keep the free fatty acid (FFA), levels less than 1 mM. This limits substrate delivery to the liver restraining hepatic ketogenesis. Ketone bodies also stimulate some insulin release from the islets. The anion gap will usually not be much elevated.

Alcoholic Ketoacidosis

This typical situation leading to alcoholic ketoacidosis is a chronic alcoholic which has a binge, then stops drinking and has little or no oral food intake. Food intake may be limited because of vomiting. The two key factors are the combination of ethanol and fasting. Presentation is typically a couple of days after the drinking binge has ceased.

The poor oral intake results in decreased glycogen stores, a decrease in insulin levels, and an increase in glucagon levels. Hepatic metabolism of ethanol to acetaldehyde and then to acetate both involve NAD^+ as a cofactor. The $NADH/NAD^+$ ratio rises and this:

- Inhibits gluconeogenesis
- Favours the production of beta-hydroxybutyrate over acetoacetate

The insulin deficiency results in increased mobilization of free fatty acids from adipose tissue. The decreased insulin/glucagon ration results in a switch in hepatic metabolism favouring increased beta-oxidation of fatty acids. This results in an increased production of acetyl-CoA which forms acetoacetate (a keto acid).

- Volume depletion is common and this can result in increased levels of counter-regulatory hormones (i.e. glucagon)
- Levels of FFA can be high (i.e. up to 3.5 mM), providing plenty of substrate for the altered hepatic lipid metabolism to produce plenty of keto-anions
- Gastrointestinal tract (GIT) symptoms are common (i.e., nausea, vomiting, abdominal pain, hematemesis, melena)

Table 2.3	Causes of metabolic acidosis (classified by anion gap)

A: High anion gap acidosis

1. Ketoacidosis
   - Diabetic ketoacidosis
   - Alcoholic ketoacidosis
   - Starvation ketoacidosis
2. Lactic acidosis
   - Type A: Lactic acidosis (impaired perfusion)
   - Type B: Lactic acidosis (impaired carbohydrate metabolism)
3. Renal failure
   - Uremic acidosis
   - Acidosis with acute renal failure
4. Drugs and toxins
   - Ethylene glycol
   - Methanol
   - Salicylates

B: Normal anion gap acidosis or hyperchloremic acidosis

1. Renal causes
   - Renal tubular acidosis
   - Carbonic anhydrase inhibitors
2. Gastrointestinal tract (GIT) causes
   - Severe diarrhea
   - Ureteroenterostomy or obstructed ileal conduit
   - Drainage of pancreatic or biliary secretions
   - Small bowel fistula
3. Other causes
   - Recovery from ketoacidosis
   - Addition of HCl, NH_4Cl

- Acidemia may be severe (i.e. pH down to 7.0)
- Plasma glucose may be depressed or normal or even elevated
- Magnesium deficiency is not uncommon
- Patients are usually not diabetic

A strong suspicion should be raised in any ill chronic alcoholic with a sweet ketone breath who presents to a hospital emergency department. Such patients are often can be noisy and generally uncooperative.

A mixed acid-base disorder may be present: High anion gap due to ketoacidosis, metabolic alkalosis due to vomiting, and a respiratory alkalosis.

Conditions Leading to Diabetic Ketoacidosis

The most common situations in patients presenting with diabetic ketoacidosis (DKA) are:

- Infection as precipitant
- Treatment non-compliance
- New diagnosis of diabetes
- No known precipitating event

The Pathogenesis Requires Two Events

- Increased mobilization of free fatty acids from adipose tissue to the liver
- A switch of hepatic lipid metabolism to ketogenesis

Free fatty acid mobilization is initiated by the effect of absolute or relative insufficient or absent of insulin on fat cells (Fig. 2.8). FFA levels can be quite high (i.e. 2.5–3.5 mmol). This provides the liver with plenty of substrates. These FFA levels are much less than ketone levels and contribute only a small amount to the metabolic acidosis.

The main switch in hepatic lipid metabolism occurs in response not just to insulin deficiency, but additionally to the concomitant rise in levels of the stress hormones (glucagon, corticosteroids, catecholamines, and growth hormone).

The role of glucagon is the most clearly established. The hepatic effects of a fall in the insulin-glucagon ratio are:

- Increased glycogenolysis
- Increased gluconeogenesis
- Increased ketogenesis

The inhibition of the enzyme acetyl CoA carboxylase is probably the key step. This enzyme is inhibited by increased FFA levels, decreased insulin levels, and particularly by the rise in glucagon. All three of these factors are present in DKA. The effect is to decrease the production and level of **malonyl CoA.** This compound has a central role in the regulation of hepatic fatty acid metabolism as it mediates the reciprocal relationship between fatty acid synthesis and oxidation. It is the first committed intermediate in fatty acid metabolism.

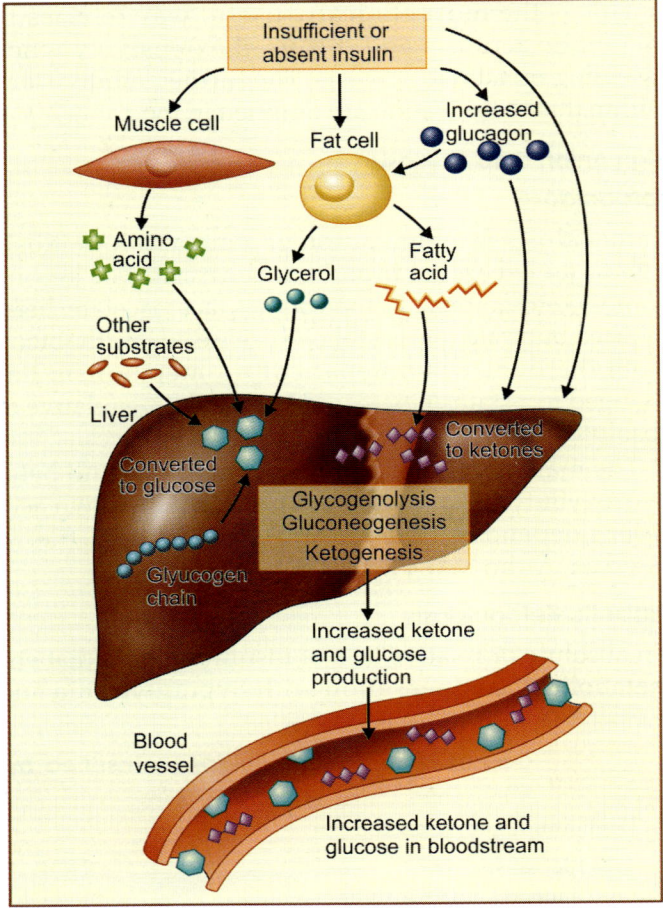

Fig. 2.8: Metabolic fate of fatty acids originating from adipose tissue by the effect of absolute or relative insulin insufficient or absent on fat cells

Malonyl CoA inhibits fatty acid oxidation by inhibiting carnitine acyltransferase I.

A fall in malonyl CoA levels removes this inhibition resulting in excessive fatty acid oxidation with excessive production of acetyl CoA and excess acetoacetate.

Two basic mechanisms underlie the pathophysiology of DKA are hyperglycemia and ketoacidosis. The above discussion shows how both these problems follow from relative insulin deficiency coupled with stress hormone excess. The problem, however, is not just of hepatic over-production of glucose and ketones, but also of peripheral underutilization of both glucose and ketones.

Acetoacetic acid (pKa 3.58) and beta-hydroxybutyric acid (pKa 4.70) dissociate producing H^+, which is buffered by HCO_3^- in the blood. For each anion produced there, is a loss of one bicarbonate. The increase in the anion gap (representing the increase in the unmeasured acid anions), should approximately equal the decrease in the $[HCO_3^-]$. A 'pure' high anion gap metabolic acidosis results.

In some cases, a hyperchloremic metabolic acidosis develops; this is the most common during the treatment phase. Why does this occur? Acetoacetate and beta-hydroxybutyrate are moderately strong acids and even at the lowest urinary pH are significantly ionized. They are excreted with a cation (usually Na^+ or K^+) to maintain electroneutrality. The net effect is the loss of 'potential bicarbonate' equal to the level of urinary ketone body loss. The HCO_3^- is replaced in the blood by Cl^- derived from renal reabsorption, gut absorption or (particularly) intravenous (IV) saline administered during treatment. The effect is to cause a rise in plasma $[Cl^-]$ and the anion gap returns towards normal despite the persistence of the metabolic acidosis. At presentation, both types of acidosis may be present and the elevation in the anion gap will be less than expected for the degree of depression in the bicarbonate level (resulting in Delta ratio <0.8).

A predominant hyperchloremic acidosis (defined as a DKA patient with a delta ratio <0.4) is present in about 10% of patients on arrival at hospital and in about 70% after 8 hours of treatment. Patients who are more severely dehydrated retain more keto-anions and have a lower incidence of hyperchloremic acidosis.

Administration of large volumes of normal saline in resuscitation of patients with acute DKA promotes continued diuresis (and continued loss of ketone bodies with Na^+ as the cation), and provides plenty of chloride to replace the lost keto-anions. This hyperchloremic acidosis is slower to resolve because the keto-anions needed for regeneration of bicarbonate have been lost. Patients who have been able to maintain fluid intake during development of their illness are more likely to have a hyperchloremic acidosis component present on admission.

It should not just be assumed that the patient only has a diabetic ketoacidosis. Possible complicating acid-base disorders are:

- Lactic acidosis due to hypoperfusion and anaerobic muscle metabolism
- Metabolic alkalosis secondary to excessive vomiting
- Respiratory acidosis due to pneumonia or mental obtundation
- Respiratory alkalosis with sepsis
- Renal tubular acidosis (type 4)

Renal tubular acidosis (type 4) is present in some diabetic patients and the associated urinary acidification defect can cause a hyperchloremic normal anion gap acidosis. This syndrome (known as hyporeninemic hypoaldosteronism) occurs in some elderly diabetics who have pre-existing moderate renal insufficiency but, is not a common problem in acute DKA.

Management

It can be considered in terms of emergency and routine components. It should be tailored to individual circumstances. Management of DKA has passed through three stages in the last 100 years:

- **Stage 1:** Preinsulin era (feature—mortality of 100%)
- **Stage 2:** High dose insulin regime (Feature: mortality down to 10%, but metabolic complications due to the treatment)
- **Stage 3:** The present—low dose insulin regime (Feature—low mortality)

Mortality with the low dose insulin regime is down to about 2–5% overall. In older patients with DKA precipitated by a main medical illness (i.e. acute pancreatitis, myocardial infarction, septicemia), the mortality rate is still high due to the severity of the precipitating problem.

Aims of Treatment

- Replace fluid and electrolyte losses
- Restore normal carbohydrate and lipid metabolism
- Treat the underlying cause
- Manage specific complications

Emergency Management

A. Airway

- Protect by intubation with a cuffed tube if patient is significantly obtunded.
- Consider placing a nasogastric tube in all patients.

B: Breathing

- Oxygen by mask initially in all patients
- Intubation may be necessary for airway protection or ventilation [i.e. if aspiration, coma, pneumonia, pulmonary oedema, acute pancreatitis and acute respiratory distress syndrom (ARDS)] but this is not common.

Maintain Compensatory Hyperventilation in Intubated Patients

Patients with metabolic acidosis (i.e. severe DKA) have marked hyperventilation (i.e. respiratory compensation, 'Kussmaul respirations'), and typically low arterial pCO_2 levels. If intubated and ventilated, ventilatory parameters (tidal volume and rate), need to be set to continue high minute ventilation. If this is not done and pCO_2 is inappropriately high, a severe acidemia and consequent severe cardiovascular collapse may occur. This is a particular problem in all situations where, a patient with a compensated metabolic acidosis is intubated and ventilated. The rule of thumb is to aim for a pCO_2 level of 1.5 times the bicarbonate level plus eight as this mimics the normal response by the body. As bicarbonate levels recover, adjust ventilation downwards.

C: Circulation

- If shock is present, this requires urgent colloid infusion to restore intravascular volume and tissue perfusion
- Arrhythmias require urgent clinical management dependent on the type and the clinical situation (i.e. hyperkalemia, myocardial infarction)
- The typical patient who presents with poor peripheral perfusion, but normotension can be adequately managed initially with ECF replacement fluids (i.e. Hartmann's solution or normal saline)

Other Specific Emergency Treatment

Cerebral edema is a dangerous complication that occurs in about 1% of children and adolescents with DKA. Onset of headache and deteriorating level of consciousness typically occurs between 2 hours and 24 hours after onset of treatment. Onset of symptoms is often sudden. Mortality is about 70% in this group. Recommended treatment is immediate IV mannitol in a dose of 0.5–2.0 g/kg body weight. Dexamethasone or hyperventilation have no proven benefit.

Routine Management

1. **General**
   - Oxygen by mask
   - Urinary catheter
   - Consider low dose calcium heparin to decrease risk of arterial thrombosis
   - Investigate for underlying illness (history, examination, cultures of blood, urine or sputum, chest X-ray, ECG, etc.)

2. **Fluids:** Immediate aim is to restore intravascular volume to improve tissue perfusion.

   Replacement solutions (i.e. normal saline or Hartmann's solution) are appropriate for initial management. Subsequently, fluids need to be adjusted to provide 'free water' to replenish intracellular fluid and to provide glucose. Maintenance fluids, such as dextrose-saline or oral fluid intake are appropriate at this later stage depending on the individual circumstances, but such solutions should not be used initially.

   Colloids are necessary only in shocked patients. Colloids are expensive and have a low, but significant risk of reactions. Albumin solutions are not required.

3. **Potassium:** Serum level is commonly normal or high (due to the acidosis) at presentation despite the presence of a large total body potassium deficit (due to renal losses). The best approach is to commence therapy with fluid and insulin and monitor the serum [K$^+$].

   Potassium replacement can be commenced when the [K$^+$] falls below 5 mmol/L. Infuse at 10–30 mmol/h dependent on [K$^+$]. Rates greater than 20 mmol/h are reserved for severe hypokalemia and require at least hourly [K$^+$] monitoring. Never commence a potassium infusion without checking the level.

4. **Insulin:** Fluid resuscitation is necessary to deliver insulin to its sites of action in liver, muscle, and adipose tissue. Rehydration itself will cause a fall in blood glucose level.

   A typical regime would be to give a stat dose initially (say 10–20 U IV) and commence the patient on a continuous insulin infusion at 5–10 U/hr decreasing to 1–3 U/hr to maintain blood glucose at 5–10 mmol/L. A pediatric regime would be insulin at 0.1U/kg IV loading dose, then infusion at 0.1U/kg/h.

   The blood glucose always falls on this regime and control of blood glucose is almost never a problem. Insulin reverses the peripheral mobilization of FFA and alters hepatic metabolism to switch off ketone body production. These effects are maximal at insulin levels of 100 μmol/L and this level is achieved with the low dose regime. The average rate of fall of plasma glucose at this insulin level is about 4.5 mmol/L/hr. There is no advantage in giving more insulin once the ceiling level is reached. This absence of additional effectiveness with very high insulin levels has been referred to in the past as insulin resistance.

5. **Phosphate:** Though a total body deficiency is always present, it has not been possible to show that acute phosphate administration makes any difference to outcome. However, the occasional patient develops extremely low phosphate levels and phosphate administration is undoubtedly necessary in these patients and must be given. Phosphate level on presentation is typically high, so phosphate administration should be delayed.

   By 12 hours after commencement of treatment, the majority (90%) of patients are hypophosphatemic. Ampoules of phosphate available in my hospital contain about 15 mmol of phosphate and 20 mmol of potassium and one ampoule can be diluted in the IV fluids and infused over an hour.

6. **Bicarbonate:** Sodium bicarbonate in DKA has arguably a minor role is in urgent management of serious arrhythmias due to hyperkalemia in DKA. However, glucose-insulin is the preferred treatment in this patient group.

None of the studies done in DKA have shown any benefit of bicarbonate treatment. Potential problems are sodium overload, CSF acidosis, intracellular acidosis, exacerbation of hypokalemia, rebound alkalosis and impaired tissue oxygen delivery (shift of oxyhemoglobin dissociation curve). After treatment of DKA starts, the slowest biochemical parameter to recover is usually the serum bicarbonate; this is especially so when substantial amounts of ketones have been lost in the urine. New bicarbonate is generated when the condition is reversed and the ketones are metabolized. Bicarbonate administration is not necessary.

7. **Monitoring:** It should include observations of airway, breathing, circulation and level of consciousness, serial blood gases and electrolytes, urinary ketones and urine output. Serum lactate is occasionally useful.

Cerebral edema presents 2–12 hours after start of treatment.

Cerebral edema is the commonest single cause of mortality, particularly in children. It typically develops after treatment has commenced. A headache or decreasing level of consciousness is the usual initial sign. Onset may be sudden. Treat urgently with IV mannitol. Intubation for airway protection may be required. Maintain hyperventilation in ventilated patients.

8. **Treat the underlying cause:** The commonest precipitants in young diabetics are inadequate insulin (i.e., first presentation of diabetes, omission of doses) and infection. Often no specific cause can be found. In older diabetics, DKA may be precipitated by a main medical illness (expecially infection). Antibiotics or surgical management are necessary in some cases. Patient education to prevent further episodes is very important.

LACTIC ACIDOSIS

Lactic acidosis is a common cause of metabolic acidosis, each day the body has an excess production of about 1500 mmol of lactate (about 20 mmol/kg/day) which enters the blood stream and is subsequently metabolized mostly in the liver. This internal cycling with production by the tissues and transport to and metabolism by the liver and kidney is known as the Cori cycle (Fig. 2.9). This normal process does not represent any net fixed acid production which requires excretion from the body.

All tissues can produce lactate under anaerobic conditions, but tissues with active glycolysis produce excess lactate from glucose under normal conditions and this lactate tends to spillover into the blood. Lactate is produced from pyruvate in a reaction catalyzed by lactate dehydrogenase:

$$\text{Pyruvate} + \text{NADH} + \text{H}^+ \leftrightarrow \text{Lactate} + \text{NAD}^+$$

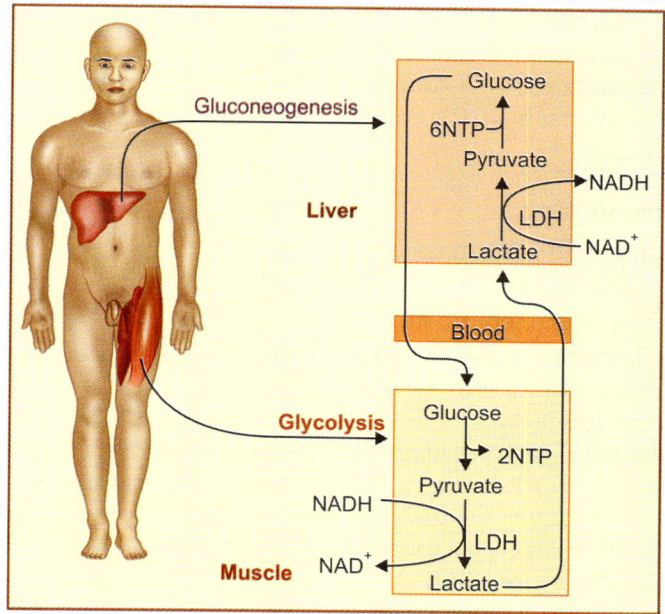

Fig. 2.9: Cori cycle; the body is very efficient in that lactic acid is sent in the blood to the liver which can convert it back to pyruvic acid and then to glucose through gluconeogenesis. The glucose can enter the blood and be carried to muscles and immediately used. If by this time the muscles have ceased activity, the glucose can be used to rebuild supplies of glycogen through glycogenesis

This reaction is so rapid that pyruvate and lactate can be considered to be always in an equilibrium situation. Normally, the ratio of lactate to pyruvate in the cell is 10 to 1. The ratio [NADH/NAD$^+$] by the law of mass action determines the balance between lactate and pyruvate. This ratio is also used to denote the redox state within the cytoplasm. Lactic acid has a pK value of about 4, so it is fully dissociated into lactate and H$^+$ at body pH. In the extracellular fluid (ECF), the H$^+$ titrates bicarbonate on a one for one basis.

Tissue Production

Lactate is released from cells into the interstitial fluid (ISF) and blood. It metabolized predominantly in the liver (60%) and kidney (30%). Half is converted to glucose (gluconeogenesis) and half is further metabolized to CO_2 and water in the citric acid cycle. The result is no net

> **Note**
> - The balance between release into the bloodstream and hepatorenal uptake maintains plasma lactate at about one mmol/L.
> - The renal threshold for lactate is about 5–6 mmol/L so at normal plasma levels, no lactate is excreted into the urine.
> - The small amount of lactate that is filtered (180 mmol/day) is fully reabsorbed.

production of H^+ (or of the lactate anion) for excretion from the body. Other tissues can use lactate as a substrate and oxidize it to CO_2 and water, but it is only the liver and kidney that have the enzymes that can convert lactate to glucose.

Mechanisms

Lactic acidosis can occur due to:
- Excessive tissue lactate production
- Impaired hepatic metabolism of lactate

In most clinical cases it is probable that both processes are contributing to the development of the acidosis. The liver has a large capacity to metabolize lactate so increased peripheral production alone is unlikely to lead to other than transient acidosis. The situation is analogous to a respiratory acidosis where increased CO_2 production alone is rarely responsible because of the efficient ventilatory regulation of pCO_2. Impaired ventilation (impaired excretion of CO_2) is almost invariably present and responsible for a respiratory acidosis.

In situations where lactic acidosis is clearly due to excessive production alone (such as severe exercise or convulsions), the acidosis usually resolves (due to hepatic metabolism) within about an hour once the precipitating disorder is no longer present. In severe exercise, lactate levels can rise to very high levels, e.g. up to 30 mmol/L. Respiratory compensation for the acidosis may not be significant because of the short time involved. However, there are other causes of hyperventilation present and arterial pCO_2 is typically reduced providing partial compensation. For example, exercise results in markedly increased ventilation and the cause of this is largely unknown. The arterial pCO_2 usually falls with exercise and this is not considered to be due to the lactic acidosis as it occurs even in less severe exercise where there is little excess lactate produced.

A continuing lactic acidosis means that there is continuing production of lactate that exceeds the liver's capacity to metabolize it. This may be due to clearly very excessive production (i.e. convulsions) with a normal liver at one extreme, or to increased production in associated with greatly impaired hepatic capacity to metabolize it (i.e. due to cirrhosis, sepsis, hypoperfusion due hypovolemia or hypotension, hypothermia, or some combinations of adverse factors) at the other extreme.

- *Hyperlactemia:* A level from 2–5 mmol/L.
- *Severe lactic acidosis:* When levels are greater than 5 mmol/L

Lactate can be converted to glucose in the liver and kidney. This part of the Cori cycle is an example of gluconeogenesis. Anaerobic glycolysis produces lactate and equivalent amounts of H^+ from ATP hydrolysis. If both these reactions are combined, then there is effectively a net production of equal amounts of lactate and H^+, but the low pKa of lactic acid dissociation means that lactic acid (the undissociated form) is present only in miniscule amounts.

Etiology

Lactic acidosis is commonly classified into either type A or type B (Table 2.4), with the main differentiating point being the adequacy of tissue oxygen delivery. In both types, the fundamental problem is the inability of the mitochondria to deal with the amount of pyruvate with which they are presented.

1. **Type A:** Lactic acidosis refers to circumstances where the clinical assessment is that tissue oxygen delivery is inadequate. This is the most common clinical situation. The inadequate oxygen supply slows mitochondrial metabolism and pyruvate is converted to lactate (and NADH to NAD^+). The conversion of NADH to NAD^+ is important as it regenerates NAD^+ needed for glycolysis to continue. This situation is known as anaerobic metabolism and results in a small net ATP production: two moles of ATP per mole of glucose. The mitochondrial reactions are presumed to be intact, but unable to function because of inadequate oxygen. If hypoxemia is the only factor present, it needs to be severe (i.e. pO_2 <35 mmHg) to precipitate lactic acidosis because of the protection

Table 2.4   Classification of some causes of lactic acidosis

Type A: Lactic acidosis—clinical evidence of inadequate tissue oxygen delivery

- Anaerobic muscular activity (i.e. sprinting, generalized convulsions)
- Tissue hypoperfusion (i.e. shock-septic, cardiogenic or hypovolemic, hypotension, cardiac arrest, acute heart failure; regional hypoperfusion especially mesenteric ischemia and malaria)
- Reduced tissue oxygen delivery or utilization (i.e. hypoxemia, carbon monoxide poisoning, and severe anemia)

Type B: Lactic acidosis—no clinical evidence of inadequate tissue oxygen delivery

- Type B1: Associated with underlying diseases (i.e. ketoacidosis, leukemia, lymphoma, and AIDS)
- Type B2: Associated with drugs and toxins (i.e. phenformin, cyanide, beta-agonists, methanol, nitroprusside infusion, ethanol intoxication in chronic alcoholics, antiretroviral drugs)
- Type B3: Associated with inborn errors of metabolism (i.e. congenital forms of lactic acidosis with various enzyme defects, i.e. pyruvate dehydrogenase deficiency)

Note: This Table does not include all causes of lactic acidosis

afforded by the body's compensatory mechanisms, which increase tissue blood flow. Similarly, anemia needs to be severe (i.e. [Hb] <5g%) if present alone because tissue blood flow is increased in compensation.

Reduced perfusion is the most important factor in causing impaired oxygen delivery in type (A) lactic acidosis.

Anemia or hypoxemia alone is not sufficient unless severe or associated with reduced perfusion.

2. **Type B:** Lactic acidosis refers to situations in which there is no clinical evidence of reduction in tissue oxygen delivery. Carbohydrate metabolism is disordered for some reason and excess lactic acid is formed.

An ischemic bowel can produce large amounts of lactate. Mesenteric ischemia can cause a severe lactic acidosis even if perfusion in the rest of the body is adequate. This situation can easily be overlooked especially in those cases where abdominal clinical signs are minimal.

Phenformin is a biguanide oral hypoglycemic agent which was associated with a severe form of type B lactic acidosis. The incidence was highest among diabetics with renal insufficiency where blood levels are highest. The mechanism of action is not fully established, but the drug probably interferes with mitochondrial function. High levels of phenformin significantly depress myocardial contractility. The decrease in cardiac output undoubtedly contributes a main component of tissue hypoperfusion to many cases.

Other factors predisposing to development of lactic acidosis are sepsis, liver failure, and some malignancies.

Patients with cirrhosis often have a much reduced ability to take up and metabolize lactate. Despite this, patients with chronic hepatic disease alone do not commonly develop lactic acidosis unless other factors, such as sepsis, shock, bleeding or ethanol abuse are also present. So, the development of lactic acidosis in patients with cirrhosis suggests severe liver damage and the presence of other factors. In this setting, death rates are high.

Any factor which stimulates glycolysis (i.e. catecholamine administration, cocaine), will lead to an increased lactate production. Lactic acidosis occurs in up to 10% of patients presenting with diabetic ketoacidosis. This may be due to poor peripheral perfusion or phenformin administration, but may occur without the presence of these factors.

Diagnosis

The condition is often suspected on the history and examination (i.e. shock, heart failure) and is easily confirmed and quantified by measuring the blood lactate level. A particular problem is the diagnosis of the condition when present as part of a mixed acid-base disorder. It may be associated with other causes of a high anion gap acidosis (i.e. ketoacidosis, uremic acidosis) and not be suspected. Coexistent lactic acidosis and metabolic alkalosis may result in minimally altered plasma bicarbonate level. A high anion gap may be a clue in this later situation, but the anion gap is not invariably elevated out of the reference range.

The main reason is that traditionally a lactate level was an uncommon investigation and the diagnosis of lactic acidosis was by exclusion in patients with a high anion gap metabolic acidosis and some evidence of impaired perfusion. Other factors were a low index of clinical suspicion and a tendency to not appreciate the significance of an elevated lactate result.

The basic investigations needed to supplement the history, examination and electrolyte results in differentiating the causes of a high anion gap acidosis are:
- Blood glucose level
- Urinary ketones
- Urea and creatinine
- Urine output
- Blood lactate level
- Calculation of osmolar gap

Management

The principles of management of patients with lactic acidosis are:
- Diagnose and correct the underlying condition (if possible)
- Restore adequate tissue oxygen delivery (especially restore adequate perfusion)
- Avoid sodium bicarbonate (except possibly for treatment of associated severe hyperkalemia)

When the circulation is restored, the liver can metabolize the circulating lactate. If lactic acidosis is severe and the cause cannot be corrected, the mortality can be quite high. Metabolic alkalosis induced by administration of sodium bicarbonate can lead to a substantial increase in the production of lactate. This may be because the intracellular acidosis strongly inhibits phosphofructokinase, which is the rate-limiting enzyme in glycolysis. This suggests that bicarbonate therapy could result in induction of alkalosis intracellularly, which could release this inhibition and increase pyruvate and lactate production.

ACIDOSIS AND RENAL FAILURE

Metabolic acidosis occurs with both acute and chronic renal failure and with other types of renal damage. The anion gap may be normal or may be elevated.

A generalization that can be made is:

- If the renal damage affects both glomeruli and tubules, the acidosis is a high anion gap acidosis. It is due to failure of adequate excretion of various acid anions due to the greatly reduced number of functioning nephrons.
- If the renal damage predominantly affects the tubules with minimal glomerular damage, a different type of acidosis may occur. This is called renal tubular acidosis (RTA) and this is a normal anion gap or hyperchloremic type of acidosis. The GFR may be normal or only minimally affected.

Uremic Acidosis

The acidosis occurring in uremic patients is due to failure of excretion of acid anions (particularly phosphate and sulphate), because of the decreased number of nephrons. There is a main decrease in the number of tubule cells, which can produce ammonia and this contributes to uremic acidosis.

Serious acidosis does not occur until the GFR has decreased to about 20 mL/min. This corresponds to a creatinine level of about 0.30–0.35 mmol/L.

The plasma bicarbonate in renal failure with acidosis is typically between 12 mmol/L and 20 mmol/L. Intracellular buffering and bone buffering are important in limiting the fall in bicarbonate. This bone buffering will cause loss of bone mineral (osteomalacia).

Most other forms of metabolic acidosis are of relatively short duration as the patient is either treated with resolution of the disorder or the patient dies. Uremic acidosis is a main exception as these patients survive with significant acidosis for many years. This long duration is the reason why loss of bone mineral (and bone buffering) is significant in uremic acidosis but is not a feature of other causes of metabolic acidosis.

Retention of metabolic acids occurs with acute renal failure. The clinical details in these patients are often complex and the actual severity of acidosis is variable. Some other complicating factors are catabolism (increased metabolic acid production), vomiting, diarrhea, lactic acidosis due to poor perfusion, bicarbonate therapy and dialysis. Hyperkalemia is often present and is often the factor determining the need for acute dialysis.

DRUGS AND TOXINS

Several drugs and toxins have been implicated as direct or indirect causes of a high anion gap metabolic acidosis. The three most common ones to consider are methanol, ethylene glycol, and salicylates. Other toxins which can cause acidosis are isopropyl alcohol and butoxyethanol. Toluene also causes an acidosis and the anion gap may be normal or elevated. The acidosis caused by these toxins may sometimes present as a normal anion gap hyperchloremic acidosis.

Coingestion of ethanol delays the metabolism of the more toxic methanol and ethylene glycol, but can also delays the diagnosis. In this situation, the osmolar gap will be even more elevated and can be explained by the measured ethanol level alone.

Ethylene Glycol Poisoning

Ethylene glycol is a colorless sweet tasting solvent which is used in antifreeze solutions. It is nontoxic itself but is converted to toxic metabolites in the liver:

- Glycolic acid (>glycolate anion) is the main contributor to the often severe high anion gap acidosis that develops
- Oxalic acid (>oxalate anion), is one of the final metabolic products which is excreted in the urine. Precipitation of calcium oxalate crystals in the kidney causes renal failure, if a sufficient dose has been ingested.

Ingestion of only 30–60 mL may be sufficient to cause permanent organ damage or death. The osmolar gap may be raised (to > 10) early in the course but this is variable.

The detection of calcium oxalate crystals in the urine is often stated to be a useful guide but this is wrong. Certainly, these crystals have a characteristic appearance and a urine analysis will easily detect them. The problem is that oxalate crystals in urine are generally very common (80% of specimens) and their presence alone means nothing for a diagnosis of ethylene glycol ingestion. Oddly, cases of ethylene glycol ingestion have also been reported without oxalate crystals in the urine. There is also no point in differentiating between the monohydrate and the dihydrate crystals.

Toxicity is usually considered as occurring in three stages: intoxication, cardiorespiratory changes, and renal toxicity as following:

Stages of Ethylene Glycol Toxicity

Stage 1: Intoxication (up to 12 hours post-ingestion)
- An ethanol-like intoxicated state (without an appropriate odour on the breath) progressing to central nervous system (CNS) depression
- Fits and coma may occur
- A high anion gap metabolic acidosis develops
- Nausea, vomiting, arrhythmias and tetany (due to hypocalcaemia) may occur

Stage 2: Cardiorespiratory changes (from 12 to 24 hours post-ingestion).
- Tachycardia, tachypnea. Shock may occur in main ingestions

Stage 3: Renal toxicity (at 24–72 hours post-ingestion)

- Acute anuric renal failure may occur due to precipitation of calcium oxalate crystals in the renal tubules.

Principles of Treatment of Ethylene Glycol Poisoning

1. **Emergency management**

   Resuscitation: Airway, breathing, and circulation. Obtunded patients require intubation for airway protection and ventilation.

2. **Ethylene glycol removal from body**
   - Hemodialysis is the most effective technique; it also removes ethanol so ethanol, infusion rate must be increased during periods of dialysis.
   - *Avoid lavage:* Lavage is effective only if used within the first hour after ingestion and patients do not present within this interval.
   - *Avoid activated charcoal:* This is not effective.

3. **Blocking of metabolism**
   - *Ethanol:* 'Ethanol blocking' treatment is the traditional treatment, but has the disadvantage of causing intoxication (CNS depression). It is also irritant and should be given via a central line.
   - *Fomepizole:* This is currently approved for this use in some countries; its advantages are effectiveness, ease of administration, and absence of intoxication. Its use may obviate the need for hemodialysis in patients without severe acidosis.

4. **Intensive supportive care and monitoring**

   Intubation and mechanical ventilation may be indicated if there is inadequate airway protection (i.e. CNS depression) or inadequate ventilation.

Methanol Poisoning

Ingestion of methanol can occur accidentally or deliberately if used as an ethanol substitute.

Methanol itself is non-toxic. Onset of symptoms is delayed until the toxic metabolites are produced by liver. Because the hepatic metabolism is slow, there is usually a considerable latent period (12–48 hours) before any toxic effects develop. Patients presenting early with a history of ingestion will be asymptomatic.

Patients presenting late are often deeply comatose and bradycardic with depressed respirations. Survivors have a high incidence of irreversible blindness. Abdominal pain is a common symptom and may be due to acute pancreatitis.

Diagnosis may be delayed if the history is not available (i.e. obtunded patient) or because of the significant delay between ingestion and symptoms. Early diagnosis is important because prompt and effective treatment can decrease mortality and decrease the incidence of blindness. A useful screening test is determination of the osmolar gap. If the osmolar gap is greater than 10, it indicates the presence of appreciable quantities of low molecular weight substances such as methanol. This can alert you to the diagnosis before the acidosis (due to metabolites) develops. As the methanol is metabolized, the osmolar gap returns toward normal and the anion gap increases. A patient presenting late after a significant ingestion may have a normal osmolar gap and a high anion gap acidosis. The osmolar gap is more likely to be elevated in methanol ingestion than with ethylene glycol ingestions because of the lower molecular weight of methanol. Osmolar gaps of >100 have been reported.

The ideal way to assess and monitor response to treatment is to measure methanol blood levels. This test is not readily available in laboratories because of infrequent need and because the test is labour intensive. Treatment should not be delayed by delays in obtaining a blood methanol level. Methanol levels >20 mg/dL are associated with severe toxicity.

The most serious toxic manifestations are:
- Metabolic acidosis
- Visual impairment up to permanent blindness
- CNS depression 'intoxication' up to coma
- Death

In patients with severe acidosis (indicating high formic acid levels), the mortality rate may be 50% or more.

Pathophysiology

Methanol is slowly converted to formaldehyde (by alcohol dehydrogenase) and then to formic acid in the liver. Methanol is nontoxic, but both the main metabolites interfere with oxidative phosphorylation and it is these metabolites that cause the toxic effects. The acidosis is due to formic acid. As methanol is converted to its metabolites the osmolar gap falls and the anion gap rises.

Some patients ingest ethanol as well as methanol and this is protective as it further delays the metabolism and limits the peak levels of the toxic metabolites. Such coingestion of ethanol can cause diagnostic problems. Clinicians are typically alerted to the possibility of ingestion of methanol (or ethylene glycol) by the combination of an acidosis and CNS symptoms (i.e. intoxication). Ethanol can mislead the clinician because it further delays the onset of the acidosis, 'explains' the presence of intoxication, and also explains the presence of an osmolar gap.

Acid-base Disorders in Methanol Toxicity

- Initially no acid-base disorder due to long latent period while methanol is metabolized
- Later, typically develop a high anion gap metabolic acidosis due to formic acid

- May also develop a respiratory acidosis secondary to CNS depression (with depression of respiratory center and/or airway obstruction)
- May occasionally present with normal anion gap acidosis if smaller ingestion
- If patient is an alcoholic, there may other types of acidosis present as well (i.e. alcoholic ketoacidosis, starvation ketoacidosis, lactic acidosis, respiratory acidosis due to aspiration, respiratory alkalosis due to chronic liver disease.)

Treatment

General principles of treatment are outlined below. Treatment must be individualized to individual patient circumstances. The best outcome is obtained with patients who present early, particularly during the latent period.

Principles of Treatment of Methanol Poisoning

1. **Emergency management:** *Resuscitation*—airway, breathing, circulation. Obtunded patients require intubation for airway protection and ventilation.
2. **Methanol removal from body:** *Hemodialysis* is the most effective technique; it also removes ethanol so ethanol infusion rate must be increased during periods of dialysis.
3. **Blocking of metabolism:** This involves competitive inhibition of alcohol dehydrogenase (ADH). The aim is to delay the production of the toxic metabolites and limit the peak concentrations achieved. Two agents are currently in use:
   - *Ethanol:* 'Ethanol blocking' treatment is the traditional treatment, but has the disadvantage of causing intoxication (CNS depression). It is also irritant and should be given via a central line.
   - *Fomepizole (aka 4-methylpyrazole):* Its advantages are effectiveness, ease of administration and absence of intoxication. Its use may obviate the need for hemodialysis in patients without visual impairment or severe acidosis.
4. **Intensive supportive care and monitoring:** Intubation and mechanical ventilation may be indicated if there is inadequate airway protection (i.e. CNS depression) or inadequate ventilation; Monitor response to treatment with methanol levels.

Normal Anion Gap Acidosis (or Hyperchloremic Acidosis)

It is a form of metabolic acidosis associated with a normal anion gap, a decrease in plasma bicarbonate concentration, and in an increase in plasma chloride concentration. Although plasma anion gap is normal, this condition is often associated with an increased urine anion gap, due to the kidney's inability to secrete ammonia.

RENAL CAUSES

Renal Tubular Acidosis

Renal tubular acidosis (RTA) is a syndrome due to either a defect in proximal tubule bicarbonate reabsorption, or a defect in distal tubule hydrogen ion secretion, or both. This results in a hyperchloremic metabolic acidosis with normal to moderately decreased GFR. Anion gap is normal. A typical situation where RTA would be suspected is if urine pH is greater than 7.0 despite the presence of a metabolic acidosis. In contrast, the acidosis that occurs with acute, chronic, or acute on chronic renal failure is a high anion gap metabolic acidosis.

Renal tubular acidosis is a form of hyperchloremic metabolic acidosis which occurs when the renal damage primarily affects tubular function without much effect on glomerular function. The result is a decrease in H^+ excretion which is greater, then can be explained by any change in GFR. In contrast, if glomerular function (i.e. GFR) is significantly depressed (hence renal failure), the retention of fixed acids results in a high anion gap acidosis.

Acidosis and Location of Renal Damage

- Predominantly tubular damage → Normal anion gap acidosis (RTA)
  - Distal (or type 1) RTA
  - Proximal (or type 2) RTA
  - Type 4 RTA
- Predominantly glomerular damage → High anion gap acidosis
  - Acidosis of acute renal failure
  - Uremic acidosis

Three main clinical categories or 'types' of renal tubular acidosis are now recognised but the number of possible causes is large. The mechanism causing the defect in ability to acidify the urine and excrete acid is different in the three types (Table 2.5).

Type (1): Distal Renal Tubular Acidosis

This is also referred to as classic RTA or distal RTA. The problem here is an inability to maximally acidify the urine. Typically urine pH remains >5.5 despite severe acidemia ($[HCO_3^-] < 15$ mmol/L). Some patients with less severe acidosis require acid loading tests (i.e. with NH_4Cl) to assist in the diagnosis. If the acid load drops the plasma $[HCO_3^-]$, but the urine pH remains >5.5, this establishes the diagnosis.

There are many different causes, but the majority of cases can be placed into one of several groups:

General Classification of Causes

- Hereditary (genetic)
- Autoimmune diseases [i.e. Sjogren's syndrome, systemic lupus erythematosus (SLE), thyroiditis]
- Disorders which cause nephrocalcinosis (i.e. primary hyperparathyroidism, vitamin D intoxication)
- Drugs or toxins (i.e. amphotericin B, toluene inhalation)
- Miscellaneous—other renal disorders (i.e. obstructive uropathy)

Typical findings are an inappropriately high urine pH (usually >5.5), low acid secretion and urinary bicarbonate excretion despite severe acidosis. Renal sodium wasting is common and results in depletion of ECF volume and secondary hyperaldosteronism with increased loss of K^- in the urine. The diagnosis of type 1 RTA is suggested by finding a hyperchloremic acidosis in association with alkaline urine particularly if there is evidence of renal stone formation.

Treatment with $NaHCO_3$ corrects the Na^+ deficit, restores the ECF volume and results in correction of the hypokalemia. Typical alkali requirements are in the range of 1–4 mmol/kg/day. K^+ supplements are only rarely required. Sodium and potassium citrate solutions can be useful particularly if hypokalemia is present. Citrate will bind Ca^{2+} in the urine and this assists in preventing renal stones.

Diagnosis of Distal Renal Tubular Acidosis

Hyperchloremic metabolic acidosis associated with a urine pH > 5.5 despite plasma $[HCO_3^-] < 15$ mmol/L, and the supportive findings are hypokalemia, nephrocalcinosis, presence of a disorder known to be associated with RTA.

Type (2): Proximal Renal Tubular Acidosis

It is called proximal RTA because the main problem is greatly impaired reabsorption of bicarbonate in the proximal tubule. At normal plasma $[HCO_3^-]$, more than 15% of the filtered HCO_3^- load is excreted in the urine. When acidosis is severe and HCO_3^- levels are low (i.e. <17 mmol/L), the urine may become bicarbonate free. Symptoms are precipitated by an increase in plasma $[HCO_3^-]$. The defective proximal tubule cannot reabsorb the increased filtered load and the distal delivery of bicarbonate is greatly increased. The H^+ secretion in the distal tubule is now overwhelmed by attempting to reabsorb bicarbonate and the net acid excretion decreases. This results in urinary loss of HCO_3^- resulting in systemic acidosis with inappropriately high urine pH. The bicarbonate is replaced in the circulation by Cl^-.

The increased distal Na^+ delivery results in hyperaldosteronism with consequent renal K^+ wasting. The hypokalemia may be severe in some cases, but as hypokalemia inhibits adrenal aldosterone secretion, this often limits the severity of the hypokalemia.

Hypercalciuria does not occur and this type of RTA is not associated with renal stones. During the NH_4Cl loading test, urine pH will drop below 5.5. The acidosis in proximal RTA is usually not as severe as in distal RTA and the plasma $[HCO_3^-]$ is typically greater than 15 mmol/L.

Etiology

There are many causes but most are associated with multiple proximal tubular defects, i.e. affecting reabsorption of glucose, phosphate, and amino acids. Some causes are hereditary. Other causes include vitamin D deficiency, cystinosis, lead nephropathy, amyloidosis, and medullary cystic disease.

Treatment

Treatment is directed towards the underlying disorder if possible. Alkali therapy ($NaHCO_3$) and supplemental K^+ are not always necessary. If alkali therapy is required, the dose is usually large (up to 10 mmol/kg/day), because of the increased urine bicarbonate wasting associated with normal plasma levels. K^+ loss is much increased in treated patients and supplementation is required. Some patients respond to thiazide diuretics which cause slight volume contraction and this result in increased proximal bicarbonate reabsorption so less bicarbonate is needed.

Type (3): Renal Tubular Acidosis

Renal tubular acidosis is now considered a subtype of type 1 where there is a proximal bicarbonate leak in addition to a distal acidification defect.

Type (4): Renal Tubular Acidosis

A number of different conditions have been associated with this type, but most patients have renal failure associated with disorders affecting the renal interstitium and tubules. In contrast to uremic acidosis, the GFR is greater than 20 mL/min, hyperkalemia occurs in type 4 RTA, but not in the other types.

The underlying defect is impairment of cation exchange in the distal tubule with reduced secretion of both H^+ and K^+. This is a similar finding to what occurs with aldosterone deficiency and type 4 RTA can occur with Addison's disease or following bilateral adrenalectomy. Acidosis is not common with aldosterone deficiency alone, but requires some degree of associated renal damage (nephron loss), especially affecting the distal tubule. The H^+ pump in the tubules is not abnormal so patients with this disorder are able to decrease urine pH to < 5.5 in response to the acidosis. The Table 2.5

Table 2.5	Comparison of main types of renal tubular acidosis		
	Type 1	**Type 2**	**Type 4**
Hyperchloremic acidosis	Yes	Yes	Yes
Minimum urine pH	>5.5	<5.5 (but usually >5.5 before the acidosis becomes established)	<5.5
Plasma potassium	Low-normal	Low-normal	High
Renal stones	Yes	No	No
Defect	Reduced H^+ excretion in distal tubule	Impaired HCO_3^- reabsorption in proximal tubule	Impaired cation exchange in distal tubule

provides a useful summary of some of the key points in differentiating the types of renal tubular acidosis.

GASTROINTESTINAL TRACT CAUSES

Secretions into the large and small bowel are mostly alkaline with a bicarbonate level higher than that in plasma. Excessive loss of these fluids can result in a normal anion gap metabolic acidosis.

Some typical at risk clinical situations are:

- Severe diarrhea
- Villous adenoma
- External drainage of pancreatic or biliary secretions (i.e. fistulas)
- Chronic laxative abuse
- Administration of acidifying salts

Severe Diarrhea

This can cause either a metabolic acidosis or a metabolic alkalosis. Development of a significant acid-base disturbance requires a significant increase in stool water loss above its normal value of 100–200 mL/day. The more fluid and anions lost, the more marked the problem.

Hyperchloremic metabolic acidosis tends to be associated with acute infective diarrhea. This is the classical finding in patients with cholera. The problem is an excessive loss of bicarbonate in the diarrheal fluid. Diarrheas which are caused by predominantly colonic pathology may cause a metabolic alkalosis; this includes chronic diarrheas due to ulcerative colitis, colonic Crohn's disease, and chronic laxative abuse.

The acid-base situation with severe diarrhea can be complicated by other factors (Table 2.6) and it may not be possible to completely sort out all the factors in the acid-base disturbance in an individual case.

OTHER CAUSES

Recovery Phase of Diabetic Ketoacidosis

Hyperchloremic metabolic acidosis commonly develops during therapy of diabetic ketoacidosis. The mechanism is effectively renal loss of base even though it is not bicarbonate which is lost in the urine. The actual loss is of ketoacids (keto-anions) and water. When therapy commences, the ketoacids are metabolized in the liver resulting in the production of equal amounts of bicarbonate. If excessive ketoacids have been lost in the urine and fluid therapy is initially with normal saline, there is a deficiency of bicarbonate precursors and a surfeit of chloride to replace bicarbonate. Correction of the acidosis will now involve renal excretion of chloride and its replacement with bicarbonate. This is a slower process than metabolism of ketoacids to regenerate bicarbonate. The net result then is that full correction of the acidosis is much slower when a hyperchloremic acidosis develops.

Chronic Administration of Carbonic Anhydrase Inhibitors

Normally, 85% of filtered bicarbonate is reabsorbed in the proximal tubule and the remaining 15% is reabsorbed in the rest of the tubule. In patients receiving acetazolamide (or other carbonic anhydrase inhibitors), proximal reabsorption of bicarbonate is decreased and distal delivery is increased. The distal tubule has only a limited capacity to reabsorb bicarbonate and when exceeded bicarbonate appears in the urine.

Table 2.6	Multiple factors which affect acid-base homeo-stasis in patients with severe diarrhea
Situation	**Comment**
Acute infective diarrhea (small bowel origin)	Normal anion gap (hyperchloremic) metabolic acidosis due to loss of bicarbonate
Chronic colonic diarrhea	May be metabolic alkalosis due predominant loss of Cl^-
Hypovolemia causing prerenal renal failure	High anion gap acidosis due to renal retention of phosphate and sulphate.
Hypovolemia causing peripheral circulatory failure	Type A lactic acidosis
Hypovolemia causing an increase in plasma protein concentration (increased unmeasured anion)	Increased anion gap
Vomiting	Metabolic alkalosis due to loss of gastric HCl
Abdominal pain	Hyperventilation (respiratory alkalosis)

Oral Ingestion of Acidifying Salts

Oral administration of $CaCl_2$ or NH_4Cl is equivalent to giving an acid load. Both of these salts are used in acid loading tests for the diagnosis of renal tubular acidosis. $CaCl_2$ reacts with bicarbonate in the small bowel resulting in the production of insoluble $CaCO_3$ and H^+. The hepatic metabolism of NH_4^+ to urea results in an equivalent production of H^+.

Symptoms and Signs

Symptoms and signs are primarily those of the cause. Mild acidemia is itself asymptomatic. More severe acidemia (pH < 7.10), may cause nausea, vomiting, and malaise. Symptoms may appear at higher pH if acidosis develops rapidly. The most characteristic sign is hyperpnea (long, deep breaths at a normal rate), reflecting a compensatory increase in alveolar ventilation; this hyperpnea is not accompanied by a feeling of dyspnea.

Severe, acute acidemia predisposes to cardiac dysfunction with hypotension and shock, ventricular arrhythmias, and coma. Chronic acidemia causes bone demineralization disorders (e.g. rickets, osteomalacia, osteopenia).

Maintenance

The disorder is maintained as long as the primary cause persists. Additionally, in many cases the acid-base disturbance tends to increase in severity while the problem causing it persists though this is not absolute.

In diabetic ketoacidosis, the pH will remain low as long as the problem (relative or absolute insulin deficiency) persists and the levels of plasma keto-anions continue to rise. However, these increased plasma levels of keto-anions exceed the renal threshold and are excreted in the urine. This will limit the rate of rise, as long as this additional mechanism of excreting the acid anions persists. This renal excretion also means that once treatment commences, there is now a deficiency of keto-anions to be metabolized to regenerate bicarbonate and consequently there can be a significant delay in the return of the plasma pH to normal.

Metabolic Effects

A metabolic acidosis can cause significant physiological effects, particularly affecting the respiratory and cardiovascular systems (Table 2.7).

The cardiac stimulatory effects of sympathetic activity and release of catecholamines usually counteract the direct myocardial depression while plasma pH remains above 7.2. At systemic pH values less than this, the direct depression of contractility usually predominates.

The direct vasodilatation is offset by the indirect sympathetically-mediated vasoconstriction and cardiac stimulation during a mild acidosis. The venoconstriction

Table 2.7	Main effects of a metabolic acidosis
Respiratory effects	

Respiratory effects
- Hyperventilation (Kussmaul respirations)—this is the compensatory response
- Shift of oxyhemoglobin dissociation curve (ODC) to the right
- Decreased 2, 3 DPG levels in red cells (shifting the ODC back to the left)

Cardiovascular effects
- Depression of myocardial contractility
- Sympathetic over activity (tachycardia, vasoconstriction, decreased arrhythmia threshold)
- Resistance to the effects of catecholamines
- Peripheral arteriolar vasodilatation
- Venoconstriction of peripheral veins
- Vasoconstriction of pulmonary arteries
- Effects of hyperkalemia on heart

Other Effects
- Increased bone resorption (chronic acidosis only)
- Shift of K^+ out of cells causing hyperkalemia

DPG, diphosphoglycerate

shifts blood centrally and this causes pulmonary congestion. Pulmonary artery pressure usually rises during acidosis.

The shift of the oxygen dissociation curve to the right due to the acidosis occurs rapidly. After 6 hours of acidosis, the red cell levels of 2, 3 DPG have declined enough to shift the oxygen dissociation curve (ODC) back to normal.

Acidosis is commonly said to cause hyperkalemia by a shift of potassium out of cells. The effect on potassium levels is extremely variable and indirect effects due to the type of acidosis present are much more important. For example hyperkalemia is due to renal failure in uremic acidosis rather than the acidosis. Significant potassium loss due to osmotic diuresis occurs during diabetic ketoacidosis and the potassium level at presentation is variable (though total body potassium stores are invariably depleted). Treatment with fluid and insulin can cause a prompt and marked fall in plasma potassium. Hypokalemia may then be a problem.

Compensation

The metabolic acidosis is detected by both the peripheral and central chemoreceptors and the respiratory center is stimulated. The initial stimulation of the central chemoreceptors is due to small increases in brain ISF $[H^+]$. The subsequent increase in ventilation causes a fall in arterial pCO_2, which inhibits the ventilatory response.

The chemoreceptor inhibition acts to limit and delay the full ventilatory response until bicarbonate shifts have stabilized across the blood brain barrier. The increase in ventilation usually starts within minutes and is usually well-advanced at 2 hours of onset, but maximal compensation may take 12–24 hours to develop. This is 'maximal' compensation rather than 'full' compensation as it does not return the extracellular pH to normal.

In situations where a metabolic acidosis develops rapidly and is short-lived there is usually little time for much compensatory ventilatory response to occur. An example is acute and sometimes severe lactic acidosis due to a prolonged generalized convulsion; this corrects due to rapid hepatic uptake and metabolism of the lactate following cessation of convulsive muscular activity, and hyperventilation due to the acidosis does not occur.

The arterial pCO_2 at maximal compensation has been measured in many patients with a metabolic acidosis. A consistent relationship between bicarbonate level and pCO_2 has been found. It can be estimated from the following equation:

Expected pCO_2 = 1.5 (Actual [HCO_3^-]) + 8 mmHg
(Units: mmol/L for [HCO_3^-], and mmHg for pCO_2).

The limiting value of compensation is the lowest level to which the pCO_2 can fall; this is typically 8–10 mmHg, though lower values are occasionally seen.

Correction

The most important approach to manage a metabolic acidosis is to treat the underlying disorder. Then with supportive management, the body will correct the acid-base disorder. Accurate analysis and diagnosis essential to ensure the correct treatment are used. Fortunately, in most cases this is not particularly difficult in principle.

Management and Treatment

1. Emergency management of immediately life-threatening conditions always has the highest priority. For example, intubation and ventilation for airway or ventilatory control; cardiopulmonary resuscitation; severe hyperkalemia.
2. Treat the underlying disorder as the primary therapeutic goal. Consequently, accurate diagnosis of the cause of the metabolic acidosis is very important. In some cases (i.e. methanol toxicity) there may be a substantial delay become the diagnosis can be confirmed so management must be based on suggestive evidence otherwise it will be too late.
3. Replace losses (e.g. of fluids and electrolytes), where appropriate. Other supportive care (oxygen administration) is useful. In most cases, intravenous (IV) sodium bicarbonate is not necessary, not helpful, and may even be harmful so is not generally recommended.

4. There are often specific problems or complications associated with specific causes or specific cases which require specific management. i.e. ethanol blocking treatment with methanol ingestion; rhabdomyolysis requires management for preventing acute renal failure; hemodialysis can remove some toxins.

Some examples of specific treatments for underlying disorders:

- Fluid, insulin, and electrolyte replacement is necessary for diabetic ketoacidosis
- Administration of bicarbonate and/or dialysis may be required for acidosis associated with renal failure
- Restoration of an adequate intravascular volume and peripheral perfusion is necessary in lactic acidosis.

Treatment of the underlying disorder will result in correction of the metabolic acidosis (i.e. the bicarbonate level will return to normal).

Bicarbonate Deficit Repair

1. **Kidney:** Renal generation of new bicarbonate—this usually occurs as a consequence of an increase in ammonium excretion.
2. **Liver:** Hepatic metabolism of acid anions to produce bicarbonate: The normal liver has a large capacity to metabolize many organic acid anions (i.e. lactate, keto-anions) with the result that bicarbonate is regenerated in the liver. In severe ketoacidosis there is often a large loss of keto-anions due to the hyperglycemia induced osmotic diuresis. This leaves a shortfall of keto-anions to be used to regenerate bicarbonate as a consequence of their metabolism in the kidney.
3. **Exogenous administration of sodium bicarbonate:** This is the time honored method to 'speed up' the return of bicarbonate levels to normal. Indeed, this may be useful in mineral acidosis (hyperchloremic metabolic acidosis) where there are no endogenous acid anions which can be metabolized by the liver. However, in most other cases of metabolic acidosis this administration is either not helpful or may be disadvantageous.

Sodium bicarbonate solutions should not be given on a routine basis no matter what the arterial pH is.

Administration of sodium bicarbonate may be useful in treatment of severe hyperkalemia. Such hyperkalemia may be immediately life-threatening. Calcium gluconate will be more rapidly protective against serious arrhythmias.

It should be noted that correction of a metabolic acidosis does not necessarily involve renal excretion of acid or renal regeneration of bicarbonate because of the role of hepatic metabolism of some anions. For example in lactic acidosis and ketoacidosis, treatment results in significant correction because of predominantly hepatic metabolism of the acid anions to regenerate bicarbonate. If acid anions have been lost in the urine, then renal regeneration of bicarbonate is very important for correction of the acid-base disorder.

In a severe ketoacidosis, there is a large loss of keto-anions in the urine. When the disorder is treated (fluids and insulin) there is a relative deficiency of acid anions which can be metabolized in the liver with regeneration of bicarbonate. Consequently, it is common to find that treatment results in a rapid correction (few hours) of the hyperglycemia and the hypovolemia, but the acidosis may take over 24 hours to return to normal. This is because 'new' bicarbonate has to be regenerated by the kidneys and this takes longer to correct the bicarbonate deficit. There has been a past tendency to speed up the process by administration of IV $NaHCO_3$ solution, but this is not necessary and has not been shown to have any advantage.

Points to be Considered About Bicarbonate Administration

1. Ventilation must be adequate to eliminate the CO_2 produced from bicarbonate

    Bicarbonate decreases H^+ by reacting with it to produce CO_2 and water. For this reaction to continue the product (CO_2) must be removed. So bicarbonate therapy can increase extracellular pH, only if ventilation is adequate to remove the CO_2. Indeed if hypercapnia occurs then as CO_2 crosses cell membranes easily, intracellular pH may decrease even further with further deterioration of cellular function.

2. Bicarbonate may cause clinical deterioration if tissue hypoxia is present.

    If tissue hypoxia is present, then the use of bicarbonate may be particularly disadvantageous due to increased lactate production (removal of acidotic inhibition of glycolysis) and the impairment of tissue oxygen unloading (left shift of ODC due increased pH). This means that with lactic acidosis or cardiac arrest then bicarbonate therapy may be dangerous.

3. Bicarbonate is probably not useful in most cases of high anion gap acidosis.

    Lactic acidosis can get worse if bicarbonate is given. Clinical studies have shown no benefit from bicarbonate in diabetic ketoacidosis. In these cases, the only indication for bicarbonate use is for the emergency management of severe hyperkalemia.

4. The preferred management of metabolic acidosis is to correct the primary cause and to use specific treatment for any potentially dangerous complications

    The organic acid anions serve as bicarbonate precursors to regenerate new bicarbonate once the primary cause is treated. In some forms of acidosis specific treatment to prevent problems is possible (i.e. ethanol blocking therapy in ethylene glycol poisoning.)

    If hyperkalemia is present then $[K^+]$ can be decreased by bicarbonate therapy. Also, bicarbonate therapy can cause an alkaline diuresis which hastens renal salicylate excretion.

5. Bicarbonate therapy may be useful for correction of acidemia due to non-organic (or mineral) acidosis (i.e. normal anion gap acidosis)

    In non-organic acidosis, there is no organic anion which can be metabolized to regenerate bicarbonate. Once the primary cause is corrected, resolution of the acidemia occurs more rapidly if bicarbonate therapy is used. Amounts sufficient for only partial correction of the disorder should be given. The aim is to increase arterial pH to above 7.2 to minimize adverse effects of the acidemia and to avoid the adverse effects of bicarbonate therapy. If the patient is improving without serious clinical problems then waiting (for renal bicarbonate regeneration) and watching (for clinical improvement), is a better strategy than giving bicarbonate.

Assessment

A metabolic acidosis is often strongly suspected because of the clinical presentation of the patient (i.e. diabetes, renal failure, and severe diarrhea). Check a biochemical profile of:

1. Low 'bicarbonate' (or low 'total CO_2'), this is often reported as part of the laboratory's biochemical profile on a venous blood sample. It represents the total concentration of all the species in the sample which can be converted to carbon dioxide gas. This is:

    Total $CO_2 = [HCO_3^-] + [H_2CO_3] + [$carbamino $CO_2] + [$dissolved $CO_2]$

    Apart from bicarbonate, all the other species are present in only small concentrations. The usefulness of the 'total CO_2' is as an estimate of the arterial bicarbonate and which can be obtained without collecting an arterial sample. The value will usually be several mmol/L higher than the actual arterial value due to the inclusion of carbamino and dissolved CO_2 and because of the higher CO_2 content of venous blood.

2. High chloride

3. High anion gap

Arterial blood gases are important for diagnosis, but should always be interpreted in conjunction with the clinical details. In addition to arterial blood gases, some other investigations useful for indicating a metabolic acidosis and for differentiating between the various main causes are:

4. Urine tests for glucose and ketones
5. Electrolytes (chloride, anion gap, and 'bicarbonate')
6. Plasma glucose
7. Urea and creatinine
8. Lactate

Ancillary Indices

There are several indices (which can be calculated from pathology results) which may be useful in assessing a metabolic acidosis:

- Anion gap
- Delta ratio
- Urinary anion gap (UAG)
- Osmolar gap

The Anion Gap

The term anion gap (AG) represents the concentration of all the unmeasured anions in the plasma. The negatively charged proteins account for about 10% of plasma anions and make up the majority of the unmeasured anion represented by the anion gap under normal circumstances. The acid anions (e.g. lactate, acetoacetate, sulphate) produced during a metabolic acidosis are not measured as part of the usual laboratory biochemical profile. The H^+ produced reacts with bicarbonate anions (buffering) and the CO_2 produced is excreted via the lungs (respiratory compensation). The net effect is a decrease in the concentration of measured anions (i.e. HCO_3^-) and an increase in the concentration of unmeasured anions (the acid anions) so the anion gap increases. AG is calculated from the following formula:

$$\text{Anion gap} = ([Na^+] + [K^+]) - ([Cl^-] - [HCO_3^-])$$

In health, the anion gap has a value of 14–18 mmol/L and mainly represents the unmeasured net negative charge on plasma proteins.

In an acidosis in which anions other than chloride are increased, the anion gap is increased. In contrast, in an acidosis due to loss of bicarbonate, e.g. in renal tubular acidosis, plasma chloride concentration is increased and the anion gap is normal. It has therefore been suggested that calculation of the anion gap is of value in the diagnosis of acidosis. In the majority of cases of acidosis, however, the cause is obvious clinically and can be confirmed by the results of simple tests. The anion gap may be useful in the analysis of complex acid-base disorders, some laboratories do not routinely measure chloride as part of an 'electrolyte profile' and the anion gap cannot then be calculated.

Main clinical uses of the anion gap

- To signal the presence of a metabolic acidosis and confirm other findings
- Help differentiate between causes of a metabolic acidosis, i.e. high anion gap versus normal anion gap metabolic acidosis. In an inorganic metabolic acidosis (e.g. due HCl infusion), the infused Cl^- replaces HCO_3^- and the anion gap remains normal. In an organic acidosis, the lost bicarbonate is replaced by the acid anion which is not normally measured. This means that the AG is increased.
- To assist in assessing the biochemical severity of the acidosis and follow the response to treatment

It is determined from a calculation involving three other measured ions, so the error with an AG is much higher than that of a single electrolyte determination. The commonest cause of a low anion gap is laboratory error in the electrolyte determinations. The 95% error range for the AG is about +/−5 mmol/L (i.e. 10 mmol/L range).

- If the AG is greater than 30 mmol/L, then it invariably means that a metabolic acidosis is present.
- If the AG is in the range 20–29 mmol/L, then about one-third of these patients will not have a metabolic acidosis.

Other clinical guides should also be used in deciding on the presence and severity of a metabolic acidosis. Significant lactic acidosis may be associated with an anion gap which remains in the reference range. Lactate levels of 5–10 mmol/L are associated with a high mortality if associated with sepsis, but the AG may be reported as within the reference range in as many as 50% of these cases. The anion gap is useful especially if very elevated or used to confirm other findings. Causes of a high anion-gap acidosis can be sorted out more specifically by using other investigations in addition to the history and examination of the patient. Investigations which may be very useful are:

- Lactate
- Creatinine
- Plasma glucose
- Urine ketone test

The Delta Ratio

The delta ratio is useful in the assessment of metabolic acidosis, the concept is related to the anion gap and buffering, it defined as:

Delta ratio = (Increase in anion gap/Decrease in bicarbonate)

Others have used the delta gap (defined as rise in AG minus the fall in bicarbonate), but this uses the same information as the delta ratio and has does not offer any advantage over it.

If one molecule of metabolic acid (HA) is added to the ECF and dissociates, the one H^+ released will react with one molecule of HCO_3^- to produce CO_2 and H_2O. This is the process of buffering. The net effect will be an increase in unmeasured anions by the one acid anion A^- (i.e. anion gap increases by one) and a decrease in the bicarbonate by one.

If all the acid dissociated in the ECF and all the buffering was by bicarbonate, then the increase in the AG should be equal to the decrease in bicarbonate, so the ratio between these two changes should be equal to one. The delta ratio quantifies the relationship between the changes in these two quantities.

Some general guidelines for use of the delta ratio when assessing metabolic acid-base disorders in provided in the (Table 2.8).

- A high delta ratio can occur in the situation where the patient had quite an elevated bicarbonate value at the onset of the metabolic acidosis. Such an elevated level could be due to a pre-existing metabolic alkalosis, or to compensation for a pre-existing respiratory acidosis (i.e. compensated chronic respiratory acidosis). With onset of a metabolic acidosis, using the 'standard' value of 24 mmol/L as the reference value for comparison when determining the 'decrease in bicarbonate' will result in an odd result.
- A low ratio occurs with hyperchloremic (or normal anion gap) acidosis. The reason here is that the acid involved is effectively hydrochloric acid (HCl) and the rise in plasma (chloride) is accounted for in the calculation of anion gap (i.e. chloride is a 'measured anion'). The result is that the 'rise in anion gap' (the numerator in the delta ration calculation) does not

occur but the 'decrease in bicarbonate' (the denominator) does rise in numerical value. The net of both these changes then is to cause a marked drop in delta ratio, commonly to <0.4.

- In lactic acidosis, the average value of the delta ratio in patients has been found to be is 1.6 due to intracellular buffering with extracellular retention of the anion. As a general rule, in uncomplicated lactic acidosis, the rise in the AG should always exceed the fall in bicarbonate level.
- In diabetic ketoacidosis, there is a special case as the urinary loss of ketones decreases the anion gap and this returns the delta ratio downwards towards one. A further complication is that these patients are often fluid resuscitated with 'normal saline' solution which results in an increase in plasma chloride and a decrease in anion gap and development of a 'hyperchloremic normal anion gap acidosis' superimposed on the ketoacidosis. The result is a further drop in the delta ratio.

The Urinary Anion Gap

The cations normally present in urine are Na^+, K^+, NH_4^+, Ca^{2+}, and Mg^{2+}. The anions normally present are Cl^-, HCO_3^-, sulphate, phosphate, and some organic anions. Only Na^+, K^+, and Cl^- are commonly measured in urine so the other charged species are the unmeasured anions (UA) and unmeasured cations (UC).

Because of the requirement for macroscopic electroneutrality, total anion charge always equals total cation charge, so:

Urinary anion gap = $(UA - UC) = [Na^+] + [K^+] - [Cl^-]$

The urinary anion gap (UAG), can help to differentiate between GIT and renal causes of a hyperchloremic metabolic acidosis. It has been found that the urinary anion gap provides a rough index of urinary ammonium excretion. Ammonium is positively charged so a rise in its urinary concentration (i.e. increased unmeasured cations) will cause a fall in UAG, as can be appreciated by inspection of the formula above. The following steps should be considered:

1. **Metabolic acidosis can be divided into two groups based on the anion gap:**
   - High anion gap acidosis
   - Normal anion gap (or hyperchloremic) acidosis.

   It is easy to calculate the anion gap so this differentiation is easy and indeed clinically useful.
2. **Consider the hyperchloremic group for further analysis. Hyperchloremic acidosis can be caused by:**
   - Loss of base via the kidney (e.g. renal tubular acidosis)
   - Loss of base via the bowel (e.g. diarrhea).
   - Gain of mineral acid (e.g. HCl infusion).

Table 2.8	General guidelines for use of the delta ratio
Delta ratio	Assessment guideline
<0.4	Hyperchloremic normal anion gap acidosis
0.4–0.8	Consider combined high AG and normal AG acidosis, but note that the ratio is often <1 in acidosis associated with renal failure
1–2	Usual for uncomplicated high AG acidosis—lactic acidosis—average value 1.6 DKA more likely to have a ratio closer to 1 due to urine ketone loss (especially if patient not dehydrated)
>2	Suggests a pre-existing elevated HCO_3^- level so consider: • A concurrent metabolic alkalosis, or • A pre-existing compensated respiratory acidosis

3. **Bowel or kidney as the cause:** Diagnosis between the above three groups of causes is usually clinically obvious, but occasionally it may be useful to have an extra aid to help in deciding between a loss of base via the kidneys or the bowel.
   - If the acidosis is due to loss of base via the bowel then the kidneys can response appropriately by increasing ammonium excretion to cause a net loss of H^+ from the body. The UAG would tend to be decreased, i.e. increased NH_4^+ (with presumably increased Cl^-) → increased UC → decreased UAG.
   - If the acidosis is due to loss of base via the kidney, then as the problem is with the kidney, it is not able to increase ammonium excretion and the UAG will not be increased.

Osmolar Gap

- An osmole is the amount of a substance that yields, in ideal solution, that number of particles (Avogadro's number) that would depress the freezing point of the solvent by 1.86 K.
- Osmolality of a solution is the number of osmoles of solute per kilogram of solvent.
- Osmolarity of a solution is the number of osmoles of solute per liter of solution.

So osmolality is a measure of the number of particles present in a unit weight of solvent. It is independent of the size, shape, or weight of the particles. It can only be measured by use of a property of the solution that is dependent on the particle concentration. These properties are collectively referred to as colligative properties. Osmolality is measured in the laboratory by machines called osmometers. The units of osmolality are mOsm/kg of solute.

Osmolarity is calculated from a formula which represents the solutes which under ordinary circumstances contribute nearly all of the osmolality of the sample.

Calculated osmolarity = 2 Na + Glucose + Urea (all in mmol/L).

or

Calculated osmolarity = 2 Na + 2 K + Glucose + Urea (all in mmol/L).

The osmolar gap is the difference between the two values—the osmolality (which is measured) and the osmolarity (which is calculated from measured solute concentrations).

Osmolar gap = Osmolality – Osmolarity

The Advantages of Anion Gap

- *Alerting role:* An elevated anion gap (especially if AG > 20 mmol/L) will alert the clinician to the presence of a high anion gap metabolic acidosis. This can be extremely useful in sorting out complicated mixed disorders.
- *Classification role:* It is used to divide metabolic acidosis into two main subgroups. The next step then is to consider either the four main categories of high anion gap acidosis (ketoacidosis, lactic acidosis, uremic acidosis, acidosis due toxins) or the two main categories of normal anion gap acidosis (renal group, GIT group). History and a few pertinent investigations will usually distinguish the cause.

The Advantages of Delta Ratio

It is useful particularly in the difficult situation of a metabolic acidosis due to two processes where one elevates the anion gap and the other does not. An example is the hyperchloremic normal anion gap acidosis which may develop in patients who have diabetic ketoacidosis (high anion gap). The ratio gives an indication of the relative contribution of the two processes. Unfortunately, its interpretation is limited somewhat by the wide error margin in this derived variable.

Prevention

Prevent accidental ingestion of (i.e. salicylates) by young children.

RESPIRATORY ALKALOSIS

Respiratory alkalosis is an alkali imbalance in the body caused by a lower than normal level of carbon dioxide in the blood. In the lungs, oxygen from inhaled air is exchanged for carbon dioxide from the blood. This process takes place between the alveoli (tiny air pockets in the lungs), and the blood vessels that connect to them. When a person hyperventilates, this exchange of oxygen for carbon dioxide is speeded up, and the person exhales too much carbon dioxide. This lowered level of carbon dioxide causes the pH of the blood to increase, leading to alkalosis.

Etiology

The primary cause of respiratory alkalosis is hyperventilation; rapid, deep breathing can be caused by conditions related to the lungs like pneumonia, lung disease, or asthma. More commonly, hyperventilation is associated with anxiety, fever, drug overdose, carbon monoxide poisoning, or serious infections. Tumors or swelling in the brain or nervous system can also cause this type of respiration. Other stresses to the body, including pregnancy, liver failure, high elevations, or metabolic acidosis can also trigger hyperventilation leading to respiratory alkalosis.

Other Miscellaneous Notes on Causes

- Hyperventilation due to respiratory center stimulation is a feature of salicylate toxicity, especially in adults, and results in a mixed disorder (metabolic acidosis and respiratory alkalosis).
- Propanidid was once used as an anesthetic induction agent, it caused prominent hyperventilation.
- A respiratory alkalosis is the commonest acid-base disorder found in patients with chronic liver disease.
- Hyperventilation syndrome related to anxiety can cause alkalosis severe enough to cause carpopedal spasm.
- A mild fairly well-compensated respiratory alkalosis is the usual finding in pregnancy.

Symptom is accompanied by dizziness, light headedness, agitation, and tingling or numbing around the mouth and in the fingers and hands. Muscle twitching, spasms, and weakness may be noted. Seizures, irregular heartbeats, and tetany (muscle spasms so severe that the muscle locks in a rigid position) can result from severe respiratory alkalosis.

Hyperventilation (i.e. increased alveolar ventilation) is the mechanism responsible for the lowered arterial pCO_2 in all cases of respiratory alkalosis. This low arterial pCO_2 will be sensed by the central and peripheral chemoreceptors and the hyperventilation will be inhibited unless the patient's ventilation is controlled (Table 2.9).

Table 2.9	Causes of respiratory alkalosis

1. **Central causes (direct action via respiratory centre)**
   - Head injury
   - Stroke
   - Anxiety-hyperventilation syndrome (psychogenic)
   - Other 'supratentorial' causes (pain, fear, stress, and voluntary)
   - Various drugs (i.e. analeptics, propanidid, and salicylate intoxication)
   - Various endogenous compounds (i.e. progesterone during pregnancy, cytokines during sepsis, toxins in patients with chronic liver disease)
2. **Hypoxemia (act via peripheral chemoreceptors)**
   - Respiratory stimulation via peripheral chemoreceptors
3. **Pulmonary causes (act via intrapulmonary receptors)**
   - Pulmonary embolism
   - Pneumonia
   - Asthma
   - Pulmonary edema (all types)
4. **Iatrogenic (act directly on ventilation)**
   - Excessive controlled ventilation

Symptoms and Signs

Symptoms and signs depend on the rate and degree of fall in pCO_2. Acute respiratory alkalosis causes light-headedness, confusion, peripheral, and circumoral paresthesias, cramps, and syncope. Mechanism is thought to be change in cerebral blood flow and pH. Tachypnea or hyperpnea is often the only sign; carpopedal spasm may occur in severe cases. Chronic respiratory alkalosis is usually asymptomatic and has no distinctive signs.

Maintenance

The alkalosis persists as long as the initiating disorder persists unless some other disorder or complication causing impairment of the hyperventilation intervenes. Hyperventilation due to anxiety may be relieved by having the patient breath into a paper bag. By rebreathing the air that was exhaled, the patient will inhale a higher amount of carbon dioxide than he or she would normally. Antibiotics may be used to treat pneumonia or other infections. Other medications may be required to treat fever, seizures, or irregular heartbeats. If the alkalosis is related to a drug overdose, the patient may require treatment for poisoning. Use of mechanical ventilation like a respirator may be necessary. If the respiratory alkalosis has triggered the body to compensate by developing metabolic acidosis, symptoms of that condition may need to be treated, as well.

Compensation

A decreased $[HCO_3^-]$ will counteract the effect of a decreased pCO_2 on the pH. Mathematically, it returns the value of the $([HCO_3^-]/0.03 \times pCO_2)$ ratio towards normal.

$$pH = pK'a + \log_{10}[(HCO_3^-)/0.03 \times pCO_2]$$

Key points regarding compensation in respiratory alkalosis:

- **Physicochemical effect:** Initially there is an immediate physicochemical change which lowers the bicarbonate slightly.
- **Role of kidney:** The effector organ for compensation is the kidney.
- **Slow response:** The renal response has a slow onset and the maximal response takes 2–3 days to be achieved.
- **Outcome:** The drop in bicarbonate results in the extracellular pH returning only partially towards its normal value.

Compensation in an Acute Respiratory Alkalosis

- *Mechanism:* Changes in the physicochemical equilibrium occur due to the lowered pCO_2 and this result in a slight decrease in HCO_3^-. There is insufficient time for the kidneys to respond, so this is the only change in an acute respiratory alkalosis. The buffering is predominantly by protein and occurs intracellularly; this alters the equilibrium position of the bicarbonate system.

- *Magnitude:* There is a drop in HCO_3^- by 2 mmol/L for every 10 mmHg decrease in pCO_2 from the reference value of 40 mmHg.

Limit: The lower limit of 'compensation' for this process is 18 mmol/L, so bicarbonate levels below that in an acute respiratory alkalosis indicate a coexisting metabolic acidosis.

Correction

Hypoxemia is an important cause of respiratory stimulation and consequent respiratory alkalosis. The decrease in arterial pCO_2 inhibits the rise in ventilation. The hypocapnic inhibition of ventilation (acting via the central chemoreceptors) may leave the patient with an impaired state of tissue oxygen delivery. Adaptation occurs over a few days and the central chemoreceptor inhibition is lessened and ventilation increases. Correction of hypoxemia is the most urgent concern and is many times more important than correction of the respiratory alkalosis. Administration of oxygen in sufficient concentrations and sufficient amounts is essential. Attention to other aspects necessary to improve oxygen delivery and minimize tissue oxygen consumption is important. In most cases correction of the underlying disorder will resolve the problem. In some cases this is easy (i.e. adjustment of ventilator settings, rebreathing via a paper bag with psychogenic hyperventilation) but in some cases it is a slow process.

Assessment

The severity of a respiratory alkalosis is determined by the difference between the actual pCO_2 and the expected pCO_2. The actual pCO_2 is the measured value from the blood gas results.

Prevention

Hyperventilation of the anaesthetized patient is common and preventable. Monitoring by capnography allows early recognition and correction. In main operations, serial arterial gases for assessment of oxygenation and ventilation is appropriate especially as the size of the endtidal-arterial pCO_2 gradient can be determined and this is useful for determining ventilation settings between blood-gas analyses.

METABOLIC ALKALOSIS

Metabolic alkalosis is a primary acid-base disorder which causes the plasma bicarbonate to rise to a level higher than expected. The severity of a metabolic alkalosis

is determined by the difference between the actual $[HCO_3^-]$ and the expected $[HCO_3^-]$. A secondary or compensatory process which causes an elevation in plasma bicarbonate should not be confused with the primary processes. An elevation in bicarbonate occurring in response to a chronic respiratory acidosis should be referred to as a 'compensatory response' and never as a 'secondary metabolic alkalosis'.

Etiology

Whenever the plasma bicarbonate rises above 24 mmol/L, bicarbonate is excreted by the kidney. This response is reasonably prompt and effective so a metabolic alkalosis will be rapidly corrected. If you infuse say 100 mL of 8.4%, sodium bicarbonate into a healthy person with normal renal function, the rise in plasma bicarbonate is brief because of prompt bicarbonaturia. This is one way to alkalinize the urine. An infusion of alkali causes only a brief metabolic alkalosis due to this rapid renal excretion. This ability of the kidney to rapidly excrete bicarbonate if its level is high is in complete contrast to its powerful ability to reabsorb the entire filtered load if plasma $[HCO_3^-]$ is low or normal. The persistence of a metabolic alkalosis requires an additional process which acts to impair renal bicarbonate excretion:

1. **The initiating process:** Normally, plasma bicarbonate is kept at a steady level of about 24 mmol/L by two renal processes:
   - Tubular reabsorption of nearly all of the large daily filtered load of bicarbonate
   - Excretion of the net daily production of the fixed acid (which results in regeneration of the titrated plasma bicarbonate)

   Causes of a metabolic alkalosis can be classified into several groups as outlined in the (Table 2.10).

   Excessive intravenous administration of alkali alone will cause a metabolic alkalosis which is only short-lived because of rapid renal excretion of bicarbonate (as mentioned previously).

   Hepatic metabolism of citrate, lactate, acetate, or certain other organic acid anions to bicarbonate can

Table 2.10	Causes of a metabolic alkalosis: classification of initiating processes for metabolic alkalosis
Gain of alkali in the ECF	
• From an exogenous source (i.e. IV $NaHCO_3$ infusion, citrate in transfused blood) • From an endogenous source (i.e. metabolism of keto-anions to produce bicarbonate)	
Loss of H+ from ECF	
• Via kidneys (i.e. use of diuretics) • Via gut [i.e. vomiting, nasogastric (NG) suction]	

cause a brief metabolic alkalosis. This may occur after a massive blood transfusion because of the metabolism of the administered citrate. The kidneys excrete the bicarbonate and the urine will be relatively alkaline.

2. **Processes responsible for maintenance of the alkalosis:** 'Causes' of clinically significant chronic metabolic alkalosis are usefully divided into two main groupings based on the main factor involved in the maintenance of the disorder:
   - The chloride depletion group
   - The potassium depletion group

Maintenance of the alkalosis requires a process which greatly impairs the kidney's ability to excrete bicarbonate and prevent the return of the elevated plasma level to normal. Chloride deficiency leads to a situation where the kidney reabsorbs more bicarbonate anion than usual, because there is not sufficient chloride anion present. Reabsorption of an anion is necessary to maintain electroneutrality as Na^+ and K^+ are reabsorbed so the deficiency of chloride leads to a resetting upwards of the maintained plasma bicarbonate level. Chloride and bicarbonate are the only anions present in appreciable quantities in extracellular fluid, so a deficiency of one must lead to an increase in the other because of the strict requirement for macroscopic electroneutrality.

CHLORIDE DEPLETION

Administration of chloride is necessary to correct these disorders. The four main subgroups of metabolic alkalosis are listed in the Table 2.11. The two commonest causes of chronic metabolic alkalosis are loss of gastric juice and diuretic therapy. The gastric secretion of H^+ results in generation of new bicarbonate which is returned to the blood.

Gastric alkalosis is most marked with vomiting due to pyloric stenosis or obstruction because the vomitus is acidic gastric juice only. Vomiting in other conditions may involve a mixture of acid gastric loss and alkaline duodenal contents and the acid-base situation that results is more variable. Histamine H2-blockers also decrease gastric H^+ losses despite continued vomiting or nasogastric drainage and alkalosis will not occur if the fluid lost is not particularly acidic, indeed loss of alkaline small intestinal contents can even result in an acidosis if gastric acid secretion is suppressed.

Diuretics such as frusemide and thiazides interfere with reabsorption of chloride and sodium in the renal tubules. Urinary losses of chloride exceed those of bicarbonate. The patients on diuretics who develop an alkalosis are those who are also volume depleted (increasing aldosterone levels) and have a low dietary

Table 2.11	Causes of a metabolic alkalosis—a common hybrid classification
A. Addition of base to ECF	
• Milk—alkali syndrome	
• Excessive $NaHCO_3$ intake	
• Recovery phase from organic acidosis (excess regeneration of HCO_3^-)	
• Massive blood transfusion (due metabolism of citrate)	
B. Chloride depletion	
• Loss of acidic gastric juice	
• Diuretics	
• Post-hypercapnia	
• Excess fecal loss (i.e. villous adenoma)	
C. Potassium depletion	
• Primary hyperaldosteronism	
• Cushing's syndrome	
• Secondary hyperaldosteronism	
• Some drugs (i.e. carbenoxolone)	
• Kaliuretic diuretics	
• Excessive licorice intake (glycyrrhizic acid)	
• Bartter's syndrome	
• Severe potassium depletion	
D. Other disorders	
• Laxative abuse	
• Severe hypoalbuminemia	

chloride intake ('salt restricted' diet). Hypokalemia is common in these patients. If dietary chloride intake is adequate then an alkalosis is unlikely to develop. This is the main reason why every patient taking diuretics such as thiazides or Lasix does not develop a metabolic alkalosis. The effect of diuretic use on urinary chloride levels depends on the relationship of the time of urine collection to diuretic effect: it is high while the diuretic is acting, but drops to low levels afterwards.

Villous adenomas typically excrete bicarbonate and can cause a hyperchloremic metabolic acidosis. Sometimes, they excrete chloride predominantly and the result is then a metabolic alkalosis.

Chloride diarrhea is a rare congenital condition due to an intestinal transport defect, where the chronic fecal chloride loss can (if associated with volume depletion and K^+ loss as maintenance factors) result in a metabolic alkalosis.

Potassium Depletion

Potassium depletion occurs with situations of mineralocorticoid excess. Bicarbonate reabsorption in both the proximal and distal tubules is increased in the presence of potassium depletion. Potassium depletion decreases aldosterone release by the adrenal cortex.

Urinary Chloride Measurements

In most cases the cause is obvious (i.e. vomiting, diuretic use) but if not then measurement of a spot urinary chloride can be useful (Table 2.12). Two things to be aware of when interpreting the result:

- Recent diuretic use can acutely elevate the urinary chloride level, but as the diuretic effect passes the urinary chloride level will fall to low levels. So seek information on the timing of diuretic use when assessing the result (this variability in urine chloride levels has been used as an indicator of surreptitious diuretic use).
- A 'spot' urine chloride may be misleading if bladder urine contains a mixture of urine from during and after diuretic effect.

Symptoms and Signs

Symptoms and signs of mild alkalemia are usually related to the underlying disorder. More severe alkalemia increases protein binding of ionized Ca^{2+}, leading to hypocalcemia and subsequent headache, lethargy, and neuromuscular excitability, sometimes with delirium, tetany, and seizures. Alkalemia also lowers threshold for anginal symptoms and arrhythmias. Concomitant hypokalemia may cause weakness.

Maintenance

1. **Maintenance factors:** The alkalosis would be only transitory. Since the kidney normally has a large capacity to excrete bicarbonate and return the plasma level to normal. This rise in urinary bicarbonate loss occurs relatively promptly (i.e., onset within an hour) but excretion takes 24 hours to peak unless some abnormal condition is causing renal retention of bicarbonate. The factors involved in maintenance of the disorder are very important not only because they are necessary to develop a persisting (i.e. chronic) alkalosis but also because they can maintain the alkalosis even after the primary process generating it has resolved.

Table 2.12   Metabolic alkalosis based on urinary chloride
Urine Cl⁻ <10 mmol/L
• Often associated with volume depletion (increased proximal tubular reabsorption of HCO_3^-)
• Respond to saline infusion (replaces chloride and volume) Common causes: Previous thiazide diuretic therapy, vomiting (90% of cases)
Urine Cl⁻ >20 mmol/L
• Often associated with volume expansion and hypokalemia· Resistant to therapy with saline infusion
• Cause: Excess aldosterone, severe K^+ deficiency
• Other causes: Diuretic therapy (current), Bartter's syndrome

2. **Abnormal maintenance factors:** The four factors that cause maintenance of the alkalosis (by increasing bicarbonate reabsorption in the tubules or decreasing bicarbonate filtration at the glomerulus) are:
   - Chloride depletion (is the most common factor)
   - Reduced glomerular filtration rate
   - Potassium depletion
   - ECF volume depletion

Volume depletion and potassium depletion may coexist in some disorders (i.e. vomiting). Severe potassium depletion alone can cause a metabolic alkalosis, but this is typically only of mild to moderate degree. The mechanism seems to be related to an intracellular shift of H^+ ('intracellular acidosis') in exchange for K^+. The alkalosis is generated predominantly due to non-renal mechanisms. Renal mechanisms are frequently involved in causing the potassium depletion (i.e. in syndromes of mineralocorticoid excess).

Volume depletion has long been implicated in maintenance of an alkalosis. The idea is that hypovolemic is associated with increased fluid and sodium reabsorption in the proximal tubule and bicarbonate is reabsorbed in preference to chloride; the alkalosis thus being maintained. The role of volume depletion has probably been overemphasized—the coexisting chloride depletion is the most important factor responsible for persistence of the alkalosis. Correction of the volume deficit without correction of the chloride deficit will not result in correction of the alkalosis. These deficits are often corrected together with a saline infusion.

Diuretics can cause excess renal loss of fixed acid anions and result in alkalosis. Their use can also cause depletion of chloride, water (hypovolemic) and potassium. These factors together maintain the alkalosis. For an alkalosis to develop in patients on diuretic therapy, there generally has to some decrease in chloride intake as well (i.e. if the patient is on a 'salt-restricted' diet). A continued normal oral chloride intake (usually as NaCl) prevents patients on diuretics from getting an alkalosis.

Metabolic Effects

1. **Adverse effects of alkalosis**
   - Decreased myocardial contractility
   - Arrhythmias
   - Decreased cerebral blood flow
   - Confusion
   - Mental obtundation
   - Neuromuscular excitability

Impaired peripheral oxygen unloading (due shift of oxygen dissociation curve to left).

2. **Risk of hypoxemia:** Hypoxemia may occur and oxygen delivery to the tissues may be reduced. Factors involved in impaired arterial oxygen content are:

- Hypoventilation (due respiratory response to metabolic alkalosis)
- Pulmonary microatelectasis (consequent to hypoventilation)
- Increased ventilation-perfusion mismatch (as alkalosis inhibits hypoxic pulmonary vasoconstriction).

Peripheral oxygen unloading may be impaired because of the alkalotic shift of the hemoglobin oxygen dissociation curve to the left. The body's main compensatory response to impaired tissue oxygen delivery is to increase cardiac output but this ability is impaired if hypovolemic and decreased myocardial contractility are present.

Compensation

The hypoventilation causes a compensatory rise in arterial pCO_2, but the magnitude of the response has generally been found to be quite variable. The expected pCO_2 due to appropriate hypoventilation in simple metabolic alkalosis can be estimated from the following formula:

Expected $pCO_2 = 0.7\,[HCO_3^-] + 20\,mmHg$ (range: +/– 5)

Correction

The main principles are:

- Correct the primary cause of the disorder
- Correct those factors which maintain the disorder (especially chloride administration in the common Cl^- deficient cases)

Repletion of chloride, potassium, and ECF volume will promote renal bicarbonate excretion and return plasma bicarbonate to normal. Chloride administration is essential for correction of chloride-depletion metabolic alkalosis and the alkalosis can be corrected with chloride even if volume depletion persists. Because of electroneutrality requirements it is not possible to give chloride alone, so 'giving chloride' is equivalent to 'giving saline' in most cases.

Volume administration will not correct the alkalosis unless the administered fluid contains chloride. This is not difficult though as all available ECF replacement fluids contain chloride so administering these IV fluids to correct the volume deficiency must necessarily replenish chloride.

HYDROCHLORIC ACID INFUSION

An infusion of hydrochloric acid can be given via a central line. The infusion will selectively correct the chloride deficiency and the infusion can be titrated to an end-point of a specific bicarbonate level of pH level. The H^+ will consume HCO_3^- provided the excess CO_2 can be ventilated off.

The correction of alkalosis will result in a right shift in the oxygen dissociation curve which will improve peripheral oxygen unloading. An HCl infusion is a dramatic way of administering chloride but published reports attest to its safety and successful use. An increase in arterial pO_2 and a decrease in pCO_2 generally occur and may assist with weaning from mechanical ventilation. The administration of chloride in a small volume may be useful in patients who are at risk of volume overload.

Use of Acetazolamide

Acetazolamide is a carbonic anhydrase inhibitor which has also been used to speed the rapidity of correction of alkalosis. It is usually more readily available than sterile hydrochloric acid solutions and is a more acceptable therapeutic option. It causes renal bicarbonate loss to increase and plasma bicarbonate levels fall. Only one or two doses probably should be used. Some problems with acetazolamide are:

- Renal losses of water, Na^+ and K^+ increase (so appropriate adjustments in IV fluids and K^+ supplementation are necessary)
- It interferes with CO_2 transport
- It is slower acting and more difficult to titrate to a given bicarbonate level

Other sources of HCl have been used (i.e. lysine HCl, ammonium chloride). Hepatic metabolism of the ammonium generates hydrogen ions.

These ancillary measures may prove useful in a small number of patients but are not generally recommended.

Treatment

1. Correct cause if possible (i.e. correct pyloric obstruction, cease diuretics)
2. Correct the deficiency which is impairing renal bicarbonate excretion (e.g. give chloride, water and K^+)
3. Expand ECF volume with normal/saline (and KCl if K^+ deficiency)
4. Rarely ancillary measures such as:
   - HCl infusion
   - Acetazolamide (one or two doses only)
   - Oral lysine hydrochloride
5. Supportive measures (e.g. give O_2 in view of hypoventilation; appropriate monitoring and observation)
6. Avoid hyperventilation as this worsens the alkalemia.

Assessment

The pattern of high values of $[HCO_3^-]$ and pCO_2 occurring together suggests either a metabolic alkalosis or a respiratory acidosis (or both). If pCO_2 is over 60 mmHg, the metabolic alkalosis is either very severe or there is a mixed disorder with a respiratory acidosis.

Metabolic alkalosis is suspected if one of the known causes of the disorder is present especially vomiting, nasogastric suction, pyloric obstruction, excess mineralocorticoid syndromes, or diuretic use.

The delta ratio can be a useful adjunct in detecting the presence of a second acid-base disorder in patients with a metabolic acidosis. In patients who have a metabolic acidosis and a chronic metabolic alkalosis the delta ratio has a value greater than 2. Such a high value can also occur in patients with a pre-existing chronic respiratory acidosis because the bicarbonate is also elevated in that disorder as well. Because of potential errors, the delta ratio should be assessed cautiously.

Prevention

There are two aspects of prevention for a metabolic alkalosis:

- Prevention of the primary or initiating process, and/or
- Prevention of the factors that are involved in maintaining the alkalosis.

Patients with nasogastric drainage and pyloric obstruction should receive adequate fluid replacement using a chloride containing fluid. Patients receiving thiazide diuretics likewise need to have adequate chloride intake. Proton pump inhibitors can be used to greatly decrease gastric acid loss despite continuing nasogastric drainage.

Mixed Acid-base Disorders

Mixed acid-base disorders are defined as independently coexisting disorders, not merely compensatory responses are often seen in patients in critical care units and can lead to dangerous extremes of pH. A patient with diabetic ketoacidosis (metabolic acidosis), may develop an independent respiratory problem leading to respiratory acidosis or alkalosis. Patients with underlying pulmonary disease may not respond to metabolic acidosis with appropriate ventilatory response because of insufficient respiratory reserve. Such imposition of respiratory acidosis on metabolic acidosis can lead to severe acidemia and a poor outcome. When metabolic acidosis and metabolic alkalosis coexist in the same patient the pH may be normal or near normal. When the pH is normal, an elevated anion gap denotes the presence of a metabolic acidosis. A diabetic patient with ketoacidosis may have renal dysfunction resulting in simultaneous metabolic acidosis. Patients who have ingested an overdose of drug combinations, such as sedatives and salicylates may have mixed disturbances as a result of the acid-base response to the individual drugs (metabolic acidosis mixed with respiratory acidosis or respiratory alkalosis, respectively). Even more complex are triple acid-base disturbances. For example, patients with metabolic acidosis due to alcoholic ketoacidosis may develop metabolic alkalosis due to vomiting and superimposed respiratory alkalosis due to the hyperventilation of hepatic dysfunction or alcohol withdrawal.

Correct diagnosis requires a logical approach and a clear understanding both of the relevant pathophysiology and of the quantitative relationships between $[H^+]$ and pCO_2. The biochemical changes that are characteristic of the various acid-base disturbances are shown in Table 2.13. With this physiological approach, calculated parameters, such as 'standard bicarbonate' and 'base excess' are redundant.

The standard bicarbonate is a calculated estimate of the bicarbonate concentration that would be present if the pCO_2 were normal, and thus reflects only the metabolic influences on bicarbonate. The base excess is a calculated estimate of the metabolic influences on total buffering capacity. These parameters were introduced with a view to distinguishing between the respiratory and metabolic components in acid-base disorders, but they take no account of normal physiological responses. An abnormal standard bicarbonate or base excess indicates the presence of a metabolic acidosis or alkalosis. It does not, however, indicate whether this is either part of a mixed

Table 2.13	Biochemical changes characteristic of disturbances of acid-base homoeostasis							
	Acidosis				**Alkalosis**			
	Respiratory		*Metabolic*		*Respiratory*		*Metabolic*	
	Acute	*Chronic*			*Acute*	*Chronic*		
H^+	↑	(S, N, H) ↑	↑		↓	(S, N, L) ↓	↓	
pH	↓	(S, N, L) ↓	↓		↑	(S, N, H) ↑	↑	
pCO_2	↑	↑	↓		↓	↓	↑	
HCO_3	S ↑	↑↑	↓↓		S ↓	↓	↑↑	

S, slight; L, low; N, normal; H, high.

disturbance of acid-base homoeostasis or related to normal physiological compensation.

INTERPRETATION OF ACID-BASE DATA

A thorough understanding of the pathophysiology of acid-base homoeostasis is essential for the correct interpretation of laboratory data, but these data should always be considered in the clinical context.

The starting point in any evaluation should be the hydrogen ion concentration or pH. This will indicate whether the predominant disturbance is an acidosis or an alkalosis. However, a normal value does not exclude an acid-base disorder. There may be either a fully compensated disturbance or two primary disturbances which effects on hydrogen ion concentration cancel each other out.

If the pCO_2 is abnormal, there must be a respiratory component to the disturbance. If the pCO_2 is raised in an acidosis, the acidosis is respiratory and comparison of the hydrogen ion concentration with that predicted for an acute change in pCO_2 (bearing in mind that an increase (decrease) in pCO_2 of 1 kPa typically causes an increase (decrease) in $[H^+]$ of 5.5 nmol/L) will indicate whether there is an additional metabolic component although it is important to appreciate that this may be a compensatory change. If the pCO_2 is low in an acidosis, the acidosis is metabolic and there is an additional respiratory component, which will often reflect compensation. A similar rationale applies to alkalotic states.

As the derived bicarbonate is calculated from the pCO_2 and $[H^+]$, it does not provide any more information than these two measurements alone. However, knowing the bicarbonate concentration may simplify the interpretation of acid-base data. Its concentration is always decreased in metabolic acidosis and increased in metabolic alkalosis, regardless of whether or not there is compensation.

Oxygen Transport and its Disorders

In patients with respiratory disorders, a disturbance of the arterial partial pressure of oxygen (pO_2) may be of greater clinical significance than either an abnormal pCO_2 or abnormal $[H^+]$. Although, both oxygen and carbon dioxide are transported between the alveoli and the bloodstream, albeit in opposite directions, their respective partial pressures do not necessarily change in a reciprocal fashion. There are two reasons for this; first, carbon dioxide is generally more diffusible than oxygen, with the result that, in pulmonary edema and interstitial lung disease, hypoxemia develops but the pCO_2 may not increase; second, very little oxygen is carried in physical solution in the blood, and hemoglobin is normally nearly fully saturated with oxygen. As a result, hyperventilation

cannot increase pO_2 significantly, but can reduce the pCO_2. A raised pO_2 is only seen in patients given supplementary oxygen, which increases the proportion of oxygen in the inspired gas [fraction of inspired oxygen (FiO_2)] and results in an increased inspired pO_2. It is essential to know the FiO_2 in order to interpret pO_2 correctly.

The Oxyhemoglobin Dissociation Curve

The oxyhemoglobin dissociation curve (ODC) is an important tool for understanding how our blood carries and releases oxygen. Specifically, the ODC relates oxygen saturation (sO_2) and partial pressure of oxygen in the blood (pO_2), and is determined by what is called "hemoglobin's affinity for oxygen," that is, how readily hemoglobin (Hb) acquires and releases oxygen molecules from its surrounding tissue.

Hemoglobin, an intracellular protein, is the primary vehicle for transporting oxygen in the blood. Oxygen is also carried (dissolved) in plasma, but to a much lesser degree. Hemoglobin is contained in erythrocytes, more commonly referred to as red blood cells.

Under certain conditions, oxygen bound to the hemoglobin is released into the body tissue, and under others, it is absorbed from the tissue into the blood. Each hemoglobin molecule has a limited capacity for holding oxygen molecules. How much of that capacity that is filled by oxygen bound to the hemoglobin at any time is called the oxygen saturation. Expressed as a percentage, the oxygen saturation is the ratio of the amount of oxygen bound to the hemoglobin, to the oxygen carrying capacity of the hemoglobin. The oxygen carrying capacity is determined by the amount of hemoglobin present in the blood.

The amount of oxygen bound to the hemoglobin at any time is related, in large part, to the partial pressure of oxygen to which the hemoglobin is exposed. In the lungs, at the alveolar-capillary interface, the partial pressure of oxygen is typically high, and, therefore, the oxygen binds readily to hemoglobin that is present. As the blood circulates to other body tissue in which the partial pressure of oxygen is less, the hemoglobin releases the oxygen into the tissue because the hemoglobin cannot maintain its full bound capacity of oxygen in the presence of lower oxygen partial pressures.

UNDERSTANDING THE OXYHEMOGLOBIN DISSOCIATION CURVE

In its basic form, the oxyhemoglobin dissociation curve describes the relation between the partial pressure of oxygen (x-axis) and the oxygen saturation (y-axis). Hemoglobin's affinity for oxygen increases as successive molecules of oxygen bind. More molecules bind as the oxygen partial pressure increases until the maximum amount that can be bound is reached. As this limit is approached, very little additional binding occurs and the curve levels out as the hemoglobin becomes saturated with oxygen. Hence the curve has a sigmoidal or S-shape (Fig. 2.10). At pressures above about 60 mmHg, the standard dissociation curve is relatively flat, which means that the oxygen content of the blood does not change significantly even with large increases in the oxygen partial pressure. To get more oxygen to the tissue would require blood transfusions to increase the hemoglobin count (and hence the oxygen carrying capacity), or supplemental oxygen that would increase the oxygen dissolved in plasma.

Although binding of oxygen to hemoglobin continues to some extent for pressures below about 60 mmHg, as oxygen's partial pressures decrease in this steep area of the curve, the oxygen is unloaded to peripheral tissue readily as the hemoglobin's affinity diminishes.

The partial pressure of oxygen in the blood at which the hemoglobin is 50% saturated, typically about 26.6 mmHg for a healthy person, is known as the P_{50}. The P_{50} is a conventional measure of hemoglobin affinity for oxygen. In the presence of disease or other conditions that change the hemoglobin's oxygen affinity and, consequently, shift the curve to the right or left, the P_{50} changes accordingly. An increased P_{50} indicates a rightward shift of the standard curve, which means that a larger partial pressure is necessary to maintain 50% oxygen saturation. This indicates a decreased affinity. Conversely, a lower P_{50} indicates a leftward shift and a higher affinity.

Factors that Affect the Standard Dissociation Curve

The effectiveness of hemoglobin-oxygen binding can be affected by several factors. The factors can be viewed as having the effect of shifting or reshaping the oxyhemoglobin curve ('the standard curve') of a typical, healthy person. The standard curve is shifted to the right by an **increase** in temperature, 2, 3-DPG, or pCO_2, or a **decrease** in pH. The curve is shifted to the left by the opposite of these conditions. A rightward shift, by definition, causes a decrease in the affinity of hemoglobin for oxygen. This makes it harder for the hemoglobin to bind to oxygen (requiring a higher partial pressure to achieve the same oxygen saturation), but it makes it easier for the hemoglobin to release bound oxygen. Conversely, a leftward shift increases the affinity, making the oxygen easier for the hemoglobin to pick up but harder to release.

We list several of the factors here and indicate how the curve is affected:

- **Variation of the hyrogen ion concentration:** This changes the blood pH. A decrease in pH shifts the standard curve to the right, while an increase shifts it to the left. This is known as the Bohr effect.

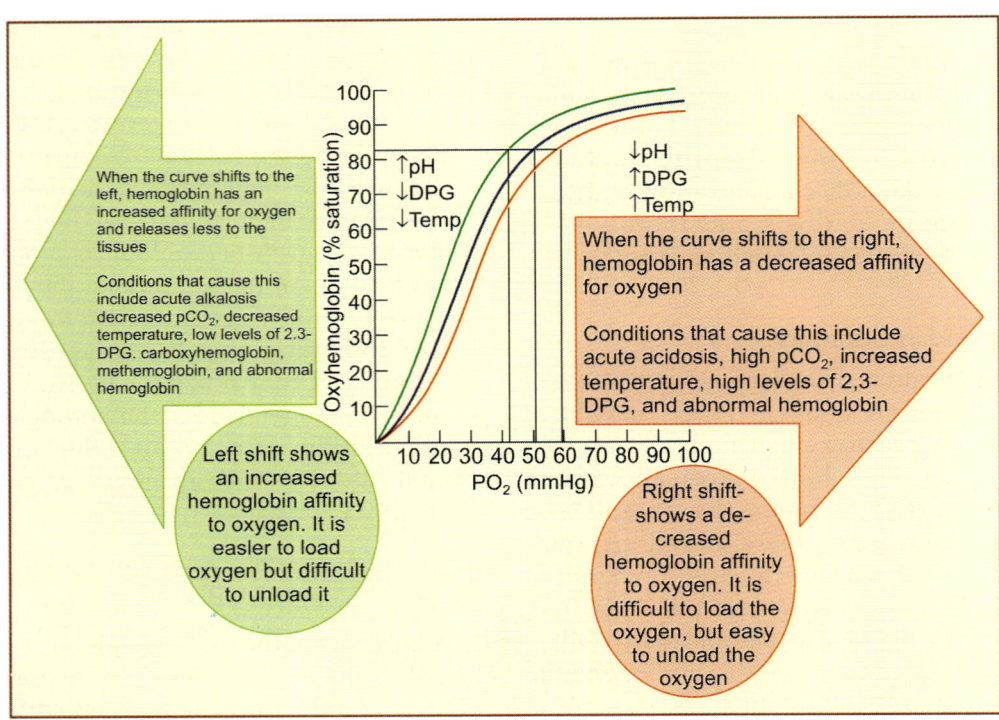

Fig. 2.10: The oxyhemoglobin dissociation curve. Normal arterial and venous pO_2 are shown. The effect of a right or left shift in the amount of oxygen delivered to tissues is indicated. A right shift causes an increase, a left shift a decrease. P_{50} is the pO_2 at which hemoglobin is 50% saturated with oxygen. DPG, diphosphoglycerate

- **Effects of carbon dioxide:** Carbon dioxide affects the curve in two ways; first, it influences intracellular pH (the Bohr effect), and second, CO_2 accumulation causes carbamino compounds to be generated through chemical interactions. Low levels of carbamino compounds have the effect of shifting the curve to the right, while higher levels cause a leftward shift.

- **Effects of 2, 3-DPG:** 2, 3-diphosphoglycerate, or 2, 3-DPG, is an organophosphate, which is created in erythrocytes during glycolysis. The production of 2,3-DPG is likely an important adaptive mechanism, because the production increases for several conditions in the presence of diminished peripheral tissue O_2 availability, such as hypoxemia, chronic lung disease, anemia, and congestive heart failure, among others. High levels of 2, 3-DPG shift the curve to the right, while low levels of 2, 3-DPG cause a leftward shift, seen in states, such as septic shock and hypophosphatemia.

- **Temperature:** Temperature does not have so dramatic effect as the previous factors, but hyperthermia causes a rightward shift, while hypothermia causes a leftward shift.

- **Carbon monoxide:** Hemoglobin binds with carbon monoxide 240 times more readily than with oxygen, and, therefore, the presence of carbon monoxide can interfere with the hemoglobin's acquisition of oxygen. In addition to lowering the potential for hemoglobin to bind to oxygen, carbon monoxide also has the effect of shifting the curve to the left. With an increased level of carbon monoxide, a person can suffer from severe hypoxemia while maintaining a normal PO_2.

- **Effects of methemoglobinemia (a form of abnormal hemoglobin):** Methemoglobinemia causes a leftward shift in the curve.

- **Fetal hemoglobin:** Fetal hemoglobin (HbF) is structurally different from normal hemoglobin. The fetal dissociation curve is shifted to the left relative to the curve for the normal adult. Typically, fetal arterial oxygen pressures are low, and hence the leftward shift enhances the placental uptake of oxygen.

DISSOCIATION CURVE'S CLINICAL USES

Dissociation curve (DOC) and the role of hemoglobin are important clinically in understanding the relationship of arterial oxygen saturation to the partial pressure of oxygen in arterial blood, particularly as it relates to disease. For example, it is useful to observe in healthy patients that the slope of the curve increases significantly from the mid-sixties (pO_2) downward, which indicates to the health professional that decreases in pO_2 in this region will have dramatic effects on arterial oxygen saturation.

Also, it is useful to have a good grasp on the influence of factors that can affect the curve or the affinity of hemoglobin to oxygen. For example, it is useful to remember the powerful effects of carbon monoxide in trying to explain hypoxemia in the presence of a normal pO_2 and SaO_2.

Understanding the elements of the dissociation curve, such as the basis of oxygen saturation, can also help explain clinical problems. For example, the differential diagnosis of a patient that presents with shortness of breath in the presence of adequate ventilation and SaO_2 should include hemoglobin deficiency, because routine SaO_2 calculations are based on normal hemoglobin values.

Arterial pCO_2 Adjustment

Carbon dioxide is produced in huge quantities by cells: typically 12,000 (basally) to as much as 15,000– 20,000 mmol/day with typical levels of activity. An efficient system exists for its removal. The arterial pCO_2 is of critical importance for intracellular acid-base homeostasis because of both its potential to change rapidly and because of its effectiveness in altering intracellular $[H^+]$.

Carbon dioxide crosses cell membranes easily. A change in ventilation affects the arterial pCO_2 level and the intracellular pCO_2 throughout the body. The compensatory response to a metabolic acid-base disorder is to increase alveolar ventilation and, thus, decrease arterial pCO_2 levels. This changed pCO_2 will affect intracellular pH and this effect is rapid. For example, an acute metabolic acidosis will be compensated by a fall in pCO_2, which will minimize the intracellular effects of the acidosis.

Blood-gas Analysis

Blood-gas analysis is a collective term applied to three separate measurements pH, pCO_2, and pO_2, generally made together to evaluate acid-base status which can reveal important clues about lung and kidney function and the body's general metabolic state, adequacy of ventilation, arterial oxygenation and respiratory diseases and conditions that affect the lungs.

Oxygen (O_2) and carbon dioxide (CO_2) are the most important respiratory gases, and their partial pressures in arterial blood reflect the overall adequacy of gas exchange. pO_2 is affected by age and altitude. pCO_2 by altitude. Therefore, pO_2 must be individually calculated for each patient, and both determinations must be interpreted against local normal values. Hydrogen is not present in blood as a gas and, therefore, does not exert a partial pressure. However, pH, which measures hydrogen ion activity, is a conventional part of every arterial blood gas determination. The normal range for blood pH is 7.35–7.45.

Arterial Puncture

Blood is usually withdrawn from the radial artery as it is easy to palpate and has a good collateral supply. The patient's arm is placed palm-up on a flat surface, with the wrist dorsiflexed at 45° (Fig. 2.11). A towel may be placed under the wrist for support. The puncture site should be cleaned with alcohol or iodine, and a local anesthetic (such as 2% lignocaine) should be infiltrated. Local anesthetic makes arterial puncture less painful for the patient and does not increase the difficulty of the procedure. The radial artery should be palpated for a pulse, and a preheparinized syringe with a 23 or 25 gauge needle should be inserted at an angle just distal to the palpated pulse. A small quantity of blood is sufficient. After the puncture, sterile gauze should be placed firmly over the site and direct pressure applied for several minutes to obtain hemostasis. If repeated arterial blood gas analysis is required, it is advisable to use a different site (such as the other radial artery) or insert an arterial line.

To ensure accuracy, it is important to deliver the sample for analysis promptly. If there is any delay in processing the sample, the blood can be stored on ice for approximately 30 minutes with little effect on the accuracy of the results. Complications of arterial puncture are infrequent. They include prolonged bleeding, infection, thrombosis, or arteriospasm.

Venous Blood Gases

It is easier to obtain a venous sample than an arterial sample. In some situations analysis of venous blood can provide enough information to assist in clinical decisions. In general, the pH, CO_2, and HCO_3^- values are similar in venous and arterial blood. The main difference is the partial pressure of oxygen in venous blood is less than half that of arterial blood. Venous blood should not therefore be used to assess oxygenation.

Blood Gas Normal and Abnormal Values

These results shown in (Tables 2.14 and 2.15) are for sea level arterial blood gas results. At altitudes 3,000 feet and above, the oxygen results are lower.

Factors Influencing Blood-gas Results

A number of sampling and environmental factors may affect the result of the analysis. Delayed processing of the sample may yield a falsely low pO_2, as the delay allows leucocytes to consume oxygen. This can be avoided by prompt transport of the sample on ice.

Air bubbles introduced when performing the arterial puncture can also cause a falsely high pO_2 and a falsely low pCO_2.

This can be avoided by gently removing the air bubbles within the specimen immediately after collection without agitating the sample.

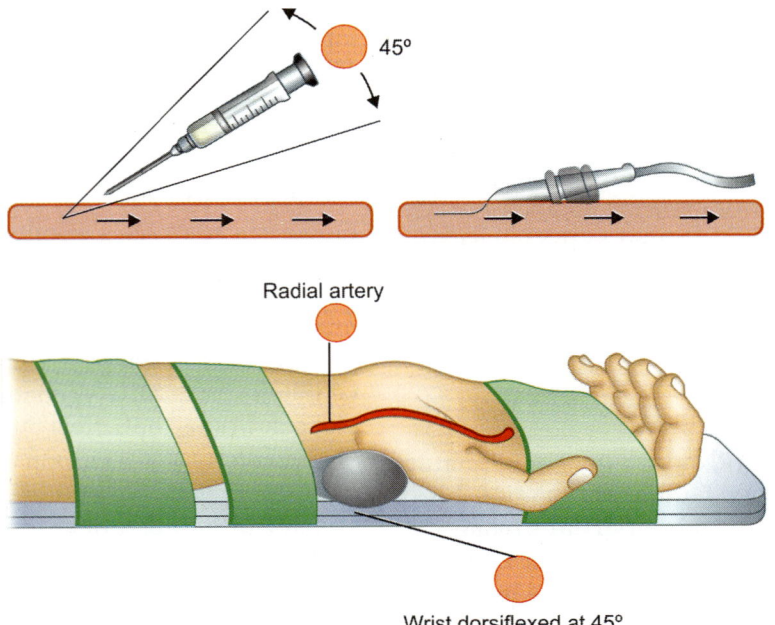

45°

Radial artery

Wrist dorsiflexed at 45°

Fig. 2.11: The wrist dorsiflexed at 45° during arterial puncture

Table 2.14 | Sea level arterial blood gas normal values

	Arterial	Venous
pH	7.35–7.45	7.32–7.42

Not a gas, but a measurement of acidity or alkalinity, based on the hydrogen (H$^+$) ions present. The pH of a solution is equal to the negative log of the hydrogen ion concentration in that solution: $pH = -\log [H^+]$

	Arterial	Venous
PO$_2$	80–100 mmHg	28–48 mmHg

The partial pressure of oxygen that is dissolved in arterial blood. Newborn—acceptable range 40–70 mmHg. Elderly—subtract 1 mmHg from the minimal 80 mmHg level for every year over 60 years of age: 80 – (age –60) (Note: up to age 90)

	Arterial	Venous
HCO$_3^-$	22–26 mmol/L	19–25 mmol/L
	(21–28 mmol/L)	

The calculated value of the amount of bicarbonate in the bloodstream. Not a blood gas but the anion of carbonic acid.

	Arterial	Venous
PCO$_2$	35–45 mmHg	38–52 mmHg

The amount of carbon dioxide dissolved in arterial blood. Measured—partial pressure of arterial CO$_2$. (Note: Large A = alveolar CO$_2$). CO$_2$ is called a 'volatile acid' because it can combine reversibly with H$_2$O to yield a strongly acidic H$^+$ ion and a weak basic bicarbonate ion (HCO$_3^-$) according to the following equation: $CO_2 + H_2O \leftrightarrow H^+ + HCO_3^-$

	Arterial	Venous
BE	–2 to +3 mmol/L	

The base excess indicates the amount of excess or insufficient level of bicarbonate in the system. (A negative base excess indicates a base deficit in the blood.) A negative base excess is equivalent to an acid excess. A value outside of the normal range (–2 to +3 mmol) suggests a metabolic cause for the abnormality. Calculated value—the base excess is defined as the amount of H$^+$ ions that would be required to return the pH of the blood to 7.35, if the pCO$_2$ were adjusted to normal.

It can be estimated by the equation:

Base excess = 0.93 (HCO$_3^-$ 24.4 + 14.8 (pH – 7.4))

Alternatively: Base excess = 0.93 × HCO$_3^-$ + 13.77 × pH – 124.53

A base excess > +3 = Metabolic alkalosis a base excess < –3 = Metabolic acidosis

	Arterial	Venous
SaO$_2$	95–100%	50–70%

The arterial oxygen saturation.

Abnormal Values: Acid-base Disorders

Table 2.15 | Sea level arterial blood gas abnormal values—acid-base disorders

Respiratory alkalosis (chronic alveolar hyperventilation)	pH:	7.44
	PCO$_2$:	12
	HCO$_3^-$:	16
	BE:	–6
Respiratory acidosis (chronic ventilation failure)	pH:	7.38
	PCO$_2$:	76
	HCO$_3^-$:	42
	BE:	+14
Uncompensated metabolic alkalosis	pH:	7.56
	PCO$_2$:	44
	HCO$_3^-$:	38
	BE:	+14
Respiratory acidosis (acute ventilation failure)	pH:	7.26
	PCO$_2$:	56
	HCO$_3^-$:	24
	BE:	–4
Uncompensated metabolic alkalosis	pH:	7.56
	PCO$_2$:	40
	HCO$_3^-$:	34
	BE:	+11

Contd.

Table 2.15	Sea level arterial blood gas abnormal values—acid-base disorders *(Contd.)*
Respiratory alkalosis (chronic alveolar hyperventilation)	pH: 7.44 PCO_2: 26 HCO_3^-: 18 BE: −4
Respiratory acidosis (chronic ventilation failure)	pH: 7.40 PCO_2: 56 HCO_3^-: 34 BE: +7
Respiratory alkalosis (chronic alveolar hyperventilation)	pH: 7.44 PCO_2: 20 HCO_3^-: 16 BE: −7
Uncompensated metabolic acidosis	pH: 7.24 PCO_2: 36 HCO_3^-: 14 BE: −13
Respiratory alkalosis (acute alveolar hyperventilation)	pH: 7.52 PCO_2: 28 HCO_3^-: 22 BE: +1
Acute respiratory acidosis	Heroin overdose Breathing-shallow, slow ABGs: pH: 7.30 PCO_2: 55 mm/Hg HCO_3^-: 27 mmol/L
Chronic respiratory acidosis	Emphysema, labored breathing at rest ABGs: pH: 7.36 PCO_2: 64 mm $HgHCO_3^-$: 35 mmol/L
Acute respiratory alkalosis	Anxiety, psychosomatic origin Rapid breathing and slurred speech ABGs: pH: 7.57 PCO_2: 23 mm $HgHCO_3^-$: 21 mmol/L
Compensated respiratory alkalosis	Persistent bacterial pneumonia Mild cyanosis and labored breathing ABGs: pH: 7.44 PCO_2: 26 mm $HgHCO_3^-$: 17 mmol/L PO_2: 53 mmHg
Metabolic alkalosis	Diuretic ABGs: pH: 7.58 PCO_2: 48 mm $HgHCO_3^-$: 44 mmol/L BE: +19 mmol/L Serum CL—95 mmol/L

Body temperature can also affect arterial blood gas tensions. This is relevant in febrile or hypothermic patients, so body temperature should be recorded at the time of collection.

Respiratory Failure and Respiratory Support

The respiratory apparatus consists of the lungs (where gas exchange takes place) and a ventilatory pump (the respiratory muscles acting on the thorax). Respiratory failure (that is, inadequate oxygenation of or removal of carbon dioxide from the blood) is conventionally divided into type 1 (hypoxemic, where the primary problem is with gas exchange) and type 2 (hypercapnic or ventilatory failure). Typically, in type 1 (caused by parenchymal lung damage, e.g. pneumonia, pulmonary edema), pO_2 is low and pCO_2 is normal or low; in type 2 (causes include chronic obstructive pulmonary disease and diseases causing respiratory muscle weakness), pO_2 is low and pCO_2 is high. Note, however, that there is often overlap and patients with some conditions (notably severe asthma) can progress from type 1 to type 2 or develop either type of respiratory failure.

If a patient is unable to maintain an adequate pO_2 by breathing room air, it may be possible to overcome this by increasing the oxygen supply, for example by using some form of facemask or nasal cannula. This increases alveolar pO_2 in poorly ventilated areas but is of no value in hypoxemia caused by shunts. The efficacy can be checked by pulse oximetry and measurement of pO_2. High concentrations (40–60%) using a high flow rate mask are typically prescribed in acute type 1 respiratory failure (e.g. as a result of pneumonia), but lower concentrations (24% or 28%, achieved using Venturi-type low flow rate) are preferred in type 2 respiratory failure.

If adequate oxygenation (i.e. $pO_2 > 8.0$) cannot be achieved using supplementary oxygen alone, even when augmented by, e.g. the use of aggressive physiotherapy to remove secretions and bronchodilators to reduce airways resistance, some form of respiratory support will be required. Other factors that are taken into consideration are the presence of acidosis, tachypnea and the use of accessory muscles of respiration.

BIBLIOGRAPHY

1. Adrogue HE, Adrogue HJ. Acid-base physiology. Respir Care. 2001 A; 46(4): 328–41.
2. Adrogué HJ. Mixed acid-base disturbances. J Nephrol. 2006; 19 Suppl. 9: S97–103.
3. Andritsch RF, Muravchick S, Gold MI. Temperature correction of arterial blood gas parameters: a comparative review of methodology. Anesthesiology. 1981; 55: 311–6.
4. Badrick T, Hickman PE. The anion gap. A reappraisal. Am J Clin Pathol. 1992; 98(2): 249–52.
5. Banga A, Khilnani GC. Post-hypercapnic alkalosis is associated with ventilator dependence and increased ICU stay. COPD. 2009; 6: 437–40.
6. Bellomo R. Bench-to-bedside review: lactate and the kidney. Crit Care. 2002; 6(4) 322–6.
7. Bernards WC Interpretation of Clinical Acid-Base Data. Regional Refresher Courses in Anesthesiology. 1973; 1: 17–26.
8. Brimacombe JR, Breen DP. Anesthesia and Bartter's syndrome: a case report and review. AANA J. 1993; 61(2): 193–7.
9. Brimioulle S, Kahn RJ. Effects of metabolic alkalosis on pulmonary gas exchange. Am Rev Respir Dis. 1990; 141 (5 Pt 1): 1185-9.
10. Brimioulle S, Berre J, Dufaye P, et al. Hydrochloric acid infusion for treatment of metabolic alkalosis associated with respiratory acidosis. Crit Care Med. 1989; 17(3): 232–6.
11. Brimioulle S, Vincent JL, Dufaye P, et al. Hydrochloric acid infusion for treatment of metabolic alkalosis: effects on acid-base homeostasis and oxygenation. Crit Care Med. 1985; 13(9): 738–42.
12. Buchanan IB, Campbell BT, Peck MD, et al. Chest wall necrosis and death secondary to hydrochloric acid infusion for metabolic alkalosis. South Med J. 2005; 98(8) 822–4.
13. Bushinsky DA. Acidosis and bone. Miner Electrolyte Metab 1994; 20(1–2): 40–52.
14. Carvounis CP, Feinfeld DA. A simple estimate of the effect of the serum albumin level on the anion Gap. Am J Nephrol. 2000; 20(5): 369–72.
15. Chillar RK, Belman MJ, Farbstein M. Explanation for apparent hypoxemia associated with extreme leukocytosis: leukocytic oxygen consumption. Blood. 1980; 55: 922–24.
16. Dorwart W, Chambers L. Comparison of Methods for Calculating Serum Osmolality from Chemical Concentrations, and the Prognostic Value of Such Calculations. Clin Chem. 1975; 21: 190–194.
17. Dorwart WV, Chalmers L. Comparison of methods for calculating serum osmolality form chemical concentrations, and the prognostic value of such calculations. Clin Chem. 1975 Feb; 21(2).
18. Editorial: Hydrochloric acid for metabolic alkalosis. Lancet. 1974; 20; 1(7860) 720. pmid: 4132434.
19. Emmett M, Narins RG. Clinical use of the anion gap. Medicine (Baltimore). 1977; 56(1): 38–54.
20. Figge J, Jabor A, Kazda A, et al. Anion gap and hypoalbuminemia. Crit Care Med. 1998; 26(11) 1807–10.
21. Fox MJ, Brody JS, Weintraub LR. et al. Leukocyte larceny: a cause of spurious hypoxemia. Am J Med. 1979;67: 742–46.
22. Ganong, WF. Review of Medical Physiology, 16th edition, Appleton and Lange, Norwalk, CT, 1993.
23. Glaser DS. Utility of the Serum Osmol Gap in the Diagnosis of Methanol or Ethylene Glycol Ingestion. Ann Emerg Med. 1996: 343–346.
24. Goodkin DA, Krishna GG, Narins RG. The role of the anion gap in detecting and managing mixed metabolic acid-base disorders. Clin Endocrinol Metab. 1984; 13(2): 333–49.
25. Grippi, MA, Pulmonary Pathophysiology, JB Lippincott Company, Philadelphia, 1995.

26. Hess CE, Nichols AB, Hunt WB. et al. Pseudohypoxemia secondary to leukemia and thrombocytosis. N Engl J Med. 1979; 301:361–63.

27. Hixson R, Christmas D. Use of omeprazole in life-threatening metabolic alkalosis. Intensive Care Med. 1999; 25(10): 1201.

28. Hixson R, Christmas D. Use of omeprazole in life-threatening metabolic alkalosis. Intensive Care Med. 1999; 25(10): 1201.

29. Hsu SC, Wang MC, Liu HL, Tsai MC, et al. Extreme metabolic alkalosis treated with normal bicarbonate hemodialysis. Am J Kidney Dis. 2001; 37(4): E31.

30. Igarashi T, Sekine T, Watanabe H. Molecular basis of proximal renal tubular acidosis. J Nephrol. 2002; 15 Suppl 5 S135–41.

31. Iida R, Otsuka Y, Matsumoto K, Kuriyama S, et al. Pseudoaldosteronism due to the concurrent use of two herbal medicines containing glycyrrhizin: interaction of glycyrrhizin with angiotensin-converting enzyme inhibitor. Clin Exp Nephrol. 2006; 10(2): 131–5.

32. Juel C. Lactate-proton cotransport in skeletal muscle. Physiol Rev. 1997; 77(2): 321–58.

33. Juel C. Muscle pH regulation: role of training. Acta Physiol Scand. 1998; 162(3): 359–66.

34. Kelman GR, Nunn JF. Nomograms for correction of blood PO_2, PCO2, pH and base excess for time and temperature. J Appl Physiol. 1966; 21:1484–90.

35. Kim HY, Han JS, Jeon US, et al. Clinical significance of the fractional excretion of anions in metabolic acidosis. Clin Nephrol. 2001; 55(6): 448–52.

36. Kinahan TJ, Khoury AE, McLorie GA, et al. Omeprazole in post-gastrocystoplasty metabolic alkalosis and aciduria. J Urol. 1992; 147(2): 435–7.

37. Kinahan TJ, Khoury AE, McLorie GA, and Churchill BM. Omeprazole in post-gastrocystoplasty metabolic alkalosis and aciduria. J Urol. 1992; 147(2) 435–7.

38. Korkmaz A, Yildirim E, Aras N, et al. Hydrochloric acid for treating metabolic alkalosis. JPN J Surg. 1989; 19(5): 519–23.

39. Kraut JA abd Madias NE. Serum Anion Gap: Its Uses and Limitations in Clinical Medicine Clin J Am Soc Nephrol. 2007; 2: 162–174.

40. Kraut JA, Kurtz I. Metabolic acidosis of CKD: diagnosis, clinical characteristics, and treatment. Am J Kidney Dis. 2005; 45(6): 978–93.

41. Kruse JA, Carlson RW. Lactate metabolism. Crit Care Clin. 1987; 3(4): 725–46.

42. Kryger MH, ed. Pathophysiology of respiration. New York: Wiley, 1981.

43. Kwun KB, Boucherit T, Wong J, et al. Treatment of metabolic alkalosis with intravenous infusion of concentrated hydrochloric acid. Am J Surg. 1983; 146(3): 328–30.

44. Laing CM, Unwin RJ. Renal tubular acidosis. J Nephrol. 2006; 19 Suppl 9 S46–52.

45. Laing CM, Toye AM, Capasso G, et al. Renal tubular acidosis: developments in our understanding of the molecular basis. Int J Biochem Cell Biol. 2005; 37(6) 1151–61.

46. Luft FC. Lactic acidosis update for critical care clinicians. J Am Soc Nephrol 2001; 12 Suppl. 17 S15–9.

47. Maitland K and Newton CR. Acidosis of severe falciparum malaria: heading for a shock?. Trends Parasitol. 2005; 21(1): 11–6.

48. Marik PE, Kussman BD, Lipman J, et al. Acetazolamide in the treatment of metabolic alkalosis in critically ill patients. Heart Lung. 1991; 20(5 Pt 1): 455–9.

49. Martinu T, Menzies D, Dial S. Re-evaluation of acid-base prediction rules in patients with chronic respiratory acidosis. Can Respir J. 2003; 10(6): 311–5.

50. McAuliffe JJ, Lind LJ, Leith DE, et al. Hypoproteinemic alkalosis. Am J Med. 1986; 81(1): 86–90.

51. Mellemgaard K. The alveolar-arterial oxygen difference: its size and components in normal man. Acta Physiol Scand. 1966;67: 10–20.

52. Mitchell JE, Pyle RL, Eckert ED, et al. Electrolyte and other physiological abnormalities in patients with bulimia. Psychol Med. 1983; 13(2): 273–8.

53. Moe OW, Fuster D. Clinical acid-base pathophysiology: disorders of plasma anion gap. Best Pract Res Clin Endocrinol Metab. 2003; 17(4): 559–74.

54. Narins RG, Emmett M. Simple and mixed acid-base disorders: a practical approach. Medicine (Baltimore). 1980; 59(3): 161–87.

55. Narins RG, Emmett M. Simple and mixed acid-base disorders: a practical approach. Medicine (Baltimore). 1980; 59: 161–87.

56. Nicoletta JA, Schwartz GJ. Distal renal tubular acidosis. Curr Opin Pediatr. 2004; 16(2): 194–8.

57. Oster JR, Materson BJ, Rogers AI. Laxative abuse syndrome. Am J Gastroenterol. 1980; 74(5): 451–8.

58. Oster JR, Perez GO, Materson BJ. Use of the anion gap in clinical medicine. South Med J. 1988; 81(2): 229–37.

59. Pagana KD, Pagana TJ (2005). Mosby's Manual of Diagnostic and Laboratory Tests, 7th ed. St. Louis: Mosby.

60. Pasvol G. The treatment of complicated and severe malaria. Br Med Bull. 2005; 75–76: 29–47.

61. Paulson WD, Gadallah MF. Diagnosis of mixed acid-base disorders in diabetic ketoacidosis. Am J Med Sci. 1993; 306(5): 295–300.

62. Pitts RF. Mechanisms for stabilizing the alkaline reserves of the body. Harvey Lect. 1952–1953; 48: 172–209.

63. Powner DJ, Kellum JA, Darby JM. Concepts of the Strong Ion Difference applied to Large Volume Resuscitation J Intensive Care Med. 2001; 16: 169–176.

64. Robergs RA, Ghiasvand F, Parker D. Biochemistry of exercise-induced metabolic acidosis. Am J Physiol Regul Integr Comp Physiol. 2004; 287(3): R502–16.

65. Rosen RA, Julian BA, Dubovsky EV, et al. On the mechanism by which chloride corrects metabolic alkalosis in man. Am J Med. 1988; 84(3 Pt 1) 449–58.

66. Severinghaus JW. Blood gas calculator. J Appl Physiol. 1966; 21: 1108–16.

67. Shayakul C, Alper SL. Inherited renal tubular acidosis. Curr Opin Nephrol Hypertens. 2000; 9(5): 541–6.

68. Sorbini CA, Grassi V, Solinas E. et al. Arterial oxygen tension in relation to age in healthy subjects. Respiration. 1968; 25: 3–13.

69. Stacpoole PW. Lactic acidosis. Endocrinol Metab Clin North Am. 1993; 22(2): 221–45. pmid:8325284.

70. Vantyghem MC, Douillard C, Binaut R, et al. [Bartter's syndromes]. Ann Endocrinol (Paris). 1999; 60(6) 465–72.

71. Walmsley RN and White GH. Mixed acid-base disorders. Clin Chem. 1985; 31(2): 321–5.

72. Williamson JC. Acid-base disorders: classification and management strategies. Am Fam Physician. 1995; 52(2): 584–90.

73. Worthley LI. Hydrogen ion metabolism. Anaesth Intensive Care. 1977; 5(4): 347–60.

74. Worthley LI. Intravenous hydrochloric acid in patients with metabolic alkalosis and hypercapnia. Arch Surg. 1986; 121(10): 1195–8.

75. Wrenn K. The delta gap: an approach to mixed acid-base disorders. Ann Emerg Med. 1990; 19(11): 1310–3.

3

Water and Electrolytes

INTRODUCTION

Water is the most abundant molecule in the human body and provides the only solvent. The total amount of water in a man of average weight 70 kilograms is approximately 40 liters, averaging of 60% of his body weight and 55% of that of an adult female. This difference between the sexes primarily reflects the proportionately larger mass of adipose tissue in adult females, and the greater average muscle mass in adult In a newborn infant, this may be as high as 79% of the body weight, but it progressively decreases from birth to old age, most of the decrease occurring during the first 10 years of life. Also, obesity decreases the percentage of water in the body, sometimes to as low as 45%.

Approximately 66% of water is in the intracellular fluid (ICF) and 33% in the extracellular fluid (ECF); only 8% of body water is in the plasma. Water is not actively transported in the body. It is, in general, freely permeable through the ICF and ECF and its distribution is determined by the osmotic contents of these compartments. Except in the kidneys, the osmotic concentrations, or osmolalities, of these compartments are always equal; they are isotonic. Any change in the solute content of a compartment engenders a shift of water, which restores isotonicity.

The major contributors to the osmolality of the ECF are sodium and its associated anions, mainly chloride and bicarbonate; in the ICF the predominant cation is potassium. Other determinants of ECF osmolality include glucose and urea. Protein makes a numerically small contribution of approximately 0.5%. This is because osmolality is dependent on the molar concentrations of solutes: although; the total concentration of plasma proteins is approximately 70 g/L, their high molecular weight results in their combined molar concentrations being <1 mmol/L. However, as the capillary endothelium is relatively impermeable to protein and as the protein concentration of interstitial fluid is much less than that of plasma, the osmotic effect of proteins is an important factor in determining water distribution between these two compartments. The contribution of proteins to the osmotic pressure of plasma is known as the 'colloid osmotic pressure' or 'oncotic pressure'.

WATER DISTRIBUTION

The water in the body is contained within the numerous organs and tissues of the body. These collections are referred to as compartments. The major division is into intracellular fluid (about 23 liters) and extracellular fluid (about 19 liters) based on which side of the cell membrane the fluid lies. Exchange between the ICF and the ECF occurs across cell membranes by osmosis, diffusion, and carrier-mediated transport. Typical values for the size of the fluid compartments are listed in the Table 3.1.

Table 3.1	Typical values for the size of the fluid compartments		
Body fluid compartment (70 kg male)			
Compartment	% of body weight	% of total body water	Volume (liters)
ECF	27	45	19
Plasma	4.5	7.5	3.2
ISF	12.0	20.0	8.4
Dense CT water	4.5	7.5	3.2
Bone water	4.5	7.5	3.2
Transcellular	1.5	2.5	1.0
ICF	33	55	23
TBW	60	100	42

Intracellular Fluid

The intracellular fluid is composed of at least 1014 separate tiny cellular packages. The concept of a single united 'compartment' called intracellular fluid is clearly artificial. The intracellular fluid of the cytosol or cytoplasmic matrix is the liquid found inside cells. It is separated into compartments by membranes, i.e. the mitochondrial matrix separates the mitochondrion into compartments.

The cytosol is a complex mixture of substances dissolved in water. Although water forms the large majority of the cytosol, its structure and properties within cells is not well understood. The concentrations of ions such as sodium and potassium are different in the cytosol than in the extracellular fluid; these differences in ion levels are important in processes such, as osmoregulation and cell signaling. The cytosol also contains large amounts of macromolecules, which can alter how molecules behave, through macromolecular crowding.

Extracellular Fluid

The ECF is divided into several smaller compartments e.g. plasma, interstitial fluid, fluid of bone, and dense connective tissue and transcellular fluid. These compartments are distinguished by different locations and different kinetic characteristics. The ECF compositional similarity is in some ways, the opposite of that for the ICF, e.g. low in potassium and magnesium and high in sodium and chloride).

The extracellular fluid also includes the transcellular fluid; making up only about 2.5% of the ECF. In humans, the normal glucose concentration of extracellular fluid that is regulated by homeostasis is approximately 5 mm. The pH of extracellular fluid is tightly regulated by buffers and maintained around 7.4.

Interstitial Fluid

The ISF consists of all the bits of fluid, which lie in the interstices of all body tissues. This is also a 'virtual' fluid (e.g. it exists in many separate small bits but is spoken about as though it was a pool of fluid of uniform composition in the one location). The ISF bathes all the cells in the body and is the link between the ICF and the intravascular compartment. Oxygen, nutrients, wastes, and chemical messengers all pass through the ISF. ISF has the compositional characteristics of ECF, but in addition, it is distinguished by its usually low protein concentration (in comparison to plasma). Lymph is considered as a part of the ISF. The lymphatic system returns protein and excess ISF to the circulation. Lymph is more easily obtained for analysis than other parts of the ISF.

Plasma

Plasma is the only major fluid compartment that exists as a real fluid collection all in one location. It differs from ISF in its much higher protein content and its high bulk flow (transport function). Blood contains suspended red and white cells so plasma has been called the 'interstitial fluid of the blood'. The fluid compartment called the blood volume is interesting in that it is a composite compartment containing ECF (plasma) and ICF (red cell water).

Blood plasma is colored as pale yellow liquid component of blood that normally holds the blood cells in whole blood in suspension. It makes up about 55% of total blood volume. It is the intravascular fluid part of extracellular fluid (all body fluid outside of cells). It is mostly water (93% by volume) and contains dissolved proteins (major proteins are fibrinogens, globulins, and albumins), glucose, clotting factors, mineral ions (Na^+, Ca^{2+}, Mg^{2+}, HCO_3^-, Cl^-, etc.), hormones, and carbon dioxide (plasma being the main medium for excretory product transportation). Plasma also serves as the protein reserve of the human body. It plays a vital role in intravascular osmotic effects that keep electrolyte levels balanced and protects the body from infection and other blood disorders.

The Fluid of Bone and Dense Connective Tissue

It is a significant because it contains about 15% of the total body water. this fluid is mobilized only very slowly and this lessens its importance when considering the effects of acute fluid interventions.

Transcellular Fluid

It is a small compartment that represents all those body fluids which are formed from the transport activities of cells. It is contained within epithelial lined spaces. It includes cerebrospinal fluid (CSF), gastrointestinal tract (GIT) fluids, bladder urine, and joint fluid. It is important because of the specialized functions involved. The fluid fluxes involved with GIT fluids, can be quite significant. The electrolyte composition of the various transcellular fluids is quite dissimilar.

PROPERTIES OF WATER

Water is one of the two major solvents in the body. It is a remarkable substance with several important properties, in particular, it has:

- A very high molar concentration
- A large dielectric constant
- A very small dissociation constant

Its concentration in biological systems is very high, i.e. 55.5 Molar at 37°C. This is almost 400 times the concentration of the next most concentrated substance in the body, e.g. $[Na^+]$ in ECF = 0.14 M, [K+] in ICF = 0.15M). The significance is that water provides an inexhaustible supply of hydrogen ions for the body.

Calculation of Water Concentration

Molecular weight of H_2O = (1 + 1 + 16) = 18, so one mole is 18 grams.

One milliliter of liquid H_2O weighs about 1 gram (so, 1 liter weighs 1,000 grams)

Therefore, $[H_2O]$ = 1000/18 = 55.5 moles/liter

The large dielectric constant means that substances which molecules contain ionic bonds will tend to dissociate in water yielding solutions containing ions. This occurs because water as a solvent opposes the electrostatic attraction between positive and negative ions that would prevent ionic substances from dissolving. The ions of a salt are held together by ionic forces as defined by Coulomb's law.

Coulomb's Law

$$F = (k . q_1 . q_2)/D . r^2$$

where, F is the force between two electric charges q_1 and q_2 at a distance r apart, D the dielectric constant of the solvent and k is Coulomb's constant.

The large dielectric constant of water means that the force between the ions in a salt is very much reduced permitting the ions to separate. These separated ions become surrounded by the oppositely charged ends of the water dipoles and become hydrated. This ordering tends to be counteracted by the random thermal motions of the molecules. Water molecules are always associated with each other through as many as four hydrogen bonds and this ordering of the structure of water greatly resists the random thermal motions. In fact, it is this hydrogen bonding which is responsible for its large dielectric constant.

WATER REGULATION

Intake Regulation

Fluid can enter the body as preformed water, ingested food and drink, and to a lesser extent, as metabolic water, which is produced as a by-product of aerobic respiration (cellular respiration) and dehydration synthesis. A constant supply is needed to replenish the fluids lost through normal physiological activities, such as respiration, sweating, and urination. Water generated from the biochemical metabolism of nutrients provides a significant proportion of the daily water requirements for some arthropods and desert animals, but it provides only a small fraction of a human's necessary intake. In the normal resting state, input of water through ingested fluids is approximately 1200 mL/day, from ingested

foods 1000 mL/day, and from aerobic respiration 300 mL/day, totaling 2500 mL/day.

Body water homeostasis is regulated mainly through ingested fluids, which in turn, depends on thirst. An insufficiency of water results in an increased osmolarity in the extracellular fluid. This is sensed by osmoreceptors which trigger the sensation of thirst. Thirst can be voluntarily resisted to some degree, as during fluid restriction.

Output Regulation

Fluid can leave the body in several ways, i.e. urination, excretion (feces), and perspiration (sweating).

The majority of fluid output occurs via the urine, at approximately 1500 mL/day in a normal adult at resting state.

Some fluid is lost through perspiration (part of the body's temperature control mechanism) and as water vapor in expired air. These are termed 'insensible fluid losses' as they cannot be measured easily. Some sources say insensible losses account for 500– 650 mL/day of water in adults, while other sources put the minimum value at 800 mL. In children, one calculation used for insensible fluid loss is 400 mL/m^2 body surface area.

In addition, an adult loses approximately 100 mL/day of fluid through feces. For females, an additional 50 mL/day is lost through vaginal secretions. These outputs are in balance with the input of ~2500 mL/day.

The bodies homeostatic control mechanisms, which maintain a constant internal environment, ensure that a balance between fluid gain and fluid loss is maintained. The hormones ADH (antidiuretic hormone, also known as vasopressin) and aldosterone play a major role in this. If the body is becoming fluid-deficient, there will be an increase in the secretion of these hormones, causing fluid to be retained by the kidneys and urine output to be reduced. Conversely, if fluid levels are excessive, secretion of these hormones is suppressed, resulting in less retention of fluid by the kidneys and a subsequent increase in the volume of urine produced.

If the body is becoming fluid-deficient, this will be sensed by osmoreceptors in the organum vasculosum of lamina terminalis and subfornical organ. These areas project to the supraoptic nucleus and paraventricular nucleus, which contain neurons that secrete the antidiuretic hormone, vasopressin, from their nerve endings in the posterior pituitary. Thus, there will be an increase in the secretion of antidiuretic hormone, causing fluid to be retained by the kidneys and urine output to be reduced.

A fluid-insufficiency causes a decreased perfusion of the juxtaglomerular apparatus in the kidneys, activating the renin-angiotensin system. Among other actions, this causes renal tubules (e.g. the distal convoluted tubules and the cortical collecting ducts) to reabsorb more sodium and water from the urine. Potassium is secreted into the tubule in exchange for the sodium, which is reabsorbed. The activated renin-angiotensin system stimulates zona glomerulosa of the adrenal cortex, which in turn secretes hormone aldosterone. This hormone stimulates the reabsorption of sodium ions from distal tubules and collecting ducts. Water in the tubular lumen follows the sodium reabsorption osmotically.

MOVEMENT OF WATER AMONG COMPARTMENTS
Formation of Interstitial Fluid

Hydrostatic pressure is generated by the systolic force of the heart. It pushes water out of the capillaries. The water potential is created due to the ability of small solutes to pass through the walls of capillaries. This buildup of solutes induces osmosis. The water passes from a high concentration outside of the vessels to a low concentration inside of the vessels, in an attempt to reach equilibrium. The osmotic pressure drives water back into the vessels. Because the blood in the capillaries is constantly flowing, equilibrium is never reached.

The balance between the two forces differs at different points on the capillaries. At the arterial end of a vessel, the hydrostatic pressure is greater than the osmotic pressure, so the net movement favors water and other solutes being passed into the tissue fluid. At the venous end, the osmotic pressure is greater, so the net movement favors substances being passed back into the capillary. This difference is created by the direction of the flow of blood and the imbalance in solutes created by the net movement of water favoring the tissue fluid.

Removal of Interstitial Fluid

To prevent a buildup of tissue fluid surrounding the cells in the tissue, the lymphatic system plays a part in the transport of tissue fluid. Tissue fluid can pass into the surrounding lymph vessels, and eventually ends up rejoining the blood. Sometimes, the removal of tissue fluid does not function correctly, and there is a build-up. This can cause swelling, often around the feet and ankles, which is generally known as edema. The position of swelling is due to the effects of gravity.

Constituents of Body Fluids

Electrolytes are ionized molecules found throughout the blood, tissues, and cells of the body. These molecules, which are either positive (cations) or negative (anions), conduct an electric current and help to balance pH and acid-base levels in the body. Electrolytes also facilitate the passage of fluid between and within cells through a process known as osmosis and play a part in regulating the function of the neuromuscular, endocrine, and excretory systems.

Stabilizing the volumes, solute concentrations, and pH of the ECF and the ICF involves three interrelated processes:

1. **Fluid balance:** Fluid balance is when the amount of gained-water each day is equal to the amount that is lose to the environment. The maintenance of normal fluid balance involves regulating the content and distribution of body water in the ECF and the ICF. The digestive system is the primary source of water gains; a small amount of additional water is generated by metabolic activity. The urinary system is the primary route for water loss under normal conditions. Although cells and tissues cannot transport water, they can transport ions and create concentration gradients that are then eliminated by osmosis.

2. **Electrolyte balance:** Electrolytes are ions released through the dissociation of inorganic compounds; they are so named because they can conduct an electrical current in a solution. If the gains and losses for every electrolyte are in balance, you are said to be in electrolyte balance. Electrolyte balance primarily involves balancing the rates of absorption across the digestive tract with rates of loss at the kidneys, although losses at sweat glands and other sites can play a secondary role.

3. **Acid-base balance:** When acid-base balance exists, the pH of body fluids remains within normal limits. Preventing a reduction in pH is the primary problem, because your body generates a variety of acids during normal metabolic operations. The kidneys play a major role by secreting hydrogen ions into the urine and generating buffers that enter the bloodstream. Such secretion occurs primarily in the distal segments of the distal convoluted tubule (DCT) and along the collecting system. The lungs also play a key role through the elimination of carbon dioxide.

WATER AND ECF OSMOLALITY

Changes in body water content independent of the amount of solute will alter the osmolality. The osmolality of the ECF is normally maintained in the range 282–295 mmol/kg of water. Any loss of water from the ECF, such as occurs with water deprivation, will increase its osmolality and results in movement of water from the ICF to the ECF. However, a slight increase in ECF osmolality will still occur, stimulating the hypothalamic thirst centre, causing thirst and, thus, promoting a desire to drink, and stimulation of the hypothalamic osmoreceptors, which causes the release of antidiuretic hormone hormone (vasopressin).

Vasopressin renders the renal collecting ducts permeable to water [its combination with V2-receptors results in the insertion of aquaporins (water channels) into the normally impermeable apical membrane of the cells of the collecting tubules], permitting water reabsorption and concentration of the urine; the maximum urine concentration that can be achieved in humans is about 1200 mmol/kg. The osmoreceptors are highly sensitive to osmolality, responding to a change of as little as 1%. Plasma vasopressin concentration falls to very low values at an osmolality of 282 mmol/kg, but rises sharply if osmolality increases above this level. However, if an increase in ECF osmolality occurs as a result of the presence of a solute, such as urea that diffuses readily across cell membranes, ICF osmolality also increases and osmoreceptors are not stimulated.

If ECF osmolality falls, there is no sensation of thirst and vasopressin secretion is inhibited. Dilute urine is produced, allowing water excretion and restoration of ECF osmolality to normal. The vasopressin responses to changes in osmolality occur rapidly. In health, the ingestion of water surplus to requirements leads to a rapid diuresis, and water depletion to a rapid increase in the concentration of the urine.

Other stimuli affecting vasopressin secretion include angiotensin II, arterial, and venous baroreceptors and volume receptors (which sense blood pressure and volume, respectively). Hypovolemia and hypotension increase the slope of the vasopressin response to an increase in osmolality and lower the threshold osmolality for vasopressin secretion. The vasopressin response to a fall in blood pressure is exponential; it is relatively small with small decreases in plasma volume, but greater falls cause a massive increase in vasopressin secretion. Osmolar controls are overridden, so that ECF volume is defended (by stimulating water retention) at the expense of a decrease in osmolality.

ANTIDIURETIC HORMONE

Antidiuretic hormone, also known as 'vasopressin', is produced by the hypothalamus and stored in the posterior pituitary gland. When the water level in the blood decreases, in response to eating salty food or losing water from sweat, i.e. osmoreceptors in the hypothalamus will detect this increase in blood osmolarity. This stimulates the pituitary gland to release ADH to the blood and, eventually, to the target organs, the kidneys. The ADH causes the collecting tubules of the kidneys' nephrons to become more permeable to water. This increased permeability implies that more water is retained by the nephrons, and the kidneys produce concentrated urine with a low volume of water. When blood osmolarity returns to lower values, a negative feedback mechanism in the hypothalamus reduces the release of ADH.

If the water content of the blood is high, ADH is held back in the pituitary, and the collecting duct is less permeable to water. Only a little water is reabsorbed, and a large amount of dilute urine is created. Increased urination, called 'diuresis', occurs. ADH is called 'antidiuretic', because it inhibits diuresis and the production of dilute urine. ADH works by binding to receptor cells that cause an increase in aquaporin proteins. These proteins create the channels that make the collecting duct membrane porous to water, so that water diffuses out of the collecting ducts into the medulla interior and blood, thereby, reducing the volume of urine.

Certain disorders and diseases cause severe dehydration or severe solute imbalances as a result of mutations in ADH production or recognition. Diabetes insipidus (DI) is a condition associated with abnormal ADH metabolism. DI is characterized by excessive thirst and excretion of large amounts of severely diluted urine, with reduction of fluid intake having no effect on the latter. Some substances, such as alcohol, inhibit the release of ADH and cause excessive urination which leads to dehydration.

WATER DEPLETION

Water depletion will occur if water intake is inadequate or if losses are excessive. Excessive loss of water without any sodium loss is unusual, except in diabetes insipidus, but, even if there is loss of sodium as well, provided that this is small, the clinical consequences will be related primarily to the water depletion.

Loss of water from the ECF causes an increase in osmolality, which in turn causes movement of water from the ICF to the ECF, thus lessening the increase. Nevertheless, the increase in ECF osmolality will be sufficient to stimulate the thirst centre and vasopressin secretion. Plasma sodium concentration is increased; plasma protein concentration and the hematocrit are usually only slightly elevated. Unless water depletion is due to uncontrolled loss through the kidneys, the urine becomes highly concentrated and there is a rapid decrease in its volume. Because water loss is borne by the total body water pool, and not just the ECF, signs of a reduced ECF volume are not usually present. Furthermore, the increased colloid osmotic pressure of the plasma tends to hold extracellular water in the vascular compartment. Circulatory failure is a very late feature of water depletion; it is much more likely to occur if sodium depletion is also present.

Severe water depletion induces cerebral dehydration, which may cause cerebral hemorrhage through tearing of blood vessels. In the short term, cerebral shrinkage is mitigated somewhat by movement of extracellular ions into cerebral cells, causing an osmotic intracellular shift of water. If dehydration persists, brain cells adapt by synthesizing osmotically active organic compounds (osmolytes), and cerebral edema may then follow rapid fluid replacement.

The treatment for minor water depletion often considered the most effective, is drinking water and stopping fluid loss. Plain water restores only the volume of the blood plasma, inhibiting the thirst mechanism before solute levels can be replenished. Solid foods can contribute to fluid loss from vomiting and diarrhea. In more severe cases, correction of a water-depletion state is accomplished by the replenishment of necessary water and electrolytes through oral rehydration therapy or fluid replacement by intravenous therapy. As oral rehydration is less painful, less invasive, less expensive, and easier to provide; it is the treatment of choice for mild dehydration. Solutions used for intravenous rehydration must be isotonic or hypotonic. Pure water injected into the veins will cause the breakdown (lysis) of red blood cells (erythrocytes).

WATER EXCESS

This is usually related to an impairment of water excretion. However, the limit to the ability of the healthy kidneys to excrete water is about 20 mL/min and, occasionally, excessive intake is alone sufficient to cause water intoxication. This can sometimes occur in patients with psychiatric disorders. It has also been described in people drinking large amounts of beer with a low solute content, because this results in a low osmotic load for excretion and there is a minimum osmolality below which the urine cannot be diluted further. Increased thirst can occur in organic brain disease (particularly trauma, and following surgery), although decreased thirst is more common. Hyponatremia is invariably present in water overload. The increased water load is shared by the ICF and ECF.

The clinical features of water overload are related to cerebral over hydration; their incidence and severity depend upon the extent of the water excess and its time course. Thus, a patient with a plasma sodium concentration of 120 mmol/L, in whom water retention has occurred gradually over several days, may be asymptomatic; while one in whom this is an acute phenomenon may show signs of severe water intoxication. In the short term, the effects of hypotonicity are mitigated to some extent by a movement of ions out of cerebral glial cells; more chronically (days), a decrease in intracellular organic 'osmolytes' further reduces intracellular water content. As is the case with water depletion, this adaptation necessitates a cautious approach to treatment, particularly in chronic water overload.

ELECTROLYTES

The serum electrolytes include (as shown in Fig. 3.1):
1. **Sodium (Na⁺):** A positively charged electrolyte that helps to balance fluid levels in the body and facilitates neuromuscular functioning.

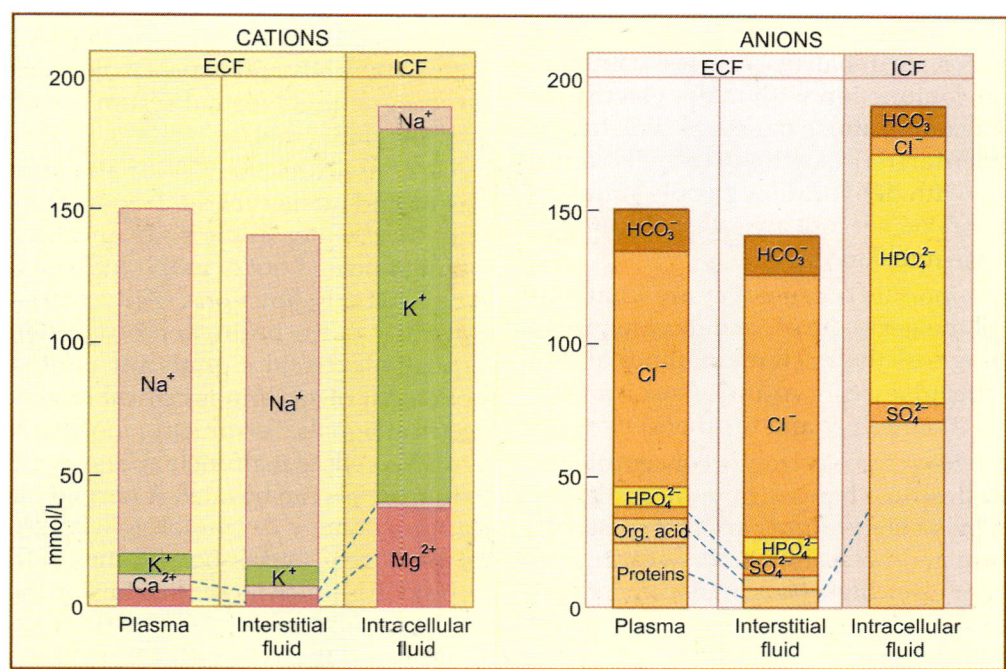

Fig. 3.1: Electrolyte composition of body fluid

2. **Potassium (K^+):** A main component of cellular fluid, this positive electrolyte helps to regulate neuro-muscular function and osmotic pressure.

3. **Chloride (Cl^-):** An anion, or negative electrolyte, that regulates blood pressure.

4. **Calcium (Ca^{2+}):** A cation, or positive electrolyte, that affects neuromuscular performance and contributes to skeletal growth and blood coagulation.

5. **Phosphate (HPO_4^{-3}):** Negative electrolyte that impacts metabolism and regulates acid-base balance and calcium levels.

6. **Magnesium (Mg^{2+}):** A cation that influences muscle contractions and intracellular activity.

7. **Bicarbonate (HCO_3^-):** A negatively charged electrolyte that assists in the regulation of blood pH levels. Bicarbonate insufficiencies and elevations cause acid-base disorders (e.g. acidosis, alkalosis).

Electrolyte Balance

Electrolytes play a vital role in maintaining homeostasis within the body; they help to regulate myocardial and neurological function, fluid balance, oxygen delivery, acid-base balance, and much more.

Electrolyte imbalances can develop by the following mechanisms

- Excessive ingestion
- Diminished elimination of an electrolyte
- Diminished ingestion or excessive elimination of an electrolyte
- Renal failure

The most serious electrolyte disturbances involve abnormalities in the levels of sodium, potassium, and/or calcium. Other electrolyte imbalances are less common, and often occur in conjunction with major electrolyte changes. Chronic laxative abuse or severe diarrhea or vomiting (gastroenteritis) can lead to electrolyte disturbances along with dehydration. People suffering from bulimia or anorexia nervosa are especially at high risk for an electrolyte imbalance.

Electrolytes are important because they are what cells (especially those of the nerve, heart, and muscle) use to maintain voltages across their cell membranes and to carry electrical impulses (nerve impulses, muscle contractions) across themselves and to other cells.

Kidneys work to keep the electrolyte concentrations in blood constant despite changes in your body, e.g. during heavy exercise electrolytes are lost in sweat, particularly sodium and potassium, and sweating can increase the need for electrolyte (salt) replacement. It is necessary to replace these electrolytes to keep their concentrations in the body fluids constant.

There are three types of dehydration: Hypotonic or hyponatremic (primarily a loss of electrolytes, sodium in particular), hypertonic or hypernatremic (primarily a loss of water), and isotonic or isonatremic (equal loss of water and electrolytes).

In humans, the most common type of dehydration by far is isotonic (isonatremic) dehydration which effectively equates with hypovolemia; but the distinction of isotonic from hypotonic or hypertonic dehydration may be important when treating people with dehydration. Physiologically, and despite the name, dehydration does not simply mean loss of water, as both water and solutes (mainly sodium) are usually lost in roughly equal quantities as to how they exist in blood plasma. In hypotonic dehydration, intravascular water shifts to the extravascular space, exaggerating intravascular volume depletion for a given amount of total body water loss. Neurological complications can occur in hypotonic and hypertonic states. The former can lead to seizures, while the latter can lead to osmotic cerebral edema upon rapid rehydration.

In more severe cases, correction of a dehydrated state is accomplished by the replenishment of necessary water and electrolytes (through oral rehydration therapy or fluid replacement by intravenous therapy). As oral rehydration is less painful, less invasive, less expensive, and easier to provide, it is the treatment of choice for mild dehydration. Solutions used for intravenous rehydration must be isotonic or hypotonic (as shown in Fig. 3.2).

SODIUM

Sodium (Na^+) is the major cation (positively charged ion) found outside the cell. It regulates the total amount of water in the body and plays a major role in neuronal and nerve signaling. Normal serum sodium values range from 135–145 mmol/L.

Na^+ constitutes 90–95% of all cations in the blood plasma and interstitial fluid. Sodium regulates the total amount of water in the body and the transmission of sodium into and out of individual cells also plays a role in critical body functions. Many processes in the body, especially in the brain, nervous system, and muscles, require electrical signals for communication. The movement of sodium is critical in generation of these electrical signals. Too much or too little sodium therefore can cause cells to malfunction, and extremes in the blood sodium levels can be fatal. A normal plasma osmolality is approximately 295 mmol/L, with 270 mmol/L being the result of Na^+ and associated anions. Na^+ concentration in the ECF is much larger than inside the cells. Because a small amount of Na^+ can diffuse through the cell membrane, the two sides would eventually reach

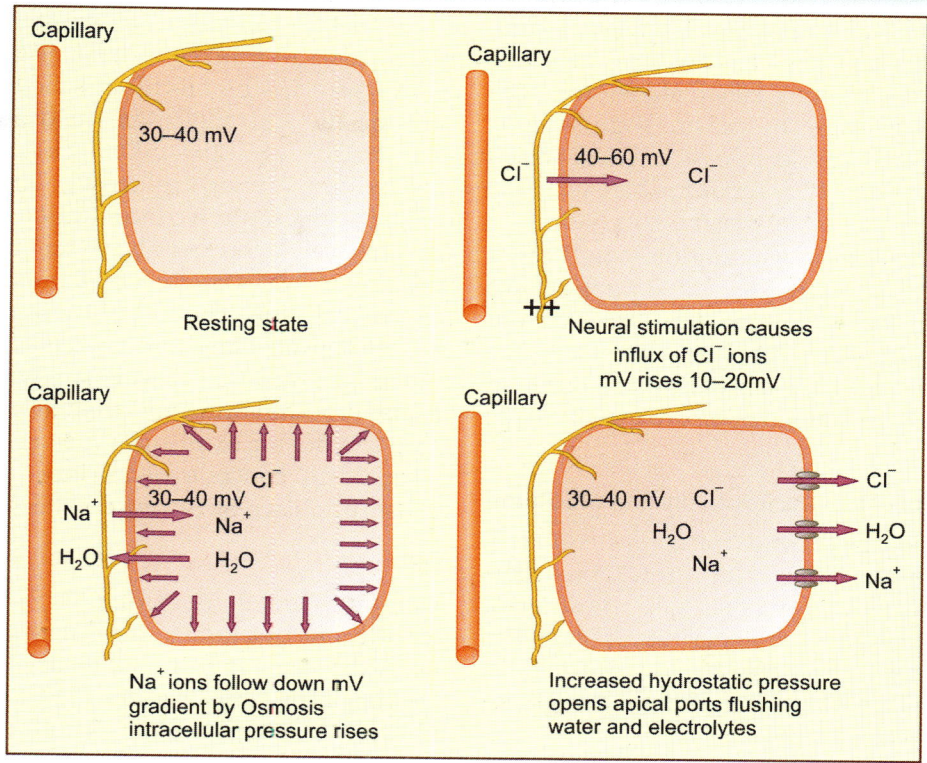

Capillary

30–40 mV

Resting state

Capillary

Cl⁻   40–60 mV   Cl⁻

++

Neural stimulation causes
influx of Cl⁻ ions
mV rises 10–20mV

Capillary

Cl⁻
Na⁺   30–40 mV
Na⁺
H₂O   H₂O

Na⁺ ions follow down mV
gradient by Osmosis
intracellular pressure rises

Capillary

30–40 mV   Cl⁻   Cl⁻
H₂O   H₂O
Na⁺   Na⁺

Increased hydrostatic pressure
opens apical ports flushing
water and electrolytes

Fig. 3.2: Mechanism for transportation of water and electrolytes across epithelial cells in secretory glands

equilibrium. To prevent equilibrium from occurring, active transport systems, such as ATPase ion pumps, are present in all cells. Potassium is the major intracellular cation. Like Na^+, K^+ would eventually diffuse across the cell membrane until equilibrium is reached. The Na^+- K^+ ATPase ion pump moves three Na^+ ions out of the cell in exchange for two K^+ ions moving into the cell as ATP is converted to ADP. Because water follows electrolytes across cell membranes, the continual removal of Na^+ from the cell prevents osmotic rupture of the cell by also drawing water from the cell.

Sodium Regulation

Sodium is an important cation distributed primarily outside the cell. The cell sodium concentration is about 15 mmol/L but varies in different organs and with an intracellular volume of 30 liters about 400 mmol are inside the cell. The plasma and interstitial sodium is about 140 mmol/L with an extracellular volume of about 13 liters, 1800 mmol are in the extracellular space. The total body sodium, however, is about 3700 mmol as there is about 1500 mmol stored in bones (listed in the Table 3.2).

Extra sodium is lost from the body by reducing the activity of the renin-angiotensin-aldosterone system which leads to increased sodium loss from the body. Sodium is lost through the kidneys, sweat, and feces.

In states of sodium depletion aldosterone levels increase. In states of sodium excess aldosterone levels decrease. The major physiological controller of aldosterone secretion is the plasma angiotensin II level, which increases aldosterone secretion. High plasma potassium also increases aldosterone secretion because besides retaining Na^+ high plasma aldosterone causes K^+ loss by the kidney. Plasma Na^+ levels have little effect on aldosterone secretion.

A low renal perfusion pressure stimulates the release of renin, which forms angiotensin I which is converted to angiotensin II. Angiotensin II will correct the low perfusion pressure by causing constriction of blood vessels and by increasing sodium retention by a direct effect on the proximal renal tubule and by an effect operated through aldosterone. The perfusion pressure to the adrenal gland has little direct effect on aldosterone secretion and the low blood pressure operates to

Table 3.2	Sodium distribution	
Different organs	**Amount**	**Concentration**
Amount in body	3700 mmol	
Intracellular	400 mmol	15 mmol/L
Extracellular	1800 mmol	140 mmol/L
Plasma	420 mmol	140 mmol/L
Interstitial	1400 mmol	140 mmol/L
Bone	1500 mmol	

control aldosterone via the renin angiotensin system. Aldosterone also acts on the sweat ducts and colonic epithelium to conserve sodium. When aldosterone has been activated to retain sodium the plasma sodium tends to rise. This immediately causes release of ADH which causes water to be retained, thus retaining Na^+ and H_2O in the right proportion to restore plasma volume.

In addition to aldosterone and angiotensin II other factors influence sodium excretion. Atrial peptide also causes loss of sodium by the kidneys; it is secreted from the heart in high sodium states due either to excess intake or cardiac disease. Elevated blood pressure will also tend to cause Na^+ loss and a low blood pressure usually leads to sodium retention.

Intrinsic Renal Control of Tubular Reabsorption of Sodium

Under normal physiological conditions, approximately 80% of the sodium in the glomerular filtrate is reabsorbed in the proximal tubule. The protein concentration of the blood within the postglomerular peritubular capillary bed is believed to exert a strong oncotic pressure on fluid in the proximal tubules, and this in turn helps to regulate the volume of fluid reabsorbed.

This process contributes to the autoregulation of filtration and reabsorption known as glomerulotubular balance. Despite a considerable physiological interest in the control of proximal tubular sodium reabsorption and other intrinsic renal control mechanisms, such as redistribution of filtering activity from superficial nephrons (relatively salt-losing) to juxtamedullary nephrons (relatively salt-retaining), the major humoral influences on sodium reabsorption reside in the distal tubules and collecting ducts.

SODIUM AND EXTRACELLULAR FLUID

The sodium content of a normal adult is 55–65 mmol/kg body weight. The concentration of sodium in plasma is approximately 140 mmol/L (152 mmol/kg). Under physiological conditions, the control of the ECF volume is through the control of functioning or effective plasma volume (that part of the plasma volume actively per fusing tissues). There are a variety of afferent mechanisms to monitor effective plasma volume (and thus ECF volume), which include intrathoracic volume receptors such as atrial stretch receptors, hepatic volume receptors, arterial baroreceptors, intrarenal baroreceptors, and possibly, tissue receptors monitoring tissue perfusion. Whatever the actual or relative function of all these sensory systems, their resultant influence is fine control over the renal conservation of sodium and the appetite for oral sodium intake.

Under normal conditions, plasma sodium concentrations are finely maintained within the narrow range of 135–145 mmol/L despite great variations in water and salt intake. Sodium and its accompanying anions, principally chloride and bicarbonate, account for 86% of the extracellular fluid osmolality, which is normally 285–295 mOsm/kg and calculated as (2× [sodium]+ [urea]+ [glucose]). The main determinant of the plasma sodium concentration is the plasma water content, itself determined by water intake (thirst or habit), 'insensible' losses (such as metabolic water, sweat), and urinary dilution. The last of these undermost circumstances, the most important and is predominantly determined by arginine vasopressin, which is synthesized in the hypothalamus and then stored in and released from the posterior pituitary. In response to arginine vasopressin, concentrated urine is produced by water reabsorption across the renal collecting ducts.

ATRIAL NATRIURETIC PEPTIDE HORMONES

Atrial natriuretic peptide (ANP) is a 28 amino acid peptide, one of a family of similar peptides, secreted by the cardiac atria in response to atrial stretch following a rise in atrial pressure (e.g. due to ECF volume expansion). It has a role in controlling sodium excretion. ANP acts both directly by inhibiting distal tubular sodium reabsorption and through decreasing renin (and hence aldosterone) secretion. It also antagonizes the pressor effects of norepinephrine (noradrenaline) and angiotensin II [and thus tends to increase glomerular filtration rate (GFR) and has a systemic vasodilatory effect. It appears to provide 'fine tuning' of sodium homoeostasis but is probably more important in pathological states than physiologically. Two other structurally similar peptides have been identified, i.e. one (brain natriuretic peptide, BNP) is secreted by the cardiac ventricles in response to ventricular stretching and has similar properties to ANP; the other (C-type natriuretic peptide, CNP) is present in high concentrations in vascular endothelium and is a vasodilator. Measurement of BNP is of value in the management of patients with suspected cardiac failure. Increased secretion of natriuretic peptides has been postulated to be at least in part responsible for the natriuresis seen in cerebral salt-wasting.

Sodium-potassium Pump in the Body

Inside the cells, the sodium-potassium pump does not appear particularly significant. The sodium-potassium pump is anchored in the cell membrane and pumps sodium ions and potassium ions out of and into the cell, respectively. The intracellular Na^+ concentration is lower than the extracellular. To equalize the difference, Na^+ automatically flows into the cell via channels in the cell membrane, but it is continuously pumped out again by means of the sodium-potassium pump. For each round of this pumping action, a high-energy molecule called ATP is broken down (ATPase activity takes place), whereby three Na^+ are transported out of the cell and two K^+ in (as shown in Fig. 3.3). The difference in the intracellular and extracellular concentrations forms the basis for the electrical potential difference across the cell membrane that is released by nerve impulses in muscles and the brain.

The sodium-potassium pump is the key to functions such as cardiac and renal activity, as well as all general transport processes into and out of the cell. The pump thus forms the basis for our ability to absorb a considerable number of nutrients, excrete waste products from the kidneys and regulate the water balance in the cells. If this little pump stopped pumping sodium ions out of the cells, the latter would rapidly swell up because of the infiltration of water and finally burst.

Sodium Depletion and Hyponatremia

Hyponatremia is defined as serum sodium below 135 mmol/L as a result of an accumulation of total body water greater than the body's accumulation of electrolytes (sodium and potassium); it is the most common electrolyte abnormality and is often a marker of underlying disease. Severe hyponatremia defined as serum sodium of less than 120 mmol/L, occurs in 2.5–6% of inpatients. Hyponatremia is associated with increased morbidity and mortality in hospitalized patients. It is also associated with increased mortality in patients in intensive care, patients with hepatic cirrhosis, congestive heart failure and community acquired pneumonia, and liver transplant patients who were hyponatremic at the time of transplantation. Severe hyponatremia is also associated with prolonged hospitalization and its treatment can cause adverse outcomes including death. Severe hyponatremia is therefore a medical emergency, requiring intensive care. Decreased levels may be caused by increased Na^+ loss, increased water retention, or water imbalance.

Total body sodium is primarily extracellular, and any increase results in increased tonicity, which stimulates the thirst center and arginine vasopressin secretion. Arginine vasopressin then acts on the V2-receptors in the renal tubules, causing increased water reabsorption. The opposite occurs with decreased extracellular sodium; a decrease inhibits-the thirst center and arginine vasopressin secretion, resulting in diuresis. In most cases, hyponatremia results when the elimination of total body water decreases.

Etiology

Hyponatremia reflects an excess of total body water (TBW) relative to total body Na^+ content. Because total body Na^+ content is reflected by ECF volume status, hyponatremia must be considered along with status of the ECF volume; hypovolemia, euvolemia, and hypervolemia (listed in the Table 3.3).

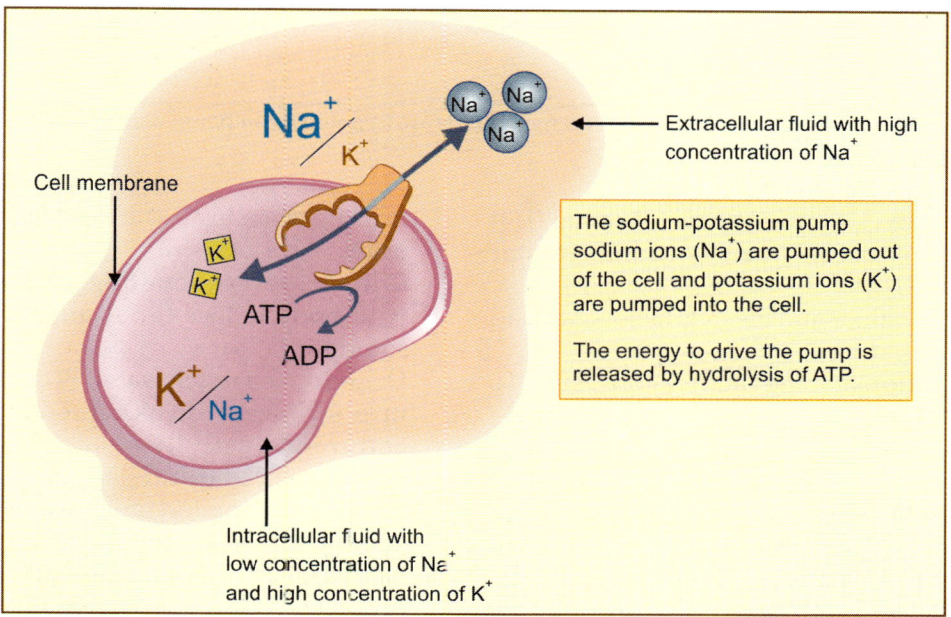

Fig. 3.3: Sodium-potassium pump shows (the intracellular Na^+ concentration is lower than the extracellular. To equalize the difference, Na^+ automatically flows into the cell via channels in the cell membrane, but it is continuously pumped out again by means of the sodium-potassium pump and it is very important that the pump continuously maintains the (unequal) intracellular and extracellular Na^+ balance because the flow of Na^+ into a nerve cell forms the basis for the nerve impulses that make it possible for us to move

Table 3.3	Principal causes of hyponatremia	
Mechanism	**Category**	**Examples**
Hypovolemic hyponatremia Decreased TBW and Na$^+$, with a relatively greater decrease in Na$^+$	GI losses*	Diarrhea Vomiting
	Third space losses*	Burns Pancreatitis Peritonitis Rhabdomyolysis Small-bowel obstruction
	Renal losses	Diuretics Mineralocorticoid deficiency Osmotic diuresis (glucose, urea, and mannitol) Salt-losing nephropathies (e.g. interstitial nephritis, medullary cystic disease, partial urinary tract obstruction, and polycystic kidney disease)
Euvolemic hyponatremia Increased TBW with near normal total body Na$^+$	Drugs	Diuretics, barbiturates, carbamazepine, chlorpropamide, clofibrate, opioids, tolbutamide, and vincristine Possibly cyclophosphamide, NSAIDs, oxytocin
	Disorders	Adrenal insufficiency as in Addison's disease Hypothyroidism Syndrome of inappropriate ADH secretion
	Increased intake of fluids	Primary polydipsia
	States that increase nonosmotic release of ADH	Emotional stress Pain Postoperative states
Hypervolemic hyponatremia Increased total body Na with a relatively greater increase in TBW	Extrarenal disorders	Cirrhosis Heart failure
	Renal disorders	Acute kidney dysfunction Chronic kidney disease Nephrotic syndrome

*GI and third space losses cause hyponatremia, if replacement fluids are hypotonic compared with losses.
TBW, total body water.

A normal sodium level is between 135–145 mmol/L of sodium. Hyponatremia occurs when the sodium in your blood falls below 135 mmol/L.

Many possible conditions and lifestyle factors can lead to hyponatremia, including:
- **Certain medications:** Some medications, such as some water pills (diuretics), antidepressants and pain medications, can cause you to urinate or perspire more than normal.
- **Heart, kidney, and liver problems:** Congestive heart failure and certain diseases affecting the kidneys or liver can cause fluids to accumulate in your body, which dilutes the sodium in your body, lowering the overall level.
- **Syndrome of inappropriate antidiuretic hormone (SIADH):** In this condition, high levels of the antidiuretic hormone are produced, causing your body to retain water instead of excreting it normally in your urine.
- **Chronic, severe vomiting, or diarrhea:** This causes your body to lose fluids and electrolytes, such as sodium.
- **Drinking too much water:** Because you lose sodium through sweat, drinking too much water during endurance activities, such as marathons and triathlons, can dilute the sodium content of your blood. Drinking too much water at other times can also cause low sodium.
- **Dehydration:** Taking in too little fluid can also be a problem. If you get dehydrated, your body loses fluids and electrolytes.
- **Hormonal changes:** Adrenal gland insufficiency (Addison's disease) affects your adrenal glands' ability to produce hormones that help maintain your

body's balance of sodium, potassium, and water. Low levels of thyroid hormone also can cause a low blood-sodium level.

- **The recreational drug ecstasy:** This amphetamine increases the risk of severe and even fatal cases of hyponatremia.

CLASSIFICATION OF HYPONATREMIA

There are several methods of classifying hyponatremia, and classification based on the volume status as follows:

- **Euvolemic hyponatremia:** Normal body sodium with increase in total body water.
- **Hypovolemic hyponatremia:** Decrease in total body water with greater decrease in total body sodium.
- **Hypervolemic hyponatremia:** Increase in total body sodium with greater increase in total body water.

Euvolemic Hyponatremia

A dilutional form of hyponatremia occurs when the total serum sodium is normal or near normal, but the total body water is increased without clinically evident edema. The syndrome of inappropriate antidiuretic hormone (SIADH) is the most common cause of euvolemic hyponatremia. Patients with euvolemic hyponatremia have no signs of volume depletion or volume expansion. It is the most common form of hyponatremia as following:

Urine sodium >30 mmol/L

- Syndrome of inappropriate antidiuretic hormone secretion (SIADH)
  - **Drugs:** Particularly, thiazide diuretics including combinations with angiotensin converting enzyme inhibitors and angiotensin receptor antagonists
    1. *Antidepressants:* Tricyclics, selective serotonin reuptake inhibitors, monoamine oxidase inhibitors, venlafaxine
    2. *Antipsychotics:* Phenothiazines, haloperidol
    3. *Antiepileptics:* Carbamazepine, oxcarbazepine, valproate, lamotrigine
    4. *Antidiabetics:* Chlorpropamide, tolbutamide
    5. *Antibiotics:* Ciprofloxacin, trimethoprim-sulfamethoxazole, rifabutin
    6. *Antiarrhythmics:* Amiodarone
    7. *Antihypertensives:* Angiotensin converting enzyme inhibitors (angiotensin receptor antagonists), amlodipine
    8. *Anticancer/Chemotherapeutic drugs:* Vincristine/vinblastine, cisplatin/carboplatin, alkylating agents, methotrexate, levamisole
    9. Proton pump inhibitors
    10. Nonsteroidal anti-inflammatory drugs
    11. Oxytocin, antidiuretic hormone analogues
    12. *Amphetamines:* 3,4-Methylenedioxymethamphetamine (MDMA) (commonly known as ecstasy)

- **Tumors with ectopic hormone production**
  1. Small cell and other pulmonary carcinomas
  2. Pancreatic and duodenal carcinoma
  3. Head and neck malignancies
  4. Mesothelioma
  5. Lymphoma

- **Central nervous system disorders**
  1. Infections
  2. Cerebral tumors
  3. Stroke or intracerebral hemorrhage with raised intracranial pressure
  4. Hydrocephalus
  5. Guillain-Barré syndrome
  6. Multiple sclerosis

- **Pulmonary disease**
  1. Pneumonia and other infections
  2. Acute respiratory failure with or without positive pressure ventilation
  3. Asthma
  4. Pneumothorax

- **Miscellaneous**
  1. Major thoracic or abdominal surgery
  2. Transphenoidal pituitary surgery
  3. Postoperative pain
  4. Positive pressure ventilation
  5. HIV/AIDS
  6. Extreme exercise
  7. Hereditary

- Hypothyroidism
- Hypopituitarism (glucocorticoid deficiency)
- Water intoxication:
  1. Primary polydipsia
  2. Excessive administration of parenteral hypotonic fluids
  3. Post-transurethral prostatectomy

Hypovolemic Hyponatremia

In hypovolemic hyponatremia the extracellular fluids volume is reduced as following:

Extrarenal loss, urine sodium <30 mmol/L

- Dermal losses, such as burns, sweating
- Gastrointestinal losses, such as vomiting, diarrhea
- Pancreatitis

Renal loss, urine sodium >30 mmol/L

- Diuretics
- Salt-wasting nephropathy
- Cerebral-salt wasting
- Mineralocorticoid deficiency (Addison's disease)

Hypervolemic Hyponatremia

A dilutional form of hyponatremia occurs when there is an increase in total body water, but a relatively smaller increase in the total serum sodium, so the available sodium is effectively diluted. The three main causes of hypervolemic hyponatremia are congestive heart failure, liver cirrhosis, and renal diseases such as renal failure and nephrotic syndrome. These disorders usually are obvious from the clinical history and physical examination alone. The clinical signs of hypervolemic hyponatremia include signs of volume expansion, such as the presence of clinically evident edema, ascites, and pulmonary edema. Extracellular fluids is increased as following:

- **Urine sodium <30 mmol/L**
  - Congestive cardiac failure
  - Cirrhosis with ascites
  - Nephrotic syndrome
- **Urine sodium >30 mmol/L**
  - Chronic renal failure

Hyponatremia can be further subclassified according to effective osmolality, as follows:
  - Hypotonic hyponatremia
  - Isotonic hyponatremia
  - Hypertonic hyponatremia

Because Na^+ is a major contributor to osmolality, both levels can assist in identifying the cause of hyponatremia. There are three categories of hyponatremia low osmolality, normal osmolality, or high osmolality. Most instances of hyponatremia occur with decreased osmolality. This may be a result of Na^+ loss or water retention, as previously mentioned.

HYPONATREMIA BY OSMOLALITY

Hyponatremia can be further subclassified according to effective osmolality (listed in the Table 3.4), as follows:

Hypotonic Hyponatremia

Hypotonic hyponatremia is a condition where hyponatremia associated with a low plasma osmolality is also known as hypoosmolar hyponatremia. It occurs by two mechanisms—(1) usual (or greater than usual) water intake in the setting of impaired renal water excretion leading to dilution of body solutes or less commonly, (2) water intake in excess of the normal renal ability to excrete water. Hypotonic hyponatremia can be classified as hypovolemic, euvolemic and hypervolemic on the basis of ECF volume as assessed clinically (orthostatic changes

Table 3.4	Classification of hyponatremia by osmolality	
Type	**Serum osmolality (mOsm/kg)**	**Description**
Hypotonic hyponatremia	<280	When the plasma osmolality is low, the extracellular fluid volume status may be in one of three states: low volume, normal volume, or high volume.
Isotonic hyponatremia	Between 280 and 295	Certain conditions that interfere with laboratory tests of serum sodium concentration (such as extraordinarily high blood levels of lipid or protein) may lead to an erroneously low "measurement" of sodium. This is called pseudohyponatremia.
Hypertonic hyponatremia	>295	Hypertonic hyponatremia can be associated with shifts of fluid due to osmotic pressure.

in blood pressure and heart rate, edema, jugular venous distension, skin turgor, mucous membranes, and ascites).

Isotonic Hyponatremia

Isotonic hyponatremia is a form of hyponatremia with osmolality measured between 280 and 295. It can be associated with pseudo hyponatremia, or with isotonic infusion of glucose or mannitol with normal osmolality, such as:

- Increased non-sodium cations
- Lithium excess
- Increased-globulins-cationic (multiple myeloma)
- Severe hyperkalemia
- Severe hypermagnesemia
- Severe hypercalcemia
- Pseudohyponatremia
- Hyperlipidemia
- Hyperproteinemia
- Pseudohyperkalemia as a result of in vitro hemolysis
- With high osmolality
- Hyperglycemia
- Mannitol infusion

Hypertonic Hyponatremia

Hypertonic hyponatremia is caused by resorption of water drawn by molecules, such as:

- **Excess water loss**
  - Diabetes insipidus
  - Renal tubular disorder
  - Prolonged diarrhea
  - Profuse sweating
  - Severe burns

■ **Decreased water intake**
- Older persons
- Infants
- Mental impairment

■ **Increased intake or retention**
- Hyperaldosteronism
- Sodium bicarbonate excess
- Dialysis fluid excess

In multiple myeloma, the cationic gamma globulins replace some Na^+ to maintain the electroneutrality; however, because it is a multivalent cation, it has little effecton osmolality.

PSEUDOHYPONATREMIA

Pseudohyponatremia is a falsely low serum sodium measurement, it occurs in cases of extreme hyperlipidemia or hyperproteinemia, when serum from patients with hyperviscosity analyzed by techniques, such as flame photometry or indirect potentiometry. The serum sample should be diluted before analysis by the flame photometry or indirect potentiometry, the serum sodium values would be expected to below in the presence of hyperproteinemia and hyperviscosity. With direct potentiometry no sample dilution is required, and sodium measurements are unaffected by hyperlipidemia and hyperproteinemia where no sample dilution takes place, no interference would be expected since the activity of sodium in the water phase only is being measured. Pseudohyponatremia may also be seen with *in vitro* hemolysis, considered the most common cause for a false decrease. When red blood cells (RBCs) lyse, Na^+, K^+, and water are released. Na^+ concentration is lower in RBCs, resulting in a false decrease.

Specific Clinical Hyponatremia

■ **Alcohol abuse:** Hyponatremia in this setting is beer potomania syndrome, and the diagnostic criteria include a history of binge drinking, poor dietary solute intake, and decreased sodium concentrations in the absence of other causes. Urine osmolarity is <100 mOsm/kg in this situation, indicating ADH suppression. In addition to alcoholic liver disease, traumatic cerebral injury plus all the other disorders mentioned above may affect the alcoholic patient.

■ **Hyponatremia in psychiatric disorders:** Syndrome of inappropriate antidiuretic hormone (SIADH), can occur in the setting of acute psychosis and also after use of psychotropic medication. Excessive water intake is often seen in association with psychiatric illness and is commonly referred to as psychogenic polydipsia. High-volume water intake eventually overburdens the renal diluting mechanism. It is unclear what causes such compulsive drinking, but proposed mechanisms include hyperactivity of the hypothalamic thirst centre, neuroleptic drugs, and resetting of the hypothalamic osmostat.

■ **Marathon runners:** Marathoninduced hyponatremia is now emerging as a cause of racerelated death. Hyponatremia is caused by the consumption of high volumes >3 liters of fluid in excess of sodium losses.

■ **Postoperative hyponatremia:** Careful assessment of admission notes, premedication, intraoperative records, fluid balance charts and anesthetic records is imperative. Drug therapy, surgical procedures and pain are all causes of SIADH. Sodium picosulphate bowel preparation before colonic surgery may cause dehydration and electrolyte disorders, including hyponatremia. As previously mentioned, irrigation solutions, such as mannitol, sorbitol and glycine may cause hypertonic hyponatremia when absorbed. The intravenous administration of large volumes of 5% dextrose is a common cause of postoperative hyponatremia.

■ **Hyponatremia in primary adrenal insufficiency (Addison's disease) and secondary adrenal insufficiency:** Primary adrenal insufficiency is associated with glucocorticoid deficiency, which impairs renal water excretion and mineralocorticoid deficiency, which causes renal sodium loss. Secondary adrenal insufficiency may be due to hypopituitarism. Glucocorticoid deficiency is the predominant cause of hyponatremia in this setting, as mineralocorticoid activity is preserved. In addition, SIADH induced by hypothyroidism may contribute. Hyponatremia may resolve after correction of cortisol deficiency.

PATIENT HISTORY

The key diagnostic factors are the hydration status of the patient and the urine 'spot sodium' concentration, which is available quickly and allows the crucial distinction in Hypovolemic hyponatremia between renal >30 mmol/L and extrarenal low; <30 mmol/L salt loss. Urinary sodium is similarly helpful in patients, in whom volume status is difficult to assess, as patients with dilutional hyponatremia by and large have a urinary sodium >30 mmol/L, whereas those with extracellular fluid depletion (unless the source is renal) will have a urinary sodium <30 mmol/L. Plasma osmolality is almost always low in hyponatremia, and urine is less than maximally dilute (inappropriately concentrated); so, although usually measured, plasma and urine osmolalities are rarely discriminant.

Evaluation of Volume Status

■ Skin turgor
■ Pulse rate

- Postural blood pressure
- Jugular venous pressure
- Consider central venous pressure monitoring
- Examination of fluid balance charts

General Examination for Underlying Illness

- Congestive cardiac failure
- Cirrhosis
- Nephrotic syndrome
- Addison's disease
- Hypopituitarism
- Hypothyroidism

Investigations

- Urinary sodium
- Plasma glucose and lipids
- Renal function
- Thyroid function
- Peak cortisol during short synacthen test
- Plasma and urine osmolality
- If indicated: Chest X-ray, computed tomography and magnetic resonance imaging of head and thorax.

SYMPTOMS AND SIGNS

The symptoms of hyponatremia are related to both the severity and the rapidity of the fall in the plasma sodium concentration. A decrease in plasma sodium concentration creates an osmotic gradient between extracellular and intracellular fluid in brain cells, causing movement of water into cells, increasing intracellular volume, and resulting in tissue edema, raised intracranial pressure, and neurological symptoms.

Acute hyponatremia is defined as occurring within <48 hours. There are usually no symptoms if serum sodium is 130–135 mmol/L. Patients with mild hyponatremia (plasma sodium 130–135 mmol/L) are usually asymptomatic. Nausea and malaise are typically seen when plasma sodium concentration falls below 125–130 mmol/L.

Headache, lethargy, restlessness, and disorientation follow, as the sodium concentration falls below 115–120 mmol/L. With severe and rapidly evolving hyponatremia, seizure, coma, permanent brain damage, respiratory arrest, brain stem herniation, and death may occur.

Severe cerebral edema may occur in premenopausal women with acute hyponatremia, perhaps because estrogen and progesterone inhibit brain $Na^+ K^+ ATPase$ and decrease solute extrusion from brain cells. Sequelae include hypothalamic and posterior pituitary infarction and occasionally osmotic demyelination syndrome or brain stem herniation.

In chronic hyponatremia present for >48 hours, the brain self regulates to prevent swelling over hours to days by transport of, firstly, sodium, chloride, and potassium and, later, organic solutes including glutamate, taurine, myoinositol, and glutamine from intracellular to extracellular compartments. This induces water loss and ameliorates brain swelling, and hence leads to few symptoms in patients with chronic hyponatremia.

DIAGNOSIS

After sampling error, hyperglycemia, and pseudo-hyponatremia have been ruled out, the diagnosis of hyponatremia begins with careful examination of the patient's extracellular fluid volume status (listed in the Table 3.5). Patients are classified as hypovolemic, euvolemic, or hypervolemic according to features of the history (e.g. emesis, diarrhea) and physical examination findings (e.g. flat or distended neck veins, dry, or moist skin or mucosa, heart rate, blood pressure, orthostatic vital signs, presence of edema or ascites).

Patients with edema or ascites are, by definition, hypervolemic. Patients with hypotension, flat neck veins, dry mucosa, and no edema are hypovolemic. Other patients may be euvolemic or might have clinically undetectable forms of hypovolemia. Additional testing using determination of spot urine sodium, blood urea nitrogen (BUN), and serum uric acid levels and response to isotonic intravenous fluids may be helpful in this patient subgroup.

The presence of low urinary spot sodium (<10 mmol/L), normal or elevated serum uric acid, and elevated BUN levels suggest hypovolemia, whereas levels of urinary spot sodium higher than 10–20 mmol/L, low serum uric

Table 3.5	Causes of hyponatremia based on extracellular fluid volume status
Hypovolemia	
Gastrointestinal solute loss (diarrhea, emesis)	
Third-spacing (ileus, pancreatitis)	
Diuretic use	
Addison's disease	
Salt-wasting nephritis	
Euvolemic	
Syndrome of inappropriate antidiuretic hormone (SIADH)	
Diuretic use	
Glucocorticoid deficiency	
Hypothyroidism	
Beer drinker's potomania, psychogenic polydipsia	
Reset osmostat	
Hypervolemia with decreased effective circulating blood volume	
Decompensated heart failure	
Advanced liver cirrhosis	
Renal failure with or without nephrosis	

acid, and normal BUN imply that the ECF volume is not decreased. Additionally, the response of the serum sodium concentration to volume replacement may be helpful. In patients with hypovolemia, the serum sodium level should increase following administration of 1–2 L of normal saline. In patients with euvolemia, the serum sodium level will decrease further (e.g. syndrome of inappropriate antidiuretic hormone) as water is reclaimed by the nephron, or the level will remain unchanged.

Urine osmolality is inappropriately >100 mOsm/kg in almost every patient with hyponatremia. It should be checked to confirm inappropriate urinary dilution, but it does not help delineate the cause of hyponatremia, except in patients found to have diluted urine (psychogenic polydipsia and reset osmostat). Plasma osmolality (posm) is almost always <270 mOsm/kg in patients with hyponatremia, because serum sodium is the major determinant of posm. If measured posm is more than 10 mOsm/kg higher than calculated osmolality ($[2\,Na^+ + BUN/2.8] + [glucose/18]$), there is an effective osmole in the plasma other than sodium or glucose (e.g. mannitol, glycine, or sorbitol), or high levels of plasma protein or lipid causing pseudohyponatremia.

In euvolemic patients, or those with clinical suspicion of endocrine disorders, measures of thyroid function [thyroid-stimulating hormone (TSH) and free thyroid hormone level determination] and adrenal function [cosyntropin (Cortrosyn) stimulation test] can be assessed. Euvolemic patients with normal thyroid, adrenal, and renal function might have SIADH. This syndrome is associated with various drugs and clinical disorders including pulmonary infections, ectopic production by certain cancers (particularly small cell lung carcinoma), various CNS disorders, and pain.

Laboratory Testing

There are three essential laboratory tests in the evaluation of patients with hyponatremia that together with the history and the physical examination help to establish the primary underlying etiologic mechanism, these tests are as follow:

- Urine osmolality helps to differentiate between conditions associated with impaired free water excretion and primary polydipsia, in which water excretion should be normal (provided intact kidney function). With primary polydipsia, as with malnutrition (severe decreased solids intake) and reset osmostat, the urine osmolality is maximally dilute, generally less than 100 mOsm/kg. A urine osmolality greater than 100 mOsm/kg indicates impaired ability of the kidneys to dilute the urine. This usually is secondary to elevated vasopressin (ADH) levels, appropriate or inappropriate.

- Serum osmolality readily differentiates between true hyponatremia and pseudohyponatremia secondary to hyperlipidemia, hyperproteinemia, or hypertonic hyponatremia associated with elevated glucose, mannitol, glycine, sucrose, or maltose.

Serum osmolality is governed by contributions from all molecules in the body that cannot easily move between the intracellular and extracellular space. Sodium is the most abundant electrolyte, but glucose, urea, plasma proteins, and lipids are also important. A patient with diabetic ketoacidosis may have hyponatremia, but normal osmolality, due to hyperglycemia, hypertriglyceridemia and ketonemia. Patients with acute renal failure may have hyponatremia due to uremia. If a patient has hyponatremia, with low measured and calculated serum osmolality, we call this hypotonic hypernatremia. If serum osmolality is normal or high, this is isotonic or hypotonic hyponatremia or pseudohyponatremia.

- Urinary sodium concentration helps to differentiate between hyponatremia secondary to hypovolemia and SIADH. With SIADH (and salt-wasting syndrome), the urine sodium is greater than 20–40 mmol/L. With hypovolemia, the urine sodium typically measures less than 20 mmol/L. However, if sodium intake in a patient with SIADH (or salt-wasting) happens to be low, then urine sodium may fall below 20 mmol/L.

Ancillary Tests

Serum uric acid levels can be important supportive information (typically reduced in SIADH and also reduced in salt wasting). After correction of hyponatremia, the hypouricemia corrects in SIADH, but remains with a salt-wasting process.

Thyroid-stimulating hormone (TSH) and serum cortisol levels; if hypothyroidism or hypoadrenalism is suspected.

Serum albumin, triglycerides, and a serum protein electrophoresis; also may be indicated for particular patients.

MANAGEMENT AND TREATMENT OF HYPONATREMIA

Initial evaluation of any patient with hyponatremia involves identification of the onset of the condition (acute or chronic), the presence of symptoms and assessment of volume status.

A clinical history of renal, liver or cardiac disease should be noted, as well as previous electrolytes to distinguish acute from chronic hyponatremia. Any loss of blood or extracellular fluid should be determined. A precise drug history, which includes recreational drug use, is necessary. Symptoms of headache, nausea, seizures, and confusion suggest raised intracranial pressure.

The biochemical parameters in salt-wasting conditions and those in SIADH can be identical and are differentiated by determining volume status (listed in the Table 3.6), i.e. distinguishing cerebral salt wasting from SIADH is of vital importance, as fluid restriction in a volume depleted patient may worsen ischemic cerebral injury in subarachnoid hemorrhage. Measurement of central venous pressure may be required.

The presence or absence of edema, skin turgor and postural drop in systolic blood pressure of >20 mmHg should all be recorded. When the patient cannot stand upright, sitting blood pressure can be used as an estimate. Examination may also reveal signs of an underlying illness causing hyponatremia, such as hypoadrenalism, hypopituitarism, chronic liver disease or nephrotic syndrome.

The recommendations for treatment of hyponatremia rely on the current understanding of the central nervous system adaptation to an alteration in serum osmolality. In the setting of an acute fall in the serum osmolality, neuronal cell swelling occurs due to the water shift from the extracellular space to the intracellular space (e.g. Starling forces). Therefore, correction of hyponatremia should take into account the limited capacity of this adaptation mechanism to respond to acute alteration in the serum tonicity, because the degree of brain edema and consequent neurologic symptoms depend as much on the rate and duration of hypotonicity as they do on its magnitude.

Intravenous Fluids and Water Restriction

Hypotonic hyponatremia accounts for most clinical cases of hyponatremia. The first step in the approach and evaluation of hypotonic hyponatremia is to determine

Table 3.6	Biochemical parameters in hyponatremia
EABV low	
Urine Na$^+$ >20 mmol/L	
High low serum osmolarity	
Urine osmolarity	
Diuretics	
Cerebral salt wasting	
Salt-losing nephropathy	
Mineralocorticoid deficiency	
EABV normal	
Urine Na$^+$ >20 mmol/L	
High urine osmolarity	
Low serum osmolarity	

EABV, effective arterial blood volume; SIADH, syndrome of inappropriate ADH

whether emergency therapy is warranted. Guide treatment by the three following factors:
- Patient's volume status
- Duration and magnitude of the hyponatremia
- Degree and severity of clinical symptoms

For the asymptomatic patient, the following treatments may be of use:
- Hypovolemic hyponatremia: Administer isotonic saline to patients who are hypovolemic to replace the contracted intravascular volume (thereby treating the cause of vasopressin release). Patients with hypovolemia secondary to diuretics may also need potassium repletion, which, like sodium, is osmotically active. Correction of volume repletion turns off the stimulus to ADH secretion, so a large water diuresis may ensue, leading to a more rapid correction of hyponatremia than desired. If so, hypotonic fluid, such as normal saline may need to be administered.
- Hypervolemic hyponatremia: Treat patients who are hypervolemic with salt and fluid restriction, plus loop diuretics, and correction of the underlying condition. The use of a V2-receptor antagonist may be considered.
- Euvolemic asymptomatic hyponatremic patients, free water restriction <1 L/d are generally the treatment of choice. There is no role for hypertonic saline in these patients. Base the volume of restriction on the patient's renal diluting capacity. For instance, a fluid restriction to 1 L/d, enough to raise the serum sodium in some patients may exceed the renal free water excretion capacity in others, necessitating more severe restriction. This approach is recommended as initial treatment for patients with asymptomatic SIADH. However, many patients will not adhere to fluid restriction. Further, the definition of asymptomatic is changing due to the recognition that subtle but significant deficits such as in gait may be present. Therefore, pharmacologic treatment may be considered.

During therapy, closely monitoring serum electrolytes (e.g. every 2–4 hours) to avoid overcorrection is essential.

Acute hyponatremia (duration <48 hours) can be safely corrected more quickly than chronic hyponatremia. A severely symptomatic patient with acute hyponatremia is in danger from brain edema. In contrast, a symptomatic patient with chronic hyponatremia is more at risk from rapid correction of hyponatremia. Correction of serum sodium that is too rapid can precipitate severe neurologic complications, such as central pontine myelinosis, which can produce spastic quadriparesis, swallowing dysfunction, pseudobulbar palsy, and mutism. A symptomatic patient with unknown duration of hyponatremia is the most challenging, warranting a prompt, but controlled and limited correction of hyponatremia, until symptoms resolve. However, excessive therapy and fear of osmotic demyelination should not deter prompt and definitive treatment.

With patients who are acutely symptomatic (duration <48 hours, such as after surgery), the treatment goal is to increase the serum sodium level by approximately 1–2 mmol/L/h for 3–4 hours, until the neurologic symptoms subside or until plasma Na$^+$ is over 120 mmol/L.

In chronic, severe symptomatic hyponatremia, the rate of correction should not exceed 0.5–1 mmol/L/h, with a total increase not to exceed 8–12 mmol/L/d and no more than 18 mmol/L in the first 48 h. It is necessary to correct the hyponatremia to a safe range (usually to no greater than 120 mmol/L) rather than to a normal value. As noted above, spontaneous diuresis secondary to ADH suppression with intravascular volume repletion could lead to unintended overcorrection.

Sodium Excess and Hypernatremia

Hypernatremia is defined as a serum sodium concentration greater than 145 mmol/L, occurs in patients with inadequate access to water or impaired thirst mechanism usually in infants or elderly adults. It is much less common than hyponatremia. It reflects a net water loss or a hypertonic sodium gain, with inevitable hyper osmolality. Severe symptoms are usually evident only with acute and large increases in plasma sodium concentrations to above 158–160 mmol/L. Importantly, the sensation of intense thirst that protects against severe hypernatremia in health may be absent or reduced in patients with altered mental status or with hypothalamic lesions affecting their sense of thirst (adipsia) and in infants and elderly people. Non-specific symptoms, such as anorexia, muscle weakness, restlessness, nausea, and vomiting tend to occur early. More serious signs follow, with altered mental status, lethargy, irritability, stupor, or coma. Acute brain shrinkage can induce vascular rupture, with cerebral bleeding and subarachnoid hemorrhage.

ETIOLOGY OF HYPERNATREMIA

Hypernatremia reflects a deficit of total body water (TBW) relative to total body Na$^+$ content. Because total body Na$^+$ content is reflected by ECF volume status, hypernatremia must be considered along with status of the ECF volume, i.e. hypovolemia, euvolemia, and hypervolemia.

Hypernatremia usually implies either an impaired thirst mechanism or limited access to water. The severity of the underlying disorder that results in an inability to drink in response to thirst and the effects of hyperosmolality on the brain are thought to be responsible for a high mortality rate in hospitalized adults with hypernatremia. There are several common causes of hypernatremia (listed in the Table 3.7).

Several risk factors exist for hypernatremia. The greatest risk factor is age older than 65 years. In addition, mental or physical disability may result in impaired thirst sensation, an impaired ability to express thirst, and/or decreased access to water.

Table 3.7	Principal causes of hypernatremia	
Description	**Category**	**Examples**
Hypovolemic hypernatremia		
Decreased TBW and Na$^+$ with a relatively greater decrease in TBW	GI losses	Diarrhea
		Vomiting
	Skin losses	Burns
		Excessive sweating
	Renal losses	Intrinsic renal disease
		Loop diuretics
		Osmotic diuresis (glucose, urea, and mannitol)
Euvolemic hypernatremia		
Decreased TBW with near normal total body Na$^+$	Extrarenal losses from the respiratory tract	Tachypnea
	Extrarenal losses from the skin	Excessive sweating
		Fever
	Renal losses	Central diabetes insipidus
		Nephrogenic diabetes insipidus
	Other	Inability to access water
		Primary hypodipsia
		Reset osmostat

Contd.

Table 3.7	Principal causes of hypernatremia *(Contd.)*		
Description		**Category**	**Examples**
Hypervolemic hypernatremia Increased Na⁺ with normal or increased TBW		Hypertonic fluid administration	Hypertonic saline $NaHCO_3$ TPN
		Mineralocorticoid excess	Adrenal tumors secreting deoxycorticosterone Congenital adrenal hyperplasia (caused by 11-hydroxylase defect)
TBW, total body water			

Hypernatremia often is the result of several concurrent factors. The most prominent is poor fluid intake. Again, developing hypernatremia is virtually impossible if the thirst response is intact and water is available. Normally, an increase in osmolality of just 1–2% stimulates thirst, as do hypovolemia and hypotension. For clinical purposes, hypernatremia can, in a simplified view, be classified on the basis of the concurrent water loss or electrolyte gain and on corresponding changes in extracellular fluid volume:

- Hypotonic fluid deficits (loss of water and electrolytes)
- Nearly pure-water deficits
- Hypertonic sodium gain (gain of electrolytes in excess of water).

Loss of Hypotonic Fluid (Loss of Water in Excess of Electrolytes)

Patients who lose hypotonic fluid have a deficit in free water and electrolytes (low total body sodium and potassium) and have decreased extracellular volume. In these patients, hypovolemia may be more life threatening than hypertonicity. When physical evidence of hypovolemia is present, fluid resuscitation with normal saline is the first step in therapy.

- **Renal hypotonic fluid loss:** Results from anything that will interfere with the ability of the kidney to concentrate the urine or osmotic diuresis
  - Diuretic drugs (loop and thiazide diuretics)
  - Osmotic diuresis [hyperglycemia, mannitol, urea (high-protein tube feeding)]
  - Postobstructive diuresis
  - Diuretic phase of acute tubular necrosis
- **Nonrenal hypotonic fluid loss**
  - Gastrointestinal: Vomiting, diarrhea, lactulose, cathartics, nasogastric suction, gastrointestinal fluid drains, and fistulas
  - Cutaneous: Sweating (extreme sports, marathon runs), burn injuries

Pure-water Deficits

Patients with pure-water deficits in the majority of cases have a normal extracellular volume with normal total body sodium and potassium. This condition most commonly develops when impaired intake is combined with increased insensible (e.g. respiratory) or renal water losses.

Free-water loss will also result from an inability of the kidney to concentrate the urine. The cause of that can be either from failure of the hypothalamic-pituitary axis to synthesize or release adequate amounts of arginine vasopressin (AVP), (central diabetes insipidus) or a lack of responsiveness of the kidney to AVP (nephrogenic diabetes insipidus). Patients with diabetes insipidus and intact thirst mechanisms most often present with normal plasma osmolality and serum Na⁺, but with symptoms of polyuria and polydipsia.

- Water intake less than insensible losses
  - Lack of access to water (through incarceration, restraints, intubation, immobilization)
  - Altered mental status (through medications, disease)
  - Neurologic disease (dementia, impaired motor function)
  - Abnormal thirst
    - Geriatric hypodipsia
    - Osmoreceptor dysfunction (reset of the osmotic threshold).
    - Injury to the thirst centers by any lesions to the hypothalamus, including from metastasis, granulomatous diseases, vascular abnormalities, and trauma.
    - Autoantibodies to the sodium-level sensor in the brain
  - Loss of water through the respiratory tract

Vasopressin Deficiency (Diabetes Insipidus)

Central diabetes insipidus can be caused by any pathologic process that destroys the anatomic structures of the hypothalamic-pituitary axis involved in AVP production and secretion. Such processes include the following:

- **Pituitary injury:** Post-traumatic, neurosurgical, hemorrhage, ischemia (Sheehan's), idiopathic-autoimmune, lymphocytic hypophysitis, immunoglobulin (Ig) G4-related disease
- **Tumors:** Craniopharyngioma, pinealoma, meningioma, germinoma, lymphoma, metastatic disease, cysts
- **Aneurysms:** Particularly anterior communicating
- **Inflammatory states and granulomatous disease:** Acute meningitis/encephalitis, langerhans cell histiocytosis, neurosarcoidosis, tuberculosis
- **Drugs:** Ethanol (transient), phenytoin
- **Genetic:** Neurophysin II (AVP carrier protein) gene defect

Nephrogenic Diabetes Insipidus (Decreased Responsiveness of the Kidney to Vasopressin)

- **Genetic:** V2-receptor defects, aquaporin defects (AQP2 and AQP1); 90% by AVPR2 mutations (X-liked recessive), AQP2 gene mutation
- **Structural:** Urinary tract obstruction, papillary necrosis, sickle-cell nephropathy
- **Tubulointerstitial disease:** Medullary cystic disease, polycystic kidney disease, nephrocalcinosis, Sjögren's syndrome, lupus, analgesic-abuse nephropathy, sarcoidosis, M-protein disease, cystinosis, nephronophthisis
- **Others:** Distal renal tubular acidosis, Bartter syndrome, apparent mineralocorticoid excess
- **Electrolyte disorders:** Hypercalcemia, hypokalemia
- **Any prolonged state of severe polyuria:** By washing out the renal medullary-intramedullary concentration gradient needed for urinary concentration, and by down-regulating kidney AQP2 water channels (partial diabetes insipidus)
- Medications that induce nephrogenic diabetes insipidus
  - Lithium (40% of patients)
  - Amphotericin B
  - Demeclocycline
  - Dopamine
  - Ofloxacin
  - Orlistat
  - Ifosfamide
- Medications that possibly cause nephrogenic diabetes insipidus
  - Contrast agents
  - Cyclophosphamide
  - Cidofovir

- Ethanol
- Foscarnet
- Indinavir
- Libenzapril
- Mesalazine
- Methoxyflurane
- Pimozide
- Rifampin
- Streptozocin
- Tenofir
- Triamterene hydrochloride
- Cholchicine

Adipsic Diabetes Insipidus (Central Diabetes Insipidus with Deficient Thirst)

This is caused by a combination of damage to the osmoreceptors regulating thirst sensation and central diabetes insipidus (see above).

- Congenital conditions (septo-optic dysplasia, germinoma)
- Vascular (anterior communicating artery aneurysm clipping/rupture)
- Others (craniopharyngioma, pinealoma, Langerhans cell histiocytosis, neurosarcoidosis, head trauma, cytomegalovirus encephalitis)

GESTATIONAL DIABETES INSIPIDUS

In this form of diabetes insipidus, AVP is rapidly degraded by a high circulating level of oxytocinase/vasopressinase. It is a rare condition, because increased AVP secretion will compensate for the increased rate of degradation. Gestational diabetes insipidus occurs only in combination with impaired AVP production.

Hypertonic Sodium Gain

Patients with hypertonic sodium gain have high total-body sodium and an extracellular volume overload (rare, mostly iatrogenic). When thirst and renal function are intact, this condition is transient.

- Administration of hypertonic electrolyte solutions, i.e. sodium bicarbonate solutions, hypertonic alimentation solutions, normal saline with or without potassium supplements
- Sodium ingestion—NaCl tablets, seawater ingestion
- Sodium modeling in hemodialysis

Water Shift (Transient)

Water shift occurs into muscle cells during extreme exercise or seizures (caused by increased intracellular osmoles).

In clinical practice, a combination of the above may be present, i.e. an intubated patient in the ICU develops hypernatremia due to hypertonic sodium gain caused by normal saline volume resuscitation and, in addition, increased free water excretion due to recovering renal failure and/or osmotic urea-diuresis caused by high-protein tube feeding.

CLASSIFICATION OF HYPERNATREMIA

A hyperosmolar condition caused by a decrease in total body water relative to electrolyte content. Hypernatremia is classified according to the patient's state of hydration and on the content of sodium as hypovolemic, euvolemic, and hypervolemic. Even the concentrations of sodium in urine are often of great importance for a correct diagnosis

Hypovolemic Hypernatremia

Hypernatremia associated with hypovolemia occurs with Na^+ loss accompanied by a relatively greater loss of water from the body. Common extrarenal causes include most of those that cause hyponatremia and volume depletion. Either hypernatremia or hyponatremia can occur with severe volume loss, depending on the relative amounts of Na^+ and water lost and the amount of water ingested before presentation.

Renal causes of hypernatremia and volume depletion include therapy with diuretics. Loop diuretics inhibit Na^+ reabsorption in the concentrating portion of the nephrons and can increase water clearance. Osmotic diuresis can also impair renal concentrating capacity because of a hypertonic substance present in the tubular lumen of the distal nephron. Glycerol, mannitol, and occasionally urea can cause osmotic diuresis resulting in hypernatremia. The most common cause of hypernatremia due to osmotic diuresis is hyperglycemia in patients with diabetes. Because glucose does not penetrate cells in the absence of insulin, hyperglycemia further dehydrates the ICF compartment. The degree of hyperosmolality in hyperglycemia may be obscured by the lowering of serum Na^+ resulting from movement of water out of cells into the ECF (translational hyponatremia, see hyponatremia). Patients with renal disease can also be predisposed to hypernatremia when their kidneys are unable to maximally concentrate urine.

Euvolemic Hypernatremia

Hypernatremia with euvolemia is a decrease in total body water with near normal total body Na^+ (pure water deficit). Extrarenal causes of water loss, such as excessive sweating, result in some Na^+ loss, but because sweat is hypotonic, hypernatremia can result before significant hypovolemia. A deficit of almost purely water also occurs in central and nephrogenic diabetes insipidus.

Essential hypernatremia (primary hypodipsia) occasionally occurs in children with brain damage and in chronically ill elderly adults. It is characterized by an impaired thirst mechanism, e.g. caused by lesions of the brain's thirst center). Altered osmotic trigger for ADH release is another possible cause of euvolemic hyper-natremia; some lesions cause both an impaired thirst mechanism and an altered osmotic trigger. The nonosmotic release of ADH appears intact, and these patients are generally euvolemic.

Hypervolemic Hypernatremia

Hypernatremia in rare cases is associated with volume overload. In this case, hypernatremia results from a grossly elevated Na^+ intake associated with limited access to water. One example is the excessive administration of hypertonic $NaHCO_3$ during treatment of lactic acidosis. Hypernatremia can also be caused by the administration of hypertonic saline or incorrectly formulated hyper-alimentation.

Hypernatremia in the Elderly

Hypernatremia is common among the elderly, particularly postoperative patients and those receiving tube feedings or parenteral nutrition. Other contributing factors may include the following:
- Dependence on others to obtain water
- Impaired thirst mechanism
- Impaired renal concentrating capacity (due to diuretics, impaired ADH release, or nephron loss accompanying aging or other renal disease)
- Impaired angiotensin II production (which may contribute directly to the impaired thirst mechanism)

PATIENT HISTORY

Patients developing hypernatremia outside of the hospital setting are generally elderly and debilitated, and often present with an intercurrent acute (febrile) illness. Hospital-acquired hypernatremia affects patients of all ages.

The history should be used to discover why the patient was unable to prevent hypernatremia with adequate oral fluid intake, e.g. it should be determined whether the patient is suffering from an altered mental status or whether there are any factors causing increased fluid excretion (e.g. the use of diuretic therapy, the existence of diabetes mellitus, or the occurrence of fever, diarrhea, and vomiting). The history should also cover the symptoms and causes of possible diabetes insipidus (e.g. the presence of pre-existing polydipsia or polyuria, a history of cerebral pathology, or medication use like lithium).

It is important to find out if the hypernatremia developed acutely or over time, because this will guide treatment decisions.

Risk factors for hypernatremia include the following:

- Advanced age
- Mental or physical impairment
- Uncontrolled diabetes (solute diuresis)
- Underlying polyuria disorders
- Diuretic therapy
- Residency in nursing home, inadequate nursing care
- Hospitalization
  - Decreased baseline levels of consciousness
  - Tube feeding
  - Hypertonic infusions
  - Osmotic diuresis
  - Lactulose
  - Mechanical ventilation
  - Medication (e.g. diuretics, sedatives)

SYMPTOMS AND SIGNS

The major symptom of hypernatremia is thirst. The absence of thirst in conscious patients with hyper-natremia suggests an impaired thirst mechanism. Patients with difficulty communicating may be unable to express thirst or obtain access to water.

The major signs of hypernatremia result from CNS dysfunction due to brain cell shrinkage. Confusion, neuromuscular excitability, hyperreflexia, seizures, or coma may result. Cerebrovascular damage with subcortical or subarachnoid hemorrhage and venous thrombosis are common among patients who died of severe hypernatremia.

In chronic hypernatremia, osmotically active substances occur in CNS cells (idiogenic osmoles) and increase intracellular osmolality. Therefore, the degree of brain cell dehydration and resultant CNS symptoms are less severe in chronic than in acute hypernatremia.

When hypernatremia occurs with abnormal total body Na^+, the typical symptoms of volume depletion or overload are present. Patients with renal concentrating defects typically excrete a large volume of hypotonic urine. When losses are extrarenal, the route of water loss is often evident (e.g. vomiting, diarrhea, excessive sweating), and the urinary Na^+ concentration is low.

Diagnosis

Figure 3.4 illustrates important causes of hypernatremia correlating with the bedside determination of the ECF volume status. Patients with euvolemia usually have had a pure water loss. Patients with evidence of reduced ECF volume and hypernatremia have predominantly developed a water loss; however, they have also had some loss of sodium from the ECF to account for the clinical signs of hypovolemia.

Accurate diagnosis requires that the clinician uncover the source of water loss or sodium gain. A careful assessment of the patient's volume status, access to water, ongoing water losses, and renal response to water loss are also important. Additionally, if impaired thirst is present, the clinician should inquire into possible causes, such as delirium (e.g. from any cause) or the development of a new lesion in the CNS (e.g. stroke).

Whereas the cause of hypernatremia is usually apparent (e.g. diarrhea), the urine osmolality may be useful in clarifying the cause in patients without obvious

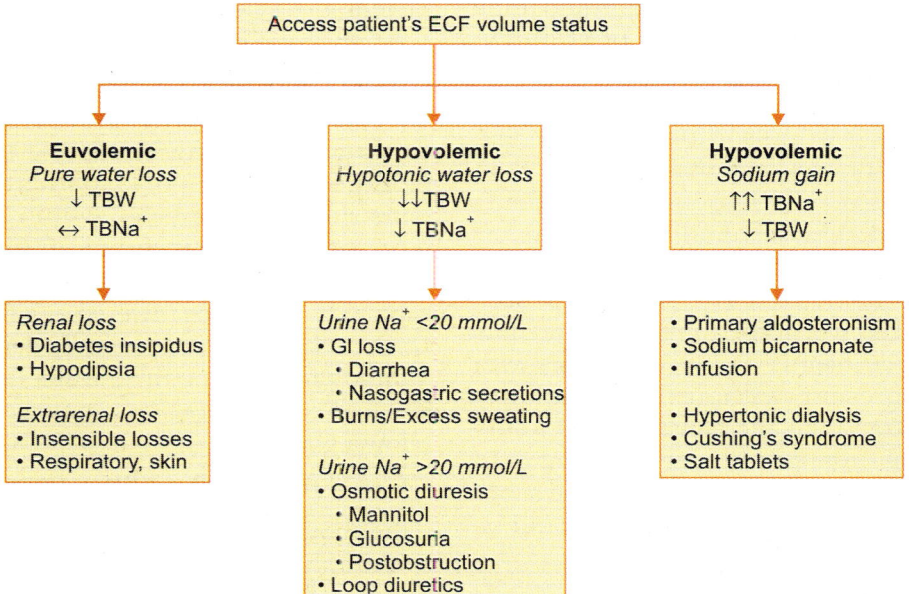

Fig. 3.4: Important causes of hypernatremia correlating with the bedside determination of the ECF volume status

GI or insensible water losses. During hypernatremia caused by extrarenal water losses, the renal response should be to generate hypertonic urine with an osmolality of 700–800 mOsm/kg.

If the urine osmolality (uOsm) is lower than 300 mOsm/kg, then water loss is occurring via the kidneys, secondary to decreased hypothalamic release of ADH (central diabetes insipidus) or impaired sensation in the cortical collecting tubule (nephrogenic diabetes insipidus). In central diabetes insipidus, provision of ADH results in an increase in uOsm, whereas in nephrogenic diabetes insipidus, it results in little to no increase in uOsm.

If uOsm is between 300 mOsm and 800 mOsm/kg, patients might have partial forms of nephrogenic or central diabetes insipidus or an osmotic diuresis from urea or glucose. In patients believed to have diabetes insipidus, a water deprivation test can be performed to assess the integrity of pituitary release and renal response to ADH.

LABORATORY TESTING

An assessment of clinical circumstances, acuity, and volume status is of paramount importance in the management of hypernatremia. Patients with hypotonic fluid loss can be more hypovolemic if potassium is also lost concurrently. Pure water loss is associated with a lesser degree of ECF volume contraction than hypotonic fluid loss as most of the lost water comes from ICF compartment. As a result hypovolemia may not be evident clinically in patients who have lost pure water, i.e. diabetes insipidus and insensible losses. Serum glucose should be checked in all patients to rule out osmotic diuresis. Measurement of urine output and urine osmolality helps in the determination of etiology. Measurement of urine Na^+ can help in the assessment of the volume status of the patient. Diuretic use can confuse the picture by altering urine sodium. A low urine Na^+ (<10 mmol/L) with urine osmolality greater than 800 mOsm/kg H_2O is seen in hypovolemic patients with extra renal and remote renal fluid losses or inadequate water intake. An elevation of urine osmolality with urine sodium greater than 100 mmol/L can be seen in patients who have received hypertonic fluids and thus have developed hypervolemia. Polyuric patients with osmotic diuresis present with urine osmolality greater than 300 mOsmol/kg and elevated total solute excretion. A 24 hours urine solute output greater than 900 mOsmol/day suggests osmotic diuresis or the use of diuretics. Urine glucose and urea nitrogen should be measured if osmotic diuresis is suspected.

In diabetes insipidus total daily solute excretion is normal. Water deprivation test can differentiate between different types of DI. In complete central and nephrogenic DI, urine osmolality is generally less than 300 mOsmol/kg. It can be differentiated further. More than 50% rise in urine osmolality by desmopressin administration indicates complete central DI, whereas a lack of response indicates complete nephrogenic DI. In partial diabetes insipidus, urine osmolality can be between 300 mOsmol and 800 mOsmol/kg in response to a water deprivation test. A distinction between partial central and partial nephrogenic DI can be made during water deprivation test by the concurrent measurements of plasma osmolality, urine osmolality and vasopressin level. It may require the administration of hypertonic saline.

Serum creatinine, potassium, calcium, osmolality, and blood urea nitrogen should also be checked in all patients. Further laboratory and radiological tests may be needed for specific etiologies especially, if an abnormality in hypothalamic neurohypophyseal region is suspected.

Management and Treatment

The management and treatment of hypernatremia involves the following principles:
- Replacement of intravascular volume and of free water
- Correction of the underlying cause of water loss

Importantly, if hypovolemia is present, plasma volume should be restored with isotonic saline or colloid before the correction of the water deficit. Correction of the underlying cause of the water losses can include withdrawal of loop diuretics or mannitol, treatment of diarrhea with antimotility agents or antibiotics, provision of ADH to correct central diabetes insipidus, or use of pharmacologic agents to treat nephrogenic diabetes insipidus.

Oral hydration is effective in conscious patients without significant GI dysfunction. In severe hypernatremia or in patients unable to drink because of continued vomiting or mental status changes, IV hydration is preferred. Hypernatremia that lasts <24 hours should be corrected within 24 hours. However, hypernatremia that is chronic or of unknown duration should be corrected over 48 hours, and the serum osmolality should be lowered at a rate of no faster than 2 mOsm/L/h to avoid cerebral edema caused by excess brain solute. The amount of water (in liters) necessary to replace existing deficits may be estimated by the following formula:

$$\text{Free water deficit} = TBW \times [(\text{serum } Na^+/140) - 1]$$

In the above equation, TBW is in liters and is estimated by multiplying weight in kilograms by 0.6; serum Na^+ is in mmol/L. This formula assumes constant total body Na^+ content. In patients with hypernatremia and depletion of total body Na^+ content (i.e. who have volume depletion), the free water deficit is greater than that estimated by the formula.

In patients with hypernatremia and ECF volume overload (excess total body Na^+ content), the free water deficit can be replaced with 5% D/W, which can be supplemented with a loop diuretic. However, too rapid infusion of 5% D/W may cause glucosuria, thereby increasing salt-free water excretion and hypertonicity, especially in patients with diabetes mellitus. Other electrolytes, including serum K^+, should be monitored and should be replaced as needed.

In patients with hypernatremia and euvolemia, free water can be replaced using either 5% D/W or 0.45% saline.

Treatment of patients with central diabetes insipidus is discussed in discussed in Treatment. Acquired nephrogenic diabetes insipidus is also discussed in discussed in Nephrogenic Diabetes Insipidus.

In patients with hypernatremia and hypovolemia, particularly in patients with diabetes with nonketotic hyperglycemic coma, 0.45% saline can be given as an alternative to a combination of 0.9% normal saline and 5% D/W to replenish Na^+ and free water. Alternatively, ECF volume and free water can be replaced separately, using the formula given previously to estimate the free water deficit. When severe acidosis (pH < 7.10) is present, $NaHCO_3$ solution can be added to 5% D/W or 0.45% saline, as long as the final solution remains hypotonic.

Laboratory Assessment of Water and Sodium Status

Plasma sodium concentration is dependent on the relative amounts of sodium and water in the plasma. In isolation, therefore, plasma sodium concentration provides no information about the sodium content of the ECF. It may be raised, normal or low, in states of sodium excess or depletion, according to the amount of water in the ECF.

The plasma sodium concentration is one of the most frequent measurements made in clinical chemistry laboratories (largely for historical reasons), but definite indications for its measurement are few and results are often misinterpreted. Plasma sodium concentration should be measured in the following:

1. Patients with dehydration or excessive fluid loss, as a guide to appropriate replacement
2. Patients on parenteral fluid replacement who are unable to indicate or respond to thirst (e.g. the comatose, infants, and the elderly)
3. Patients with unexplained confusion, abnormal behavior, or signs of CNS irritability

In the assessment of a patient's water and sodium status, clinical observations, such as measurements of central venous pressure, fluid balance and body weight, may all provide vital information. An increase in the concentration of plasma proteins or in the hematocrit suggests hemoconcentration. Other abnormal results may suggest specific conditions; i.e. hyperkalemia in a hyponatremic patient with clinical evidence of sodium depletion suggests adrenal failure.

Analysis of urine can provide valuable information, but results may be misleading. It should be established whether the urine volume and composition are physiologically appropriate for the patient's water and sodium status. If they are not, the reason should be sought, i.e. a low urinary sodium excretion is to be expected in a patient with hyponatremia who is sodium depleted (unless this is due to renal sodium loss; natriuresis in such a patient would imply either a failure of aldosterone secretion or a failure of the kidney to respond to the hormone.

MEASUREMENT OF SODIUM

Through the years, Na^+ has been measured in various ways, including chemical methods, flame emission spectrophotometry (FES), atomic absorption spectro-photometry (AAS), and ion-selective electrodes (ISEs). Chemical methods are outdated because of large sample volume requirements and lack of precision. ISEs are the most routinely used method in clinical laboratories.

Ion-selective electrode method uses a semipermeable membrane to develop a potential produced by having different ion concentrations on either side of the membrane. In this type system, two electrodes are used. One electrode has a constant potential, making it the reference electrode. The difference in potential between the reference and measuring electrodes can be used to calculate the 'concentration' of the ion in solution. However, it is the activity of the ion, not the concentration that is being measured.

Most analyzers use a glass ion-exchange membrane in its ISE system for Na^+ measurement. There are two types of ISE measurement, based on sample preparation, i.e. direct and indirect. Direct measurement provides an undiluted sample to interact with the ISE membrane. With the indirect method, a diluted sample is used for measurement. There is no significant difference in results, except when samples are hyperlipidemic or hyper-proteinemic. Excess lipids or proteins displace plasma water, which leads to a falsely decreased measurement of ionic activity in millimoles per liter of plasma, whereas the direct method measures in plasma water only. In these cases, direct ISE is more accurate.

One source of error with ISEs is protein buildup on the membrane through continuous use. The protein-coated membranes cause poor selectivity, which results in poor reproducibility of results.

Specimen Requirements

Serum, plasma, and urine are all acceptable for Na^+ measurements. When plasma is used, lithium heparin, ammonium heparin, and lithium oxalate are suitable anticoagulants. Hemolysis does not cause a significant change in serum or plasma values as a result of decreased levels of intracellular Na^+. However, with marked hemolysis, levels may be decreased as a result of a dilutional effect.

Whole blood samples may be used with some analyzers. Consult the instrument operation manual for acceptability. The specimen of choice in urine Na^+ analyses is a 24-hour collection.

POTASSIUM

Potassium (K^+) is the major intracellular cation found inside the cells. Potassium is essential for the proper functioning of the heart, kidneys, muscles, nerves, and digestive system. The normal blood potassium level is 3.5–5.0 mmol/L.

Total body potassium content is approximately 50 mmol per kilogram body weight. Therefore, a 70 kilogram person has about 3500 mmol total body potassium, 98% of which is in the intracellular compartment. The sodium potassium ATPase is the major cellular enzyme responsible for maintaining very low intracellular Na^+ concentration and increased potassium intracellular concentration.

Although, only 2% of total body potassium (70–100 mmol) remains in the extracellular compartment; the extracellular potassium concentration plays a critical role in maintaining cell membrane resting potential. This is particularly important for electrically excitable cells, (muscle and nervous system activity). The proper level of potassium is essential for normal cell function. Among the many functions of potassium in the body are regulation of the heartbeat and the function of the muscles.

A seriously abnormal increase or decrease in potassium can profoundly affect the nervous system and increases the chance of irregular heartbeats (arrhythmias), which, when extreme, can be fatal.

In combination with other minerals in the body, potassium forms alkaline salts that are important in body processes and play an essential role in maintenance of the acid-base and water balance in the body. All body cells, especially muscle tissue, require a high content of potassium. A proper balance between sodium, calcium, and potassium in the blood plasma is necessary for proper cardiac function.

Potassium intake and excretion determine the total body potassium content. Equally important is the distribution of potassium between extracellular and intracellular fluid. If potassium intake were not matched by excretion, high serum potassium would soon result. Under normal circumstances salivary and gastro-intestinal potassium losses are minor; therefore, excretion of potassium by the kidneys is vital.

On the other hand, the fluid that is filtered by the kidneys contains much more potassium than is present in the extra cellular fluid. Therefore, reabsorption of potassium by the kidneys is also vital to normal potassium balance.

Regulation

K^+ is a major determinant of intracellular osmolality. The ratio between K^+ concentration in the ICF and ECF strongly influences cell membrane polarization, which in turn influences important cell processes, such as the conduction of nerve impulses and muscle (including myocardial) cell contraction. Thus, relatively small alterations in serum K^+ concentration can have significant clinical manifestations.

In the absence of factors that shift K^+ in or out of cells (K^+ shifts), the serum K^+ concentration correlates closely with total body K^+ content. Once intracellular and extracellular concentrations are stable, a decrease in serum K^+ concentration of about 1 mmol/L indicates a total K deficit of about 200–400 mmol. Patients with $K^+ < 3$ mmol/L typically have a significant K^+ deficit.

K^+ Shifts

Factors that shift K^+ in or out of cells include the following:
1. **Insulin concentrations:** Insulin moves K^+ into cells; high concentrations of insulin thus lower serum K^+ concentration. Low concentrations of insulin, as in diabetic ketoacidosis, cause K^+ to move out of cells, thus raising serum K^+, sometimes even in the presence of total body K^+ deficiency.
2. **β-adrenergic activity:** β-adrenergic agonists, especially selective β_2-agonists, move K^+ into cells, whereas β-blockade and β-agonists promote movement of K^+ out of cells.
3. **Acid-base status:** Acute metabolic acidosis causes K^+ to move out of cells, whereas acute metabolic alkalosis causes K^+ to move into cells. However, changes in serum HCO_3^- concentration may be more important than changes in pH; acidosis caused by accumulation of mineral acids (non-anion gap, hyperchloremic acidosis) is more likely to elevate serum K^+. In contrast, metabolic acidosis due to accumulation of organic acids (increased anion gap (AG) acidosis) does not cause hyperkalemia. Thus, the hyperkalemia common in diabetic ketoacidosis results more from insulin deficiency than from acidosis. Acute respiratory acidosis and alkalosis affect serum K^+ concentration

less than metabolic acidosis and alkalosis. Nonetheless, serum K^+ concentration should always be interpreted in the context of the serum pH (and HCO_3^- concentration).

The kidneys are important in the regulation of K^+ balance. Initially, the proximal tubules reabsorb nearly all the K^+. Then, under the influence of aldosterone, additional K^+ is secreted into the urine in exchange for Na^+ in both the distal tubules and the collecting ducts. Thus, the distal nephron is the principal determinant of urinary K^+ excretion. Most individuals consume far more K^+ than needed; the excess is excreted in the urine but may accumulate to toxic levels if renal failure occurs.

K^+ uptake from the ECF into the cells is important in normalizing an acute rise in plasma K^+ concentration due to an increased K^+ intake. Excess plasma K^+ rapidly enters the cells to normalize plasma K^+. As the cellular K^+ gradually returns to the plasma, it is removed by urinary excretion. Note that chronic loss of cellular K^+ may result in cellular depletion before there is an appreciable change in the plasma K^+ concentration because excess K^+ is normally excreted in the urine.

Dietary K^+ intake normally varies between 40 mmol/day and 150 mmol/day. In the steady state, fecal losses are usually close to 10% of intake. The remaining 90% is excreted in the urine so alternations in renal K^+ secretion greatly affect K^+ balance.

When K^+ intake is >150 mmol/day, about 50% of the excess K^+ appears in the urine over the next several hours. Most of the remainder is transferred into the intracellular compartment, thus minimizing the rise in serum K^+. When elevated K^+ intake continues, aldosterone secretion is stimulated and thus renal K^+ excretion rises. In addition, K^+ absorption from stool appears to be under some regulation and may fall by 50% in chronic K^+ excess.

When K^+ intake falls, intracellular K^+ again serves to buffer wide swings in serum K+ concentration. Renal K^+ conservation develops relatively slowly in response to decreases in dietary K^+ and is far less efficient than the kidneys' ability to conserve Na^+. Thus, K^+ depletion is a frequent clinical problem. Urinary K^+ excretion of 10 mmol/day represents near maximal renal K^+ conservation and implies significant K^+ depletion.

Acute acidosis impairs K^+ excretion, whereas chronic acidosis and acute alkalosis can promote K^+ excretion. Increased delivery of Na^+ to the distal nephrons, as occurs with high Na^+ intake or loop diuretic therapy, promotes K^+ excretion.

Dietary deficiency or excess is rarely a primary cause of hypokalemia or hyperkalemia. However, with a pre-existing condition, dietary deficiency or excess can enhance the degree of hypokalemia or hyperkalemia.

POTASSIUM DEPLETION AND HYPOKALEMIA

Hypokalemia is probably the most common electrolyte abnormality in hospitalized patients. It is usually defined as serum potassium of less than 3.5 mmol/L. Patients with mild hypokalemia (serum potassium 3.0–3.5 mmol/L), usually have no symptoms. However, with more severe hypokalemia (serum potassium of <2.5 mmol/L), generalized weakness can occur. In addition, patients with severe hypokalemia can develop muscle necrosis (rhabdomyolysis) and paralysis. Both mild and severe hypokalemia can increase the incidence of cardiac arrhythmias.

The most common causes are excess losses from the kidneys or GI tract. Clinical features include muscle weakness and polyuria; cardiac hyper excitability may occur with severe hypokalemia.

Etiology

Hypokalemia can result from increased loss, transcellular shift, or decreased intake of potassium. Increased potassium loss (through the kidney or gastrointestinal tract) is the most common cause of hypokalemia. Less frequently, hypokalemia can occur as a result of shift of potassium from the extracellular space into cells. Rarely, hypokalemia can result from decreased intake of potassium. Increased potassium loss, which is the most common cause of hypokalemia, occurs mostly in patients who are on diuretics (thiazide or loop diuretics) or in patients with gastrointestinal diseases (diarrhea).

GI Tract Losses

Abnormal GI K^+ losses occur in all of the following:
- Chronic diarrhea, including chronic laxative abuse and bowel diversion
- Clay (bentonite) ingestion, which binds K^+ and greatly decreases absorption
- Vomiting
- Protracted gastric suction (which removes volume and HCl, causing the kidneys to excrete HCO_3^- and, to electrically balance lost HCO_3^-, K^+)
- Rarely, villous adenoma of the colon, which causes massive K secretion

GI K^+ losses may be compounded by concomitant renal K^+ losses due to metabolic alkalosis and stimulation of aldosterone due to volume depletion.

Intracellular Shift

The transcellular shift of K^+ into cells may also cause hypokalemia. This shift can occur in any of the following:
- Glycogenesis during total parenteral nutrition (TPN) or enteral hyper alimentation (stimulating insulin release)
- After administration of insulin

- Stimulation of the sympathetic nervous system, particularly with β_2-agonists (e.g. albuterol, terbutaline), which may increase cellular K^+ uptake
- Thyrotoxicosis (occasionally) due to excessive β-sympathetic stimulation (hypokalemic thyrotoxic periodic paralysis)
- Familial periodic paralysis

Familial periodic paralysis which is a rare autosomal dominant disorder characterized by transient episodes of profound hypokalemia thought to be due to sudden abnormal shifts of K^+ into cells. Episodes frequently involve varying degrees of paralysis. They are typically precipitated by a large carbohydrate meal or strenuous exercise.

RENAL LOSSES

Various disorders can increase renal K^+ excretion. Excess mineralocorticoid effect can directly increase K^+ secretion by the distal nephrons and occurs in any of the following:

- Adrenal steroid excess that is due to Cushing syndrome, primary hyperaldosteronism, rare renin-secreting tumors, glucocorticoid-remediable aldosteronism (a rare inherited disorder involving abnormal aldosterone metabolism), and congenital adrenal hyperplasia.
- Ingestion of substances, such as glycyrrhizin (present in natural licorice and used in the manufacture of chewing tobacco), which inhibits the enzyme 11β-hydroxysteroid dehydrogenase (11β-HSDH), preventing the conversion of cortisol, which has some mineralocorticoid activity, to cortisone, which does not, resulting in high circulating concentrations of cortisol and renal K^+ wasting.
- Bartter syndrome, an uncommon genetic disorder that is characterized by renal K^+ and Na^+ wasting, excessive production of renin and aldosterone, and normotension. Bartter syndrome which is caused by mutations in a loop diuretic-sensitive ion transport mechanism in the loop of Henle.
- Gitelman syndrome is an uncommon genetic disorder characterized by renal K^+ and Na^+ wasting, excessive production of renin and aldosterone, and normotension. Gitelman syndrome is caused by loss of function mutations in a thiazide-sensitive ion transport mechanism in the distal nephron.

Liddle syndrome which is a rare autosomal dominant disorder characterized by severe hypertension and hypokalemia. Liddle syndrome is caused by unrestrained Na^+ reabsorption in the distal nephron due to one of several mutations found in genes encoding for epithelial Na^+ channel subunits. Inappropriately high reabsorption of Na^+ results in both hypertension and renal K^+ wasting.

Renal K^+ wasting can also be caused by numerous congenital and acquired renal tubular diseases, such as the renal tubular acidosis and Fanconi syndrome, an unusual syndrome resulting in renal wasting of K^+, glucose, phosphate, uric acid, and amino acids.

Magnesium depletion, which is caused by either decreased dietary intake or increased loss, is a common electrolyte disorder in hospitalized patients. It can cause severe hypokalemia by increasing renal potassium loss. The exact mechanism is, however, remains unclear. Hypokalemia is also a common finding in patients with raised serum aldosterone either secondary to the activation of the renin-angiotensin system (Bartter syndrome or Gitelman syndrome) or due to overproduction by aldosterone-producing tumors (primary aldosteronism).

DRUGS

Diuretics are by far the most commonly used drugs that cause hypokalemia. K^+ wasting diuretics that block Na^+ reabsorption proximal to the distal nephron include:

- Thiazides
- Loop diuretics
- Osmotic diuretics

By inducing diarrhea, laxatives, especially when abused, can cause hypokalemia. Surreptitious diuretic or laxative use or both is a frequent cause of persistent hypokalemia, particularly among patients preoccupied with weight loss and among health care practitioners with access to prescription drugs.

Other drugs that can cause hypokalemia include:

- Amphotericin B
- Antipseudomonal penicillins, e.g. carbenicillin)
- Penicillin in high doses
- Theophylline (both acute and chronic intoxication)

Pseudohypokalemia

Pseudohypokalemia or falsely low serum K^+ occasionally is found when blood specimens from patients with chronic myelocytic leukemia and a WBC count >10^5/μL remain at room temperature before being processed because of uptake of serum K^+ by abnormal leukocytes in the sample. It is prevented by prompt separation of plasma or serum in blood samples.

Symptoms and Signs

Hypokalemia is often asymptomatic; this is specifically true in patients with mild hypokalemia (serum potassium 3.0–3.5 mmol/L). Patients with more severe hypokalemia (serum potassium less than 2.5 mmol/L) usually present with generalized weakness and, in some cases, ascending paralysis. In addition, severe hypokalemia can precipitate rhabdomyolysis, which manifests as muscle tenderness and swelling. Cardiac arrhythmias are common in hypokalemia, specifically in patients with underlying heart disease or on digoxin. In moderate to severe hypokalemia changes in ECG are minimal and are often limited to the presence of a U wave.

Renal Syndromes Associated with Hypokalemia

In addition to the above clinical symptoms, hypokalemia can cause several distinct renal syndromes as the following:

Nephrogenic Diabetes Insipidus

Hypokalemia can impair urinary concentrating mechanism and result in nephrogenic diabetes insipidus. Patients with nephrogenic diabetes insipidus due to hypokalemia present with polyuria and polydipsia. Molecular studies have demonstrated that potassium depletion causes down regulation of the water channel aquaporin 2 in the collecting duct, therefore impairing the renal concentrating mechanism and resulting in polyuria.

Metabolic Alkalosis

Hypokalemia can contribute to the maintenance of metabolic alkalosis in several disease states (such as vomiting) by enhancing bicarbonate absorbing ability of renal tubules. This in turn decreases the ability of the kidney to excrete the excess bicarbonate and as a result maintains the plasma bicarbonate at a raised level. Functional and molecular studies in luminal and basolateral membranes of kidney proximal tubules and in microperfused kidney nephrons have demonstrated that hypokalemia up regulates the expression of bicarbonate absorbing transporters in proximal tubules and cortical and medullary collecting ducts. There is also evidence in support of hypokalemia being involved in the generation of metabolic alkalosis in human by increasing ammoniagenesis.

ENHANCED RENAL CHLORIDE EXCRETION

Hypokalemia increases urinary chloride excretion. Functional and molecular studies in the kidney have demonstrated that renal chloride wasting in hypokalemia is due to suppression of the apical sodium potassium chloride cotransporter in the thick limb of Henle and the apical sodium chloride cotransporter in the distal convoluted tubule. It is possible that by increasing renal chloride excretion, hypokalemia can result in hypochloremia, which in turn can contribute to the maintenance of metabolic alkalosis in pathophysiological states.

Diagnosis

When hypokalemia is reported, the initial step is to ascertain whether it is associated with clinical symptoms or arrhythmias that would require prompt intervention. In the absence of compelling indications for immediate therapy, a careful history and physical examination should be performed. Important clinical clues, such as medication, vomiting, and hypertension should be specifically sought. Factitious or spurious hypokalemia, which can occur in patients with leukemia or elevated white cell counts because K^+ is taken up by these metabolically active cells in the test tube, should be ruled out. If true hypokalemia is present, then determine whether it was caused by a transcellular shift or a decrease in total body potassium. Hypokalemia from transcellular shift is managed by treating the underlying condition or removing the offending agent. Decreased total body K^+ requires further diagnostic workup. Urine potassium, chloride, creatinine, and serum aldosterone levels are determined to distinguish the causes of extrarenal and renal losses of K^+, so that the primary condition can be treated, in addition to replacement therapy (as shown in Fig. 3.5).

Hypokalemia is usually diagnosed by the following: Serum K^+ measurement of less than 3.5 mmol/L, may be found on routine serum electrolyte measurement. It should be suspected in patients with typical changes on an ECG or who have muscular symptoms and risk factors and confirmed by blood testing.

Electrocardiography (ECG) should be done on patients with hypokalemia. Cardiac effects of hypokalemia are usually minimal until serum K^+ concentrations are <3 mmol/L. Hypokalemia causes sagging of the ST segment, depression of the T wave, and elevation of the U wave. With marked hypokalemia, the T wave becomes progressively smaller and the U wave becomes increasingly larger. Sometimes, a flat or positive T wave merges with a positive U wave, which may be confused with QT prolongation (as shown in Fig. 3.6). Hypokalemia may cause premature ventricular and atrial contractions, ventricular and atrial tachyarrhythmias, and second- or third-degree atrioventricular block. Such arrhythmias become more severe with increasingly severe hypokalemia; eventually, ventricular fibrillation may occur. Patients with significant pre-existing heart disease and patients receiving digoxin, when the mechanism not evident clinically, 24-hour urinary K^+ excretion and serum Mg^{2+} concentration is measured.

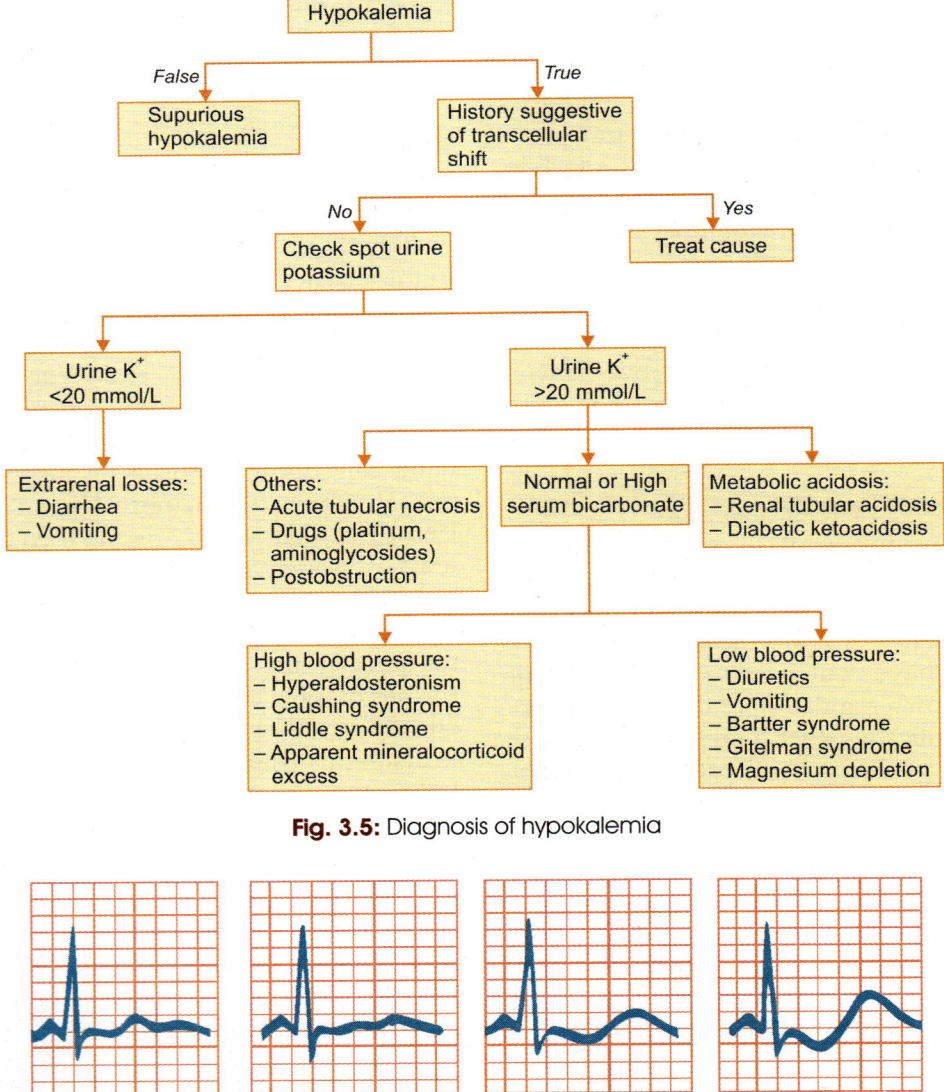

Fig. 3.5: Diagnosis of hypokalemia

Fig. 3.6: ECG patterns in hypokalemia

Management of Hypokalemia

The management of hypokalemia is almost always by potassium replacement, with the amount of potassium supplement depending on the severity of hypokalemia (listed in the Table 3.8).

Table 3.8	Treatment of hypokalemia

1. **Intravenous potassium (as potassium chloride)**
   - Usually, reserved for severe hypokalemia (serum potassium of <2.6 mmol/L).
   - The rate of should not exceed 20 mmol/hour.
2. **Oral potassium**
   - Potassium chloride: 40–100 mmol/day in divided doses
   - Potassium phosphate (in patients with hypokalemia and hypophosphatemia).
   - Potassium bicarbonate (in patients with acidosis)

The potassium can be given orally (in mild to moderate hypokalemia) or intravenously (in severe hypokalemia). When given intravenously, the rate of potassium administration should not exceed 20 mmol/hour. To calculate the amount of potassium supplement, one should have an estimate of the potassium deficit. On average, a reduction of serum potassium by 0.3 mmol/L suggests a total body deficit of 100 mmol. Based on this formula, a patient with serum potassium of 2.6 mmol/L needs at least 300 mmol of potassium for the correction of the deficit. In calculating the total body potassium deficit one has to consider factors that can independently affect serum potassium. A patient with serum potassium of 2.6 mmol/L has less total body deficit at blood pH of 7.5 than 7.3. The reason is that alkaline serum pH (that is, 7.5) can independently lower the serum potassium by intracellular shift. Potassium phosphate and potassium bicarbonate can be used in certain conditions. Potassium phosphate can be used in patients with combined potassium and phosphate depletion, e.g. in patients with liver cirrhosis or diabetic ketoacidosis). Potassium bicarbonate can be used in patients with potassium depletion and metabolic acidosis, e.g. in distal renal tubular acidosis). Aside from intravenous potassium chloride for severe hypokalemia, mild or moderate hypokalemia can be treated with oral potassium chloride. Usually, 50–100 mmol of potassium chloride is required per day to maintain serum potassium concentration within the normal range in patients with increased potassium loss (that is, in patients receiving a diuretic).

POTASSIUM EXCESS AND HYPERKALEMIA

Potassium excess can be due to excessive intake or decreased excretion. A normal intake may be excessive if excretion is decreased, e.g. in renal failure). Hyperkalemia is defined as a serum potassium concentration higher than 5.0 mmol/L, and severe hyperkalemia is defined as a serum potassium concentration higher than 6.5 mmol/L. An elevated potassium level occurs, when potassium homeostasis is disrupted. Pseudohyperkalemia can occur with thrombocytosis, hemolysis, and extremely high white blood cell counts. In these cases, lysis of the cells in the test tube releases potassium into the serum and increases potassium concentrations. Repeated fist clenching with a tourniquet can also release K^+ from muscle cells and increase potassium concentrations factitiously. Excessive intake is otherwise virtually always iatrogenic and the result of parenteral administration. Drugs are frequently implicated as causes of hyperkalemia; combinations of a potassium-sparing diuretic with either an angiotensin-converting enzyme inhibitor (ACEI) or a non-steroidal anti-inflammatory drug (NSAID) are particularly hazardous. NSAIDs tend to decrease renal potassium excretion through their effect on eicosanoid synthesis.

Hyperkalemia can result from potassium excess but can also be a result of redistribution of potassium from the intracellular to the extracellular compartment. This mechanism can sometimes give rise to hyperkalemia even in a patient who is potassium depleted, e.g. in diabetic ketoacidosis). As with hypokalemia, more than one cause of hyperkalemia may be present. Spurious hyperkalemia, due to the leakage of potassium from blood cells *in vitro*, often occurs. If hyperkalemia is found unexpectedly, the possibility that it is spurious should be explored by repeating the measurement on a fresh sample. Spurious hyperkalemia may be present in the absence of frank hemolysis. Loss of potassium from cells into plasma can occur rapidly in patients with high white blood cell or platelet counts, e.g. in patients with leukemia).

Etiology

The most common cause of increased serum K^+ concentration is probably Pseudohyperkalemia caused by hemolysis of RBCs in the blood sample. Normal kidneys eventually excrete K^+ loads, so sustained, non-artifactual hyperkalemia usually implies diminished renal K^+ excretion. However, other factors usually contribute the causes:

1. **Excessive intake:** In patients with unimpaired renal function and intact other regulatory mechanisms, large amounts of potassium are needed to achieve hyperkalemia. Whereas in patients with impaired renal function, especially when GFR is <15 mL/min, a slight increase in potassium intake can cause severe hyperkalemia.

2. **Impaired elimination of potassium:**
   - Renal insufficiency acute or chronic: reduced GFR (especially <15 mL/min/1.73 m^2) with low urine flow (and, therefore, low sodium delivery to the distal tubule) lead to decreased renal excretion of potassium.
   - Medications interfering with urinary potassium excretion of special clinical relevance are potassium-sparing diuretics (amiloride or spironolactone), cyclosporine, trimetoprim. Non-steroidal anti-inflammatory drugs NSAIDs; (ibuprofen, naproxen) and ACEI (angiotensin converting enzyme inhibitors) as well as angiotensin-receptor inhibitors can cause a decrease in aldosterone and GFR and thereby lead to hyperkalemia. Combined treatment with spironolactone and ACE inhibitors, especially in patients with renal impairment or heart failure, has to be monitored very carefully.
   - Hypoaldosteronism may either be primary, e.g. M. Addison (or secondary, e.g. chronic renal failure), resulting in hyperkalemia accompanied by urinary salt wasting, leading to volume depletion and hypotension. A similar picture can be seen in patients with obstructive uropathy and renal tubular acidosis.
   - Pseudohypoaldosteronism (PHA) refers to a heterogeneous group of disorders of electrolyte metabolism characterized by hyperkalemia, metabolic acidosis, and normal GRF. PHA type I caused by autosomal dominant mutations in the human mineralocorticoid receptor (MR) gene is limited to the kidneys. PHA type I secondary to loss of function mutations of the ENaC not only affects the kidney but also the lungs, colon, and sweat and

salivary glands. PHA-II (also known as Gordon syndrome) is a rare familial renal tubular defect caused by loss of function mutations in WNK1 or WNK4. Gordon syndrome is characterized by volume expansion, suppressed renin, and reduced mineralocorticoid-induced renal clearance of potassium leading to hypertension and hyperkalemia, and hyperchloremic acidosis with normal glomerular filtration rate.

- *Congenital adrenal hyperplasia:* It is caused by mutation or deletion of any of the genes that code for enzymes involved in cortisol or aldosterone synthesis results. Approximately 90% of cases of congenital adrenal hyperplasia (CAH) are due to 21-hydroxylase deficiency. The particular phenotype and degree of hyperkalemia depends on the sex of the individual, the location of the block in synthesis, and the severity of the genetic deletion or mutation.

- *Congestive heart failure:* Reduced renal function and treatment with drugs interfering with renal potassium excretion often lead to hyperkalemia.

- *Constipation:* Enteral elimination of potassium can be decreased and therefore lead to hyperkalemia, which again might lead to reduced bowel movements. Patients with bowel emptying problems secondary to myelodysplasia are at special risk.

3. **Increased shift of potassium from intracellular space to extracellular space:**
   - *Acidosis:* Mineral acidosis is more likely to cause a shift of potassium from intracellular space into extracellular space than organic acidosis.
   - *Acute:* Increase in osmolality secondary to hyperglycemia or mannitol infusion causes potassium to exit from cells.
   - *Acute cell-tissue breakdown:* If extensive cell damage occurs, intracellular potassium is released into extracellular space. This can be the case in patients with rhabdomyolysis, tumorlyis, hemolysis, or after massive transfusion.
   - *Drugs:* Digoxin and beta-blockers (especially non-selective ones) inhibit the basolateral Na^+-K^+ ATPase. Succinylcholine, especially when given to patients with burn injuries, immobilization, or inflammation.
   - *Hyperkalemic periodic paralysis:* Rare condition with mutations of the muscular sodium channel, resulting in paralytic episodes associated with elevated K^+ levels.

Pseudohyperkalemia

Pseudo hyperkalemia or falsely elevated serum K^+, is more common, typically occurring due to hemolysis and release of intracellular K^+.

Signifies an *in vitro* phenomenon, e.g. the *in vivo* serum potassium is normal. This is caused by the release of potassium from cellular components of blood during the process of clotting and, less commonly, by the release of potassium from ischemic muscle cells due to tight tourniquet or hand/arm exercise during the blood-drawing process. If the latter is suspected, blood should be drawn in a proper manner again and serum potassium repeated. If the former is suspected, the platelet and white blood cell counts should be checked, and serum should be inspected for significant hemolysis. Hyperkalemia occurs, when there is thrombocytosis (platelet count greater than 600,000), leukocytosis (WBC greater than 200,000) or significant hemolysis. If thrombocytosis or severe leukocytosis is present, then plasma potassium should be measured. If hemolysis is present, blood drawing should be carefully repeated.

Symptoms and Signs

Hyperkalemia is usually asymptomatic until cardiac toxicity develops. Hyperkalemia is less common than hypokalemia, but is more dangerous; through its effect on the heart, it can kill without warning. It lowers the resting membrane potential, shortens the cardiac action potential and increases the speed of repolarization. Cardiac arrest in asystole or slow ventricular fibrillation may be the first sign of hyperkalemia. The risk increases significantly with potassium concentrations exceeding 6.5 mmol/L (particularly if the increase has occurred rapidly); a true potassium concentration of >7.0 mmol/L is a medical emergency. It is therefore necessary to be alert for this disorder in appropriate circumstances, for instance in acute kidney injury, to ensure that effective early management is instituted. Characteristic ECG changes (initially peaking of T waves, followed by loss of P waves and, finally, the development of abnormal QRS complexes) may precede cardiac arrest. Other clinical features of hyperkalemia include muscle weakness; in hyperkalemia associated with acidosis, hyperventilation may be present. In the rare disorder hyperkalemic familial periodic paralysis, weakness frequently develops during attacks and can progress to frank paralysis.

Diagnosis

Hyperkalemia is rarely associated with symptoms, occasionally patients complain of palpitations, nausea, muscle pain, or paresthesia. However, moderate and especially severe hyperkalemia can lead to disturbances of cardiac rhythm, which can be fatal. Electrocardiography monitoring is mandatory in patients with serum potassium >6.5 mmol/L. ECG changes may present as non-specific repolarization abnormalities, 'peaked' T-waves, and QRS widening as well as depression of ST-segment.

Examination and investigations should be systematic and should include the following:

Serum K measurement: Hyperkalemia (serum K > 5.5 mmol/L) may be found on routine serum electrolyte measurement. It should be suspected in patients with typical changes on an ECG or patients at high risk, such as those with renal failure, advanced heart failure, or urinary obstruction, or treated with ACE inhibitors and K^+ sparing diuretics.

ECG should be done on patients with hyperkalemia. ECG changes (as shown in Fig. 3.7), are frequently visible when serum K^+ is >5.5 mmol/L. Slowing of conduction characterized by an increased PR-interval and shortening of the QT-interval as well as tall, symmetric, peaked T waves are visible initially. K^+ > 6.5 mmol/L causes further slowing of conduction with widening of the QRS-interval, disappearance of the P wave, and nodal and escape ventricular arrhythmias. Finally, the QRS-complex degenerates into a sine wave pattern, and ventricular fibrillation or asystole ensues.

Pseudohyperkalemia should be considered in patients without risk factors or ECG abnormalities. Hemolysis may be reported by the laboratory. When pseudo-hyperkalemia is suspected, K^+ concentration should be repeated, taking measures to avoid hemolysis of the sample.

Diagnosis of the cause of hyperkalemia requires a detailed history, including a review of drugs, a physical examination with emphasis on volume status, and measurement of electrolytes, BUN, and creatinine. In cases in which renal failure is present, additional tests, including renal ultrasonography to exclude obstruction, are needed.

MANAGEMENT AND TREATMENT

Intravenous calcium gluconate (10 mL of a 10% solution given over 1 minute and repeated as necessary) affords some degree of immediate protection to the myocardium by antagonizing the effect of hyperkalemia on myocardial excitability. Intravenous glucose and insulin, i.e. 500 mL of 20% dextrose with 20 units of soluble insulin given over 30 minutes, promotes intracellular potassium uptake. Salbutamol, which activates Na^+-K^+ATPase, has a similar effect. If insulin is used, blood glucose must be monitored for the subsequent 6 hours because of the risk of hypo-glycemia. In an acidotic patient, hyperkalemia can be controlled temporarily by bicarbonate infusion (using a 1.26% solution, not 8.4%, which risks causing ECF volume expansion because of the high sodium concentration).

In acute kidney injury and in other circumstances where the hyperkalemia is uncontrollable, dialysis or hemofiltration will be required. In chronic kidney disease, restriction of potassium intake and the administration of oral ion-exchange resins are often successful in preventing dangerous hyperkalemia until such time as dialysis becomes necessary for other reasons.

ECG monitoring can be valuable in patients with hyperkalemia. Changes in the plasma potassium concentration are reflected by changes in the ECG waveform more rapidly than could be determined by biochemical measurement.

Measurement of Potassium

It is used to diagnose and manage disorders that affect the potassium balance in the body. Renal disorders are the most common type of disorders affecting the body's potassium balance.

Serum potassium is measured by the use of ion-selective electrode, atomic absorption, spectrophotometry and flame photometry. ISE procedure is rapid, simple, and reproducible. In interpreting serum potassium, it should be kept in mind that because the intracellular potassium concentration is approximately forty fold greater than the extracellular concentration, any manoeuvre that would result in the release of a small amount of intracellular potassium will erroneously raise serum potassium. These include (1) tight tourniquet, (2) vigorous exercise of the extremity during blood drawing, (3) hemolysis due to vigorous shaking of the test tube, (4) thrombocytosis (platelet count greater than 600,000), and (5) leukocytosis (WBC greater than 200,000). In the last two situations, the longer the blood stands, the greater the rise in serum potassium will be.

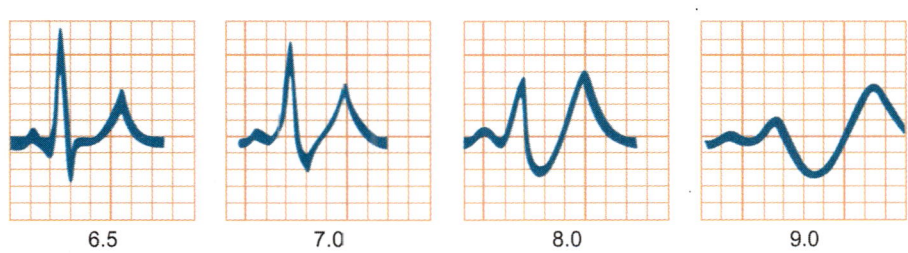

| 6.5 | 7.0 | 8.0 | 9.0 |

Fig. 3.7: ECG patterns in hyperkalemia

Specimen Requirements

Serum or plasma, free from hemolysis, is the recommended specimen. Specimen can be collected in plain silicone coated glass/plastic tubes, gel separator tubes with or without clot activator for serum estimations (with thrombin-based clot activator for stat estimations) or in tubes containing lithium/sodium/ammonium heparin as an anticoagulant for plasma estimations with or without gel separator. Platelets release potassium during the clotting process, resulting in higher (0.36 ± 0.18 mmol/L) potassium concentrations in the serum as compared to plasma. Plasma should be centrifuged at 1100–2000 g for a minimum of 10 minutes. And allow the serum to clot, and then centrifuge it at 1100–2000 g for a minimum of 10 minutes.

Urine samples should be collected in a clean, leak-proof container and should not be acidified. If transport is delayed, specimens should be kept refrigerated at 2–8°C. A 24-hour collection is the recommended specimen to determine the urine potassium.

CHLORIDE

Chloride (Cl^-) is the major anion in the extracellular fluid (as shown in Fig. 3.8) and thus makes a major contribution to its osmolarity. Chloride plays a critical role in keeping

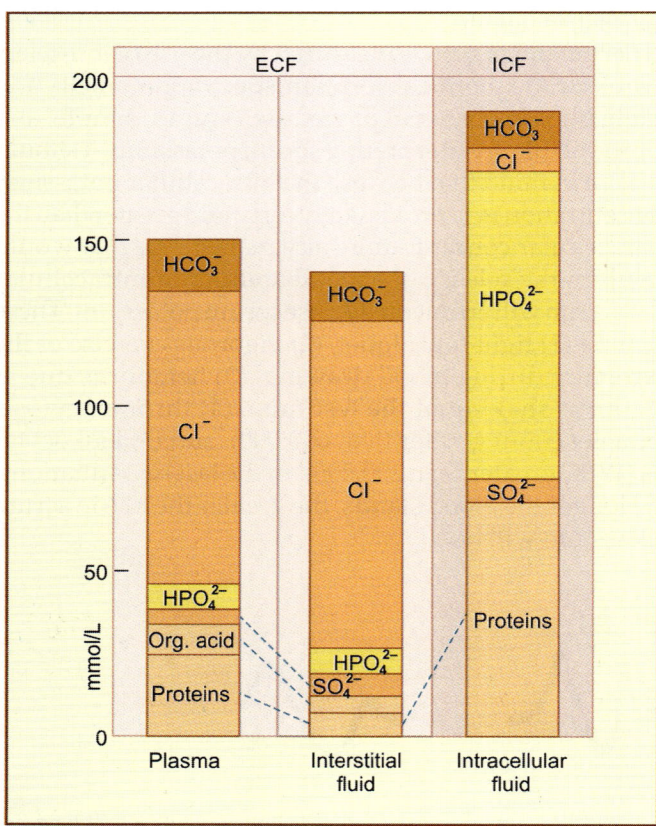

Fig. 3.8: Chloride distribution

the proper balance of body fluids and maintaining the body's acid-base balance. The normal chloride values are 96–106 mmol/L.

Chloride represents 70% of the body's total negative ion content. On average, an adult human body contains approximately 115 grams of chloride, making up about 0.15% of total body weight. Chloride ions are strongly attracted to Na^+, K^+, and Ca^{2+}. It would require great expenditure of energy to keep it separate from these cations, so chloride homeostasis is achieved primarily as an effect of sodium homeostasis, as sodium is retained or excreted, chloride ions passively follow.

In addition to its functions as an electrolyte, chloride combines with hydrogen in the stomach to make hydrochloric acid, a powerful digestive enzyme that is responsible for the breakdown of proteins, absorption of other metallic minerals, and activation of intrinsic factor, which in turn absorbs vitamin. Chloride ions play a major role in the regulation of body pH.

Regulation

The suggested amount of chloride intake ranges from 750–900 milligrams per day, based on the fact that total obligatory loss of chloride in the average person is close to 530 milligrams per day. As the principle negatively charged ion in the body, chloride serves as one of the main electrolytes of the body. Chloride, in addition to potassium and sodium, assist in the conduction of electrical impulses when dissolved in bodily water. Potassium and sodium become positive ions as they lose an electron when dissolved and chloride becomes a negative ion as it gains an electron when dissolved. A positive ion is always accompanied by a negative ion, hence the close relationship between sodium, potassium and chloride. The electrolytes are distributed throughout all body fluids including the blood, lymph, and the fluid inside and outside cells. The negative charge of chloride balances against the positive charges of sodium and potassium ions in order to maintain serum osmolarity.

In addition chloride is specially transported into the gastric lumen, in exchange for another negatively charged electrolyte (bicarbonate), in order to maintain electrical neutrality across the stomach membrane. After utilization in hydrochloric acid, some chloride is reabsorbed by the intestine, back into the bloodstream where it is required for maintenance of extracellular fluid volume. Chloride is both actively and passively absorbed by the body, depending on the current metabolic demands. A constant exchange of chloride and bicarbonate, between red blood cells and the plasma helps to govern the pH balance and transport of carbon dioxide, a waste product of respiration, from the body. With sodium and potassium, chloride works in the nervous system to aid in the transport of electrical impulses throughout the body, as movement of negatively charged chloride into the cell propagates the nervous electrical potential.

Chloride Depletion and Hypochloremia

Total body chloride depletion can result from both extra-renal and renal causes (listed in the Table 3.9). Extrarenal causes include inadequate sodium chloride intake, losses of certain gastrointestinal fluids, e.g. vomiting and nasogastric suction associated with loss of HCl, or diarrhea as a result of abnormalities in small bowel transport), and loss of fluids through the skin occurring as a result of trauma, e.g. burns). Severe vomiting may lead to the most disproportionate loss of chloride compared to sodium since gastric chloride content is greater than 100 mmol/L and gastric sodium content is relatively low (20–30 mmol/L). In individuals with protracted vomiting or nasogastric suction, the serum sodium concentration may be only mildly depressed (130 mmol/L), whereas the serum chloride concentration is usually markedly lowered (80–90 mmol/L). The most reduced levels of serum chloride (range 45–70 mmol/L) are associated with pernicious forms of vomiting due to gastric outlet obstruction, protracted vomiting in alcoholics, or self-induced vomiting. Individuals with hypochloremia secondary to total body chloride depletion will have physical findings that indicate ECF volume contraction, e.g. hypotension, tachycardia, and orthostatic changes in blood pressure). Further support of total body chloride and sodium depletion is the finding of low concentrations of sodium and chloride in the urine. Renal causes of chloride and sodium losses include diuretic abuse, particularly loop diuretics; osmotic diuresis, e.g. mannitol, diabetic ketoacidosis, or hyper-osmolar nonketotic coma); renal diseases associated with a salt-losing nephropathy including interstitial nephritis, chronic renal failure, postobstructive diuresis, and conditions associated with adrenal insufficiency, e.g. lack of endogenous or exogenous glucocorticoids or mineralocorticoids). The physical findings in individuals with hypochloremia as a result of renal losses of sodium and chloride will be similar to individuals with extrarenal chloride losses. In these individuals, however, the concentration of chloride and sodium in the urine will be elevated, indicating renal losses of chloride and sodium despite evidence of ECF volume contraction.

Metabolic alkalosis (blood pH greater than 7.45), is also associated with total chloride depletion. The reabsorption of sodium bicarbonate ($NaHCO_3$) in the proximal and distal tubule is augmented because total body chloride depletion results in both ECF volume contraction (which stimulates HCO_3^- reabsorption) and decreased quantities of filtered chloride available to the tubules for reabsorption with sodium. The virtual absence of chloride in the urine in the presence of a metabolic alkalosis is a strong indication that total body chloride depletion is present. Augmented reabsorption of $NaHCO_3$ will persist until adequate quantities of chloride are administered and/or the volume of the ECF compartment is normalized. Metabolic alkalosis also increases potassium excretion by the kidneys which can lead to hypokalemia.

A number of chloride-containing solutions can be used to correct total body chloride depletion including isotonic sodium chloride (normal saline, physiologic saline) for replacement of just sodium and chloride, potassium chloride for replacement of potassium and chloride, and lysine monochloride, arginine monochloride, ammonium chloride, or HCl, when acid replacement is necessary in conditions associated with chloride deple-tion and severe metabolic alkalosis.

Clinical conditions associated with excess water retention can cause a dilutional hyponatremia with a proportionate decrease in the chloride concentration (listed in the Table 3.9). This form of hypochloremia does

Table 3.9	Conditions associated with hypochloremia
Total body chloride depletion	

Extrarenal
  Inadequate NaCl intake
  Losses of gastrointestinal fluids
    Vomiting
    Nasogastric suction
    Small bowel fistulas
  Burns
Renal
  Diuretic abusers
  Salt-losing nephropathy
    Interstitial nephritis
    Adrenal insufficiency
Dilutional (decreased chloride concentration)
Increased effective circulatory blood volume
    Hypertonic infusions
    Hyperglycemia (early stages)
Normal effective circulatory blood volume
  Pathologic water drinkers
  Intrinsic renal diseases
  Hypothyroidism
  Syndrome of inappropriate antidiuretic hormone (SIADH)
  Drugs
    Barbiturates
    Chlorpropamide
    Clofibrate
    Morphine
    Nicotine
    Tricyclics

Contd.

Table 3.9	Conditions associated with hypochloremia *(Contd.)*
Total body chloride depletion	

Decreased effective circulatory blood volume
- Edema states
  - Congestive heart failure
  - Cirrhosis of the liver
  - Nephrotic syndrome
Acid-base abnormalities
Compensated respiratory acidosis
Metabolic alkalosis

Table 3.10	Conditions associated with hyperchloremia
Loss of electrolyte free fluids (pure water loss)	

Skin losses
- Fever
- Hypermetabolic states
- Increased ambient room temperature
Inadequate water intake
- Loss of thirst perception
Renal losses
- Central diabetes insipidus
- Nephrogenic diabetes insiuidos
Loss of hypotonic fluids (water deficit in excess of sodium and chloride deficits)
Extrarenal
- Diarrhea
- Burns
Renal losses
- Osmotic diuresis
- Diuretics
- Postobstructive diuresis
- Intrinsic renal disease
Sodium gain
Administration of 3–5% NaCl
Saltwater drowning
Saline abortion
Hyperchloremic metabolic acidosis
Renal tubular acidosis
- Interstitial renal disease
- Multiple myeloma
- Idiopathic
- Drugs
  - Carbonic anhydrase inhibitors-acetazolamide
  - Topical sulfamylon acetate and metabolites
Small bowel diarrhea
Ureteral diversion procedures
- Ureterosigmoidostomy
- Ileal bladder
- Ileal ureter
Administration of acidic salts
- NH_4Cl
- Arginine HCl
- Lysine HCl
- Hyperalimentation
Early renal failure
Primary hyperparathyroidism
Recovery from diabetic ketoacidosis
Respiratory alkalosis

not reflect total body chloride or sodium depletion, and, in fact, many of the conditions associated with dilutional hypochloremia have a normal or increased total body content of chloride and sodium. Individuals with dilutional hypochloremia generally have a normal or elevated blood pressure and evidence of ECF volume expansion. The sodium and chloride urine concentrations are variable depending on the underlying medical condition.

Specific acid-base abnormalities may also be associated with hypochloremia. Conditions associated with a respiratory acidosis, e.g. retention of CO_2 as with chronic obstructive lung disease) cause the proximal tubule to increase its secretion of hydrogen ion. This results in sodium being retained preferrentially as sodium bicarbonate and not sodium chloride. Although this is a compensatory mechanism to help ameliorate the acidemia, the end result is increased concentrations of serum bicarbonate (greater than 30 mmol/L) and decreased serum chloride concentrations. Conditions causing dilutional hyponatremia and hypochloremia do not require chloride-containing fluids, since they do not have total body chloride depletion. However, respiratory acidosis associated with hypochloremia may need chloride-containing fluids if a metabolic alkalosis and/or hypokalemia is also present.

Chloride Excess and Hyperchloremia

Hyperchloremia is also associated with a variety of clinical conditions (Table 3.10). Conditions causing an elevation of the serum chloride concentration and a concomitant elevation of the serum sodium concentration result primarily from disorders associated with loss of electrolyte-free fluids (pure water loss), hypotonic fluids (water deficit in excess of sodium, and chloride deficits), or administration of NaCl-containing fluids. Loss of electrolyte-free fluids occurs in conditions with increased insensible losses as a result of increased sweating, (e.g. fever), hyper metabolic states (thyrotoxicosis), increased ambient room temperature and inadequate water replacement (as a result of loss of thirst perception as seen in the elderly); in ill infants; and in individuals with altered mental status (stroke patients, postanesthesia, and narcotic medications). This results in hypotonic dehydration, e.g. loss of TBW and contraction of the ICF and ECF compartments) and an elevation in both the serum sodium and chloride concentration—hypernatremia and hyperchloremia. Loss of electrolyte-free fluids, also occurs in clinical conditions associated with central or nephrogenic diabetes insipidus. Both the conditions are associated with an inability to concentrate the urine and large volumes of dilute urine (urine osmolality less than plasma osmolality). However, hypernatremia and hyperchloremia will not develop in association with either of these latter abnormalities as long as individuals drink adequate amounts of fluid or are given adequate quantities of electrolyte-free intravenous fluids to replace the daily urine losses. Loss of hypotonic fluids occurs with certain types of diarrhea states and burns; in conditions associated with an osmotic diuresis, e.g. diabetic glycosuria, mannitol, glycerol), diuretics, following a postobstructive diuresis, and in association with some intrinsic renal diseases. Since more water is lost relative to sodium, the serum sodium chloride concentration rises. But since some sodium and chloride are excreted into the urine, the serum sodium and chloride concentrations will not be as elevated as that occurring in conditions associated with loss of electrolyte-free fluids. Administration of NaCl-containing fluids can also result in hypernatremia and hyperchloremia if excessive quantities of hypertonic solutions of sodium chloride (3% or 5%) are given iatrogenically in place of 5% D5/W or inadvertently administered during instillation *in utero* for a second semester abortion. It can also be found in association with saltwater drowning. Administration of hypertonic tube feedings without the concurrent administration of adequate quantities of free water to dilute the feedings to isotonicity can also cause hypernatremia and hyperchloremia.

Individuals with hyperchloremia secondary to electrolyte-free fluid losses will have physical findings of dehydration—dry mucous membranes, coated tongue, and no axillary sweat. Urine chloride and sodium concentrations may or may not be helpful. However, the finding of a dilute urine (uOsm less than 100 mOsm with low chloride and sodium concentrations), in the presence of hyperchloremia and hypernatremia most likely confirms the diagnosis of diabetes insipidus. With the loss of hypotonic fluids, individuals will have findings of both dehydration (a result of electrolyte-free fluid losses) and sodium depletion. As a consequence of the latter, such individuals will have evidence of ECF contraction (hypotension, tachycardia, orthostatic hypotension) in addition. In contrast, individuals with hyperchloremia secondary to administration of NaCl containing solutions will have physical findings indicative of an expanded ECF volume—hypertension, edema, congestive heart failure, and pulmonary edema.

Elevated levels of serum chloride without increased levels of serum sodium occur as a result of clinical conditions that predispose to a hyperchloremic metabolic acidosis. Individuals with this acid-base disturbance have a serum chloride concentration above 110 mmol/L (and a low bicarbonate concentration) in association with an acidemic blood pH (pH lower than 7.35). Hyperchloremic metabolic acidosis can occur when the kidney tubules (either proximal or distal) do not reabsorb adequate quantities of the bicarbonate filtered by the glomerulus. Disorders causing intrinsic damage to the tubules (e.g. interstitial nephritis); drugs that block bicarbonate reabsorption (e.g. carbonic anhydrase inhibitors acetazolamide, and topically applied sulfur drugs and their metabolites used as a topical antibiotic in burn patients) result in the condition called renal tubular acidosis (RTA). A diagnosis of RTA can frequently be made if one finds a blood pH that is acidemic in association with nonacidic urine (a urine pH above 5.5). Other causes of hyperchloremic metabolic acidosis include conditions associated with severe diarrhea having losses of bicarbonate equivalents (e.g. lactate and acetate), ureteral diversion procedures, which often have hyper reabsorption of chloride by the interposed bowel segment, and ingestion of acidic chloride-containing salts (NH_4Cl, arginine chloride, and lysine chloride), or acidic salts of amino acids found in some hyper alimentation solutions. Hyperchloremic metabolic acidosis can also be seen in the early stages of chronic renal failure, especially secondary to conditions resulting from interstitial renal damage; in the recovery phase of diabetic ketoacidosis (loss of ketone bodies in the urine prevents them from being converted to bicarbonate in the liver and results in bicarbonate deficits), and in primary hyperparathyroidism (which is associated with renal bicarbonate losses). In addition, respiratory alkalosis, a condition seen in individuals with hyperventilation (e.g sepsis, pregnancy, pulmonary infections, anxiety), is associated with an elevated serum chloride concentration and a low bicarbonate concentration. An arterial blood pH will help distinguish between hyperchloremic metabolic acidosis and respiratory alkalosis.

Hyperchloremia is also seen with bromide intoxication because bromide is measured as a chloride equivalent by certain chloride measurement techniques. This results in the finding of an anion gap (as measured by the difference of sodium plus potassium minus chloride plus the total CO_2 content being less than 8 mmol/L). Although the use of medications with bromide has decreased, cases of bromide intoxications still occur. It is unusual to see acute bromide intoxication, since bromide causes significant gastrointestinal irritation, resulting in nausea and vomiting, making toxic levels difficult to achieve. Slow chronic ingestion of bromide, however, can lead to toxic levels, since bromide is excreted by the kidneys, and accumulation can occur if intake exceeds output. The clinical features of bromide intoxication include fever, neurologic disturbances, skin rash, and history of ingesting proprietary bromide-containing drugs. Toxic manifestations include irritability, delirium, sedation, psychic disturbances, tremors, motor incoordination, and increases in CSF pressure and protein. Spuriously increased levels of serum chloride concentration appear in bromism, but the degree of elevation is dependent on the chloride methodology employed. There may be a poor correlation between the severity of bromide intoxication and serum bromide levels. However, bromide intoxication will cause mental and neurologic symptoms when the serum levels of bromide exceed 9 mmol/L. Most patients show signs of bromide poisoning when the serum bromide concentrations are in the range of 19–25 mmol/L.

MEASUREMENT OF CHLORIDE

Chloride is determined by (1) mercurimetric titration, (2) spectrophotometry, (3) coulometric-amperometric titration, or most commonly today, (4) ISE.

Specimen Requirements

Chloride most often is measured in serum or plasma, urine, and sweat. Cl^- is stable in serum and plasma. Even gross hemolysis does not significantly alter serum or plasma Cl^- concentration because the erythrocyte concentration of Cl^- is approximately half of that in plasma. Because very little Cl^- is protein bound, change in posture or stasis, or the use of tourniquets, has little effect on its plasma concentration. Measurement of Cl^- loss in gastric aspirates or intestinal drainages is an adjunct to parenteral replacement therapy. Fecal Cl^- determination may be useful for the diagnosis of congenital hypochloremic alkalosis with hyper-chloridorrhea (increase dexcretion of Cl^- in stool). In this condition, the concentration of Cl^- in feces may reach 180 mmol/L, with undetectable Cl^- in urine.

Calcium

Calcium (Ca^{2+}) is the most abundant electrolyte in the body, 99% or more is deposited in bone and the remainder plays a vital role in nerve conduction, muscle contraction, hormone release and cell signaling, blood clotting and maintaining normal heart function. Normal total serum Ca^{2+} concentration ranges from (2.20–2.60 mmol/L).

Forty percen of the total blood Ca^{2+} is bound to plasma proteins, primarily albumin. The remaining 60% includes ionized Ca plus Ca^{2+} complexed with phosphate (HPO_4^{-3}) and citrate. Total Ca^{2+} (e.g. protein-bound, complexed, and ionized Ca^{2+}) is usually what is determined by clinical laboratory measurement. Ideally, ionized or free Ca^{2+} should be determined because it is the physiologically active form of Ca^{2+} in plasma; this determination, because of its technical difficulty, is usually restricted to patients in whom significant alteration of protein binding of serum Ca^{2+} is suspected. Ionized Ca^{2+} is generally assumed to be about 50% of the total serum Ca^{2+}.

Calcium Regulation

Absorption is controlled by vitamin D, while excretion is controlled by parathyroid hormones. However, the distribution from bone to plasma is controlled by both the parathyroid hormones and vitamin D. There is also a constant loss of calcium via the kidneys even if there is none in the diet. This excretion of calcium by the kidneys and its distribution between bone and the rest of the body is primarily controlled by parathyroid hormone (as shown in Fig. 3.9).

Calcium in plasma exists in three forms—ionized, nonionized, and protein bound. It is the ionized calcium concentration that is monitored by the parathyroid gland and if low, parathyroid hormone secretion is increased. This increases ionized calcium levels by increasing bone reabsorption, decreasing renal excretion and acting on the kidney to increase the rate of formation of active vitamin D, thereby increasing gut absorption of calcium.

The usual amount of phosphate in the diet is about 1 g/d, but not all is absorbed. Any excess is excreted by

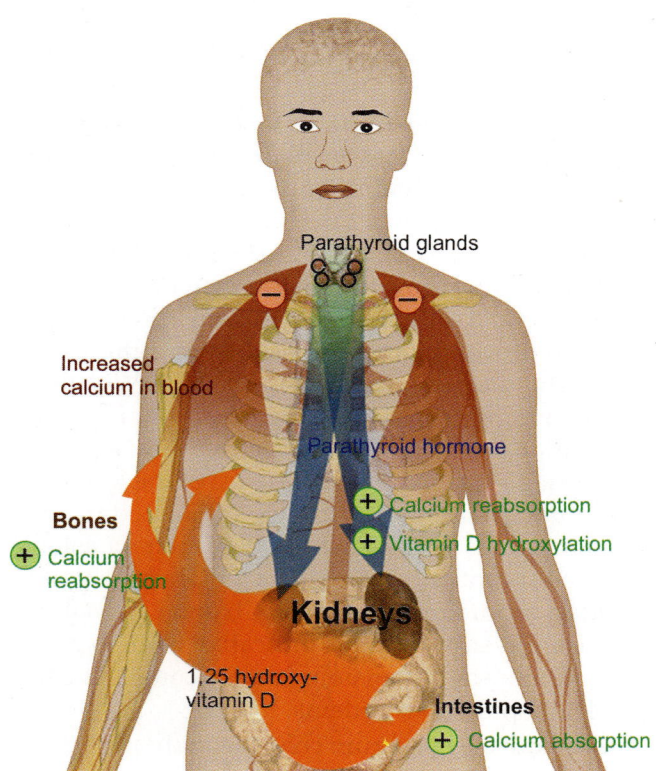

Fig. 3.9: Calcium regulation

the kidney and this excretion is increased by the parathyroid hormone. This hormone also causes phosphate to leach out of bone. Plasma phosphate has no direct effect on parathyroid hormone secretion; however, if it is elevated it combines with Ca^{2+}, decreasing ionized Ca^{2+} in plasma, and thereby increasing parathyroid hormone secretion.

Calcium Depletion and Hypocalcemia

Hypocalcemia is total serum Ca^{2+} concentration <2.20 mmol/L in the presence of normal plasma protein concentrations or a serum ionized Ca^{2+} concentration <1.17 mmol/L. Causes include hypoparathyroidism, vitamin D deficiency, and renal disease. Manifestations include paresthesias, tetany, and, when severe, seizures, encephalopathy, and heart failure. Diagnosis involves measurement of serum Ca^{2+} with adjustment for serum albumin concentration. Treatment is administration of Ca^{2+}, sometimes with vitamin D.

Hypocalcemia has a number of causes, including the following:
- Hypoparathyroidism
- Pseudohypoparathyroidism
- Vitamin D deficiency and dependency
- Renal disease
- Mg^{2+} depletion [can cause relative parathyroid hormone (PTH)] deficiency and end-organ resistance to PTH action, usually when serum Mg^{2+} concentrations are <0.5 mmol/L; Mg^{2+} repletion increases PTH concentrations and improves renal Ca^{2+} conservation).
- Acute pancreatitis (when lipolytic products released from the inflamed pancreas chelate Ca^{2+}).
- Hypoproteinemia (reduces the protein-bound fraction of serum Ca^{2+}; hypocalcemia due to diminished protein binding is asymptomatic, because ionized Ca^{2+} is unchanged, this entity has been termed factitious hypocalcemia).
- Hungry bone syndrome (persistent hypocalcemia and hypophosphatemia occurring after surgical or medical correction of moderate to severe hyperparathyroidism in patients in whom serum Ca^{2+} concentrations had been supported by high bone turnover induced by greatly elevated PTH, hungry bone syndrome has been described after parathyroidectomy, after renal transplantation, and rarely in patients with end-stage renal disease treated with calcimimetics).
- Septic shock (due to suppression of PTH release and decreased conversion of 25(OH)D to 1,25(OH)$_2$D).
- Hyperphosphatemia (causes hypocalcemia by poorly understood mechanisms; patients with renal failure and subsequent $HPO4^{-3}$ retention are particularly prone).

- Drugs including anticonvulsants, e.g. phenytoin, phenobarbital) and rifampin, which alter vitamin D metabolism, and drugs generally used to treat hypercalcemia.
- Transfusion of >10 units of citrate-anticoagulated blood and use of radiocontrast agents containing the divalent ion-chelating agent ethylenediaminetetraacetate (EDTA can decrease the concentration of bioavailable ionized Ca^{2+} while total serum Ca^{2+} concentrations remain unchanged).
- Infusion of gadolinium (may spuriously lower Ca^{2+} concentration).

Although, excessive secretion of calcitonin might be expected to cause hypocalcemia, low serum Ca^{2+} concentrations rarely occur in patients with large amounts of circulating calcitonin due to medullary carcinoma of the thyroid.

Calcium Excess and Hypercalcemia

Hypercalcemia is total serum Ca^{2+} concentration >2.60 mmol/L or ionized serum Ca^{2+}>1.30 mmol/L. Principal causes include hyperparathyroidism, vitamin D toxicity, and cancer. Clinical features include polyuria, constipation, muscle weakness, confusion, and coma. Diagnosis is by serum ionized Ca^{2+} and parathyroid hormone concentrations. Treatment to increase Ca^{2+} excretion and reduce bone resorption of Ca^{2+} involves saline, Na^+ diuresis, and drugs, such as pamidronate.

Hypercalcemia usually results from excessive bone resorption. There are many causes of hypercalcemia but the most common are hyperparathyroidism and cancer.

PHOSPHATE

Phosphate (HPO_4^{-3}) makes up 1% of a person's total body weight. A majority of the body's phosphate is found in the bones and teeth where it promotes their formation. It also plays an important role in the body's utilization of carbohydrates and fats. Phosphates are also critical to the synthesis of proteins that promote the growth, maintenance, and repair of cells and tissues. The normal serum inorganic HPO_4^{-3} concentration in adults ranges from 0.81–1.45 mmol/L, HPO_4^{-3} concentration is 50% higher in infants and 30% higher in children, possibly because of the important roles these HPO_4^{-3} dependent processes play in growth.

Phosphate Regulation

Phosphate ions are required for bone mineralization, and roughly 740 g of HPO_4^{-3} is bound up in the mineral salts of the skeleton. In body fluids, the most important functions of HPO_4^{-3} involve the ICF, where the ions are required for the formation of high-energy compounds, the activation of enzymes, and the synthesis of nucleic acids. Phosphate ions are reabsorbed from tubular fluid along the proximal convoluted tubule; fecal losses vary depending on the amount of HPO_4^{-3} binding compounds (mainly Ca^{2+}) in the diet. Also, like Ca^{2+}, GI HPO_4^{-3} absorption is enhanced by vitamin D. Renal HPO_4^{-3} excretions roughly equals GI absorption to maintain HPO_4^{-3} balance. HPO_4^{-3} depletion can occur in various disorders and normally results in conservation of HPO_4^{-3} by the kidneys. Bone HPO_4^{-3} serves as a reservoir, which can buffer changes in plasma and intracellular HPO_4^{-3}.

Phosphate Depletion and Hypophosphatemia

Hypophosphatemia is serum phosphate (HPO_4^{-3}) concentration <0.81 mmol/L. Causes include alcoholism, burns, starvation, and diuretic use. Clinical features include muscle weakness, respiratory failure, and heart failure; seizures and coma can occur. Diagnosis is by serum HPO_4^{-3} concentration. Treatment consists of HPO_4^{-3} supplementation.

Hypophosphatemia occurs in 2% of hospitalized patients, but is more prevalent in certain populations, e.g. it occurs in up to 10% of hospitalized patients with alcoholism).

Hypophosphatemia has numerous causes, but clinically significant acute hypophosphatemia occurs in relatively few clinical settings, including the following:

- The recovery phase of diabetic ketoacidosis
- Acute alcoholism
- Severe burns
- When receiving total parenteral nutrition (TPN)
- Refeeding after prolonged undernutrition
- Severe respiratory alkalosis

Acute severe hypophosphatemia with serum HPO_4^{-3} < 0.32 mmol/L is most often caused by transcellular shifts of HPO_4^{-3}, often superimposed on chronic HPO_4^{-3} depletion.

Chronic hypophosphatemia usually is the result of decreased renal HPO_4^{-3} reabsorption. Causes include the following:

- Hyperparathyroidism
- Other hormonal disturbances, such as Cushing syndrome and hypothyroidism
- Electrolyte disorders, such as hypomagnesemia and hypokalemia
- Theophylline intoxication
- Long-term diuretic use

Severe chronic hypophosphatemia usually results from a prolonged negative HPO_4^{-3} balance. Causes include:

- Chronic starvation or malabsorption, especially when combined with vomiting or copious diarrhea
- Long-term ingestion of large amounts of HPO_4^{-3} binding aluminum, usually in the form of antacids

Ingestion of aluminum is particularly prone to cause HPO_4^{-3} depletion when combined with decreased dietary intake and dialysis losses of HPO_4^{-3} in patients with end-stage renal disease.

Phosphate Excess and Hyperphosphatemia

Hyperphosphatemia is serum phosphate concentration >1.46 mmol/L. Causes include chronic kidney disease, hypoparathyroidism, and metabolic or respiratory acidosis. Clinical features may be due to accompanying hypocalcemia and include tetany. Diagnosis is by serum HPO_4^{-3}. Treatment includes restriction of HPO_4^{-3} intake and administration of HPO_4^{-3} binding antacids, such as Ca^{2+} carbonate.

The usual cause of hyperphosphatemia is a decrease in renal excretion of HPO_4^{-3}. Advanced renal insufficiency (GFR < 30 mL/min) reduces excretion sufficiently to increase serum HPO_4^{-3}. Defects in renal excretion of HPO_4^{-3} in the absence of renal failure also occur in pseudo hypoparathyroidism and hypoparathyroidism. Hyperphosphatemia can also occur with excessive oral HPO_4^{-3} administration and occasionally with overzealous use of enemas containing HPO_4^{-3}.

Hyperphosphatemia occasionally results from a transcellular shift of HPO_4^{-3} into the extracellular space that is so large that the renal excretory capacity is overwhelmed. This transcellular shift occurs most frequently in diabetic ketoacidosis (despite total body HPO_4^{-3} depletion), crush injuries, and non-traumatic rhabdomyolysis as well as in overwhelming systemic infections and tumor lysis syndrome.

Major Causes of Hyperphosphatemia

- GFR < 30 mL/min
- Hypo parathyroidism
- Pseudohypoparathyroidism
- Excessive oral HPO_4^{-3} administration
- Overzealous use of enemas containing HPO_4^{-3}
- Shifts of HPO_4^{-3} into the extracellular space, e.g. in diabetic ketoacidosis, rhabdomyolysis, overwhelming systemic infections, and tumor lysis syndrome)

Hyperphosphatemia plays a critical role in the development of secondary hyperparathyroidism and renal osteodystrophy in patients with advanced chronic kidney disease as well as in patients on dialysis. Lastly, hyperphosphatemia can be spurious in cases of hyperproteinemia (multiple myeloma or Waldenström's macroglobulinemia), hyperlipidemia, hemolysis, or hyper bilirubinemia.

Hyperphosphatemia can lead to Ca^{2+} precipitation into soft tissues, especially when the serum $Ca^{2+} \times HPO_4^{-3}$ product is chronically >55 in patients with chronic kidney disease. Soft-tissue calcification in the skin is one cause of excessive pruritis in patients with end-stage renal disease on chronic dialysis. Vascular calcification also occurs in dialysis patients with a chronically elevated $Ca^{2+} \times HPO_4^{-3}$ product; this vascular calcification is a major risk factor for cardiovascular morbidity including stroke, myocardial infarction (MI), and claudication.

MAGNESIUM

Magnesium (Mg^{2+}) is the fourth most abundant mineral in the body. Half of the body's magnesium is found in the bone and the other half is found mainly within the cells of body tissues and organs. Magnesium is needed for more than 300 biochemical reactions in the body. It helps maintain normal muscle and nerve function, keeps the heart rhythm steady, supports a healthy immune system, and keeps bones strong. Magnesium also helps regulate blood sugar levels, promotes normal blood pressure, and is also involved in energy metabolism. Normal serum values of magnesium are 0.70–1.05 mmol/L.

Magnesium Regulation

The adult body contains about 29 g of magnesium; almost 60% of it is deposited in the skeleton, the magnesium in body fluids is contained primarily in the ICF. Magnesium is required as a cofactor for several important enzymatic reactions, including the phosphorylation of glucose within cells and the use of ATP by contracting muscle fibers. Magnesium is also important as a structural component of bone.

The Mg^{2+} concentration of the ECF averages about considerably lower than levels in the ICF. The proximal convoluted tubule reabsorbs magnesium very effectively. Keeping pace with the daily urinary loss requires a minimum dietary intake of only 0.3–0.4 g per day.

The maintenance of serum Mg^{2+} concentration is largely a function of dietary intake and effective renal and intestinal conservation. Within 7 days of initiation of Mg^{2+}-deficient diet, renal and stool Mg^{2+} excretion each fall to about 0.5 mmol/day.

About 70% of serum Mg^{2+} is ultrafiltered (filtered through minute pores) by the kidney; the remainder is bound to protein. Protein binding of Mg^{2+} is pH dependent. Serum Mg^{2+} concentration is not closely related to either total body Mg^{2+} or intracellular Mg^{2+} content. However, severe serum hypomagnesemia may reflect diminished total body Mg.

Many enzymes are activated by or are dependent on Mg^{2+}. Mg^{2+} is required by all enzymatic processes involving ATP and by many of the enzymes involved in nucleic acid metabolism. Mg^{2+} is required for thiamine pyrophosphate cofactor activity and appears to stabilize the structure of macromolecules, such as DNA and RNA. Mg^{2+} is also related to Ca^{2+} and K^+ metabolism in an intimate, but poorly understood way.

Magnesium Depletion and Hypomagnesemia

Hypomagnesemia is serum Mg^{2+} concentration <0.70 mmol/L. Causes include inadequate Mg^{2+} intake and absorption or increased excretion due to hypercalcemia or drugs such as furosemide. Symptoms and signs are often due to accompanying hypokalemia and hypocalcemia and include lethargy, tremor, tetany, seizures, and arrhythmias. Treatment is with Mg^{2+} replacement.

Serum Mg^{2+} concentration, even when free Mg^{2+} ion is measured, may be normal even with decreased intracellular or bone Mg^{2+} stores.

Causes of Hypomagnesemia

Inadequate intake plus impairment of renal conservation or GI absorption, chronic alcoholism, pancreatitis, aldosteronism, burns, and hyperparathyroidism.

Magnesium Excess and Hypermagnesemia

Hypermagnesemia is a serum Mg^{2+} concentration >1.05 mmol/L. The major cause is renal failure. Symptoms include hypotension, respiratory depression, and cardiac arrest. Diagnosis is by serum Mg^{2+} concentration. Treatment includes IV administration of Ca^{2+} gluconate and possibly furosemide; hemodialysis can be helpful in severe cases.

Symptomatic hypermagnesemia is fairly uncommon. It occurs most commonly in patients with renal failure after ingestion of Mg^{2+} containing drugs, such as antacids or purgatives. Symptoms and signs include hyporeflexia, hypotension, respiratory depression, and cardiac arrest.

Causes of Hypermagnesemia

Excessive magnesium levels may occur with end-stage renal disease, Addison's disease, or an overdose of magnesium salts.

BICARBONATE

This electrolyte is an important ion acts as a buffer to maintain the normal levels of acidity (pH) in blood and other fluids in the body. The lungs regulate the amount of carbon dioxide, and the kidneys regulate bicarbonate.

This electrolyte helps buffer the acids that build up in the body as normal by products of metabolism, i.e. when muscles are working, they produce lactic acid as a by product of energy formation. Bicarbonate is required to be available to bind the hydrogen released from the acid to form carbon dioxide and water. When the body malfunctions, too much acid may also be produced, e.g. diabetic ketoacidosis, renal tubular acidosis and bicarbonate is needed to try to compensate for the extra acid production.

The bicarbonate test is usually performed along with tests for other blood electrolytes. Disruptions in the normal bicarbonate level may be due to diseases that interfere with respiratory function, kidney diseases, metabolic conditions, or other causes. The normal serum range for bicarbonate is 22–30 mmol/L.

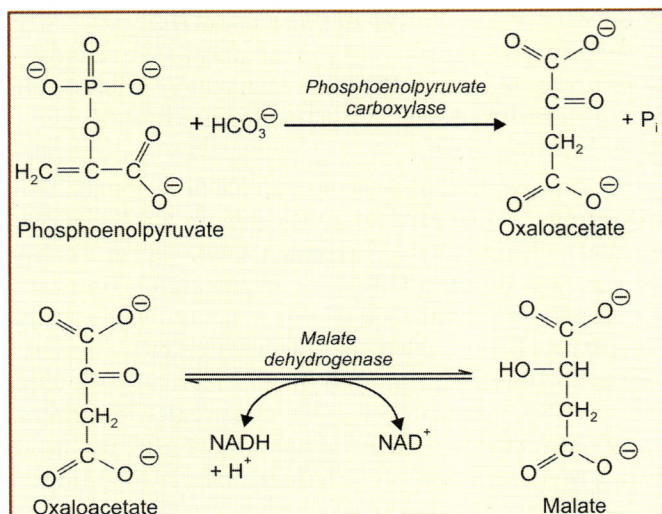

Fig. 3.10: Decreased absorbance of NADH at 340 nm is proportional to the total CO_2 content

Serum or Plasma Total Carbon Dioxide Measurement

One of the earliest methods for determining total CO_2 was the manometric method for total CO_2 content, using the Natelson microgasometer. This has been supplanted in clinical laboratories by automated methods. The first step in automated methods is acidification or alkalinization of the sample. Acidifying the sample converts the various forms of CO_2 in plasma to gaseous CO_2 by dilution with an acid buffer. Alkalinizing the sample converts all CO_2 and carbonic acid to HCO_3. Methods for total CO_2 measurement with today's automated instruments may be electrode based or enzymatic. In indirect electrode-based methods, the amount of released gaseous CO_2 after acidification is determined by a PCO_2 electrode in the reaction chamber of the CO_2 module. Direct ISE methods for total CO_2 are no longer common on automated analyzers. Direct methods for total CO_2 had problems with specificity and are no longer in use. For instance, one direct total CO_2 electrode reacted almost equivalently with nitrate. In enzymatic methods for CO_2, the specimen is first alkalinized to convert all CO_2 and carbonic acid to $HCO\}$. The enzymatic reactions are shown in Fig. 3.10.

Specimens Requirements

The same sample types used for Na^+ or K^+ may be assayed. Given a specimen in a vacuum-draw tube, the concentration of total CO_2 is most accurately determined, when the assay is done as promptly as possible after collection and centrifugation of the blood in the unopened tube. Ambient air contains far less CO_2 than does plasma, and gaseous dissolved CO_2 will escape from the specimen into the air, with a consequent decrease in the CO_2 value of up to 4–5 mmol/L in the course of 1 hour. In practical terms, the logistics of high volume processing and automated analysis of specimens almost ensures that most CO_2 measurements are done on specimens that have lost some dissolved gaseous CO_2 simply because preservation of anaerobic conditions is not practical between the time plasma is placed on an instrument and the time it is sampled. Thus the term *bicarbonate* may be preferable to total CO_2, On the other hand, a sample that is rapidly processed and promptly analyzed has a much smaller error.

BIBLIOGRAPHY

1. Adrogue HJ, Madias NE. Aiding fluid prescription for the dysnatraemias. Intensive Care Med. 1997; 23309–316.316.
2. Adrogue H, Madias NE. Hyponatremia. N Engl J Med. 2000; 342: 1581–9.
3. Adrogué HJ, Chap Z, Ishida T, et al. Role of the endocrine pancreas in the kalemic response to acute metabolic acidosis in conscious dogs. J Clin Invest. 1985; 75:798.
4. Adrogué HJ, Madias NE. Changes in plasma potassium concentration during acute acid-base disturbances. Am J Med. 1981; 71:456.
5. Adrogue HJ, Madias NE. Hypernatremia. N Engl J Med. 2000; 342: 1493–99.
6. Adrogue HJ, Madias NE. Hyponatremia. N Engl J Med. 2000; 342:1581–89.
7. Agarwal M, Lynn KL, Richards AM, et al. Hyponatremic-hypertensive syndrome with renal ischemia: an under-recognized disorder. Hypertension. 1999; 33: 1020–4.
8. Agarwal R, Emmett M. The post-transurethral resection of prostate syndrome: therapeutic proposals. Am J Kidney Dis. 1994; 24:108–11.
9. Allon M, Dansby L, Shanklin N. Glucose modulation of the disposal of an acute potassium load in patients with end-stage renal disease. Am J Med. 1993; 94:475.

10. Almond CS, Shin AY, Fortescue EB, et al. Hyponatremia among runners in the Boston Marathon. N Engl J Med. 2005; 352(15):1550–6.

11. Anderson R J, Chung H M, Kluge R, et al Hyponatraemia: a prospective analysis of its epidemiology and the role of vasopressin. Ann Intern Med. 1985. 102164–168.168.

12. Anderson RJ. Hospital acquired hyponatremia. Kidney Int. 1986;29: 1237–47.

13. Arieff AI, Guisado R. Effects on the central nervous system of hypernatraemic and hyponatraemic states. Kidney Int. 1976: 10104–106.106.

14. Arieff A, Llach F, Massry S G. Neurological manifestations and morbidity of hyponatraemia: correlation with brain water and electrolytes. Medicine. 1976: 55121–129.129.

15. Arieff AI, Ayus JC, Fraser CL. Hyponatremia and death or permanent brain damage in healthy children. BMJ. 1992; 304: 1218–22.

16. Arieff AI, Carroll HJ. Nonketotic hyperosmolar coma with hyperglycemia: clinical features, pathophysiology, renal function, acid-base balance, plasma-cerebrospinal fluid equilibria and the effects of therapy in 37 cases. Medicine (Baltimore). 1972; 51:73.

17. Arieff AI, Llach F, Massry SG. Neurological manifestations and morbidity of hyponatremia: correlation with brain water and electrolytes. Medicine (Baltimore). 1976;55:121–9.

18. Arieff AI. Hyponatremia, convulsions, respiratory arrest, and permanent brain damage after elective surgery in healthy women. N Engl J Med. 1986;314:1529–35.

19. Arseneau JC, Bagley CM, Anderson T, et al. Hyperkalemia, a sequel to chemotherapy of Burkitt's lymphoma. Lancet. 1973; 1:10.

20. Asadollahi K, Beeching N, Gill G. Hyponatraemia as a risk factor for hospital mortality. QJM. 2006; 99(12): 877–80.

21. Ayus JC, Arieff AI. Chronic hyponatremic encephalopathy in postmenopausal women—association of therapies with morbidity and mortality. JAMA. 1999; 281: 2299–304.

22. Ayus JC, Krothapalli RK, Arieff AI. Treatment of symptomatic hyponatremia and its relation to brain damage. A prospective study. N Engl J Med. 1987;317: 1190–5.

23. Ayus JC, Wheeler JM, Arieff AI. Postoperative hyponatraemic encephalopathy in menstruant women. Ann Int Med. 1992; 117: 891–7.

24. Beck LH. Hypouricemia in the syndrome of inappropriate secretion of antidiuretic hormone. N Engl J Med. 1979;301: 528–30.

25. Berendes E, Walter M, Cullen P, et al. Secretion of brain natriuretic peptide in patients with aneurysmal subarachnoid haemorrhage. Lancet. 1997. 349245–249.249.

26. Bibl D, Lampl C, Gabriel C, et al. Treatment of central pontine myelinolysis with therapeutic plasmapheresis. Lancet. 1999; 353:1155.

27. Bilbrey GL, Carter NW, White MG, et al. Potassium deficiency in chronic renal failure. Kidney Int. 1973; 4:423.

28. Blumberg A, Weidmann P, Shaw S, et al. Effect of various therapeutic approaches on plasma potassium and major regulating factors in terminal renal failure. Am J Med. 1988; 85:507.

29. Blume RS, MacLowry JD, Wolff SM. Limitations of chloride determination in the diagnosis of bromism. N Engl J Med. 1968; 279:593–5.

30. Braden GL, von Oeyen PT, Germain MJ, et al. Ritodrine- and terbutaline-induced hypokalemia in preterm labor: mechanisms and consequences. Kidney Int. 1997; 51:1867.

31. Brown MJ, Brown DC, Murphy MB. Hypokalemia from beta2-receptor stimulation by circulating epinephrine. N Engl J Med. 1983; 309:1414.

32. Brown RS. Extrarenal potassium homeostasis. Kidney Int. 1986; 30:116.

33. Castello L, Pirisi M, Sainagh P P, et al. Quantative treatment of the hyponatraemia of cirrhosis. Dig Liver Dis. 2005. 37176–180.180.

34. Chan TY. Drug-induced syndrome of inappropriate antidiuretic hormone secretion. Causes, diagnosis and management. Drugs Aging. 1997;11:27–44.

35. Chapman MD, Hanrahan R, McEwen J, et al. Hyponatremia and hypokalaemia due to indapamide. Med J Aust. 2002; 176:219–21.

36. Chung H-M, Kluge R, Schrier RW, et al. Clinical assessment of extracellular fluid volume in hyponatremia. Am J Med. 1987;83: 905–8.

37. Clausen T, Everts ME. Regulation of the Na,K-pump in skeletal muscle. Kidney Int 1989; 35:1.

38. Clausen T, Flatman JA. Effects of insulin and epinephrine on Na^+-K^+ and glucose transport in soleus muscle. Am J Physiol. 1987; 252:E492.

39. Cohn, Jay N., et al. "New Guidelines for Potassium Replacement in Clinical Practice: A Contemporary Review by the National Council on Potassium in Clinical Practice." Archives of Internal Medicine 160, no.16 (September 11, 2000): 2429–36.

40. Conte G, Dal Canton A, Imperatore P, et al. Acute increase in plasma osmolality as a cause of hyperkalemia in patients with renal failure. Kidney Int. 1990; 38:301.

41. Cotlove E, Nishi HH. Automatic titration with direct read out of chloride concentration. Clin Chem. 1961;7:285–91.

42. Cox M, Sterns RH, Singer I. The defense against hyperkalemia: the roles of insulin and aldosterone. N Engl J Med. 1978; 299:525.

43. Curtis NJ, van Heyningen C, Turner JJ. Irreversible nephrotoxicity from demeclocycline in the treatment of hyponatremia. Age Ageing. 2002;31:151–2.

44. Daut J, Maier-Rudolph W, von Beckerath N, et al. Hypoxic dilation of coronary arteries is mediated by ATP-sensitive potassium channels. Science. 1990; 247:1341.

45. Decaux G, Soupart A, Vassart G. Non-peptide arginine-vasopressin antagonists: the vaptans. Lancet. 2008; 371(9624): 1624–32.

46. DeFronzo RA, Bia M, Birkhead G. Epinephrine and potassium homeostasis. Kidney Int. 1981; 20:83.

47. DeFronzo RA, Lee R, Jones A, et al. Effect of insulinopenia and adrenal hormone deficiency on acute potassium tolerance. Kidney Int. 1980; 17:586.

48. DeFronzo RA, Sherwin RS, Dillingham M, et al. Influence of basal insulin and glucagon secretion on potassium and

sodium metabolism. Studies with somatostatin in normal dogs and in normal and diabetic human beings. J Clin Invest. 1978; 61:472.

49. DeFronzo RA, Taufield PA, Black H, et al. Impaired renal tubular potassium secretion in sickle cell disease. Ann Intern Med. 1979; 90:310.

50. DeVita MV, Gardenswartz MH, Konecky A, et al. Incidence and etiology of hyponatremia in an intensive care unit. Clin Nephrol. 1990;34:163–6.

51. DeVoe RD, Maloney PC. Principles of cell homeostasis. In Medical Physiology, 1980. 14th edition Mountcastle, VB (ed). Mosby, St. Louis.

52. Diederich S, Franzen N. F, Bähr V, et al. Severe hyponatremia due to hypopituitarism with adrenal insufficiency: report on 28 cases, Eur J Endocrinol. 2003; 148609–617.617.

53. Dluhy RG, Axelrod L, Williams GH. Serum immunoreactive insulin and growth hormone response to potassium infusion in normal man. J Appl Physiol. 1972; 33:22.

54. Don BR, Sebastian A, Cheitlin M, et al. Pseudohyperkalemia caused by fist clenching during phlebotomy. N Engl J Med. 1990; 322:1290.

55. Doucet A. Function and control of Na-K-ATPase in single nephron segments of the mammalian kidney. Kidney Int. 1988; 34:749.

56. Drakos P, Bar-Ziv J, Catane R. Tumor lysis syndrome in nonhematologic malignancies. Report of a case and review of the literature. Am J Clin Oncol. 1994; 17:502.

57. Edmondson RP, Thomas RD, Hilton PJ, et al. Leucocyte electrolytes in cardiac and non-cardiac patients receiving diuretics. Lancet. 1974; 1:12.

58. Ellis SJ. Severe hyponatremia: complications and treatment. QJM. 1995;88: 905-9.

59. Ellison DH, Berl T. Clinical practice. The syndrome of inappropriate antidiuresis. N Engl J Med. 2007;356: 2064–72.

60. Ferguson JW, Therapondos G, Newby DE, et al. Therapeutic role of vasopressin receptor antagonism in patients with liver cirrhosis. Clin Sci. 2003;105: 1–8.

61. Fernandez JA, Lopez P, Orozco D, et al. Clinical study of an outbreak of Legionnaire's disease in Alcoy, Southeastern Spain. Eur J ClinMicrobiol Infect Dis. 2002; 21:729–35.

62. Forrest JN Jr, Cox M, Hong C, et al. Superiority of demeclocycline over lithium in the treatment of chronic syndrome of inappropriate secretion of antidiuretic hormone. N Engl J Med. 1978;298:173–7.

63. Freda BJ, Davidson MB, Hall PM. Evaluation of hyponatremia. A little physiology goes a long way. Cleve Clin J. Med. 2004;71:639–50.

64. Frizelle F A, Colls B M. Hyponatraemia and seizures after bowel preparation: report of 3 cases. Dis Colon Rectum. 2005. 48393–396.396.

65. Fulop M. Serum potassium in lactic acidosis and ketoacidosis. N Engl J Med. 1979; 300:1087.

66. Gennari F J. Serum osmolality: uses and limitations. N Engl J Med. 1984. 310102–105.105.

67. Gennari FJ. Hypo–hypernatraemia: disorders of water balance. In: Davison AM, Cameron JS, Grünfeld JP, Kerr DNS, Ritz E, Winearls CG, eds. Oxford Textbook of Clinical Nephrology, 2nd Edition. Oxford University Press, Oxford, New York, Tokyo: 1998: 175-89.

68. Gerbes A, Gulberg, V, Gines P, et al. Therapy of hyponatraemia in cirrhosis with a vasopressin receptor antagonist: a randomised double blind multicentre trial. Gastroenterology. 2003; 124933–939.939.

69. Goh, Kian Ping. "Management of Hyponatremia." American Family Physician May 15, 2004: 2387.

70. Goldenberg IF, Olivari MT, Levine TB, et al. Effect of dobutamine on plasma potassium in congestive heart failure secondary to idiopathic or ischemic cardiomyopathy. Am J Cardiol. 1989; 63:843.

71. Goldman MB, Robertson GL, Luchins DJ, et al. Psychotic exacerbations and enhanced vasopressin secretion in schizophrenic patients with hyponatremia and polydipsia. Arch Gen Psychiatry. 1997; 54443–449.449.

72. Goldsmith SR, Gheorghiade M. Vasopressin antagonism in heart failure. J Am Coll Cardiol. 2005; 46: 1785–91.

73. Graber M. A model of the hyperkalemia produced by metabolic acidosis. Am J Kidney Dis. 1993; 22:436.

74. Gross P, Reimann D, Neidel J, et al. The treatment of severe hyponatremia. Kidney Int. 1998; Suppl 64:S6–S11.

75. Gross P. Treatment of severe hyponatremia. Kidney Int. 2001; 60: 2417–27.

76. Hande KR, Garrow GC. Acute tumor lysis syndrome in patients with high-grade non-Hodgkin's lymphoma. Am J Med. 1993; 94:133.

77. Hantman D, Rossier B, Zohlman R, et al. Rapid correction of hyponatremia in the syndrome of inappropriate antidiuretic hormone: an alternative treatment to hypertonic saline. Ann Int Med. 1973;78: 870–5.

78. Harrigan M R. Cerebral salt wasting syndrome: a review. Neurosurgery. 1996. 38152–160.160.

79. Hartung TK, Schofield E, Short AI, et al. Hyponatraemic states following 3,4-methylene-dioxymethamphetamine (MDMA, 'ecstasy') ingestion. QJM. 2002; 95:431–7.

80. Hilden T, Svendsen TL. Electrolyte disturbances in beer drinkers. A specific hypoosmolality syndrome. Lancet. 1975; 2245–246.246.

81. Hillier TA, Abbott R D, Barrett E J. Hyponatremia evaluating the correction factor for hyperglycaemia. Am J Med. 1999. 106399–403.403.

82. Illowsky BP, Kirch DG. Polydipsia and hyponatremia in psychiatric patients. Am J Psychol. 1988; 145675–683.683.

83. Almond C S, Shin A Y, Fortescue E B. et al Hyponatremia among runners in the Boston marathon. N Engl J Med. 2005; 3521550–1556.1556.

84. Ishikawa S, Schrier R. Pathophysiological roles of arginine vasopressin and aquaporin-2 in impaired water excretion. ClinEndocrinol (Oxf). 2003; 581–17.17.

85. Ishikawa S, Schrier RW. Pathophysiological roles of arginine vasopressin and aquaporin-2 in impaired water excretion. Clin Endocrinol. 2003;58: 1–17.

86. Janicic N, Verbalis JG. Evaluation and management of hypoosmolality in hospitalized patients. Endocrinol Metab Clin North Am. 2003; 32:459–81.

87. Johnson BE, Damodaran A, Rushin J, et al. Ectopic production and processing of atrial natriuretic peptide in a small cell lung carcinoma cell line and tumor from a patient with hyponatremia. Cancer. 1997; 79: 35–44.

88. Kaji D, Thomas K. Na^+-K^+ pump in chronic renal failure. Am J Physiol. 1987; 252:F785.

89. Karp B, Laureno R. Pontine and extrapontinemyelinolysis: a neurologic disorder following rapid correction of hyponatraemia. Medicine. 1993. 72359–373.373.

90. Klein L, O'Connor CM, Leimberger JD, et al. Lower serum sodium is associated with increased short-term mortality in hospitalized patients with worsening heart failure: results from the outcomes of a prospective trial of intravenous milrinone for exacerbations of chronic heart failure (OPTIME-CHF) study. Circulation. 2005;111: 2454–60.

91. Kleinfeld M, Casimir M, Borra S. Hyponatremia as observed in a chronic disease facility. J Am Geriatr Soc. 1979;27: 156–61.

92. Knochel JP, Blachley JD, Johnson JH, et al. Muscle cell electrical hyperpolarization and reduced exercise hyperkalemia in physically conditioned dogs. J Clin Invest. 1985; 75:740.

93. Knochel JP, Schlein EM. On the mechanism of rhabdomyolysis in potassium depletion. J Clin Invest. 1972; 51:1750.

94. Knochel JP. Neuromuscular manifestations of electrolyte disorders. Am J Med. 1982; 72:521.

95. Koay ES, Walmsley RN. A primer of chemical pathology. Singapore: World Scientific. 1996:20.

96. Kokko JP, Jacobson HR. Renal chloride transport. In: Selden DW, Giebisch G, eds. The kidney: physiology and pathophysiology. New York: Raven Press, 1985;1097–117.

97. Konstam MA, Gheorghiade M, Burnett JC Jr, et al. Effects of oral tolvaptan in patients hospitalized for worsening heart failure. The EVEREST Outcome Trial. JAMA. 2007;297: 1319–31.

98. Kumar S, Berl T. Sodium. Lancet. 1998;352:220–8.

99. Kunhle U, Lewicka S, Fuller P J. Endocrine disorders of sodium regulation. Horm Res. 2004; 6168–83.83.

100. Kunin As, Surawicz B, Sims EA. Decrease in serum potassium concentrations and appearance of cardiac arrhythmias during infusion of potassium with glucose in potassium-depleted patients. N Engl J Med. 1962; 266:228.

101. Kurtzman NA, Gonzalez J, DeFronzo R, Giebisch G. A patient with hyperkalemia and metabolic acidosis. Am J Kidney Dis. 1990; 15:333.

102. Lauriat SM, Berl T. The hyponatremic patient: practical focus on therapy. J Am Soc Nephrol. 1997;8:1599–607.

103. Lauriat SM, Berl T: The hyponatremic patient: Practical focus on therapy. J Am SocNephrol. 1997;8:1599–1607.

104. Lawson DH, Murray RM, Parker JL. Early mortality in the megaloblasticanaemias. Q J Med. 1972; 41:1

105. Lee CT, Guo HR, Chen JB. Hyponatremia in the emergency department. Am J Emerg Med. 2000;18:264–8.

106. Lehrich RW, Greenberg A. When is it appropriate to use vasopressin receptor antagonists? J Am SocNephrol. 2008; 19:1054–58.

107. Liamis G, Kalogirou M, Saugos V, et al. Therapeutic approach in patients with dysnatraemias. Nephrol Dial Transplant. 2006. 211564–1569.1569.

108. Liamis G, Milionis H, Elisaf M. A review of drug-induced hyponatremia. Am J Kidney Dis. 2008; 52 (1): 144–53.

109. Liberopoulos EN, Alexandridis GH, Christidis DS, et al. SIADH and hyponatremia with theophylline. Ann Pharmacother. 2002;36:1180–2.

110. Lien YH, Shapiro JI. Hyponatremia: clinical diagnosis and management. Am J Med. 2007;120(8):653–8.

111. Lim M, Linton RA, Wolff CB, et al. Propranolol, exercise, and arterial plasma potassium. Lancet. 1981; 2:591.

112. Lindinger MI, Heigenhauser GJ, McKelvie RS, et al. Blood ion regulation during repeated maximal exercise and recovery in humans. Am J Physiol. 1992; 262:R126.

113. Lindner G, Funk GC, Schwarz C, et al. Hypernatremia in the critically ill is an independent risk factor for mortality. Am J Kidney Dis. 2007;50:952–7.

114. Lindner G, Schwarz C, Kneidinger N, et al. Can we really predict the change in serum sodium levels? An analysis of currently proposed formulae in hypernatraemic patients. Nephrol Dial Transplant. 2008; 23:3501–8.

115. Lipworth BJ, McDevitt DG, Struthers AD. Prior treatment with diuretic augments the hypokalemic and electrocardiographic effects of inhaled albuterol. Am J Med. 1989; 86:653.

116. Lytton J, Lin JC, Guidotti G. Identification of two molecular forms of (Na^+, K^+)-ATPase in rat adipocytes. Relation to insulin stimulation of the enzyme. J BiolChem. 1985; 260: 1177.

117. Madias NE, Adrogue HJ. Hypo–hypernatraemia: disorders of water balance. In: Davidson AM, Cameron JS, Grünfeld J-P, et al. (eds.), Oxford Textbook of Clinical Nephrology, 3rd edition Oxford University Press, 2005, pp. 213–29.

118. Maesaka JK, Imbriano LJ, Ali NM, et al. Is it cerebral or renal salt wasting? Kidney Int. 2009;76:934-8.

119. Magner PO, Robinson L, Halperin RM, et al. The plasma potassium concentration in metabolic acidosis: a reevaluation. Am J Kidney Dis. 1988; 11:220.

120. McGee S, Abernethy WB 3d, Simel DL. The rational clinical examination. Is this patient hypovolemic?. JAMA. 1999;281:10229.

121. Milionis HJ, Liamis GL, Elisaf MS. The hyponatremic patient: a systematic approach to laboratory diagnosis. CMAJ. 2002;166:1056–62.

122. Miller M, Morley JE, Rubenstein LZ. Hyponatremia in a nursing home population. J Am Geriatr Soc. 1995;43: 1410–3.

123. Mohmand HK, Issa D, Ahmad Z, et al. Hypertonic saline for hyponatremia: risk of inadvertent overcorrection. Clin J Am Soc Nephrol. 2007;2:1110–7.

124. Moreno M, Murphy C, Goldsmith C. Increase in serum potassium resulting from the administration of hypertonic mannitol and other solutions. J Lab Clin Med. 1969; 73:291.

125. Moritz, Michael L., Juan Carlos Ayus. "Hospital-acquired Hyponatremia: Why are There Still Deaths?" Pediatrics. 2004: 1395-1397.

126. Narins RG, Emmett M. Simple and mixed acid–base disorders: a practical approach. Medicine. 1980;50:161–87.

127. Nguyen MK, Kurtz I. Analysis of current formulas used for treatment of the dysnatremias. ClinExpNephrol. 2004; 8: 12–16.

128. Nicolis GL, Kahn T, Sanchez A, et al. Glucose-induced hyperkalemia in diabetic subjects. Arch Intern Med. 1981; 141:49.

129. Nzerue CM, Baffoe-Bonnie H, You W, et al. Predictors of outcome in hospitalized patients with severe hyponatremia. J Natl Med Assoc. 2003; 95:335–43.

130. Oren R M. Hyponatremia in congestive heart failure. Am J Cardiol. 2005; 95(95A)2B–7B.7B.

131. Orringer CE, Eustace JC, Wunsch CD, et al. Natural history of lactic acidosis after grand-mal seizures. A model for the study of an anion-gap acidosis not associated with hyperkalemia. N Engl J Med. 1977; 297:796.

132. Oster JR, Singer I: Hyponatremia, hyposmolality, and hypotonicity: Tables and fables. Arch Intern Med. 1999; 159:333–336.

133. Palevsky PM, Bhagrath R, Greenberg A. Hypernatremia in hospitalized patients. Ann Intern Med. 1996;124:197–203.

134. Patel GP, Kasiar JB. Syndrome of inappropriate antidiuretic hormone-induced hyponatremia associated with amiodarone. Pharmacotherapy. 2002;22:649–51.

135. Perez GO, Oster JR, Vaamonde CA. Serum potassium concentration in acidemic states. Nephron. 1981; 27:233.

136. Perianayagam A, Sterns RH, Silver SM, et al. DDAVP is effective in preventing and reversing inadvertent over-correction of hyponatremia. Clin J Am Soc Nephrol. 2008;3: 331–6.

137. Peters J P, Welt L G, Sims E A. et al. A saltwasting syndrome associated with cerebral disease. Trans Assoc Am Physicians. 1950. 6357–64.64.

138. Pham PC, Pham PM, Pham PT. Vasopressin excess and hyponatremia. Am J Kidney Dis. 2006;47: 727–37.

139. Pitts RF. Physiology of the Kidney and Body Fluids,. Year Book, Chicago. 1974; Chap 11.

140. Reddy P, Mooradian AD. Diagnosis and management of hyponatremia in hospitalised patients. Int J ClinPract. 2009;63: 1494–508.

141. Reynolds R, Secki J R. Hyponatraemia for the clinical endocrinologist. ClinEndocrinol (Oxf). 2005; 63366–374.374.

142. Reza MJ, Kovick RB, Shine KI, et al. Massive intravenous digoxin overdosage. N Engl J Med. 1974; 291:777.

143. Robertson GL. Regulation of arginine vasopressin in the syndrome of inappropriate antidiuresis. Am J Med. 2006;119(7 Suppl 1): S36-42.

144. Rosa RM, Silva P, Young JB, et al. Adrenergic modulation of extrarenal potassium disposal. N Engl J Med. 1980; 302:431.

145. Rose BD, Black RM (eds). Clinical Problems in Nephrology, 1st edition Boston, Little, Brown. 1996; pp 3–17.

146. Saito T, Ishikawa S, Abe K, et al. Acute aquaresis by the nonpeptide arginine vasopressin (AVP) antagonist OPC-31260 improves hyponatremia in patients with syndrome of inappropriate secretion of antidiuretic hormone (SIADH). J Clin Endocrinol Metab. 1997;82:1054–7.

147. Sands JM, Bichet DG. Nephrogenic diabetes insipidus. Ann Intern Med. 2006; 144:186–194.

148. Sassard J, Vincent M, Annat G, et al. A kinetic study of plasma renin and aldosterone during changes of posture in man. J Clin Endocrinol Metab. 1976; 42:20.

149. Schnack C, Podolsky A, Watzke H, et al. Effects of somatostatin and oral potassium administration on terbutaline-induced hypokalemia. Am Rev Respir Dis. 1989; 139:176.

150. Schrier RW, Gross P, Gheorghiade M, et al. Tolvaptan, a selective oral vasopressin V2 receptor antagonist for hyponatremia. N Engl J Med. 2006; 3552099–2112.2112.

151. Schrier RW. Body fluid volume regulation in health and disease: A unifying hypothesis. Ann Intern Med. 1990;113: 155–9.

152. Scwartz WB, Bennett W, Curelop S. et al. A syndrome of renal sodium loss and hyponatremia probably resulting from inappropriate secretion of antidiuretic hormone. Am J Med 1957. 13529–542.542.

153. Seckl JR, Williams TD, Lightman S L. Oral hypertonic saline causes transient fall of vasopressin in humans. Am J Physiol1986. 251R214–R217.R217.

154. Seifter JR. Acid-base disorders. In: Goldman L, Schafer AI, (eds.). Cecil Medicine. 24th edition. Philadelphia, Pa: Saunders Elsevier; 2011:chap 120.

155. Seldin DW, Rector RC Jr. The generation and maintenance of metabolic alkalosis. Kidney Int. 1972;1:306–21.

156. Sivakumar V, Rajshekar V, Chandy M J. Management of neurosurgical patients with hyponatraemia and natriuresis. Neurosurgery. 1994; 34269–274.274.

157. Smith AF, Beckett GJ, Walker SW, et al. Lecture notes on clinical biochemistry. 6th ed. Oxford: Blackwell Science, 1998:22.

158. Smith DM, McKenna K, Thompson CJ. Hyponatremia. Clin Endocrinol. 2000;52: 667–78.

159. Spital A. Diuretic-induced hyponatremia. Am J Nephrol. 1999; 19:447–52.

160. Springate, James E., Mary F. Carroll. "HAdditional Causes of Hypercalcemia in Infants." American Family Physician. 2004: 2766.

161. Sterns RH, Cappuccio JD, Silver SM, et al. Neurologic sequelae after treatment of severe hyponatremia: a multi-center perspective. J Am SocNephrol. 1994;4:1522–30.

162. Sterns RH, Cox M, Feig PU, et al. Internal potassium balance and the control of the plasma potassium concentration. Medicine (Baltimore) 1981; 60:339.

163. Sterns RH, Hix JK. Overcorrection of hyponatremia is a medical emergency. Kidney Int. 2009;76:587–9.

164. Sterns RH, Nigwekar SU, Hix JK. The treatment of hyponatremia. Semin Nephrol. 2009;29:282–99.

165. Sterns RH, Riggs JE, Schochet SS Jr. Osmotic demyelination syndrome following correction of hyponatremia. N Engl J Med. 1986;314:1535–42.

166. Struthers AD, Quigley C, Brown MJ. Rapid changes in plasma potassium during a game of squash. Clin Sci (Lond). 1988; 74:397.

167. Struthers AD, Whitesmith R, Reid JL. Prior thiazide diuretic treatment increases adrenaline-induced hypokalaemia. Lancet. 1983; 1:1358.

168. Szatalowicz VL, Miller PD, Lacher JW, et al. Comparative effect of diuretics on renal water excretion in hyponatremic oedematous disorders. Clin Sci [Lond]. 1982;62:235–8.

169. Thomas DR, Tariq SH, Makhdomm S, et al. Physician misdiagnosis of dehydration in older adults. J Am Med Dir Assoc. 2003;4:251–4.

170. Thomson A, Kelly DT. Exercise stress-induced changes in systemic arterial potassium in angina pectoris. Am J Cardiol. 1989; 63:1435.

171. Tietz textbook of clinical chemistry 3rd edition, Philadelphia, WB Saunders company (1995).

172. Tietz textbook of clinical chemistry and molecular biology, 5th edition, Philadelphia, W.B. Saunders company (2012).

173. Udelson JE, Smith WB, Hendrix GH, et al. Acute haemo-dynamic effects of conivaptan, a dual V1a and V2 vasopressin receptor antagonist in patients with advanced heart failure. Circulation. 2001; 1042417–2423.2423.

174. Upadhyay A, Jaber BL, Madias NE. Epidemiology of hyponatremia. Semin Nephrol. 2009;29:227–38.

175. Upadhyay A, Jaber BL, Madias NE. Incidence and prevalence of hyponatremia. Am J Med. 2006;119:S30–5.

176. Verbalis JG, Goldsmith SR, Greenberg A, Schrier RW, Sterns RH. Hyponatremia treatment guidelines 2007: expert panel recommendations. Am J Med. 2007;120:S1–21.

177. Verbalis JG. Whole-body volume regulation and escape from antidiuresis. Am J Med 2006;119(7 Suppl 1):S21-9.

178. Viberti GC. Glucose-induced Hyperkalemia: A hazard for diabetics? Lancet. 1978; 1:690.

179. Walmsley RN, Watkinson LR, Koay ES. Cases in chemical pathology: a diagnostic approach, 3rd edtion. Singapore: World Scientific, 1992:22.

180. Weiss-Guillet EM, Takala J, Jakob SM. Diagnosis and management of electrolyte emergencies. Best Pract Res Clin Endocrinol Metab. 2003;17: 623–51.

181. Wilkinson TJ, Begg EJ, Winter AC, et al. Incidence and risk factors for hyponatremia following treatment with fluoxetine or paroxetine in elderly people. Br J Clin Pharmacol. 1999; 47:211–7.

182. William Marshall, Stephen K. Clinical Chemistry book, 6th edition, London, Mosby (2008).

183. Williams ME, Gervino EV, Rosa RM, et al. Catecholamine modulation of rapid potassium shifts during exercise. N Engl J Med. 1985; 312:823.

184. Wong F, Blei AT, Blendis LM, et al. A vasopressin receptor antagonist (VPA-985) improves serum sodium concentration in patients with hyponatremia: a multicentre, randomised, placebo-controlled trial. Hepatology. 2003;37: 182–91.

185. Wong LL, Verbalis JG. Vasopressin V2 receptor antagonists. Cardiovasc Res. 2001;51:391–402.

186. Woo MH, Smythe MA. Association of SIADH with selective serotonin reuptake inhibitors. Ann Pharmacother. 1997;31: 108–10.

187. Zhang ZW, Kang Y, Deng LJ, et al. Therapy of central pontine myelinolysis following liver transplantation: report of three cases. World J Gastroenterol. 2009;15:3960–3.

188. Zierler Kl, Rabinowitz D. Effect of very small concentrations of insulin on forearm metabolism. persistence of its action on potassium and free fatty acids without its effect on glucose. J Clin invest. 1964; 43:950.

4

The Kidneys

INTRODUCTION

The **kidneys** are a pair of bean-shaped organs found along the posterior wall of the abdominal cavity. The left kidney is located slightly higher than the right kidney because the right side of the liver is much larger than the left side. The kidneys, unlike the other organs of the abdominal cavity, are located posterior to the peritoneum and touch the muscles of the back. The kidneys are surrounded by a layer of adipose that holds them in place and protects them from physical damage.

The kidneys are essential for homeostasis (maintaining a constant internal environment) of the body's extracellular fluids. Their basic functions include:

1. Regulation of extracellular fluid (ECF) volume: The kidneys work to ensure an adequate quantity of plasma to keep blood flowing to vital organs.
2. Regulation of osmolarity: The kidneys help keep extracellular fluid from becoming too dilute or concentrated with respect to the solutes carried in the fluid.
3. Regulation of ion concentrations: The kidneys are responsible for maintaining relatively constant levels of key ions including sodium, potassium, and calcium.
4. Regulation of pH: The kidneys prevent blood plasma from becoming too acidic or basic by regulating ions.
5. Excretion of wastes and toxins: The kidneys filter out a variety of water-soluble waste products and environmental toxins into the urine for excretion.
6. Production of hormones: The kidneys produce erythropoietin, which stimulates red blood cell synthesis, and renin, which helps control salt and water balance and blood pressure. They are also involved in regulating plasma calcium and glucose levels.

The kidneys purify toxic metabolic waste products from the blood in several hundred thousand functionally independent units called **nephrons**. A nephron consists of one glomerulus and one double hairpin-shaped tubule that drain the filtrate into the renal pelvis (Fig. 4.1). The glomeruli located in the kidney cortex are bordered by the Bowman's capsule. They are lined with parietal epithelial cells and contain the mesangium with many capillaries to filter the blood. The glomerular filtration barrier consists of endothelial cells, the glomerular basement membrane and visceral epithelial cells (also known as podocytes).

The glomerular filtrate is an ultrafiltrate of plasma; that is, it has a similar composition to plasma except that it is almost free of large proteins. This is because the endothelium provides a barrier to red and white blood cells, and the basement membrane, although permeable to water and low molecular weight substances, is largely impermeable to macromolecules. This impermeability is related to both molecular size and electrical charge. Proteins with molecular weights lower than that of albumin (68 kDa) are filterable; negatively charged molecules are less easily filtered than those bearing a positive charge. Almost all the protein in the glomerular filtrate is reabsorbed and catabolized by proximal convoluted tubular cells, with the result that normal urinary protein excretion is <150 mg/24 h.

Filtration is a passive process. The total filtration rate of the kidneys is mainly determined by the difference between the blood pressure in the glomerular capillaries and the hydrostatic pressure in the lumen of the nephron, the nature of the glomerular basement membrane and the number of glomeruli. The difference in the osmotic pressures of the plasma and the ultrafiltrate provides a

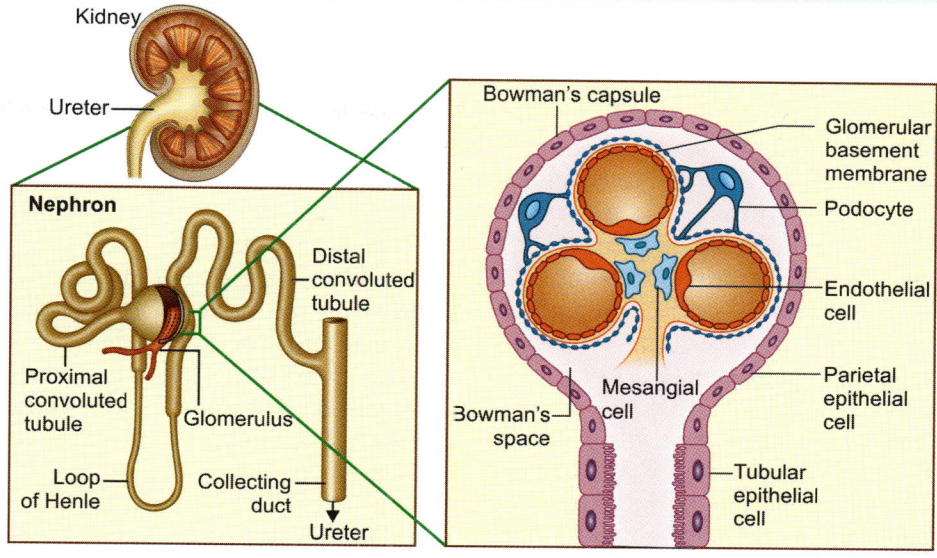

Fig. 4.1: The structure of a nephron

small force that opposes filtration. The amount of filtrate formed decreases along the length of the glomerular capillaries as the difference in hydrostatic pressures falls and that in osmotic pressures rises. The normal glomerular filtration rate (GFR) is approximately 120 mL/min, equivalent to a volume of about 170 L/24 h. However, urine production is only 1–2 L/24 h, depending on fluid intake; the bulk of the filtrate is reabsorbed further along the nephron.

The glomerular filtrate passes into the proximal convoluted tubules, where much of it is reabsorbed. Under normal circumstances, all the glucose, amino acids, potassium and bicarbonate, and about 75% of the sodium, is reabsorbed isotonically here by energy-dependent mechanisms.

Medullary hyperosmolality, which is vital for the further reabsorption of water, is generated by the counter-current system, summarized in (Fig. 4.2). Chloride ions,

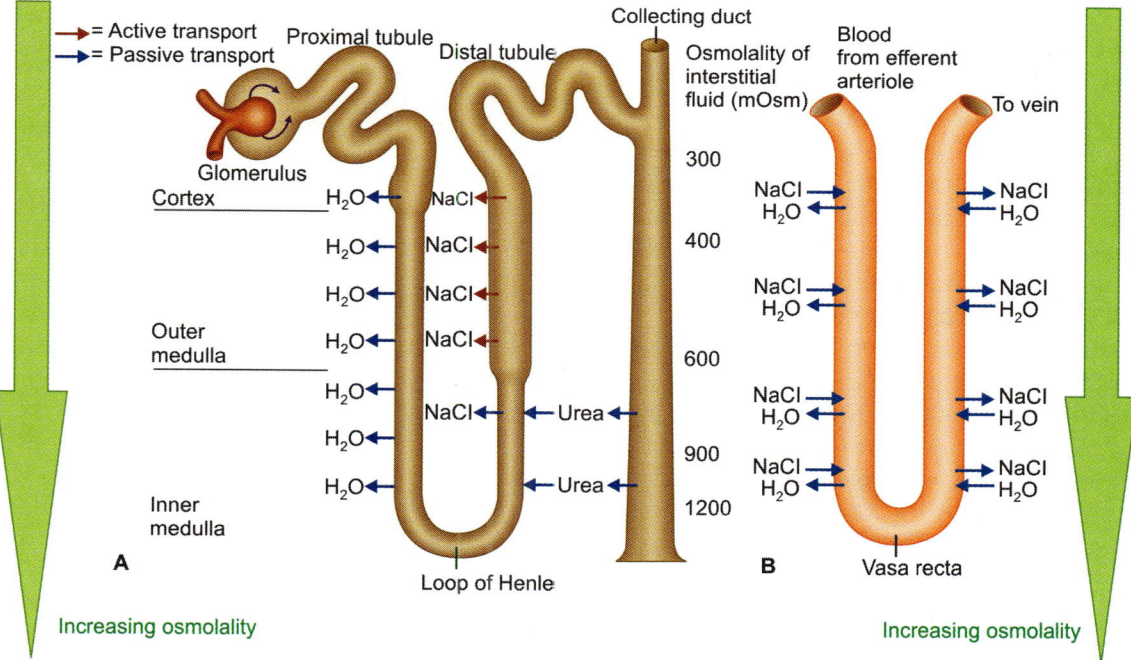

Fig. 4.2: Movements of major ions, passive movement of water and changes in osmolality in the nephron. In the ascending loop of Henle, chloride ions are actively transported and sodium ions accompany them to maintain electrochemical neutrality

accompanied by sodium, are pumped out of the ascending limbs of the loops of Henle into the surrounding interstitial fluid, and thence diffuse into the descending limbs. As the ascending limbs of the loops of Henle are impermeable to water, the net effect is an exchange of sodium and chloride ions between the ascending and descending limbs. This alters the osmolality of both the fluid within the nephrons and the surrounding interstitial fluid. A gradient of osmolality is setup between the isotonic corticomedullary junction and the extremely hypertonic (approximately 1200 mmol/L) deep medulla. Diffusion of urea from the collecting ducts into the interstitium and thence into the loops of Henle also makes an important contribution to medullary hypertonicity. It is noteworthy that urinary concentrating ability is impaired in malnourished children, but can be restored by increasing their dietary protein intake or (experimentally) by adding urea to their diets.

The tubular fluid becomes increasingly dilute as it passes-up the ascending limbs of the loops of Henle, as a result of the continued removal of chloride and sodium ions. Fluid entering the distal convoluted tubules is hypotonic (approximately 150 mmol/L) with respect to the glomerular filtrate. Further dilution takes place in the early part of the distal convoluted tubules.

Approximately 90% of the filtered sodium and 80% of the filtered water has been reabsorbed from the glomerular filtrate by the time it reaches the beginning of the distal convoluted tubules. In the distal tubules, further sodium reabsorption takes place, in part controlled by aldosterone; this generates an electro-chemical gradient that is balanced by the secretion of potassium and hydrogen ions. Ammonia is also secreted in the distal tubule and buffers hydrogen ions, being excreted as ammonium ions.

Whereas the proximal tubules are responsible for bulk reabsorption of the glomerular filtrate, the distal tubules exert fine control over the composition of the tubular fluid, depending on the requirements of the body.

Tubular fluid then passes into the collecting ducts, which extend through the hypertonic renal medulla and discharge urine into the renal pelvices. The cells lining the collecting ducts are normally impermeable to water. Vasopressin (antidiuretic hormone, ADH) renders them permeable by stimulating the incorporation of aquaporins (water channels) into the cell membranes and allows water to be reabsorbed passively in response to the osmotic gradient between the duct lumen and the interstitial fluid. Thus, in the absence of vasopressin, dilute urine is produced; in its presence, the urine is concentrated. Some reabsorption of sodium also occurs in the collecting ducts under the stimulus of aldosterone.

The collecting ducts drain into the renal pelvices, from which urine passes through the ureters to the bladder.

As the normal GFR is approximately 120 mL/min, a volume of fluid equivalent to the entire ECF is filtered every 2 hours. Disease processes affecting the kidney therefore have a considerable potential for affecting water, salt, and hydrogen ion homoeostasis and the excretion of waste products.

The kidneys are also important endocrine organs, producing renin, erythropoietin, and calcitriol. The secretion of these hormones may be altered in renal disease. In addition, several other hormones are either inactivated or excreted by the kidneys and hence their concentrations in the blood can also be affected by renal disease.

The Biochemical Investigation of Renal Function

Diseases affecting the kidneys can selectively damage glomerular or tubular function, but isolated disorders of tubular function are relatively uncommon. In acute and chronic renal failure, there is effectively a loss of function of whole nephrons and, as the process of filtration is essential to the formation of urine, tests of glomerular function are almost invariably required in the investigation and management of any patient with renal disease. The principal function of the glomeruli is to filter water and low molecular weight components of the blood while retaining cells and high molecular weight components. The most frequently used tests are those that assess either the GFR or the integrity of the glomerular filtration barrier.

It should be noted that the GFR declines with age (to a greater extent in males than in females) and this must be taken into account when interpreting results.

MEASUREMENT OF GLOMERULAR FILTRATION RATE

Glomerular filtration rate is defined as the volume of plasma that can be completely cleared of a particular substance by all the renal corpuscles in both kidneys per minute. The 'gold standard' for determining GFR is to measure the clearance of exogenous substances such as inulin, iohexol, ^{51}Cr-ethylenediaminetetraacetic acid (EDTA), ^{99m}Tc-labeled diethylenetriamine pentaacetic acid (DTPA), or ^{125}I-labeled iothalamate. These techniques, however, are time-consuming, labor-intensive, expensive, and require administration of substances that make them incompatible with routine monitoring. Thus, the measurement of endogenous blood substances to estimate GFR is a common practice. Properties of an ideal endogenous blood substance to estimate GFR should include release into the bloodstream at a constant rate, free filtration by the glomerulus, no reabsorption or secretion by the renal tubules, and exclusive elimination via the kidneys.

The glomerular filtration rate is directly proportional to the net filtration pressure, so a fluctuation in pressure will change the GFR. Prolonged changes in normal GFR will cause either too much or too little water and solutes to be removed from the blood. Conditions that can affect GFR include arterial pressure, afferent arteriole constriction, efferent arteriole constriction, plasma protein concentration, and colloid osmotic pressure. The glomerular blood pressure provides the driving force for fluid and solutes to be filtered out of the blood and into the space made by Bowman's capsule. The remainder of the blood not filtered into the glomerulus passes into the narrower efferent arteriole.

Glomerular filtration rate is the volume of fluid filtered from the renal (kidney) glomerular capillaries into the Bowman's capsule per unit time. Central to the physiologic maintenance of GFR is the differential basal tone of the afferent and efferent arterioles. GFR is equal to the clearance rate when any solute is freely filtered and is neither reabsorbed nor secreted by the kidneys.

Therefore, the rate measured is the quantity of the substance in the urine that originated from a calculable volume of blood. Relating this principle to the below equation for the substance used, the product of urine concentration and urine flow equals the mass of substance excreted during the time that urine has been collected. This mass equals the mass filtered at the glomerulus as nothing is added or removed in the nephron. Dividing this mass by the plasma concentration gives the volume of plasma, which the mass must have originally come from, and thus the volume of plasma fluid that has entered Bowman's capsule within the aforementioned period of time. The GFR is typically recorded in units of volume per time, e.g. milliliters per minute (mL/min).

$$GFR = \frac{\text{Urine concentration} \times \text{Urine flow}}{\text{Plasma concentration}}$$

This equation applies to GFR calculation when it is equal to the clearance rate. In the physiology of the kidneys, tubuloglomerular feedback (TGF) is one of several mechanisms the kidneys use to regulate glomerular filtration rate. Changes in GFR are detected by the renal tubule, which sends feedback signals to the glomerulus, initiating a cascade of events that ultimately brings GFR to an appropriate level. The macula densa serves as the detector, while the glomerulus acts as the effector.

Proper function of the kidney requires that it receives and adequately filters blood. This is performed at a microscopic level by many hundreds of thousands of filtration units called renal corpuscles, each of which is composed of a glomerulus and a Bowman's capsule. A universally accepted way to assess efficient renal function is to estimate the rate of filtration, called the GFR.

Tubular reabsorption is the process by which solutes and water are removed from the tubular fluid and transported into the blood. It is called reabsorption (not absorption), because these substances have already been absorbed previously, usually in the intestines.

Reabsorption is a two-step process beginning with the active or passive extraction of substances from the tubular fluid into the renal interstitium (the connective tissue that surrounds the nephrons); then these substances are transported from the interstitium into the bloodstream. These transport processes are driven by Starling forces, diffusion, and active transport.

Within the peritubular capillary network, molecules, and ions are reabsorbed back into the blood. The sodium chloride that is reabsorbed into the system increases the osmolarity of blood in comparison to the glomerular filtrate.

This reabsorption process allows water to pass from the glomerular filtrate, back into the circulatory system. Glucose and various amino acids are also reabsorbed into the circulatory system. Glomerular filtrate is then separated into two forms—reabsorbed filtrate and non-reabsorbed filtrate. The non-reabsorbed filtrate is then known as tubular fluid as it passes through the collecting duct to be processed into urine.

CLEARANCE

An estimate of the GFR can be made by measuring the urinary excretion of a substance that is completely filtered from the blood by the glomeruli and is not secreted, reabsorbed, or metabolized by the renal tubules. Experimentally, inulin (a plant polysaccharide) has been found to meet these requirements. The volume of blood from which inulin is cleared or completely removed in 1 minute is known as the inulin clearance, and is equal to the GFR.

Measurement of inulin clearance requires the infusion of inulin into the blood and is not suitable for routine clinical use. The most widely used biochemical clearance test is based on measurements of creatinine in plasma and urine. This endogenous substance is derived mainly from the turnover of creatine in muscle and daily production is relatively constant, being a function of total muscle mass. A small amount of creatinine is derived from meat in the diet.

Creatinine-clearance Test

A test that helps determines whether the kidneys are functioning normally. Specifically, the creatinine-clearance test gauges the rate at which a waste, creatinine, is 'cleared' from the blood by the kidneys. Creatinine is produced from the metabolism of protein as when muscles burn energy. Most creatinine is then filtered out of the blood by the kidneys and excreted in urine.

The rate of creatinine clearance is measured by first noting the volume of urine excreted in a given time period, such as 24 hours. Then the amount of creatinine in the excreted urine is measured and compared with the amount of creatinine circulating in the blood. If the kidneys are not removing enough creatinine, the level of creatinine in the urine will fall. And consequently the level of creatinine in the blood will rise.

When the kidneys fail to clear enough creatinine and other wastes from the blood, the wastes buildup in the bloodstream. Symptoms of kidney disease, including swelling (edema), nausea, and high blood pressure may develop.

However, the creatinine-clearance test can usually detect waste buildup in the blood before it threatens the body. Doctors can then have an opportunity to eliminate the cause of the buildup and restore blood creatinine to normal levels. A creatinine-clearance test, thus, plays a key role in preventive medicine as well as in diagnostic and therapeutic medicine.

Creatinine clearance is calculated using the formula:

$$\text{Clearance} = \frac{\text{Urinary creatinine concentration} \times \text{Urine flow rate}}{\text{Plasma creatinine}}$$

U = Urinary creatinine concentration (μmol/L)
V = Urine flow rate (mL/min or (L/24 h)/1.44)
P = Plasma creatinine concentration (μmol/L)

Creatinine clearance in adults is normally of the order of 120 mL/min, corrected to a standard body surface area of 1.73 m^2. It should be noted that the clearance formula is only valid for a steady state, that is, when renal function is not changing rapidly.

The accurate measurement of creatinine clearance is difficult, especially in outpatients, as it is necessary to obtain a complete and accurately timed sample of urine. The usual collection time is 24 hours, but patients may forget the time or forget to include some urine in the collection. Incontinent patients, may find it impossible to make a urine collection. Patients have been known to add water or some other person's urine to their own collection, hoping to gain the doctor's approval for having been so prolific.

It may be more convenient and reliable to base the collection period on a patient's normal habits (e.g. overnight). The time at which the bladder is emptied before retiring to bed is noted; any urine passed during the night is collected, as is the urine voided when the patient rises. The time is noted and a blood sample is taken that morning for the measurement of plasma creatinine. As long as the time over which the urine collection is made is known, and the collection is complete, any suitable time period can be used.

Creatinine is actively secreted by the renal tubules and, as a result, the creatinine clearance is higher than the true GFR. The difference is of little significance when the GFR is normal, but when the GFR is low (<10 mL/min), tubular secretion makes a major contribution to creatinine excretion and creatinine clearance significantly overestimates the GFR. The effect of creatinine breakdown in the gut also becomes significant when the GFR is very low. Certain drugs, including spironolactone, cimetidine, fenofibrate, trimethoprim and amiloride, decrease creatinine secretion and thus can reduce creatinine clearance. Lastly, in the calculation of creatinine clearance, two measurements of creatinine concentration and one of urine volume are required. Each of these has an inherent imprecision that can affect the accuracy of the overall result. Even in well-motivated subjects, studied under ideal conditions, the coefficient of variation of measurements of creatinine clearance can be as high as 10%, and it can be two or three times greater than this in ordinary patients.

Thus, although hitherto widely used, measurements of creatinine clearance are potentially unreliable and no longer recommended in routine practice. Alternative methods should be used if a reliable calculation of GFR is required, for example in the assessment of potential kidney donors, investigation of patients with minor abnormalities of renal function and calculation of the initial doses of potentially toxic drugs that are eliminated from the body by renal excretion.

There are two main alternative approaches to determining the GFR in clinical practice. These are to use exogenous markers of clearance or to derive an estimated GFR (eGFR) from the plasma creatinine concentration. GFR can be measured by measuring the disappearance from the blood of a test substance that is completely filtered by the glomeruli and neither secreted nor reabsorbed by the tubules, following a single injection. This approach has the advantage that a urine collection is not required. Suitable substances for this purpose include ^{51}Cr-labeled EDTA, ^{125}I-iothalamate (for which the decline in plasma radioactivity is monitored) and iohexol, a non-radioactive X-ray contrast medium that is simple to measure using high performance liquid chromatography. Typically, blood samples are taken at 2, 3 and 4 hours after injection, although samples taken over a longer period may be required in renal impairment.

Plasma Creatinine

Plasma creatinine concentration is the most reliable simple biochemical test of glomerular function. Ingestion of a meat-rich meal can increase plasma creatinine concentration by as much as 20 µmol/L for up to 10 hours afterwards, so ideally blood samples should be collected after an overnight fast. Strenuous exercise also causes a transient, slight increase in plasma creatinine concentrations. Plasma creatinine concentration is related to muscle bulk and, therefore, a value of 120 µmol/L could be normal for an athletic young man, but would suggest renal impairment in a thin, 70-year-old woman. Although muscle bulk tends to decline with age, so too does the GFR, and hence plasma creatinine concentrations remain fairly constant.

Some commonly used laboratory methods for the measurement of creatinine can suffer from interference, for example from bilirubin and ketones. The laboratory should be able to advise on whether this may be a problem in individual cases.

The reference range for plasma creatinine in the adult population is 60–120 µmol/L, but the day-to-day variation in an individual is much less than this range. Creatinine clearance equation indicates that plasma creatinine concentration is inversely related to the GFR. GFR can decrease by 50% before plasma creatinine concentration rises beyond the normal range; plasma creatinine concentration doubles for each further 50% fall in GFR. Consequently, a normal plasma creatinine does not necessarily imply normal renal function, although a raised creatinine does usually indicate impaired renal function (Fig. 4.3). Furthermore, a change in creatinine concentration, provided that it is outside the limits of normal biological and analytical variation, does suggest a change in GFR, even if both the values are within the population reference range.

Changes in plasma creatinine concentration can occur, independently of renal function, owing to changes in muscle mass. Thus, a decrease can occur as a result of starvation and in wasting diseases, immediately after surgery and in patients treated with corticosteroids; an increase can occur during refeeding. However, changes in creatinine concentration for these reasons rarely lead to diagnostic confusion.

In pregnancy, the GFR increases. This usually more than balances the effect of increased creatinine synthesis during pregnancy, and results in a decrease in plasma creatinine concentration.

Estimated Glomerulus Filtration Rate

The eGFR is used to screen for and detect early kidney damage, and to monitor kidney status. It is performed by ordering a creatinine test and calculating the eGFR. The creatinine test is ordered frequently as part of a routine comprehensive metabolic panel (CMP) or basic metabolic panel (BMP), or along with a blood urea nitrogen (BUN) test, whenever a health practitioner wants to evaluate the status of a patient's kidneys. It is ordered to monitor those with known chronic kidney disease (CKD), and those with conditions such as diabetes and hypertension that may lead to kidney damage.

A creatinine test and eGFR may be ordered any time to evaluate a person's kidney function as part of a health checkup, or if kidney disease is suspected. Various formulas have been derived for this purpose, including factors, such as age, body weight, sex (creatinine production tends to be lower in women than men with the same body weight, because of their relatively smaller muscle mass) and racial origin. Several formulas have been derived from the modification of diet in renal disease (MDRD) study. **The 'four-variable' formula** is:

$$eGFR = 175 \times [sCr \times 0.011312]^{-1.154} \times age^{-0.203} \times [0.742 \text{ if female}] \times [1.21 \text{ for African black people}]$$

sCr: serum creatinine concentration (µmol/L)

A six-variable formula includes serum urea and albumin concentrations in addition. Because different laboratories may measure creatinine using different techniques, correction factors can be used to relate the estimated GFR to the reference method for creatinine measurement, thus supposedly ensuring that all eGFR values are comparable.

It is recommended that values of eGFR greater than 60 mL/min should be reported as '>60 mL/min' and regarded as normal in the absence of clinical or laboratory evidence of renal disease (e.g. abnormalities on imaging,

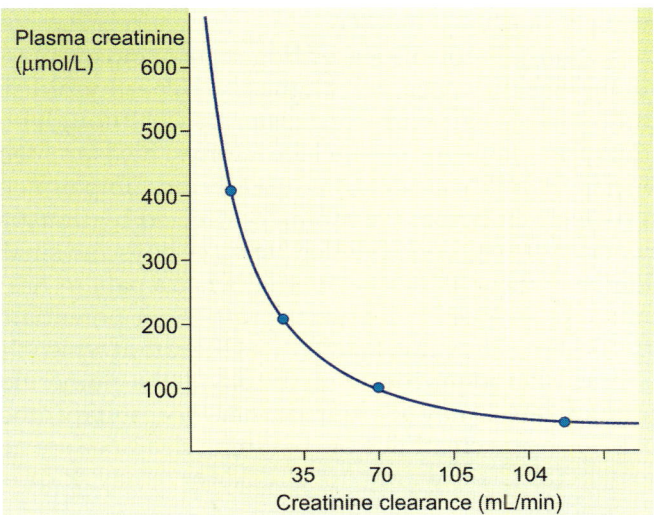

Fig. 4.3: Relationship between creatinine clearance and plasma creatinine concentration

proteinuria or hematuria). Neither it is applicable in acute kidney disease, pregnancy, in conditions in which there is severe muscle wasting, edematous conditions, amputees nor in children. A major use of the MDRD eGFR is as a tool for screening for chronic kidney disease (CKD). A more recent formula, the chronic kidney disease epidemiology collaboration (CKD-EPI), is based on pooled data from several studies and correlates better with measured GFR than the original MDRD formula, especially at values above 60 mL/min.

Although, now less widely used and not validated for use in screening for CKD, the Cockcroft–Gault formula, which is applicable over a wider range of GFRs, also provides an estimate of the creatinine clearance and hence GFR. Many drug dosing regimens, such as some of those used in cancer chemotherapy, are based on this, despite lack of adjustment for local creatinine calibration. The formula takes into account body weight in addition to sex, age and serum creatinine concentration:

Estimated clearance (mL/min) =

$$\frac{(140\text{-age in years} \times (\text{Weight in kg})}{\text{Serum [Creatinine] (}\mu\text{mol/L)} \times 0.81 \times (\text{For female}) \, 0.85}$$

PLASMA UREA

Urea is synthesized in the liver, primarily as a by-product of the deamination of amino acids. Its elimination in the urine represents the major route for nitrogen excretion. It is freely filtered by the glomerulus and not secreted by the tubules. However, a large portion (40–70%) is passively reabsorbed from the renal tubules; thus, its concentration will underestimate GFR in settings of decreased renal perfusion because some of the urea that is filtered will return to the bloodstream.

Urea was the first endogenous substance measured in serum or plasma to assess renal function. It is a major by-product of protein metabolism, and >90% of urea is cleared by the kidneys.

Plasma urea concentration is a less reliable indicator of renal glomerular function than creatinine. Urea production is increased by a high protein intake, in catabolic states, and by the absorption of amino acids and peptides after gastrointestinal hemorrhage. Conversely, production is decreased in patients with a low protein intake and sometimes in patients with liver disease. Tubular reabsorption increases at low rates of urine flow (e.g. in fluid depletion), and this can cause increased plasma urea concentration even when renal function is normal.

Factors affecting the ratio of plasma urea to creatinine are summarized in Table: 4.1. Changes in plasma urea concentration are a feature of renal impairment, but it is

Table 4.1	Causes of an abnormal plasma urea to creatinine ratio	
Increased	**Decreased**
High protein intake	Low protein intake
Gastrointestinal bleeding	Dialysis
Hypercatabolic state	Severe liver disease
Dehydration	
Urinary stasis	
Muscle wasting	
amputation	

important to consider possible extrarenal influences on urea concentrations before ascribing any changes to an alteration in renal function.

Urea diffuses readily across dialysis membranes and, during renal dialysis; a fall in plasma urea concentration is a poor guide to the efficacy of the process in removing other toxic substances from the blood.

Cystatin C

This low molecular weight peptide (13 kDa) is produced by all nucleated cells. It is a member of the family of cysteine proteinase inhibitors. It is the product of a 'housekeeping' gene expressed in all nucleated cells and is produced at a constant rate. Because of its small size is freely filtered by the glomerulus. It is not secreted, but is reabsorbed by tubular epithelial cells and subsequently catabolized so that it does not return to the blood flow. This latter property negates calculation of a Cystatin C (CysC) clearance using urine concentrations of CysC. The use of serum CysC to estimate GFR is based on the same logic as the use of blood urea and creatinine, but because it does not return to the bloodstream and is not secreted by renal tubules, it has been suggested to be closer to the 'ideal' endogenous marker.

Cystatin C is not influenced by gender or muscle mass, but may be increased in malignancy, hyperthyroidism and by treatment with corticosteroids. Although not widely available in routine laboratories, measurement may have a role in the detection of early renal impairment in patients in whom creatinine is affected by unusual muscle bulk (e.g. body builders, teenage boys and small, elderly women). It may be ordered when a patient has a known or suspected disease that affects or potentially affects kidney function and reduces the rate at which the kidneys filter impurities from the blood, the glomerular filtration rate. It may be ordered when the results of other tests, such as a creatinine or creatinine clearance are not satisfactory, or wants to check for early kidney dysfunction.

High level of cystatin C in the blood corresponds to a decreased glomerular filtration rate and hence to kidney dysfunction. Since cystatin C is produced throughout the body at a constant rate and removed and broken down by the kidneys, it should remain at a steady level in the blood if the kidneys are working efficiently and the GFR is normal.

Recent studies suggest that increased levels of CysC may also indicate an increased risk of heart disease, heart failure, stroke, and mortality. CysC has been associated with hyperhomocysteinemia (increased homocysteine), which is often found in kidney transplant patients, and it has been shown to increase with the progression of liver disease. In the absence of kidney disease, CysC levels may be elevated in rheumatic diseases and in malignant diseases, although they are not affected by tumor burden, the amount of cancer that someone has.

ASSESSMENT OF GLOMERULAR INTEGRITY

Impairment of glomerular integrity results in the filtration of large molecules that are normally retained and is manifest as proteinuria. Clinical proteinuria is proteinuria that can be reliably detected by dipstick testing of urine, and is >300 mg/L. The significance of microalbuminuria (increased urinary albumin excretion, but not to an extent that can be detected by conventional dipsticks).

With severe glomerular damage, red blood cells are detectable in the urine (hematuria). While hematuria can occur as a result of lesions anywhere in the urinary tract, the red cells often have an abnormal morphology in glomerular disease, owing to their passage through the basement membrane. The presence of red cell casts (cells embedded in a proteinaceous matrix) in urinary sediment is strongly suggestive of glomerular dysfunction.

TESTS OF RENAL TUBULAR FUNCTION

Formal tests of renal tubular function are performed less frequently than tests of glomerular function. Many rely on the detection of increased quantities of substances in the urine that are normally reabsorbed by the tubules.

Proximal tubule: Analysis of excretion of the following substances can assist in the diagnosis of proximal tubular disorders:

1. **Glucose:** The maximum reabsorption rate for glucose (T_mG) in the proximal tubule can be determined following infusion of 20% dextrose and it is usually around 15 mmol/litre (T_mG/GFR).
2. **Phosphate:** The theoretical maximum tubular threshold of phosphate (T_MP/GFR) can be estimated by formula from the plasma and urinary phosphate and

creatinine concentrations, or can be measured directly following infusion of phosphate.

3. **Amino acids:** Five types of renal aminoaciduria are distinguished—dibasic amino acids, neutral amino acids (monoaminomonocarboxylic acids), glycine and imino acids, dicarboxylic amino acids, and generalized amino aciduria (Fanconi syndrome).

Distal tubule: a water-deprivation test can help to distinguish patients with primary or secondary nephrogenic or cranial diabetes insipidus from those with primary polydipsia, who may all present with polyuria.

Renal-induced Electrolyte and Acid-base Imbalances

1. Estimation of urinary free-water clearance is useful in the analysis of patients with hyponatremia.
2. Estimation of transtubular potassium gradient (TTKG) is advocated by some as useful in analysis of disorders of potassium homeostasis.
3. Tests of urinary acidification to diagnose distal renal tubular acidosis.

Renal Imaging

Ultrasonography: This non-invasive, safe, versatile, and (relatively) inexpensive technique is the first-line method for imaging the kidney and urinary tract in many clinical circumstances.

Ultrafast multislice CT scanning, this allows resolution of 2–3 mm or less and has become the mainstay of renal imaging. CT urography can be performed with a combination of unenhanced, nephrogenic-phase, and excretory-phase imaging—the unenhanced images are ideal for detecting urinary calculi; renal masses can be detected and characterized with the combination of unenhanced, nephrogenic- and excretory-phase imaging; the excretory phase provides imaging of the urothelium. CT angiography is the first-line investigation in the evaluation of acute renal trauma, assessment of tumor blood supply in cases of nephron-sparing surgery, and for the diagnosis of renal artery stenosis and/or aneurysms.

Magnetic resonance imaging (MRI): This is an alternative to CT scanning in patients who are allergic to conventional iodine-based radiocontrast media and has particular value in the staging of renal carcinoma and assessment of complex renal cysts. Magnetic resonance angiography (MRA) tends to overemphasize the significance of stenoses. Gadolinium contrast scanning should be carefully considered in patients with eGFR below 30 mL/min, because of the risk of nephrogenic systemic fibrosis, which limits the utility of magnetic resonance techniques for many renal patients.

Renal Nuclear Medicine Scanning

1. Dimercaptosuccinic acid (DMSA), used in estimation of differential renal function and detection of scarring (usually associated with reflux).
2. Mercaptoacetyltriglycine (MAG3), used in detection of functionally significant obstruction, estimation of differential renal function, screening for renal artery stenosis, and monitoring of renal transplants.

Fluorodeoxyglucose-position emission tomography (FDG-PET) scanning combines the functional aspects of a nuclear medicine scan with the anatomical definition of CT scanning and is used to investigate renal tumors and to diagnose and monitor large vessel vasculitis.

Invasive techniques: These can allow therapeutic intervention as well as diagnosis, including antegrade or retrograde ureteropyelography (insertion of stents to relieve urinary obstruction) and angiography (angioplasty or stenting of the renal artery).

Renal Biopsy

A renal biopsy should be considered in any patient with disease affecting the kidney when the clinical information and other laboratory investigations have failed to establish a definitive diagnosis or prognosis, or when there is doubt as to the optimal therapy. However, renal biopsy has the potential to cause morbidity and (on rare occasions) mortality, hence its risk must be outweighed by the potential advantages of the result to the individual patient. Biopsies which would be 'of interest', but 'not in the patient's interest' should not be performed.

Laboratory Testing of the Urine

Midstream urine (MSU) sample: This standard investigation requires consideration of:

1. Macroscopic appearance—this may be suggestive of a diagnosis, e.g. frothy urine suggests heavy proteinuria.
2. Stick testing including for pH (<5.3 in an early-morning specimen makes a renal acidification defect unlikely), glycosuria, specific gravity (should be >1.024 in an early-morning or concentrated sample), nitrite (>90% of common urinary pathogens produce nitrite) and leucocyte esterase.
3. Microscopy for cellular elements (in particular red cells, with the presence of dysmorphic red cells detected by experienced observers indicative of glomerular bleeding), casts (cellular casts indicate renal inflammation), and crystals.

Quantification of proteinuria: This is important because the risk for progression of underlying kidney disease to end-stage renal failure is related to the amount of protein in the urine. Quantification by 24 hours urinary collection is cumbersome and unreliable in many patients, and has been replaced by estimation of the urinary albumin-creatinine ratio (ACR; normal is <2.5 mg/mmol for men and less than 3.5 mg/mmol for women) or protein-creatinine ratio (PCR; normal is <13 mg/mmol) on a spot sample. An ACR of 100 mg/mmol approximately corresponds to proteinuria of 1.5 g/day, and 350 mg/mmol to nephrotic-range proteinuria.

Low molecular weight proteinuria is caused by proximal tubular injury and can be detected with markers including α-glutathione-S-transferase, α_1-macroglobulin, and retinol-binding protein.

Renal Disorders

Kidney disease is an increasing global problem, with a significant economic impact, especially in the developed world. Several organizations have produced guidelines to improve detection and treatment of kidney disorders using internationally agreed nomenclature for describing the stage and type of disease. The standardization of nomenclature allows better comparison of data between different countries and healthcare organizations. Thus, the older terms 'chronic renal failure' and 'acute renal failure' have been largely replaced with 'chronic kidney disease', and 'acute kidney injury'. Similarly, the term 'end-stage renal failure' has been replaced with 'established renal failure'.

Failure of renal function may occur rapidly, producing the syndrome of acute kidney injury (AKI). This is potentially reversible as, if the patient survives the acute illness, normal renal function can be regained. However, chronic kidney disease often develops insidiously over many years, and is irreversible, leading eventually to established (end-stage) renal failure (ERF). Patients with ERF require either long-term renal replacement treatment (i.e. dialysis) or a successful renal transplant in order to survive. Biochemical tests are essential to the diagnosis and management of renal failure, but seldom provide information of help in determining its cause.

The term 'glomerulonephritis' encompasses a group of renal diseases that are characterized by pathological changes in the glomeruli, usually with an immunological basis, such as immune complex deposition. Glomerulonephritis may present in many ways, e.g. as an acute nephritic syndrome with hematuria, hypertension and oedema, as acute or chronic kidney disease, or as proteinuria leading to the nephrotic syndrome (proteinuria, hypoproteinemia, and edema).

Many disorders primarily affect renal tubular function, but most are rare. Their metabolic and clinical consequences range from being trivial (as in isolated renal glycosuria) to being serious.

ACUTE KIDNEY INJURY

Acute kidney injury is a rapid decrease in renal function over days to weeks, causing an accumulation of nitrogenous products in the blood (azotemia). It often results from severe trauma, illness, or surgery, but is sometimes caused by a rapidly progressive, intrinsic renal disease. Symptoms include anorexia, nausea, and vomiting. Seizures and coma may occur if the condition is untreated. Fluid, electrolyte, and acid-base disorders develop quickly. Diagnosis is based on laboratory tests of renal function, including serum creatinine. Urinary indices, urinary sediment examination, and often imaging and other tests are needed to determine the cause. Treatment is not only directed at the cause, but also includes fluid and electrolyte management and sometimes dialysis.

In all cases of acute kidney injury, creatinine and urea build-up in the blood over several days, and fluid and electrolyte disorders develop. The most serious of these disorders are hyperkalemia and fluid overload (possibly causing pulmonary edema). Phosphate retention leads to hyperphosphatemia. Hypocalcemia is thought to occur because the impaired kidney no longer produces calcitriol and because hyperphosphatemia causes Ca phosphate precipitation in the tissues. Acidosis develops because hydrogen ions cannot be excreted. With significant uremia, coagulation may be impaired, and pericarditis may develop. Urine output varies with the type and cause of AKI.

Etiology

The causes of AKI can be divided into three categories (Fig. 4.4); prerenal which caused by decreased renal perfusion, often because of volume depletion, renal which caused by a process within the kidneys and postrenal which caused by inadequate drainage of urine distal to the kidneys (Table 4.2):

1. **Prerenal:** Azotemia is due to inadequate renal perfusion. The main causes are ECF volume depletion and cardiovascular disease. Prerenal conditions cause about 50–80% of AKI, but do not cause permanent kidney damage (and hence are potentially reversible) unless hypoperfusion is severe enough to cause tubular ischemia. Hypoperfusion of an otherwise functioning kidney leads to enhanced reabsorption of Na and water, resulting in oliguria with high urine osmolality and low urine Na.

2. **Renal:** Causes of AKI involve intrinsic kidney disease or damage. Renal causes are responsible for about 10–40% of cases. Overall, the most common causes are prolonged renal ischemia and nephrotoxins. Disorders may involve the glomeruli, tubules, or interstitium.

Glomerular disease reduces GFR and increases glomerular capillary permeability to proteins; it may be inflammatory (glomerulonephritis) or the result of vascular damage from ischemia or vasculitis. Tubules also may be damaged by ischemia and may become obstructed by cellular debris, protein or crystal deposition, and cellular or interstitial edema. Tubular damage impairs reabsorption of Na, so urinary Na tends to be elevated, which is helpful diagnostically. Interstitial inflammation (nephritis) usually involves an immunologic or allergic phenomenon. These mechanisms of tubular damage are complex and interdependent, rendering the previously popular term acute tubular necrosis an inadequate description.

3. **Postrenal** azotemia is due to various types of obstruction in the voiding and collecting parts of the urinary system and is responsible for about 5–10% of cases. Obstruction can also occur within the tubules when crystalline or proteinaceous material precipitates. This form of renal failure is often grouped with postrenal failure because the mechanism is obstructive. Obstructed ultrafiltrate flow in tubules or more distally increases pressure in the urinary space of the glomerulus, reducing GFR. Obstruction also affects renal blood flow, initially increasing the flow and pressure in the glomerular capillary by reducing afferent arteriolar resistance. However, within 3–4 hours, the renal blood flow is reduced, and by 24 hours, it has fallen to <50% of normal because of increased resistance of renal vasculature. Renovascular resistance may take up to a week to return to normal after relief of a 24 hours obstruction. To

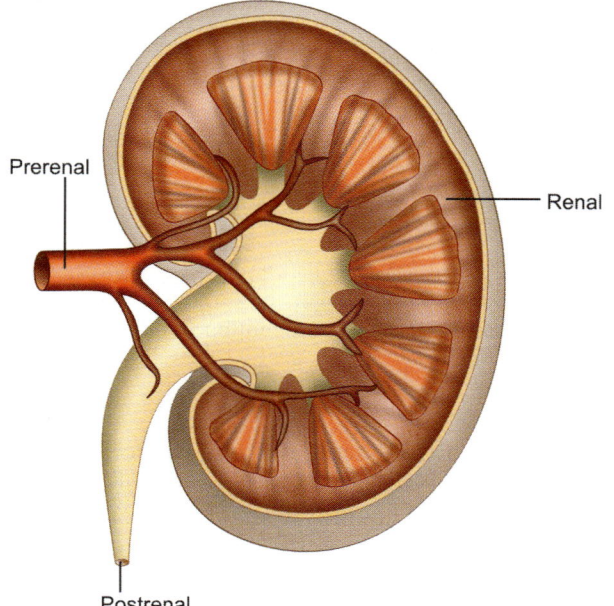

Fig. 4.4: The causes of acute kidney injury

Table 4.2	Major causes of acute kidney injury
Cause	**Examples**
Prerenal ECF volume depletion	Excessive diuresis, hemorrhage, GI losses, loss of intravascular fluid into the extravascular space (due to ascites, peritonitis, pancreatitis, or burns), loss of skin and mucus membranes, renal salt- and water-wasting states
Low cardiac output	Cardiomyopathy, MI, cardiac tamponade, pulmonary embolism, pulmonary hypertension, positive-pressure mechanical ventilation
Low systemic vascular resistance	Septic shock, liver failure, antihypertensive drugs
Increased renal vascular resistance	NSAIDs, cyclosporine, tacrolimus, hypercalcemia, anaphylaxis, some anesthetics, renal artery obstruction, renal vein thrombosis, sepsis, and hepatorenal syndrome
Decreased efferent arteriolar tone (leading to decreased GFR from reduced glomerular transcapillary pressure, especially in patients with bilateral renal artery stenosis)	ACE inhibitors or angiotensin II receptor blockers
Renal acute tubular injury	Ischemia (prolonged or severe prerenal state): Surgery, hemorrhage, arterial or venous obstruction, NSAIDs, cyclosporine, tacrolimus, and amphotericin B
	Toxins: Aminoglycosides, amphotericin B, foscarnet, ethylene glycol, hemoglobin (as in hemoglobinuria), myoglobin (as in myoglobinuria), ifosfamide, heavy metals, methotrexate, radiopaque contrast agents, and streptozotocin
Acute glomerulonephritis	ANCA-associated: Crescentic glomerulonephritis, polyarteritis nodosa, and granulomatosis with polyangiitis (formerly Wegener granulomatosis)
	Anti-GBM glomerulonephritis: Goodpasture syndrome
	Immune-complex: Lupus glomerulonephritis, postinfectious glomerulonephritis, and cryoglobulinemic glomerulonephritis
Acute tubulointerstitial nephritis	Drug reaction (e.g. β-lactams, NSAIDs, sulfonamides, ciprofloxacin, thiazide diuretics, furosemide, cimetidine, phenytoin, and allopurinol), pyelonephritis, and papillary necrosis
Acute vascular nephropathy	Vasculitis, malignant hypertension, thrombotic microangiopathies, systemic sclerosis, and atheroembolism
Infiltrative diseases	Lymphoma, sarcoidosis, and leukemia
Postrenal tubular precipitation	Uric acid (tumor lysis), sulfonamides, triamterene, acyclovir, indinavir, methotrexate, Ca oxalate (ethylene glycol ingestion), myeloma protein, and myoglobin
Ureteral obstruction	Intrinsic: Calculi, clots, sloughed renal tissue, fungus ball, edema, cancer, and congenital defects
	Extrinsic: Cancer, retroperitoneal fibrosis, ureteral trauma during surgery, or high impact injury
Bladder obstruction	Mechanical: Benign prostatic hyperplasia, prostate cancer, bladder cancer, urethral strictures, phimosis, paraphimosis, urethral valves, and obstructed indwelling urinary catheter
	Neurogenic: Anticholinergic drugs, upper, or lower motor neuron lesion

ANCA, antineutrophil cytoplasmic antibody; GBM, glomerular basement membrane; ACE inhibitors, angiotensin-converting enzyme inhibitor.

produce significant azotemia, obstruction at the level of the ureter requires involvement of both ureters unless the patient has only a single functioning kidney. Bladder outlet obstruction is probably the most common cause of sudden, and often total, cessation of urinary output in men.

Urine Output

Prerenal causes typically manifest with oliguria, not anuria. Anuria usually occurs only in obstructive uropathy, or less commonly, in bilateral renal artery occlusion, acute cortical necrosis, or rapidly progressive glomerulonephritis.

A relatively preserved urine output of 1–2.4 L/day is initially present in most renal causes. In acute tubular injury, output may have three phases:

- The **prodromal phase,** with usually normal urine output, varies in duration depending on causative factors (e.g. the amount of toxin ingested, the duration and severity of hypotension).
- The **oliguric phase,** with output typically between 50 mL/day and 400 mL/day, lasts an average of 10–14 days, but varies from 1 day to 8 week. However, many patients are never oliguric. Non-oliguric patients have lower mortality and morbidity and less need for dialysis.
- In the **postoliguric phase,** urine output gradually returns to normal, but serum creatinine and urea levels may not fall for several more days. Tubular dysfunction may persist and is manifested by Na wasting, polyuria (possibly massive) unresponsive to vasopressin, or hyperchloremic metabolic acidosis.

Symptoms and Signs

Initially, weight gain and peripheral edema may be the only findings. Often, predominant symptoms are those of the underlying illness or those caused by the surgical complication that precipitated renal deterioration. Later, as nitrogenous products accumulate, symptoms of uremia may develop, including anorexia, nausea, vomiting, weakness, myoclonic jerks, seizures, confusion, and coma; asterixis and hyperreflexia may be present on examination. Chest pain (typically worse with inspiration or when recumbent), a pericardial friction rub, and findings of pericardial tamponade may occur if uremic pericarditis is present. Fluid accumulation in the lungs may cause dyspnea and crackles on auscultation.

Other findings depend on the cause. Urine may be cola-colored in glomerulonephritis or myoglobinuria. A palpable bladder may be present with outlet obstruction. The costovertebral angle may be tender if the kidney is acutely enlarged.

Diagnosis

Acute kidney injury is suspected when urine output falls or serum BUN and creatinine rise. Evaluation should determine the presence and type of AKI and seek a cause. Blood tests generally include complete blood count (CBC), BUN, creatinine, and electrolytes (including Ca and phosphate). Urine tests include Na and creatinine concentration and microscopic analysis of sediment. Early detection and treatment increase the chances of reversing renal failure and in some cases preventing it.

A progressive daily rise in serum creatinine is diagnostic of AKI. Serum creatinine can increase by as much as 180 µmol/L/day, depending on the amount of creatinine produced (which varies with lean body mass) and total body water. A rise of > 2 mg/dL/day, suggests overproduction due to rhabdomyolysis.

Urea nitrogen may increase by 3.6–7.1 mmol urea/L/day, but BUN may be misleading, because it is frequently elevated in response to increased protein catabolism resulting from surgery, trauma, corticosteroids, burns, transfusion reactions, parenteral nutrition or gastrointestinal (GI) or internal bleeding.

When creatinine is rising, 24 hours urine collection for creatinine clearance and the various formulas used to calculate creatinine clearance from serum creatinine are inaccurate and should not be used in estimating GFR, because the rise in serum creatinine concentration is a delayed function of GFR decline.

Other laboratory findings are progressive acidosis, hyperkalemia, hyponatremia, and anemia. Acidosis is ordinarily moderate, with a plasma HCO_3 content of 15–20 mmol/L. Serum K concentration increases slowly, but when catabolism is markedly accelerated, it may rise by 1–2 mmol/L/day. Hyponatremia usually is moderate (serum Na, 125–135 mmol/L) and correlates with a surplus of water. Normochromic-normocytic anemia with an hematocrit (Hct) of 25–30% is typical.

Hypocalcemia is common and may be profound in patients with myoglobinuric AKI, apparently because of the combined effects of Ca deposition in necrotic muscle, reduced calcitriol production, resistance of bone to parathyroid hormone (PTH), and hyperphosphatemia. During recovery from AKI, hypercalcemia may supervene as renal calcitriol production increases, the bone becomes responsive to PTH, and Ca deposits are mobilized from damaged tissue.

DETERMINATION OF CAUSE

Immediately reversible prerenal or postrenal causes must be excluded first. ECF volume depletion and obstruction are considered in all patients. The drug history must be accurately reviewed and all potentially renal toxic drugs stopped. Urinary diagnostic indices (Table 4.3) are helpful in distinguishing prerenal azotemia from acute tubular injury, which are the most common causes of AKI in hospitalized patients.

Prerenal causes are often apparent clinically. If so, correction of an underlying hemodynamic abnormality should be attempted.

Postrenal causes should be sought in most cases of AKI. Immediately after the patient voids, bedside ultrasonography of the bladder is done (or, alternatively,

Table 4.3	Urinary diagnostic indices in prerenal azotemia and acute tubular injury		
Index		Prerenal	Tubular injury
U/P osmolality		> 1.5	1–1.5
Urine Na (mmol/L)		< 10	> 40
Fractional excretion of Na (FE$_{Na}$)*		< 1%	> 1%
Renal failure index†		< 1	> 2
BUN/Creatinine ratio		> 20	< 10

*U/P Na ÷ U/P creatinine.

†Urine Na ÷ U/P creatinine ratio.

U/P, urine-to-plasma ratio

a urinary catheter is placed) to determine the residual urine in the bladder. A postvoid residual urine volume > 200 mL, suggests bladder outlet obstruction, although detrusor muscle weakness and neurogenic bladder may also cause residual volume of this amount. The catheter may be kept in for the first day to monitor hourly output, but is removed once oliguria is confirmed (if bladder outlet obstruction is not present) to decrease risk of infection. Renal ultrasonography is then done to diagnose more proximal obstruction. However, sensitivity for obstruction is only 80–85%, when ultrasonography is used because the collecting system is not always dilated, especially when the condition is acute, an intrarenal pelvis is present, the ureter is encased (e.g. in retroperitoneal fibrosis or neoplasm), or the patient has concomitant hypovolemia. If obstruction is strongly suspected, non-contrast CT can establish the site of obstruction and guide therapy.

The urinary sediment may provide etiologic clues. Normal urine sediment occurs in prerenal azotemia and sometimes in obstructive uropathy. With renal tubular injury, the sediment characteristically contains tubular cells, tubular cell casts, and many granular casts (often with brown pigmentation). Urinary eosinophils suggest allergic tubulointerstitial nephritis. Red blood cell (RBC) casts indicate glomerulonephritis or vasculitis.

Renal causes are sometimes suggested by clinical findings. Patients with glomerulonephritis often have edema, marked proteinuria (nephrotic syndrome), or signs of arteritis in the skin and retina, often without a history of intrinsic renal disease. Hemoptysis suggests granulomatosis with polyangiitis (formerly Wegener granulomatosis) or Goodpasture syndrome. Certain rashes (e.g. erythema nodosum, cutaneous vasculitis, discoid lupus) suggest polyarteritis, cryoglobulinemia, systemic lupus erythematosus (SLE), or Henoch-Schönlein purpura. Tubulointerstitial nephritis and drug allergy are suggested by a history of drug ingestion and a maculopapular or purpuric rash.

To further differentiate renal causes, antistreptolysin-O and complement titers, antinuclear antibodies, and antineutrophil cytoplasmic antibodies are determined. Renal biopsy may be done if the diagnosis remains elusive (Table 4.4).

Prognosis

Although, many causes are reversible if diagnosed and treated early, the overall survival rate remains about 50% because many patients with AKI have significant underlying disorders (e.g. sepsis, respiratory failure). Death is usually the result of these disorders rather than AKI itself. Most survivors have adequate kidney function. About 10% require dialysis or transplantation—half right away and the others as renal function slowly deteriorate.

Table 4.4	Causes of acute kidney injury based on laboratory findings	
Blood test	Finding	Possible diagnosis
Antiglomerular basement membrane antibodies	Positive	Goodpasture syndrome
Antineutrophil cytoplasmic antibodies	Positive	Small-vessel vasculitis (granulomatosis with polyangiitis [formerly Wegener granulomatosis] or polyarteritis nodosa)
Antinuclear antibodies or antibodies to double-stranded DNA	Positive	SLE
Antistreptolysin-O or antibodies to streptokinase or hyaluronidase	Positive	Poststreptococcal glomerulonephritis
CK or myoglobin level	Markedly elevated	Rhabdomyolysis
Complement titers	Low	Postinfectious glomerulonephritis, SLE, subacute bacterial endocarditis, cholesterol embolization
Protein electrophoresis (serum)	Monoclonal spike	Multiple myeloma
Uric acid level	Elevated	Cancer or tumor lysis syndrome (leading to uric acid crystals) Prerenal acute renal failure

SLE, systemic lupus erythematosus

Management and Treatment
Emergency Treatment

Life-threatening complications are addressed, preferably in a critical care unit. Pulmonary edema is treated with O_2, intravenous (IV) vasodilators (e.g. nitroglycerin), and diuretics (often ineffective in AKI). Hyperkalemia is treated as needed with IV infusion of 10 mL of 10% Ca gluconate, 50 g of dextrose, and 5–10 units of insulin. These drugs do not reduce total body K, so further (but slower acting) treatment with 30 g of oral or rectal Na polystyrene sulfonate is begun. Although, correction of an anion gap metabolic acidosis with $NaHCO_3$ is controversial, correction of the non-anion gap portion of severe metabolic acidosis (pH < 7.20) is less controversial. The nonanion gap portion may be treated with IV $NaHCO_3$ in the form of a slow infusion ($\leq$150 mEq $NaHCO_3$ in 1 L of 5% D/W at a rate of 50–100 mL/h). The non-anion gap portion of metabolic acidosis is determined by calculating the increase in anion gap above normal and then subtracting this number from the decrease in HCO_3 from 24 mmol/L. HCO_3 is given to raise the serum HCO_3 by this difference. Because variations in body buffer systems and the rate of acid production are hard to predict, calculating the amount of HCO_3 needed to achieve a full correction is usually not recommended. Instead, HCO_3 is given via continuous infusion and the anion gap is monitored serially.

Hemodialysis is Initiated When

- Severe electrolyte abnormalities cannot otherwise be controlled (e.g. K > 6 mmol/L)
- Pulmonary edema persists despite drug treatment
- Metabolic acidosis is unresponsive to treatment
- Uremic symptoms occur (e.g. vomiting thought to be due to uremia, asterixis, encephalopathy, pericarditis, and seizures)

Blood urea nitrogen (BUN) and creatinine levels are probably not the best guides for initiating dialysis in AKI. In asymptomatic patients who are not seriously ill, particularly those in whom return of renal function is considered likely, dialysis can be deferred until symptoms occur, thus avoiding placement of a central venous catheter with its attendant complications.

CHRONIC KIDNEY DISEASE

Chronic kidney disease is long-standing, progressive deterioration of renal function. Symptoms develop slowly and include anorexia, nausea, vomiting, stomatitis, dysgeusia, nocturia, lassitude, fatigue, pruritus, decreased mental acuity, muscle twitches and cramps, water retention, undernutrition, peripheral neuropathies, and seizures. Diagnosis is based on laboratory testing of renal function, sometimes followed by renal biopsy. Treatment is primarily directed at the underlying condition, but includes fluid and electrolyte management, erythropoietin for anemia, and often dialysis or transplantation.

Etiology

Chronic kidney disease may result from any cause of renal dysfunction of sufficient magnitude (Table 4.5). The most common cause in the United State is diabetic nephropathy, followed by hypertensive nephroangiosclerosis, and various primary and secondary glomerulopathies. Metabolic syndrome, in which hypertension and type 2 diabetes are present, is a large and growing cause of renal damage.

Table 4.5	Major causes of chronic kidney disease
Cause	Examples
Chronic tubulointerstitial nephropathies	Balkan nephropathy, cystic diseases, drugs, granulomatous, hematologic, hereditary nephropathy associated with hyperuricemia and gout, idiopathic, immunologic, and radiation nephritis
Glomerulopathies (primary)	Focal glomerulosclerosis, idiopathic crescentic glomerulonephritis, IgA nephropathy, membranoproliferative glomerulonephritis, and membranous nephropathy
Glomerulopathies associated with systemic disease	Amyloidosis, diabetes mellitus, granulomatosis with polyangiitis (formerly Wegener granulomatosis), hemolytic-uremic syndrome, mixed cryoglobulinemia, postinfectious glomerulonephritis, SLE
Hereditary nephropathies	Autosomal dominant interstitial kidney disease (medullary cystic kidney disease), hereditary nephritis (Alport syndrome), Nail-patella syndrome, and polycystic kidney disease
Hypertension	Malignant glomerulosclerosis, nephroangiosclerosis
Obstructive uropathy	Benign prostatic hyperplasia, posterior urethral valves, retroperitoneal fibrosis, ureteral obstruction (congenital, calculi, and cancer), and vesicoureteral reflux
Renal macrovascular disease (vasculopathy of renal arteries and veins)	Renal artery stenosis caused by atherosclerosis or fibromuscular dysplasia

Pathophysiology

Chronic kidney disease can be roughly categorized as diminished renal reserve, renal insufficiency, or renal failure (end-stage renal disease). Initially, as renal tissue loses function, there are few abnormalities because the remaining tissue increases its performance (renal functional adaptation); a loss of 75% of renal tissue causes a fall in GFR to only 50% of normal.

Decreased renal function interferes with the kidneys' ability to maintain fluid and electrolyte homeostasis. Changes proceed predictably, but considerable overlap and individual variation exist. The ability to concentrate urine declines early and is followed by decreases in ability to excrete phosphate, acid, and K. When renal failure is advanced (GFR ≤ 10 mL/min/1.73 m^2), the ability to dilute urine is lost; thus urine osmolality is usually fixed close to that of plasma (300–320 mOsm/kg), and urinary volume does not respond readily to variations in water intake.

Plasma concentrations of creatinine and urea (which are highly dependent on glomerular filtration) begin a hyperbolic rise as GFR diminishes. These changes are minimal early on. When the GFR falls below 10 mL/min/1.73 m^2 (normal = 100 mL/min/1.73 m^2), their levels increase rapidly and are usually associated with systemic manifestations (uremia). Urea and creatinine are not major contributors to the uremic symptoms; they are markers for many other substances (some not yet well defined) that cause the symptoms.

Despite a diminishing GFR, Na, and water balance is well maintained by increased fractional excretion of Na and a normal response to thirst. Thus, the plasma Na concentration is typically normal, and hypervolemia is infrequent unless dietary intake of Na or water is very restricted or excessive. Heart failure can occur from Na and water overload, particularly in patients with decreased cardiac reserve.

For substances whose secretion is controlled mainly through distal nephron secretion (e.g. K), adaptation usually maintains plasma levels at normal until renal failure is advanced. K-sparing diuretics, angiotensin-converting enzyme inhibitor (ACE inhibitor), β-blockers, nonsteroidal anti-inflammatory drugs (NSAIDs), cyclosporine, tacrolimus, trimethoprim /sulfamethoxazole, pentamidine, or angiotensin II receptor blockers may raise plasma K levels in patients with less advanced renal failure.

Abnormalities of Ca, phosphate, parathyroid hormone. vitamin-D metabolism, and renal osteodystrophy can occur. Decreased renal production of calcitriol contributes to hypocalcemia. Decreased renal excretion of phosphate results in hyperphosphatemia. Secondary hyperparathyroidism is common and can develop in renal failure before abnormalities in Ca or phosphate concentrations occur. For this reason, monitoring PTH in patients with moderate CKD, even before hyperphosphatemia occurs, has been recommended.

Renal osteodystrophy (abnormal bone mineralization resulting from hyperparathyroidism, calcitriol deficiency, elevated serum phosphate, or low or normal serum Ca), usually takes the form of increased bone turnover due to hyperparathyroid bone disease (osteitis fibrosa), but can also involve decreased bone turnover due to adynamic bone disease (with increased parathyroid suppression) or osteomalacia. Calcitriol deficiency may cause osteopenia or osteomalacia.

Moderate acidosis (plasma HCO$_3$ content 15–20 mmol/L) and anemia are characteristic. The anemia of CKD is normochromic-normocytic, with an Hct of 20–30% (35–40% in patients with polycystic kidney disease). It is usually caused by deficient erythropoietin production due to a reduction of functional renal mass. Other causes include deficiencies of iron, folate, and vitamin B$_{12}$.

Symptoms and Signs

Patients with mildly diminished renal reserve are asymptomatic. Even patients with mild to moderate renal insufficiency may have no symptoms despite elevated BUN and creatinine. Nocturia is often noted, principally due to a failure to concentrate the urine. Lassitude, fatigue, anorexia, and decreased mental acuity often are the earliest manifestations of uremia.

With more severe renal insufficiency (e.g. creatinine clearance < 10 mL/min for patients without diabetes and <15 mL/min for those with diabetes), neuromuscular symptoms may be present, including coarse muscular twitches, peripheral sensory and motor neuropathies, muscle cramps, hyperreflexia, restless legs syndrome, and seizures (usually the result of hypertensive or metabolic encephalopathy). Anorexia, nausea, vomiting, weight loss, stomatitis, and an unpleasant taste in the mouth are almost uniformly present. The skin may be yellow-brown. Occasionally, urea from sweat crystallizes on the skin (uremic frost). Pruritus may be especially uncomfortable. Undernutrition leading to generalized tissue wasting is a prominent feature of chronic uremia.

In advanced CKD, pericarditis and GI ulceration and bleeding are common. Hypertension is present in > 80% of patients with advanced CKD, is usually related to hypervolemia, and is occasionally the result of activation of the renin-angiotensin-aldosterone system. Heart failure caused by hypertension or coronary artery disease and renal retention of Na and water may lead to dependent edema.

Diagnosis

Chronic kidney disease is usually first suspected when serum creatinine rises. The initial step is to determine whether the renal failure is acute, chronic, or acute superimposed on chronic (i.e. an acute disease that further compromises renal function in a patient with CKD (Table 4.6). The cause of renal failure is also determined. Sometimes, determining the duration of renal failure helps determine the cause; sometimes it is easier to determine the cause than the duration, and determining the cause helps determine the duration.

Testing includes urinalysis with examination of the urinary sediment, electrolytes, urea nitrogen, and creatinine, phosphate, Ca, and CBC. Sometimes, specific serologic tests are needed to determine the cause. Distinguishing acute from chronic renal failure is most helped by a history of an elevated creatinine level or abnormal urinalysis. Urinalysis findings depend on the nature of the underlying disorder, but broad (> 3 WBC diameters wide) or especially waxy (highly refractile) casts often, are prominent in advanced renal failure of any cause.

An ultrasound examination of the kidneys, is usually helpful in evaluating for obstructive uropathy and in distinguishing acute from chronic renal failure based on kidney size. Except in certain conditions (Table 4.5), patients with chronic renal failure have small shrunken kidneys (usually <10 cm in length) with thinned, hyperechoic cortex. Obtaining a precise diagnosis becomes increasingly difficult as renal function reaches values close to those of end-stage renal disease. The definitive diagnostic tool is renal biopsy, but it is not recommended when ultrasonography indicates small, fibrotic kidneys.

Prognosis

Progression of CKD is predicted in most cases by the degree of proteinuria. Patients with nephrotic-range proteinuria (>3 g/24 hours or urine protein/creatinine >3), usually have a poorer prognosis and progress to renal failure more rapidly. Progression may occur even if the underlying disorder is not active. In patients with urine protein <1.5 g/24 h, progression usually occurs more slowly if at all. Hypertension, acidosis, and hyperparathyroidism are associated with more rapid progression as well.

Management and Treatment

If the cause of CKD can be determined, appropriate treatment may reduce the rate of further loss of renal function, but rarely prevents it. Patients usually progress inexorably to ERF but considerable amelioration of symptoms and biochemical abnormalities can be obtained by conservative measures before renal replacement therapy becomes necessary.

As the kidneys become unable to control water and sodium balance, it is essential that intake is matched to obligatory losses. Diuretics are often used to promote sodium excretion, as adequate dietary salt restriction may be unacceptable to the patient. At the same time, volume depletion must be avoided; it decreases renal blood flow and thus, the GFR.

Hypertension

Hypertension is a frequent complication of CKD and also exacerbates it. Angiotensin-converting enzyme inhibitors have been shown to reduce the rate of progression of renal impairment in patients with diabetic nephropathy

Table 4.6	Distinction between acute kidney injury and chronic kidney disease	
Finding	**Comment**
Prior known increase in serum creatinine	Most reliable evidence of CKD
Renal sonogram showing small kidneys	Usually CKD
Renal sonogram showing normal or enlarged kidneys	May be AKI or some forms of CKD [diabetic nephropathy, PCKD, myeloma, malignant nephroangiosclerosis, rapidly progressive glomerulonephritis, infiltrative diseases (e.g. lymphoma, leukemia, amyloidosis), obstruction]
Oliguria, daily increases in serum creatinine and BUN	Probably AKI or AKI superimposed on CKD
Eye-band keratopathy	Probably CKD
No anemia	Probably AKI or CKD due to PCKD
Severe anemia, hyperphosphatemia, and hypocalcemia	Possibly CKD, but may be AKI
Subperiosteal erosions on radiography	Probably CKD
Chronic symptoms or signs (e.g. fatigue, nausea, pruritus, nocturia, hypertension)	Usually CKD

PCKD, polycystic kidney disease

independently of their effect on blood pressure, and may be beneficial in CKD from other causes. However, in patients with renal artery stenosis or advanced CKD, ACE inhibitors can cause deterioration in function and hyperkalemia. Patients' plasma creatinine and potassium concentrations should be checked 1–2 weeks after starting treatment or increasing the dose.

Nutrition

Some limitation of dietary protein is beneficial to reduce the formation of nitrogenous waste products, but the limitation should not usually be so severe as to cause negative nitrogen balance (in practice, the anorectic effect of uremia may itself threaten adequate nutrition). In patients who are not candidates for maintenance dialysis or transplantation, however, a very low protein intake can cause considerable symptomatic improvement in the terminal stage of renal failure, and may even slow the rate of decline in renal function. It is important to maintain an adequate intake of essential amino acids and carbohydrate.

Fluid and Electrolytes

1. **Water intake** is restricted only when serum Na concentration is < 135 mmol/L or there is heart failure or severe edema.
2. **Na restriction** of 1.5 g/day benefits patients, especially, those with edema, heart failure, or hypertension.
3. **K intake** is closely related to meat, vegetable, and fruit ingestion and usually does not require adjustment. However, foods (especially salt substitutes) rich in K should generally be avoided. Hyperkalemia is infrequent (unless there is hyporeninemic hypoaldosteronism or K-sparing diuretic therapy) until end-stage renal failure, when K intake may need to be restricted to ≤ 50 mmol/day. Mild hyperkalemia (< 6 mmol/L) can be treated by reducing K intake and correcting metabolic acidosis. More severe hyperkalemia (> 6 mmol/L) warrants urgent treatment

4. **Phosphate** restriction to < 1 g/day is often sufficient to maintain phosphate level in the target range during the early phase of stages 3 and 4 CKD. However, in the later phases, phosphate binders, such as Ca salts (acetate or carbonate but avoid citrate) or non–Ca-containing phosphate binders are often necessary. No more than 1500 mg/day of elemental Ca should be given as binders (2000 mg/day of total Ca; binders plus dietary Ca).
5. **Bicarbonate** can be given orally to control acidosis; hyperkalemia is usually of less significance in CKD than in AKI, because it develops more slowly. However, most patients with chronic metabolic acidosis, who have a pH < 7.3 have plasma HCO_3 content <15 mmol/L and symptoms of anorexia, lassitude, dyspnea, and exaggerated protein catabolism and renal osteodystrophy. $NaHCO_3$ 1–2 g potwice daily, is given and amount is increased gradually until HCO_3 concentration is about 20 mmol/L or until evidence of Na overloading prevents further therapy.

ANEMIA AND COAGULATION DISORDERS

Anemia is treated to keep the Hb between 11 and 12 g/dL. Anemia slowly responds to recombinant human erythropoietin. Because of increased iron utilization with stimulated erythropoiesis, iron stores must be replaced, often requiring parenteral iron. Iron concentrations, iron-binding capacity, and ferritin concentrations should be followed closely. Target transferrin saturation (TSAT), calculated by dividing serum iron by total iron binding capacity and multiplying by 100%, should be > 20%, target ferritin in patients not on dialysis is >100 ng/mL. Transfusion should not be done unless anemia is severe (Hb <8 g/dL) or causes symptoms. The bleeding tendency in CKD rarely needs treatment. Cryoprecipitate, RBC transfusions, desmopressin 0.3–0.4 mcg/kg (20 mcg maximum) in 20 mL of isotonic saline IV over 20–30 minutes, or conjugated estrogens 2.5–5 mg by mouth once a day help when needed. The effects of these treatments last 12–48 hours, except for conjugated estrogens, which may last for several days.

Bone Disease

Bone disease should be monitored by regular measurements of serum calcium, phosphate and PTH concentrations, alkaline phosphatase activity, and imaging as required. PTH concentrations should ideally be 2–4 times normal, reflecting the resistance to PTH that is characteristic of uremia. Lower values indicate an increased risk of a dynamic bone disease. The basis of prevention and treatment is to attempt to prevent hyperphosphatemia and hypocalcaemia. This usually requires a combination of an oral phosphate binder and oral calcitriol or another active form of vitamin D. Occasionally, the parathyroids become autonomous (tertiary hyperparathyroidism): the massively elevated concentrations of PTH can produce severe hypercalcaemia, necessitating parathyroidectomy.

Heart Failure

Symptomatic heart failure is treated with Na restriction and diuretics. If left ventricular function is depressed, ACE inhibitors and β-blockers (carvedilol or metoprolol) should be used. Digoxin may be added, but the dosage must be reduced. Diuretics such as furosemide usually are effective even when renal function is markedly reduced, although large doses may be needed. Moderate or severe hypertension should be treated to avoid its deleterious effects on cardiac and renal function. Patients who do not respond to sodium restriction (1.5 g/day), should receive diuretic therapy (furosemide 80–240 mg by mouth twice daily). Hydrochlorothiazide 12.5 mg (starting dose) to 25 mg (rarely up to 50 mg) by mouth once a day or metolazone 5–10 mg by mouth once a day or twice daily may be added to high-dose furosemide therapy, if hypertension or edema is not controlled. Even in renal failure, the combination of a thiazide with a loop diuretic is quite potent and must be used with caution to avoid overdiuresis. Occasionally, dialysis may be required to control heart failure. If reduction of the ECF volume does not control BP, conventional anti-hypertensives are added. Azotemia may increase with such treatment and may be necessary for adequate control of heart failure and/or hypertension.

Drugs

Renal excretion of drugs is often impaired in patients with renal failure. Common drugs that require revised dosing include penicillins, cephalosporins, aminoglycosides, fluoroquinolones, vancomycin, and digoxin. Hemodialysis reduces the serum concentrations of some drugs, which should be supplemented after hemodialysis. It is strongly recommended that physicians consult a reference on drug dosing in renal failure before prescribing drugs to these very vulnerable patients. Certain drugs should be avoided entirely in patients undergoing dialysis. They include nitrofurantoin, metformin and phenazopyridine.

Renal Replacement Therapy

Renal replacement therapy (RRT) may be required for patients with AKI and for patients with ERF. Techniques include dialysis, hemofiltration, and combinations of the two and, in patients with ERF, transplantation. Dialysis-related techniques do not replace the endocrine functions of the kidney; patients on long-term dialysis require treatment with erythropoietin and vitamin D derivatives, and must follow a special diet. Patients who successfully undergo renal transplantation are free of these restrictions, but must take immunosuppressive drugs to prevent rejection.

The principle of dialysis is that blood is exposed to dialysis fluid from which it is separated by a semipermeable membrane. In hemodialysis, an extracorporeal circuit and artificial membrane are used and substances move from the plasma to the dialysate by diffusion. A controlled pressure gradient can be used to remove fluid. In peritoneal dialysis, dialysate is instilled into the peritoneal cavity, and the peritoneum acts as the semipermeable membrane. Haemodialysis is usually performed intermittently; peritoneal dialysis is often performed continuously.

In hemofiltration, a membrane capable of a high rate of fluid transfer is used, but there is no dialysis fluid. A pressure gradient drives fluid and solutes across the membrane by a process called convection. Fluid and electrolyte balance is maintained by infusion of a suitable fluid into the extracorporeal circuit. Hemofiltration is usually performed continuously. The technique of hemodiafiltration removes fluid and solutes by a combination of diffusion and convection and provides greater urea and middle molecule (molecular weight >1000 Da) clearance than hemodialysis alone. Accumulation of middle molecules, such as β_2-microglobulin, can lead to widespread deposition in tissues, causing a form of amyloidosis.

The factors governing the choice of renal replacement technique are complex. In AKI, the preferred technique is usually semicontinuous hemofiltration or hemodiafiltration; most patients with ERF requiring chronic renal replacement are treated by intermittent hemodialysis (typically three times weekly) or peritoneal dialysis. Peritoneal dialysis is usually performed continuously (continuous ambulatory peritoneal dialysis, CAPD) and typically involves exchanges of 2 L of fluid 4 times daily. CAPD is a relatively simple technique and can be performed without specialized equipment. In CAPD, the dialysate is made hypertonic with glucose to facilitate removal of fluid, but diffusion of this glucose into the bloodstream can lead to diabetes and hypertrigly-ceridemia. Peritoneal dialysis can also lead to loss of protein. All renal replacement techniques can lead to loss of amino acids, trace minerals, and vitamins.

Clearance rates by diffusion fall off rapidly with increasing molecular weight, but convection, which more nearly reflects normal glomerular function, allows fairly uniform clearance of all substances that can pass through the semipermeable membrane, typically decreasing significantly only with molecular weights exceeding 10 kDa. However, as the 'uremic toxins' are primarily low molecular weight substances, dialysis is an effective technique for renal replacement.

The efficacy of dialysis in ERF can be measured by calculating the function Kt/V, where K is the urea clearance of the dialyzer (mL/min), t is the dialysis time (min), and V is the volume of distribution of urea (mL) (equal to the total body water). Kt/V correlates with outcome—effective symptom control requires a value of Kt/V of 1 or more; that is, the urea clearance per session should be equal to total body water. Current targets in the

United Kingdom are a value of Kt/V of >1.2 in patients on thrice weekly hemodialysis, and >1.7 in patients on CAPD.

Patients who have undergone transplantation require careful clinical and biochemical monitoring to assess graft function and to provide warning of incipient graft rejection. Features of graft rejection include oliguria and pyrexia, but these may not be present and a rise in plasma creatinine concentration may be the first sign. However, an increase in creatinine can also occur with nephrotoxicity due to cyclosporine, a frequently used immunosuppressive drug. Indicators of tubular damage, e.g. the urinary activity of the tubular enzyme N-acetyl-β-d-glucosaminidase, have been studied as possible indicators of early rejection, but none is specific to the process and they are not widely used.

ALUMINUM TOXICITY

Toxicity is a risk in hemodialysis patients who are exposed to aluminum-contaminated dialysate (now uncommon) and aluminum-based phosphate binders. Manifestations are osteomalacia, microcytic anemia (iron-resistant), and probably dialysis dementia (a constellation of memory loss, dyspraxia, hallucinations, facial grimaces, myoclonus, seizures, and a characteristic EEG). Aluminum toxicity should be considered in patients receiving RRT who develop osteomalacia, iron-resistant microcytic anemia, or neurologic manifestations such as memory loss, dyspraxia, hallucinations, facial grimaces, myoclonus, or seizures. Diagnosis is by measurement of plasma aluminum before and 2 days after IV infusion of deferoxamine 5 mg/kg. Deferoxamine chelates aluminum, releasing it from tissues and increasing the blood level among patients with aluminum toxicity. A rise in aluminum level of $\geq 50\,\mu g/L$ suggests toxicity. Aluminum-related osteomalacia can also be diagnosed by needle biopsy of bone (requires special stains for aluminum). Treatment is avoidance of aluminum-based binders plus IV or intraperitoneal deferoxamine.

Proteinuria

The glomeruli normally filter 7–10 g of protein per 24 hours, but almost all is reabsorbed by endocytosis and subsequently catabolized in the proximal tubules. Normal urinary protein excretion is <150 mg/24 hours approximately half of this is Tamm–Horsfall protein, a glycoprotein secreted by tubular cells; <30 mg is albumin.

The presence or absence of proteinuria is usually assessed using a reagent-impregnated strip (dipstick), which is dipped into the urine. This reliably detects albumin at concentrations >200 mg/L, but is less sensitive to other proteins. False positive results are obtained with urine, i.e. alkaline, contaminated by various antiseptics or contains X-ray contrast media. It should be appreciated that a particular concentration of protein will be more significant if a large volume of urine is being produced, as it will represent a greater total excretion than if urine volume is low. For this reason, urine protein concentration can be compared to that of creatinine in a 'spot' urine sample; a concentration of >50 mg/mmol creatinine (approximately equivalent to 500 mg/24 hours) reliably predicts significant proteinuria.

The mechanisms of proteinuria are categorized as:

1. **Glomerular proteinuria** results from glomerular disorders, which typically involve increased glomerular permeability; this permeability allows increased amounts of plasma proteins (sometimes very large amounts) to pass into the filtrate.

2. **Tubular proteinuria** results from renal tubulointerstitial disorders that impair reabsorption of protein by the proximal tubule, causing proteinuria (mostly from smaller proteins, such as immunoglobulin light chains rather than albumin). Causative disorders are often accompanied by other defects of tubular function (e.g. HCO_3 wasting, glucosuria, aminoaciduria) and sometimes by glomerular pathology (which also contributes to the proteinuria).

3. **Overflow proteinuria** occurs when excessive amounts of small plasma proteins (e.g. immunoglobulin light chains produced in multiple myeloma) exceed the reabsorptive capacity of the proximal tubules.

5. **Functional proteinuria** occurs when increased renal blood flow (e.g. due to exercise, fever, high-output heart failure) delivers increased amounts of protein to the nephron, resulting in increased protein in the urine (usually <1 g/day). Functional proteinuria reverses when renal blood flow returns to normal.

Orthostatic proteinuria is a benign condition (most common among children and adolescents) in which proteinuria occurs mainly when the patient is upright. Thus, urine typically contains more protein during waking hours (when people are more often upright) than during sleep. It has a very good prognosis and requires no special intervention.

Etiology

Causes can be categorized by mechanism. The most common causes of proteinuria are glomerular disorders, typically manifesting as nephrotic syndrome (Table 4.7).

The most common causes of proteinuria (and nephrotic syndrome) in adults are:
- Focal segmental glomerulosclerosis
- Membranous nephropathy
- Diabetic nephropathy

Table 4.7	Causes of proteinuria
Mechanism	**Examples**
Glomerular	Primary glomerular disorders (e.g. membranous nephropathy, minimal change disease, focal segmental glomerulosclerosis)
	Secondary glomerular disorders (e.g. diabetic nephropathy, preeclampsia, postinfectious glomerulonephritis, lupus nephritis, and amyloidosis)
Tubular	Fanconi syndrome
	Acute tubular necrosis
	Tubulointerstitial nephritis
	Polycystic kidney disease
Overflow	Acute monocytic leukemia with lysozymuria
	Monoclonal gammopathy
	Multiple myeloma
	Myelodysplastic syndromes
Functional	Fever
	Heart failure
	Intense exercise or activity
Unknown	Orthostatic

The most common causes in children are:
- Minimal change disease (in young children)
- Focal segmental glomerulosclerosis (in older children)

NEPHROTIC SYNDROME

Nephrotic syndrome is urinary excretion of >3 g of protein/day due to a glomerular disorder plus edema and hypoalbuminemia. It is more common among children and has both primary and secondary causes. Diagnosis is by determination of urine protein/creatinine ratio in a random urine sample or measurement of urinary protein in a 24 hours urine collection; cause is diagnosed based on history, physical examination, serologic testing, and renal biopsy. Prognosis and treatment vary by cause.

Etiology

Nephrotic syndrome occurs at any age but is more prevalent in children, mostly between ages 1½ year and 4 years. Congenital nephrotic syndromes appear during the first year of life. At younger ages, boys are affected more often than girls, but both are affected equally at older ages. Causes differ by age and may be primary or secondary (Table 4.8).

The **most common primary causes** are the following:
- Minimal change disease
- Focal segmental glomerulosclerosis
- Membranous nephropathy

Secondary causes account for <10% of childhood cases, but >50% of adult cases, most commonly the following:
- Diabetic nephropathy
- Preeclampsia

Table 4.8	Causes of nephrotic syndrome
Primary causes	**Examples**
Idiopathic	Fibrillary and immunotactoid GN
	Focal segmental glomerulosclerosis
	IgA nephropathy*
	Membranoproliferative GN*
	Membranous nephropathy
	Minimal change disease
	Rapidly progressive GN*
Secondary causes metabolic	Amyloidosis
	Diabetes mellitus
Immunologic	Cryoglobulinemia
	Erythema multiforme
	Immunoglobulin
	A—associated vasculitis (Henoch-Schönlein purpura)*
	Microscopic polyangiitis
	Polyarteritis nodosa
	Serum sickness
	Sjögren syndrome
	SLE*
Idiopathic	Castleman disease
	Sarcoidosis
Neoplastic	Carcinoma (e.g. bronchus, breast, colon, stomach, and kidney)
	Leukemia
	Lymphomas
	Melanoma
	Multiple myeloma
Drug-related	Gold
	Heroin
	Lithium
	NSAIDs
	Mercury
	Pamidronate
	Penicillamine
Bacterial†	Infective endocarditis
	Leprosy
	Syphilis
Protozoan†	Filariasis
	Helminthic infections
	Malaria
	Schistosomiasis
Viral†	Epstein-Barr virus infection
	Hepatitis B and C
	Herpes zoster
	HIV infection

Contd.

Table 4.8	Causes of nephrotic syndrome *(Contd.)*
Primary causes	**Examples**
Allergic	Antitoxins
	Insect stings
	Poison ivy or oak
	Snake venoms
Genetic syndromes	Congenital nephrotic syndrome (Finnish type)
	Corticosteroid-resistant nephrotic-syndrome
	Deny–Drash syndrome
	Fabry disease
	Familial FSGS
	Hereditary nephritis (Alport syndrome)*
Physiologic	Adaptation to reduced nephrons
	Morbid obesity oligomeganephronia
Miscellaneous	Chronic allograft nephropathy
	Malignant hypertension
	Preeclampsia

*More commonly manifests as part of nephritic syndrome.
†Infectious and postinfectious causes.
FSGS, focal segmental glomerulonephritis;
GN, glomerulonephritis.

Amyloidosis, an underrecognized cause, is responsible for 4% of cases.

Human immunodeficiency virus (HIV) associated nephropathy is a type of focal segmental glomerulosclerosis that occurs in patients with acquired immune deficiency syndrome (AIDS).

Pathophysiology

Proteinuria occurs because of changes to capillary endothelial cells, the glomerular basement membrane (GBM), or podocytes, which normally filter serum protein selectively by size and charge.

The mechanism of damage to these structures is unknown in primary and secondary glomerular diseases, but evidence suggests that T cells may up-regulate a circulating permeability factor or down-regulate an inhibitor of permeability factor in response to unidentified immunogens and cytokines. Other possible factors include hereditary defects in proteins that are integral to the slit diaphragms of the glomeruli, activation of complement leading to damage of the glomerular epithelial cells and loss of the negatively charged groups attached to proteins of the GBM and glomerular epithelial cells.

Symptoms and Signs

Primary symptoms include anorexia, malaise, and frothy urine (caused by high concentrations of protein). Fluid retention may cause dyspnea (pleural effusion or laryngeal edema), arthralgia (hydrarthrosis), or abdominal pain (ascites or, in children, mesenteric edema). Corresponding signs may develop, including peripheral edema and ascites. Edema may obscure signs of muscle wasting and cause parallel white lines in fingernail beds (Muehrcke lines). Other symptoms and signs are attributable to the many complications of nephrotic-syndrome.

Diagnosis

Diagnosis is suspected in patients with edema and proteinuria on urinalysis and confirmed by random (spot) urine protein and creatinine levels or 24 hours measurement of urinary protein. The cause may be suggested by clinical findings (e.g. SLE, preeclampsia, cancer); when the cause is unclear, additional (e.g. serologic) testing and renal biopsy are indicated.

LABORATORY URINE TESTING

A finding of significant **proteinuria** (3 g protein in a 24 hours urine collection) is diagnostic (normal excretion is <150 mg/day). Alternatively, the protein/creatinine ratio in a random urine specimen usually reliably estimates grams of protein/1.73 m^2 body surfcae area in a 24 hours collection (e.g. values of 40 mg/dL protein and 10 mg/dL creatinine in a random urine sample are equivalent to the finding of 4 g/1.73 m^2 in a 24 hours specimen). Calculations based on random specimens may be less reliable when creatinine excretion is high (e.g. during athletic training) or low (e.g. in cachexia). However, calculations based on random specimens are usually preferred to 24 hours collection because random collection is more convenient and less prone to error (e.g. due to lack of adherence); more convenient testing facilitates monitoring changes that occur during treatment.

Besides proteinuria, urinalysis may demonstrate casts (hyaline, granular, fatty, waxy, or epithelial cell). Lipiduria, the presence of free lipid or lipid within tubular cells (oval fat bodies), within casts (fatty casts), or as free globules, suggests a glomerular disorder causing nephrotic syndrome. Urinary cholesterol can be detected with plain microscopy and demonstrates a Maltese cross pattern under crossed polarized light; Sudan staining must be used to show triglycerides.

Adjunctive Testing

Adjunctive testing helps characterize severity and complications.
- BUN and creatinine concentrations vary by degree of renal impairment.
- Serum albumin often is <2.5 g/dL.
- Total cholesterol and triglyceride levels are typically increased.

It is not routinely necessary to measure levels of α- and γ-globulins, immunoglobulins, hormone-binding proteins, ceruloplasmin, transferrin, and complement components, but these levels may also be low.

Renal Biopsy

Renal biopsy is indicated in adults to diagnose the disorder causing idiopathic nephroticsyndrome. Idiopathic nephroticsyndrome in children is most likely minimal change disease and is usually presumed without biopsy unless the patient fails to improve during a trial of corticosteroids. Specific biopsy findings are discussed under the individual disorders.

Management and Treatment

There are two aspects to **management**—treatment of the underlying disorder, where the disorder can be identified and treatment is possible, and treatment of the consequences of protein loss. Minimal change glomerulonephritis often responds to corticosteroids or immunosuppressive drugs, but other types of glomerulonephritis are generally much less responsive to treatment.

General measures to counteract the consequences of protein loss include a high protein, low salt diet, although decreased appetite and impaired absorption of nutrients owing to oedema of the gut may be limiting factors. A high protein intake must be introduced with caution, when there is concurrent renal failure. It is important not to cause too rapid a diuresis as this can lead to hypovolaemia and thus impair renal function; potassium depletion must also be avoided. Spironolactone is the diuretic of first choice, but thiazides or loop diuretics may be necessary in addition. Prevention of infection is vital and hypertension requires careful control. The risk of thrombosis, especially renal vein thrombosis, which may cause a rapid increase in proteinuria, may warrant the prophylactic use of anticoagulants.

Renal Tubular Disorders

Renal tubular disorders can be congenital or acquired; they can involve single or multiple aspects of tubular function. The congenital conditions are inherited and all are rare; their clinical abnormality relate to the consequences of loss of substances that are normally completely or partially reabsorbed by the tubules. Some are discussed here; others, e.g. Liddle's syndrome, a cause of hypertension.

The Fanconi Syndrome

This is a generalized disorder of the proximal tubule and not the other nephron segments. Fanconi syndrome may be inherited or acquired and leads to aminoaciduria, glycosuria, phosphaturia, renal tubular acidosis (RTA) type 2 (proximal), hypophosphatemic rickets (children) or osteomalacia (adults), and renal glycosuria.

Etiology

Renal fanconi syndrome is caused by a variety of predominantly causes:

1. **Hereditary fanconi syndrome:** This disorder usually accompanies another genetic disorder, particularly cystinosis. Cystinosis is an inherited (autosomal recessive) metabolic disorder in which cystine accumulates within cells and tissues (and is not excreted to excess in the urine as occurs in cystinuria). Besides renal tubular dysfunction, other complications of cystinosis include eye disorders, hepatomegaly, hypothyroidism, and other manifestations.Fanconi syndrome may also accompany Wilson disease, hereditary fructose intolerance, galactosemia, glycogen storage disease, oculocerebrorenal syndrome (Lowe syndrome), mitochondrial cytopathies, and tyrosinemia. Inheritance patterns vary with the associated disorder.

2. **Acquired Fanconi syndrome:** This disorder may be caused by various drugs, including certain cancer chemotherapy drugs (e.g. ifosfamide, streptozocin), antiretrovirals (e.g. didanosine, cidofovir), and outdated tetracycline. All of these drugs are nephrotoxic. Acquired Fanconi syndrome also may occur after renal transplantation and in patients with multiple myeloma, amyloidosis, intoxication with heavy metals or other chemicals, or vitamin D deficiency.

Pathophysiology

Various defects of proximal tubular transport function occur, including impaired resorption of glucose, phosphate, amino acids, HCO_3, uric acid, water, K, and Na. The aminoaciduria is generalized, and, unlike that in cystinuria, increased cystine excretion is a minor component. The basic pathophysiologic abnormality is unknown, but may involve a mitochondrial disturbance. Low levels of serum phosphate cause rickets, which is worsened by decreased proximal tubular conversion of vitamin D to its active form.

Symptoms and Signs

In hereditary Fanconi syndrome, the chief clinical features, e.g. proximal tubular acidosis, hypophosphatemic rickets, hypokalemia, polyuria, and polydipsia, usually appear in infancy.

When Fanconi syndrome occurs because of cystinosis, failure to thrive and growth retardation are common. The retinas show patchy depigmentation. Interstitial nephritis develops, leading to progressive renal failure that may be fatal before adolescence.

In acquired Fanconi syndrome, adults present with the laboratory abnormalities of renal tubular acidosis (proximal type 2), hypophosphatemia, and hypokalemia. They may present with symptoms of bone disease (osteomalacia) and muscle weakness.

Diagnosis

Diagnosis is made by showing the abnormalities of renal function, particularly glucosuria (in the presence of normal serum glucose), phosphaturia, and amino-aciduria. In cystinosis, slit-lamp examination may show cystine crystals in the cornea.

Management and Treatment

The main aim of treatment for fanconi syndrome is replacement of the substances that have been lost in urine. Dehydration as a result of loss of urea through urine needs to be stopped by way of adequate hydration and prevention of dehydration. Metabolic acidosis as a result of Fanconi syndrome can be corrected by administering alkaline solutions. Along with correcting metabolic acidosis supplementing phosphorus and vitamin D is also important. The phosphate levels can be corrected by supplementing phosphates.

Renal Tubular Acidosis

Renal tubular acidosis (RTA) is a disease that occurs when the kidneys fail to excrete acids into the urine, which causes a person's blood to remain too acidic. Without proper treatment, chronic acidity of the blood leads to growth retardation, kidney stones, bone disease, chronic kidney disease, and possibly total kidney failure.

Renal tubular acidosis is acidosis and electrolyte disturbances due to impaired renal hydrogen ion excretion (type 1), impaired HCO_3 resorption (type 2), or abnormal aldosterone production or response (type 4) (Table 4.9) type 3 is extremely rare and it is now thought to be a combination of types 1 and 2.

Patients may be asymptomatic, display symptoms and signs of electrolyte derangements, or progress to chronic kidney disease. Diagnosis is based on characteristic changes in urine pH and electrolytes in response to provocative testing. Treatment corrects pH

and electrolyte imbalances using alkaline agents, electrolytes and rarely drugs.

RTA defines a class of disorders in which excretion of hydrogen ions or reabsorption of filtered HCO_3 is impaired, leading to a chronic metabolic acidosis with a normal anion gap. Hyperchloremia is usually present, and secondary derangements may involve other electrolytes, such as K (frequently) and Ca (rarely). Chronic RTA is often associated with structural damage to renal tubules and may progress to chronic kidney disease.

Type 1: (Classic Distal) Renal Tubular Acidosis

Type 1 is impairment in hydrogen ion secretion in the distal tubule, resulting in a persistently high urine pH (> 5.5) and systemic acidosis. Plasma HCO_3 is usually <15 mmol/L, and hypokalemia, hypercalciuria, and decreased citrate excretion are often present. Hyper-calciuria is the primary abnormality in some familial cases, with Ca-induced tubulointerstitial damage causing distal RTA. Nephrocalcinosis and nephrolithiasis are possible complications of hypercalciuria and hypo-citraturia if urine is relatively alkaline.

This syndrome is rare. Sporadic cases occur most often in adults and may be primary (nearly always in women) or secondary. Familial cases usually first manifest in childhood and are most often autosomal dominant. Secondary type 1 RTA may result from various disorders, drugs, or kidney transplantation:

- Autoimmune disease with hypergammaglobulinemia, particularly Sjögren syndrome or RA
- Kidney transplantation
- Nephrocalcinosis
- Medullary sponge kidney
- Chronic obstructive uropathy
- Drugs (mainly amphotericin B, ifosfamide, and lithium)
- Cirrhosis
- Sickle cell anemia

Table 4.9	Comparison of major types of RTA		
	Type 1	**Type 2**	**Type 4**
Incidence	Rare	Very rare	Common
Plasma HCO_3 (mmol/L)	Usually < 15, often < 10	Usually 12–20	Usually > 17
Urine pH	>5.5	> 7 if plasma HCO_3 is normal < 5.5 if plasma HCO_3 is depleted (e.g. < 15 mmol/L)	<5.5
Plasma potassium	Low-normal	Low-normal	**High**
Renal stones	**Yes**	No	No
Defect	Reduced H^+ excretion in distal tubule	Impaired HCO_3 reabsorption in proximal tubule	Impaired cation exchange in distal tubule

K level may be high in patients with chronic obstructive uropathy or sickle cell anemia.

Type 2: (Proximal) Renal Tubular Acidosis

Type 2 RTA is also called proximal RTA because the main problem is greatly impaired reabsorption of bicarbonate in the proximal tubule.

At normal plasma (HCO_3), more than 15% of the filtered HCO_3 load is excreted in the urine. When acidosis is severe and HCO_3 levels are low (e.g. <17 mmols/L), the urine may become bicarbonate free. Symptoms are precipitated by an increase in plasma [HCO_3]. The defective proximal tubule cannot reabsorb the increased filtered load and the distal delivery of bicarbonate is greatly increased. The H^+ secretion in the distal tubule is now overwhelmed by attempting to reabsorb bicarbonate and the net acid excretion decreases. This results in urinary loss of HCO_3 resulting in systemic acidosis with inappropriately high urine pH. The bicarbonate is replaced in the circulation by Cl^-. The increased distal Na^+ delivery results in hyperaldosteronism with consequent renal K^+ wasting. The hypokalemia may be severe in some cases, but as hypokalemia inhibits adrenal aldosterone secretion, this often limits the severity of the hypokalemia.

Hypercalciuria does not occur and this type of RTA is not associated with renal stones. During the NH_4Cl loading test, urine pH will drop below 5.5. The acidosis in proximal RTA is usually not as severe as in distal RTA and the plasma [HCO_3] is typically greater than 15 mmol/L.

There are many causes, but most are associated with multiple proximal tubular defects, e.g. affecting reabsorption of glucose, phosphate, and amino acids. Type 2 RTA is very rare and most often occurs in patients who have one of the following:

- Fanconi syndrome
- Light chain nephropathy due to multiple myeloma
- Various drug exposures (usually acetazolamide, sulfonamides, ifosfamide, outdated tetracycline, or streptozocin)

It sometimes has other etiologies, including vitamin D deficiency, chronic hypocalcemia with secondary hyperparathyroidism, kidney transplantation, heavy metal exposure, and other inherited diseases [e.g. fructose intolerance, Wilson disease, oculocerebrorenal syndrome (Lowe syndrome), cystinosis].

Type 3: Renal Tubular Acidosis

This term is no longer used. Type 3 RTA is now considered to be a combination of type 1 and type 2, where there is a proximal bicarbonate leak in addition to a distal acidification defect.

Type 4: (Hyperkalemic) Renal Tubular Acidosis

Type 4 results from aldosterone deficiency or unresponsiveness of the distal tubule to aldosterone. Because aldosterone triggers Na resorption in exchange for K and hydrogen, there is reduced K excretion, causing hyperkalemia, and reduced acid excretion. Hyperkalemia may decrease ammonia excretion, contributing to metabolic acidosis. Urine pH is usually appropriate for serum pH (usually <5.5, when there is serum acidosis). Plasma HCO_3 is usually >17 mmol/L. This disorder is the most common type of RTA. It typically occurs sporadically secondary to impairment in the renin-aldosterone-renal tubule axis (hyporeninemic hypoaldosteronism), which occurs in patients with the following:

- Diabetic nephropathy
- Chronic interstitial nephritis

Other factors that can contribute to type 4 RTA include the following:

- ACE inhibitor use
- Aldosterone synthase type I or II deficiency
- Angiotensin II receptor blocker use
- Chronic kidney disease, usually due to diabetic nephropathy or chronic interstitial nephritis
- Congenital adrenal hyperplasia, particularly 21-hydroxylase deficiency
- Critical illness
- Cyclosporine use
- Heparin use (including low molecular weight heparins)
- HIV nephropathy (due, possibly in part, to infection with mycobacterium avium complex or cytomegalovirus)
- Interstitial renal damage (e.g. due to SLE, obstructive uropathy, or sickle cell disease)
- K-sparing diuretics (e.g. amiloride, eplerenone, spironolactone, and triamterene)
- NSAID use
- Obstructive uropathy
- Other drugs (e.g. pentamidine and trimethoprim)
- Primary adrenal insufficiency
- Pseudohypoaldosteronism (type I or II)
- Volume expansion (e.g. in acute glomerulonephritis or chronic kidney disease)

Symptoms and Signs

Renal tubular acidosis is usually asymptomatic. However, bony involvement (e.g. bone pain and osteomalacia in adults and rickets in children) may occur in type 2 and sometimes in type 1 RTA. Nephrolithiasis and nephrocalcinosis are possible, particularly with type 1 RTA.

Severe electrolyte disturbances are rare, but can be life threatening. People with type 1 or type 2 RTA may show symptoms and signs of hypokalemia, including muscle weakness, hyporeflexia, and paralysis. Type 4 RTA is usually asymptomatic with only mild acidosis, but cardiac arrhythmias or paralysis may develop if hyperkalemia is severe. Signs of ECF volume depletion may develop from urinary water loss accompanying electrolyte excretion in type 2 RTA.

Diagnosis

Renal tubular acidosis is suspected in any patient with unexplained metabolic acidosis (low plasma HCO_3 and low blood pH) with normal anion gap. Type 4 RTA should be suspected in patients who have persistent hyperkalemia with no obvious cause, such as K supplements, K-sparing diuretics, or chronic kidney disease. Atrial blood gas (ABG) sampling is done to help confirm RTA and to exclude respiratory alkalosis as a cause of compensatory metabolic acidosis. Serum electrolytes, BUN, creatinine, and urine pH are measured in all patients. Further tests and sometimes provocative tests are done, depending on which type of RTA is suspected:

1. **Type 1 RTA** is confirmed by a urine pH that remains > 5.5 during systemic acidosis. The acidosis may occur spontaneously or be induced by an acid load test (administration of ammonium Cl, 100 mg/kg by mouth). Normal kidneys reduce urine pH to <5.2 within 6 hours of acidosis.

2. **Type 2 RTA** is diagnosed by measurement of the urine pH and fractional HCO_3 excretion during an HCO_3 infusion. In type 2, urine pH rises above 7.5, and the fractional excretion of HCO_3 is >15%. Because IV HCO_3 can contribute to hypokalemia, K supplements should be given in adequate amounts before infusion.

3. **Type 4 RTA** is confirmed by a transtubular K concentration gradient of <5 (normal value >10 if serum K is high), which indicates inappropriately low urinary K excretion, suggesting hypoaldosteronism or tubular unresponsiveness to aldosterone. Calculation of the gradient assumes that the urine sodium is >25 mmol/L and urine osmolality is greater than serum. It is calculated by:

$$\text{Transtubular K gradient} = \frac{\text{Urine K/Plasma K}}{\text{Urine osmolality/Plasma osmolality}}$$

Definitive diagnosis of hyporeninemic hypoaldosteronism can be obtained by measuring plasma renin and aldosterone levels after provocation (e.g. administering a loop diuretic and having the patient remain upright for 3 hours), but is usually not necessary.

Management and Treatment

Treatment consists of correction of pH and electrolyte balance with alkali therapy. Failure to treat RTA in children slows growth.

Alkaline agents such as $NaHCO_3$, $KHCO_3$, or Na citrate help achieve a relatively normal plasma HCO_3 concentration (22–24 mmol/L). K citrate can be substituted when persistent hypokalemia is present or, because Na increases Ca excretion, when Ca calculi are present. Vitamin D (e.g. ergocalciferol 800 IU by mouth once a day) and oral Ca supplements (elemental Ca 500 mg by mouth three times a day, e.g. as Ca carbonate, 1250 mg by mouth 3 times a day) may also be needed to help reduce skeletal deformities resulting from osteomalacia or rickets.

DEFECTS OF URINARY CONCENTRATION

Impairment of urinary concentration is a feature of nephrogenic diabetes insipidus, a group of primary tubular disorders. It is also a feature of cranial diabetes insipidus and CKD and can occur with hypercalcaemia, hypokalemia and certain drugs, notably lithium. In inherited nephrogenic diabetes insipidus, vasopressin secretion is normal, but there is a mutation either affecting its receptor (the V2 receptor) or aquaporin 2. Hypercalcemia and hypokalemia interfere with the intracellular cyclic AMP-mediated signaling pathway that leads to the insertion of aquaporins into the cell membranes of the collecting ducts.

Glucosuria

Virtually all the glucose that is filtered through the glomeruli is reabsorbed by the proximal renal tubule and so glucosuria represents an abnormal state. The amount of glucose not reabsorbed by the kidneys is usually less than 0.1%. Renal glucosuria is results from either an acquired or an inherited, isolated defect in glucose transport or occurs with other renal tubule disorders.

Renal glucosuria is the excretion of glucose in the urine in the presence of normal plasma glucose levels. The inherited form usually involves a reduction in the glucose transport maximum (the maximum rate at which glucose can be resorbed) and subsequent escape of glucose in the urine. The acquired form of renal glucosuria occurs primarily in advanced chronic kidney disease.

The inherited disorder is usually transmitted as an autosomal dominant trait, but is occasionally recessive. Renal glucosuria may occur without any other abnormalities of renal function or as part of a generalized defect in proximal tubule function (Fanconi syndrome). It also may occur with various systemic disorders, including cystinosis, Wilson disease, hereditary tyrosinemia, and oculocerebrorenal syndrome (Lowe syndrome).

Renal glucosuria is asymptomatic and without serious sequelae. However, if there is an associated generalized defect in proximal tubular function, symptoms, and signs may include hypophosphatemic rickets, volume depletion, short stature, muscle hypotonia, and ocular changes of cataracts or glaucoma (oculocerebrorenal syndrome) or Kayser-Fleischer rings (Wilson disease). With such findings, transport defects other than glucosuria should be sought.

The disorder is typically initially noted on routine urinalysis. Diagnosis is based on finding glucose in a 24 hours urine collection (when the diet contains 50% carbohydrate) in the absence of hyperglycemia. To confirm that the excreted sugar is glucose and to exclude pentosuria, fructosuria, sucrosuria, maltosuria, galactosuria, and lactosuria, the glucose oxidase method should be used for all laboratory measurements. Some experts require a normal result on an oral glucose tolerance test for the diagnosis.

Amino Aciduria

Three distinct groups of inherited aminoacidurias are distinguished, based on the net charge of the target amino acids at neutral pH:
- Acidic (negative charge)
- Basic (positive charge)
- Neutral (no charge)

Transient aminoacidurias may occur during the diuretic phase after acute renal insufficiency, or as a result of a deficiency of potassium. Aminoacidurias of longer duration occur as a result of poisoning with heavy metals, particularly cadmium and uranium, but also with lead or mercury. There is aminoaciduria found in patients with Wilson's disease; it is associated with the toxic effect of copper on the renal tubule, which characteristically accumulates in patients with this disease.

Pathogenesis

Under normal circumstances, the renal tubules reabsorb in excess of 93% of the amino acids filtered from the plasma, influenced by the glomerular filtration rate. When the filtered load of amino acids is increased, there is an increase in both the amounts reabsorbed and those excreted. However, the ability of the renal tubule to respond to an increased filtered load of amino acids is so great that a maximum rate of reabsorption has not been found in the human.

In some instances, the aminoaciduria is generalized; there is increased excretion of all of the amino acids occurring in the plasma. In other instances, the aminoaciduria is more specific, in that there are increased amounts of some amino acids in the urine while all others are excreted in normal amounts. Secondary or 'overflow'

aminoaciduria can also be seen in conditions in which there is hyperaminoacidemia.

Fanconi syndrome is the most frequently studied inherited aminoaciduria. The syndrome is characterised by a generalized aminoaciduria and by other renal tubular defects affecting reabsorption of phosphate and glucose.

Cystinuria

In this condition, the glomerulus fails to resorb cystine, ornithine, lysine, and arginine into the tubule and they are excreted into the urine. There are three types of cystinuria, distinguished by the mode of inheritance and by the pattern of the tubular amino-acid transport.

It usually presents with cystine stone formation in the kidneys; a quarter of patients experience symptoms in the first decade of life. There may be pain, hematuria, renal obstruction, and infection. Renal failure can sometimes occur.

The diagnosis is suspected when stone analysis reveals a cystine stone. Cystine stones are pale yellow. Diagnosis can be confirmed by an amino-acid chromatogram and quantification of cystine excretion. This is worth doing even when the stone is mainly composed of calcium, which can occur in cystinuria, due to predisposing infection. For a patient with cystinuria who does not have a stone, first-line therapy in most cases is a conservative approach. This includes:

1. **Large-volume fluid intake (at least 3 litres/day in adults):** This must include 500 mL before retiring to bed, with a nocturnal rise to pass urine and drink a further 500 mL. Keeping the urine dilute over the 24 hours period is the difficult part, but may be sufficient treatment for those without stones.
2. **Regular:** Urine pH monitoring (urine pH level of 7.5 and <8).
3. **Dietary restrictions:** Reduced protein intake diminishes cystine excretion, but this is not often used in treatment.
4. **Urinary alkalinisation with potassium citrate:** Cystine is much more soluble at alkaline pH (>7.5). Use of sodium bicarbonate is limited by the large doses (6 g/day or more) needed to raise urine pH significantly. These are contraindicated in hypertension or renal failure. In addition, alkaline urine may predispose to the precipitation of calcium salts.

Glycinuria

This is a rare autosomal recessive neutral aminoaciduria. It is a clinically benign disorder where the defective protein has not yet been identified. There is no defect in reabsorption of other amino acids. The renal tubular defect produces renal oxalate stones. Glycinuria has been described more often in the Ashkenazi Jewish population. Glycine shares its renal tubular reabsorption mechanism with the imino acids (proline and hydroxyproline). Iminoglycinuria is also a benign inborn error of amino acid transport and a normal finding in neonates and infants under 6 months of age.

Hartnup Disease

Hartnup (H) disease is a rare autosomal recessive metabolic disorder where renal tubular transport is defective and causes gross aminoaciduria. Tryptophan and other neutral amino acids are not absorbed in the small intestine and are converted by gut bacteria into indolic compounds that are toxic to the CNS. The renal loss of amino acids plus poor absorption from the gut cause protein malnutrition. Abnormal tryptophan transport leads to niacin deficiency, or pellagra. The mutated gene (SLC6A19) is located on chromosome locus 5p.15.33 and is known to encode an abnormal neutral amino-acid transporter. Heterozygotes have no abnormality. Differing mutations may be associated with different phenotypic expression. Symptoms tend to arise between the ages of 3 years and 9 years, although sometimes in infancy. It occasionally presents in adults. Episodes of neurological and dermatological problems progress for several days and last from a week to a month before spontaneous remission. Skin problems usually precede neurological features. Psychiatric symptoms including anxiety, emotional instability, and changes of mood are common. Psychosis and delirium are rare.

Photosensitivity occurs and the skin becomes red after exposure to sunlight. Continuing exposure leads to dry, scaly, well-delineated eruptions, sometimes resembling chronic eczema. These eruptions tend to affect the forehead, cheeks, periorbital regions, the dorsum of the hands, and other light-exposed areas. Lesions on the face may be similar to the butterfly rash of systemic lupus erythematosus. Skin changes cause permanent hypo-pigmentation and/or hyperpigmentation, made worse by further exposure to sunlight.

Mental development is usually normal, but mild learning difficulties described in a few patients. Neurological symptoms may vary and are fully reversible. They include:
- Intermittent cerebellar ataxia
- Wide-based gait
- Spasticity
- Delayed motor development
- Tremor
- Headaches
- Hypotonia

Ocular manifestations include diplopia, nystagmus, photophobia, and strabismus. Gingivitis, stomatitis, and glossitis suggest niacin deficiency. Diarrhea occasionally precedes or follows attacks of the disease. Short stature has been described, but is not marked.

Urine chromatography shows increased levels of neutral amino acids. Urinary 5-hydroxyindoleacetic acid may be found after an oral tryptophan load. Urine excretion of proline, hydroxyproline, and arginine is normal. Skin biopsy may, rarely, be required.

General measures include a high-protein diet, avoidance of sunlight, use of sun protection and neurological and psychiatric treatment, where there is CNS involvement. Nicotinic acid or Nicotinamide at 50–300 mg daily can provide remission from both the skin and neurological manifestations. Maternal Hartnup disease does not have an adverse effect on the fetus.

LYSINURIC PROTEIN INTOLERANCE

This is a relatively rare autosomal recessive disease causing a defect in diamino acid transport. There is defective ornithine, lysine, and arginine transport affecting the renal tubule and intestine with only minor defects of cystine transport. It is characterised chemically by renal hyperdibasic aminoaciduria and by impaired formation of urea with hyperammonemia after protein ingestion. Patients thrive during breastfeeding but ingestion of cows' milk causes diarrhea and vomiting. Failure to thrive and poor appetite are common with poor growth. Stones do not form. Occasionally, intermittent hyperammonemic encephalopathy occurs. Osteoporosis is an important part of the clinical picture, with vertebral collapse.

Diagnosis depends upon the demonstration of a failure to increase plasma lysine levels after oral lysine loads or the ingestion of lysyl peptides. Long-term management includes dietary protein restriction, oral supplementation with citrulline and nitrogen scavenger drugs, low-dose lysine, and carnitine:

1. Symptoms can be largely prevented by a low-protein diet. However, adequate calorie intake is difficult to sustain in infancy and appetite often remains poor.
2. Protein restriction does not correct lysine deficiency. Long-term low-dose oral lysine supplementation has been found to be beneficial and well-tolerated.
3. Oral citrulline (2.5–8.5 g/day) absorbed via a different transport system, corrects ornithine and arginine deficiency and lowers plasma ammonia by priming the urea cycle. Citrulline treatment should be maintained, but IV citrulline is not readily available.
4. During acute hyperammonemic crises
5. Arginine chloride and nitrogen scavenger drugs (sodium benzoate, sodium phenylacetate) to block ammonia production.

6. Reduction of excess nitrogen in the diet.
7. Providing energy as carbohydrates to reduce catabolism.

Hypophosphatemic Rickets

This condition, also known as vitamin-D-resistant rickets, has a dominant X-linked pattern of inheritance. A defect in tubular phosphate reabsorption leads to severe rickets and growth retardation. This does not respond to treatment with vitamin D alone, even if administered in massive doses, but can be treated effectively with a combination of oral phosphate supplements and vitamin D, usually given as a 1α-hydroxylated derivative. An autosomal dominant variety has also been described.

Hypophosphatemic rickets should not be confused with inherited vitamin-D-dependent rickets type I, an autosomal recessive condition. The defect is in the 1α-hydroxylation of 25-hydroxycholecalciferol. This condition can be treated with 1α-hydroxylated derivatives of vitamin D alone, and is discussed, together with vitamin-D-dependent rickets type II.

Renal Calculi

Renal calculi are formed when the urine is supersaturated with salt and minerals, such as calcium oxalate, struvite (ammonium magnesium phosphate), uric acid and cystine 60–80% of stones contain calcium. They vary considerably in size from small 'gravel-like' stones, to large staghorn calculi. The calculi may stay in the position in which they are formed, or migrate down the urinary tract, producing symptoms along the way.

The other factor that leads to stone production is the formation of Randall's plaques. Calcium oxalate precipitates form in the basement membrane of the thin loops of Henle; these eventually accumulate in the sub-epithelial space of the renal papillae, leading to a Randall's plaque and eventually a calculus.

TYPES OF STONES

There are four major classifications of kidney stones (Table 4.10). The most common type contains calcium. Struvite stones contain magnesium, ammonia, and phosphate. Other less common ones are composed of uric

Table 4.10	Major classifications of kidney stones			
Type	Frequency	Crystal shape	X-ray characteristic	Risk factors
Calcium oxalate +/– phosphate	75%	Envelope	Radiopaque	Low urine volume Hypercalciuria Hyperuricosuria Hyperoxaluria Hypocitraturia
Calcium phosphate (Brushite)	5%	Amorphous	Radiopaque	Hypercalciuria Hyperphosphaturia Raised urine pH
Uric acid	10%	Diamond or barrel	Radiolucent	Hyperuricosuria Low urine pH Low urine volume
Struvite	10%	Coffin-lid	Radiopaque	Urinary tract infection (Urease splitting organism)
Cystine	1%	Hexagon	Faintly radiopaque	Autosomal recessive disorder

acid and cystine. Kidney stones may be as small as a grain of sand or as large as a pea. Some stones are even as big as golf balls. Stones may be smooth or jagged, and they usually are yellow or brown.

Calcium Stones

A majority of calcium stones consist of >90% oxalate with trace amounts of phosphate. Several factors contribute to formation of this type of stone. An estimated 40–60% of all calcium stone formers have hypercalciuria, which is either idiopathic or secondary to conditions that increase calcium excretion in urine, including primary hyperparathyroidism, vitamin-D toxicity, and sarcoidosis. Idiopathic hypercalciuria, with a prevalence rate ranging from 2.9–6.5%, is defined as increased urinary calcium excretion in patients with an unrestricted calcium diet and no evidence of secondary causes.

There are three types of hypercalciuria (1) absorptive, caused by increased absorption of calcium in the jejunum; (2) resorptive, caused by increased bone demineralization and turnover; and (3) renal, caused by a primary defect in renal tubular calcium excretion. All three can coexist and contribute to each other.

Calcium stones occur primarily in individuals who excrete excess levels of oxalate in urine. Hyperoxaluria arises from either increased oxalate absorption from the gut or increased dietary intake of oxalate. Because calcium binds with oxalate in the gut and hinders its absorption, oxalate is more readily absorbed when dietary calcium is low. Besides decreased dietary calcium intake, hyperoxaluria can be due to unusually high intake of oxalate-rich food products, such as spinach, rhubarb, and nuts.

Enteric hyperoxaluria is a consequence of fat malabsorption, such as that seen in inflammatory bowel diseases or short bowel syndrome. In malabsorption, increased amounts of intraluminal fat and bile salt bind readily with calcium, leaving excess oxalate to be reabsorbed and excreted in the urine. In addition, bile salts and fat also increase colonic absorption of oxalate.

Primary hyperoxaluria, a rare autosomal recessive condition, causes disturbances in the oxalate biosynthetic pathway, leading to very high oxalate excretion.

An estimated 20–60% of calcium stone formers have reduced citrate excretion, leading to excess citrate. The citrate build-up reduces calcium oxalate supersaturation in urine by forming complexes with calcium and directly inhibiting crystal growth and aggregation.

Calcium Phosphate Stones

Hypercalciuria and alkaline urine lead to formation of calcium phosphate stones. Patients with these types of stones have a significantly lower threshold of renal phosphate reabsorption. The ensuing hypophosphatemia stimulates calcitriol synthesis, resulting in hypercalciuria. Researchers believe that phosphaturia is due to defects in the sodium-phosphate transporter found in the proximal renal tubule. This defect contributes to increased concentration of both calcium and phosphate in the renal loop of Henle and creates conditions that favor stone formation.

Uric Acid Stones

Uric acid (UA) is an end product of purine metabolism that the body excretes in urine. Both purine overproduction and excess purine ingestion favor formation of UA stones. The three major risk factors for UA stones are low urine pH (<5.5), low urine volume, and hyperuricosuria. These factors result in undissociated UA, a poorly soluble molecule that contributes to precipitation and crystallization. As pH rises, it dissociates into a more soluble urate ion.

Patients without any obvious underlying congenital or acquired conditions are known as idiopathic UA stone formers. In these individuals, low urinary pH may be due to a defect in renal ammonium excretion that reduces the buffer for H^+ and results in a pH increase. Some studies have suggested a link between this defect and insulin resistance.

Struvite Stones

Struvite stones consist of a mixture of magnesium, ammonium, and phosphate. They are associated with chronic urinary tract infections and are more prevalent in women. Several urea-splitting microorganisms are responsible for struvite stone formation, including proteus, staphylococcus, klebsiella, and pseudomonas. These bacteria hydrolyze urea to produce NH_4^+ and OH^- ions that contribute to the alkalinity of urine. Both ammonium and alkaline urine are essential for struvite supersaturation of urine.

Cystine Stones

Cystinuria is an inheritable autosomal recessive disorder of amino acids transport, specifically cystine, arginine, ornithine, and lysine, that affects epithelial cells of the renal tubules and GI tract. Stone formation usually is the only clinical manifestation of this disorder, which can occur at any age, although the mean is 20–40 years.

Biochemical Investigations of Risk Factors

Biochemical investigations help identify risk factors associated with stone formation, and help clinicians determine the most appropriate treatment and monitor its effectiveness. The goal of such efforts is to prevent stone recurrence. Analyses involve three components—blood, urine, and the actual stone.

Blood investigations assess levels of electrolytes, calcium, phosphate, uric acid, and parathyroid hormone, as well as renal and thyroid functions and vitamin D status.

Analysis of urine is probably the most important element of assessing patients, irrespective of stone type. Urine pH plays a critical role in stone composition. Acidic urine promotes UA and cystine stones, whereas alkaline urine promotes calcium phosphate and struvite stones. A simple test performed during an outpatient visit is all it takes to measure urine pH. However, urinary pH fluctuates over a 24 hours period, typically increasing after meals, and dropping <5.5 in periods of fasting. Therefore, urine normally is alkaline during the day and slightly acidic in the early morning and late at night.

Patients who form UA stones most commonly have persistently low urine pH <5.5, along with a loss of the normal postprandial alkaline tide. To measure alkaline tide, labs should check the pH of fresh urine periodically over a 24 hours period. If the patient's urine pH is 4.5–6, alkali therapy is indicated. This type of assessment also is used to monitor therapy.

Urine culture is another important element of assessing patients. The presence of infection can lead to struvite stones and low urine citrate.

The cornerstone of kidney stone biochemical evaluations is a 24 hours urine analysis. The results provide important prognostic information, guide preventive recommendations, and aide in monitoring therapy. Generally speaking, labs should obtain two 24 hours urine collections for comparison, as mineral excretion varies from day-to-day.

A patient's urine output is also an important indicator. Low urine volume increases the risk of stone formation. Between 12–25% of first-time stone formers have low urine excretion volume, defined as <1 L/24 hours.

Wet chemical analysis (WA), is the most widely employed technique. Although, quantitative WA identifies the common stone components, it may miss rare and unidentified materials. Sophisticated techniques, such as X-ray diffraction crystallography, infrared spectroscopy, and scanning electron microscopy with energy dispersion, provide highly accurate stone analysis. Infrared spectroscopy also has the ability to generate accurate quantitative analysis.

Biochemical investigations of patients with kidney stones are important for discovering underlying risk factors for stone formation (Table 4.11), as well as for directing appropriate treatment and monitoring it. While surgical treatments for kidney stones, such as

Table 4.11	Biochemical investigations of patients with kidney stone risk factors
Investigation	**Risk factor for stone formation**
Blood	
Calcium	Hypercalcemia (primary hyperparathyroidism, vitamin-D toxicity, sarcoidosis)
Urate	Hyperuricemia (gout)
Potassium bicarbonate	Hyperchloremia with hypokalemia and low bicarbonate (distal renal tubular acidosis)
Chloride Phosphate	Hypophosphatemia (renal phosphate leak)
Creatinine	Chronic kidney disease
24 hours urine	
Urine volume	Low urine volume promotes urine supersaturation
Calcium	Hypercalciuria
Phosphate	Phosphaturia
Sodium	High urinary sodium
Oxalate	Hyperoxaluria
Citrate	Hypocitraturia
Uric acid	Hyperuricosuria
Magnesium	Hypermagnesiuria
Cystine	High urinary cystine

extracorporal shock wave lithotripsy® (ESWL) and endoscopic laser stone fragmentation, attempt to remove the stone, these procedures do not tackle the underlying cause of stone formation or prevent recurrence.

In the urology community today, the general consensus is that patients with a high risk of stone recurrence should undergo extensive metabolic stone evaluation. Various studies have shown that such efforts not only reduce stone recurrence but also are cost-effective. In fact, many hospitals now have dedicated metabolic stone clinics.

Clearly, over the last few decades, much progress has been made in understanding the pathophysiology, diagnosis, and management of kidney stones. Both clinically and economically, metabolic stone evaluation plays a vital role in the treatment and prevention of kidney stones.

BIBLIOGRAPHY

1. ADAM Medical Encyclopedia (2012). "Acute kidney failure". US National Library of Medicine. Retrieved 1 Jan. 2013.
2. American Society of Nephrology. "Five Things Physicians and Patients Should Question". Choosing Wisely: an initiative of the ABIM Foundation (American Society of Nephrology).
3. Appel LJ, Wright JT, Greene T, et al. "Long-term effects of renin-angiotensin system-blocking therapy and a low blood

pressure goal on progression of hypertensive chronic kidney disease in African Americans". Arch Intern Med. 168 (8): 832–9.

4. Asplin JR. Uric acid stones. SeminNephrol. 1996;16:412–24

5. Asselman M, Verhulst A, De Broe ME, et al. Calcium oxalate crystal adherence to hyaluronan–, osteopontin–, and CD44– expressing injured/regenerating tubular epithelial cells in rat kidneys. J Am SocNephrol. 2003;14:3155–66

6. Asselman M, VerhulstA,VanBallegooijen ES, et al. Hyaluronan is apically secreted and expressed by proliferating or regenerating renal tubular cells. Kidney Int. 2005;68:71–83.

7. Bacchetta J, Sea JL, Chun RF, et al. "FGF23 inhibits extra-renal synthesis of 1, 25-dihydroxy vitamin D in human monocytes". J Bone Miner Res. 2012;28(1):46–55.

8. Bauer C, Melamed ML, Hostetter TH. "Staging of Chronic Kidney Disease: Time for a Course Correction". American Society of Nephrology. 2008;19(5): 844–46.

9. Bellomo R, Cass A, Cole L, et al. "Intensity of continuous renal-replacement therapy in critically ill patients". The New England Journal of Medicine. 2009;361(17):1627–38.

10. Bellomo R, Ronco C, Kellum JA, et al. "Acute renal failure - definition, outcome measures, animal models, fluid therapy and information technology needs: the Second International Consensus Conference of the Acute Dialysis Quality Initiative (ADQI) Group". Crit Care. 2004;8(4):R204–12.

11. Borghi L, Meschi T, Amato F, et al. Urinary volume, water and recurrences in idiopathic calcium nephrolithiasis: a 5– year randomized prospective study. J Urol. 1996;155:839–43.

12. Borghi L, Schianchi T, Meschi T, et al. Comparison of two diets for the prevention of recurrent stones in idiopathic hypercalciuria. N Engl J Med. 2002; 346:77–84

13. Bostrom, M.A., Freedman, B.I. "The Spectrum of MYH9-Associated Nephropathy". Clinical Journal of the American Society of Nephrology. 2010; 5(6): 1107–13.

14. Brady HR, Brenner BM. "Chronic renal failure". In Kasper DL, Braunwald E, Fauci AS et al. Harrison's Principles of Internal Medicine (16th edition). New York, NY: McGraw-Hill. 2005; pp. 1644–53. ISBN 0-07-139140-1.

15. Brenner and Rector's The Kidney. Philadelphia: Saunders. 2007; ISBN 1-4160-3110-3.

16. Brenner BM, Cooper ME, de Zeeuw D, et al. "Effects of losartan on renal and cardiovascular outcomes in patients with type 2 diabetes and nephropathy". N Engl J Med. 2001; 345 (12): 861–9.

17. Buckalew VM Jr. Nephrolithiasis in renal tubular acidosis. J Urol 1989;141(3 Pt 2)731–7

18. Bywaters EG, Beall D (1941). "Crush injuries with impairment of renal function.". Br Med J. 1(4185): 427–32.

19. Castle SM, Cooperberg MR, Sadetsky N, et al. Adequacy of a single 24 hours urine collection for metabolic evaluation of recurrent nephrolithiasis. J Urol. 2010; 184:579–83.

20. Chertow GM, Paltiel AD, Owen WF, et al. "Cost-effectiveness of Cancer Screening in End-Stage Renal Disease". Archives of Internal Medicine. 1996; 156 (12): 1345–1350.

21. Cheung CK, Bhandari S; Perspectives on eGFR reporting from the interface between primary and secondary Clin J Am SocNephrol. 2009; 4(2): 258–60.

22. Cicerello E, Merlo F, Gambaro G, et al. Effect of alkaline citrate therapy on clearance of residual renal stone fragments after extracorporeal shock wave lithotripsy in sterile calcium and infection nephrolithiasis patients. J Urol. 1994;151:5–9.

23. Cockcroft DW, Gault MH. "Prediction of creatinine clearance from serum creatinine". Nephron. 1976; 16(1): 31–41.

24. Connolly JO, Woolfson RG; A critique of clinical guidelines for detection of individuals with chronic Nephron ClinPract. 2009; 111(1):c69-73. Epub. 2008; Dec 5.

25. Curhan GC, Willett WC, Rimm EB, et al. A prospective study of dietary calcium and other nutrients and the risk of symptomatic kidney stones. N Engl J Med. 1993; 328:833–8.

26. Curhan GC, Willett WC, Speizer FE, et al. Comparison of dietary calcium with supplemental calcium and other nutrients as factors affecting the risk for kidney stones in women. Ann Intern Med. 1997;126:497–504.

27. Dan Longo, Anthony Fauci, Dennis Kasper, et al. Harrison's Principles of Internal Medicine, 18th edition. 2011.

28. Davis A, Gooch I. "The use of loop diuretics in acute renal failure in critically ill patients to reduce mortality, maintain renal function, or avoid the requirements for renal support". Emergency Medicine Journal. 2006; 23(7): 569–70.

29. Eknoyan G. Chronic kidney disease definition and classification: no need for a rush to kidney. Int. 2009 75(10):1015-8. Epub 2009 Mar 4.

30. Gault MH, Chafe LL, Morgan JM, et al. Comparison of patients with idiopathic calcium phosphate and calcium oxalate stones. Medicine Baltimore. 1991; 70: 345–59

31. Gault MH, Longerich LL, Harnett JD, et al. "Predicting glomerular function from adjusted serum creatinine". Nephron. 1992; 62(3): 249–56.

32. Genovese, Giulio; Friedman, David J.; Ross, Michael D, et al. "Association of Trypanolytic ApoL1 Variants with Kidney Disease in African Americans". Science. 2010; 329 (5993): 841–5.

33. Gerber GS, Brendler CB. Evaluation of the urologic patient: history, physical examination, and urinalysis. In: Wein AJ, Kavoussi LR, Novick AC, et al., eds. Campbell-Walsh Urology, 10th edtion. Philadelphia, Pa: Elsevier Saunders; 2011:chap 3.

34. Giri M. "Choice of renal replacement therapy in patients with diabetic end stage renal disease". Edtna Erca J. 2004; 30 (3): 138–42.

35. Goldfarb DS, Fischer ME, Keich Y, et al. A twin study of genetic and dietary influences on nephrolithiasis: a report from the Vietnam Era Twin (VET) Registry. Kidney Int. 2005; 67:1053–61

36. Guyton, Arthur; Hall, John (2006). "Chapter 26: Urine Formation by the Kidneys: I. Glomerular Filtration, Renal Blood Flow, and Their Control". In Gruliow, Rebecca. Textbook of Medical Physiology 11th edtion. Philadelphia, Pennsylvania: Elsevier Inc. pp. 308–25. ISBN 0-7216-0240-1.

37. Heidenheim AP, Kooistra MP, Lindsay RM. "Quality of life". ContribNephrol. Contributions to Nephrology. 2004; 145: 99–105.

38. Holmes CL, Walley KR. "Bad medicine: low-dose dopamine in the ICU". Chest. 2003; 123(4): 1266–75.

39. Hruska KA, Mathew S, Lund R, Qiu P, Pratt R. "Hyper-phosphatemia of chronic kidney disease". Int. 2008; 74(2): 148–57.

40. Israni AK, Kasiske BL. Laboratory assessment of kidney disease: glomerular filtration rate, urinalysis, and proteinuria. In: Taal MW, Chertow GM, Marsden PA, et al., eds. Brenner and Rector's The Kidney. 9th edtion. Philadelphia, Pa: Elsevier Saunders; 2011:chap 25.

41. Jim Cassidy, Donald Bissett, Roy A. J. Spence, Miranda Payne (1 January 2010). Oxford Handbook of Oncology. Oxford University Press. p. 706.

42. Johri N, Cooper B, Robertson W, et al. An update and practical guide to renal stone management. Nephron Clin Pract. 2010; 116:c159–71

43. Kallner A, Ayling PA, Khatami Z. "Does eGFR improve the diagnostic capability of S-Creatinine concentration results? A retrospective population based study". International Journal of Medical Sciences. 2008; 5 (1): 9–17.

44. Katzung, Bertram G. Basic and Clinical Pharmacology (10th ed.). New York, NY: McGraw Hill Medical. 2007; p. 733. ISBN 978-0-07-145153-6.

45. Keener, James; Sneyd, James. "20: Renal Physiology". In Marsden, J.E. Mathematical Physiology (Book). Inter-disciplinary Mathematics. Mathematical Biology Vol. 8. Sirovich, Wiggins (1st ed.). New York, NY: Springer Science +Business Media LLC. 2004; pp. 612–636. ISBN 0-387-98381-3.

46. Keevil BG, Owen L, Thornton S, et al. Measurement of citrate in urine using liquid chromatography tandem mass spectrometry: Comparison with an enzymatic method. Ann Clin Biochem. 2005; 42:357–63.

47. Keevil BG, Thornton S. Quantification of urinary oxalate by liquid chromatography tandem mass spectrometry with online weak anion exchange chromatography. Clin Chem. 2006; 52:2296–99.

48. Kes, Petar; Basiæ-Jukiæ, Nikolina; Ljutiæ, Dragan; Brunetta-Gavraniæ, Bruna. "Ulogaarterijskehipertenzije u nastankukroniè

nogzatajenjabubrega" [The role of arterial hypertension in the development of chronic renal failure]. ActaMedicaCroatica (in Croatian). 2011; 65 (Suppl 3): 78–84.

49. Kidney Disease: Improving Global Outcomes (KDIGO) Acute Kidney Injury Work Group. KDIGO Clinical Practice Guideline for Acute Kidney Injury. Kidney inter.

50. Klag MJ, Whelton PK, Randall BL, et al. "End-stage renal disease in African-American and white men. 16-year MRFIT findings". JAMA. 277 1997; (16): 1293–8.

51. Klahr, Saulo; Miller, Steven B. (1998). "Acute Oliguria". New England Journal of Medicine 338 (10): 671–5.

52. Lameire N, Van Biesen W, Vanholder R (2005). "Acute renal failure". Lancet 365 (9457): 417–30.

53. Lee A. Hebert, M.D., Jeanne Charleston, R.N. and Edgar Miller, M.D. (2009). "Proteinuria".

54. Levin A, Hemmelgarn B, Culleton B, et al. "Guidelines for the management of chronic kidney disease". CMAJ 2008; 179 (11): 1154–62.

55. Lewis EJ, Hunsicker LG, Clarke WR, et al. "Renoprotective effect of the angiotensin-receptor antagonist irbesartan in patients with nephropathy due to type 2 diabetes". N Engl J Med. 2001; 345(12): 851–60.

56. Liao, Min-Tser; Sung, Chih-Chien; Hung, Kuo-Chin; et al. "Insulin Resistance in Patients with Chronic Kidney Disease". Journal of Biomedicine and Biotechnology. 2012: 1–5.

57. Lieske JC, Pena de la Vega LS, Slezak JM, et al. Renal stone epidemiology in Rochester, Minnesota: an update. Kidney Int 2006;69:760–4.

58. Lifshitz DA, Shalhav AL, Lingeman JE, et al. Metabolic evaluation of stone disease patients: A practical approach. J Endourol. 1999;13:669–78.

59. Locatelli F, Aljama P, Canaud B, et al. "Target haemoglobin to aim for with erythropoiesis-stimulating agents: a position statement by ERBP following publication of the Trial to reduce cardiovascular events with Aranesp therapy (TREAT) study". Nephrol Dial Transplant. 2010; 25 (9): 2846–50.

60. Longo et al. Harrison's Principles of Internal Medicine, 18th edition: p. 3109.

61. Maisonneuve P, Agodoa L, Gellert R, et al. "Cancer in patients on dialysis for end-stage renal disease: An international collaborative study". Lancet. 1999; 354 (9173): 93–99.

62. McPherson RA, Ben-Ezra J. Basic examination of urine. In: McPherson RA, Pincus MR, eds. Henry's Clinical Diagnosis and Management by Laboratory Methods. 22nd edition Philadelphia, Pa: Elsevier Saunders; 2011:chap 28.

63. Medline Plus (2011). "Chronic kidney disease". A.D.A.M. Medical Encyclopedia. National Institutes of Health.

64. Medline Plus (2012). "Kidney Failure". National Institutes of Health. Retrieved 1 January 2013.

65. Mehta RL, Kellum JA, Shah SV, et al. "Acute Kidney Injury Network: report of an initiative to improve outcomes in acute kidney injury". Critical Care (London, England) 2007; 11(2): R31.

66. Meyer, Timothy W.; Hostetter, Thomas H. "Uremia". New England Journal of Medicine. 2007; 357(13): 1316–25.

67. Moe OW. Kidney stones: pathophysiology and medical management. Review. Lancet. 2006;367:333–44

68. Moore, EM; Bellomo, R; Nichol, AD. "The meaning of acute kidney injury and its relevance to intensive care and anaesthesia". Anaesthesia and intensive care. 2012; 40(6): 929–48.

69. Morrison NA, Qi JC, Tokita A, et al. Prediction of bone density from vitamin D receptor alleles. Nature. 1994; 367: 284–7.

70. Muldowney FP, Freaney R, Barnes E. Dietary chloride and urinary calcium in stone disease. QJM. 1994; 87:501–9.

71. National Institute for Health and Clinical Excellence. Clinical guideline 73: Chronic kidney disease. London, 2008.

72. National Kidney and Urologic Diseases Information Clearinghouse (2012). "The Kidneys and How They Work". National Institute of Diabetes and Digestive and Kidney Diseases.

73. Nguyen QV, Kälin A, Drouve U, et al. Sensitivity to meat protein intake and hyperoxaluria in idiopathic calcium stone formers. Kidney Int. 2001; 59:2273–81.

74. Orantes CM, Herrera R, Almaguer M, et al. "Chronic kidney disease and associated risk factors in the BajoLempa region of El Salvador: Nefrolempa study, 2009" (PDF). MEDICC Rev. 2011; 13(4): 14–22.

75. Orantes CM, Herrera R, Almaguer M, et al. "Epidemiology of chronic kidney disease in adults of Salvadoran agricultural communities". MEDICC Rev. 2014; 16(2): 23–30.

76. Palevsky PM, Zhang JH, O'Connor TZ, et al. "Intensity of renal support in critically ill patients with acute kidney injury". The New England Journal of Medicine. 2008; 359(1): 7–20.

77. Papadakis MA, McPhee SJ. Current Medical Diagnosis and Treatment. McGraw-Hill Professional. ISBN 0-07-159 124–9.

78. Park C, Ha YS, Kim YJ, et al. Comparison of Metabolic Risk Factors in Urolithiasis Patients according to Family History. Korean J Urol. 2010;51:50–3

79. Parks JH, Coe FL. An increasing number of calcium oxalate stone events worsens treatment outcome. Kidney Int. 1994; 45: 1722–30

80. Pearle MS, Roehrborn CG, Pak CY. Meta–analysis of randomized trials for medical prevention of calcium oxalate nephrolithiasis. J Endourol. 1999;13:679–85

81. Perneger, Thomas V.; Whelton, Paul K.; Klag, Michael J. (1994). "Risk of Kidney Failure Associated with the Use of Acetaminophen, Aspirin, and Nonsteroidal Antiinflammatory Drugs". New England Journal of Medicine. 331(25): 1675–9.

82. Qutb A, Syed G, Tamim HM, et al; Cystatin C-based formula is superior to MDRD, Cockcroft-Gault and NankivellExpClin Transplant. 2009 Dec. 7(4):197–202.

83. Randall A. Recent Advances in Knowledge Relating to the Formation,Recognition and Treatment of Kidney Calculi. Bull N Y Acad Med. 1944; 20:473–84.

84. Reddy ST, Wang CY, Sakhaee K, et al. Effect of low–carbohydrate high–protein diets on acid–base balance, stone–forming propensity, and calcium metabolism. Am J Kidney Dis. 2002;40:265–74

85. Redmon JH, Elledge MF, Womack DS. "Additional perspectives on chronic kidney disease of unknown aetiology (CKDu) in Sri Lanka – lessons learned from the WHO CKDu population prevalence study". BMC Nephrology. 2014. 15 (1): 125.

86. Rendina D, Esposito T, Mossetti G, et al. A functional allelic variant of the FGF23 gene is associated with renal phosphate leak in calcium nephrolithiasis. J Clin Endocrinol Metab. 2012; 97:E840–4

87. Resnick M, Pridgen DB, Goodman HO. Genetic predisposition to formation of calcium oxalate renal calculi. N Engl J Med. 1968; 278:1313–8.

88. Reynolds TM, Burgess N, Matanhelias S, et al. The frusemide test: Simple screening test for renal acidification defect in urolithiasis. Br J Urol 1993;72:153–6.

89. Robertson WG, Peacock M. The cause of idiopathic calcium stone disease: hypercalciuria or hyperoxaluria? Nephron. 1980; 26:105–10.

90. Robijn S, Hoppe B, Vervaet BA, et al. Hyperoxaluria: a gut–kidney axis? Kidney Int. 2011; 80:1146–58

91. Roncal Jimenez CA, Ishimoto T, Lanaspa MA, et al. "Fructokinase activity mediates dehydration-induced renal injury". Kidney Int. 2014; 86 (2): 294–302.

92. Ruggenenti P, Perna A, Gherardi G, et al. "Renoprotective properties of ACE-inhibition in non-diabetic nephropathies with non-nephrotic proteinuria". Lancet. 1998; 354(9176): 359–64.

93. Ruggenenti P, Perna A, Gherardi G, et al. "Renal function and requirement for dialysis in chronic nephropathy patients on long-term ramipril: REIN follow-up trial. GruppoItaliano di StudiEpidemiologici in Nefrologia (GISEN). Ramipril Efficacy in Nephropathy". Lancet. 1998; 352(9136): 1252–6.

94. Rule AD, Larson TS, Bergstralh EJ,et al. "Using serum creatinine to estimate glomerular filtration rate: accuracy in good health and in chronic kidney disease". J. Annals of Internal Medicine. 2004; 141(12): 929–37.

95. Samuell CT, Kasidas GP. Biochemical investigations in renal stone formers. Ann Clin Biochem. 1995;32:112–22.

96. Sarnak MJ, Levey AS, Schoolwerth AC, et al. "Kidney disease as a risk factor for development of cardiovascular disease: a statement from the American Heart Association Councils on Kidney in Cardiovascular Disease, High Blood Pressure Research, Clinical Cardiology, and Epidemiology and Prevention". Circulation. 2003; 108(17): 2154–69.

97. Schrier RW, Wang W, Poole B, et al. "Acute renal failure: definitions, diagnosis, pathogenesis, and therapy". J Clin Invest. 2004; 114(1): 5–14.

98. Schwartz GJ, Furth SL; Glomerular filtration rate measurement and estimation in chronic kidney disease. Pediatr Nephrol. 2007; 22(11):1839-48. Epub 2007 Jan 10.

99. Shekarriz B, Stoller ML. Uric acid nephrolithiasis: Current concepts and controversies. J Urol. 2002; 168:1307–14.

100. Siew ED, Davenport A. "The growth of acute kidney injury: a rising tide or just closer attention to detail?". Kidney International (Review). 2015; 87(1): 46–61.

101. Silver J, Rubinger D, Friedlaender MM, et al. Sodium–dependent idiopathic hypercalciuria in renal–stone formers. Lancet 1983; 2:484–6

102. Skorecki K, Green J, Brenner BM. "Chronic renal failure". In Kasper DL, Braunwald E, Fauci AS et al. Harrison's Principles of Internal Medicine. 16th edtion 2005; New York, NY: McGraw-Hill. pp. 1653–63. ISBN 0-07-139140-1.

103. Stamatelou KK, Francis ME, Jones CA, et al. Time trends in reported prevalence of kidney stones in the United States: 1976-1994. Kidney Int. 2003;63:1817–23.

104. Stoller ML, Chi T, Eisner BH, et al. Changes in urinary stone risk factors in hypocitraturic calcium oxalate stone formers treated with dietary sodium supplementation. J Urol. 2009;181:1140–4

105. Strohmaier WL. Economic aspects of evidence-based metaphylaxis. Urologe A. 2006; 45:1406–9.

106. Sugiyama T, Wang JC, Scott DK, et al. Transcription activation by the orphan nuclear receptor, chicken ovalbumin upstream promoter–transcription factor I (COUP–TFI). Definition of the domain involved in the glucocorticoid response of the phosphoenolzpyruvate-carboxy kinase gene. J BiolChem. 2000; 275: 3446–54.

107. The Merck Manuals, www.merckmanuals.com/...kidney

108. Tierney, Lawrence M.; Stephen J. McPhee; Maxine A. Papadakis. "22". CURRENT Medical Diagnosis and Treatment2005. 44th edtion. 2004.McGraw-Hill. p. 871. ISBN 0-07-143692-8.

109. Tomson CR. Prevention of recurrent calcium stones: a rational approach. Review. Br J Urol. 1995; 76:419–24

110. Tonelli M, Wiebe N, Culleton B, et al. "Chronic kidney disease and mortality risk: a systematic review". J Am Soc Nephrol. 2006; 17(7): 2034–47.

111. Torio CM, Andrews RM. National Inpatient Hospital Costs: The Most Expensive Conditions by Payer, 2011. HCUP Statistical Brief #160. Agency for Healthcare Research and Quality, Rockville, MD. 2013. [1]

112. Traynor J, Mactier R, Geddes CC, et al; How to measure renal function in clinical practice. BMJ. 2006; 7;333(7571): 733–7.

113. Tzur, Shay; Rosset, Saharon; Shemer, Revital; et al. "Missense mutations in the APOL1 gene are highly associated with end stage kidney disease risk previously attributed to the MYH9 gene". Human Genetics. 2010; 128(3): 345–50.

114. Uchino S, Doig GS, Bellomo R, et al. "Diuretics and mortality in acute renal failure". Crit. Care Med. 2004; 32(8): 1669–77.

115. UK Guidelines for the management of Chronic Kidney Disease, The Renal Association, January 2009.

116. Vecchio M, Navaneethan SD, Johnson DW, et al. "Interventions for treating sexual dysfunction in patients with chronic kidney disease". Cochrane Database Syst Rev. 2010; (12): CD007747.

117. Vezzoli G, Terranegra A, Arcidiacono T, et al. Calcium kidney stones are associated with a haplotype of the calcium–sensing receptor gene regulatory region. Nephrol Dial Transplant. 2010; 25:2245–52.

118. Vezzoli G, Terranegra A, Arcidiacono T, et al. Genetics and calcium nephrolithiasis. Review. Kidney Int. 2011;80: 587–93.

119. Wenzel RR, Littke T, Kuranoff S, et al. "Avosentan reduces albumin excretion in diabetics with macroalbuminuria". J Am Soc Nephrol. 2009; 20(3): 655–64.

120. Wesseling C, Crowe J, Hogstedt C, et al. "The epidemic of chronic kidney disease of unknown etiology in Mesoamerica: a call for interdisciplinary research and action". Am J Public Health. 2013; 103(11): 1927–30.

121. William Marshall, Márta Lapsley, Stephen K Bangert. Clinical Chemistry, 7th Edition . Elsevier.com: Clinical Chemistry, ISBN-9780723437031

122. Zuckerman JM, Assimos DG. Hypocitraturia: pathophysiology and medical management. Rev Urol 2009; 11: 134–44.

123. Praught ML, Shlipak MG. Are small changes in serum creatinine an important risk factor? Curr Opin Nephrol Hypertens. 2005; 14, 265–270.

124. Bellomo R, Ronco C, Kellum JA, et al. Acute renal failure – definition, outcome measures, animal models, fluid therapy and information technology needs. The second international consensus conference of Acute Dialysis Quality Initiative (ADQI) Group. Crit Care. 2004; 8: R204-R212.

125. Mehta RL, Kellum JA, Shah SV, et al. Acute Kidney Injury Network (AKIN): report of an initiative to improve outcomes in acute kidney injury. Critical care. 2007; 11, R 31.

126. Molitoris BA, Levin A, Warnock D, et al. Improving outcomes of acute kidney injury: report of an initiative. Nat ClinPractNephrol. 2007; 3(8): 439–42.

127. Kidney Disease: Improving Global Outcomes. Clinical practice guideline on acute kidney injury. 2011. www. kdigo.org.

128. Nash K, Hafeez A, Hou S. Hospital-acquired renal insufficiency. Am J Kidney Dis. 2002; 39: 930–36

129. Kaufman J, Dhakal M, Patel B, et al. Community-acquired acute renal failure. Am J Kidney Dis. 1991; 17: 191–8.

130. Feest TG, Round A, Hamad S. Incidence of severe acute renal failure in adults: results of a living community based study. BMJ. 1993; 306: 481–83.

131. Stevens PE, Tamimi NA, Al Hasani MK, et al. Non-specialist management of acute renal failure. QJM. 2001; 94: 533–40.

132. Metcalfe W, Simpson KM, Khan IH, et al. Acute renal failure requiring renal replacement therapy: incidence and outcome. QJM. 2002; 95: 579–83.

133. Hegarty J, Middleton R, Krebs M, et al. Severe acute renal failure. Place of care, incidence and outcomes. QJM. 2005; 98: 661–66

134. Metnitz PGH, Krenn CG, Steltzer H, et al. Effect of acute renal failure requiring renal replacement therapy on outcome in critically ill patients. Crit Care Med. 2002; 30: 2051–58.

135. Intensive-Care National Audit Research Centre. 2005 www.icnarc.org.

136. Hou SH, Bushinsky DA, Wish JB, et al. Hospital-acquired renal insufficiency: a prospective study. Am J Med. 1983; 74:243–8

137. Shusterman N, Strom BL, Murray TG, Morrison G, West SL, Maislin G. Risk factors and outcome of hospital-acquired acute renal failure. Clinical epidemiologic study. Am J Med 1987; 83:65–71

138. Liaño F, Junco E, Pascual J, et al. The spectrum of acute renal failure in the intensive care unit compared with that seen in other settings. The Madrid Acute Renal Failure Study Group. Kidney Int. 1998; 53:S16–24.

139. Cosentino F, Chaff C, Piedmonte M. Risk factors influencing survival in ICU acute renal failure. Nephrol Dial Transplant. 1994; 9:179–82.

140. Chertow GM, Levy EM, Hammermeister KE, et al. Independent association between acute renal failure and mortality following cardiac surgery. Am J Med. 104: 343–8, 1998.

141. Levy EM, Viscoli CM, Horwitz RI. The effect of acute renal failure on mortality: a cohort analysis. JAMA. 1996; 275: 1489–1494.

142. Uchino S, Bellomo R, Goldsmith D, et al. An assessment of the RIFLE criteria for acute renal failure in hospitalized patients. Crit Care Med. 2006; 34: 1913–1917

143. Li X, Hassoun HT, Santora R, et al. Organ crosstalk: the role of the kidney. Curr Opin Crit Care. 2009; 15(6): 481–7.

144. National Confidential Enquiry into Patient Outcome and Death, Adding Insult to Injury 2009. www.ncepod.org - See more at: http://www.renal.org/guidelines/modules/acute-kidney-injury#sthash.MQF5tpR8.dpuf

145. Schwartz GJ, Haycock GB, Edelmann CM, et al. "A simple estimate of glomerular filtration rate in children derived from body length and plasma creatinine". Pediatrics. 1976; 58(2): 259–63.

146. Adrogué HJ, Madias NE. "Changes in plasma potassium concentration during acute acid-base disturbances". Am J Med. 1981; 71 (3): 456–67.

147. Schwartz GJ, Feld LG, Langford DJ. "A simple estimate of glomerular filtration rate in full-term infants during the first year of life". The Journal of Pediatrics. 1981; 104(6): 849–54.

148. Brion LP, Fleischman AR, McCarton C, et al. "A simple estimate of glomerular filtration rate in low birth weight infants during the first year of life: noninvasive assessment of body composition and growth". The Journal of Pediatrics. 1986; 109(4): 698–707.

149. Haenggi MH, Pelet J, Guignard JP (February 1999). "[Estimation of glomerular filtration rate by the formula GFR = K x T/Pc]". Archives De Pédiatrie (in French). 1999; 6(2): 165–72.

150. National Kidney Foundation. "K/DOQI clinical practice guidelines for chronic kidney disease: evaluation, classification, and stratification". American Journal of Kidney Diseases. 2002; 39(2 Suppl 1): S1–266.

151. Pierratos A, McFarlane P, Chan CT. "Quotidian dialysis–update 2005". Curr. Opin. Nephrol. Hypertens. 2005; 14 (2): 119–24.

152. DrPerGrinsted (2005-03-02). "Kidney failure (renal failure with uremia, or azotaemia)".

153. Joint Specialty Committee on Renal Disease (June 2005). "Chronic kidney disease in adults: UK guidelines for identification, management and referral" (PDF).

154. Groothoff JW. "Long-term outcomes of children with end-stage renal disease". Pediatr Nephrol. 2005; 20(7): 849–53.

155. Davey RX. "Chronic kidney disease and automatic reporting of estimated glomerular filtration rate". The Medical Journal of Australia. 2006; 184 (1): 42–3.

156. Perazella MA, Khan S. "Increased mortality in chronic kidney disease: a call to action". Am J Med Sci. 2006; 331 (3): 150–3.

157. Stevens LA, Coresh J, Greene T, et al. "Assessing kidney function—measured and estimated glomerular filtration rate". The New England Journal of Medicine. 2006; 354 (23): 2473–83.

158. Levey AS, Coresh J, Greene T, et al. "Using standardized serum creatinine values in the modification of diet in renal disease study equation for estimating glomerular filtration rate". Annals of Internal Medicine. 2006; 145 (4): 247–54.

159. Twomey PJ, Reynolds TM. "The MDRD formula and validation". QJM. 2006; 99 (11): 804–5.

160. Mathew TH, Johnson DW, Jones GR. "Chronic kidney disease and automatic reporting of estimated glomerular filtration rate: revised recommendations". The Medical Journal of Australia. 2007; 187 (8): 459–63.

161. Webb S, Dobb G. "ARF, ATN or AKI? It's now acute kidney injury". Anaesthesia and Intensive Care. 2007; 35(6): 843–4.

162. Pannu N, Klarenbach S, Wiebe N, et al. "Renal replacement therapy in patients with acute renal failure: a systematic review". JAMA: the Journal of the American Medical Association. 2008; 299(7): 793–805.

163. Stevens LA; Coresh J; Schmid CH et al. "Estimating GFR using serum cystatin C alone and in combination with serum creatinine: a pooled analysis of 3,418 individuals with CKD". American Journal of Kidney Diseases. 2008; 51(3): 395–406.

164. MedicineNet, Inc. (2008-07-03). "Hyperkalemia".

165. Weisberg LS. "Management of severe hyperkalemia". Crit. Care Med. 2008; 36(12): 3246–51.

166. Schwartz GJ; Muñoz A; Schneider MF, et al. "New equations to estimate GFR in children with CKD". Journal of the American Society of Nephrology. 2009; 20(3): 629–37.

167. Levey AS; Stevens LA; Schmid CH, et al. "A new equation to estimate glomerular filtration rate". Annals of Internal Medicine. 2009; 150 (9): 604–12.

168. Eckardt K-U, Berns JS, Rocco MV, et al. "Definition and Classification of CKD: The Debate Should Be About Patient Prognosis—A Position Statement From KDOQI and KDIGO" (PDF). American Journal of Kidney Diseases. 2009; 53 (6): 915–20.

169. Chauhan V, Vaid M, et al. "Dyslipidemia in chronic kidney disease: managing a high-risk combination". Postgrad Med. 2009; 121(6): 54–61.

170. Matsushita K, Selvin E, Bash LD, et al. "Risk implications of the new CKD Epidemiology Collaboration (CKD-EPI) equation compared with the MDRD Study equation for estimated GFR: the Atherosclerosis Risk in Communities (ARIC) Study". American Journal of Kidney Diseases. 2010; 55(4): 648–59.

171. Johnson, David. "Chapter 4: CKD Screening and Management: Overview". In: Daugirdas, John. Handbook of Chronic Kidney Disease Management. 2011; Lippincott Williams and Wilkins. pp. 32–43. ISBN 1-58255-893-0.

172. Chavkin, Sasha; Greene, Ronnie (12 December 2011). "Thousands of sugar cane workers die as wealthy nations stall on solutions". International Consortium of Investigative Journalists. 2011.

173. Chawla LS, Kellum JA. "Acute kidney injury in 2011: Biomarkers are transforming our understanding of AKI.". Nature Reviews Nephrology. 2012; 8(2): 68–70.

174. Johnson RJ, Sánchez-Lozada LG. "Chronic kidney disease: Mesoamerican nephropathy—new clues to the cause". Nat Rev Nephrol. 2013; 9(10): 560–1.

175. Levey AS, Bosch JP, Lewis JB, et al. "A more accurate method to estimate glomerular filtration rate from serum creatinine: a new prediction equation. Modification of Diet in Renal Disease Study Group". Annals of Internal Medicine. 1999; 130(6): 461–70.

176. Clement FM, Klarenbach S, Tonelli M, et al. "The impact of selecting a high hemoglobin target level on health-related quality of life for patients with chronic kidney disease: a systematic review and meta-analysis". Archives of Internal Medicine. 2009; 169(12): 1104–12.

177. Qaseem A, Hopkins RH, Sweet DE, et al. "Screening, Monitoring, and Treatment of Stage 1 to 4 Chronic Kidney Disease: A Clinical Practice Guideline From the Clinical Guidelines Committee of the American College of Physicians." Annals of internal medicine. 2013; 159(12): 835–47.

5

The Liver

INTRODUCTION

The liver is the largest glandular organ in the body and performs many vital functions to keep the body pure of toxins and harmful substances. It is of vital importance in intermediary metabolism and in the detoxification and elimination of toxic substances. Damage to the organ may not obviously affect its activity, as the liver has considerable functional reserve and, as a consequence, simple tests of liver function (e.g. plasma bilirubin and albumin concentrations) are insensitive indicators of liver disease. Tests reflecting liver cell damage (particularly the measurement of the activities of hepatic enzymes in plasma) are often superior in this respect. The categorization of such tests as 'liver function tests' is clearly a misnomer, but seems likely to endure.

LIVER STRUCTURE

The liver is a roughly triangular organ that extends across the entire abdominal cavity just inferior to the diaphragm. Most of the liver's mass is located on the right side of the body where it descends inferiorly toward the right kidney. The liver is made of very soft, pinkish-brown tissues encapsulated by a connective tissue capsule (Fig. 5.1). This capsule is further covered and reinforced by the peritoneum of the abdominal cavity, which protects the liver and holds it in place within the abdomen.

The peritoneum connects the liver in four locations: The are coronary ligament, the left and right triangular ligaments, and the falciform ligament. These connections are not true ligaments in the anatomical sense; rather, they

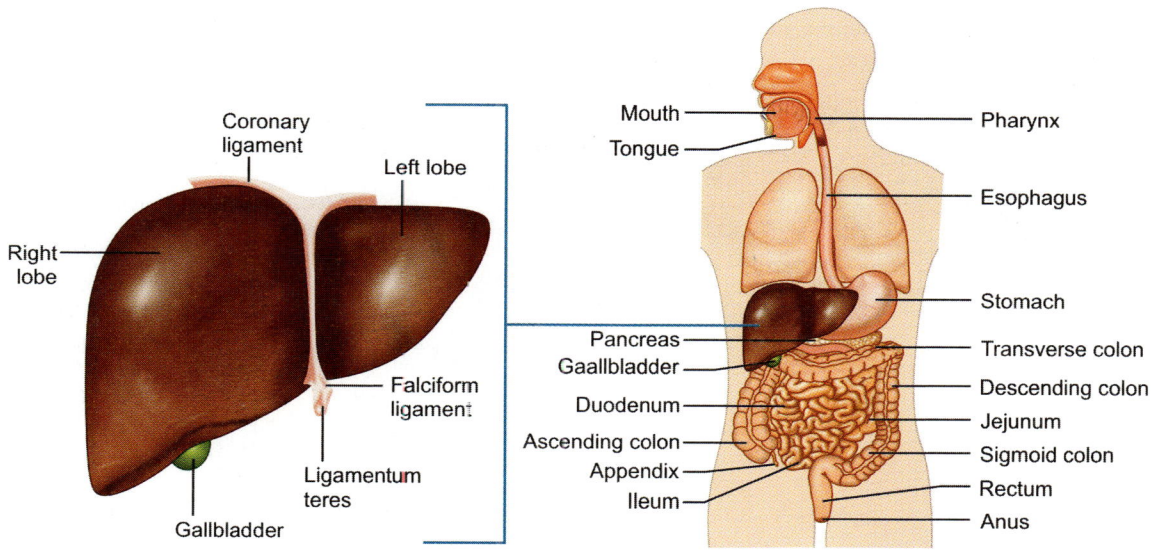

Fig. 5.1: The liver anatomy

are condensed regions of peritoneal membrane that support the liver.

- The wide coronary ligament connects the central superior portion of the liver to the diaphragm.
- Located on the lateral borders of the left and right lobes, respectively, the left and right triangular ligaments connect the superior ends of the liver to the diaphragm.
- The falciform ligament runs inferiorly from the diaphragm across the anterior edge of the liver to its inferior border. At the inferior end of the liver, the falciform ligament forms the round ligament (ligamentum teres) of the liver and connects the liver to the umbilicus. The round ligament is a remnant of the umbilical vein that carries blood into the body during fetal development.

The liver consists of four distinct lobes—the left, right, caudate, and quadrate lobes.

- The left and right lobes are the largest lobes and are separated by the falciform ligament. The right lobe is about 5–6 times larger than the tapered left lobe.
- The small caudate lobe extends from the posterior side of the right lobe and wraps around the inferior vena cava.
- The small quadrate lobe is inferior to the caudate lobe and extends from the posterior side of the right lobe and wraps around the gallbladder.

Bile Ducts

The tubes that carry bile through the liver and gallbladder are known as bile ducts and form a branched structure known as the biliary tree. Bile produced by liver cells drains into microscopic canals known as bile canaliculi.

The countless bile canaliculi join together into many larger bile ducts found throughout the liver.

These bile ducts next join to form the larger left and right hepatic ducts, which carry bile from the left and right lobes of the liver. Those two hepatic ducts join to form the common hepatic duct that drains all bile away from the liver. The common hepatic duct finally joins with the cystic duct from the gallbladder to form the common bile duct, carrying bile to the duodenum of the small intestine. Most of the bile produced by the liver is pushed back up the cystic duct by peristalsis to arrive in the gallbladder for storage, until it is needed for digestion.

Blood Vessels

The blood supply of the liver is unique among all organs of the body due to the hepatic portal vein system. Blood traveling to the spleen, stomach, pancreas, gallbladder, and intestines passes through capillaries in these organs and is collected into the hepatic portal vein. The hepatic portal vein then delivers this blood to the tissues of the liver where the contents of the blood are divided up into smaller vessels and processed before being passed on to the rest of the body. Blood leaving the tissues of the liver collects into the hepatic veins that lead to the vena cava and return to the heart. The liver also has its own system of arteries and arterioles that provides oxygenated blood to its tissues just like any other organ.

Lobules

The internal structure of the liver is made of around 100,000 small hexagonal functional units known as lobules (Fig. 5.2). Each lobule consists of a central vein

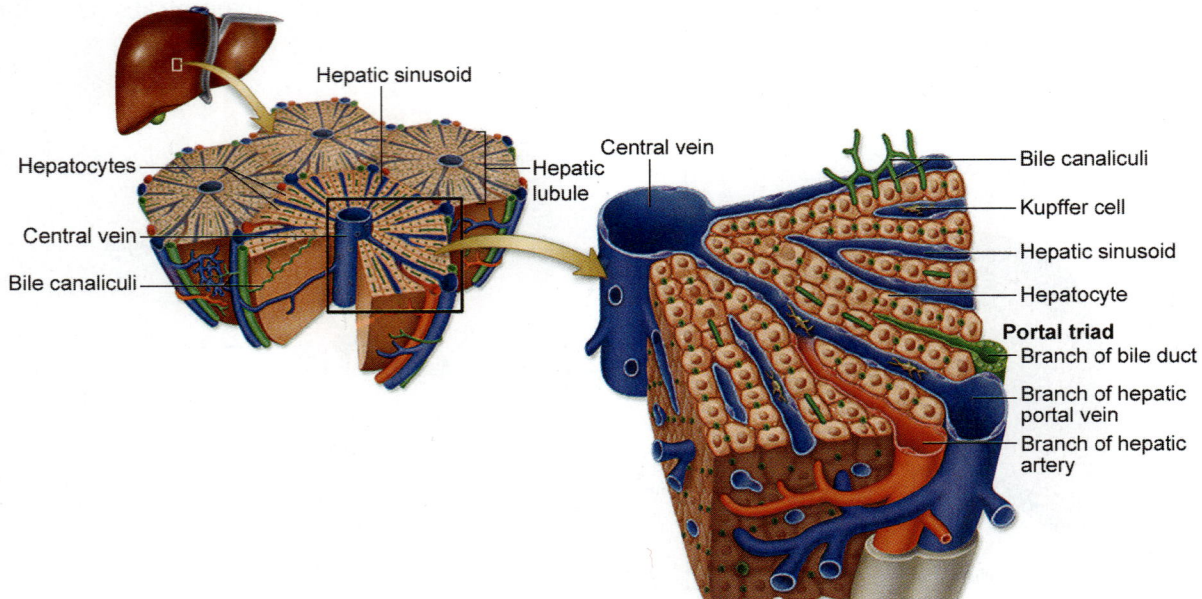

Fig. 5.2: Liver lobule structure

surrounded by 6 hepatic portal veins and 6 hepatic arteries. These blood vessels are connected by many capillary-like tubes called sinusoids, which extend from the portal veins and arteries to meet the central vein like spokes on a wheel.

Each sinusoid passes through liver tissue containing two main cell types: Kupffer cells and hepatocytes.

- Kupffer cells are a type of macrophage that capture and break down old, worn out red blood cells passing through the sinusoids.
- Hepatocytes are cuboidal epithelial cells that line the sinusoids and make up the majority of cells in the liver. Hepatocytes perform most of the liver's functions—metabolism, storage, digestion, and bile production. Tiny bile collection vessels known as bile canaliculi run parallel to the sinusoids on the other side of the hepatocytes and drain into the bile ducts of the liver.

LIVER FUNCTION

Digestion

The liver plays an active role in the process of digestion through the production of *bile*. Bile is a mixture of water, bile salts, cholesterol, and the pigment bilirubin. Hepatocytes in the liver produce bile, which then passes through the bile ducts to be stored in the gallbladder. When food containing fats reaches the duodenum, the cells of the duodenum release the hormone cholecystokinin to stimulate the gallbladder to release bile. Bile travels through the bile ducts and is released into the duodenum where it emulsifies large masses of fat. The emulsification of fats by bile turns the large clumps of fat into smaller pieces that have more surface area and are therefore easier for the body to digest.

Bilirubin present in bile is a product of the liver's digestion of worn out red blood cells. Kupffer cells in the liver catch and destroy old, worn out red blood cells and pass their components on to hepatocytes. Hepatocytes metabolize hemoglobin, the red oxygen-carrying pigment of red blood cells, into the components *heme* and *globin*. Globin protein is further broken down and used as an energy source for the body. The iron-containing heme group cannot be recycled by the body and is converted into the pigment bilirubin and added to bile to be excreted from the body. Bilirubin gives bile its distinctive greenish color. Intestinal bacteria further convert bilirubin into the brown pigment stercobilin, which gives feces its brown color.

Metabolism

The hepatocytes of the liver are tasked with many of the important metabolic jobs that support the cells of the body. Because all of the blood leaving the digestive system passes through the hepatic portal vein, the liver is responsible for metabolizing carbohydrate, lipids, and proteins into biologically useful materials.

Our digestive system breaks down carbohydrates into the monosaccharide glucose, which cells use as a primary energy source. Blood entering the liver through the hepatic portal vein is extremely rich in glucose from digested food. Hepatocytes absorb much of this glucose and store it as the macromolecule glycogen, a branched polysaccharide that allows the hepatocytes to pack away large amounts of glucose and quickly release glucose between meals. The absorption and release of glucose by the hepatocytes helps to maintain homeostasis and protects the rest of the body from dangerous spikes and drops in the blood glucose level.

Fatty acids in the blood passing through the liver are absorbed by hepatocytes and metabolized to produce energy in the form of ATP. Glycerol, another lipid component, is converted into glucose by hepatocytes through the process of gluconeogenesis. Hepatocytes can also produce lipids like cholesterol, phospholipids, and lipoproteins that are used by other cells throughout the body. Much of the cholesterol produced by hepatocytes gets excreted from the body as a component of bile.

Dietary proteins are broken down into their component amino acids by the digestive system before being passed on to the hepatic portal vein. Amino acids entering the liver require metabolic processing before they can be used as an energy source. Hepatocytes first remove the amine groups of the amino acids and convert them into ammonia and eventually urea. Urea is less toxic than ammonia and can be excreted in urine as a waste product of digestion. The remaining parts of the amino acids can be broken down into ATP or converted into new glucose molecules through the process of gluconeogenesis.

Detoxification

As blood from the digestive organs passes through the hepatic portal circulation; the hepatocytes of the liver monitor the contents of the blood and remove many potentially toxic substances before they can reach the rest of the body. Enzymes in hepatocytes metabolize many of these toxins, such as alcohol and drugs into their inactive metabolites. And in order to keep hormone levels within homeostatic limits, the liver also metabolizes and removes from circulation hormones produced by the body's own glands.

Storage

The liver provides storage of many essential nutrients, vitamins, and minerals obtained from blood passing through the hepatic portal system. Glucose is transported into hepatocytes under the influence of the hormone insulin and stored as the polysaccharide glycogen. Hepatocytes also absorb and store fatty acids from digested triglycerides. The storage of these nutrients allows the liver to maintain the homeostasis of blood glucose. Our liver also stores vitamins and minerals-such as vitamins A, D, E, K, and B12, and the minerals iron and copper, in order to provide a constant supply of these essential substances to the tissues of the body.

Production

The liver is responsible for the production of several vital protein components of blood plasma—prothrombin, fibrinogen, and albumins. Prothrombin and fibrinogen proteins are coagulation factors involved in the formation of blood clots. Albumins are proteins that maintain the isotonic environment of the blood, so that cells of the body do not gain or lose water in the presence of body fluids.

Immunity

The liver functions as an organ of the immune system through the function of the Kupffer cells that line the sinusoids. Kupffer cells are a type of fixed macrophage that form part of the mononuclear phagocyte system along with macrophages in the spleen and lymph nodes. Kupffer cells play an important role by capturing and digesting bacteria, fungi, parasites, worn-out blood cells, and cellular debris. The large volume of blood passing through the hepatic portals.

BILIRUBIN METABOLISM

Bilirubin is derived mainly from the heme moiety of hemoglobin molecules and is liberated when senescent red cells are removed from the circulation by the reticuloendothelial system (Fig. 5.3); the iron in heme is reutilized but the tetrapyrrole ring is degraded to bilirubin. Other sources of bilirubin include myoglobin and the cytochromes.

Bilirubin, which is bound to albumin in the plasma, is taken up into hepatocytes, conjugated in the smooth endoplasmic reticulum and excreted via the bile ducts into the gut, where it is converted to urobilinogen. Most of the urobilinogen is oxidized to stercobilin in the colon and excreted in the stool. Some urobilinogen is absorbed from the small intestine and enters the enterohepatic circulation. While most is excreted in the bile, some reaches the systemic circulation and is excreted in the urine.

Unconjugated bilirubin is not water soluble: It is transported in the bloodstream bound to albumin. In the liver, it is taken up by hepatocytes in a process involving

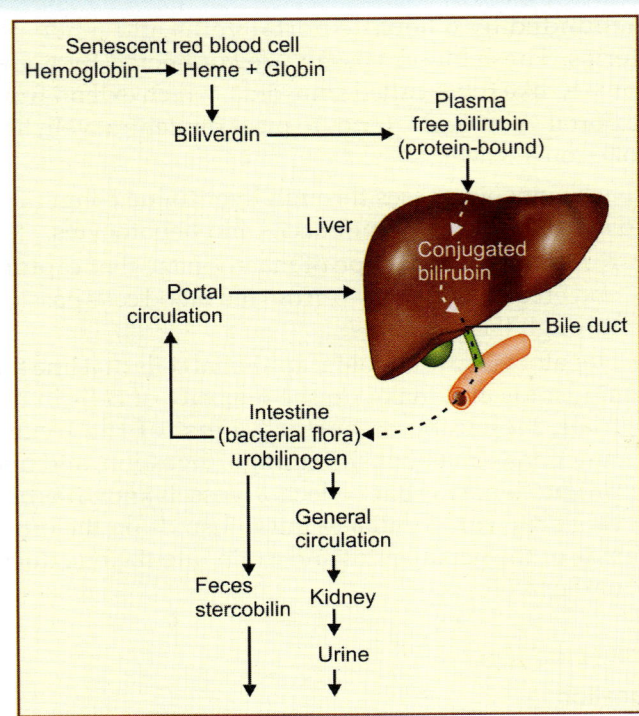

Fig. 5.3: Excretion of bilirubin by the liver

specific carrier proteins. It is then transported to the smooth endoplasmic reticulum, where it undergoes conjugation, principally with glucuronic acid, to form mono- and diglucuronides; this process is catalyzed by the enzyme bilirubin-uridyl diphosphate (UDP) glucuronosyl transferase. The resulting conjugated bilirubin is water soluble and is secreted into the biliary canaliculi, eventually reaching the small intestine via the ducts of the biliary system. Secretion into the biliary canaliculi is the rate-limiting step in bilirubin metabolism. In the gut, bilirubin is converted by bacterial action into urobilinogen, a colorless compound. Some urobilinogen is absorbed from the gut into the portal blood. Hepatic uptake of this is incomplete; a small quantity reaches the systemic circulation and is excreted in the urine. Most of the urobilinogen in the gut is oxidized in the colon to a brown pigment, stercobilin, which is excreted in the stool.

Some 300 mg of bilirubin is produced daily but the healthy liver can metabolize and excrete ten times this amount. The measurement of plasma bilirubin concentration is thus an insensitive test of liver function; it is frequently normal in early or mild liver disease.

The bilirubin normally present in the plasma is mainly (approximately 95%) unconjugated; because it is protein bound, it is not filtered by the renal glomeruli and, in health; bilirubin is not detectable in the urine. Bilirubinuria reflects an increase in the plasma concentration of conjugated bilirubin, and is always pathological.

Although jaundice is a frequent feature of liver disease, it may not be obvious clinically unless the plasma bilirubin concentration is more than two and half times the upper limit of normal, i.e. more than 50 μmol/L. Hyperbilirubinemia can be caused by increased production of bilirubin, impaired metabolism, decreased excretion or a combination of these.

The Liver Diseases

Because of the liver's complexity, liver disease is often reflected by abnormalities of different hepatic 'systems', i.e. hepatocytes (hepatocellular dysfunction), the biliary excretory apparatus (cholestasis) and the vascular system (portal hypertension). In addition, the liver often is involved in systemic disease by virtue of its rich metabolic and reticuloendothelial activity and its large blood supply.

Patterns of disproportionate involvement often provide an important clue to the underlying disorder. For example, viral hepatitis characteristically produces predominantly hepatocellular dysfunction; primary biliary cirrhosis, predominantly cholestasis; cryptogenic cirrhosis, predominantly portal hypertension; and alcoholic liver disease, variable dysfunction of any of these three systems. The clinician can often take advantage of these general patterns to help establish a diagnosis, though overlap and exceptions are frequent.

The most common disease processes affecting the liver are:

- **Hepatitis**, which may be acute or chronic or a combination of both, in which there is damage to and destruction of liver cells.
- **Cirrhosis**, in which increased fibrous tissue formation leads to shrinkage of the liver, decreased numbers of hepatocytes and hence decreased hepatocellular function, hypertension in the portal venous system and cholestasis.
- **Tumors**, both primary and more frequently, secondary; for example, metastases from cancers of the large bowel, stomach, and bronchus.

Patients with liver disease often present with characteristic symptoms and signs, particularly jaundice, the yellow-orange discoloration of the skin caused by a high plasma concentration of bilirubin, but the clinical features may be non-specific and, in some patients, liver disease is discovered incidentally. Because of the intimate relationship between the liver and biliary system, extrahepatic biliary disease may present with clinical features suggestive of liver disease or may have secondary effects on the liver. For instance, obstruction to the common bile duct may cause jaundice and, if prolonged, a form of cirrhosis.

Acute Liver Failure

Acute liver failure is caused most often by drugs and hepatitis viruses, Cardinal manifestations are jaundice, coagulopathy, and encephalopathy. Diagnosis is clinical. Treatment is mainly supportive, sometimes with liver transplantation and/or specific therapies (e.g. N-acetylcysteine for acetaminophen toxicity). Liver failure can be classified in several ways, but no system is universally accepted (Table 5.1).

Etiology

Overall, the most common viral cause is hepatitis B; hepatitis C is not a common cause. Other possible viral causes include cytomegalovirus, Epstein-Barr virus, herpes simplex virus, human herpesvirus 6, parvovirus B19, varicella-zoster virus, hepatitis A virus (rarely), hepatitis E virus (especially if contracted during pregnancy), and viruses that cause hemorrhagic fever. The most common toxin is acetaminophen; toxicity is dose-related. Predisposing factors for acetaminophen-induced liver failure include preexisting liver disease, chronic alcohol use, and use of drugs that induce the cytochrome P-450 enzyme system (e.g. anticonvulsants). Other toxins include amoxicillin/clavulanate, halothane, iron compounds, isoniazid, nonsteroidal anti-inflammatory drugs (NSAIDs), some compounds in herbal products, and *Amanita phalloides* mushrooms.

Vascular causes include hepatic vein thrombosis (Budd-Chiari syndrome), ischemic hepatitis, portal vein thrombosis, and hepatic sinusoidal obstruction syndrome (also called hepatic veno-occlusive disease),

Table 5.1	Classification of liver failure	
Severity	Description	Common findings
Acute (fulminant)	Portosystemic encephalopathy develops within • 2 weeks after jaundice appears· • 8 weeks in a patient with no prior liver disease	Often cerebral edema
Subacute (sub-fulminant)	Encephalopathy develops within 6 months but later than in acute liver failure.	Renal failure, portal hypertension (more common than in acute liver failure)
Chronic	Encephalopathy develops after 6 months.	Often caused by cirrhosis

Note: No classification system is universally accepted.

which is sometimes drug- or toxin-induced. Metabolic causes include acute fatty liver of pregnancy, HELLP syndrome (hemolysis, elevated liver function tests, and low platelets), Reye syndrome, and Wilson disease. Other causes include autoimmune hepatitis, metastatic liver infiltration, heatstroke, and sepsis. The cause cannot be determined in up to 20% of cases.

Pathophysiology

In acute liver failure, multiple organ systems malfunction, often for unknown reasons and by unknown mechanisms. Affected systems include:

- **Hepatic:** Hyperbilirubinemia is almost always present at presentation. The degree of hyperbilirubinemia is one indicator of the severity of liver failure. Coagulopathy due to impaired hepatic synthesis of coagulation factors is common. Hepatocellular necrosis, indicated by increased aminotransferase levels, is present.
- **Cardiovascular:** Peripheral vascular resistance and BP decrease, causing hyperdynamic circulation with increased heart rate and cardiac output.
- **Cerebral:** Portosystemic encephalopathy occurs, possibly secondary to increased ammonia production by nitrogenous substances in the gut. Cerebral edema is common among patients with severe encephalopathy secondary to acute liver failure; uncal herniation is possible and usually fatal.
- **Renal:** For unknown reasons, acute kidney injury occurs in up to 50% of patients. Because blood urea nitrogen (BUN) level depends on hepatic synthetic function, the level may be misleadingly low; thus, the creatinine level better indicates kidney injury. As in hepatorenal syndrome, urine Na and fractional Na excretion decrease even when diuretics are not used and tubular injury is absent (as may occur when acetaminophen toxicity is the cause).
- **Immunologic:** Immune system defects develop; they include defective opsonization, deficient complement, and dysfunctional WBCs and killer cells. Bacterial translocation from the gastrointestinal (GI) tract increases. Respiratory and urinary tract infections and sepsis are common; pathogens can be bacterial, viral, or fungal.
- **Metabolic:** Metabolic and respiratory alkalosis may occur early. If shock develops, metabolic acidosis can supervene. Hypokalemia is common, in part because sympathetic tone is decreased and diuretics are used. Hypophosphatemia and hypomagnesemia can develop. Hypoglycemia may occur because hepatic glycogen is depleted and gluconeogenesis and insulin degradation are impaired.
- **Pulmonary:** Noncardiogenic pulmonary edema may develop.

Symptoms and Signs

Characteristic manifestations are altered mental status, bleeding, purpura, jaundice, and ascites. Other symptoms may be nonspecific (e.g. malaise, anorexia) or result from the causative disorder. Fetor hepaticus (a musty or sweet breath odor) and motor dysfunction are common. Tachycardia, tachypnea, and hypotension may occur with or without sepsis. Signs of cerebral edema can include obtundation, coma, bradycardia, and hypertension. Patients with infection sometimes have localizing symptoms (e.g. cough, dysuria), but these symptoms may be absent.

Diagnosis

Acute liver failure should be suspected if patients have acute jaundice, unexplained bleeding, or changes in mental status (possibly suggesting encephalopathy) or if patients with known liver disease quickly deteriorate in any way.

Laboratory tests to confirm the presence and severity of liver failure include liver enzyme and bilirubin levels and prothrombin time (PT). Acute liver failure is usually considered confirmed if sensorium is altered or PT is prolonged by >4 sec or if international normalized ratio (INR) is >1.5 in patients who have clinical and/or laboratory evidence of acute liver injury. Evidence of cirrhosis suggests that liver failure is chronic.

Patients with acute liver failure should be tested for complications. Tests usually did during the initial evaluation include complete blood count (CBC), serum electrolytes (including Ca, PO_4 and Mg), renal function tests, and urinalysis. If acute liver failure is confirmed, arterial blood gases (ABGs), amylase and lipase, and blood type and screen should also be done. Plasma ammonia is sometimes recommended for diagnosing encephalopathy or monitoring its severity. If patients have hyperdynamic circulation and tachypnea, cultures (blood, urine, ascitic fluid) and chest X-ray should be done to rule out infection. If patients have impaired or worsening mental status, particularly those with coagulopathy, head CT should be done to rule out intracranial bleeding.

To determine the cause of acute liver failure, clinicians should take a complete history of toxins ingested, including prescription and over-the-counter (OTC) drugs, herbal products, and dietary supplements. Tests done routinely to determine the cause include.

- Viral hepatitis serologic tests [e.g. IgM antibody to hepatitis A virus (IgM anti-HAV), hepatitis B surface antigen (HBsAg), IgM antibody to hepatitis B core antigen (IgM anti-HBcAg), antibody to hepatitis C virus (anti-HCV)]
- Autoimmune markers [e.g. antinuclear antibodies (ANA), anti-smooth muscle antibodies, immunoglobulin levels].

Other testing is done based on findings and clinical suspicion, as for the following:

- *Recent travel to developing countries:* Tests for hepatitis A, B, D, and E.
- *Females of child-bearing age:* Pregnancy testing.
- *Age < 40 and relatively normal aminotransferase levels:* Ceruloplasmin level to check for Wilson disease.
- *Suspicion of a disorder with structural abnormalities (e.g. Budd-Chiari syndrome, portal vein thrombosis, liver metastases).* Ultrasonography and sometimes other imaging.

Patients should be monitored closely for complications (e.g., subtle changes in vital signs compatible with infection), and the threshold for testing should be low. For example, clinicians should not assume worsening mental status is due to encephalopathy; in such cases, head CT and often bedside glucose testing should be done. Routine laboratory testing (e.g., daily PT, serum electrolytes, renal function tests, blood glucose, and ABGs) should be repeated frequently in most cases.

Prognosis

Prediction of prognosis can be difficult. Important predictive variables include

- *Degree of encephalopathy:* Worse when encephalopathy is severe.
- *Patient age:* Worse when age is < 10 or > 40 years.
- *PT:* Worse when PT is prolonged.
- *Cause of acute liver failure:* Better with acetaminophen toxicity, hepatitis A, or hepatitis B than with idiosyncratic drug reactions or Wilson disease.

Treatment

Whenever possible, patients should be treated in an ICU at a center capable of liver transplantation. Patients should be transported as soon as possible because deterioration can be rapid and complications (e.g. bleeding, aspiration, worsening shock) become more likely as liver failure progresses.

Intensive supportive therapy is the mainstay of treatment. Drugs that could worsen manifestations of acute liver failure (e.g. hypotension, sedation) should be avoided or used in the lowest possible doses.

For **hypotension** and **acute kidney injury,** the goal of treatment is maximizing tissue perfusion. Treatment includes IV fluids and usually, until sepsis is excluded, empiric antibiotics. If hypotension is refractory to about 20 mL/kg of crystalloid solution, clinicians should consider measuring pulmonary capillary wedge pressure to guide fluid therapy. If hypotension persists despite adequate filling pressures, clinicians should consider using pressors (e.g. dopamine, epinephrine, and norepinephrine).

For encephalopathy, the head of the bed is elevated 30° to reduce risk of aspiration; intubation should be considered early. When selecting drugs and drug doses, clinicians should aim to minimize sedation, so that they can monitor the severity of encephalopathy. Propofol is the usual induction drug for intubation because it protects against intracranial hypertension and has a brief duration of action, allowing rapid recovery from sedation. Lactulose may be helpful for encephalopathy, but it is not given orally or nasogastric tube to patients who have altered mental status unless they are intubated. Measures are taken to avoid increasing intracranial pressure (ICP) and avoid decreasing cerebral perfusion pressure:

- To avoid sudden increases in ICP: Stimuli that could trigger a Valsalva maneuver are avoided (e.g. lidocaine is given before endotracheal suctioning to prevent the gag reflex).
- To temporarily decrease cerebral blood flow: Mannitol (0.5–1 g/kg, repeated once or twice as needed), can be given to induce osmotic diuresis, and possibly brief hyperventilation can be used, particularly when herniation is suspected.
- To monitor ICP: It is not clear whether or when the risks of ICP monitoring (e.g. infection, bleeding) outweigh the benefits of being able to detect cerebral edema early and being able to use ICP to guide fluid and pressor therapy; some experts recommend such monitoring if encephalopathy is severe. Goals of treatment are ICP of < 20 mmHg and a cerebral perfusion pressure of > 50 mmHg.

Seizures are treated with phenytoin; benzodiazepines are avoided or used only in low doses because they cause sedation.

Infection is treated with antibacterial and/or antifungal drugs; treatment is started as soon as patients show any sign of infection (e.g. fever localizing signs, deterioration of hemodynamics, mental status, or renal function). Because signs of infection overlap with those of acute liver failure, infection is likely to be overtreated pending culture results.

Electrolyte deficiencies may require supplementation with K, PO_4, or Mg.

Hypoglycemia is treated with continuous glucose infusion (e.g. 10% dextrose), and blood glucose should be monitored frequently because encephalopathy can mask the symptoms of hypoglycemia.

Coagulopathy is treated with fresh frozen plasma if bleeding occurs, if an invasive procedure is planned, or possibly if coagulopathy is severe (e.g. INR > 7). Fresh frozen plasma is otherwise avoided because it may result in volume overload and worsening of cerebral edema. Also, when it is used, clinicians cannot follow changes in

PT, which are important because PT is an index of severity of acute liver failure and is thus sometimes a criterion for transplantation. Recombinant factor VII is sometimes used instead of or with fresh frozen plasma in patients with volume overload.

Nutritional support may be necessary if patients cannot eat. Severe protein restriction is unnecessary; 60 g/day is recommended.

Acute acetaminophen overdose is treated with *N*-acetylcysteine. Because chronic acetaminophen toxicity can be difficult to diagnose, use of *N*-acetylcysteine should be considered, if no cause for acute liver failure is evident. Whether *N*-acetylcysteine has a slight beneficial effect on patients with acute liver failure due to other conditions is under study.

Liver transplantation is thus recommended, if prognosis without transplantation is worse.

Ascites

Ascites is free fluid in the peritoneal cavity. The most common cause is portal hypertension. Symptoms usually result from abdominal distention. Diagnosis is based on physical examination and often ultrasonography or CT. Treatments include bed rest, dietary Na restriction, diuretics, and therapeutic paracentesis. Ascitic fluid can become infected (spontaneous bacterial peritonitis), often with pain and fever. Diagnosis of infection involves analysis and culture of ascitic fluid. Infection is treated with antibiotics.

Etiology

Ascites can result from hepatic disorders, usually chronic but sometimes acute; conditions unrelated to the liver can also cause ascites.

Hepatic Causes

Include the following:

- Portal hypertension (accounts for > 90% of hepatic cases), usually due to cirrhosis.
- Chronic hepatitis.
- Severe alcoholic hepatitis without cirrhosis.
- Hepatic vein obstruction (e.g. Budd–Chiari syndrome).

Portal vein thrombosis does not usually cause ascites unless hepatocellular damage is also present.

Nonhepatic Causes

Include the following:

- Generalized fluid retention associated with systemic diseases (e.g. heart failure, nephrotic syndrome, severe hypoalbuminemia, constrictive pericarditis).
- Peritoneal disorders (e.g. carcinomatous or infectious peritonitis, biliary leak due to surgery or another medical procedure).
- Less common causes, such as renal dialysis, pancreatitis, systemic lupus erythematosus (SLE), and endocrine disorders (e.g. myxedema).

Pathophysiology

Mechanisms are complex and incompletely understood. Factors include altered Starling forces in the portal vessels (low oncotic pressure due to hypoalbuminemia plus increased portal venous pressure), avid renal Na retention (urinary Na concentration is typically < 5 mmol/L), and possibly increased hepatic lymph formation.

Mechanisms that seem to contribute to renal Na retention include activation of the renin-angiotensin-aldosterone system; increased sympathetic tone; intrarenal shunting of blood away from the cortex; increased formation of nitric oxide; and altered formation or metabolism of antidiuretic hormone (ADH), kinins, prostaglandins, and atrial natriuretic factor. Vasodilation in the splanchnic arterial circulation may be a trigger, but the specific roles and interrelationships of these abnormalities remain uncertain.

Symptoms and Signs

Small amounts of ascitic fluid cause no symptoms. Moderate amounts cause increased abdominal girth and weight gain. Massive amounts may cause nonspecific diffuse abdominal pressure, but actual pain is uncommon and suggests another cause of acute abdominal pain. If ascites results in elevation of the diaphragm, dyspnea may occur. Symptoms of spontaneous bacterial peritonitis may include new abdominal discomfort and fever.

Signs include shifting dullness (detected by abdominal percussion) and a fluid wave. Volumes < 1500 mL may not cause physical findings. Massive ascites causes tautness of the abdominal wall and flattening of the umbilicus. In liver diseases or peritoneal disorders, ascites is usually isolated or disproportionate to peripheral edema; in systemic diseases (e.g. heart failure), the reverse is usually true.

Diagnosis

Diagnosis may be based on physical examination if there is a large amount of fluid, but imaging tests are more sensitive. Ultrasonography and CT reveal much smaller volumes of fluid (100–200 mL) then does physical examination. Spontaneous bacterial peritonitis (SBP) is suspected if a patient with ascites also has abdominal pain, fever, or unexplained deterioration.

Diagnostic paracentesis should be done if any of the following occur:

About 50–100 mL of fluid is removed and analyzed for gross appearance, protein content, cell count and differential cytology, culture, and as clinically indicated, acid-fast stain, amylase, or both. In contrast to ascites due to inflammation or infection, ascites due to portal hypertension produces fluid that is clear and straw-colored, has a low protein concentration, a low polymorphonuclear (PMN) count (<250 cells/μL), and, most reliably, a high serum-to-ascites albumin concentration gradient, which is the serum albumin concentration minus the ascitic albumin concentration. Gradients ≥1.1 g/dL are relatively specific for ascites due to portal hypertension. In ascitic fluid, turbidity and a PMN count of >250 cells/μL indicate SBP, whereas bloody fluid can suggest a tumor or TB. The rare milky (chylous) ascites is most common with lymphoma or lymphatic duct occlusion.

Treatment

Bed rest and dietary Na restriction (2000 mg/day) are the first and least risky treatments for ascites due to portal hypertension. Diuretics should be used if rigid Na restriction fails to initiate diuresis within a few days. Spironolactone is usually effective (in oral doses ranging from 50 mg once/day to 200 mg bid). A loop diuretic (e.g. furosemide 20–160 mg orally usually once/day or 20–80 mg orally bid), should be added if spironolactone is insufficient. Because spironolactone can cause K retention and furosemide can cause K depletion, the combination of these drugs often provides optimal diuresis with a lower risk of K abnormalities. Fluid restriction is indicated only for treatment of hyponatremia (serum Na <120 mmol/L). Changes in body weight and urinary Na determinations reflect response to treatment. Weight loss of about 0.5 kg/day is optimal because the ascitic compartment cannot be mobilized much more rapidly. More aggressive diuresis depletes fluid from the intravascular compartment, especially when peripheral edema is absent; this depletion may cause renal failure or electrolyte imbalance (e.g., hypokalemia) that may precipitate portosystemic encephalopathy. Inadequate dietary Na restriction is the usual cause of persistent ascites.

Therapeutic paracentesis is an alternative. Removal of 4 L/day is safe; many clinicians infuse IV salt-poor albumin (about 40 g/paracentesis) at about the same time to prevent intravascular volume depletion. Even single total paracentesis may be safe. Therapeutic paracentesis shortens the hospital stay with relatively little risk of electrolyte imbalance or renal failure; nevertheless, patients require ongoing diuretics and tend to re-accumulate fluid more rapidly than those treated without paracentesis.

Techniques for the autologous infusion of ascitic fluid (e.g. the LeVeen peritoneovenous shunt) often cause complications and are generally no longer used. Transjugular intrahepatic portosystemic shunting (TIPS) can lower portal pressure and successfully treat ascites resistant to other treatments, but TIPS is invasive and may cause complications, including portosystemic encephalopathy and worsening hepatocellular function.

NONALCOHOLIC STEATOHEPATITIS

Nonalcoholic steatohepatitis (NASH) is a syndrome that develops in patients who are not alcoholic; it causes liver damage that is histologically indistinguishable from alcoholic hepatitis. It develops most often in patients with at least one of the following risk factors: obesity, dyslipidemia, and glucose intolerance. Pathogenesis is poorly understood but seems to be linked to insulin resistance (e.g. as in obesity or metabolic syndrome). Most patients are asymptomatic. Laboratory findings include elevations in aminotransferase levels. Biopsy is required to confirm the diagnosis. Treatment includes elimination of causes and risk factors.

NASH (sometimes called steatonecrosis) is diagnosed most often in patients between 40 years and 60 years, but can occur in all age groups. Many affected patients have obesity, type 2 diabetes mellitus (or glucose intolerance), dyslipidemia, and/or metabolic syndrome.

Pathophysiology

Pathophysiology involves fat accumulation (steatosis), inflammation, and variably, fibrosis. Steatosis results from hepatic triglyceride accumulation. Possible mechanisms for steatosis include reduced synthesis of very low density lipoprotein (VLDL) and increased hepatic triglyceride synthesis (possibly due to decreased oxidation of fatty acids or increased free fatty acids being delivered to the liver). Inflammation may result from lipid peroxidative damage to cell membranes. These changes can stimulate hepatic stellate cells, resulting in fibrosis. If advanced, NASH can cause cirrhosis and portal hypertension.

Symptoms and Signs

Most patients are asymptomatic. However, some have fatigue, malaise, or right upper quadrant abdominal discomfort. Hepatomegaly develops in about 75% of patients. Splenomegaly may develop if advanced hepatic fibrosis is present and is usually the first indication that portal hypertension has developed. Patients with cirrhosis due to NASH can be asymptomatic and may lack the usual signs of chronic liver disease.

Diagnosis

The diagnosis should be suspected in patients with risk factors, such as obesity, type 2 diabetes mellitus, or dyslipidemia and in patients with unexplained laboratory abnormalities suggesting liver disease. The most common laboratory abnormalities are elevations in aminotransferase levels. Unlike in alcoholic liver disease, the ratio of aspartate aminotransferase (AST), alanine transferase (ALT) in NASH is usually <1. Alkaline phosphatase and γ-glutamyl transpeptidase (GGT) occasionally increase. Hyperbilirubinemia, prolongation of PT, and hypoalbuminemia are uncommon.

For diagnosis, strong evidence (such as a history corroborated by friends and relatives) that alcohol intake is not excessive (e.g. is <20 g/day) is needed, and serologic tests should show absence of hepatitis B and C (i.e. hepatitis B surface antigen and hepatitis C virus antibody should be negative). Liver biopsy reveals damage similar to that seen in alcoholic hepatitis, usually including large fat droplets (macrovesicular fatty infiltration). Indications for biopsy include unexplained signs of portal hypertension (e.g. splenomegaly, cytopenia) and unexplained elevations in aminotransferase levels that persist for >6 months in a patient with diabetes, obesity, or dyslipidemia.

Imaging tests, including ultrasonography, CT, and particularly MRI, may identify hepatic steatosis. However, these tests cannot identify the inflammation typical of NASH and cannot differentiate NASH from other causes of hepatic steatosis.

Prognosis

Prognosis is hard to predict. Probably, most patients do not develop hepatic insufficiency or cirrhosis. However, some drugs (e.g. cytotoxic drugs) and metabolic disorders are associated with acceleration of NASH. Prognosis is often good unless complications develop.

Treatment

Elimination of causes and control of risk factors, the only widely accepted treatment goal is to eliminate potential causes and risk factors. Such a goal may include discontinuation of drugs or toxins, weight loss, and treatment for dyslipidemia or hyperglycemia. Preliminary evidence suggests that thiazolidinediones and vitamin E can help correct biochemical and histologic abnormalities in NASH. Many other treatments (e.g. ursodeoxycholic acid, metronidazole, metformin, betaine, glucagon, glutamine infusion) have not been proved effective.

ALCOHOLIC LIVER DISEASE

Alcohol is a common cause of liver disease. There are three main categories. Fat accumulation in the liver (hepatic steatosis) occurs frequently in people who abuse alcohol; it may give rise to asymptomatic hepatomegaly, with modest increases in plasma aminotransferases, a more marked increase in GGT activity, but a normal bilirubin concentration. This is a benign condition if patients abstain completely from alcohol. Frank alcoholic hepatitis often develops after a bout of heavy drinking in patients with a history of excessive alcohol ingestion; if severe, it is life-threatening. Third, chronic alcohol ingestion is a common cause of cirrhosis. This risk is greater for women than for men, but cirrhosis is not inevitable even in heavy drinkers: only about 10% of heavy drinkers develop cirrhosis.

Pathophysiology

Alcohol absorption and Metabolism

Alcohol (ethanol) is readily absorbed from the stomach, but most is absorbed from the small intestine. Alcohol cannot be stored. A small amount is degraded in transit through the gastric mucosa, but most is catabolized in the liver, primarily by alcohol dehydrogenase (ADH), but also by cytochrome P-450 2E1 (CYP2E1) and the microsomal enzyme oxidation system (MEOS).

Metabolism via the ADH pathway involves the following:

- ADH, a cytoplasmic enzyme, oxidizes alcohol into acetaldehyde. Genetic polymorphisms in ADH account for some individual differences in blood alcohol levels after the same alcohol intake but not in susceptibility to alcoholic liver disease.

- Acetaldehyde dehydrogenase (ALDH), a mitochondrial enzyme, then oxidizes acetaldehyde into acetate. Chronic alcohol consumption enhances acetate formation. Asians, who have lower levels of ALDH, are more susceptible to toxic acetaldehyde effects (e.g. flushing); the effects are similar to those of disulfiram, which inhibits ALDH.

- These oxidative reactions generate hydrogen, which converts nicotinamide-adenine dinucleotide (NAD) to its reduced form (NADH), increasing the redox potential (NADH/NAD) in the liver.

- The increased redox potential inhibits fatty acid oxidation and gluconeogenesis, promoting fat accumulation in the liver.

Chronic alcoholism induces the MEOS (mainly in endoplasmic reticulum), increasing its activity. The main enzyme involved is CYP2E1. When induced, the MEOS pathway can account for 20% of alcohol metabolism. This pathway generates harmful reactive O_2 species, increasing oxidative stress and formation of O_2-free radicals.

Hepatic Fat Accumulation

Fat (triglycerides) accumulates throughout the hepatocytes for the following reasons:

- Export of fat from the liver is decreased because hepatic fatty acid oxidation and lipoprotein production decrease.
- Input of fat is increased because the decrease in hepatic fat export increases peripheral lipolysis and triglyceride synthesis, resulting in hyperlipidemia.

Hepatic fat accumulation may predispose to subsequent oxidative damage.

Endotoxins in the Gut

Alcohol changes gut permeability, increasing absorption of endotoxins released by bacteria in the gut. In response to the endotoxins (in which will impair liver and it can not longer detoxify), liver macrophages (Kupffer cells) release free radicals, increasing oxidative damage.

Oxidative Damage

Oxidative stress is increased by:

- Liver hypermetabolism, caused by alcohol consumption
- Free radical-induced lipid peroxidative damage
- Reduction in protective antioxidants (e.g. glutathione, vitamins A and E), caused by alcohol-related undernutrition
- Binding of alcohol oxidation products, such as acetaldehyde, to liver cell proteins, forming neoantigens and resulting in inflammation
- Accumulation of neutrophils and other WBCs, which are attracted by lipid peroxidative damage and neoantigens
- Inflammatory cytokines secreted by WBCs

Accumulation of hepatic iron, if present, aggravates oxidative damage. Iron can accumulate in alcoholic liver disease through ingestion of iron-containing fortified wines; most often, the iron accumulation is modest. This condition must be differentiated from hereditary hemochromatosis.

Resultant Inflammation, Cell Death, and Fibrosis

A vicious circle of worsening inflammation occurs: Cell necrosis and apoptosis result in hepatocyte loss, and subsequent attempts at regeneration result in fibrosis. Stellate cells, which line blood channels (sinusoids) in the liver, proliferate and transform into myofibroblasts, producing an excess of type I collagen and extracellular matrix. As a result, the sinusoids narrow, limiting blood flow. Fibrosis narrows the terminal hepatic venules, compromising hepatic perfusion and thus contributing to portal hypertension. Extensive fibrosis is associated with an attempt at regeneration, resulting in liver nodules. This process culminates in cirrhosis.

Pathology

Fatty liver, alcoholic hepatitis and cirrhosis are often considered separate, progressive manifestations of alcoholic liver disease. However, their features often overlap.

Fatty liver (steatosis) is the initial and most common consequence of excessive alcohol consumption. Fatty liver is potentially reversible. Macrovesicular fat accumulates as large droplets of triglyceride and displaces the hepatocyte nucleus, most markedly in perivenular hepatocytes. The liver enlarges.

Alcoholic hepatitis (steatohepatitis) is a combination of fatty liver, diffuse liver inflammation, and liver necrosis, all in various degrees of severity. The damaged hepatocytes are swollen with a granular cytoplasm (balloon degeneration) or contain fibrillar protein in the cytoplasm (Mallory or alcoholic hyaline bodies). Severely damaged hepatocytes become necrotic. Sinusoids and terminal hepatic venules are narrowed. Cirrhosis may also be present.

Alcoholic cirrhosis is advanced liver disease characterized by extensive fibrosis that disrupts the normal liver architecture. The amount of fat present varies. Alcoholic hepatitis may coexist. The feeble compensatory attempt at hepatic regeneration produces relatively small nodules (micronodular cirrhosis). As a result, the liver usually shrinks. In time, even with abstinence, fibrosis forms broad bands, separating liver tissue into large nodules.

Symptoms and Signs

Symptoms usually become apparent in patients during their 30s or 40s; severe problems appear about a decade later.

Fatty liver is often asymptomatic. In one-third of patients, the liver is enlarged and smooth, but it is not usually tender.

Alcoholic hepatitis ranges from mild and reversible to life threatening. Most patients with moderate disease are undernourished and present with fatigue, fever, jaundice, right upper quadrant pain, tender hepatomegaly, and sometimes a hepatic bruit. About 40% deteriorate soon after hospitalization, with consequences ranging from mild (e.g. increasing jaundice) to severe (e.g. ascites, portosystemic encephalopathy, variceal bleeding, liver failure with hypoglycemia, coagulopathy). Other manifestations of cirrhosis may be present.

Cirrhosis, if compensated, may be asymptomatic. The liver is usually small; when the liver is enlarged, fatty liver or hepatoma should be considered. Symptoms range from those of alcoholic hepatitis to the complications of end-stage liver disease, such as portal hypertension (often with esophageal varices and upper GI bleeding, splenomegaly, ascites, and portosystemic encephalopathy). Portal hypertension may lead to intrapulmonary arteriovenous shunting with hypoxemia (hepatopulmonary syndrome), which may cause cyanosis and nail clubbing. Acute renal failure secondary to progressively decreasing renal blood flow (hepatorenal syndrome) may develop. Hepatocellular carcinoma develops in 10–15% of patients with alcoholic cirrhosis.

Chronic alcoholism, rather than liver disease, causes Dupuytren's contracture of the palmar fascia, vascular spiders, myopathy, and peripheral neuropathy. In men, chronic alcoholism causes signs of hypogonadism and feminization (e.g. smooth skin, lack of male-pattern baldness, gynecomastia, testicular atrophy, changes in pubic hair). Undernutrition may lead to multiple vitamin deficiencies (e.g. of folate and thiamin), enlarged parotid glands, and white nails. In alcoholics, Wernicke encephalopathy and Korsakoff psychosis result mainly from thiamin deficiency. Pancreatitis is common. Hepatitis-C occurs in >25% of alcoholics; this combination markedly worsens the progression of liver disease.

Rarely, patients with fatty liver or cirrhosis present with Zieve syndrome (hyperlipidemia, hemolytic anemia, and jaundice).

Diagnosis

Alcohol is suspected as the cause of liver disease in any patient who chronically consumes excess alcohol, particularly >80 g/day. When the patient's alcohol consumption is in doubt, history should be confirmed by family members. There is no specific test for alcoholic liver disease, but if the diagnosis is suspected, liver function tests (PT; serum bilirubin, aminotransferase, and albumin levels) and CBC are done to detect signs of liver injury and anemia.

Elevations of aminotransferases are moderate (<300 IU/L) and do not reflect the extent of liver damage. The ratio of AST to ALT is ≥2. The basis for low ALT is a dietary deficiency of pyridoxal phosphate (vitamin B_6), which is needed for ALT to function. Its effect on AST is less pronounced. Serum γ-glutamyl transpeptidase (GGT) increases, more because ethanol induces this enzyme than because patients have cholestasis or liver injury or use other drugs. Serum albumin may be low, usually reflecting undernutrition, but occasionally reflecting otherwise obvious liver failure with deficient synthesis. Macrocytosis with a mean corpuscular volume (MCV) >100 fL reflects the direct effect of alcohol on bone marrow as well as macrocytic anemia resulting from

folate deficiency, which is common among undernourished alcoholics. Indexes of the severity of liver disease are:
- Serum bilirubin, which represents secretory function
- PT or INR, which reflects synthetic ability

Thrombocytopenia can result from the direct toxic effects of alcohol on bone marrow or from splenomegaly, which accompanies portal hypertension. Neutrophilic leukocytosis may result from alcoholic hepatitis, although coexisting infection (particularly pneumonia and spontaneous bacterial peritonitis) should also be suspected.

Imaging tests are not routinely needed for diagnosis. If done for other reasons, abdominal ultrasonography or CT may suggest fatty liver or show splenomegaly, evidence of portal hypertension, or ascites. Ultrasound elastrography measures liver stiffness and thus detects advanced fibrosis. This valuable adjunct can obviate the need for liver biopsy to check for cirrhosis and help assess prognosis. If abnormalities suggest alcoholic liver disease, screening tests for other treatable forms of liver disease, especially viral hepatitis, should be done.

Because features of fatty liver, alcoholic hepatitis, and cirrhosis overlap, describing the precise findings is more useful than assigning patients to a specific category, which can only be determined by liver biopsy.

Not all experts agree on the indications for liver biopsy. Proposed indications include the following:
- Unclear clinical diagnosis (e.g. equivocal clinical and laboratory findings, unexplained persistent elevations of aminotransferase levels)
- Clinical suspicion of > 1 cause of liver disease (e.g. alcohol plus viral hepatitis)
- Desire for a precise prediction of prognosis

Liver biopsy confirms liver disease, helps identify excessive alcohol use as the likely cause, and establishes the stage of liver injury. If iron accumulation is observed, measurement of the iron content and genetic testing can eliminate hereditary hemochromatosis as the cause.

For stable patients with cirrhosis, α-fetoprotein measurement and liver ultrasonography should be done every 6 months to screen for hepatocellular carcinoma.

Prognosis

Prognosis is determined by the degree of hepatic fibrosis and inflammation. Fatty liver and alcoholic hepatitis without fibrosis are reversible if alcohol is avoided. With abstinence, fatty liver completely resolves within 6 weeks. Fibrosis and cirrhosis are irreversible.

Certain biopsy findings (e.g. neutrophils, perivenular fibrosis) indicate a worse prognosis. Proposed quantitative indexes to predict severity and mortality use primarily laboratory features of liver failure, such as PT, creatinine (for hepatorenal syndrome), and bilirubin levels.

Treatment

Abstinence is the mainstay of treatment; it prevents further damage from alcoholic liver disease and thus prolongs life. Because compliance is problematic, a compassionate team approach is essential. Behavioral and psychosocial interventions can help motivated patients; they include rehabilitation programs and support groups, brief interventions by primary care physicians, and therapies that explore and clarify the motivation to abstain (motivational enhancement therapy).

Drugs, if used, should only supplement other interventions. Opioid antagonists (naltrexone or nalmefene) and drugs that modulate γ-aminobutyric acid receptors (baclofen or acamprosate) appear to have a short-term benefit by reducing the craving and withdrawal symptoms. Disulfiram inhibits aldehyde dehydrogenase, allowing acetaldehyde to accumulate; thus, drinking alcohol within 12 hours of taking disulfiram causes flushing and has other unpleasant effects. However, disulfiram has not been shown to promote abstinence and consequently is recommended only for certain patients.

General management emphasizes supportive care. A nutritious diet and vitamin supplements (especially B vitamins) are important during the first few days of abstinence. Alcohol withdrawal requires use of benzodiazepines (e.g. diazepam). In patients with advanced alcoholic liver disease, excessive sedation can precipitate portosystemic encephalopathy and thus must be avoided.

Severe acute alcoholic hepatitis commonly requires hospitalization, often in an ICU, to facilitate enteral feeding (which can help manage nutritional deficiencies) and to manage specific complications (e.g., infection, bleeding from esophageal varices, specific nutritional deficiencies, Wernicke encephalopathy, Korsakoff psychosis, electrolyte abnormalities, portal hypertension, ascites, and portosystemic encephalopathy.

Corticosteroids (e.g. prednisolone 40 mg/day by mouth for 4 weeks, followed by tapered doses) improve outcome in patients who have severe acute alcoholic hepatitis and who do not have infection, GI bleeding, renal failure, or pancreatitis.

Other than corticosteroids and enteral feeding, few specific treatments are clearly established. Antioxidants (e.g. S-adenosyl-L-methionine, phosphatidylcholine, metadoxine) show promise in ameliorating liver injury during early cirrhosis but require further study. Therapies directed at cytokines, particularly tumor necrosis factor-α (TNF-α), and aiming to reduce inflammation have had mixed results in small trials.

Pentoxifylline, a phosphodiesterase inhibitor that inhibits TNF-α synthesis, has some benefit. In contrast, when biologic agents that inhibit TNF-α (e.g. infliximab, etanercept) are used, risk of infection outweighs benefit. Drugs given to decrease fibrosis (e.g. colchicine, penicillamine) and drugs given to normalize the hypermetabolic state of the alcoholic liver (e.g. propylthiouracil) have no proven benefit. Antioxidant remedies, such as silymarin (milk thistle) and vitamins A and E, are ineffective.

Liver transplantation can be considered if disease is severe. With transplantation, 5-year survival rates are comparable to those for nonalcoholic liver diseases as high as 80% in patients without active liver disease and 50% in those with acute alcoholic hepatitis. Because up to 50% of patients resume drinking after transplantation, most programs require 6 months of abstinence before transplantation is done; recent data suggest that earlier transplantation may offer a survival advantage, but currently, this approach is not standard of care.

JAUNDICE

Jaundice is a yellowish discoloration of the skin and mucous membranes caused by hyperbilirubinemia. Jaundice becomes visible when the bilirubin level is about 34–51 μmol/L. Bilirubin arises primarily from the physiologic breakdown of senescent red blood cells, with a minor contribution from other heme sources. It is not water-soluble and is therefore transported in plasma attached to albumin.

Pathophysiology

Most bilirubin is produced when Hb is broken down into unconjugated bilirubin (and other substances). Unconjugated bilirubin binds to albumin in the blood for transport to the liver, where it is taken up by hepatocytes and conjugated with glucuronic acid to make it water soluble. Conjugated bilirubin is excreted in bile into the duodenum. In the intestine, bacteria metabolize bilirubin to form urobilinogen. Some urobilinogen is eliminated in the feces, and some is reabsorbed, extracted by hepatocytes, reprocessed, and re-excreted in bile.

Mechanisms of Hyperbilirubinemia

Hyperbilirubinemia may involve predominantly unconjugated or conjugated bilirubin.

Unconjugated Hyperbilirubinemia

It is most often caused by more than of the following:
- Increased production
- Decreased hepatic uptake
- Decreased conjugation

Conjugated Hyperbilirubinemia

It is most often caused by more than of the following:

- Dysfunction of hepatocytes (hepatocellular dysfunction)
- Slowing of bile egress from the liver (intrahepatic cholestasis)
- Obstruction of extrahepatic bile flow (extrahepatic cholestasis)

Consequences

Outcome is determined primarily by the cause of jaundice and the presence and severity of hepatic dysfunction. Hepatic dysfunction can result in coagulopathy, encephalopathy, and portal hypertension (which can lead to GI bleeding).

Etiology

Although, hyperbilirubinemia can be classified as predominantly unconjugated or conjugated, many hepatobiliary disorders cause both forms.

Many conditions (Table 5.2), including use of certain drugs (Table 5.3), can cause jaundice, but the most common causes overall are:

- Inflammatory hepatitis (viral hepatitis, autoimmune hepatitis, toxic hepatic injury)
- Alcoholic liver disease
- Biliary obstruction

Table 5.2	Mechanisms and some causes of jaundice in adults	
Mechanism	**Examples**	**Suggestive findings***
Unconjugated hyperbilirubinemia		
Increased bilirubin production	Common: Hemolysis Less common: Resorption of large hematomas, ineffective erythropoiesis	Few or No clinical manifestations of hepatobiliary disease; sometimes anemia, ecchymoses Serum bilirubin level usually <3.5 mg/dL (<59 μmol/L), no bilirubin in urine, normal aminotransferase levels
Decreased hepatic bilirubin uptake	Common: Heart failure Less common: Drugs, fasting, portosystemic shunts	—
Decreased hepatic conjugation	Common: Gilbert syndrome Less common: Ethinyl estradiol, Crigler-Najjar syndrome, hyperthyroidism	—
Conjugated hyperbilirubinemia[†]		
Hepatocellular dysfunction	Common: Drugs, toxins, viral hepatitis Less common: Alcoholic liver disease, hemochromatosis, primary biliary cirrhosis, primary sclerosing cholangitis, steatohepatitis, Wilson disease	Aminotransferase levels usually >500 U/L
Intrahepatic cholestasis	Common: Alcoholic liver disease, drugs, toxins, viral hepatitis Less common: Infiltrative disorders (e.g. amyloidosis, lymphoma, sarcoidosis, TB), pregnancy, primary biliary cirrhosis, steatohepatitis	Gradual onset of jaundice, sometimes pruritus If severe, clay-colored stools, steatorrhea If long-standing, weight loss Alkaline phosphatase and GGT usually >3 times normal Aminotransferase levels <200 U/L
Extrahepatic cholestasis	Common: Common bile duct stone, pancreatic cancer Less common: Acute cholangitis, pancreatic pseudocyst, primary sclerosing cholangitis, common duct strictures caused by previous surgery, other tumors	Depending on cause, manifestations possibly similar to those of intrahepatic cholestasis or a more acute disorder (e.g. abdominal pain or vomiting due to a common bile duct stone or acute pancreatitis) Alkaline phosphatase and GGT usually >3 times normal Aminotransferase levels <200 U/L
Other, less common mechanisms	Hereditary disorders (mainly Dubin-Johnson syndrome and Rotor syndrome)	Normal liver enzymes

*Symptoms and signs of the causative disorder may be present.
[†]Bilirubin is present in urine.
GGT, γ-glutamyl transferase

Mechanism	Drugs or toxins
Increased bilirubin production	Drugs that cause hemolysis (common among patients with G6PD deficiency), such as sulfa drugs and nitrofurantoin
Decreased hepatic uptake	Chloramphenicol, probenecid, rifampin

Table 5.3 Some drugs and toxins that can cause jaundice

Symptoms and Signs

Hyperbilirubinemia can cause urine to darken before jaundice is visible. Therefore, the onset of dark urine indicates onset of hyperbilirubinemia more accurately than onset of jaundice. Important associated symptoms include fever, prodromal symptoms (e.g. fever, malaise, and myalgias) before jaundice, changes in stool color, pruritus, steatorrhea, and abdominal pain (including location, severity, duration, and radiation). Important symptoms suggesting severe disease include nausea and vomiting, weight loss, and possible symptoms of coagulopathy (e.g. easy bruising or bleeding, tarry or bloody stools).

Vital signs are reviewed for fever and signs of systemic toxicity (e.g. hypotension, tachycardia). Mild jaundice is best seen by examining the sclerae in natural light; it is usually detectable when serum bilirubin reaches 34–43 µmol/L. Breath odor should be noted (e.g. for fetor hepaticus).

The abdomen is inspected for collateral vasculature, ascites, and surgical scars. The liver is palpated for hepatomegaly, masses, nodularity, and tenderness. The spleen is palpated for splenomegaly. The abdomen is examined for umbilical hernia, shifting dullness, fluid wave, masses, and tenderness. The rectum is examined for gross or occult blood.

The skin is examined for jaundice, palmar erythema, needle tracks, vascular spiders, excoriations, xanthomas (consistent with primary biliary cirrhosis), and paucity of axillary and pubic hair, hyperpigmentation, ecchymoses, petechiae, and purpura.

Diagnosis

Blood tests include measurement of total and direct bilirubin, aminotransferase, and alkaline phosphatase levels in all patients. Results help differentiate cholestasis from hepatocellular dysfunction (important because patients with cholestasis usually require imaging tests):

- *Hepatocellular dysfunction:* Marked aminotransferase elevation (>500 U/L) and moderate alkaline phosphatase elevation (<3 times normal)
- *Cholestasis:* Moderate aminotransferase elevation (<200 U/L) and marked alkaline phosphatase elevation (>3 times normal)

- *Hyperbilirubinemia without hepatobiliary dysfunction:* Mild hyperbilirubinemia [e.g. (<59 µmol/L)] with normal aminotransferase and alkaline phosphatase levels.

Also, patients with hepatocellular dysfunction or cholestasis have dark urine due to bilirubinuria because conjugated bilirubin is excreted in urine; unconjugated bilirubin is not. Bilirubin fractionation also differentiates conjugated from unconjugated forms. When aminotransferase and alkaline phosphatase levels are normal, fractionation of bilirubin can help suggest causes, such as Gilbert syndrome or hemolysis (unconjugated) vs Dubin-Johnson syndrome or Rotor syndrome (conjugated).

Other blood tests are done based on clinical suspicion and initial test findings, as for the following:

- Signs of hepatic insufficiency (e.g. encephalopathy, ascites, ecchymoses) or GI bleeding: Coagulation profile (PT/PTT, partial thromboplastin time)
- Hepatitis risk factors or a hepatocellular mechanism suggested by blood test results: Hepatitis viral and autoimmune serologic tests
- Fever, abdominal pain, and tenderness: CBC and, if patients appear ill, blood cultures

Suspicion of hemolysis can be confirmed by a peripheral blood smear.

Imaging is done if pain suggests extrahepatic obstruction or cholangitis or if blood test results suggest cholestasis.

Abdominal ultrasonography is usually done first; usually, it is highly accurate in detecting extrahepatic obstruction. CT and MRI are alternatives. Ultrasonography is usually more accurate for gallstones, and CT is more accurate for pancreatic lesions. All these tests can detect abnormalities in the biliary tree and focal liver lesions, but are less accurate in detecting diffuse hepatocellular disorders (e.g. hepatitis, cirrhosis).

If ultrasonography shows extrahepatic cholestasis, other tests may be necessary to determine the cause; usually, magnetic resonance cholangiopancreatography (MRCP), endoscopic ultrasonography (EUS), or ERCP is used. ERCP is more invasive but allows treatment of some obstructive lesions (e.g. stone removal, stenting of strictures).

Liver biopsy is not commonly required but can help diagnose certain disorders (e.g. disorders causing intrahepatic cholestasis, some kinds of hepatitis, some infiltrative disorders, Dubin-Johnson syndrome, hemochromatosis, Wilson disease). Biopsy can also help when liver enzyme abnormalities are unexplained by other tests.

Laparoscopy (peritoneoscopy) allows direct inspection of the liver and gallbladder without the trauma of a full laparotomy. Unexplained cholestatic jaundice warrants laparoscopy occasionally and diagnostic laparotomy rarely.

Treatment

Jaundice itself requires no treatment in adults, the cause and any complications are treated. Itching may be relieved with cholestyramine 2–8 g orally. However, cholestyramine is ineffective in patients with complete biliary obstruction.

INBORN METABOLIC DISORDERS

These may cause unconjugated or conjugated hyperbilirubinemia:

Unconjugated Hyperbilirubinemia
Gilbert Syndrome

Gilbert syndrome is a presumably lifelong disorder in which the only significant abnormality is asymptomatic, mild, and unconjugated hyperbilirubinemia. It can be mistaken for chronic hepatitis or other liver disorders.

Gilbert syndrome may affect as many as 5% of people. Although family members may be affected, a clear genetic pattern is difficult to establish.

Pathogenesis may involve complex defects in the liver's uptake of bilirubin. Glucuronyl transferase activity is low, though not as low as in Crigler–Najjar syndrome type II. In many patients, red blood cells (RBC) destruction is also slightly accelerated, but this acceleration does not explain hyperbilirubinemia. Liver histology is normal.

Gilbert syndrome is most often detected in young adults serendipitously by finding an elevated bilirubin level, which usually fluctuates between 2 mg/dL and 5 mg/dL (34 mmol/L and 86 mmol/L) and tends to increase with fasting and other stresses.

Gilbert syndrome is differentiated from hepatitis by fractionation that shows predominantly unconjugated bilirubin, otherwise normal liver function test results, and absence of urinary bilirubin. It is differentiated from hemolysis by the absence of anemia and reticulocytosis.

Treatment is unnecessary. Patients should be reassured that they do not have liver disease.

Crigler–Najjar Syndrome

Rare inherited disorder is caused by deficiency of the enzyme glucuronyl transferase.

Patients with autosomal recessive type I (complete) disease have severe hyperbilirubinemia. They usually die of kernicterus by age 1 year, but may survive into adulthood. Treatment may include phototherapy and liver transplantation.

Patients with autosomal dominant type II (partial) disease (which has variable penetrance) often have less severe hyperbilirubinemia [<20 mg/dL (<342 µmol/L)] and usually live into adulthood without neurologic damage. Phenobarbital 1.5–2 mg/kg orally, which induces the partially deficient glucuronyl transferase, may be effective.

Primary Shunt Hyperbilirubinemia

This rare, familial, and benign condition is characterized by overproduction of early-labeled bilirubin (bilirubin derived from ineffective erythropoiesis and nonhemoglobin heme rather than from normal RBC turnover).

Conjugated Hyperbilirubinemia

Dubin-Johnson syndrome and Rotor syndrome cause conjugated hyperbilirubinemia, but without cholestasis, causing no symptoms or sequelae other than jaundice. In contrast to unconjugated hyperbilirubinemia in Gilbert syndrome (which also causes no other symptoms), bilirubin may appear in the urine. Aminotransferase and alkaline phosphatase levels are usually normal. Treatment is unnecessary.

Dubin–Johnson Syndrome

This rare autosomal recessive disorder involves impaired excretion of bilirubin glucuronides. It is usually diagnosed by liver biopsy; the liver is deeply pigmented as a result of an intracellular melanin-like substance, but is otherwise histologically normal.

Rotor Syndrome

This rare disorder is clinically similar to Dubin–Johnson syndrome, but the liver is not pigmented and other subtle metabolic differences are present.

Hepatic Fibrosis

Hepatic fibrosis is overly exuberant wound healing in which excessive connective tissue builds up in the liver. The extracellular matrix is overproduced, degraded deficiently, or both. The trigger is chronic injury, especially if there is an inflammatory component. Fibrosis itself causes no symptoms but can lead to portal hypertension (the scarring distorts blood flow through the liver) or cirrhosis (the scarring results in disruption of normal hepatic architecture and liver dysfunction). Diagnosis is based on liver biopsy. Treatment involves correcting the underlying condition when possible.

Various types of chronic liver injury can cause fibrosis (Table 5.4), self-limited, acute liver injury (e.g. acute viral hepatitis A), even when fulminant, does not necessarily distort the scaffolding architecture and hence does not cause fibrosis, despite loss of hepatocytes. In its initial stages, hepatic fibrosis can regress if the cause is reversible (e.g. with viral clearance). After months or years of chronic or repeated injury, fibrosis becomes permanent. Fibrosis develops even more rapidly in mechanical biliary obstruction.

Table 5.4	Disorders and drugs that can cause hepatic fibrosis

Disorders with direct hepatic effects

Autoimmune hepatitis
Certain storage diseases and inborn errors of metabolism
- α_1-Antitrypsin deficiency
- Copper storage diseases (e.g. Wilson disease)
- Fructosemia
- Galactosemia
- Glycogen storage diseases (especially types III, IV, VI, IX, and X)
- Iron-overload syndromes (hemochromatosis)
- Lipid abnormalities (e.g. Gaucher disease)
- Peroxisomal disorders (e.g. Zellweger syndrome)
- Tyrosinemia

Congenital hepatic fibrosis
Infections
- Bacterial (e.g. brucellosis)
- Parasitic (e.g. echinococcosis)
- Viral (e.g. chronic hepatitis B or C*)

Nonalcoholic steatohepatitis (NASH)
Primary biliary cirrhosis
Primary sclerosing cholangitis

Disorders affecting hepatic blood flow

Budd-Chiari syndrome
Heart failure
Hepatic veno-occlusive disease†
Portal vein thrombosis

Drugs and chemicals

Alcohol*
Amiodarone
Chlorpromazine
Isoniazid
Methotrexate
Methyldopa
Oxyphenisatin
Tolbutamide

Mechanical obstruction

Scarring due to prior liver surgery
Bile duct strictures due to impacted gallstones

*Most common causes.
†Sometimes caused by pyrrolizidine alkaloids, present in herbal products such as bush teas.

Pathophysiology

Activation of the hepatic perivascular stellate cells (Ito cells, which store fat) initiates fibrosis. These and adjacent cells proliferate, becoming contractile cells termed myofibroblasts. These cells produce excessive amounts of abnormal matrix (consisting of collagen, other glycoproteins, and glycans) and matricellular proteins. Kupffer cells (resident macrophages), injured hepatocytes, platelets, and leukocytes aggregate. As a result, reactive O_2 species and inflammatory mediators (e.g. platelet-derived growth factor, transforming growth factors, and connective tissue growth factor) are released. Thus, stellate cell activation results in abnormal extracellular matrix, both in quantity and composition.

Myofibroblasts, stimulated by endothelin-1, contribute to increased portal vein resistance and increase the density of the abnormal matrix. Fibrous tracts join branches of afferent portal veins and efferent hepatic veins, bypassing the hepatocytes and limiting their blood supply. Hence, fibrosis contributes both to hepatocyte ischemia (causing hepatocellular dysfunction) and portal hypertension. The extent of the ischemia and portal hypertension determines how the liver is affected. For example, congenital hepatic fibrosis affects portal vein branches, largely sparing the parenchyma. The result is portal hypertension with sparing of hepatocellular function.

Symptoms and Signs

Hepatic fibrosis itself does not cause symptoms. Symptoms may result from the disorder causing fibrosis or, once fibrosis progresses to cirrhosis, from complications of portal hypertension. These symptoms include variceal bleeding, ascites, and portosystemic encephalopathy. Cirrhosis can result in hepatic insufficiency and potentially fatal liver failure.

Diagnosis

Hepatic fibrosis is suspected if patients have known chronic liver disease (e.g. chronic viral hepatitis C) or if results of liver function tests are abnormal; in such cases, tests are done to check for fibrosis and, if fibrosis is present, to determine its severity (stage). Knowing the stage of fibrosis can guide medical decisions. For example, screening for hepatocellular carcinoma and for gastroesophageal varices is indicated if cirrhosis is confirmed, but it is not indicated for mild or moderate fibrosis. Also, if liver biopsy does not detect advanced fibrosis in patients with hepatitis C, many clinicians defer treatment with interferons because they anticipate that more effective, less toxic drugs will be available.

Tests used to stage fibrosis include noninvasive imaging tests, blood tests, liver biopsy, and newer tests that assess liver stiffness.

Noninvasive imaging tests include ultrasonography, CT, and MRI and should include cross-sectional views. These tests can detect evidence of cirrhosis and portal hypertension, such as splenomegaly and varices. However, they are not sensitive for moderate or even advanced fibrosis if splenomegaly and varices are absent. Although, fibrosis may appear as altered echogenicity on ultrasonography or heterogeneity of signal on CT, these findings are nonspecific and may indicate only liver parenchymal fat.

Liver biopsy remains the gold standard for diagnosing and staging hepatic fibrosis and for diagnosing the underlying liver disorder causing fibrosis. However, liver biopsy is invasive, resulting in a 10–20% risk of minor complications (e.g. postprocedural pain) and a 0.5–1% risk of serious complications (e.g. significant bleeding). Also, liver biopsy is limited by sampling error and imperfect interobserver agreement in interpretation of histologic findings. Thus, liver biopsy may not always be done.

Blood tests include commercially available panels that combine indirect markers (e.g. serum bilirubin) and direct markers of hepatic function. Direct markers are substances involved in the pathogenesis of extracellular matrix deposition or cytokines that induce extracellular matrix deposition. These panels are best used to distinguish between 2 levels of fibrosis—absent to minimal vs moderate to severe; they do not accurately differentiate between degrees of moderate to severe fibrosis. Therefore, if fibrosis is suspected, one approach is to start with one of these panels and then do liver biopsy only if the panel indicates that fibrosis is moderate to severe.

Treatment

Because fibrosis represents a response to hepatic damage, primary treatment should focus on the cause (removing the basis of the liver injury). Such treatment may include eliminating hepatitis B virus or hepatitis C virus in chronic viral hepatitis, abstaining from alcohol in alcoholic liver disease, removing heavy metals such as iron in hemochromatosis or copper in Wilson disease, and decompressing bile ducts in biliary obstruction. Such treatments may stop the fibrosis from progressing and, in some patients, also reverse some of the fibrotic changes.

Treatments aimed at reversing the fibrosis are usually too toxic for long-term use (e.g. corticosteroids, penicillamine) or have no proven efficacy (e.g. colchicine). Other antifibrotic treatments are under study. Simultaneous use of multiple antifibrotic drugs may eventually prove most beneficial. Silymarin, present in milk thistle, is a popular alternative medicine used to treat hepatic fibrosis. It appears to be safe but to lack efficacy.

Cirrhosis

Cirrhosis is a late stage of hepatic fibrosis that has resulted in widespread distortion of normal hepatic architecture. Cirrhosis is characterized by regenerative nodules surrounded by dense fibrotic tissue. Symptoms may not develop for years and are often nonspecific (e.g. anorexia, fatigue, weight loss). Late manifestations include portal hypertension, ascites, and when decompensation occurs, liver failure. Diagnosis often requires liver biopsy. Cirrhosis is usually considered irreversible. Treatment is supportive.

Cirrhosis is a leading cause of death worldwide. The causes of cirrhosis are the same as those of fibrosis. In developed countries, most cases result from chronic alcohol abuse or chronic hepatitis C. In parts of Asia and Africa, cirrhosis often results from chronic hepatitis B. Cirrhosis of unknown etiology (cryptogenic cirrhosis) is becoming less common as many specific causes (e.g. chronic hepatitis C, steatohepatitis) are identified. Injury to the bile ducts also can result in cirrhosis, as occurs in mechanical bile duct obstruction, primary biliary cirrhosisand primary sclerosing cholangitis.

Pathophysiology

In response to injury and loss, growth regulators induce hepatocellular hyperplasia (producing regenerating nodules) and arterial growth (angiogenesis). Among the growth regulators are cytokines and hepatic growth factors (e.g. epithelial growth factor, hepatocyte growth factor, transforming growth factor-α, tumor necrosis factor). Insulin, glucagon, and patterns of intrahepatic blood flow determine how and where nodules develop.

Angiogenesis produces new vessels within the fibrous sheath that surrounds nodules. These vessels connect the hepatic artery and portal vein to hepatic venules, restoring the intrahepatic circulatory pathways. Such interconnecting vessels provide relatively low-volume, high-pressure venous drainage that cannot accommodate as much blood volume as normal. As a result, portal vein pressure increases. Such distortions in blood flow contribute to portal hypertension, which increases because the regenerating nodules compress hepatic venules.

The progression rate from fibrosis to cirrhosis and the morphology of cirrhosis vary from person to person. Presumably, the reason for such variation is the extent of exposure to the injurious stimulus and the individual's response.

Complications

Portal hypertension is the most common serious complication of cirrhosis, and it, in turn, causes complications, including GI bleeding from esophageal, gastric, or rectal varices and portal hypertensive gastropathy. In patients with cirrhosis, portal hypertension can also lead to ascites, acute kidney injury and pulmonary hypertension (portopulmonary hypertension). Ascites is a risk factor for spontaneous bacterial peritonitis. Portopulmonary hypertension can manifest with symptoms of heart failure. Complications of portal hypertension tend to cause significant morbidity and mortality.

Cirrhosis can cause other cardiovascular complications. Vasodilation, intrapulmonary right-to-left shunting, and ventilation/perfusion mismatch can result in hypoxia (hepatopulmonary syndrome).

Progressive loss of hepatic architecture impairs function, leading to hepatic insufficiency; it manifests as coagulopathy, acute kidney injury (hepatorenal syndrome), and hepatic encephalopathy. Hepatocytes secrete less bile, contributing to cholestasis and jaundice. Less bile in the intestine causes malabsorption of dietary fat (triglycerides) and fat-soluble vitamins. Malabsorption of vitamin D may contribute to osteoporosis. Undernutrition is common. It may result from anorexia with reduced food intake or, in patients with alcoholic liver disease, from malabsorption due to pancreatic insufficiency.

Blood disorders are common. Anemia usually results from hypersplenism, chronic GI bleeding, folate deficiency (particularly in patients with alcoholism), and hemolysis.

Cirrhosis results in decreased production of prothrombotic and antithrombotic factors. Hypersplenism and altered expression of thrombopoietin contribute to thrombocytopenia. Thrombocytopenia and decreased production of clotting factors can make clotting unpredictable, increasing risk of both bleeding and thromboembolic disease (even though INR is usually increased). Leukopenia is also common; it is mediated by hypersplenism and altered expression of erythropoietin and granulocyte-stimulating factors.

Histopatholog

Cirrhosis is characterized by regenerating nodules and fibrosis. Incompletely formed liver nodules, nodules without fibrosis (nodular regenerative hyperplasia), and congenital hepatic fibrosis (i.e. widespread fibrosis without regenerating nodules) are not true cirrhosis.

Cirrhosis can be micronodular or macronodular. Micronodular cirrhosis is characterized by uniformly small nodules (<3 mm in diameter) and thick regular bands of connective tissue. Typically, nodules lack lobular organization; terminal (central) hepatic venules and portal triads are distorted. With time, macronodular cirrhosis often develops. The nodules vary in size (3 mm to 5 cm in diameter) and have some relatively normal lobular organization of portal triads and terminal hepatic venules. Broad fibrous bands of varying thickness surround the large nodules. Collapse of the normal hepatic architecture is suggested by the concentration of portal triads within the fibrous scars. Mixed cirrhosis (incomplete septal cirrhosis) combines elements of micronodular and macronodular cirrhosis. Differentiation between these morphologic types of cirrhosis has limited clinical value.

Symptoms and Signs

Cirrhosis may be asymptomatic for years. One-third of patients never develop symptoms. Often, the first symptoms are nonspecific; they include generalized fatigue (due to cytokine release), anorexia, malaise, and weight loss. The liver is typically palpable and firm, with a blunt edge, but is sometimes small and difficult to palpate. Nodules usually are not palpable.

Clinical signs that suggest a chronic liver disorder or chronic alcohol use but are not specific for cirrhosis include muscle wasting, palmar erythema, parotid gland enlargement, white nails, clubbing, Dupuytren's contracture, spider angiomas (<10 may be normal), gynecomastia, axillary hair loss, testicular atrophy, and peripheral neuropathy.

Diagnosis
Laboratory Tests

Diagnostic testing begins with liver function tests, coagulation tests, CBC, and serologic tests for viral causes (e.g. hepatitis B and C). Laboratory tests alone may increase suspicion for cirrhosis but cannot confirm or exclude it. Liver biopsy becomes necessary if a clear diagnosis would lead to better management and outcome.

Test results may be normal or may indicate nonspecific abnormalities due to complications of cirrhosis or alcoholism. ALT and AST levels are often modestly elevated. Alkaline phosphatase and γ-GT are often normal; elevated levels indicate cholestasis or biliary obstruction. Bilirubin is usually normal but increases when cirrhosis progresses, particularly in primary biliary cirrhosis. Decreased serum albumin and a prolonged PT directly reflect impaired hepatic synthesis—usually an end-stage event. Albumin can also be low when nutrition is poor. Serum globulin increases in cirrhosis and in most liver disorders with an inflammatory component. Anemia is common and usually normocytic with a high RBC distribution width. Anemia is often multifactorial;

contributing factors may include chronic GI bleeding (usually causing microcytic anemia), folate nutritional deficiency (causing macrocytic anemia, especially in alcohol abuse), hemolysis, and hypersplenism. CBC may also detect leukopenia, thrombocytopenia, or pancytopenia.

Diagnostic Imaging

Imaging tests are not highly sensitive or specific for the diagnosis of cirrhosis by themselves, but they can often detect its complications. In advanced cirrhosis, ultrasonography shows a small, nodular liver. Ultrasonography also detects portal hypertension and ascites.

Computed tomography (CT) can detect a nodular texture, but it has no advantage over ultrasonography. Radionuclide liver scans using technetium-99m sulfur colloid may show irregular liver uptake and increased spleen and bone marrow uptake. MRI is more expensive than other imaging tests and has little advantage.

IDENTIFICATION OF THE CAUSE

Determining the specific cause of cirrhosis requires key clinical information from the history and examination, as well as selective testing. Alcohol is the likely cause in patients with a documented history of alcoholism and clinical findings, such as gynecomastia, spider angiomas (telangiectasia), and testicular atrophy plus laboratory confirmation of liver damage (AST elevated more than ALT) and liver enzyme induction (a greatly increased GGT). Fever, tender hepatomegaly, and jaundice suggest the presence of alcoholic hepatitis.

Detecting hepatitis B surface antigen and IgG antibodies to hepatitis B (IgG anti-HBc) confirms chronic hepatitis B. Identifying serum antibody to hepatitis C (anti-HCV) and HCV-RNA points to hepatitis C. Most clinicians also routinely test for the following:

- *Autoimmune hepatitis:* Suggested by a high antinuclear antibody titer (a low titer is nonspecific and does not always mandate further evaluation) and confirmed by hypergammaglobulinemia and the presence of other autoantibodies (e.g. anti-smooth muscle or anti-liver/kidney microsomal type 1 antibodies).
- *Hemochromatosis:* Confirmed by increased serum Fe and transferrin saturation and possibly results of genetic testing.
- *α_1-Antitrypsin deficiency:* Confirmed by a low serum α_1-antitrypsin level and genotyping.

If these causes are not confirmed, other causes are sought:

- Presence of antimitochondrial antibodies (in 95%) suggests primary biliary cirrhosis.

- Strictures and dilations of the intrahepatic and extrahepatic bile ducts, seen on magnetic resonance cholangiopancreatography, suggest primary sclerosing cholangitis.
- Decreased serum ceruloplasmin and characteristic copper test results suggest Wilson disease.
- The presence of obesity and a history of diabetes suggest nonalcoholic steatohepatitis.

Liver Biopsy

If clinical criteria and noninvasive testing are inconclusive, liver biopsy is usually done. For example, if well-compensated cirrhosis is suspected clinically and imaging findings are inconclusive, biopsy should be done to confirm the diagnosis. Sensitivity of liver biopsy approaches 100%. Nonalcoholic fatty liver disease (NAFLD) may be evident on ultrasound scans. However, nonalcoholic steatohepatitis (NASH), often associated with obesity, diabetes, or the metabolic syndrome, requires liver biopsy for confirmation. In obvious cases of cirrhosis with marked coagulopathy, portal hypertension, ascites, and liver failure, biopsy is not required unless results would change management. In patients with coagulopathy and thrombocytopenia, the transjugular approach to biopsy is safest. When this approach is used, pressures can be measured and thus the transsinusoidal pressure gradient can be calculated.

Monitoring

All patients with cirrhosis, regardless of cause, should be screened regularly for hepatocellular carcinoma. Currently, abdominal ultrasonography is recommended every 6 months, and if abnormalities compatible with hepatocellular carcinoma are detected, contrast-enhanced MRI or triple-phase CT of the abdomen (contrast-enhanced CT with separate arterial and venous phase images) should be done. Upper endoscopy to check for gastroesophageal varices should be done, when the diagnosis is made and then every 2–3 years. Positive findings may mandate treatment or more frequent endoscopic monitoring.

Prognosis

Prognosis is often unpredictable. It depends on factors such as etiology, severity, presence of complications, comorbid conditions, host factors, and effectiveness of therapy. Patients who continue to drink alcohol, even small amounts, have a very poor prognosis.

Treatment

In general, treatment is supportive and includes stopping injurious drugs, providing nutrition (including supplemental vitamins), and treating the underlying disorders and complications. Doses of drugs metabolized in the liver should be reduced. All alcohol and hepatotoxic substances must be avoided. Withdrawal symptoms during hospitalization should be anticipated in patients who have cirrhosis and have continued to abuse alcohol. Patients should be vaccinated against viral hepatitis A and B unless they are already immune.

Primary Biliary Cirrhosis (PBC)

Primary biliary cirrhosis (PBC) is an autoimmune liver disorder characterized by the progressive destruction of intrahepatic bile ducts, leading to cholestasis, cirrhosis, and liver failure. Patients usually are asymptomatic at presentation, but may experience fatigue or have symptoms of cholestasis (e.g. pruritus, steatorrhea) or cirrhosis (e.g. portal hypertension, ascites). Laboratory tests reveal cholestasis, increased IgM, and, characteristically, antimitochondrial antibodies in the serum. Liver biopsy may be necessary for diagnosis and staging. Treatment includes ursodeoxycholic acid, cholestyramine (for pruritus), supplementary fat-soluble vitamins, and, ultimately for advanced disease, liver transplantation.

Etiology

Primary biliary cholangitis (PBC) is the most common liver disease associated with chronic cholestasis in adults. Most (95%) cases occur in women aged 35–70. PBC also clusters in families. A genetic predisposition, perhaps involving the X chromosome, probably contributes. There may be an inherited abnormality of immune regulation. An autoimmune mechanism has been implicated; antibodies to antigens located on the inner mitochondrial membranes occur in >95% of cases. These antimitochondrial antibodies (AMAs), the serologic hallmarks of PBC, are not cytotoxic and are not involved in bile duct damage. PBC is associated with other autoimmune disorders, such as rheumatoid arthritis (RA), systemic sclerosis, Sjögren syndrome, CREST syndrome, autoimmune thyroiditis, and renal tubular acidosis.

T cells attack the small bile ducts. CD4 and CD8 T lymphocytes directly target biliary epithelial cells. The trigger for the immunologic attack on bile ducts is unknown. Exposure to foreign antigens, such as an infectious (bacterial or viral) or toxic agent, may be the instigating event. These foreign antigens might be structurally similar to endogenous proteins (molecular mimicry); then the subsequent immunologic reaction would be autoimmune and self-perpetuating. Destruction and loss of bile ducts lead to impaired bile formation and secretion (cholestasis). Retained toxic materials, such as bile acids then cause further damage, particularly to hepatocytes. Chronic cholestasis thus leads to liver cell inflammation and scarring in the periportal areas. Eventually, hepatic inflammation decreases as hepatic fibrosis progresses to cirrhosis.

Autoimmune cholangitis is sometimes considered to be a separate disorder. It is characterized by autoantibodies, such as antinuclear antibodies (ANAs), anti–smooth muscle antibodies, or both and has a clinical course and response to treatment that are similar to PBC. However, in autoimmune cholangitis, AMAs are absent.

Symptoms and Signs

About half of the patients present without symptoms. Symptoms or signs may develop during any stage of the disease and may include fatigue or reflect cholestasis (and the resulting fat malabsorption, which may lead to vitamin deficiencies and osteoporosis), hepatocellular dysfunction, or cirrhosis.

Symptoms usually develop insidiously. Pruritus, fatigue, and dry mouth and eyes are the initial symptoms in >50% of patients and can precede other symptoms by months or years. Other initial manifestations include right upper quadrant discomfort (10%); an enlarged, firm, nontender liver (25%); splenomegaly (15%); hyperpigmentation (25%); xanthelasmas (10%); and jaundice (10%). Eventually, all the features and complications of cirrhosis occur. Peripheral neuropathy and other autoimmune disorders associated with PBC may also develop.

Diagnosis

In asymptomatic patients, PBC is detected incidentally when liver function tests detect abnormalities, typically elevated levels of alkaline phosphatase and γ-glutamyl transpeptidase. PBC is suspected in middle-aged women with classic symptoms (e.g. unexplained pruritus, fatigue, right upper quadrant discomfort, jaundice) or laboratory results suggesting cholestatic liver disease: elevated alkaline phosphatase and GGT but minimally abnormal aminotransferases (ALT, AST). Serum bilirubin is usually normal in the early stages; elevation indicates disease progression and a worsening prognosis.

If PBC is suspected, liver function tests and tests to measure serum IgM (increased in PBC) and AMA should be done. Enzyme-linked immunosorbent assay (ELISA) tests are 95% sensitive and 98% specific for PBC; false-positive results can occur in autoimmune hepatitis (type 1). Other autoantibodies (e.g. ANAs, anti-smooth muscle antibodies, rheumatoid factor) may be present. Extrahepatic biliary obstruction should be ruled out.

Ultrasonography is often done first, but ultimately MRCP and sometimes ERCP are necessary. Unless life expectancy is short or there is a contraindication, liver biopsy is usually done. Liver biopsy confirms the diagnosis; it may detect pathognomonic bile duct lesions, even in early stages. As PBC progresses, it becomes morphologically indistinguishable from other forms of cirrhosis. Liver biopsy also helps stage PBC, which has four histologic stages:

- **Stage 1:** Inflammation, abnormal connective tissue, or both, confined to the portal areas
- **Stage 2:** Inflammation, fibrosis, or both, confined to the portal and periportal areas
- **Stage 3:** Bridging fibrosis
- **Stage 4:** Cirrhosis

Autoimmune cholangitis is diagnosed when AMAs are absent in a patient who otherwise would be diagnosed with PBC.

Prognosis

Usually, PBC progresses to terminal stages over 15–20 years, although the rate of progression varies. PBC may not diminish quality of life for many years. Patients who present without symptoms tend to develop symptoms over 2–7 years but may not do so for 10–15 years. Once symptoms develop, median life expectancy is 10 years. Predictors of rapid progression include the following:

- Rapid worsening of symptoms
- Advanced histologic changes
- Older patient age
- Presence of edema
- Presence of associated autoimmune disorders
- Abnormalities in bilirubin, albumin, PT, or INR

The prognosis is ominous when pruritus disappears, xanthomas shrink, jaundice develops, and serum cholesterol decreases.

Treatment

- Arresting or reversing liver damage
- Treating complications (chronic cholestasis and liver failure)
- Sometimes liver transplantation

All alcohol use and hepatotoxic drugs should be stopped. Ursodeoxycholic acid (15 mg/kg orally once/day) decreases liver damage, prolongs survival, and delays the need for liver transplantation. About 20% of patients do not have biochemical improvement after ≥4 months; they may have advanced disease and require liver transplantation in a few years. Other drugs proposed to decrease liver damage have not improved overall clinical outcomes or are controversial.

Pruritus may be controlled with cholestyramine 6–8 g orally. This anionic-binding drug binds bile salts and thus may aggravate fat malabsorption. If cholestyramine is taken long-term, supplements of fat-soluble vitamins should be considered. Cholestyramine can decrease absorption of ursodeoxycholic acid, so these drugs should not be given simultaneously. Cholestyramine can also decrease absorption of various drugs; if patients take any drug that could be affected, they should be told not to take the drug within 3 hours before or after taking cholestyramine.

Some patients with pruritus respond to ursodeoxycholic acid and ultraviolet light; others may warrant a trial of rifampin or an opioid antagonist, such as naltrexone.

Patients with fat malabsorption due to bile salt deficiency should be treated with vitamin A, D, E, and K supplements. For osteoporosis, weight-bearing exercises, bisphosphonates, or raloxifene may be needed in addition to Ca and vitamin D supplements. In later stages, portal hypertension or complications of cirrhosis require treatment.

Liver transplantation has excellent results. The general indication is decompensated liver disease (uncontrolled variceal bleeding, refractory ascites, intractable pruritus, and hepatic encephalopathy). Survival rates after liver transplantation are >90% at 1 year, >80% at 5 years, and >65% at 10 years. AMAs tend to persist after transplantation. PBC recurs in 15% of patients in the first few years and in >30% by 10 years. Recurrent PBC after liver transplantation appears to have a benign course. Cirrhosis rarely occurs.

ACUTE VIRAL HEPATITIS

Acute viral hepatitis is diffuse liver inflammation caused by specific hepatotropic viruses that have diverse modes of transmission and epidemiologies. A nonspecific viral prodrome is followed by anorexia, nausea, and often fever or right upper quadrant pain. Jaundice often develops, typically as other symptoms begin to resolve. Most cases resolve spontaneously, but some progress to chronic hepatitis. Occasionally, acute viral hepatitis progresses to acute liver failure (indicating fulminant hepatitis). Diagnosis is by liver function tests and serologic tests to identify the virus. Good hygiene and universal precautions can prevent acute viral hepatitis. Depending on the specific virus, pre-exposure and post-exposure prophylaxis may be possible using vaccines or serum globulins. Treatment is usually supportive.

Acute viral hepatitis is a common, worldwide disease that has different causes; each type shares clinical, biochemical, and morphologic features. Liver infections caused by nonhepatitis viruses (e.g. Epstein–Barr virus, yellow fever virus, and cytomegalovirus) generally are not termed acute viral hepatitis.

Etiology

At least five specific viruses appear to be responsible. Other unidentified viruses probably also cause acute viral hepatitis (Table 5.5).

Hepatitis A Virus

Hepatitis A virus (HAV) is a single-stranded RNA picornavirus. It is the most common cause of acute viral hepatitis and is particularly common among children and young adults. In some countries, >75% of adults has been exposed. HAV spreads primarily by fecal-oral contact and thus may occur in areas of poor hygiene. Waterborne and food-borne epidemics occur, especially in under-developed countries. Eating contaminated raw shellfish is sometimes responsible. Sporadic cases are also common, usually as a result of person-to-person contact.

Fecal shedding of the virus occurs before symptoms develop and usually ceases a few days after symptoms begin; thus, infectivity often has already ceased when hepatitis becomes clinically evident. HAV has no known chronic carrier state and does not cause chronic hepatitis or cirrhosis.

Hepatitis B Virus

Hepatitis B virus (HBV) is the most thoroughly characterized and complex hepatitis virus. The infective particle consists of a viral core plus an outer surface coat. The core contains circular double-stranded DNA and DNA polymerase, and it replicates within the nuclei of infected hepatocytes. A surface coat is added in the cytoplasm and, for unknown reasons, is produced in great excess.

HBV is the second most common cause of acute viral hepatitis. Prior unrecognized infection is common but is much less widespread than that with HAV. HBV is often transmitted parenterally, typically by contaminated blood or blood products. Routine screening of donor blood for hepatitis B surface antigen has nearly eliminated the previously common post transfusion transmission, but transmission through needles shared by drug users remains common. Risk of HBV is increased for patients in renal dialysis and oncology units and for hospital personnel in contact with blood. The virus may be spread through contact with other body fluids (e.g. between sex partners, both heterosexual and homosexual; in closed institutions, such as mental health institutions and prisons), but infectivity is far lower than that of HAV, and the means of transmission is often unknown. The role of insect bites in transmission is unclear. Many cases of acute hepatitis B occur sporadically without a known source.

HBV, for unknown reasons, is sometimes associated with several primarily extrahepatic disorders, including polyarteritis nodosa, other connective tissue diseases, membranous glomerulonephritis, and essential mixed cryoglobulinemia. The pathogenic role of HBV in these disorders is unclear, but autoimmune mechanisms are suggested.

Chronic HBV carriers provide a worldwide reservoir of infection. Prevalence varies widely according to several factors, including geography (e.g. <0.5% in North America and northern Europe, >10% in some regions of the Far East and Africa). Vertical transmission from mother to infant is common unless the neonate is treated with hepatitis B immune globulin (HBIG) and is vaccinated immediately after delivery.

Hepatitis C Virus

Hepatitis C virus (HCV) is a single-stranded RNA flavivirus. Six major HCV subtypes exist with varying amino acid sequences (genotypes); these subtypes vary geographically and in virulence and response to therapy.

Table 5.5	Characteristics of hepatitis viruses				
Characteristic	Hepatitis A virus	Hepatitis B virus	Hepatitis C virus	Hepatitis D virus	Hepatitis E virus
Nucleic acid	RNA	DNA	RNA	*	RNA
Serologic diagnosis	IgM anti-HA	HBsAg	Anti-HCV	Anti-HDV	Anti-HEV
Major transmission	Fecal-oral	Blood	Blood	Needle	Water
Incubation period (days)	15–45	40–180	20–120	30–180	14–60
Epidemics	Yes	No	No	No	Yes
Chronicity	No	Yes	Yes	Yes	No
Liver cancer	No	Yes	Yes	Yes	No

*Incomplete RNA; requires presence of hepatitis B virus for replication.
anti-HCV, antibody to hepatitis C virus; anti-HDV, antibody to hepatitis D virus; anti-HEV, antibody to hepatitis E virus; HBsAg, hepatitis B surface antigen; IgM anti-HAV, IgM antibody to hepatitis A virus.

HCV can also alter its amino acid pattern over time in an infected person, producing quasispecies.

Infection is most commonly transmitted through blood, primarily when parenteral drug users share needles, but also through tattoos or body piercing. Sexual transmission and vertical transmission from mother to infant are relatively rare. Transmission through blood transfusion has become very rare since the advent of screening tests for donated blood. Some sporadic cases occur in patients without apparent risk factors. HCV prevalence varies with geography and other risk factors.

HCV infection sometimes occurs simultaneously with specific systemic disorders, including essential mixed cryoglobulinemia, porphyria cutanea tarda (about 60–80% of porphyria patients have HCV infection, but only a few patients infected with HCV develop porphyria), and glomerulonephritis; the mechanisms are uncertain. In addition, up to 20% of patients with alcoholic liver disease harbor HCV. The reasons for this high association are unclear because concomitant alcohol and drug use accounts for only a portion of cases. In these patients, HCV and alcohol act synergistically to worsen liver inflammation and fibrosis.

Hepatitis D Virus

Hepatitis D virus (HDV), or delta agent, is a defective RNA virus that can replicate only in the presence of HBV. It occurs uncommonly as a coinfection with acute hepatitis B or as a superinfection in chronic hepatitis B. Infected hepatocytes contain delta particles coated with HBsAg. Prevalence of HDV varies widely geographically, with endemic pockets in several countries. Parenteral drug users are at relatively high risk, but HDV (unlike HBV) has not widely permeated the homosexual community.

Hepatitis E Virus

Hepatitis E virus (HEV) is an enterically transmitted RNA virus. Outbreaks of acute HEV infection, often waterborne and linked to fecal contamination of the water supply. HEV was not originally thought to cause chronic hepatitis, cirrhosis or chronic carrier state; however reports document chronic hepatitis E, exclusively in immunocompromised patients (including organ-transplant recipients, patients receiving cancer chemotherapy, and HIV-infected patients).

Symptoms and Signs

Acute infection tends to develop in predictable phases:

- **Incubation period:** The virus multiplies and spreads without causing symptoms.

- **Prodromal (preicteric) phase:** Nonspecific symptoms occur; they include profound anorexia, malaise, nausea and vomiting, a newly developed distaste for cigarettes (in smokers), and often fever or right upper quadrant abdominal pain. Urticaria and arthralgias occasionally occur, especially in HBV infection.

- **Icteric phase:** After 3–10 days, the urine darkens, followed by jaundice. Systemic symptoms often regress, and patients feel better despite worsening jaundice. The liver is usually enlarged and tender, but the edge of the liver remains soft and smooth. Mild splenomegaly occurs in 15–20% of patients. Jaundice usually peaks within 1–2 weeks.

- **Recovery phase:** During this 2–4 week period, jaundice fades.

Appetite usually returns after the first week of symptoms. Acute viral hepatitis usually resolves spontaneously 4–8 weeks after symptom onset.

Sometimes anicteric hepatitis, a minor flu-like illness without jaundice, is the only manifestation. It occurs more often than icteric hepatitis in patients with HCV infection and in children with HAV infection.

Recrudescent hepatitis occurs in a few patients and is characterized by recurrent manifestations during the recovery phase. Manifestations of cholestasis may develop during the icteric phase (called cholestatic hepatitis) but usually resolve. When they persist, they cause prolonged jaundice, elevated alkaline phosphatase, and pruritus, despite general regression of inflammation.

Diagnosis

Initial Diagnosis

Acute hepatitis must first be differentiated from other disorders that cause similar symptoms. In the prodromal phase, hepatitis mimics various nonspecific viral illnesses and is difficult to diagnose. Anicteric patients suspected of having hepatitis based on risk factors are tested initially with nonspecific liver function tests, including aminotransferases, bilirubin, and alkaline phosphatase. Usually, acute hepatitis is suspected only during the icteric phase. Thus, acute hepatitis should be differentiated from other disorders causing jaundice (Fig. 5.4).

Acute hepatitis can usually be differentiated from other causes of jaundice by its marked elevations of AST and ALT (typically ≥400 IU/L). ALT is typically higher than AST, but absolute levels correlate poorly with clinical severity. Values increase early in the prodromal phase, peak before jaundice is maximal, and fall slowly during the recovery phase. Urinary bilirubin usually precedes jaundice. Hyperbilirubinemia in acute viral hepatitis varies in severity, and fractionation has no

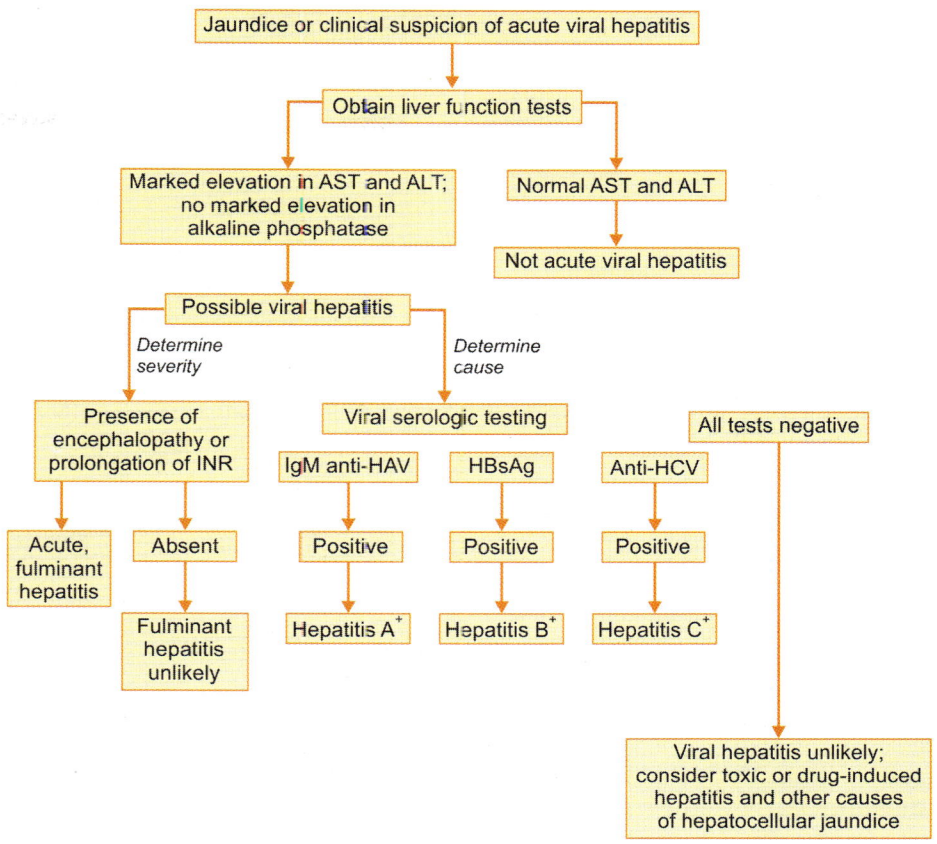

Fig. 5.4: Simplified diagnostic approach to possible acute viral hepatitis

clinical value. Alkaline phosphatase is usually only moderately elevated; marked elevation suggests extrahepatic cholestasis and prompts imaging tests (e.g. ultrasonography). Liver biopsy is usually not needed unless the diagnosis is uncertain. If laboratory results suggest acute hepatitis, particularly if ALT and AST are >1000 IU/L, PT is measured. Manifestations of portosystemic encephalopathy, bleeding diathesis, or prolongation of INR suggest acute liver failure, indicating fulminant hepatitis.

If acute hepatitis is suspected, efforts are next directed toward identifying its cause. A history of exposure may provide the only clue of drug-induced or toxic hepatitis. The history should also elicit risk factors for viral hepatitis. Prodromal sore throat and diffuse adenopathy suggest infectious mononucleosis rather than viral hepatitis. Alcoholic hepatitis is suggested by a history of drinking, more gradual onset of symptoms, and presence of vascular spiders or signs of chronic alcohol use or chronic liver disease; aminotransferase levels rarely exceed 300 IU/L, even in severe cases. Also, unlike in viral hepatitis, AST is typically higher than ALT, although this difference by itself does not reliably differentiate the two. In uncertain cases, liver biopsy usually distinguishes alcoholic from viral hepatitis.

Serology

In patients with findings suggesting acute viral hepatitis, the following studies are done to screen for hepatitis viruses A, B, and C:
- IgM antibody to HAV (IgM anti-HAV).
- HBsAg.
- IgM antibody to hepatitis B core (IgM anti-HBc).
- Antibody to HCV (anti-HCV).

If any are positive, further serologic testing may be necessary to differentiate acute from past or chronic infection. If serology suggests hepatitis B, testing for hepatitis B e antigen (HBeAg) and antibody to hepatitis B e antigen (anti-HBe) is usually done to help determine the prognosis and to guide antiviral therapy (Tables 5.6, 5.7, and 5.8). If serologically confirmed HBV infection is severe, anti-HDV is measured. If the patient has recently traveled to an endemic area, IgM antibody to HEV (IgM anti-HEV), should be measured if the test is available.

Table 5.6	Hepatitis A serology	
Marker	Acute HAV infection	Prior HAV infection*
IgM anti-HAV	+	−
IgG anti-HAV	−	+

*HAV does not cause chronic hepatitis.
HAV, hepatitis A virus; IgM anti-HAV, IgM antibody to HAV.

Table 5.7	Hepatitis B serology			
Marker	Acute HBV infection		Chronic HBV infection	Prior HBV infection[†]
HBsAg	+		+	−
Anti-HBs	−		−	+[‡]
IgM anti-HBc	+		−	−
IgG anti-HBc	−		+	±
HBeAg	±		±	−
Anti-HBe	−		±	±
HBV-DNA	+		+	−

*Antibody to hepatitis D virus (anti-HDV) levels should be measured if serologic tests confirm HBV and infection is severe.
[†] Patients have had HBV infection and recovered.
[‡] Anti-HBs is also seen as the sole serologic marker after HBV vaccination.
Anti-HBc, antibody to hepatitis B core; anti-HBe, antibody to HBeAg; anti-HBs, antibody to HBsAg; HBeAg, hepatitis B e antigen; HBsAg, hepatitis B surface antigen; HBV, hepatitis B virus.

Table 5.8	Hepatitis C serology		
Marker	Acute HCV infection	Chronic HCV infection	Prior HCV infection*
Anti-HCV	+	+	+
HCV-RNA	+	+	−

*Patients have had HCV infection and spontaneously recovered or been successfully treated.
Anti-HCV, antibody to HCV; HCV, hepatitis C virus.

HAV is present in serum only during acute infection and cannot be detected by clinically available tests. IgM antibody typically develops early in the infection and peaks about 1–2 weeks after the development of jaundice. It diminishes within several weeks, followed by the development of protective IgG antibody (IgG anti-HAV), which persists usually for life. Thus, IgM antibody is a marker of acute infection, whereas IgG anti-HAV indicates only previous exposure to HAV and immunity to recurrent infection.

HBsAg characteristically appears during the incubation period, usually 1–6 weeks before clinical or biochemical illness develops, and implies infectivity of the blood. It disappears during convalescence. However, HBsAg is occasionally transient. The corresponding protective antibody (anti-HBs) appears weeks or months later, after clinical recovery, and usually persists for life; thus, its detection indicates past HBV infection and relative immunity. In 5–10% of patients, HBsAg persists and antibodies do not develop; these patients become asymptomatic carriers of the virus or develop chronic hepatitis.

Hepatitis B core antigen (HBcAg) reflects the viral core. It is detectable in infected liver cells but not in serum except by special techniques. Antibody to HBcAg (anti-HBc) usually appears at the onset of clinical illness; thereafter, titers gradually diminish, usually over years or life. Its presence with anti-HBs indicates recovery from previous HBV infection. Anti-HBc is also present in chronic HBsAg carriers, who do not mount an anti-HBs response. In acute infection, anti-HBc is mainly of the IgM class, whereas in chronic infection, IgG anti-HBc predominates. IgM anti-HBc is a sensitive marker of acute HBV infection and occasionally is the only marker of recent infection, reflecting a window between disappearance of HBsAg and appearance of anti-HBs.

Hepatitis B e antigen (HBeAg) is a protein derived from the viral core (not to be confused with hepatitis E virus). Present only in HBsAg-positive serum, HBeAg tends to suggest more active viral replication and greater infectivity. In contrast, presence of the corresponding antibody (anti-HBe) suggests lower infectivity. Thus, e antigen markers are more helpful in prognosis than in diagnosis. Chronic liver disease develops more often among patients with HBeAg and less often among patients with anti-HBe.

Biopsy

Biopsy is usually unnecessary but, if done, usually reveals similar histopathology regardless of the specific virus: patchy cell dropout, acidophilic hepatocellular necrosis, mononuclear inflammatory infiltrate, histologic evidence of regeneration, and preservation of the reticulin framework. HBV infection can occasionally be diagnosed based on the presence of ground-glass hepatocytes (caused by HBsAg-packed cytoplasm) and using special immunologic stains for the viral components. However, these findings are unusual in acute HBV infection and are much more common in chronic HBV infection. HCV causation can sometimes be inferred from subtle morphologic clues.

Liver biopsy may help predict prognosis in acute hepatitis, but is rarely done solely for this purpose. Complete histologic recovery occurs unless extensive necrosis bridges entire acini (bridging necrosis). Most patients with bridging necrosis recover fully. However, some cases progress to chronic hepatitis.

Treatment

No treatments attenuate acute viral hepatitis except, occasionally, post-exposure immunoprophylaxis. Alcohol should be avoided because it can increase liver damage. Restrictions on diet or activity, including commonly prescribed bed rest, have no scientific basis. Most patients may safely return to work after jaundice resolves, even if AST or ALT levels are slightly elevated. For cholestatic hepatitis, cholestyramine 8 g by mouthonce/day or bid can relieve itching. Viral hepatitis should be reported to the local or state health department.

Prevention

Because treatments have limited efficacy, prevention of viral hepatitis is very important. Good personal hygiene helps prevent transmission, particularly fecal-oral transmission, as occurs with HAV and HEV. Blood and other body fluids (e.g. saliva, semen) of patients with acute HBV and HCV infection and stool of patients with HAV infection are considered infectious. Barrier protection is recommended, but isolation of patients does little to prevent spread of HAV and is of no value in HBV or HCV infection. Post-transfusion infection is minimized by avoiding unnecessary transfusions and screening all donors for HBsAg and anti-HCV. Screening has decreased the incidence of post-transfusion hepatitis, probably to about 1/100,000 units of blood component transfused.

Immunoprophylaxis can involve active immunization using vaccines and passive immunization.

CHRONIC HEPATITIS

Chronic hepatitis is hepatitis that lasts > 6 months common causes include hepatitis B and C viruses, autoimmune mechanisms (autoimmune hepatitis), and drugs. Many patients have no history of acute hepatitis, and the first indication is discovery of asymptomatic aminotransferase elevations. Some patients present with cirrhosis or its complications (e.g. portal hypertension). Biopsy is necessary to confirm the diagnosis and to grade and stage the disease. Treatment is directed toward complications and the underlying condition (e.g. corticosteroids for autoimmune hepatitis, antiviral therapy for viral hepatitis). Liver transplantation is often indicated for end-stage disease.

Etiology

Hepatitis lasting >6 months is generally defined as chronic, although this duration is arbitrary. HBV and HCV are frequent causes of chronic hepatitis; 5–10% of cases of HBV infection, with or without hepatitis D virus coinfection, and about 75% of cases of HCV infection become chronic. Rates are higher for HBV infection in children (e.g. up to 90% of infected neonates and 30–50% of young children). Hepatitis A and E viruses are not causes. Although the mechanism of chronicity is uncertain, liver injury is mostly determined by the patient's immune reaction to the infection.

Many cases are idiopathic. A high proportion of idiopathic cases have prominent features of immune-mediated hepatocellular injury (autoimmune hepatitis), including the following:

- The presence of serologic immune markers
- An association with histocompatibility haplotypes common in autoimmune disorders (e.g. HLA-B1, HLA-B8, HLA-DR3, HLA-DR4)
- A predominance of T lymphocytes and plasma cells in liver histologic lesions
- Complex *in vitro* defects in cellular immunity and immunoregulatory functions
- An association with other autoimmune disorders (e.g. RA, autoimmune hemolytic anemia, proliferative glomerulonephritis)
- A response to therapy with corticosteroids or immunosuppressants

Sometimes chronic hepatitis has features of both autoimmune hepatitis and another chronic liver disorder (e.g. primary biliary cirrhosis, chronic viral hepatitis). These conditions are called overlap syndromes.

Many drugs, including isoniazid, methyldopa, nitrofurantoin, and, rarely acetaminophen, can cause chronic hepatitis. The mechanism varies with the drug and may involve altered immune responses, cytotoxic intermediate metabolites, or genetically determined metabolic defects.

Other causes of chronic hepatitis include alcoholic hepatitis and nonalcoholic steatohepatitis. Less often, chronic hepatitis results from α_1-antitrypsin deficiency, celiac disease, a thyroid disorder, or Wilson disease.

Cases were once classified histologically as chronic persistent, chronic lobular, or chronic active hepatitis. A more useful recent classification system specifies the etiology, the intensity of histologic inflammation and necrosis (grade), and the degree of histologic fibrosis (stage). Inflammation and necrosis are potentially reversible; fibrosis usually is not.

Symptoms and Signs

Clinical features vary widely. About one-third of cases develop after acute hepatitis, but most develop insidiously de novo. Many patients are asymptomatic, especially in chronic HCV infection. However, malaise, anorexia, and fatigue are common, sometimes with low-grade fever and nonspecific upper abdominal discomfort. Jaundice is usually absent. Often, particularly with HCV, the first findings are signs of chronic liver disease (e.g. splenomegaly, spider nevi, palmar erythema) or complications of cirrhosis (e.g. portal hypertension, ascites, and encephalopathy). A few patients with chronic hepatitis develop manifestations of cholestasis (e.g. jaundice, pruritus, pale stools, and steatorrhea). In autoimmune hepatitis, especially in young women, manifestations may involve virtually any body system and can include acne, amenorrhea, arthralgia, ulcerative colitis, pulmonary fibrosis, thyroiditis, nephritis, and hemolytic anemia.

Chronic HCV is occasionally associated with lichen planus, mucocutaneous vasculitis, glomerulonephritis, porphyria cutanea tarda, and, perhaps, non-Hodgkin B-cell lymphoma. About 1% of patients develop symptomatic cryoglobulinemia with fatigue, myalgias, arthralgias, neuropathy, glomerulonephritis, and rashes (urticaria, purpura, or leukocytoclastic vasculitis); asymptomatic cryoglobulinemia is more common.

Diagnosis

Liver function tests are needed if not previously done and include serum ALT, AST, alkaline phosphatase, and bilirubin. Aminotransferase elevations are the most characteristic laboratory abnormalities. Although, levels can vary, they are typically 100–500 IU/L. ALT is usually higher than AST. Aminotransferase levels can be normal during chronic hepatitis if the disease is quiescent, particularly with HCV. Alkaline phosphatase is usually normal or only slightly elevated, but is occasionally markedly high. Bilirubin is usually normal unless the disease is severe or advanced. However, abnormalities in these laboratory tests are not specific and can result from other disorders, such as alcoholic liver disease, recrudescent acute viral hepatitis, and primary biliary cirrhosis.

If laboratory results are compatible with hepatitis, viral serologic tests are done to exclude HBV and HCV. Unless these tests indicate viral etiology, further testing is required. The first tests done include autoantibodies, immunoglobulins, thyroid tests (thyroid-stimulating hormone), tests for celiac disease (tissue trans-glutaminase antibody), and α_1-antitrypsin level. Children and young adults are screened for Wilson disease by measuring the ceruloplasmin level. Marked elevations in serum immunoglobulins suggest chronic autoimmune hepatitis but are not conclusive. Autoimmune hepatitis is normally diagnosed based on the presence of antinuclear (ANA), anti-smooth muscle, or anti-liver/kidney microsomal type 1 (anti-LKM1) antibodies at titers of 1:80 (in adults) or 1:20 (in children).

Unlike in acute hepatitis, biopsy is necessary. Mild cases may have only minor hepatocellular necrosis and inflammatory cell infiltration, usually in portal regions, with normal acinar architecture and little or no fibrosis. Such cases rarely develop into clinically important liver disease or cirrhosis. In more severe cases, biopsy typically shows periportal necrosis with mononuclear cell infiltrates (piecemeal necrosis) accompanied by variable periportal fibrosis and bile duct proliferation. The acinar architecture may be distorted by zones of collapse and fibrosis, and frank cirrhosis sometimes coexists with signs of ongoing hepatitis. Biopsy is also used to grade and stage the disease.

In most cases, the specific cause of chronic hepatitis cannot be discerned via biopsy alone, although cases caused by HBV. can be distinguished by the presence of ground-glass hepatocytes and special stains for HBV components. Autoimmune cases usually have a more pronounced infiltration by lymphocytes and plasma cells. In patients with histologic but not serologic criteria for chronic autoimmune hepatitis, variant autoimmune hepatitis is diagnosed; many have overlap syndromes.

Serum albumin, platelet count, and PT should be measured to determine severity; low serum albumin, a low platelet count, or prolonged PT may suggest cirrhosis and even portal hypertension.

If symptoms or signs of cryoglobulinemia develop during chronic hepatitis, particularly with HCV, cryoglobulin levels and rheumatoid factor should be measured; high levels of rheumatoid factor and low levels of complement suggest cryoglobulinemia.

Patients with chronic HBV infection should be screened every 6–12 months for hepatocellular cancer with ultrasonography and serum α-fetoprotein measurement, although the cost-effectiveness of this practice is debated. Patients with chronic HCV infection should be similarly screened only if advanced fibrosis or cirrhosis is present.

Prognosis

Prognosis is highly variable. Chronic hepatitis caused by a drug often regresses completely when the causative drug is withdrawn. Without treatment, cases caused by HBV can resolve (uncommon), progress rapidly, or progress slowly to cirrhosis over decades. Resolution often begins with a transient increase in disease severity and results in seroconversion from hepatitis B e antigen (HBeAg) to antibody to hepatitis B e antigen (anti-HBe). Coinfection with HDV causes the most severe form of chronic HBV infection; without treatment, cirrhosis develops in up to 70% of patients. Untreated chronic hepatitis due to HCV causes cirrhosis in 20–30% of patients, although development may take decades. Chronic autoimmune hepatitis usually responds to therapy but sometimes causes progressive fibrosis and eventual cirrhosis.

Chronic HBV infection increases the risk of hepatocellular cancer. The risk is also increased in chronic HCV infection, but only if cirrhosis has already developed.

Treatment

Treatment goals include treating the cause and managing complications (e.g. ascites, encephalopathy). Drugs that cause hepatitis should be stopped. Underlying disorders, such as Wilson disease, should be treated. In chronic hepatitis due to HBV, prophylaxis (including immunoprophylaxis) for contacts of patients may be helpful. No vaccination is available for contacts of patients with HCV infection.

Corticosteroids and immunosuppressants should be avoided in chronic hepatitis B and C, because these drugs enhance viral replication. If patients with chronic hepatitis B require treatment with corticosteroids, immunosuppressive therapies, or cytotoxic chemotherapy for other disorders, they should be treated with antiviral drugs at the same time to prevent a flare-up of acute hepatitis B or acute liver failure due to hepatitis B.

Autoimmune Hepatitis

Corticosteroids, with or without azathioprine, prolong survival. Prednisone is usually started at 30–60 mg orally once a day, and then tapered to the lowest dose that maintains aminotransferases at normal or near-normal levels. Some experts give concomitant azathioprine 1–1.5 mg/kg orally once a day; others add azathioprine only if low-dose prednisone fails to maintain suppression. Most patients require long-term, low-dose maintenance treatment. Liver transplantation may be required for end-stage disease.

HBV

Antiviral treatment is indicated for patients with elevated aminotransferase levels, clinical or biopsy evidence of progressive disease, or both. The goal is to eliminate HBV-DNA. Treatment may need to be continued indefinitely and thus may be very expensive; stopping treatment prematurely can lead to relapse, which may be severe. However, treatment may be stopped if HBeAg converts to anti-HBe or if tests for HBsAg become negative. Drug resistance is also a concern.

First-line treatment is usually with an oral antiviral drug, such as entecavir (a nucleoside analog) or tenofovir (a nucleotide analog). Oral antiviral drugs have few adverse effects and can be given to patients with decompensated liver disease. Combination therapy has not proved superior to monotherapy, but studies continue to examine their comparative usefulness. HBsAg becomes undetectable and HBeAg seroconversion occurs in patients with HBeAg-positive chronic HBV infection; these patients may be able to stop antiviral drugs. Patients with HBeAg-negative chronic HBV infection almost always need to take antiviral drugs indefinitely to maintain viral suppression; they have already developed antibodies to HBeAg, and thus the only specific criterion for stopping HBV treatment would be HBsAg that becomes undetectable.

Entecavir has a high antiviral potency, and resistance to it is uncommon; it is considered a first-line treatment for HBV infection. Entecavir is effective against adefovir-resistant strains. Dosage is 0.5 mg orally once a day; however, patients who have previously taken a nucleoside analog should take 1 mg orally once a day. Dose reduction is required in patients with renal insufficiency. Serious adverse effects appear to be uncommon, although safety in pregnancy has not been established.

Tenofovir has replaced adefovir (an older nucleotide analog) as a first-line treatment. Tenofovir is the most potent oral antiviral for hepatitis B; resistance to it is minimal. It has few adverse effects. Dosage is 300 mg orally once a day; dosing frequency may need to be reduced if creatinine clearance is reduced.

Interferon alfa (IFN-α) can be used but is no longer considered first-line treatment. Dosage is 5 million IU sc once a day or 10 million IU sc 3 times/week for 16–24 weeks in patients with HBeAg-positive chronic HBV infection and for 12–24 months in patients with HBeAg-negative chronic HBV infection. In about 40% of patients, this regimen eliminates HBV-DNA and causes seroconversion to anti-HBe; a successful response is usually presaged by a temporary increase in aminotransferase levels. The drug must be given by injection and is often poorly tolerated. The first 1 or 2 doses cause an influenza-like syndrome. Later, fatigue, malaise, depression, bone marrow suppression, and, rarely, bacterial infections or autoimmune disorders can occur. In patients with advanced cirrhosis; IFN-α can precipitate liver failure and is therefore contraindicated. Other contraindications include renal failure, immunosuppression, solid organ transplantation, and cytopenia. In a few patients, treatment must be stopped because of intolerable adverse effects. The drug should be given cautiously or not at all to patients with ongoing substance abuse or a major psychiatric disorder. Pegylated IFN-α can be used instead of IFN-α. Dosage is usually 180 mcg by injection once a week for 48 weeks. Adverse effects are similar to those of IFN-α, but may be less severe.

Lamivudine (a nucleoside analog) is no longer considered first-line treatment for HBV infection because risk of resistance is higher and efficacy is lower than those of newer antiviral drugs. Dosage is 100 mg orally once a day; it has few adverse effects.

Telbivudine is a newer nucleoside analog that has greater efficacy and potency than lamivudine, but also has a high rate of resistance; it is not considered first-line treatment. Dosage is 600 mg orally once a day.

Liver transplantation should be considered for end-stage liver disease caused by HBV. In patients with HBV infection, the long-term use of first-line oral antivirals and peritransplantation use of HBIG has improved outcomes after liver transplantation. Survival is equal to or better than that after transplantation for other indications, and recurrences of hepatitis B are minimized.

HCV

For chronic hepatitis due to HCV, treatment is indicated if aminotransferase levels are elevated and biopsy shows active inflammatory disease with evolving fibrosis. The goal of treatment is permanent elimination of HCV-RNA (sustained virologic response), which is associated with permanent normalization of aminotransferase and cessation of histologic progression. Treatment results are more favorable in patients with moderate fibrosis and a viral load of <600,000–800,000 IU/mL than in patients with cirrhosis and a viral load of >800,000 IU/mL.

HCV genotype is determined before treatment because genotype influences the course, duration, and success of treatment. Genotype 1 is more common than genotypes 2, 3, 4, 5, and 6.

Many direct-acting antivirals are being developed. These drugs affect specific HCV targets, such as proteases or polymerases. The polymerase inhibitor sofosbuvir is effective against HCV genotypes 1–6 and can be used without interferon, providing an all-oral regimen of sofosbuvir plus ribavirin for genotypes 2 and 3. This regimen is particularly useful for patients who are infected with HCV genotypes 2 or 3 (and are thus not eligible for treatment with protease inhibitors) or who have contraindications to or have not responded to treatment with interferon-based regimens.

LIVER MASSES AND GRANULOMAS

Hepatic Cysts

Isolated cysts are commonly detected incidentally on abdominal ultrasonography or CT. These cysts are usually asymptomatic and have no clinical significance. The rare congenital polycystic liver is commonly associated with polycystic disease of the kidneys and other organs. It causes progressive nodular hepato-megaly (sometimes massive) in adults. Nevertheless, hepatocellular function is remarkably well-preserved, and portal hypertension rarely develops.

Other hepatic cysts include the following:

- Hydatid (echinococcal) cysts (echinococcosis-hydatid disease)
- *Caroli disease:* This rare, autosomal recessive disorder is characterized by segmental cystic dilation of intrahepatic bile ducts; it often becomes symptomatic in adulthood, with stone formation, cholangitis, and sometimes cholangiocarcinoma.
- *Cystadenoma:* This rare disorder sometimes causes pain or anorexia and is evident on ultrasonography; treatment is cyst resection.
- *Cystadenocarcinoma:* This rare disorder is probably secondary to malignant transformation of a cystade-noma and is often multilobular; treatment is liver resection.
- *Other true cystic tumors:* These tumors are rare.

Benign Liver Tumors

Most are asymptomatic, but some cause hepatomegaly, right upper quadrant discomfort, or intraperitoneal hemorrhage. Most are detected incidentally on ultrasound or other scans. Liver function tests are usually normal or only slightly abnormal. Diagnosis is usually possible with imaging tests, but may require biopsy. Treatment is needed only in a few specific circumstances.

Hepatocellular Adenoma

Hepatocellular adenoma is the most important benign tumor to recognize. It occurs primarily in women of childbearing age, particularly those taking oral contraceptives, possibly via estrogen's effects.

Most adenomas are asymptomatic, but large ones may cause right upper quadrant discomfort. Rarely, adenomas manifest as peritonitis and shock due to rupture and intraperitoneal hemorrhage. Rarely, they become malignant.

Diagnosis is often suspected based on ultrasound or CT results, but biopsy is sometimes needed for confirmation.

Adenomas due to contraceptive use often regress if the contraceptive is stopped. If the adenoma does not regress or if it is subcapsular or >5 cm, surgical resection is often recommended.

Focal Nodular Hyperplasia

This localized hamartoma may resemble macronodular cirrhosis histologically. Diagnosis is usually based on MRI or CT with contrast, but biopsy may be necessary, treatment is rarely needed.

Hemangiomas

Hemangiomas are usually small and asymptomatic; they occur in 1–5% of adults. Symptoms are more likely if they are >4 cm; symptoms include discomfort, fullness, and, less often, anorexia, nausea, early satiety, and pain secondary to bleeding or thrombosis. These tumors often have a characteristic highly vascular appearance. Hemangiomas are found incidentally during ultrasonography, CT, or MRI. CT typically shows a well-demarcated, hypodense mass; when contrast is used, there is early peripheral enhancement, followed by later centrifugal enhancement. Treatment is usually not indicated. Resection can be considered if symptoms are troublesome or if a hemangioma is rapidly enlarging.

In infants, hemangiomas often regress spontaneously by age of 2 years. However, large hemangiomas occasionally cause arteriovenous shunting sufficient to cause heart failure and sometimes consumption coagulopathy. In these cases, treatment may include high-dose corticosteroids, sometimes diuretics and digoxin to improve heart function, interferon, surgical removal, selective hepatic artery embolization, and, rarely, liver transplantation.

Other Benign Tumors

Lipomas (usually asymptomatic) and localized fibrous tumors (e.g. fibromas) rarely occur in the liver.

Benign bile duct adenomas are rare, inconsequential, and usually detected incidentally. They are sometimes mistaken for metastatic cancer.

Hepatocellular Carcinoma (Hepatoma)

Usually occurs in patients with cirrhosis and is common in areas where infection with hepatitis B and C viruses is prevalent. Symptoms and signs are usually nonspecific. Diagnosis is based on α-fetoprotein (AFP) levels, imaging tests, and sometimes liver biopsy. Screening with periodic AFP measurement and ultrasonography is sometimes recommended for high-risk patients. Prognosis is poor when cancer is advanced, but for small tumors that are confined to the liver, ablative therapies are palliative and surgical resection or liver transplantation is sometimes curative.

Etiology

The presence of HBV increases risk of hepatocellular carcinoma by >100-fold among HBV carriers. Incorporation of HBV-DNA into the host's genome may initiate malignant transformation, even in the absence of chronic hepatitis or cirrhosis.

Other disorders that cause hepatocellular carcinoma include cirrhosis due to chronic HCV infection, hemochromatosis, and alcoholic cirrhosis. Patients with cirrhosis due to other conditions are also at increased risk.

Environmental carcinogens may play a role, e.g. ingestion of food contaminated with fungal aflatoxins is believed to contribute to the high incidence of hepatocellular carcinoma in subtropical regions.

Symptoms and Signs

Most commonly, previously stable patients with cirrhosis present with abdominal pain, weight loss, and right upper quadrant mass and unexplained deterioration. Fever may occur. In a few patients, the first manifestation of hepatocellular carcinoma is bloody ascites, shock, or peritonitis, caused by hemorrhage of the tumor. Occasionally, a hepatic friction rub or bruit develops.

Occasionally, systemic metabolic complications, including hypoglycemia, erythrocytosis, hypercalcemia, and hyperlipidemia, occur. These complications may manifest clinically.

Diagnosis

Diagnosis is based on α-fetoprotein (AFP) measurement and an imaging test. In adults, AFP signifies dedifferentiation of hepatocytes, which most often indicates hepatocellular carcinoma; 40–65% of patients with the cancer have high AFP levels. High levels are otherwise rare, except in teratocarcinoma of the testis, a much less common tumor. Lower values are less specific and can occur with hepatocellular regeneration (e.g. in hepatitis). Other blood tests, such as AFP-L3 (an AFP isoform) and des-γ-carboxyprothrombin, are being studied as markers to be used for early detection of hepatocellular carcinoma.

Depending on local preferences and capabilities, the first imaging test may be contrast-enhanced CT, ultrasonography, or MRI. Hepatic arteriography is occasionally helpful in equivocal cases and can be used to outline the vascular anatomy when ablation or surgery is planned.

If imaging shows characteristic findings and AFP is elevated, the diagnosis is clear. Liver biopsy, often guided by ultrasonography or CT, is sometimes indicated for definitive diagnosis.

Screening

An increasing number of hepatocellular carcinomas are being detected through screening programs. Screening patients with cirrhosis is reasonable, although this measure is controversial and has not been shown to reduce mortality. One common screening method is ultrasonography every 6 or 12 months. Many experts advise screening patients with long-standing hepatitis B, even when cirrhosis is absent.

Treatment

For single tumor <5 cm or ≤3 tumors that are all ≤3 cm and that are limited to the liver, liver transplantation results in as good a prognosis as liver transplantation done for noncancerous disorders. Alternatively, surgical resection may be done; however, the cancer usually recurs.

Ablative treatments [e.g. hepatic arterial chemo-embolization, yttrium-90 microsphere embolization (selective internal radiation therapy, or SIRT), drug-eluting bead transarterial embolization, radiofrequency ablation] provide palliation and slow tumor growth; they are used when patients are awaiting liver transplantation.

If the tumor is large (>5 cm), is multifocal, has invaded the portal vein, or is metastatic (i.e. stage III or higher), prognosis is much less favorable (e.g. 5-years survival rates of about 5% or less). Radiation therapy is usually ineffective. Sorafenib appears to improve outcomes.

Prevention

Use of vaccine against HBV eventually decreases the incidence, especially in endemic areas. Preventing the development of cirrhosis of any cause (e.g. via treatment of chronic hepatitis.

Liver Metastases

The first symptoms of metastases are usually nonspecific (e.g. weight loss, right upper quadrant discomfort); they are sometimes the first symptoms of the primary cancer. Liver metastases are suspected in patients with weight loss and hepatomegaly or with primary tumors likely to spread to the liver. Diagnosis is usually supported by an imaging test, most often ultrasonography, spiral CT with contrast, or MRI with contrast. Treatment usually involves palliative chemotherapy.

Metastatic liver cancer is more common than primary liver cancer and is sometimes the initial clinical manifestation of cancer originating in the GI tract, breast, lung, or pancreas.

Symptoms and Signs

Early liver metastases may be asymptomatic. Nonspecific symptoms of cancer (e.g. weight loss, anorexia, fever) often develop first. The liver may be enlarged, hard, or tender; massive hepatomegaly with easily palpable nodules signifies advanced disease. Hepatic bruits and pleuritic-type pain with an overlying friction rub are uncommon but characteristic. Splenomegaly is occasionally present, especially when the primary cancer is pancreatic. Concomitant peritoneal tumor seeding may produce ascites, but jaundice is usually absent or mild initially unless a tumor causes biliary obstruction.

In the terminal stages, progressive jaundice and hepatic encephalopathy presage death.

Diagnosis

Liver metastases are suspected in patients with weight loss and hepatomegaly or with primary tumors likely to spread to the liver. If metastases are suspected, liver function tests are often done, but results are usually not specific for the diagnosis. Alkaline phosphatase, γ-glutamyl transpeptidase, and sometimes lactate dehydrogenase (LDH) typically increase earlier or to a greater degree than do other test results; amino-transferase levels vary. Imaging tests have good sensitivity and specificity. Ultrasonography is usually helpful, but CT with contrast or MRI (Fig. 5.5) with contrast is often more accurate.

Liver biopsy guided by imaging provides the definitive diagnosis and is done if other tests are equivocal

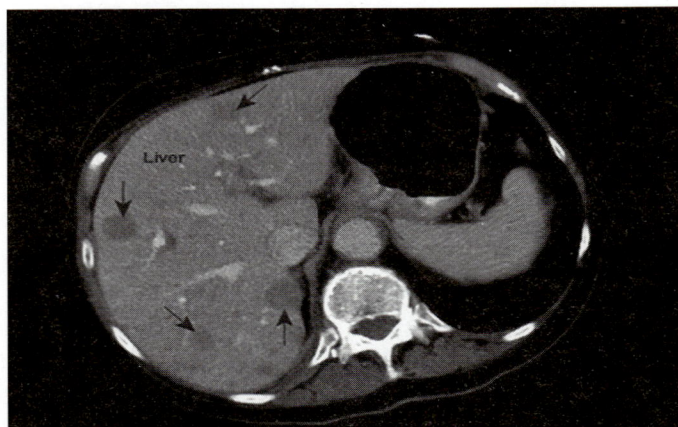

Fig. 5.5: An abnormal MRI of the chest shows areas of low attenuation (marked with arrows) inside the liver. This appearance is typical of metastatic liver cancer

or if histologic information (e.g. cell type of the liver metastasis) may help determine the treatment plan.

Treatment

Depending on characteristics of the primary tumor, systemic chemotherapy may shrink tumors and prolong life but is not curative; hepatic intra-arterial chemotherapy sometimes has the same effect but with fewer or milder systemic adverse effects.

Radiation therapy to the liver occasionally alleviates severe pain due to advanced metastases but does not prolong life. Extensive disease is fatal and is best managed by palliation for the patient and support for the family.

HEMATOLOGIC CANCERS AND THE LIVER

The liver is commonly involved in advanced leukemia and related blood disorders. Liver biopsy is not needed. In hepatic lymphoma, especially Hodgkin lymphoma, the extent of liver involvement determines staging and treatment but may be difficult to assess. Hepatomegaly and abnormal liver function tests may reflect a systemic reaction to Hodgkin lymphoma rather than spread to the liver, and biopsy often shows nonspecific focal mononuclear infiltrates or granulomas of uncertain significance. Treatment is directed at the hematologic cancer.

Hepatic Granulomas

Hepatic granulomas have numerous causes and are usually asymptomatic. However, the underlying disorder may cause extrahepatic manifestations, hepatic inflammation, fibrosis, portal hypertension, or a combination. Diagnosis is based on liver biopsy, but biopsy is necessary only if a treatable underlying disorder (e.g. infection) is suspected or if other liver disorders need to be ruled out. Treatment depends on the underlying disorder.

Hepatic granulomas, although sometimes insignificant, more often reflect clinically relevant disease. The term granulomatous hepatitis is often used to describe the condition, but the disorder is not true hepatitis, and the presence of granulomas does not imply hepatocellular inflammation.

Etiology

Hepatic granulomas have many causes (Table 5.9); drugs and systemic disorders (often infections) are more common causes than primary liver disorders. Infections must be identified because they require specific treatments. TB and schistosomiasis are the most common infectious causes worldwide; fungal and viral causes are

Table 5.9	Causes of hepatic granulomas
Cause	Examples
Drugs	Allopurinol, phenylbutazone, quinidine, sulfonamides
Infections, bacterial	Actinomycosis, brucellosis, cat-scratch fever, syphilis, TB*, other mycobacterial infections, tularemia, Q fever
Infections, fungal	Blastomycosis, cryptococcosis, histoplasmosis
Infections, parasitic	Schistosomiasis*, toxoplasmosis, visceral larva migrans
Infections, viral	Hepatitis C, cytomegalovirus infection
Liver disorders	Primary biliary cirrhosis
Systemic disorders	Hodgkin lymphoma, polymyalgia rheumatica, other connective tissue disorders, sarcoidosis*

*Most common causes.

less common. Sarcoidosis is the most common noninfectious cause; the liver is involved in about two-thirds of patients, and occasionally, clinical manifestations of sarcoidosis are predominantly hepatic.

Granulomas are much less common in primary liver disorders; primary biliary cirrhosis is the only important cause. Small granulomas occasionally occur in other liver disorders but are not clinically significant.

Idiopathic granulomatous hepatitis is a rare syndrome of hepatic granulomas with recurrent fever, myalgias, fatigue, and other systemic symptoms, which often occur intermittently for years. Some experts believe it is a variant of sarcoidosis.

Pathophysiology

A granuloma is a localized collection of chronic inflammatory cells with epithelioid cells and giant multinucleated cells. Caseation necrosis or foreign body tissue (e.g., schistosome eggs) may be present. Most granulomas occur in the parenchyma, but in primary biliary cirrhosis, granulomas may occur in the hepatic triads.

Granuloma formation is incompletely understood. Granulomas may develop in response to poorly soluble exogenous or endogenous irritants. Immunologic mechanisms are involved.

Hepatic granulomas rarely affect hepatocellular function. However, when granulomas are part of a broader inflammatory reaction involving the liver (e.g. drug reactions, infectious mononucleosis), hepatocellular dysfunction is present. Sometimes, inflammation causes progressive hepatic fibrosis and portal hypertension, typically with schistosomiasis and occasionally with extensive sarcoidal infiltration.

Symptoms and Signs

Granulomas themselves are typically asymptomatic; even extensive infiltration usually causes only minor hepatomegaly and little or no jaundice. Symptoms, if they occur, reflect the underlying condition (e.g. constitutional symptoms in infections, hepatosplenomegaly in schistosomiasis).

Diagnosis

When granulomas are suspected, liver function tests are usually done, but results are nonspecific and are rarely helpful in diagnosis. Alkaline phosphatase (and γ-glutamyl transferase) is often mildly elevated, but occasionally may be markedly elevated. Other test results may be normal or abnormal, reflecting additional hepatic damage (e.g. widespread hepatic inflammation due to a drug reaction). Usually, imaging tests, such as ultrasonography, CT, or MRI, are not diagnostic; they may show calcification (if granulomas are long-standing) or filling defects, particularly with confluent lesions.

Diagnosis is based on liver biopsy. However, biopsy is usually indicated only to diagnose treatable causes (e.g. infections) or to rule out non-granulomatous disorders (e.g. chronic viral hepatitis). Biopsy sometimes detects evidence of the specific cause (e.g. schistosome eggs, caseation of TB, fungal organisms). However, other tests (e.g., cultures, skin tests, laboratory tests, imaging tests, other tissue specimens) are often needed.

In patients with constitutional or other symptoms suggesting infection [e.g. fever of unknown origin (FUO)], specific measures are taken to increase the diagnostic sensitivity of biopsy for infections, e.g. a portion of the fresh biopsy specimen is sent for culture, or special stains for acid-fast bacilli, fungi, and other organisms are used. Often, cause cannot be established.

Prognosis

Hepatic granulomas caused by drugs or infection regress completely after treatment. Sarcoid granulomas may disappear spontaneously or persist for years, usually without causing clinically important liver disease. Progressive fibrosis and portal hypertension (sarcoidal cirrhosis) rarely develop.

In schistosomiasis, progressive portal scarring (pipestem fibrosis) is typical; liver function is usually preserved, but marked splenomegaly and variceal hemorrhage can occur.

Treatment

Treatment is directed at the underlying disorder, when the cause is unknown treatment is usually withheld, and follow-up with periodic liver function tests is instituted.

However, if symptoms of TB (e.g. prolonged fever) and deteriorating health occur, empiric antituberculous therapy may be justified.

Corticosteroids may benefit patients with progressive hepatic sarcoidosis, although whether these drugs prevent hepatic fibrosis is unclear. However, corticosteroids are not indicated for most patients with sarcoidosis and are warranted, only if TB and other infections can be excluded confidently.

LIVER INJURY CAUSED BY DRUGS

Many drugs commonly cause asymptomatic elevation of hepatic enzymes (ALT, AST, and alkaline phosphatase). However, clinically significant liver injury (e.g. with jaundice, abdominal pain, or pruritus) or impaired liver function.

The term drug-induced liver injury (DILI) may be used to mean clinically significant liver injury or all (including asymptomatic) liver injury. DILI includes injury caused by medicinal herbs, plants, and nutritional supplements as well as drugs.

Pathophysiology

The pathophysiology of DILI varies depending on the drug or other hepatotoxin. In many cases, is not entirely understood. Drug-induced injury mechanisms include covalent binding of the drug to cellular proteins resulting in immune injury, inhibition of cell metabolic pathways, blockage of cellular transport pumps, induction of apoptosis, and interference with mitochondrial function.

In general, the following are thought to increase risk of DILI:

- Age ≥18 years
- Obesity
- Pregnancy
- Concomitant alcohol consumption
- Genetic polymorphisms (increasingly recognized)

Patterns of Liver Injury

Drug-induced liver injury (DILI) can be predictable (when injury usually occurs shortly after exposure and is dose-related) or unpredictable (when injury develops after a period of latency and has no relation to dose). Predictable DILI (commonly, acetaminophen-induced), is a common cause of acute jaundice and acute liver failure. Unpredictable DILI is a rare cause of severe liver disease. Subclinical DILI may be underreported.

Biochemically, three types of liver injuries are generally noted (Table 5.10):

- **Hepatocellular:** Hepatocellular hepatotoxicity generally manifests as malaise and right upper quadrant abdominal pain, associated with marked elevation in

Table 5.10	Potentially hepatotoxic drugs
Finding	**Drug**
Hepatocellular: Elevated ALT	Acarbose
	Acetaminophen
	Allopurinol
	Amiodarone
	ART drugs
	Bupropion
	Fluoxetine
	Germander
	Green tea extract
	Baclofen isoniazid
	Kava
	Ketoconazole
	Lisinopril
	Losartan
	Methotrexate
	NSAIDs
	Omeprazole
	Paroxetine
	Pyrazinamide
	Rifampin
	Risperidone
	Sertraline
	Statins
	Tetracyclines
	Trazodone
	Trovafloxacin
	Valproate
Cholestatic: Elevated alkaline phosphatase and total bilirubin	Amoxicillin/Clavulanate
	Anabolic steroids
	Chlorpromazine
	Clopidogrel
	Oral contraceptives
	Erythromycins
	Estrogens
	Irbesartan
	Mirtazapine
	Phenothiazines
	Terbinafine
	Tricyclic antidepressants
Mixed: Elevated alkaline phosphatase and ALT	Amitriptyline
	Azathioprine
	Captopril
	Carbamazepine
	Clindamycin
	Cyproheptadine
	Enalapril
	Nitrofurantoin
	Phenobarbital
	Phenytoin
	Sulfonamides
	Trazodone
	Trimethoprim/ sulfamethoxazole
	Verapamil

ART = antiretroviral therapy.

aminotransferase levels (ALT, AST, or both), which may be followed by hyperbilirubinemia in severe cases. Hyperbilirubinemia in this setting is known as hepatocellular jaundice and, according to Hy's law, is associated with mortality rates as high as 50%. If hepatocellular liver injury is accompanied by jaundice, impaired hepatic synthesis, and encephalopathy, chance of spontaneous recovery is low, and liver transplantation should be considered. This type of injury can result from drugs, such as acetaminophen and isoniazid.

- **Cholestatic:** Cholestatic hepatotoxicity is characterized by development of pruritus and jaundice accompanied by marked elevation of serum alkaline phosphatase levels. Usually, this type of injury is less serious than severe hepatocellular syndromes, but recovery may be protracted. Substances known to lead to this type of injury include amoxicillin/clavulanate and chlorpromazine. Rarely, cholestatic hepatotoxicity leads to chronic liver disease and vanishing bile duct syndrome (progressive destruction of intrahepatic bile ducts).

- **Mixed:** In these clinical syndromes, neither amino-transferase nor alkaline phosphatase elevations are clearly predominant. Symptoms may also be mixed. Drugs such as phenytoin can cause this type of injury.

Diagnosis

Presentation varies widely, ranging from absent or nonspecific symptoms (e.g. malaise, nausea, and anorexia) to jaundice, impaired hepatic synthesis, and encephalopathy. Early recognition of DILI improves prognosis.

Identification of a potential hepatotoxin and a pattern of liver test abnormalities that is characteristic of the substance (its signature) make the diagnosis likely.

Because there is no confirmatory diagnostic test, other causes of liver disease, especially viral, biliary, alcoholic, autoimmune, and metabolic causes, need to be excluded. Drug rechallenge, although it can strengthen evidence for the diagnosis, should be avoided.

Treatment

Management emphasizes drug withdrawal, which, if done early, usually results in recovery. In severe cases, consultation with a specialist is indicated, especially if patients have hepatocellular jaundice and impaired liver function, because liver transplantation may be required. Antidotes for DILI are available for only a few hepatotoxins; such antidotes include *N*-acetylcysteine for acetaminophen toxicity and silymarin or penicillin for *Amanita phalloides* toxicity.

The Biochemical Assessment of Liver Function

Plasma Bilirubin Concentration

Hyperbilirubinemia is not always present in patients with liver disease, nor is it exclusively associated with liver disease. For example, it is not usually present in patients with well-compensated cirrhosis, but it is a common feature of advanced pancreatic carcinoma.

Unconjugated Hyperbilirubinemia

When an excess of bilirubin is unconjugated, the concentration in adults rarely exceeds 100 µmol/L. In the absence of liver disease, unconjugated hyperbilirubinemia is most often due either to hemolysis or to Gilbert syndrome, an inherited abnormality of bilirubin metabolism.

In hemolysis, hyperbilirubinemia is due to increased production of bilirubin, which exceeds the capacity of the liver to remove and conjugate the pigment. Nevertheless, more bilirubin is excreted in the bile, the amount of urobilinogen entering the enterohepatic circulation is increased and urinary urobilinogen is increased.

Activity of the hepatic conjugating enzymes is usually low at birth but increases rapidly thereafter; the transient 'physiological' jaundice of the newborn reflects this. With excessive hemolysis, as in Rhesus incompatibility or a lack of enzyme activity, as occurs in prematurity and in the Crigler–Najjar syndrome, there may be a massive rise in the plasma concentration of unconjugated bilirubin. If bilirubin concentration exceeds approximately 340 µmol/L in infants, its uptake into the brain may cause severe, irreversible brain damage (kernicterus).

Conjugated Hyperbilirubinemia

This condition is due to leakage of bilirubin from either hepatocytes or the biliary system into the bloodstream when its normal route of excretion is blocked. The water-soluble conjugated bilirubin entering the systemic circulation is excreted by the kidneys, as a result of which the urine develops a deep orange-brown color. In complete biliary obstruction, no bilirubin reaches the gut, no stercobilin is formed and the stools are pale in color.

Hyperbilirubinemia can be due to an excess of either or both conjugated and unconjugated bilirubin. The separate measurement of these entities is useful in the diagnosis of neonatal jaundice, where there may be some doubt as to the relative contribution of defective conjugation and other causes; it is less often required in adults and the chemical methods are anyway not wholly reliable at detecting small increases in either fraction. If the plasma bilirubin concentration is <100 µmol/L and other tests of liver function are normal, it can be inferred that the raised levels are due to the unconjugated form of

the pigment. The urine can be tested to confirm this because with unconjugated hyperbilirubinemia there is no bilirubin in the urine. In adults, severe jaundice is almost always a result of conjugated hyperbilirubinemia.

A third fraction of bilirubin, consisting of conjugated bilirubin bound covalently to albumin, is found in the plasma of patients with longstanding conjugated hyperbilirubinemia. This substance has a half-life similar to that of albumin. Its persistence in the plasma during the resolution of liver disease or after the relief of obstruction explains the persistence of jaundice in the absence of bilirubinuria that can occur in these circumstances.

Plasma Enzymes

Enzymes used in the assessment of the liver include aspartate and alanine aminotransferases (formerly called transaminases and still abbreviated AST and ALT, respectively), alkaline phosphatase (ALP) and γ-glutamyl transferase (GGT). In general, these enzymes are not specific indicators of liver dysfunction. The hepatic isoenzyme of ALP is an exception, and ALT is more specific to the liver than AST.

Increased aminotransferase activities reflect cell damage; plasma levels may be 20 times the upper limit of normal (ULN) in patients with hepatitis. In cholestasis (obstruction to the flow of bile), plasma ALP activity is increased. This is due mainly to increased enzyme synthesis (enzyme induction), stimulated by cholestasis. In severe obstructive jaundice, the plasma ALP activity may be up to $10 \times$ ULN.

In practice, however, increases in the plasma activities of both the aminotransferases and ALP are often present in patients with liver disease, although one may predominate. In primarily cholestatic disease, there may be secondary hepatocellular damage and increased plasma aminotransferase activities, while cholestasis frequently occurs in primarily hepatocellular disease. Increased GGT activity is found in both cholestasis and hepatocellular damage; this enzyme is a very sensitive indicator of hepatobiliary disease but is non-specific. Thus, although certain patterns of plasma enzyme activities are frequently observed in various types of liver disease, they are not reliably diagnostic.

The enzymes AST and ALT provide essentially the same information and many laboratories measure only one, but AST is sometimes disproportionately elevated in alcohol-related liver disease.

Plasma enzyme activities are very useful in following the progress of liver disease once the diagnosis has been made. Falling aminotransferase activity suggests a decrease in hepatocellular damage and falling ALP activity suggests a resolution of cholestasis. However, in severe acute hepatic failure, a decrease in amino-transferase activity may misleadingly suggest an improvement when it is actually due to almost complete destruction of parenchymal cells.

It is important to appreciate that there are many extrahepatobiliary causes of increased plasma activities of the aminotransferases, GGT, and ALP.

Plasma Proteins

Albumin is synthesized in the liver and its concentration in the plasma is in part a reflection of the functional capacity of the organ. Plasma albumin concentration tends to decrease in chronic liver disease, but is usually normal in the early stages of acute hepatitis owing to its long half-life (approximately 20 days). There are many other causes of hypoalbuminemia, but a normal plasma albumin concentration in a patient with chronic liver disease implies adequate synthetic function; a fall implies a significant deterioration.

The prothrombin time, usually expressed as a ratio (INR) to a control value, is a test of plasma clotting activity and reflects the activity of vitamin-K-dependent clotting factors synthesized by the liver, of which factor VII has the shortest half-life (4–6 hours). An increase in the prothrombin time is often an early feature of acute liver disease, but a prolonged prothrombin time may also reflect vitamin K deficiency (in which case, a single parenteral dose of vitamin K should normalize the prothrombin time within 18 hours).

A polyclonal increase in immunoglobulins is a frequent finding in patients with chronic liver disease (particularly of autoimmune origin) and may cause an increase in plasma total protein concentration even when albumin concentration is decreased. Plasma immunoglobulin A is often increased in alcoholic liver disease, IgG in autoimmune hepatitis, and IgM in primary biliary cirrhosis, but these changes are non-specific. More useful diagnostic information may be obtained from measuring individual autoantibodies; anti-mitochondrial antibody is increased in almost all patients with primary biliary cirrhosis, and anti-smooth muscle and anti-nuclear antibodies in many patients with autoimmune hepatitis. Viral infection, an important cause of both acute and chronic liver disease, can be detected by measurement of viral antigens and antibodies to them.

OTHER TESTS OF LIVER FUNCTION

Various dynamic tests, which give an indication of functional hepatic cell mass, are available, but are infrequently used. They may be considered as analogous to the use of clearance measurements for renal function. Marker substances are used that are excreted or metabolized by the liver, and either the rate of their removal from the blood or the rate of formation of a metabolite is measured. However, these processes depend on hepatic blood flow as well as hepatic metabolism, more so for substances that are efficiently extracted from the blood at first pass. Substances used include aminopyrine, antipyrine, indocyanine green, galactose and lidocaine (lignocaine). These tests are more sensitive than conventional tests, but are more time-consuming; their use is likely to remain limited to special situations (e.g. the monitoring of novel treatments, assessment of prognosis, etc.). The simplest of these quantitative tests of liver function (requiring only a single blood sample) is measurement of the formation of monoethylglycinexylidide (MEGX) after administration of a bolus of lidocaine. Unfortunately, the reference range is wide, and serial, rather than isolated, measurements are likely to prove more useful. Thus, the standard panel of biochemical tests in hepatobiliary disease continues to be, as it has been for many years, albumin and total bilirubin concentrations and the activities of one or other aminotransferase, alkaline phosphatase, and GGT, together with the prothrombin time.

Plasma bile acid concentrations are increased in liver disease but, while this is a highly specific finding, bile acid measurements are in general no more sensitive than conventional tests. They do, however, have a special role in liver disease developing during pregnancy.

Non-biochemical Investigation of Hepatobiliary Disease

Many other types of investigation can provide valuable information in patients suspected of having hepatobiliary disease. **Imaging techniques provide primarily anatomical information**. Transcutaneous ultrasound examination is low cost and safe, and is widely used as a first-line imaging investigation. It can reveal gallstones, dilatation of the biliary system, tumors and the characteristic hyper reflectivity of hepatic fatty infiltration. Endoscopic ultrasound is particularly good for visualizing the pancreas and portal vein. Cholangiography is used to examine the biliary system using an X-ray contrast medium given either endoscopically (endoscopic retrograde cholangiopancreatography, ERCP) or percutaneously into the liver (percutaneous transhepatic cholangiography, PTC); intravenous cholangiography has now been largely superseded. Arteriography can reveal the typical pathological circulation in hepatic tumors. Various techniques of computerized tomography and magnetic resonance imaging MRI can demonstrate structural abnormalities and space-occupying lesions in the hepatobiliary system. Magnetic resonance cholangiography is tending to replace contrast cholangiography where it is available.

Isotopic scanning (nuclear medicine) techniques are of limited use, but are used in the evaluation of tumors and to assess the patency of the cystic duct. The 'gold standard' of diagnosis, particularly in chronic liver disease and cancer, is histology, usually of tissue obtained by percutaneous biopsy.

BIBLIOGRAPHY

1. Addolorato G, Leggio L, Ferrulli A, et al. Effectiveness and safety of baclofen for maintenance of alcohol abstinence in alcohol-dependent patients with liver cirrhosis: randomised, double-blind controlled study. Lancet. 2007; 370: 1915–22.

2. Agabio R, Marras P, Addolorato G, et al. Baclofen suppresses alcohol intake and craving for alcohol in a schizophrenic alcohol-dependent patient: a case report. J Clin Psychopharmacol. 2007; 27:319–20.

3. Benova L, Mohamoud YA, Calvert C, et al. "Vertical transmission of hepatitis C virus: systematic review and meta-analysis". Clinical infectious diseases 2014; 59(6): 765–73.

4. Berg T, DeLanghe S, Al Alam D, et al. "β-catenin regulates mesenchymal progenitor cell differentiation during hepatogenesis". J Surg Res. 2010; 164 (2): 276–85.

5. Bien TH, Miller WR, Tonigan JS. Brief interventions for alcohol problems: a review. Addiction. 1993; 88:315–35.

6. Borowsky SA, Strome S, Lott E. Continued heavy drinking and survival in alcoholic cirrhotics. Gastroenterology. 1981; 80:1405–1409.

7. Bosma PJ, Chowdhury JR, Bakker C, et al. The genetic basis of the reduced expression of bilirubin UDP-glucuronosyl-transferase 1 in Gilbert's syndrome. N Engl J Med. 1995; 2; 333(18): 1171–5.

8. Bosma PJ. Inherited disorders of bilirubin metabolism. J Hepatol. 2003; 38(1):107–17.

9. Bramstedt K. "Living liver donor mortality: where do we stand?". Am J Gastrointestinal. 2006; 101 (4): 755–9.

10. Cabré E, Rodríguez-Iglesias P, Caballería J, et al. Short- and long-term outcome of severe alcohol-induced hepatitis treated with steroids or enteral nutrition: a multicenter randomized trial. Hepatology. 2000; 32:36–42.

11. Campillo B, Richardet JP, Scherman E, et al. Evaluation of nutritional practice in hospitalized cirrhotic patients: results of a prospective study. Nutrition. 2003; 19:515–21.

12. Chu, Jaime; Sadler, Kirsten C. "New school in liver development: Lessons from zebrafish". Hepatology. 2009; 50 (5): 1656–63.

13. Clemente, Carmin D. Anatomy a Regional Atlas of the Human Body. Philadelphia: Lippincott Williams and Wilkins. 2011; p. 243. ISBN 978-1-58255-889-9.

14. Cotran, Ramzi S.; Kumar, Vinay; Fausto, Nelson; et al. Robbins and Cotran pathologic basis of disease (7th ed.). St. Louis, MO: Elsevier Saunders. 2005; p. 878. ISBN 0-7216-0187-1.

15. Dancygier, Henryk. Clinical Hepatology Principles and Practice of. Springer. 2010; p. 895. ISBN 978-3-642-04509-7.

16. Davidoff RA. Antispasticity drugs: mechanisms of action. Ann Neurol. 1985 17:107–116.

17. De Clercq, Erik; Férir, Geoffrey; Kaptein, Suzanne; et al. "Antiviral Treatment of Chronic Hepatitis B Virus (HBV) Infections†". Viruses 2010; 2(6): 1279–305.

18. DiCecco SR, Francisco-Ziller N. Nutrition in alcoholic liver disease. Nutr Clin Pract. 2006; 21:245–254.

19. Dorland's. Dorland's Illustrated Medical Dictionary. (32nd edition). Elsevier. 2012; p. 285. ISBN 978-1-4160-6257-8.

20. European Association for the Study of Liver. EASL clinical practical guidelines: management of alcoholic liver disease. J Hepatol. 2012; 57:399–420.

21. GhamarChehreh ME, Vahedi M, Pourhoseingholi MA, et al. Estimation of diagnosis and treatment costs of non-alcoholic Fatty liver disease: a two-year observation. Hepat Mon. 2013; 13:e7382.

22. Henkel AS, Buchman AL. Nutritional support in patients with chronic liver disease. Nat Clin Pract Gastroenterol Hepatol. 2006; 3: 202–9.

23. Hirsch S, Bunout D, de la Maza P, et al. Controlled trial on nutrition supplementation in outpatients with symptomatic alcoholic cirrhosis. JPEN J Parenter Enteral Nutr. 1993 17: 119–24.

24. Hirsch S, de la Maza MP, Gattás V, et al. Nutritional support in alcoholic cirrhotic patients improves host defenses. J Am Coll Nutr. 1999; 18:434–441.

25. Hirschfield, Gideon M.; Heathcote, E. Jenny. Autoimmune Hepatitis: A Guide for Practicing Clinicians. Springer Science and Business Media. ISBN 9781607615699.(2011-12-02).

26. Hirschfield, GM; Gershwin, ME. "The immunobiology and pathophysiology of primary biliary cirrhosis." Annual review of pathology. (2013) 8: 303–30.

27. Johnston DE. "Special considerations in interpreting liver function tests". Am Fam Physician. 1999; 59(8): 2223–30.

28. Kaner EF, Dickinson HO, Beyer F, et al. The effectiveness of brief alcohol interventions in primary care settings: a systematic review. Drug Alcohol Rev. 2009; 28:301–323.

29. Kearns PJ, Young H, Garcia G, et al. Accelerated improvement of alcoholic liver disease with enteral nutrition. Gastroenterology. 1992; 102:200–205.

30. Kim WR, Brown RS, Terrault NA, et al. Burden of liver disease in the United States: summary of a workshop. Hepatology. 2002; 36:227–242.

31. Kmieae Z. "Cooperation of liver cells in health and disease". Adv Anat Embryol Cell Biol. 2001; 161: III–XIII, 1–151.

32. Komatsu H. "Hepatitis B virus: where do we stand and what is the next step for eradication?". World journal of gastroenterology. 2014; 20(27): 8998–9016.

33. Korean Association for the Study of the Liver (KASL) KASL clinical practice guidelines: management of alcoholic liver disease. Clin Mol Hepatol. 2013; 19: 216–54. (2013).

34. Lade AG, Monga SP. "Beta-catenin signaling in hepatic development and progenitors: which way does the WNT blow?". Dev Dyn. 2011; 240 (3): 486–500.

35. Lee S, Jin Y, Kee C, et al. Nutritional status in alcohol- and virus-related liver cirrhosis. Korean J Hepatol. 2000; 6:59–72.

36. Liu J, Wang L. Baclofen for alcohol withdrawal. Cochrane Database Syst Rev. 2011; (1):CD008502.

37. Louvet A, Naveau S, Abdelnour M, et al. The Lille model: a new tool for therapeutic strategy in patients with severe alcoholic hepatitis treated with steroids. Hepatology. 2007; 45:1348–54.

38. Luca A, García-Pagán JC, Bosch J, et al. Effects of ethanol consumption on hepatic hemodynamics in patients with alcoholic cirrhosis. Gastroenterology. 1997; 112:1284–1289.

39. MacSween RN, Burt AD. Histologic spectrum of alcoholic liver disease. Semin Liver Dis. 1986; 6:221–232.

40. Mann K, Lehert P, Morgan MY. The efficacy of acamprosate in the maintenance of abstinence in alcohol-dependent individuals: results of a meta-analysis. Alcohol Clin Exp Res. 2004; 28:51–63.

41. Marchesini G, Dioguardi FS, Bianchi GP, Zoli M, Bellati G, Roffi L, Martines D, Abbiati R. Long-term oral branched-chain amino acid treatment in chronic hepatic encephalopathy. A randomized double-blind casein-controlled trial. The Italian Multicenter Study Group. J Hepatol. 1990; 11: 92–101.

42. Marieb, Elaine N.; Hoehn, Katja. Human Anatomy and Physiology (9th ed.). Pearson. ISBN 2012; 0321852125.

43. Mason BJ, Lehert P. Acamprosate for alcohol dependence: a sex-specific meta-analysis based on individual patient data. Alcohol Clin Exp Res. 2012; 36:497–508.

44. Mathurin P, Mendenhall CL, Carithers RL, et al. Corticosteroids improve short-term survival in patients with severe alcoholic hepatitis (AH): individual data analysis of the last three randomized placebo controlled double blind trials of corticosteroids in severe AH. J Hepatol. 2002; 36: 480–487.

45. Maton, Anthea; Jean Hopkins; Charles William McLaughlin; et al. Human Biology and Health. Englewood Cliffs, New Jersey, USA: Prentice Hall. 1993; ISBN 0-13-981176-1.

46. Mayo-Smith MF, Beecher LH, Fischer TL, et al. Management of alcohol withdrawal delirium. An evidence-based practice guideline. Arch Intern Med. 2014; 164: 1405–12.

47. McClain CJ, Barve SS, Barve A, et al. Alcoholic liver disease and malnutrition. Alcohol Clin Exp Res. 2011; 35: 815–20. (2011).

48. McClatchey, Kenneth D. Clinical laboratory medicine. Lippincott Williams and Wilkins. 2002; pp. 288–. ISBN 978-0-683-30751-1.

49. "Medscape: Medscape Access". Emedicine.medscape.com. 03–09. (2015).

50. Mendenhall C, Roselle GA, Gartside P, et al. Relationship of protein calorie malnutrition to alcoholic liver disease: a reexamination of data from two Veterans Administration Cooperative Studies. Alcohol Clin Exp Res. 1995; 19: 635–641.

51. Mendenhall CL, Anderson S, Weesner RE, et al. Protein-calorie malnutrition associated with alcoholic hepatitis. Veterans Administration Cooperative Study Group on Alcoholic Hepatitis. Am J Med. 194; 76: 211–222.

52. Mendenhall CL, Moritz TE, Roselle GA, et al. A study of oral nutritional support with oxandrolone in malnourished patients with alcoholic hepatitis: results of a Department of Veterans Affairs cooperative study. Hepatology. 1993; 17: 564–576. (1993).

53. Mengel, Mark B.; Schwiebert, L. Peter. Family medicine: ambulatory care & prevention. McGraw-Hill Professional. pp. 268–. 2005; ISBN 978-0-07-142322-9.

54. Morgan MY. The prognosis and outcome of alcoholic liver disease. Alcohol Alcohol Suppl. 1994; 2:335–343.

55. Morgan MY. The treatment of alcoholic hepatitis. Alcohol Alcohol. 1996; 31:117–134.

56. Nageh T, Sherwood RA, Harris BM, et al. "Cardiac troponin T and I and creatine kinase-MB as markers of myocardial injury and predictors of outcome following percutaneous coronary intervention". International journal of cardiology. 2003; 92 (2–3): 285–293.

57. Nyblom H, Berggren U, Balldin J, Olsson R. "High AST/ALT ratio may indicate advanced alcoholic liver disease rather than heavy drinking". Alcohol Alcohol. 2004; 39 (4): 336–339.

58. Nyblom H, Björnsson E, Simrén M, et al. "The AST/ALT ratio as an indicator of cirrhosis in patients with PBC". Liver Int. 2006; 26 (7): 840–845.

59. O'Shea RS, Dasarathy S, McCullough AJ. Alcoholic liver disease. Hepatology. 2010; 51:307–328.

60. Pessione F, Ramond MJ, Peters L, et al. Five-year survival predictive factors in patients with excessive alcohol intake and cirrhosis. Effect of alcoholic hepatitis, smoking and abstinence. Liver Int. 2003; 23:45–53.

61. Plauth M, Cabré E, Campillo B, et al. ESPEN Guidelines on Parenteral Nutrition: hepatology. Clin Nutr. 2009; 28: 436–444.

62. Plauth M, Cabré E, Riggio O, et al. ESPEN Guidelines on Enteral Nutrition: Liver disease. ClinNutr. 2006; 25:285–294.

63. Pocock, Gillian. Human Physiology (Third ed.). Oxford University Press. 2006; p. 404. ISBN 978-0-19-856878-0.

64. Rajani R, Melin T, Björnsson E, et al. "Budd-Chiari syndrome in Sweden: epidemiology, clinical characteristics and survival - an 18-year experience". Liver International 2009; 29 (2): 253–9.

65. Rambaldi A, Saconato HH, Christensen E, et al. Systematic review: glucocorticosteroids for alcoholic hepatitis—a Cochrane Hepato-Biliary Group systematic review with meta-analyses and trial sequential analyses of randomized clinical trials. Aliment Pharmacol Ther. 2008; 27: 1167–78.

66. Rehm J, Samokhvalov AV, Shield KD. Global burden of alcoholic liver diseases. J Hepatol. 2013; 59:160–168.

67. Romer, Alfred Sherwood; Parsons, Thomas S. The Vertebrate Body. Philadelphia, PA: Holt-Saunders International. 1977; pp. 354–5. ISBN 0-03-910284-X.

68. Room R, Babor T, Rehm J. Alcohol and public health. Lancet. 2005; 365:519–530.

69. Roozen HG, de Waart R, van der Windt DA, et al. A systematic review of the effectiveness of naltrexone in the maintenance treatment of opioid and alcohol dependence. Eur Neuropsychopharmacol. 2006; 16:311–323.

70. Runyon BA. Introduction to the revised American Association for the Study of Liver Diseases Practice Guideline management of adult patients with ascites due to cirrhosis 2012. Hepatology. 2013; 57:1651–1653.

71. Saitz R, O'Malley SS. Pharmacotherapies for alcohol abuse. Withdrawal and treatment. Med Clin North Am. 1997; 81:881–907.

72. Samal J, Kandpal M, Vivekanandan P. "Molecular Mechanisms Underlying Occult Hepatitis B Virus Infection". Clinical Microbiology Reviews. 2012; 25 (1): 142–63.

73. Saxena R, Theise N; Theise. "Canals of Hering: recent insights and current knowledge". Semin. Liver Dis. 2004; 24 (1): 43–8. (2004).

74. Shaw JJ, Shah SA. Rising incidence and demographics of hepatocellular carcinoma in the USA: what does it mean? Expert Rev Gastroenterol Hepatol. 2011; 5: 365–70.

75. Sheporaitis, L; Freeny, PC. "Hepatic and portal surface veins: A new anatomic variant revealed during abdominal CT". AJR. American journal of roentgenology 1998; 171 (6): 1559–64.

76. Shneider, Benjamin L, Sherman, Philip M. Pediatric Gastrointestinal Disease. Connecticut: PMPH-USA. 2008; p.751. ISBN 1-55009-364-9.

77. Singal AK, Charlton MR. Nutrition in alcoholic liver disease. Clin Liver Dis. 2012; 16:805–26.

78. Soyka M, Rösner S. Opioid antagonists for pharmacological treatment of alcohol dependence - a critical review. Curr Drug Abuse Rev. 2008; 1:280–291.

79. Stallings W, Schrader S. Baclofen as prophylaxis and treatment for alcohol withdrawal: a retrospective chart review. J Okla State Med Assoc. 2007; 100:354–360.

80. Stickel F, Hoehn B, Schuppan D, Seitz HK. Review article: Nutritional therapy in alcoholic liver disease. Aliment Pharmacol Ther. 2003; 18:357–373.

81. Strunk, H.; Stuckmann, G.; Textor, J.; et al. "Limitations and pitfalls of Couinaud's segmentation of the liver in transaxial Imaging". European Radiology. 13(11): 2472–82. (2003).

82. Suchy, Frederick J.; Sokol, Ronald J.; Balistreri, William F. Liver Disease in Children. Cambridge University Press. ISBN 9781107729094.(2014-02-20).

83. Suk KT, Kim MY, Baik SK. "Alcoholic liver disease: treatment". World journal of gastroenterology 2014; 20 (36): 12934–44.

84. Suzuki K, Tanaka M, Watanabe N, et al. A "p75 Neurotrophin receptor is a marker for precursors of stellate cells and portal fibroblasts in mouse fetal liver". Gastroenterology 2008; 135 (1): 270–281.e3.

85. Teli MR, Day CP, Burt AD, et al. Determinants of progression to cirrhosis or fibrosis in pure alcoholic fatty liver. Lancet. 1995; 346:987–990.

86. "The Radiology Assistant : Anatomy of the liver segments". Radiologyassistant.nl. 05–07 (2006) 06–26. (2015).

87. Tietz PS, Larusso NF "Cholangiocyte biology". Current Opinion in Gastroenterology. 2006; 22 (3): 279–87.

88. Tietz textbook of clinical chemistry 3rd edition, Philadelphia, W.B Saunders company (1995).

89. Tietz textbook of clinical chemistry and molecular biology 5fifth edition, Philadelphia, W.B Saunders company (2012).

90. "Transplantation of the Liver - Ronald W. Busuttil, Goran B. Klintmalm". Books.google.co.za. Retrieved. 2015–06–26.

91. Udomuksorn W, Elliot DJ, Lewis BC, et al. Influence of mutations associated with Gilbert and Crigler-Najjar type II syndromes on the glucuronidation kinetics of bilirubin and other UDP-glucuronosyltransferase 1A substrates. Pharmacogenet Genomics. 2007; 17(12):1017-29.

92. Vasilaki EI, Hosier SG, Cox WM. The efficacy of motivational interviewing as a brief intervention for excessive drinking: a meta-analytic review. Alcohol Alcohol. 2006; 41:328–335.

93. Veldt BJ, Lainé F, Guillygomarc'h A, et al. Indication of liver transplantation in severe alcoholic liver cirrhosis: quantitative evaluation and optimal timing. J Hepatol. 2002; 36: 93–98.

94. W. Jelkmann. "The role of the liver in the production of thrombopoietin compared with erythropoietin". European journal of gastroenterology and hepatology. 2001; 13(7): 791–801. (2001).

95. William Marshall, Márta Lapsley, Stephen K Bangert. Elsevier.com: Clinical Chemistry, 7th edition. 2012; ISBN-9780723437031.

96. Williams JA, Manley S, Ding WX. "New advances in molecular mechanisms and emerging therapeutic targets in alcoholic liver diseases". World journal of gastroenterology 2014; 20(36): 12908–33.

97. Zakim, David; Boyer, Thomas D. Hepatology: A Textbook of Liver Disease. 4th edition 2002; ISBN 9780721690513.

6

The Gastrointestinal Tract

INTRODUCTION

The gastrointestinal tract (GI) is a long twisting tube that starts at the mouth through the esophagus, stomach, small and large intestine within where the nutrients are extracted for the needs of the body (Fig. 6.1). The residue then passes to the rectum where it is evacuated.

The first part of the pathway is the esophagus, which is a conduit that guides food from the mouth, where it is prepared by chewing, down to the stomach where it is stored. The stomach is both a storage space, holding as much as a quart and a half of ingested food, and a secretory organ that produces the gastric acid necessary for digestion. However, the stomach does not absorb food. When food enters the stomach from the esophagus it remains for a short period while it is mixed with gastric acid. The stomach then by involuntary muscle

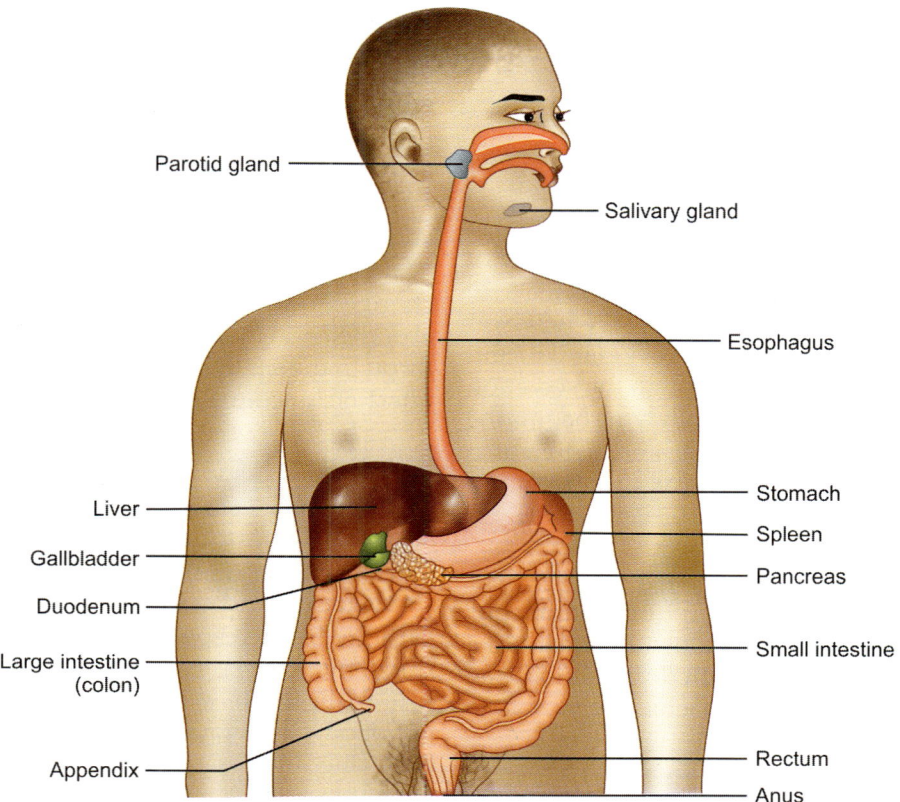

Fig. 6.1: The gastrointestinal tract (GI)

contractions (peristalsis) empties the food gradually into the duodenum, the first part of the small intestine.

The small intestine consists of three parts—the duodenum, the jejunum and the ileum. In these three parts, certain digestive secretions are mixed with food, and the nutrients are absorbed into the bloodstream.

The duodenum treats the food it receives with bile from the liver and enzymes from the pancreas. It also adds liquid duodenal fluid that comes from the wall of the duodenum itself. The food, bile, enzymes and liquids brought together in the duodenum are then passed into the jejunum. The jejunum or second portion of the small intestine is approximately 10 feet long. It lies immediately behind the duodenum and continues the process of digestion, breaking down food into essential elements.

The ileum or third portion of the small intestine, like the jejunum, is about 10 feet long. It is here that a major part of the absorption of food products and liquids occurs. Waste products of the digestive process are passed from the small intestine or terminal ileum, into the large intestine, also known as the colon. The beginning of the colon is in the right lower quadrant of the abdomen, near the appendix. The colon moves waste products through about four feet by the continuing process of undulating motions or peristalsis, which is common to all parts of the gastrointestinal tract. The primary function of the colon is to store waste products of digestion prior to evacuation. The colon absorbs small amounts of water and electrolytes.

THE STRUCTURE OF GI

Mouth

The mouth is the beginning of the digestive tract; and, in fact, digestion starts here when taking the first bite of food. The process of digestion begins in the mouth where food is chewed until it reaches a consistency, whereby it can be swallowed. In the mouth, the salivary glands begin the process of chemical digestion through the secretion of the enzyme, salivary amylase. This enzyme begins the process of breaking down carbohydrates. Saliva also moistens food which helps it to be swallowed more easily.

Esophagus

Located in throat near trachea (windpipe), the esophagus receives food from mouth after swallow. By means of a series of muscular contractions called peristalsis, the esophagus delivers food to the stomach.

Stomach

The stomach is a hollow organ, or 'container,' that holds food while it is being mixed with enzymes that continue the process of breaking down food into a usable form. Cells in the lining of the stomach secrete strong acid and powerful enzymes that are responsible for the breakdown process. When the contents of the stomach are sufficiently processed, they are released into the small intestine.

Small Intestine

The small intestine is the site where most of the chemical and mechanical digestion is carried out, and where virtually all of the absorption of useful materials is carried out. The whole of the small intestine is lined with an absorptive mucosal type, with certain modifications for each section. The intestine also has a smooth muscle wall with two layers of muscle; rhythmical contractions force products of digestion through the intestine (peristalsis). There are three main sections to the small intestine:

- **The duodenum** forms a 'C' shape around the head of the pancreas. Its main function is to neutralize the acidic gastric contents (called chyme) and to initiate further digestion; Brunner's glands in the submucosa secrete alkaline mucus which neutralizes the chyme and protects the surface of the duodenum.
- **The jejunum**.
- **The ileum**.

The jejunum and the ileum are the greatly coiled parts of the small intestine, and together are about 4–6 meters long; the junction between the two sections is not well-defined. The mucosa of these sections is highly folded (the folds are called plicae), increasing the surface area available for absorption dramatically.

Contents of the small intestine start out semisolid, and end in a liquid form after passing through the organ. Water, bile, enzymes, and mucous contribute to the change in consistency. Once the nutrients have been absorbed and the leftover food residue liquid has passed through the small intestine, it then moves on to the large intestine, or colon.

Pancreas

The pancreas consists mainly of exocrine glands that secrete enzymes to aid in the digestion of food in the small intestine. The main enzymes produced are lipases, peptidases and amylases for fats, proteins and carbohydrates respectively. These are released into the duodenum via the duodenal ampulla; the same place that bile from the liver drains into. Pancreatic exocrine secretion is hormonally regulated, and the same hormone that encourages secretion (cholesystokinin) also encourages discharge of the gall bladder's store of bile. As bile is essentially an emulsifying agent, it makes fats water soluble and gives the pancreatic enzymes lots of surface area to work on. Structurally, the pancreas has four sections—head, neck, body and tail; the tail stretches back to just in front of the spleen.

Colon (Large Intestine)

The colon is a muscular tube that connects the small intestine to the rectum. The large intestine is made up of the cecum, the ascending (right) colon, the transverse (across) colon, the descending (left) colon, and the sigmoid colon, which connects to the rectum. The appendix is a small tube attached to the cecum. The large intestine is a highly specialized organ that is responsible for processing waste, so that emptying the bowels is easy and convenient.

Stool or waste left over from the digestive process, is passed through the colon by means of peristalsis, first in a liquid state and ultimately in a solid form. As stool passes through the colon, water is removed. Stool is stored in the sigmoid (S-shaped) colon until a 'mass movement' empties it into the rectum once or twice a day. It normally takes about 36 hours for stool to get through the colon. The stool itself is mostly food debris and bacteria. These bacteria perform several useful functions, such as synthesizing various vitamins, processing waste products and food particles, and protecting against harmful bacteria. When the descending colon becomes full of stool, or feces, it empties its contents into the rectum to begin the process of elimination.

Rectum

The rectum (Latin for 'straight') is an 8-inch chamber that connects the colon to the anus. It is the rectum's job to receive stool from the colon, to let the person know that there is stool to be evacuated, and to hold the stool until evacuation happens. When anything (gas or stool) comes into the rectum, sensors send a message to the brain. The brain then decides if the rectal contents can be released or not. If they can, the sphincters relax and the rectum contracts, disposing its contents. If the contents cannot be disposed, the sphincter contracts and the rectum accommodates so that the sensation temporarily goes away.

Anus

The anus is the last part of the digestive tract. It is a 2-inch long canal consisting of the pelvic floor muscles and the two anal sphincters (internal and external). The lining of the upper anus is specialized to detect rectal contents. It lets you know whether the contents are liquid, gas, or solid. The anus is surrounded by sphincter muscles that are important in allowing control of stool.

The pelvic floor muscle creates an angle between the rectum and the anus that stops stool from coming out when it is not supposed to. The internal sphincter is always tight, except when stool enters the rectum. It keeps us continent when we are asleep or otherwise unaware of the presence of stool. When we get an urge to go to the bathroom, we rely on our external sphincter to hold the stool until reaching a toilet, where it then relaxes to release the contents.

GASTROINTESTINAL DISORDERS

Upper GI complaints include chest pain, chronic and recurrent abdominal pain, dyspepsia, lump in the throat, halitosis, hiccups, nausea and vomiting, and rumination. Some upper GI complaints represent functional illness (i.e. no physiologic cause found after extensive evaluation.

Lower GI complaints include constipation, diarrhea, gas and bloating, abdominal pain, and rectal pain or bleeding. As with upper GI complaints, lower GI complaints result from physiologic illness or represent a functional disorder (i.e. no radiologic, biochemical, or pathologic abnormalities are found even after extensive evaluation). The reasons for functional symptoms are not clear. Evidence suggests that patients with functional symptoms may have disturbances of motility, nociception, or both; i.e. they perceive as uncomfortable certain sensations (e.g. luminal distention, peristalsis) that other people do not find distressing.

No bodily function is more variable and subject to external influences than defecation. Bowel habits vary considerably from person to person and are affected by age, physiology, diet, and social and cultural influences. Some people have unwarranted preoccupation with bowel habits.

Chronic and Recurrent Abdominal Pain

Chronic abdominal pain (CAP) persists for more than 3 months either continuously or intermittently. Intermittent pain may be referred to as recurrent abdominal pain (RAP). CAP occurs any time after 5 years of age.

Pathophysiology

Functional abdominal pain syndrome (FAPS) is pain that persists >6 months without evidence of physiologic disease, shows no relationship to physiologic events (e.g. meals, defecation, menses), and interferes with daily functioning. FAPS is poorly understood but seems to involve altered nociception. Sensory neurons in the dorsal horn of the spinal cord may become abnormally excitable and hyperalgesic due to a combination of factors. Cognitive and psychologic factors (e.g. depression, stress, culture, secondary gain, coping, and support mechanisms) may cause efferent stimulation that amplifies pain signals, resulting in perception of pain with low-level inputs and persistence of pain long after the stimulus has ceased. Additionally, the pain itself may function as a stressor, perpetuating a positive feedback loop.

In addition, menopause increases GI symptoms in several disorders including irritable bowel syndrome, inflammatory bowel disease, endometriosis, and non-ulcer dyspepsia.

Etiology

Perhaps 10% of patients have an occult physiologic illness (Table 6.1); the remainder has a functional process. However, determining whether a particular abnormality (e.g. adhesions, ovarian cyst, and endometriosis) is the cause of CAP symptoms or an incidental finding can be difficult.

If the diagnosis of functional CAP is made, frequent examinations and tests should be avoided because they may focus on or magnify the physical complaints or imply that the physician lacks confidence in the diagnosis.

Table 6.1	Physiologic causes of chronic abdominal pain	
Cause	Suggestive findings*	Diagnostic approach
GU disorders		
Congenital abnormalities	Recurrent UTIs	IVU Ultrasonography
Endometriosis	Discomfort before or during menses	Laparoscopy
Ovarian cyst, ovarian cancer	Vague lower abdominal discomfort, bloating Sometimes a palpable pelvic mass	Pelvic ultrasonography Gynecologic consultation
Renal calculi	Fever, flank pain, dark or bloody urine	Urine culture IVU CT
Sequelae of acute PID	Pelvic discomfort History of acute PID	Pelvic examination Sometimes laparoscopy
GI disorders		
Celiac disease	In children, failure to thrive Abdominal bloating, diarrhea, and often steatorrhea Symptoms that worsen when gluten-containing products are ingested	Serologic markers Small-bowel biopsy
Chronic appendicitis	Several previous discrete episodes of RLQ pain	Abdominal CT Ultrasonography
Chronic cholecystitis	Recurrent colicky RUQ pain	Ultrasonography HIDA scan
Chronic hepatitis	Upper abdominal discomfort, malaise, anorexia Jaundice uncommon In about one-third of patients, a history of acute hepatitis	Liver tests Viral hepatitis titers
Chronic pancreatitis, pancreatic pseudocyst	Episodes of severe epigastric pain Sometimes malabsorption (e.g. diarrhea, fatty stool) Usually a history of acute pancreatitis	Serum amylase and lipase levels CT, MRCP
Colon cancer	Discomfort uncommon but possibly colicky discomfort if left colon is partially obstructed Often occult or visible blood in stool	Colonoscopy
Crohn disease	Episodic severe pain with fever, anorexia, weight loss, diarrhea Extraintestinal symptoms (joints, eyes, mouth, skin)	CT enterography or upper GI series with SBFT Colonoscopy and esophagogastroduodenoscopy with biopsies
Gastric cancer	Dyspepsia or mild pain Often occult blood in stool	Upper endoscopy

Contd.

Table 6.1 Physiologic causes of chronic abdominal pain *(Contd.)*		
Cause	**Suggestive findings***	**Diagnostic approach**
Granulomatous enterocolitis	Family history Recurrent infections in other sites (e.g. lungs, lymph nodes)	ESR Barium enema CT enterography
Hiatus hernia with gastroesophageal reflux	Heartburn Sometimes cough and/or hoarseness Symptoms relieved by taking antacids Sometimes regurgitation of gastric contents into mouth	Barium swallow Endoscopy
Intestinal TB	Chronic nonspecific pain Sometimes palpable RLQ mass Fever, diarrhea, weight loss	Tuberculin test Endoscopy for biopsy CT with oral contrast
Lactose intolerance	Bloating and cramps after ingesting milk products	H_2 breath test Trial of elimination of lactose-containing foods
Pancreatic cancer	Severe upper abdominal pain that • Often radiates to the back • Occurs late in disease, when weight loss is often present May cause obstructive jaundice	CT MRCP or ERCP
Parasitic infestation (particularly giardiasis)	History of travel or exposure Cramps, flatulence, diarrhea	Stool examination for ova or parasites Stool enzyme immunoassay (for Giardia)
Peptic ulcer disease	Upper abdominal pain relieved by food and antacids May awaken patient at night	Endoscopy and biopsy for *Helicobacter pylori* *H. pylori* breath test Evaluation of NSAID use Stool examination for occult blood
Postoperative adhesive bands	Previous abdominal surgery Colicky discomfort accompanied by nausea and sometimes vomiting	Upper GI series, SBFT, or enteroclysis
Ulcerative colitis	Crampy pain with bloody diarrhea	Sigmoidoscopy, colonoscopy, rectal biopsy
Systemic disorders		
Abdominal epilepsy	Very rare Episodic pain No other GI symptoms	EEG
Familial angioneurotic edema	Family history Pain often with peripheral angioedema and fever	Serum complement level (C4) during attacks
Familial Mediterranean fever	Family history Fever and peritonitis often accompanying the bouts of pain Starting in childhood or adolescence	Genetic testing
Food allergy	Symptoms developing only after consuming certain foods (e.g. seafood)	Elimination diet
Immunoglobulin A-associated vasculitis (formerly Henoch-Schönlein purpura)	Palpable purpuric rash Joint pains Occult blood in stool	Biopsy of skin lesions
Lead poisoning	Cognitive/Behavioral abnormalities	Blood lead level
Migraine equivalent	Rare variant with epigastric pain and vomiting Mainly in children Usually family history of migraine	Clinical evaluation

Contd.

Table 6.1	Physiologic causes of chronic abdominal pain (Contd.)	
Cause	Suggestive findings*	Diagnostic approach
Porphyria	Recurrent severe abdominal pain, vomiting	Urine porphobilinogen and δ-aminolevulinic acid screening
	Benign abdominal examination	RBC deaminase assay
	Sometimes neurologic symptoms (e.g. muscle weakness, seizures, mental disturbance)	
	In some types, skin lesions	
Sickle cell disease	Family history	Sickle preparation
	Severe episodes of abdominal pain lasting over a day	Hb electrophoresis
	Recurrent pain in nonabdominal sites	

*Findings are not always present and may be present in other disorders.
HIDA, hydroxyiminodiacetic acid; MRCP, magnetic resonance cholangiopancreatography; PID, pelvic inflammatory disease; RLQ, right lower quadrant; RUQ, right upper quadrant; SBFT, small-bowel follow-through; GU, genitourinary.

There are no modalities to cure functional CAP; however, many helpful measures are available. These measures rest on a foundation of a trusting, empathic relationship among the physician, patient, and family. Patients should be reassured that they are not in danger; specific concerns should be sought and addressed. The physician should explain the laboratory findings and the nature of the problem and describe how the pain is generated and how the patient perceives it (i.e. that there is a constitutional tendency to feel pain at times of stress). It is important to avoid perpetuating the negative psychosocial consequences of chronic pain (e.g. prolonged absences from school or work, withdrawal from social activities) and to promote independence, social participation, and self-reliance. These strategies help the patient control or tolerate the symptoms while participating fully in everyday activities.

Drugs such as aspirin, nonsteroidal anti-inflammatory drugs (NSAIDs), H_2 receptor blockers, proton pump inhibitors, and tricyclic antidepressants can be effective. Opioids should be avoided because they invariably lead to dependency.

Cognitive methods (e.g. relaxation training, biofeedback, hypnosis) may help by contributing to the patient's sense of well-being and control. Regular follow-up visits should be scheduled weekly, monthly, or bimonthly, depending on the patient's needs, and should continue until well after the problem has resolved. Psychiatric referral may be required if symptoms persist, especially if the patient is depressed or there are significant psychologic difficulties in the family.

Dyspepsia

Dyspepsia is a sensation of pain or discomfort in the upper abdomen; it often is recurrent. It may be described as indigestion, gassiness, early satiety, postprandial fullness, gnawing, or burning.

Etiology

There are several common causes of dyspepsia (Table 6.2).

Many patients have findings on testing (e.g. duodenitis, pyloric dysfunction, motility disturbance, *Helicobacter pylori* gastritis, lactose deficiency, cholelithiasis) that correlate poorly with symptoms

Table 6.2	Some causes of dyspepsia	
Cause	Suggestive findings	Diagnostic approach
Achalasia	Slowly progressive dysphagia	Barium swallow
	Early satiety, nausea, vomiting, bloating, and symptoms that are worsened by food	Esophageal manometry
	Sometimes nocturnal regurgitation of undigested food	Endoscopy
	Chest discomfort	
Cancer (e.g. esophageal, gastric)	Chronic, vague discomfort	Upper endoscopy
	Later, dysphagia (esophageal) or early satiety (gastric)	
	Weight loss	
Coronary ischemia	Symptoms described as gas or indigestion rather than chest pain by some patients	ECG
	May have exertional component	Serum cardiac markers
	Cardiac risk factors	Sometimes stress testing

Contd.

Table 6.2	Some causes of dyspepsia *(Contd.)*	
Cause	**Suggestive findings**	**Diagnostic approach**
Delayed gastric emptying (caused by diabetes, viral illness, or drugs)	Nausea, bloating, fullness	Scintigraphic test of gastric emptying
Drugs (e.g. bisphosphonates, erythromycin and other macrolide antibiotics, estrogens, iron, NSAIDs, potassium)	Use apparent on history Symptoms coincident with use	Clinical evaluation
Esophageal spasm	Substernal chest pain with or without dysphagia for liquids and solids	Barium swallow Esophageal manometry
Gastroesophageal reflux disease	Heartburn	Clinical evaluation
	Sometimes reflux of acid or stomach contents into mouth	Sometimes endoscopy
	Symptoms sometimes triggered by lying down Relief with antacids	Sometimes 24 hours pH testing
Peptic ulcer disease	Burning or Gnawing pain relieved by food or antacids	Upper endoscopy

(i.e. correction of the condition does not alleviate dyspepsia).

Nonulcer (functional) dyspepsia is defined as dyspeptic symptoms in a patient who has no abnormalities on physical examination and upper GI endoscopy.

PEPTIC ULCER DISEASE

A peptic ulcer is an erosion in a segment of the GI mucosa, typically in the stomach; gastric ulcer or the first few centimeters of the duodenum; duodenal ulcer (Fig. 6.2), that penetrates through the muscularis mucosae. Nearly all ulcers are caused by *Helicobacter pylori* infection or NSAID use. Symptoms typically include burning epigastric pain that is often relieved by food. Diagnosis is by endoscopy and testing for *H. pylori*. Treatment involves acid suppression, eradication of *H. pylori* (if present), and avoidance of NSAIDs.

Ulcers may range in size from several millimeters to several centimeters. Ulcers are delineated from erosions by the depth of penetration; erosions are more superficial and do not involve the muscularis mucosae. Ulcers can occur at any age, including infancy and childhood, but are most common among middle-aged adults.

Etiology

H. pylori and NSAIDs disrupt normal mucosal defense and repair, making the mucosa more susceptible to acid. *H. pylori* infection is present in 50–70% of patients with duodenal ulcers and 30–50% of patients with gastric ulcers. If *H. pylori* is eradicated, only 10% of patients have recurrence of peptic ulcer disease, compared with 70% recurrence in patients treated with acid suppression alone. NSAIDs now account for >50% of peptic ulcers.

Cigarette smoking is a risk factor for the development of ulcers and their complications. Also, smoking impairs ulcer healing and increases the incidence of recurrence. Risk correlates with the number of cigarettes smoked per day. Although, alcohol is a strong promoter of acid secretion, no definitive data link moderate amounts of alcohol to the development or delayed healing of ulcers. Very few patients have hypersecretion of gastrin (Zollinger–Ellison syndrome).

Symptoms and Signs

Symptoms depend on ulcer location and patient age; many patients, particularly elderly patients, have few or no symptoms. Pain is most common, often localized to the epigastrium and relieved by food or antacids. The

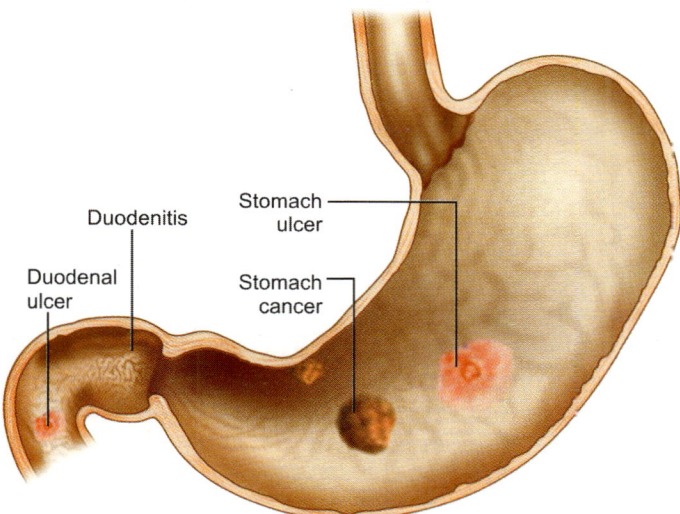

Fig. 6.2: Peptic ulcer disease

pain is described as burning or gnawing, or sometimes as a sensation of hunger. The course is usually chronic and recurrent. Only about half of patients present with the characteristic pattern of symptoms.

Gastric Ulcer

Symptoms often do not follow a consistent pattern (e.g. eating sometimes exacerbates rather than relieves pain). This is especially true for pyloric channel ulcers, which are often associated with symptoms of obstruction (e.g. bloating, nausea, vomiting) caused by edema and scarring.

Duodenal Ulcers

Duodenal ulcers tend to cause more consistent pain. Pain is absent when the patient awakens but appears in mid-morning, is relieved by food, but recurs 2–3 hours after a meal. Pain that awakens a patient at night is common and is highly suggestive of duodenal ulcer. In neonates, perforation and hemorrhage may be the first mani-festation of duodenal ulcer. Hemorrhage may also be the first recognized sign in later infancy and early childhood, although repeated vomiting or evidence of abdominal pain may be a clue.

Diagnosis

Diagnosis of peptic ulcer is suggested by patient history and confirmed by endoscopy. Empiric therapy is often begun without definitive diagnosis. However, endos-copy allows for biopsy or cytologic brushing of gastric and esophageal lesions to distinguish between simple ulceration and ulcerating stomach cancer. Stomach cancer may manifest with similar manifestations and must be excluded, especially in patients who are >45, have lost weight, or report severe or refractory symptoms. The incidence of malignant duodenal ulcer is extremely low, so biopsies of lesions in that area are generally not warranted. Endoscopy can also be used to definitively diagnose H. pylori infection, which should be sought when an ulcer is detected.

Gastrin-secreting cancer and Zollinger–Ellison syndrome should be considered when there are multiple ulcers, when ulcers develop in atypical locations (e.g. postbulbar) or are refractory to treatment, or when the patient has prominent diarrhea or weight loss. Serum gastrin levels should be measured in these patients.

Treatment

Treatment of gastric and duodenal ulcers requires eradication of H. pylori when present and a reduction of gastric acidity. For duodenal ulcers, it is particularly important to suppress nocturnal acid secretion.

Methods of decreasing acidity include a number of drugs, all of which are effective but which vary in cost, duration of therapy, and convenience of dosing. In addition, mucosal protective drugs (e.g. sucralfate) and acid-reducing surgical procedures may be used.

Gastritis

Gastritis is inflammation of the gastric mucosa caused by any of several conditions, including infection (Helicobacter pylori), drugs (NSAIDs, alcohol), stress, and autoimmune phenomena (atrophic gastritis). Many cases are asympto-matic, but dyspepsia and GI bleeding sometimes occur. Diagnosis is by endoscopy. Treatment is directed at the cause but often includes acid suppression and, for H. pylori infection, antibiotics.

Gastritis is classified as erosive or non-erosive based on the severity of mucosal injury. It is also classified according to the site of involvement (i.e. cardia, body, and antrum). Gastritis can be further classified histologically as acute or chronic based on the inflammatory cell type. No classification scheme matches perfectly with the pathophysiology; a large degree of overlap exists. Some forms of gastritis involve acid-peptic and H. pylori disease. Additionally, the term is often loosely applied to nonspecific (and often undiagnosed) abdominal discomfort and gastroenteritis.

Acute Gastritis

It is characterized by polymorphonuclear leukocytes (PMN) infiltration of the mucosa of the antrum and body.

Chronic Gastritis

Chronic gastritis implies some degree of atrophy (with loss of function of the mucosa) or metaplasia. It predominantly involves the antrum (with subsequent loss of G cells and decreased gastrin secretion) or the corpus (with loss of oxyntic glands, leading to reduced acid, pepsin, and intrinsic factor).

HELICOBACTER PYLORI INFECTION

H. pylori is a spiral-shaped, gram-negative organism that has adapted to thrive in acid. In developing countries, it commonly causes chronic infections and is usually acquired during childhood. The organism has been cultured from stool, saliva, and dental plaque, which suggests oral-oral or fecal-oral transmission. Infections tend to cluster in families and in residents of custodial institutions. Nurses and gastroenterologists seem to be at high risk because bacteria can be transmitted by improperly disinfected endoscopes.

Pathophysiology

Effects of *H. pylori* infection vary depending on the location within the stomach. Antral-predominant infection results in increased gastrin production, probably via local impairment of somatostatin release. Resultant hypersecretion of acid predisposes to prepyloric and duodenal ulcer (Fig. 6.3).

Body-predominant infection leads to gastric atrophy and decreased acid production, possibly via increased local production of IL-1β. Patients with body-predominant infection are predisposed to gastric ulcer and adenocarcinoma.

Some patients have mixed infection of both antrum and body with varying clinical effects. Many patients with *H. pylori* infection have no noticeable clinical effects.

Ammonia produced by *H. pylori* enables the organism to survive in the acidic environment of the stomach and may erode the mucus barrier. Cytotoxins and mucolytic enzymes (e.g. bacterial protease, lipase) produced by *H. pylori* may play a role in mucosal damage and subsequent ulcerogenesis.

Infected people are 3–6 times more likely to develop stomach cancer. *H. pylori* infection is associated with intestinal-type adenocarcinoma of the gastric body and antrum, but not cancer of the gastric cardia. Other associated cancers include gastric lymphoma and mucosa-associated lymphoid tissue (MALT) lymphoma, a monoclonally restricted B-cell tumor.

Diagnosis

Screening of asymptomatic patients is not warranted. Tests are done during evaluation for peptic ulcer and gastritis. Post-treatment testing is typically done to confirm eradication of the organism. Different tests are preferred for initial diagnosis and Post-treatment.

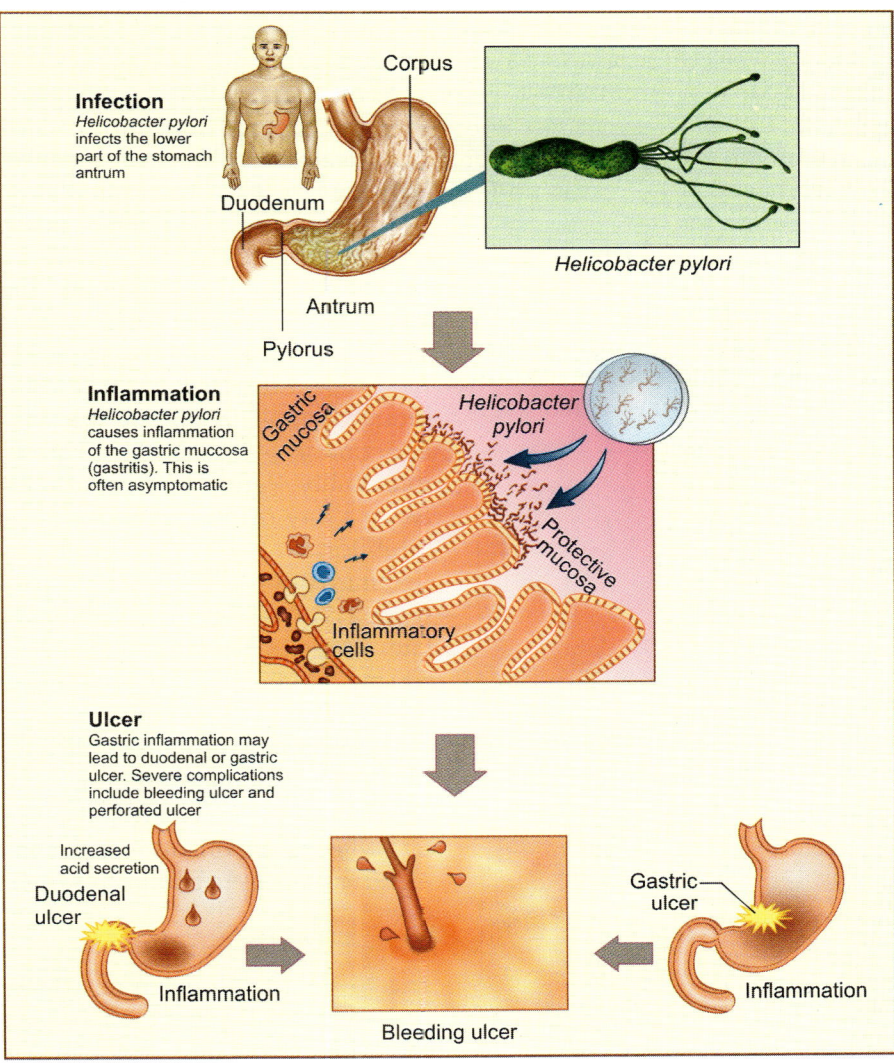

Fig. 6.3: Helicobacter pylori infection

Noninvasive Tests

Laboratory and office-based serologic assays for antibodies to *H. pylori* have sensitivity and specificity of >85% and are considered the noninvasive tests of choice for initial documentation of *H. pylori* infection. However, because qualitative assays remain positive for up to 3 years after successful treatment and because quantitative antibody levels do not decline significantly for 6–12 months after treatment, serologic assays are not usually used to assess cure.

Urea breath tests use an oral dose of $^{13}C/^{14}C$- labeled urea (Fig. 6.4). In an infected patient, the organism metabolizes the urea and liberates labeled CO_2, which is exhaled and can be quantified in breath samples taken 20–30 minutes after ingestion of the urea. Sensitivity and specificity are >90%. Urea breath tests are well-suited for confirming eradication of the organism after therapy. False-negative results are possible with recent antibiotic use or concomitant proton pump inhibitor therapy; therefore, follow-up testing should be delayed ≥4 weeks after antibiotic therapy and 1 week after proton pump inhibitor therapy. H_2 blockers do not affect the test.

Stool antigen assays seem to have a sensitivity and specificity near that of urea breath tests, particularly for initial diagnosis; an office-based stool test is under development.

Invasive Tests

Endoscopy is used to obtain mucosal biopsy samples for a rapid urease test (RUT) or histologic staining. Bacterial culture is of limited use because of the fastidious nature of the organism. Endoscopy is not recommended solely

for diagnosis of *H. pylori;* noninvasive tests are preferred unless endoscopy is indicated for other reasons.

The RUT, in which presence of bacterial urease in the biopsy sample causes a color change on a special medium, is the diagnostic method of choice on tissue samples. Histologic staining of biopsy samples should be done for patients with negative RUT results but suspicious clinical findings, recent antibiotic use, or treatment with proton pump inhibitors. RUT and histologic staining each have a sensitivity and specificity of >90%.

Treatment

Patients with complications (e.g., gastritis, ulcer, cancer) should have the organism eradicated. Eradication of *H. pylori* can even cure some cases of MALT lymphoma (but not other infection-related cancers). Treatment of asymptomatic infection has been controversial, but the recognition of the role of *H. pylori* in cancer has led to a recommendation for treatment. Vaccines, both preventive and therapeutic (i.e., as an adjunct to treatment of infected patients), are under development.

Helicobacter pylori eradication requires multidrug therapy, typically antibiotics plus acid suppressants. Proton pump inhibitors suppress *H. pylori,* and the increased gastric pH accompanying their use can enhance tissue concentration and efficacy of antimicrobials, creating a hostile environment for *H. pylori.*

Triple therapy is recommended. Oral omeprazole 20 mg twice a day or lansoprazole 30 mg twice a day, plus clarithromycin 500 mg twice a day, plus amoxicillin 1 g twice a day (or, for penicillin-allergic patients, metronidazole 500 mg twice a day) for 14 days, cures infection in >95% of cases. This regimen has excellent tolerability. Ranitidine bismuth citrate 400 mg by mouth twice a day may be substituted for the proton pump inhibitor.

Quadruple therapy with a proton pump inhibitor twice a day, tetracycline 500 mg and bismuth subsalicylate or subcitrate 525 mg 4 times a day and metronidazole 500 mg 3 times a day is also effective but more cumbersome.

Infected patients with duodenal or gastric ulcer require continuation of the acid suppression for at least 4 weeks.

Treatment is repeated if *H. pylori* is not eradicated. If two courses are unsuccessful, some authorities recommend endoscopy to obtain cultures for sensitivity testing.

THE SMALL INTESTINE DISEASES

The small intestine can be affected by many disease processes, but the major effects on function relate to the consequences of impaired absorption of nutrients and fluid, and to disruption of its barrier function.

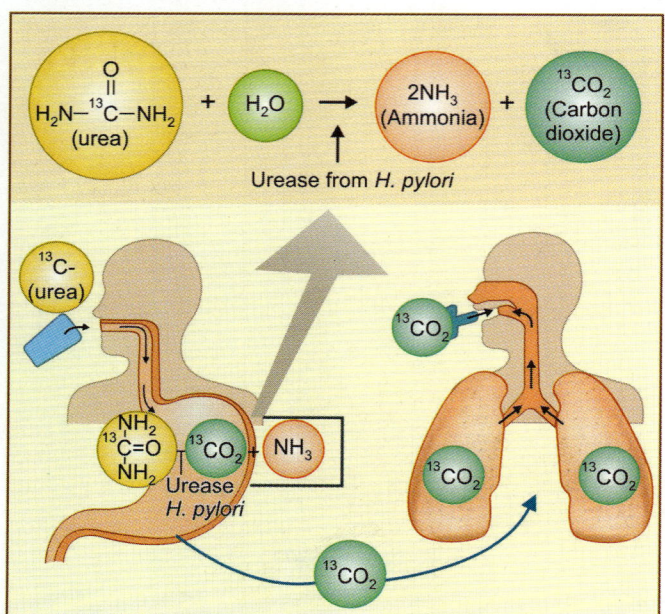

Fig. 6.4: Urea breath test

Celiac Disease

Celiac disease is an immunologically mediated disease in genetically susceptible people caused by intolerance to gluten, resulting in mucosal inflammation and villous atrophy (Fig. 6.5), which causes malabsorption. Symptoms usually include diarrhea and abdominal discomfort. Diagnosis is by small-bowel biopsies showing characteristic though not specific pathologic changes of villous atrophy that resolve with a strict gluten-free diet.

Etiology

Celiac disease is a hereditary disorder caused by sensitivity to the gliadin fraction of gluten, a protein found in wheat; similar proteins are present in rye and barley. In a genetically susceptible person, gluten-sensitive T cells are activated when gluten-derived peptide epitopes are presented. The inflammatory response causes characteristic mucosal villous atrophy in the small bowel.

Symptoms and Signs

The clinical presentation varies; no typical presentation exists. Some patients are asymptomatic or have only signs of nutritional deficiency. Others have significant GI symptoms.

Celiac disease can manifest in infancy and childhood after introduction of cereals into the diet. The child has failure to thrive, apathy, anorexia, pallor, generalized hypotonia, abdominal distention, and muscle wasting. Stools are soft, bulky, clay-colored, and offensive. Older children may present with anemia or failure to grow normally.

In adults, lassitude, weakness, and anorexia are most common. Mild and intermittent diarrhea is sometimes the presenting symptom. Steatorrhea ranges from mild to severe (7–50 g of fat/day). Some patients have weight loss, rarely enough to become underweight. Anemia, glossitis, angular stomatitis, and aphthous ulcers are usually seen in these patients. Manifestations of vitamin D and Ca deficiencies (e.g. osteomalacia, osteopenia, and osteoporosis) are common. Both men and women may have reduced fertility; women may not have menstrual periods.

About 10% of patients have dermatitis herpetiformis, an intensely pruritic papulovesicular rash that is symmetrically distributed over the extensor areas of the elbows, knees, buttocks, shoulders, and scalp. This rash can be induced by a high-gluten diet. Celiac disease is also associated with diabetes mellitus, autoimmune thyroid disease, and Down syndrome.

Diagnosis

The diagnosis is suspected clinically and by laboratory abnormalities suggestive of malabsorption. Family incidence is a valuable clue. Celiac disease should be strongly considered in a patient with iron deficiency without obvious GI bleeding.

Confirmation requires a small-bowel biopsy from the second portion of the duodenum. Findings include lack or shortening of villi (villous atrophy), increased intraepithelial cells, and crypt hyperplasia. However, such findings can also occur in tropical sprue, severe intestinal bacterial overgrowth, eosinophilic enteritis, lactose intolerance, and lymphoma.

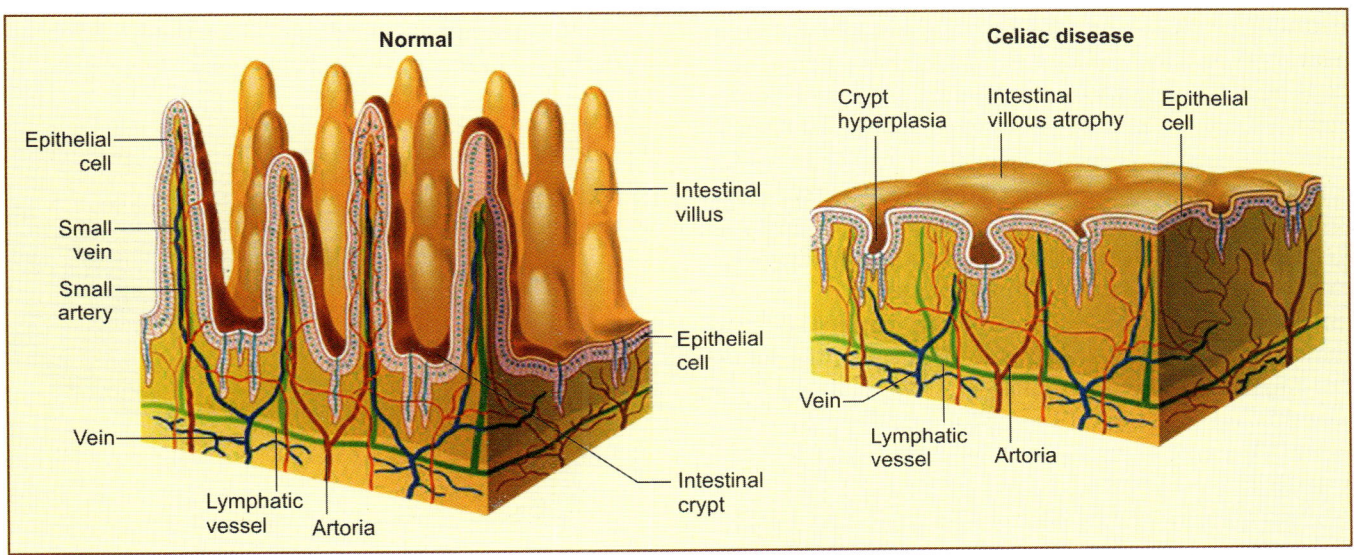

Fig. 6.5: Mucosal inflammation and villous atrophy in celiac disease

Because biopsy lacks specificity, serologic markers can aid diagnosis. Anti-tissue transglutaminase antibody (AGA) and anti-endomysial antibody (EMA; an antibody against an intestinal connective tissue protein) have sensitivity and specificity >90%. These markers can also be used to screen populations with high prevalence of celiac disease, including first-degree relatives of affected patients and patients with diseases that occur at a greater frequency in association with celiac disease. If either test is positive, the patient should have a diagnostic small-bowel biopsy. If both are negative, celiac disease is extremely unlikely. These antibodies decrease in titer in patients on a gluten-free diet and thus are useful in monitoring dietary adherence.

Other laboratory abnormalities often occur and should be sought. They include anemia (iron-deficiency anemia in children and folate-deficiency anemia in adults); low albumin, Ca, K, and Na; and elevated alkaline phosphatase and PT.

Malabsorption tests are not specific for celiac disease. If done, common findings include steatorrhea of 10–40 g/day and abnormal results with d-xylose and (in severe ileal disease) Schilling tests.

Prognosis

Complications include refractory disease, collagenous sprue, and intestinal lymphomas. Intestinal lymphomas affect 6–8% of patients with celiac disease, usually manifesting after 20–40 years of disease. The incidence of other GI cancers (e.g. carcinoma of the esophagus or oropharynx, small-bowel adenocarcinoma) also increases. Adherence to a gluten-free diet can significantly reduce the risk of cancer.

Treatment

Treatment is a gluten-free diet (avoiding foods containing wheat, rye, or barley). Gluten is so widely used (e.g. in commercial soups, sauces, ice creams, and hot dogs) that a patient needs a detailed list of foods to avoid. Patients are encouraged to consult a dietitian and join a celiac support group. The response to a gluten-free diet is usually rapid, and symptoms resolve in 1–2 weeks. Ingesting even small amounts of food containing gluten may prevent remission or induce relapse.

Small-bowel biopsy should be repeated after 3–4 months of a gluten-free diet. If abnormalities persist, other causes of villous atrophy (e.g. lymphoma) should be considered. Lessening of symptoms and improvement in small-bowel morphology are accompanied by a decrease in AGA and EMA titers.

Supplementary vitamins, minerals, and hematinics may be given, depending on the deficiencies. Mild cases may not require supplementation, whereas severe cases may require comprehensive replacement. For adults, replacement includes ferrous sulfate 300 mg by mouth once a day to 3 times a day, folate 5–10 mg by mouth once a day, Ca supplements, and any standard multivitamin. Sometimes children (but rarely adults) who are seriously ill on initial diagnosis require bowel rest and total parenteral nutrition (TPN).

If a patient responds poorly to gluten withdrawal, either the diagnosis is incorrect or the disease has become refractory. Corticosteroids can control symptoms in refractory disease.

CROHN'S DISEASE

Crohn's disease is a chronic transmural inflammatory disease that usually affects the distal ileum and colon but may occur in any part of the GI tract (Fig. 6.6).

Pathophysiology

Crohn's disease begins with crypt inflammation and abscesses, which progress to tiny focal aphthoid ulcers. These mucosal lesions may develop into deep longitudinal and transverse ulcers with intervening mucosal edema, creating a characteristic cobblestoned appearance to the bowel.

Transmural spread of inflammation leads to lymphedema and thickening of the bowel wall and mesentery. Mesenteric fat typically extends onto the serosal surface of the bowel. Mesenteric lymph nodes often enlarge. Extensive inflammation may result in hypertrophy of the muscularis mucosae, fibrosis, and stricture formation, which can lead to bowel obstruction. Abscesses are common, and fistulas often penetrate into adjoining structures, including other loops of bowel, the bladder, or psoas muscle. Fistulas may even extend to the skin of the anterior abdomen or flanks. Independently of intra-abdominal disease activity, perianal fistulas and

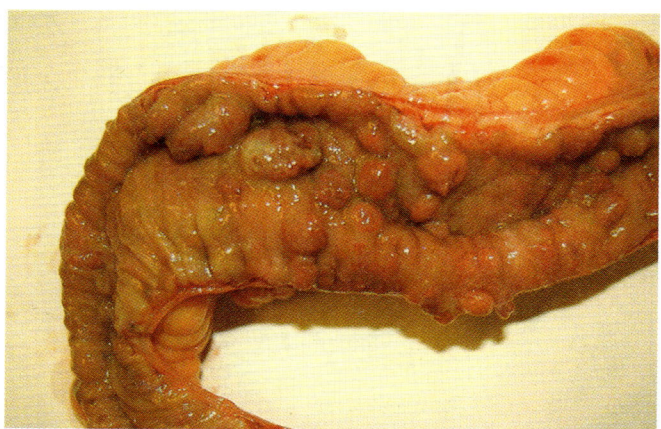

Fig. 6.6: Crohn's disease

abscesses occur in 25–33% of cases; these complications are frequently the most troublesome aspects of Crohn's disease.

Noncaseating granulomas can occur in lymph nodes, peritoneum, the liver, and all layers of the bowel wall. Although, pathognomonic when present, granulomas are not detected in about half of patients with Crohn's disease. The presence of granulomas does not seem to be related to the clinical course.

Symptoms and Signs

The abdomen is tender, and a mass or fullness may be palpable. Gross rectal bleeding is unusual except in isolated colonic disease. Some patients present with an acute abdomen that simulates acute appendicitis or intestinal obstruction. About 33% of patients have perianal disease (especially fissures and fistulas), which is sometimes the most prominent or even initial complaint.

In children, extraintestinal manifestations frequently predominate over GI symptoms; arthritis, anemia, or growth retardation may be a presenting symptom, whereas abdominal pain or diarrhea may be absent.

With recurrent disease, symptoms vary. Pain is most common and occurs with both simple recurrence and abscess formation. Patients with severe flare-up or abscess are likely to have marked tenderness, guarding, rebound, and a general toxic appearance. Stenotic segments may cause bowel obstruction, with colicky pain, distention, obstipation, and vomiting. Adhesions from previous surgery may also cause bowel obstruction, which begins rapidly, without the prodrome of fever, pain, and malaise, typical of obstruction due to a Crohn's disease flare-up. An enterovesical fistula may produce air bubbles in the urine (pneumaturia). Draining cutaneous fistulas may occur. Free perforation into the peritoneal cavity is unusual.

Chronic Disease

Chronic disease causes a variety of systemic symptoms, including fever, weight loss, undernutrition, and extraintestinal manifestations.

Diagnosis

Crohn's disease should be suspected in a patient with inflammatory or obstructive symptoms or in a patient without prominent GI symptoms but with perianal fistulas or abscesses or with otherwise unexplained arthritis, erythema nodosum, fever, anemia, or (in a child) stunted growth. A family history of Crohn's disease also increases the index of suspicion.

Patients presenting with an acute abdomen (either initially or during a relapse) should have flat and upright abdominal X-rays and an abdominal CT scan. These may show obstruction, abscesses or fistulas, and other possible causes of an acute abdomen (e.g. appendicitis). Ultrasonography may better delineate gynecologic pathology in women with lower abdominal and pelvic pain.

If initial presentation is less acute, an upper GI series with small-bowel follow-through and spot films of the terminal ileum is preferred over conventional CT. However, newer techniques of CT or MR enterography, which combine high-resolution CT or MRI with large volumes of ingested contrast, are becoming the procedures of choice in some centers. These imaging studies are virtually diagnostic if they show characteristic strictures or fistulas with accompanying separation of bowel loops. If findings are questionable, CT enteroclysis or video capsule enteroscopy may show superficial aphthous and linear ulcers. Barium enema X-ray may be used if symptoms seem predominantly colonic (e.g. diarrhea) and may show reflux of barium into the terminal ileum with irregularity, nodularity, stiffness, wall thickening, and a narrowed lumen. Differential diagnoses in patients with similar X-ray findings include cancer of the cecum, ileal carcinoid, lymphoma, systemic vasculitis, radiation enteritis, ileocecal TB, and ameboma.

In atypical cases (e.g. predominantly diarrhea, with minimal pain), evaluation is similar to suspected ulcerative colitis (UC), with colonoscopy (including biopsy, sampling for enteric pathogens, and, when possible, visualization of the terminal ileum). Upper GI endoscopy may identify subtle gastroduodenal involvement even in the absence of upper GI symptoms.

Laboratory tests should be done to screen for anemia, hypoalbuminemia, and electrolyte abnormalities. Liver function tests should be done; elevated alkaline phosphatase and γ-glutamyl transpeptidase levels in patients with major colonic involvement suggest possible primary sclerosing cholangitis. Leukocytosis or Increased levels of acute-phase reactants [e.g. erythrocyte sedimentation rate (ESR), C-reactive protein) are nonspecific but may be used serially to monitor disease activity. To detect nutritional deficiencies, levels of vitamin D and B12 should be checked every 1–2 years. Additional laboratory measurements, such as levels of water-soluble vitamins (folic acid and niacin), fat-soluble vitamins (A, D, E and K), and minerals (zinc, selenium, and copper) may be checked when deficiencies are suspected. All patients with inflammatory bowel disease (IBD), whether male or female, young or old, should have their bone mineral density monitored, usually by dual-energy X-ray absorptiometry scan.

Perinuclear antineutrophil cytoplasmic antibodies are present in 60–70% of patients with UC and in only 5–20% of patients with Crohn's disease. Anti-*Saccharomyces cerevisiae* antibodies are relatively specific for Crohn's disease. However, these tests do not reliably separate the two diseases. They have uncertain value in cases of indeterminate colitis and are not recommended for routine diagnosis. Additional antibodies, such as anti-OmpC and anti-CBir1 are now available, but the clinical value of these supplementary tests is uncertain.

Prognosis

Established Crohn's disease is rarely cured but is characterized by intermittent exacerbations and remissions. Some patients have severe disease with frequent, debilitating periods of pain. However, with judicious medical therapy and, where appropriate, surgical therapy, most patients function well and adapt successfully.

Disease-related mortality is very low. GI cancer, including cancer of the colon and small bowel, is the leading cause of excess Crohn's disease-related mortality.

Treatment

General Management

Cramps and diarrhea may be relieved by oral administration of loperamide 2–4 mg or antispasmodic drugs up to 4 times a day (ideally before meals). Such symptomatic treatment is safe, except in cases of severe, acute Crohn's colitis, which may progress to toxic megacolon.

Hydrophilic mucilloids (e.g. methylcellulose or psyllium preparations), sometimes help prevent anal irritation by increasing stool firmness. Dietary roughage is to be avoided in stricturing disease or active colonic inflammation.

Mild to Moderate Disease

This category includes ambulatory patients who tolerate oral intake and have no signs of toxicity, tenderness, mass, or obstruction.

Mesalamine or 5-aminosalicylic acid (5-ASA) is commonly used as first-line treatment, although its benefits for small-bowel disease are modest at best. Pentasa is the most effective formulation for disease proximal to the terminal ileum; Asacol is effective in distal ileal disease. All formulations are roughly equivalent for Crohn's colitis, although none of the newer preparations rival sulfasalazine for efficacy on a dose-for-dose basis.

Antibiotics are considered a first-line agent by some clinicians, or they may be reserved for patients not responding to 4 weeks of 5-ASA; their use is strictly empiric. With any of these drugs, 8–16 weeks of treatment may be required.

Moderate to Severe Disease

Patients without fistulas or abscesses but with significant pain, tenderness, fever, or vomiting, or those who have not responded to treatment for mild disease, require corticosteroids, either oral or parenteral, depending on severity of symptoms and frequency of vomiting. Oral prednisone or prednisolone may act more rapidly and reliably than oral budesonide, but budesonide has somewhat fewer adverse effects and is considered the corticosteroid of choice in many centers, especially in Europe.

Patients not responding to corticosteroids, or those whose doses cannot be tapered, should receive azathioprine, 6-mercaptopurine, or possibly methotrexate. An anti-tumor necrosis factor (TNF) agent (infliximab, adalimumab, or certolizumab pegol) is preferred by some as second-line therapy after corticosteroids, and even as first-line therapy in preference to corticosteroids, but its use is contraindicated in active uncontrolled infection.

Obstruction is managed initially with nasogastric suction and IV fluids. Obstruction due to uncomplicated Crohn's disease should resolve within a few days and therefore does not require parenteral nutrition; absence of prompt response indicates a complication or another etiology and demands immediate surgery.

Fulminant Disease or Abscess

Patients with toxic appearance, high fever, persistent vomiting, rebound, or a tender or palpable mass must be hospitalized for administration of intravenous (IV) fluids and antibiotics. Abscesses must be drained, either percutaneously or surgically. IV corticosteroids should be given only when infection has been ruled out or controlled. If there is no response to corticosteroids and antibiotics within 5–7 days, surgery is usually indicated.

FISTULAS

Fistulas are treated initially with metronidazole and ciprofloxacin. Patients who do not respond in 3–4 weeks may receive an immunomodulator (e.g. azathioprine, 6-mercaptopurine), with or without an induction regimen of infliximab or adalimumab for more rapid response. Anti-TNF therapy (infliximab or adalimumab) can also be used alone. Cyclosporine is an alternative, but fistulas often relapse after treatment.

Severe refractory perianal fistulas may require temporary diverting colostomy but almost invariably recur after reconnection; hence, diversion is more appropriately considered a preparation for definitive surgery or at best an adjunct to infliximab or adalimumab rather than a primary treatment.

Maintenance Therapy

Patients who require only 5-ASA or an antibiotic to achieve remission can be maintained on that drug. Patients requiring acute treatment with corticosteroids or anti-TNF agents typically require azathioprine, 6-mercaptopurine, methotrexate, or anti-TNF therapy for maintenance. Many, if not most patients brought into remission with an anti-TNF, will require escalation of the dose or shortening of the treatment intervals within a year or two. Systemically active corticosteroids are neither safe nor effective for long-term maintenance, although budesonide has been shown to delay relapse with fewer adverse effects. Patients who respond to anti-TNF therapy for acute disease but who are not well maintained on antimetabolites may stay in remission with repeat doses of anti-TNF agents.

Monitoring during remission can be done by following symptoms and doing blood tests and does not require routine X-rays or colonoscopy (other than regular surveillance for dysplasia after 7–8 years of disease).

SURGERY

Even though about 70% of patients ultimately require an operation, surgery is often done reluctantly. It is best reserved for recurrent intestinal obstruction or intractable fistulas or abscesses. Resection of the involved bowel may ameliorate symptoms but does not cure the disease, which is likely to recur even after resection of all clinically apparent lesions.

Malabsorption

Malabsorption is inadequate assimilation of dietary substances due to defects in digestion, absorption, or transport.

Malabsorption can affect macronutrients (e.g. proteins, carbohydrates, and fats), micronutrients (e.g. vitamins, minerals), or both, causing excessive fecal excretion, nutritional deficiencies, and GI symptoms. Malabsorption may be global, with impaired absorption of almost all nutrients, or partial (isolated), with malabsorption of only specific nutrients.

Pathophysiology

Digestion and absorption occur in three phases:
- Intraluminal hydrolysis of fats, proteins, and carbohydrates by enzymes—bile salts enhance the solubilization of fat in this phase

- Digestion by brush border enzymes and uptake of end-products
- Lymphatic transport of nutrients

The term malabsorption is commonly used when any of these phases is impaired, but, strictly speaking, impairment of phase 1 is maldigestion rather than malabsorption.

Fats

Pancreatic enzymes (lipase and colipase) split long-chain triglycerides into fatty acids and monoglycerides, which combine with bile acids and phospholipids to form micelles that pass through jejunal enterocytes. Absorbed fatty acids are resynthesized and combined with protein, cholesterol, and phospholipid to form chylomicrons, which are transported by the lymphatic system. Medium-chain triglycerides are absorbed directly.

Unabsorbed fats trap fat-soluble vitamins (A, D, E, and K) and possibly some minerals, causing deficiency. Bacterial overgrowth results in deconjugation and dehydroxylation of bile salts, limiting the absorption of fats. Unabsorbed bile salts stimulate water secretion in the colon, causing diarrhea.

Carbohydrates

The pancreatic enzyme amylase and brush border enzymes on microvilli lyse carbohydrates and disaccharides into constituent monosaccharides. Colonic bacteria ferment unabsorbed carbohydrates into CO_2, methane, H_2, and short-chain fatty acids (butyrate, propionate, acetate, and lactate). These fatty acids cause diarrhea. The gases cause abdominal distention and bloating.

Proteins

Gastric pepsin initiates digestion of proteins in the stomach (and also stimulates release of cholecystokinin that is critical to the secretion of pancreatic enzymes). Enterokinase, a brush border enzyme, activates trypsinogen into trypsin, which converts many pancreatic proteases into their active forms. Active pancreatic enzymes hydrolyze proteins into oligopeptides, which are absorbed directly or hydrolyzed into amino acids.

Etiology

Malabsorption has many causes (Table 6.3). Some malabsorptive disorders (e.g. celiac disease), impair the absorption of most nutrients, vitamins, and trace minerals (global malabsorption); others (e.g. pernicious anemia) are more selective.

Table 6.3	Causes of malabsorption
Mechanism	**Cause**
Inadequate gastric mixing, rapid emptying, or both	Billroth II gastrectomy
	Gastrocolic fistula
	Gastroenterostomy
Insufficient digestive agents	Biliary obstruction and cholestasis
	Cirrhosis
	Chronic pancreatitis
	Cholestyramine-induced bile acid loss
	Cystic fibrosis
	Lactase deficiency
	Pancreatic cancer
	Pancreatic resection
	Sucrase-isomaltase deficiency
Abnormal milieu	Abnormal motility secondary to diabetes, scleroderma, hypothyroidism, or hyperthyroidism
	Bacterial overgrowth due to blind loops (deconjugation of bile salts), diverticula in the small intestine
	Zollinger–Ellison syndrome (low duodenal pH)
Acutely abnormal epithelium	Acute intestinal infections
	Alcohol
	Neomycin
Chronically abnormal epithelium	Amyloidosis
	Celiac disease
	Crohn's disease
	Ischemia
	Radiation enteritis
	Tropical sprue
	Whipple disease
Short bowel	Intestinal resection (e.g. for Crohn's disease, volvulus, intussusception, or infarction)
	Jejunoileal bypass for obesity
Impaired transport	Abetalipoproteinemia
	Addison disease
	Blocked lacteals due to lymphoma or TB
	Intrinsic factor deficiency (as in pernicious anemia)
	Lymphangiectasia

Pancreatic insufficiency causes malabsorption if >90% of function is lost. Increased luminal acidity (e.g. Zollinger–Ellison syndrome) inhibits lipase and fat digestion. Cirrhosis and cholestasis reduce hepatic bile synthesis or delivery of bile salts to the duodenum, causing malabsorption.

Symptoms and Signs

The effects of unabsorbed substances, especially in global malabsorption, include diarrhea, steatorrhea, abdominal bloating, and gas. Other symptoms result from nutritional deficiencies. Patients often lose weight despite adequate food intake.

Chronic diarrhea is the most common symptom and is what usually prompts evaluation of the patient. Steatorrhea; fatty stool, the hallmark of malabsorption; occurs when >7 g/day of fat are excreted. Steatorrhea causes foul-smelling, pale, bulky, and greasy stools.

Severe vitamin and mineral deficiencies occur in advanced malabsorption; symptoms are related to the specific nutrient deficiency (Table 6.4). Vitamin B12 deficiency may occur in blind loop syndrome or after extensive resection of the distal ileum or stomach. Iron deficiency may be the only symptom in a patient with mild malabsorption.

Amenorrhea may result from undernutrition and is an important manifestation of celiac disease in young women.

Diagnosis

Malabsorption is suspected in a patient with chronic diarrhea, weight loss, and anemia. The etiology is sometimes obvious. For example, patients with malabsorption due to chronic pancreatitis usually have had prior bouts of acute pancreatitis. Patients with celiac disease can present with classic lifelong diarrhea exacerbated by gluten products and may have dermatitis herpetiformis. Patients with cirrhosis and pancreatic cancer can present with jaundice. Abdominal distention, excessive flatus, and watery diarrhea occurring 30–90 minutes after carbohydrate ingestion suggest deficiency of a disaccharidase enzyme, usually lactase. Previous extensive abdominal operations suggest short bowel syndrome.

If the history suggests a specific cause, testing should be directed to that condition. If no cause is readily apparent, blood tests can be used as screening tools [e.g. complete blood count, (CBC), red blood cells (RBC) indices, ferritin, vitamin B12, folate, Ca, albumin, cholesterol, prothrombin time (PT)]. Test results may suggest a diagnosis and direct further investigation.

Table 6.4	Symptoms of malabsorption
Symptom	**Malabsorbed nutrient**
Anemia (hypochromic, microcytic)	Iron
Anemia (macrocytic)	Vitamin B12, folate
Bleeding, bruising, petechiae	Vitamins K and C
Carpopedal spasm	Ca, Mg
Edema	Protein
Glossitis	Vitamins B_2 and B12, folate, niacin, iron
Night blindness	Vitamin A
Pain in limbs, bones, pathologic fractures	K, Mg, Ca, vitamin D
Peripheral neuropathy	Vitamins B_1, B_6, B12

Macrocytic anemia should prompt measurement of serum folate and B12 levels. Folate deficiency is common in mucosal disorders involving the proximal small bowel (e.g. celiac disease, tropical sprue, Whipple disease. Low B12 levels can occur in pernicious anemia, chronic pancreatitis, bacterial overgrowth, and terminal ileal disease. A combination of low B12 and high folate levels is suggestive of bacterial overgrowth, because intestinal bacteria use vitamin B12 and synthesize folate.

Microcytic anemia suggests iron deficiency, which may occur with celiac disease. Albumin is a general indicator of nutritional state. Low albumin can result from poor intake, decreased synthesis in cirrhosis, or protein wasting. Low serum carotene (a precursor of vitamin A) suggests malabsorption if intake is adequate.

INVESTIGATION OF INTESTINAL FUNCTION

Tests of Carbohydrate Absorption

A variety of tests involving the ingestion of carbohydrates and the measurement of their plasma concentrations or urinary excretion were developed for the investigation of small intestinal function, prior to the widespread use of endoscopic biopsy. The best known is the xylose absorption test, which involves the administration of a test dose of d-xylose, a plant sugar. This is absorbed from the jejunum without prior digestion. It is only partly metabolized in the body, mainly being excreted unchanged in the urine, where it can be measured. Accurately timed urine collection is essential. Misleadingly low results are obtained if the glomerular filtration rate is decreased, as occurs in renal failure and many normal elderly people. Other factors that can produce misleading results include delayed gastric emptying, edema, and obesity. An alternative approach is to measure serum xylose concentration 60 minutes after administering xylose.

The diagnostic performance of the xylose test is improved by giving the xylose (5.0 g) together with 3-O-methyl-d-glucose (2.5 g) and comparing the absorption of the two sugars by measurement of their plasma concentrations. However, pharmaceutical grade 3-O-methyl-d-glucose is now difficult to obtain. In practice, the ease with which the proximal small intestine can now be biopsied has greatly reduced the need for and use of such investigations.

Some conditions of the small intestine, including inflammatory bowel diseases, give rise to increased gut permeability. This can be assessed by measuring the fecal concentration of the neutrophil protein, calprotectin. This is increased in almost all patients with IBD, correlates well with disease activity and is predictive of relapse in patients in remission. Of great practical importance is the fact that fecal calprotectin is usually normal in patients with irritable bowel syndrome (IBS), so that the demonstration of a normal value obviates the need for more extensive investigation of patients in whom a diagnosis of IBD or IBS is being considered.

Suspected intestinal disaccharidase deficiency can be investigated by administering the appropriate disaccharide (50 g) orally and measuring the blood glucose response. If the result is abnormal, specificity can be improved by comparing the result with that obtained following administration of the equivalent quantities (25 g each) of the constituent monosaccharides. The test is unphysiological because of the large oral load of, for example, lactose, although patients who do not develop symptoms during the test are not lactose intolerant. A more reliable test is to measure breath hydrogen after giving the disaccharide (Fig. 6.7) because it is not absorbed, the disaccharide reaches the colon, where one of the products of bacterial fermentation is hydrogen. Another approach to the investigation of disaccharidase deficiencies is measurement of the appropriate enzyme in a biopsy sample.

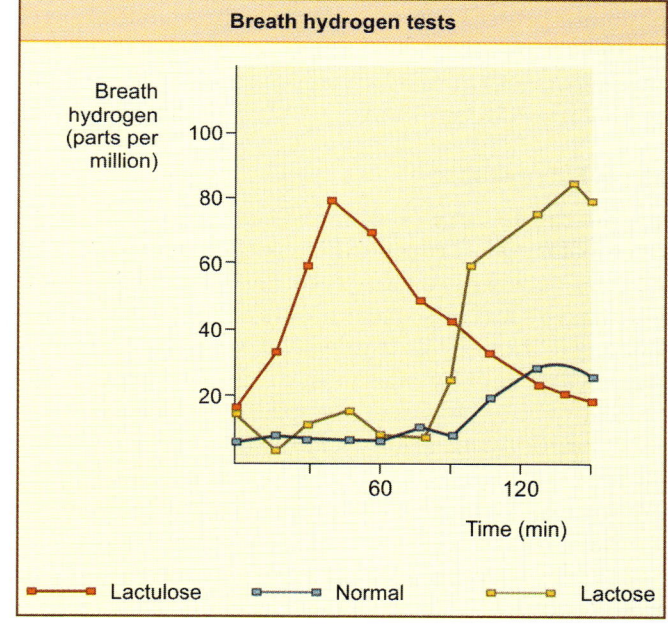

Fig. 6.7: Breath hydrogen tests. Hydrogen is not produced by mammalian cells; its presence in expired air is due to bacterial fermentation of unabsorbed carbohydrate. Typical results are shown from the test performed in a patient with bacterial colonization of the small intestine when challenged with oral lactulose (10 g), where the lactulose acts as a substrate for bacterial metabolism, and in a patient with intestinal lactase deficiency when challenged with oral lactose (50 g), compared with a normal individual given lactose. Hydrogen is generated by the fermentation of unabsorbed lactose in the colon, with the result that the increase in breath hydrogen occurs later than with small intestinal bacterial overgrowth

The most common disaccharidase deficiency affects lactase. It may be congenital or acquired; it often occurs transiently when there is damage to gut mucosa, such as after gastroenteritis. Less common are sucrase–isomaltase and maltase deficiencies.

Tests of Amino Acid Absorption

Tests of amino acid absorption from the gut are only used as research procedures. Generalized malabsorption of amino acids occurs only with extensive small bowel disease. Malabsorption of specific amino acids occurs in certain inherited metabolic disorders, e.g. deficiency of tryptophan can occur in Hartnup disease, an inherited disorder of the transport of neutral amino acids. In cystinuria, there is impaired transport of the dibasic amino acids lysine, cystine, ornithine, and arginine, but this condition is not associated with a deficiency syndrome.

Loss of protein from the gut in a protein-losing enteropathy can be assessed by measuring fecal radioactivity after parenteral administration of isotopically labelled proteins (e.g. ^{51}Cr-albumin, or polyvinylpyrrolidone), or by measuring fecal α_1-antitrypsin (which resists enzymatic proteolysis on its passage through the bowel). Such investigations are not frequently performed, however, as the cause of any hypoproteinemia is usually obvious in such conditions.

Tests of Fat Absorption

Because the absorption of fat is a complex process, the effects of fat malabsorption are often a prominent feature of generalized malabsorption. For this reason, and because fat malabsorption can occur with gastric, pancreatic, hepatic and intestinal disease, tests of fat absorption can be used to diagnose generalized malabsorption. However, the presence of generalized malabsorption can often be reliably inferred from clinical findings (particularly steatorrhea) and the results of simple tests. Further investigations will then be required to determine the cause of malabsorption, but formal tests to confirm its presence are now required only infrequently.

Fecal Fat Test

Fat absorption has traditionally been assessed by measuring the excretion of fat in faces. After digestion, dietary fat is normally absorbed completely in the small intestine; a small quantity of fat (<18 mmol/24 hours) is excreted in faces, but this fat is derived from enterocytes.

With malabsorption of fat, its excretion in the feces is increased. However, a major problem with its measurement is the need to obtain an accurately timed fecal collection. Collections should preferably be made for five consecutive days, although for practical reasons 3-day collections are more often used. This test is unpleasant for all concerned and is only of any value if performed correctly. Dietetic guidance should be sought to ensure that the patient consumes 90–100 g fat/day for 48 hours before and during the period of collection; if less fat is ingested, minor degrees of malabsorption may be missed. In practice, few laboratories now include this investigation in their repertoire and many experts consider it to be obsolete.

Triolein Breath Test

This was developed as an alternative to the measurement of fecal fat excretion. The principle of the test is that, when isotopically labelled triolein is given orally, digested and absorbed, some of the label appears in the breath as isotopically labelled carbon dioxide, which can be measured using appropriate equipment. The triolein is labelled with either ^{13}C, a stable isotope, or ^{14}C, which is radioactive. As it is the specific activity of the expired carbon dioxide that is measured, a constant rate of production of carbon dioxide from all other sources must be assumed; patients must be fasting and must rest throughout the test. This test has also largely fallen into disuse.

Tests for Bacterial Overgrowth

Bacterial overgrowth in the small intestine can occur in a number of conditions, particularly when there is stasis of gut contents, e.g. as a result of a stricture or in jejunal diverticulosis. Bacterial deconjugation of bile acids leads to failure of mixed micelle formation and malabsorption of fat.

The most reliable diagnostic test for bacterial overgrowth is aspiration and culture of duodenal contents. However, this method has disadvantages, it is an invasive procedure and the cultures are sometimes negative when other evidence of bacterial overgrowth is overwhelming.

The measurement of urinary indicans (products of the bacterial metabolism of tryptophan) was formerly widely used to screen for bacterial overgrowth, but results correlate poorly with those of duodenal aspiration.

Breath tests can be used to diagnose bacterial overgrowth. Breath hydrogen is increased in this condition, particularly after administration of a non-absorbable carbohydrate (Fig. 6.7); the breath hydrogen test has largely replaced the ^{13}C/^{14}C-labelled xylose and the ^{13}C/^{14}C-labelled glycocholic acid breath tests.

Tests of Terminal Ileal Function

Terminal ileal function can be investigated using the Schilling test of vitamin B12 absorption, as this vitamin is absorbed in the terminal ileum. The test involves giving vitamin B12 with and without intrinsic factor (necessary for its absorption) and measuring the subsequent urinary excretion. The test involves the use of radioactive isotopes and is now rarely used. Malabsorption of vitamin B12 occurs in pernicious anemia, an autoimmune disease, and suspected pernicious anemia is now usually investigated by measuring serum vitamin B12 concentration and anti-parietal cell and anti-intrinsic factor antibodies.

Non-biochemical Tests of Intestinal Function

The mucosa of the small intestine can be biopsied endoscopically under direct vision. **Wireless capsule endoscopy** can also be used to visualize the inside of the small intestine. **Small intestinal biopsy** is the definitive procedure for the diagnosis of coeliac disease. The diagnosis of disaccharidase deficiencies can also be confirmed by measuring the enzyme in an intestinal biopsy.

WHIPPLE DISEASE

Whipple disease is a rare systemic illness caused by the bacterium *Tropheryma whippelii*. Main symptoms are arthritis, weight loss, abdominal pain, and diarrhea. Diagnosis is by small-bowel biopsy. Treatment is initially with ceftriaxone or penicillin followed by a minimum 1 year of trimethoprim/sulfamethoxazole.

Whipple disease predominately affects white men aged 30–60. Although, it affects many parts of the body, (e.g. heart, lung, brain, serous cavities, joints, eye, and GI tract), the mucosa of the small bowel is almost always involved. Affected patients may have subtle defects of cell-mediated immunity that predispose to infection with *T. whippelii*. About 30% of patients have HLA-B27.

Symptoms and Signs

Clinical presentation varies depending on the organ systems affected. The four cardinal symptoms of Whipple disease are arthralgia, diarrhea, abdominal pain, and weight loss.

Usually, the first symptoms are arthritis and fever. Intestinal symptoms (e.g. watery diarrhea, steatorrhea, abdominal pain, anorexia, weight loss), usually manifest later, sometimes years after the initial complaint. Gross or occult intestinal bleeding may occur. Severe malabsorption may be present in patients diagnosed late in the clinical course. Other findings include increased skin pigmentation, anemia, lymphadenopathy, chronic cough, serositis, peripheral edema, and CNS symptoms.

Diagnosis

The diagnosis may be missed in patients without prominent GI symptoms. Whipple disease should be suspected in middle-aged white men who have arthritis and abdominal pain, diarrhea, weight loss, or other symptoms of malabsorption. Such patients should have upper endoscopy with small-bowel biopsy; the intestinal lesions are specific and diagnostic. The most severe and consistent changes are in the proximal small bowel. Light microscopy shows periodic acid-Schiff–positive macrophages that distort the villus architecture. Gram-positive, acid fast–negative bacilli (*T. whippelii*) are seen in the lamina propria and in the macrophages. Confirmation by electron microscopy is recommended.

Whipple disease should be differentiated from intestinal infection with *Mycobacterium avium-intracellulare* (MAI), which has similar histologic findings. However, MAI stains positive with acid fast. Polymerase chain reaction (PCR) testing may be useful for confirmation.

Treatment

Untreated disease is progressive and fatal. Many antibiotics are curative (e.g. tetracycline, trimethoprim/sulfamethoxazole, penicillin, cephalosporins). Treatment is initiated with ceftriaxone (2 g IV daily) or penicillin G (1.5–6 million units IV q 6 hours). This regimen is followed by a long-term course of trimethoprim sulfamethoxazole (160/800 mg by mouth twice a day for 1 year). Sulfa-allergic patients may substitute oral penicillin V potassium (K) or ampicillin. Prompt clinical improvement occurs, with fever and joint pains resolving in a few days. Intestinal symptoms usually abate within 1–4 weeks.

To confirm response to treatment, PCR testing can be done on stool, saliva, or other tissue. However, other authorities recommend repeat biopsy after 1 year with electron microscopy to document bacilli (not just macrophages, which may persist for years after successful treatment).

Relapses are common and may occur years later. If relapse is suspected, small-bowel biopsies or PCR testing should be done (regardless of affected organ systems) to determine presence of free bacilli.

PANCREATIC DISORDERS AND THEIR INVESTIGATION

The major disorders of the exocrine pancreas are acute pancreatitis, chronic pancreatitis, pancreatic cancer, and cystic fibrosis. Biochemical investigations are essential in the diagnosis and management of the first of these, of limited use in the second, and of little use in the third. Cystic fibrosis, an inherited metabolic disease causing progressive loss of pancreatic function. Clinical evidence of impaired exocrine function is usually only seen in advanced pancreatic disease. Endocrine function is usually well preserved, although glucose intolerance or frank diabetes can develop in severe or advanced disease.

Acute Pancreatitis

Acute pancreatitis is an inflammation of the pancreas and, sometimes, adjacent tissues (Fig. 6.8) caused by the release of activated pancreatic enzymes. The most common triggers are biliary tract disease and chronic heavy alcohol intake. The condition ranges from mild (abdominal pain and vomiting) to severe (pancreatic necrosis and a systemic inflammatory process with shock and multiorgan failure). Diagnosis is based on clinical presentation and serum amylase and lipase levels. Treatment is supportive, with IV fluids, analgesics, and fasting.

Etiology

Biliary tract disease and alcoholism account for ≥80% of acute pancreatitis cases. The remaining 20% result from myriad causes (Table 6.5).

Pathophysiology

The precise mechanism by which obstruction of the sphincter of Oddi by a gallstone or microlithiasis (sludge) causes pancreatitis is unclear, although it probably involves increased ductal pressure. Prolonged alcohol intake may cause the protein of pancreatic enzymes to precipitate within small pancreatic ductules. Ductal obstruction by these protein plugs may cause premature activation of pancreatic enzymes. An alcohol binge in such patients can trigger pancreatitis, but the exact mechanism is not known.

A number of genetic mutations predisposing to pancreatitis have been identified. One, an autosomal dominant mutation of the cationic trypsinogen gene, causes pancreatitis in 80% of carriers; an obvious familial pattern is present. Other mutations have lesser penetrance and are not readily apparent clinically except through genetic testing. The genetic abnormality responsible for cystic fibrosis increases the risk of recurrent acute as well as chronic pancreatitis.

Regardless of the etiology, pancreatic enzymes (including trypsin, phospholipase A_2, and elastase) become

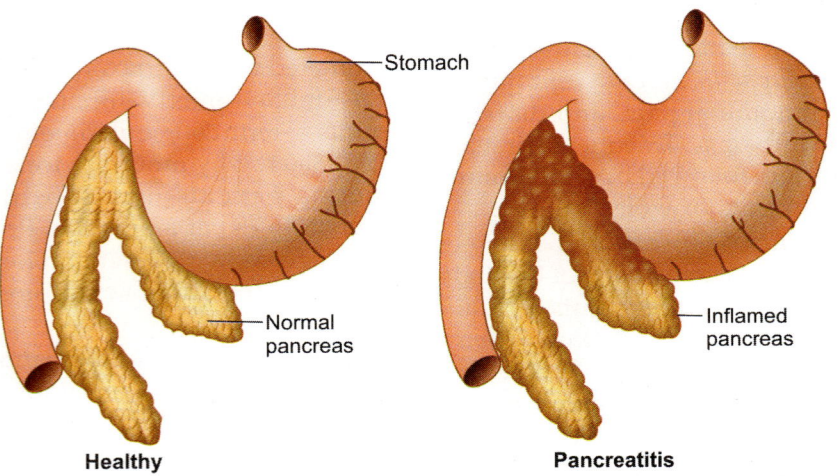

Fig. 6.8: Inflamed pancreas pancreatitis

Table 6.5	Causes of acute pancreatitis
Cause	**Examples**
Drugs	ACE inhibitors, asparaginase, azathioprine, 2′,3′-dideoxyinosine, furosemide, 6-mercaptopurine, pentamidine, sulfa drugs, valproate
Infectious	Coxsackie B virus, cytomegalovirus, mumps
Inherited	Multiple known gene mutations, including a small percentage of cystic fibrosis patients
Mechanical/Structural	Gallstones, endoscopic retrograde cholangiopancreatography (ERCP), trauma, pancreatic or periampullary cancer, choledochal cyst, sphincter of Oddi stenosis, pancreas divisum
Metabolic	Hypertriglyceridemia, hypercalcemia (including hyperparathyroidism), estrogen use associated with high lipid levels
Toxins	Alcohol, methanol
Other	Pregnancy, postrenal transplant, ischemia caused by hypotension or atheroembolism, tropical pancreatitis

ACF inhibitors, angiotensin-converting enzyme inhibitor

activated within the gland itself. The enzymes can damage tissue and activate the complement system and the inflammatory cascade, producing cytokines. This process causes inflammation, edema, and sometimes necrosis. In mild pancreatitis, inflammation is confined to the pancreas; the mortality rate is <5%. In severe pancreatitis, there is significant inflammation, with necrosis and hemorrhage of the gland and a systemic inflammatory response; the mortality rate is 10–50%. After 5–7 days, necrotic pancreatic tissue may become infected by enteric bacteria.

Activated enzymes and cytokines that enter the peritoneal cavity cause a chemical burn and third spacing of fluid; those that enter the systemic circulation cause a systemic inflammatory response that can result in acute respiratory distress syndrome and renal failure. The systemic effects are mainly the result of increased capillary permeability and decreased vascular tone, which result from the released cytokines and chemokines. Phospholipase A_2 is thought to injure alveolar membranes of the lungs.

In about 40% of patients, collections of enzyme-rich pancreatic fluid and tissue debris form in and around the pancreas. In about half, the collections resolve spontaneously. In others, the collections become infected or form pseudocysts. Pseudocysts have a fibrous capsule without an epithelial lining. Pseudocysts may hemorrhage, rupture, or become infected.

Death during the first several days is usually caused by cardiovascular instability (with refractory shock and renal failure) or respiratory failure (with hypoxemia and at times adult respiratory distress syndrome). Occasionally, death results from heart failure secondary to an unidentified myocardial depressant factor. Death after the first week is usually caused by multiorgan system failure.

Symptoms and Signs

An acute attack causes steady, boring upper abdominal pain, typically severe enough to require large doses of parenteral opioids. The pain radiates through to the back in about 50% of patients; rarely, pain is first felt in the lower abdomen. Pain usually develops suddenly in gallstone pancreatitis; in alcoholic pancreatitis, pain develops over a few days. The pain usually persists for several days. Sitting up and leaning forward may reduce pain, but coughing, vigorous movement, and deep breathing may accentuate it. Nausea and vomiting are common.

The patient appears acutely ill and sweaty. Pulse rate is usually 100–140 beats/min. Respiration is shallow and rapid. BP may be transiently high or low, with significant postural hypotension. Temperature may be normal or even subnormal at first, but may increase to 37.7–38.3°C within a few hours. Sensorium may be blunted to the point of semicoma. Scleral icterus is occasionally present. The lungs may have limited diaphragmatic excursion and evidence of atelectasis.

About 20% of patients experience upper abdominal distention caused by gastric distention or displacement of the stomach by a pancreatic inflammatory mass. Pancreatic duct disruption may cause ascites (pancreatic ascites). Marked abdominal tenderness occurs, most often in the upper abdomen. There may be mild tenderness in the lower abdomen, but the rectum is not tender and the stool is usually negative for occult blood. Mild-to-moderate muscular rigidity may be present in the upper abdomen but is rare in the lower abdomen. Rarely, severe peritoneal irritation results in a rigid and boardlike abdomen. Bowel sounds may be hypoactive. The Grey Turner sign (ecchymoses of the flanks) and the Cullen sign (ecchymoses of the umbilical region) indicate extravasation of hemorrhagic exudate.

Infection in the pancreas or in an adjacent fluid collection should be suspected if the patient has a generally toxic appearance with elevated temperature and WBC count or if deterioration follows an initial period of stabilization.

Diagnosis

Pancreatitis is suspected whenever severe abdominal pain occurs, especially in a patient with significant alcohol use or known gallstones. Conditions causing similar symptoms include perforated gastric or duodenal ulcer, mesenteric infarction, strangulating intestinal obstruction, dissecting aneurysm, biliary colic, appendicitis, diverticulitis, inferior wall myocardial infarction (MI), and hematoma of the abdominal muscles or spleen.

Diagnosis is made by clinical suspicion, serum markers (amylase and lipase), and the absence of other causes for the patient's symptoms. Thus, a broad range of tests is done, typically including CBC, electrolytes, Ca, Mg, glucose, blood urea nitrogen (BUN), creatinine, amylase, and lipase. Other routine tests include ECG and an abdominal series (chest, flat, and upright abdomen). A urine dipstick for trypsinogen-2 has sensitivity and specificity of > 90% for acute pancreatitis. Ultrasonography and CT are not generally done specifically to diagnose pancreatitis but are often used to evaluate acute abdominal pain.

LABORATORY TESTS

Serum amylase and lipase concentrations increase on the first day of acute pancreatitis and return to normal in

3–7 days. Lipase is more specific for pancreatitis, but both enzymes may be increased in renal failure and various abdominal conditions (e.g. perforated ulcer, mesenteric vascular occlusion, and intestinal obstruction). Other causes of increased serum amylase include salivary gland dysfunction, macroamylasemia, and tumors that secrete amylase. Both amylase and lipase levels may remain normal if destruction of acinar tissue during previous episodes precludes release of sufficient amounts of enzymes. The serum of patients with hypertriglyceridemia may contain a circulating inhibitor that must be diluted before an elevation in serum amylase can be detected.

Amylase

Creatinine clearance ratio does not have sufficient sensitivity or specificity to diagnose pancreatitis. It is generally used to diagnose macroamylasemia when no pancreatitis exists. In macroamylasemia, amylase bound to serum immunoglobulin falsely elevates the serum amylase level.

Fractionation of total serum amylase into pancreatic type (p-type) isoamylase and salivary-type (s-type) isoamylase increases the accuracy of serum amylase. However, the level of p-type also increases in renal failure and in other severe abdominal conditions in which amylase clearance is altered.

The WBC count usually increases to 12,000–20,000/μL. Third-space fluid losses may increase the hematocrit (Hct) to as high as 50–55%, indicating severe inflammation. Hyperglycemia may occur. Serum Ca concentration falls as early as the first day because of the formation of Ca 'soaps' secondary to excess generation of free fatty acids, especially by pancreatic lipase. Serum bilirubin increases in 15–25% of patients because pancreatic edema compresses the common bile duct.

Treatment

Adequate fluid resuscitation is essential; up to 6–8 L/day of fluid containing appropriate electrolytes may be required. Inadequate fluid therapy increases the risk of pancreatic necrosis.

Fasting is indicated until acute inflammation subsides (i.e. cessation of abdominal tenderness and pain, normalization of serum amylase, return of appetite, feeling better). Fasting can last from a few days in mild pancreatitis to several weeks. In severe cases, TPN should be initiated within the first few days to prevent undernutrition.

Pain relief requires parenteral opioids, which should be given in adequate doses. Although morphine may cause the sphincter of Oddi to contract, this is of doubtful clinical significance. Antiemetic agents (e.g., prochlorperazine 5–10 mg IV q6h), should be given to alleviate vomiting. **A nasogastric tube** (NGT) is required only if significant vomiting persists or ileus is present.

Parenteral H2 blockers or proton pump inhibitors are given. Efforts to reduce pancreatic secretion with drugs (e.g. anticholinergics, glucagon, somatostatin, octreotide) have no proven benefit. Severe acute pancreatitis should be treated in an ICU, particularly in patients with hypotension, oliguria, Ranson's score ≥3, APACHE II ≥ 8, or pancreatic necrosis on CT >30%. In the ICU, vital signs and urine output are monitored hourly; metabolic parameters (Hct, glucose, and electrolytes) are reassessed every 8 hours; arterial blood gas (ABG) is determined as needed; central venous pressure line or Swan-Ganz catheter measurements are determined every 6 hours if the patient is hemodynamically unstable or if fluid requirements are unclear. CBC, platelet count, coagulation parameters, total protein with albumin, BUN, creatinine, Ca, and Mg are measured daily.

Chronic Pancreatitis

Chronic pancreatitis is a persistent inflammation of the pancreas that results in permanent structural damage with fibrosis and ductal strictures, followed by a decline in exocrine and endocrine function. It can occur as the result of chronic alcohol abuse but may be idiopathic. Initial symptoms are recurrent attacks of pain. Later in the disease, some patients develop malabsorption and glucose intolerance. Diagnosis is usually made by imaging studies, such as endoscopic retrograde cholangiopancreatography (ERCP), endoscopic ultrasonography, or secretin pancreatic function testing. Treatment is supportive, with dietary modification, analgesics, and enzyme supplements. In some cases, surgical treatment is helpful.

Etiology

Recent data suggest that alcohol is becoming less of a cause. Less common causes include hereditary pancreatitis, autoimmune pancreatitis, hyperparathyroidism, and obstruction of the main pancreatic duct caused by stenosis, stones, or cancer. In India, Indonesia, and Nigeria, idiopathic calcific pancreatitis occurs among children and young adults (tropical pancreatitis).

Pathophysiology

Similar to acute pancreatitis, the mechanism of disease may be ductal obstruction by protein plugs. The protein plugs may result from excess secretion of glycoprotein-2 or a deficiency of lithostatin, a protein in pancreatic fluid that inhibits Ca precipitation. If obstruction is chronic, persistent inflammation leads to fibrosis and alternating areas of ductal dilation and stricture, which may become calcified. Neuronal sheath hypertrophy and perineural inflammation occur and may contribute to chronic pain.

After several years, progressive fibrosis leads to loss of exocrine and endocrine function. Diabetes develops in 20–30% of patients within 10–15 years of onset.

Symptoms and Signs

Most patients present with episodic abdominal pain. About 10–15% have no pain and present with malabsorption. Pain is epigastric, severe, and may last many hours or several days. Episodes typically subside spontaneously after 6–10 years, as the acinar cells that secrete pancreatic digestive enzymes are progressively destroyed. When lipase and protease secretions are reduced to <10% of normal, the patient develops steatorrhea, passing greasy stools or even oil droplets, and creatorrhea (the presence of undigested muscle fibers in the feces). Symptoms of glucose intolerance may appear at this time.

Diagnosis

Diagnosis can be difficult because amylase and lipase levels are frequently normal because of significant loss of pancreatic function. In a patient with a typical history of alcohol abuse and recurrent episodes of acute pancreatitis, detection of pancreatic calcification on plain X-ray of the abdomen may be sufficient. However, such calcifications typically occur late in the disease and then are visible in only about 30% of patients. In patients without a typical history, pancreatic cancer must be excluded as the cause of pain; abdominal CT is recommended. CT can show calcifications and other pancreatic abnormalities (e.g. pseudocyst or dilated ducts), but still may be normal early in the disease. MRCP is now frequently used for diagnosis and can show masses in the pancreas as well as provide more optimal visualization of ductal changes consistent with chronic pancreatitis.

The primary options for patients with normal CT findings include ERCP, endoscopic ultrasonography, and secretin pancreatic function testing. These tests are quite sensitive, but ERCP precipitates acute pancreatitis in about 5% of patients.

Late in the disease, tests of pancreatic exocrine function become abnormal. Direct tests, involving analysis of fluid aspirated from the duodenum; and indirect tests, in which intubation of the patient is not required. The former are now rarely performed. Examples include the measurement of bicarbonate concentration and amylase or trypsin activity in duodenal fluid either following a test meal (Lundh test) or the administration of secretin and cholecystokinin (CCK). Bicarbonate concentration and enzyme activities are decreased in chronic pancreatic insufficiency.

Examples of indirect tests include the fluorescein dilaurate and p-aminobenzoic acid (PABA) tests. Both utilize the same principle, measuring the excretion of an orally administered substance in a form dependent on pancreatic enzyme activity for its absorption.

Pancreatic elastase and chymotrypsin activities in feces are reduced in chronic pancreatic insufficiency. Measurements of both enzymes have been used as tests for this condition; both show high sensitivity and specificity, with elastase being slightly superior in both respects. Measurement of fecal elastase is now widely used to distinguish between diarrhea of pancreatic and non-pancreatic origin.

Treatment

A relapse requires treatment similar to acute pancreatitis with fasting, IV fluids, and analgesics. When feeding resumes, the patient must eschew alcohol and consume a low-fat (<25 g/day) diet (to reduce secretion of pancreatic enzymes). An H2 blocker or proton pump inhibitor may reduce acid-stimulated release of secretin, thereby decreasing the flow of pancreatic secretions. Too often, these measures do not relieve pain, requiring increased amounts of opioids, with the threat of addiction. Medical treatment of chronic pancreatic pain is often unsatisfactory.

Pancreatic enzyme supplementation may reduce chronic pain by inhibiting the release of cholecystokinin thereby reducing the secretion of pancreatic enzymes. Supplementation is more likely to be successful in mild idiopathic pancreatitis than in alcoholic pancreatitis. Enzymes are also used to treat steatorrhea. Various preparations are available, and a dose providing at least 30,000 U of lipase should be used. Nonenteric coated tablets should be used, and they should be taken with meals. An H2 blocker or proton pump inhibitor should be given to prevent acid breakdown of the enzymes.

Favorable clinical responses include weight gain, fewer bowel movements, elimination of oil droplet seepage, and improved well-being. Clinical response can be documented by showing a decrease in stool fat after enzyme therapy. If steatorrhea is particularly severe and refractory to these measures, medium-chain triglycerides can be provided as a source of fat (they are absorbed without pancreatic enzymes), reducing other dietary fats proportionally. Supplementation with fat-soluble vitamins (A, D, K) should be given, including vitamin E, which may minimize inflammation.

Surgical treatment may be effective for pain relief. A pancreatic pseudocyst, which may cause chronic pain, can be decompressed into a nearby structure to which it firmly adheres (e.g. the stomach) or into a defunctionalized loop of jejunum (via a Roux-en-Y cystojejunostomy). If the main pancreatic duct is dilated >5–8 mm, a lateral pancreaticojejunostomy (Puestow procedure) relieves pain in about 70–80% of patients. If the duct is not dilated, a partial resection is similarly effective; either distal pancreatectomy (for extensive disease at the tail of the pancreas) or Whipple procedure (for extensive disease at the head of the pancreas) is done. Operative approaches should be reserved for patients who have stopped using alcohol and who can manage diabetes that may be intensified by pancreatic resection.

Some pseudocysts can be drained endoscopically. Endoscopic ultrasound-guided denervation of the celiac plexus with alcohol and bupivacaine may provide pain relief. If there is significant stricture at the papilla or distal pancreatic duct, ERCP with sphincterotomy, stent placement, or dilatation may be effective.

Oral hypoglycemic drugs rarely help treat diabetes caused by chronic pancreatitis. Insulin should be given cautiously because the coexisting deficiency of glucagon secretion by α-cells means that the hypoglycemic effects of insulin are unopposed and prolonged hypoglycemia may occur.

Patients are at increased risk of pancreatic cancer. Worsening of symptoms, especially with development of a pancreatic duct stricture, should prompt an evaluation for cancer. Evaluation may include brushing strictures for cytologic analysis or measuring serum markers (e.g. CA 19-9, carcinoembryonic antigen).

PANCREATIC CANCER

Most pancreatic cancers are exocrine tumors that develop from ductal and acinar cells (Fig. 6.9). Adenocarcinomas of the exocrine pancreas arise from duct cells 9 times more often than from acinar cells; 80% occur in the head of the gland. Adenocarcinomas appear at the mean age of 55 years and occur 1.5–2 times more often in men. Prominent risk factors include smoking, a history of chronic pancreatitis, obesity, and possibly long-standing diabetes mellitus (primarily in women). Heredity plays some role. Alcohol and caffeine consumption do not seem to be risk factors.

Symptoms and Signs

Symptoms occur late. By diagnosis, 90% of patients have locally advanced tumors that have involved retroperitoneal structures, spread to regional lymph nodes, or metastasized to the liver or lung.

Most patients have severe upper abdominal pain, which usually radiates to the back. The pain may be relieved by bending forward or assuming the fetal position. Weight loss is common. Adenocarcinomas of

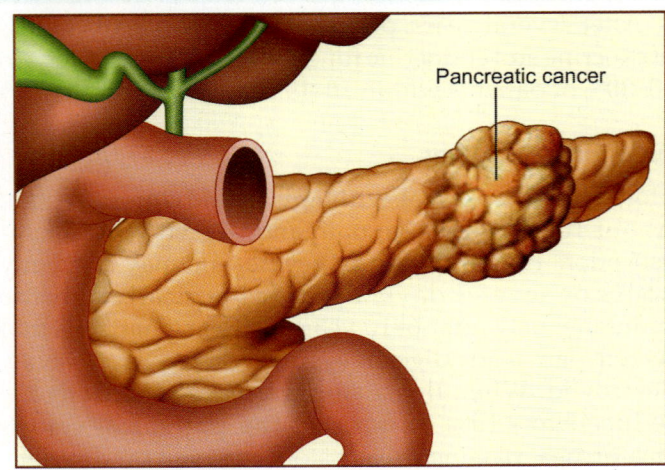

Fig. 6.9: Pancreatic cancer

the head of the pancreas cause obstructive jaundice (often causing pruritus) in 80–90% of patients. Cancer in the body and tail may cause splenic vein obstruction, resulting in splenomegaly, gastric and esophageal varices, and GI hemorrhage. The cancer causes diabetes in 25–50% of patients, leading to symptoms of glucose intolerance (e.g. polyuria and polydipsia). Pancreatic cancer can also interfere with production of digestive enzymes by the pancreas (pancreatic exocrine insufficiency) in some patients and with the ability to break down food and absorb nutrients. This malabsorption causes bloating and gas and a watery, greasy, and/or foul-smelling diarrhea, leading to weight loss and vitamin deficiencies.

Diagnosis

The preferred tests are an abdominal helical CT or MRCP. If CT or MRCP shows apparent unresectable or metastatic disease, a percutaneous needle aspiration of an accessible lesion might be considered to obtain a tissue diagnosis. If CT shows a potentially resectable tumor or no tumor, MRCP or endoscopic ultrasound may be used to stage disease or detect small tumors not visible with CT. Patients with obstructive jaundice may have ERCP as the first diagnostic procedure.

Biochemical tests of pancreatic function are rarely of any use in diagnosis, and other techniques, particularly imaging, are far more powerful diagnostic tools. The plasma concentration of the tumor markers carcinoembryonic antigen (CEA) and CA 19-9 are elevated in up to 80% of patients with pancreatic malignancy, but can be elevated with other (particularly colorectal) cancers and sometimes in non-malignant disease. Unfortunately, pancreatic cancer often presents late; by the time it is diagnosed, metastases are often present and only palliative surgical procedures are feasible.

Prognosis

Prognosis varies with stage but overall is poor (5-years survival: <2%), because many patients have advanced disease at the time of diagnosis.

Treatment

About 80–90% of cancers are considered surgically unresectable at time of diagnosis because of metastases or invasion of major blood vessels. Depending on location of the tumor, the procedure of choice is most commonly a Whipple procedure (pancreaticoduodenectomy). Adjuvant therapy with 5-fluorouracil (5-FU) and external beam radiation therapy is typically given, resulting in about 40% 2-years and 25% 5-years survival. This combination is also used for patients with localized but unresectable tumors and results in median survival of about 1 year. Newer drugs (e.g. gemcitabine, irinotecan, paclitaxel, oxaliplatin, and carboplatin) may be more effective than 5-FU–based chemotherapy, but no drug, singly or in combination, is clearly superior in prolonging survival. Patients with hepatic or distant metastases may be offered chemotherapy as part of an investigational program, but the outlook is dismal with or without such treatment and some patients may choose to forego it.

If an unresectable tumor is found at operation and gastroduodenal or bile duct obstruction is present or pending, a double gastric and biliary bypass operation is usually done to relieve obstruction. In patients with inoperable lesions and jaundice, endoscopic placement of a bile duct stent relieves jaundice. However, surgical bypass should be considered in patients with unresectable lesions if life expectancy is >6–7 months because of complications associated with stents.

Symptomatic Treatment

Ultimately, most patients experience pain and die. Thus, symptomatic treatment is as important as controlling disease.

Patients with moderate to severe pain should receive an oral opioid in doses adequate to provide relief. Concern about addiction should not be a barrier to effective pain control. For chronic pain, long-acting preparations (e.g. transdermal fentanyl, oxycodone, oxymorphone) are usually best. Percutaneous or operative splanchnic (celiac) block effectively controls pain in most patients. In cases of intolerable pain, opioids given SC or by IV, epidural, or intrathecal infusion provides additional relief.

If palliative surgery or endoscopic placement of a biliary stent fails to relieve pruritus secondary to obstructive jaundice, the patient can be managed with cholestyramine 4 g by mouth once a day to 4 times a day.

Phenobarbital 30–60 mg by mouth 3 times a day to 4 times a day may be helpful.

Exocrine pancreatic insufficiency is treated with tablets of porcine pancreatic enzymes (pancrelipase). The patient should take enough to supply 16,000–20,000 lipase units before each meal or snack. If a meal is prolonged (as in a restaurant), some of the tablets should be taken during the meal. Optimal intraluminal pH for the enzymes is 8; thus, some clinicians give a proton pump inhibitor or H2 blocker 2 times a day. Diabetes mellitus should be closely monitored and controlled.

CYSTIC FIBROSIS

Cystic fibrosis (CF) is an inherited disease of the exocrine glands affecting primarily the GI and respiratory systems. It leads to chronic lung disease, exocrine pancreatic insufficiency, hepatobiliary disease, and abnormally high sweat electrolytes. Diagnosis is by sweat test or identification of 2 cystic fibrosis-causing mutations in patients with characteristic symptoms or a positive newborn screening test result. Treatment is supportive through aggressive multidisciplinary care.

Etiology

Cystic fibrosis (CF) is carried as an autosomal recessive trait by about 3% of the white population. The responsible gene has been localized on the long arm of chromosome 7. It encodes a membrane-associated protein called the cystic fibrosis transmembrane conductance regulator (CFTR). The most common gene mutation, F508del, occurs in about 70% of CF alleles; >1900 less common CFTR mutations have been identified. CFTR is a cyclic adenosine monophosphate (cAMP) regulated Cl channel, regulating Cl and Na transport across epithelial membranes. A number of additional functions are considered likely. Disease manifests only in homozygotes. Heterozygotes may show subtle abnormalities of epithelial electrolyte transport but are clinically unaffected. The CFTR mutations have been divided into 5 classes, each of which causes different severity of disease. However, there is no strict relationship between specific mutations and disease manifestation, so clinical testing (i.e. of organ function) rather than genotyping is a better guide to prognosis.

Pathophysiology

Respiratory

Although the lungs are generally histologically normal at birth, most patients develop pulmonary disease beginning in infancy or early childhood. Mucus plugging and chronic bacterial infection, accompanied by a pronounced inflammatory response, damage the airways, ultimately leading to bronchiectasis and respiratory insufficiency. The course is characterized by episodic exacerbations with infection and progressive decline in pulmonary function.

Pulmonary damage is probably initiated by diffuse obstruction in the small airways by abnormally thick mucus secretions. Bronchiolitis and mucopurulent plugging of the airways occur secondary to obstruction and infection (Fig. 6.10). Airway changes are more common than parenchymal changes, and emphysema is not prominent. About 50% of patients have bronchial hyperreactivity that responds to bronchodilators. In patients with advanced pulmonary disease, chronic hypoxemia results in muscular hypertrophy of the pulmonary arteries, pulmonary hypertension, and right ventricular hypertrophy. Much of the pulmonary damage may be caused by inflammation secondary to the release of proteases and proinflammatory cytokines by cells in the airways.

The lungs of most patients are colonized by pathogenic bacteria. Early in the course, *Staphylococcus aureusis* the most common pathogen, but as the disease progresses, *Pseudomonas aeruginosa* is most frequently isolated. A mucoid variant of *P. aeruginosa* is uniquely associated with CF and results in a worse prognosis than nonmucoid Pseudomonas. The prevalence of methicillin-resistant *S. aureus* (MRSA) in the respiratory tract is now >25%; patients who are infected with MRSA have lower survival rates than those who are not. Colonization with Burkholderia cepacia complex occurs in about 3% of patients and may be associated with more rapid pulmonary deterioration. Nontuberculous mycobacteria, including *Mycobacterium avium* complex and *M. abscessus,* are potential respiratory pathogens. Prevalence varies with age and geographic location and probably exceeds 10%. Differentiating infection from colonization can be challenging. Other common respiratory pathogens include *Stenotrophomonas maltophilia, Achromobacter xylosoxidans,* and *Aspergillus sp.*

Gastrointestinal

The pancreas, intestines, and hepatobiliary system are frequently affected. Exocrine pancreatic function is compromised in 85–95% of patients. An exception is a subset of patients who have certain 'mild' CF mutations, in whom pancreatic function is unaffected. Patients with pancreatic insufficiency have malabsorption of fats (and fat-soluble vitamins) and protein. Duodenal fluid is abnormally viscid and shows absence or diminution of enzyme activity and decreased HCO_3^- concentration; stool trypsin and chymotrypsin are absent or diminished. Endocrine pancreatic dysfunction is less common, but diabetes mellitus is present in about 2% of children, 20% of adolescents, and at least 40% of adults.

Bile duct involvement with bile stasis and biliary plugging leads to asymptomatic hepatic fibrosis in 30% of patients. About 2–3% of patients progress to irreversible multinodular biliary cirrhosis with varices and portal hypertension, usually by 12 years of age. Hepatocellular failure is a rare and late event. There is an increased incidence of cholelithiasis, which is usually asymptomatic.

Abnormally viscid intestinal secretions often cause meconium ileus in neonates and sometimes meconium plugging of the colon. Older children and adults, also may have intermittent or chronic constipation and intestinal obstruction.

Other GI problems include intussusception, volvulus, rectal prolapse, periappendiceal abscess, pancreatitis, an increased risk of cancer of the hepatobiliary and GI tracts, gastroesophageal reflux, and esophagitis.

Other

Infertility occurs in 98% of adult men secondary to maldevelopment of the vas deferens or to other forms of

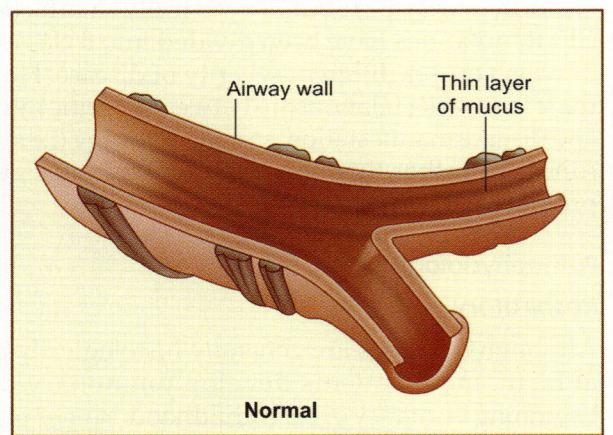
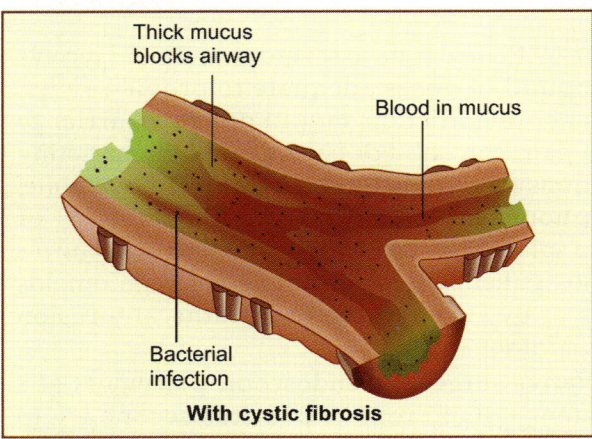

Fig. 6.10: Cross section of airway—normal versus cystic fibrosis

obstructive azoospermia. In women, fertility is somewhat decreased secondary to viscid cervical secretions, although many women have carried pregnancies to term. Pregnancy outcome for both the mother and neonate is related to the mother's health.

Other complications include osteopenia/osteoporosis, renal stones, iron deficiency anemia, and episodic arthralgias/arthritis.

Symptoms and Signs
Respiratory

Fifty percent of patients not diagnosed through newborn screening present with pulmonary manifestations, often beginning in infancy. Recurrent or chronic infections manifested by cough, sputum production, and wheezing are common. Cough is the most troublesome complaint, often accompanied by sputum, gagging, vomiting, and disturbed sleep. Intercostal retractions, use of accessory muscles of respiration, a barrel-chest deformity, digital clubbing, and cyanosis occur with disease progression. Upper respiratory tract involvement includes nasal polyposis and chronic or recurrent sinusitis. Adolescents may have retarded growth, delayed onset of puberty, and a declining tolerance for exercise. Pulmonary complications include pneumothorax, infection with nontuberculous mycobacteria, hemoptysis, allergic bronchopulmonary aspergillosis, and right heart failure secondary to pulmonary hypertension.

Gastrointestinal

Meconium ileus due to obstruction of the ileum by viscid meconium may be the earliest sign and is present in 15–20% of CF-affected neonates. It typically manifests with abdominal distention, vomiting, and failure to pass meconium. Some infants have intestinal perforation, with signs of peritonitis and shock. Infants with meconium plug syndrome have a delayed passage of meconium. They can have similar signs of obstruction or very mild and transient symptoms that go unnoticed. Older patients may have episodes of constipation or develop recurrent and sometimes chronic episodes of partial or complete small- or large-bowel obstruction (distal intestinal obstruction syndrome). Symptoms include crampy abdominal pain, change in stooling pattern, decreased appetite, and sometimes vomiting.

In infants without meconium ileus, disease onset may be heralded by a delay in regaining birth weight and inadequate weight gain at 4–6 weeks of age.

Occasionally, infants who are undernourished, especially if on hypoallergenic formula or soy formula,

present with generalized edema secondary to protein malabsorption.

Pancreatic insufficiency is usually clinically apparent early in life and may be progressive. Manifestations include the frequent passage of bulky, foul-smelling, oily stools; abdominal protuberance; and poor growth pattern with decreased subcutaneous tissue and muscle mass despite a normal or voracious appetite. Clinical manifestations may occur secondary to deficiency of fat-soluble vitamins.

Rectal prolapse occurs in 20% of untreated infants and toddlers. Gastroesophageal reflux is relatively common among older children and adults.

Other

Excessive sweating in hot weather or with fever may lead to episodes of hyponatremic/hypochloremic dehydration and circulatory failure. In arid climates, infants may present with chronic metabolic alkalosis. Salt crystal formation and a salty taste on the skin are highly suggestive of CF.

Diagnosis

Universal newborn screening for CF is now standard; >90% of cases are first identified by newborn screening, but about 10% are not diagnosed until adolescence or early adulthood. Despite advances in genetic testing, the sweat Cl test remains the standard for confirming a CF diagnosis in most cases because of its sensitivity and specificity, simplicity, and availability.

Sweat Testing

In cystic fibrosis, the CFTR chloride channel is faulty which inhibits chloride to be reabsorbed into sweat duct cells (Fig. 6.11). Since this reabsorbtion does not occur, it is secreted in the sweat in higher levels than normal. In this test, localized sweating is stimulated with pilocarpine, the amount of sweat is measured, and the Cl concentration is determined. The results are valid after 48 hours of life, but an adequate sweat sample (>75 mg on filter paper or >15 µL in microbore tubing) may be difficult to obtain before 2 weeks of age. False-negative results are rare but may occur in the presence of edema and hypoproteinemia or an inadequate quantity of sweat. False-positive results are usually due to technical error. Transient elevation of sweat Cl concentration can occur from psychosocial deprivation (e.g. child abuse, neglect) and in patients with anorexia nervosa. Although the sweat Cl concentration increases slightly with age, the sweat test is valid at all ages. A positive sweat test result should be confirmed by a second sweat test or by identification of two CF-causing mutations. A chloride

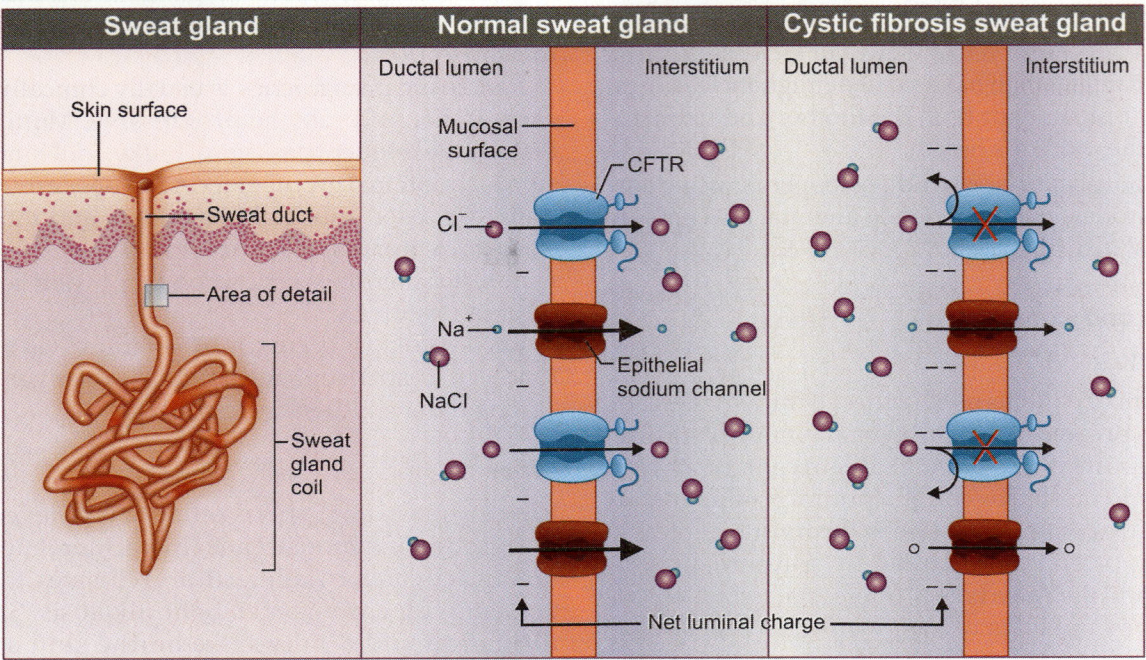

Fig. 6.11: Sweat gland normal versus cystic fibrosis

concentration of >60 mmol/L is indicative of cystic fibrosis (Table 6.6).

INTERMEDIATE SWEAT TEST RESULTS

A small subset of patients have a mild or partial CF phenotype and sweat Cl values that are persistently in the intermediate or even normal range. In addition, there are patients who have single-organ manifestations, such as pancreatitis, chronic sinusitis, or congenital bilateral absence of the vas deferens that may be due to partial CFTR protein dysfunction. In some of these patients, the diagnosis of CF can be confirmed by the identification of two CF-causing mutations, one in each of the CFTR genes. If two CF-causing mutations are not identified, ancillary evaluations such as pancreatic function testing and pancreatic imaging, high-resolution chest CT, sinus CT, pulmonary function testing, urogenital evaluation in males, and bronchoalveolar lavage including assessment of microbial flora may be useful. Additional potentially helpful diagnostic tests include expanded CFTR genetic analysis and measurement of nasal transepithelial potential difference (based on the observation of increased Na reabsorption across epithelium that is relatively impermeable to Cl in patients with CF).

Pancreatic Tests

Pancreatic function should be assessed at the time of diagnosis, usually by measuring 72 hours fecal fat excretion or the concentration of human pancreatic elastase in stool. This latter test is valid even in the presence of exogenous pancreatic enzymes. Infants who are initially pancreatic sufficient and who carry two 'severe' mutations should have serial measurements to detect progression to pancreatic insufficiency.

RESPIRATORY ASSESSMENT

Chest X-rays are done at times of pulmonary deterioration or exacerbations and routinely every 1–2 years. High-resolution chest CT may be helpful to more precisely define the extent of lung damage and to detect subtle airway abnormalities (Fig. 6.11). Both may show hyperinflation and bronchial wall thickening as the earliest findings. Subsequent changes include areas of infiltrate, atelectasis, and hilar adenopathy. With advanced disease, segmental or lobar atelectasis, cyst formation, bronchiectasis, and pulmonary artery and right ventricular hypertrophy occur. Branching, finger-like opacifications that represent mucoid impaction of dilated bronchi are characteristic.

Sinus CT studies are indicated in patients with significant sinus symptoms or nasal polyps in whom endoscopic sinus surgery is being considered (Fig. 6.12). These studies almost always show persistent opacification of the paranasal sinuses.

Table 6.6	Sweat Cl concentration ranges		
Age	Normal (mmol/L)	Intermediate (mmol/L)	Abnormal (mmol/L)
≤6 months	≤ 29	30–59	≥ 60
>6 months	≤ 39	40–59	≥ 60

patients have evidence of reversible airway obstruction as shown by improvement in pulmonary function after aerosol administration of a bronchodilator.

Screening oropharyngeal or sputum cultures should be done 4 times/year, especially in patients not yet colonized with *Pseudomonas aeruginosa*. Bronchoscopy/bronchoalveolar lavage is indicated when it is important to precisely define the patient's lower airway microbial flora (e.g. to direct antibiotic selection) or to remove inspissated mucus plugs.

NEWBORN SCREENING

Newborn screening for CF is now universal in the United States. Screening is based on detecting an elevated concentration of immunoreactive trypsinogen (IRT) in the blood. There are two methods of following up on an elevated IRT level. In one method, a second IRT test is done, which, if also elevated, is followed by a sweat test. In the other, more commonly used method, an elevated IRT level is followed by CFTR mutation testing and, if 1 or 2 mutations are identified, then a sweat test is done. For diagnosis, both strategies have about 90–95% sensitivity.

Prognosis

The course is largely determined by the degree of pulmonary involvement. Deterioration is inevitable, leading to debilitation and eventual death, usually due to a combination of respiratory failure and cor pulmonale. Prognosis has improved steadily over the past 5 decades, mainly because of aggressive treatment before the onset of irreversible pulmonary changes. Long-term survival is significantly better in patients without pancreatic insufficiency. Outcomes are also affected by CFTR mutation profile, modifier genes, airway microbiology, ambient temperature, exposure to air pollutants (including tobacco smoke), adherence to prescribed therapies, and socioeconomic status. The FEV_1, adjusted for age and sex, is the best predictor of survival.

Treatment

Comprehensive and intensive therapy should be directed by an experienced physician working with a multidisciplinary team that includes other physicians, nurses, dieticians, physical and respiratory therapists, counselors, pharmacists, and social workers. The goals of therapy are maintenance of normal nutritional status, prevention or aggressive treatment of pulmonary and other complications, encouragement of physical activity, and provision of psychosocial support. With appropriate support, most patients can make an age-appropriate adjustment at home and school. Despite myriad

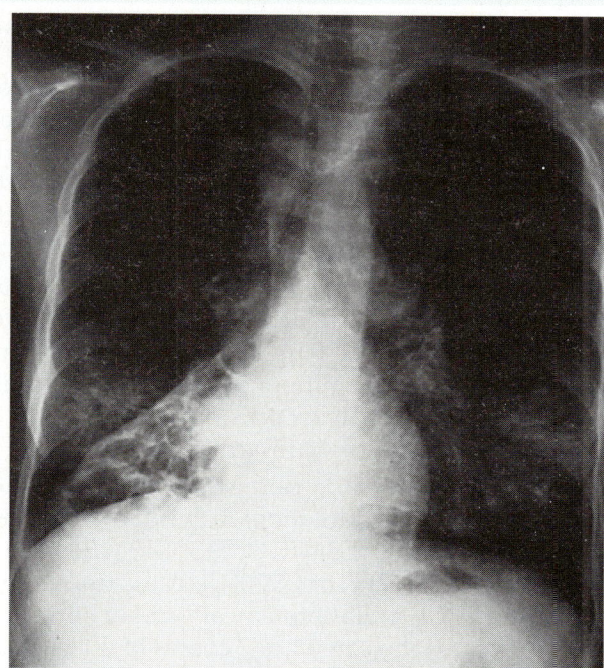

Fig. 6.12: Cystic fibrosis (chest X-ray)

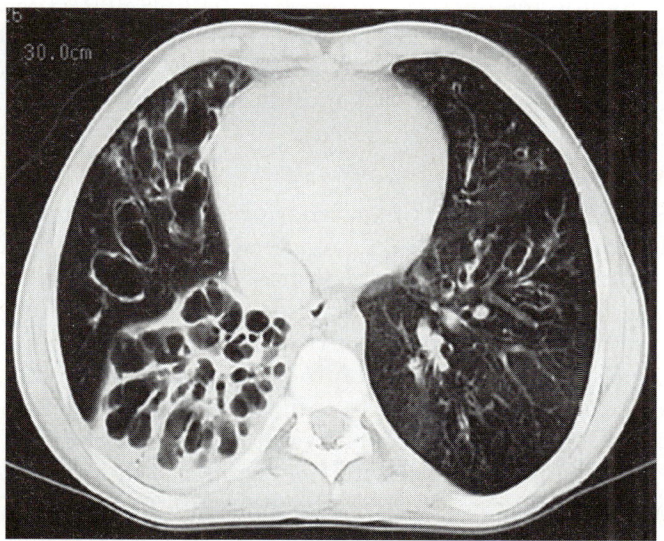

Fig. 6.13: Cystic fibrosis (CT scan)

Pulmonary function tests are the best indicators of clinical status and should be done routinely 4 times/year and at times of clinical decline. Pulmonary function can now be evaluated in infants by using a raised volume rapid thoracoabdominal compression technique. Pulmonary function tests indicate hypoxemia; reduction in forced vital capacity (FVC), forced expiratory volume in 1 sec (FEV_1), forced expiratory flow between 25% and 75% expired volume (FEF_{25-75}), and FEV_1/FVC ratio; and an increase in residual volume and the ratio of residual volume to total lung capacity. Fifty percent of

problems, the educational, occupational, and marital successes of patients are impressive.

Respiratory

Treatment of pulmonary problems centers on prevention of airway obstruction and prophylaxis against and control of pulmonary infection. Prophylaxis against pulmonary infections includes maintenance of pertussis, *Hemophilus influenzae*, varicella, *Streptococcus pneumoniae*, and measles immunity and annual influenza vaccination. In patients exposed to influenza, a neuraminidase inhibitor can be used prophylactically. Giving palivizumab to infants with CF for prevention of respiratory syncytial virus infection has been shown to be safe, but efficacy has not been documented.

Airway clearance measures consisting of postural drainage, percussion, vibration, and assisted coughing are recommended at the time of diagnosis and should be done on a regular basis. In older patients, alternative airway clearance measures, such as active cycle of breathing, autogenic drainage, positive expiratory pressure devices, and high-frequency chest wall oscillation, may be effective. Regular aerobic exercise is recommended; it may also help airway clearance.

For patients with reversible airway obstruction, bronchodilators may be given by aerosol. Corticosteroids by aerosol usually are not effective O_2 therapy is indicated for patients with severe pulmonary insufficiency and hypoxemia.

Mechanical ventilation is typically not indicated for chronic respiratory failure. Its use should be restricted to patients with good baseline status in whom acute reversible respiratory complications develop, in association with pulmonary surgery, or to patients in whom lung transplantation is imminent. Noninvasive positive pressure ventilation nasally or by face mask also can be beneficial. Oral expectorants are widely used, but few data support their efficacy. Cough suppressants should be discouraged. Long-term daily aerosol therapy with dornase alfa (recombinant human deoxyribonuclease) as well as 7% hypertonic saline (in patients >6 years) has been shown to slow the rate of decline in pulmonary function and to decrease the frequency of respiratory tract exacerbations.

Pneumothorax can be treated with closed chest tube thoracostomy drainage. Open thoracotomy or thoracoscopy with resection of pleural blebs and mechanical abrasion of the pleural surfaces is effective in treating recurrent pneumothoraces.

Massive or Recurrent hemoptysis is treated by embolizing involved bronchial arteries.

Oral corticosteroids are indicated in infants with prolonged bronchiolitis and in patients with refractory bronchospasm, allergic bronchopulmonary aspergillosis, and inflammatory complications (e.g. arthritis, vasculitis). Long-term use of alternate-day corticosteroid therapy can slow the decline in pulmonary function, but because of corticosteroid-related complications, it is not recommended for routine use. Patients receiving corticosteroids must be closely monitored for evidence of diabetes and linear growth retardation.

Ibuprofen, when given over several years at a dose sufficient to achieve a peak plasma concentration between 50 µg/mL and 100 µg/mL, has been shown to slow the rate of decline in pulmonary function, especially in children 5–13 years. The appropriate dose must be individualized based on pharmacokinetic studies.

Ivacaftor is a drug that potentiates the CFTR ion channel in patients with mutations in the following genes: G551D , G178R, S549N , S549R, G551S, G1244E, S1251N, S1255P, G1349D, R117H , or G970R; it is the first drug to target a specific CF mutation. Ivacaftor may be used in patients ≥6 years who carry 1 or 2 copies of that specific mutation. The drug is given orally twice a day and can improve pulmonary function, increase weight, decrease CF symptoms and pulmonary exacerbations, and reduce and sometimes normalize sweat Cl concentrations. Other drugs that may correct defective CFTR or potentiate CFTR function in other CF mutations are under study.

ANTIBIOTICS

For **mild pulmonary exacerbations,** a short course of antibiotics should be given based on culture and sensitivity testing. A penicillinase-resistant penicillin (e.g., cloxacillin or dicloxacillin), a cephalosporin (e.g. cephalexin), or trimethoprim/sulfamethoxazole is the drug of choice for staphylococci. Erythromycin, amoxicillin/clavulanate, ampicillin, tetracycline, linezolid, or occasionally chloramphenicol may be used. For patients colonized with *P. aeruginosa*, a short course of inhaled tobramycin or aztreonam lysine (e.g. 4 weeks) and/or an oral fluoroquinolone (e.g. 2–3 weeks) may be effective. Fluoroquinolones have been used safely in young children.

For **moderate-to-severe pulmonary exacerbations,** especially in patients colonized with *P. aeruginosa*, IV antibiotic therapy is advised. Patients often require hospital admission, but carefully selected patients can safely receive the therapy at home. Combinations of an aminoglycoside (e.g. tobramycin, gentamicin) and an antipseudomonal penicillin are given IV. IV administration of cephalosporins and monobactams with antipseudomonal activity may also be useful. The usual starting dose of tobramycin or gentamicin is 2.5–3.5 mg/kg 3 times a day, but higher doses

(3.5–4 mg/kg 3 times a day) may be required to achieve acceptable serum concentrations [peak level 8–10 µg/mL (11–17 µmol/L), trough value of <2 µg/mL (<4 µmol/L)]. Alternatively, tobramycin can be given safely and effectively in one daily dose (10–12 mg/kg). Because of enhanced renal clearance, large doses of some penicillins may be required to achieve adequate serum levels. For patients colonized with methicillin-resistant *S. aureus*, vancomycin or linezolid can be added to the IV regimen.

In patients who are chronically colonized with *P. aeruginosa*, antibiotics delivered by aerosol improve clinical parameters and possibly reduce the bacterial burden in the airways. The long-term use of alternate-month aerosol tobramycin or aztreonam lysine therapy along with continuous (every month) oral azithromycin given 3 times a weeks may be effective in improving or stabilizing pulmonary function and decreasing the frequency of pulmonary exacerbations.

Eradication of chronic *Pseudomonas* colonization is not usually possible. It has been shown, however, that early antibiotic treatment around the time the airways are initially infected with nonmucoid strains of *P. aeruginosa* may be effective in eradicating the organism for some period of time. Treatment strategies vary but usually consist of aerosol tobramycin or colistin sometimes along with an oral fluoroquinolone. Patients who have a clinically significant nontuberculous mycobacterium infection may require long-term therapy with a combination of oral, aerosol, and IV antibiotics.

Gastrointestinal

Neonatal intestinal obstruction can sometimes be relieved by enemas containing a hyperosmolar or iso-osmolar radiopaque contrast material; otherwise, surgical enterostomy to flush out the viscid meconium in the intestinal lumen may be necessary. After the neonatal period, episodes of partial intestinal obstruction (distal intestinal obstruction syndrome) can be treated with enemas containing a hyperosmolar or iso-osmolar radiopaque contrast material or acetylcysteine, or by oral administration of a balanced intestinal lavage solution. A stool softener such as dioctyl sodium sulfosuccinate or lactulose may help prevent such episodes. Ursodeoxycholic acid, a hydrophilic bile acid, is often used in patients with liver disease caused by CF, but there is little evidence to support its efficacy in preventing progression from bile stasis to cirrhosis.

PANCREATIC ENZYME REPLACEMENT

It should be given with all meals and snacks to patients with pancreatic insufficiency. The most effective enzyme preparations contain pancrelipase in pH-sensitive, enteric-coated microspheres or microtablets. Infants are usually started at a dose of 2000–4000 IU lipase per 120 mL of formula or per breastfeeding session. For infants, the capsules are opened and the contents are mixed with food. After infancy, weight-based dosing is used starting at 1000 IU lipase/kg/meal for children <4 years and at 500 IU lipase/kg/meal for those >4 years. Usually, half the standard dose is given with snacks. Doses >2,500 IU lipase/kg/meal or >10,000 IU lipase/kg/day should be avoided because high enzyme dosages have been associated with fibrosing colonopathy. In patients with high enzyme requirements, acid suppression with an H2 blocker or proton pump inhibitor may improve enzyme effectiveness.

Diet therapy also includes a normal-to-high total fat intake to increase the caloric density of the diet, a water-miscible multivitamin supplement in double the recommended daily allowance, and salt supplementation during infancy and periods of thermal stress and increased sweating. Infants receiving broad-spectrum antibiotics and patients with liver disease and hemoptysis should be given additional supplemental vitamin K. Formulas containing protein hydrolysates and medium-chain triglycerides may be used instead of modified whole-milk formulas for infants with severe malabsorption. Glucose polymers and medium-chain triglyceride supplements can be used to increase caloric intake. In patients who fail to maintain adequate nutritional status, enteral supplementation via nasogastric tube (NGT), gastrostomy, or jejunostomy may restore normal growth and stabilize pulmonary function. The use of appetite stimulants to enhance growth may be helpful in some patients.

Other

Cystic fibrosis-related diabetes (CFRD) is caused by insulin insufficiency and shares features of both type 1 and type 2 diabetes. Insulin is the only recommended treatment. Management includes an insulin regimen, nutrition counseling, a diabetes self-management education program, and monitoring for microvascular complications. The plan should be carried out in conjunction with an endocrinologist with experience in treating both CF and diabetes.

Patients with symptomatic right heart failure should be treated with diuretics, salt restriction, and O_2.

RECOMBINANT HUMAN GROWTH HORMONE (RHGH)

It may improve pulmonary function, increase height and weight and bone mineral content, and reduce the rate of hospitalization. However, because of the added cost and inconvenience, RHGH is not commonly used.

Surgery

Surgery may be indicated for localized bronchiectasis or atelectasis that cannot be treated effectively with drugs, nasal polyps, and chronic sinusitis, bleeding from esophageal varices secondary to portal hypertension, gallbladder disease, and intestinal obstruction due to a volvulus or an intussusception that cannot be medically reduced. Liver transplantation has been done successfully in patients with end-stage liver disease. Bilateral cadaveric lung and live donor lobar transplantation has been done successfully in patients with advanced pulmonary disease, as well as combined liver-lung transplantation for patients with end-stage liver and lung disease. Bilateral lung transplantation for severe lung disease is becoming more routine and more successful with experience and improved techniques. About 60% of people are alive 5 years after transplantation of both lungs, and their condition is much improved.

End-of-life Care

The patient and family deserve sensitive discussions of prognosis and preferences for care throughout the course of illness, especially as the patient's pulmonary reserves become increasingly limited. Most people facing the end of life with CF will be older adolescents or adults and will be appropriately responsible for their own choices. Thus, they must know what is in store and what can be done. One mark of respect for patients living with CF is to ensure that they are given the information and opportunity to make life choices, including having a substantial hand in determining how and when to accept dying. Often, discussion of transplantation is needed. In considering transplantation, patients need to weigh the merits of longer survival with a transplant against the uncertainty of getting a transplant and the ongoing (but different) burden of living with an organ transplant.

Deteriorating patients need to discuss the eventuality of dying. Patients and their families need to know that most often dying is actually gentle and not profoundly symptomatic. When appropriate, palliative care, including sufficient sedation, should be offered to ensure peaceful dying. A useful strategy for the patient to consider is to accept a time-limited trial of fully aggressive treatment when needed, but to agree in advance to parameters that indicate when to stop aggressive measures.

BIBLIOGRAPHY

1. A, Sonnenberg, Müller-Lissner SA, Vogel E, et al. "Predictors of duodenal ulcer healing and relapse." Journal of Gastroenterology 1981; 81(6): 1061–7.

2. Abraham L. Kierszenbaum. Histology and cell biology: an introduction to pathology. 2002; St. Louis: Mosby. ISBN 0-323-01639-1.

3. Adams F, translator "On The Cœliac Affection". The extant works of Aretaeus, The Cappadocian. 1956. London: Sydenham Society. pp. 350–1. Retrieved 12 December 2009.

4. Adams, Scott. "Bishops in Italy Approve a German-made Low Gluten Eucharistic Host". 2002. Celiac.com.

5. Agrawal G, Borody TJ, Chamberlin W; Borody; Chamberlin. "'Global warming' to Mycobacterium avium subspecies paratuberculosis". Future Microbiology. 2014; 9 (7): 829–832.

6. Akobeng AK, Ramanan AV, Buchan I, et al. "Effect of breast feeding on risk of coeliac disease: a systematic review and meta-analysis of observational studies". Arch Dis Child. 2006; 91 (1): 39–43.

7. Alton, EW; Armstrong, DK. "Repeated nebulisation of non-viral CFTR gene therapy in patients with cystic fibrosis: a randomised, double-blind, placebo-controlled, phase 2b trial.". The Lancet. Respiratory medicine. 2015; 3: 684–91.

8. Alves Cde A, Aguiar RA, Alves AC, Santana MA . "Diabetes mellitus in patients with cystic fibrosis". J Bras Pneumol. 2007; 33 (2): 213–21.

9. American College of Obstetricians and Gynecologists; American College of Medical Genetics. Preconception and prenatal carrier screening for cystic fibrosis. Clinical and laboratory guidelines. Washington DC: American College of Obstetricians and Gynecologists. 2001; ISBN 0-915473-74-7.

10. American Gastroenterological Association medical position statement: Celiac Sprue. Gastroenterology. 2001; 120(6): 1522–5.

11. Andersen DH. "Cystic fibrosis of the pancreas and its relation to celiac disease: a clinical and pathological study". Am J Dis Child. 1938; 56: 344–399.

12. Anderson CM, French JM, Sammons HG, et al. "Coeliac disease; gastrointestinal studies and the effect of dietary wheat flour". Lancet. 1952; 1 (17): 836–42.

13. Apte MV, Pirola RC, Wilson JS. "Pancreas: alcoholic pancreatitis—it's the alcohol, stupid". Nature Reviews Gastroenterology & Hepatology. 2009; 6(6): 321–2.

14. Yadav D, Hawes RH, Brand RE, et al. "Alcohol consumption, cigarette smoking, and the risk of recurrent acute and chronic pancreatitis". Arch. Intern. Med. 2009; 169 (11): 1035–45.

15. Assael BM, Castellani C, Ocampo MB, et al. "Epidemiology and survival analysis of cystic fibrosis in an area of intense neonatal screening over 30 years". American Journal of Epidemiology. 2002; 156(5): 397–401.

16. Augarten A, Yahav Y, Kerem BS, et al. "Congenital bilateral absence of vas deferens in the absence of cystic fibrosis". Lancet. 1994; 344 (8935): 1473–4.

17. Balfour-Lynn, IM; Welch, K. "Inhaled corticosteroids for cystic fibrosis." The Cochrane database of systematic reviews. 2014; 10: CD001915.

18. Barker JM, Liu E. "Celiac disease: pathophysiology, clinical manifestations, and associated autoimmune conditions". Adv Pediatr. 2008; 55: 349–65.

19. Barnich N, Darfeuille-Michaud A . "Adherent-invasive Escherichia coli and Crohn's disease". Current Opinion in Gastroenterology. 2007; 23(1): 16–20.

20. Baumgart DC, Sandborn WJ. "Inflammatory bowel disease: clinical aspects and established and evolving therapies.". The Lancet. 2007; 369 (9573): 1641–57.

21. Baumgart DC, Sandborn WJ; Sandborn. "Crohn's disease". The Lancet. 2012; 380 (9853): 1590–605.

22. Baumgart M, Dogan B, Rishniw M, et al. "Culture independent analysis of ileal mucosa reveals a selective increase in invasive Escherichia coli of novel phylogeny relative to depletion of Clostridiales in Crohn's disease involving the ileum". The ISME Journal. 2007; 1(5): 403–18.

23. Beattie RM, Croft NM, Fell JM, et al. "Inflammatory bowel disease". Archives of Disease in Childhood. 2006; 91 (5): 426–32.

24. Bebb JR, Bailey-Flitter N, Ala'Aldeen D, et al. "Mastic gum has no effect on Helicobacter pylori load in vivo". J. Antimicrob. Chemother. 2003; 52 (3): 522–3.

25. Belkin RA, Henig NR, Singer LG, et al. "Risk factors for death of patients with cystic fibrosis awaiting lung transplantation". Am. J. Respir. Crit. Care Med. 2006; 173 (6): 659–66.

26. Ben MH, Thabet H, Zaghdoudi I, et al. "Metformin associated acute pancreatitis". Veterinary and human toxicology. 2002; 44 (1): 47–8.

27. Bernstein M, Irwin S, Greenberg GR. "Maintenance Infliximab Treatment is Associated with Improved Bone Mineral Density in Crohn's Disease". The American Journal of Gastroenterology. 2005; 100 (9): 2031–5.

28. Blackman SM, Deering-Brose R, McWilliams R, et al. "Relative contribution of genetic and nongenetic modifiers to intestinal obstruction in cystic fibrosis". Gastroenterology. 2006; 131 (4): 1030–9.

29. Bobadilla JL, Macek M, Fine JP, et al. "Cystic fibrosis: a worldwide analysis of CFTR mutations—correlation with incidence data and application to screening". Hum. Mutat. 2002; 19(6): 575–606.

30. Boorom KF, Smith H, Nimri L, et al. "Oh my aching gut: irritable bowel syndrome, Blastocystis, and asymptomatic infection". Parasit Vectors. 2008; 1(1): 40.

31. Borobio E, Arín A, Valcayo A, et al. "[Isotretinoin and ulcerous colitis]". An Sist Sanit Navar (in Spanish). 2004; 27 (2): 241–3.

32. Braat H, Peppelenbosch MP, Hommes DW. "Immunology of Crohn's disease". Annals of the New York Academy of Sciences. 2006; 1072 (1): 135–54.

33. Broomé U, Bergquist A. "Primary sclerosing cholangitis, inflammatory bowel disease, and colon cancer". Seminars in Liver Disease. 2006; 26 (1): 31–41.

34. Bruce M. Carlson (2004). Human Embryology and Developmental Biology. 3rd edtion. 2004; Saint Louis: Mosby. ISBN 0-323-03649-X.

35. Buchanan N. Child and Adolescent Health for Practitioners. Williams & Wilkins. 1987; p. 164. ISBN 0-86433-015-4.

36. Buckingham, Lela. Molecular diagnostics fundamentals, methods, and clinical applications. 2nd edtion 2012. Philadelphia: F.A. Davis Co. p. 351.

37. Bull TJ, Gilbert SC, Sridhar et al. "A novel multi-antigen virally vectored vaccine against Mycobacterium avium subspecies paratuberculosis". PLoS ONE. 2007; 2 (11): e1229.

38. Büller HA . "Problems in diagnosis of IBD in children". The Netherlands Journal of Medicine. 1997; 50 (2): S8–11.

39. Burgess, L; Southern, KW. "Pneumococcal vaccines for cystic fibrosis.". The Cochrane database of systematic reviews. 2014; 8: CD008865.

40. Busch R. "On the history of cystic fibrosis". Acta Univ Carol Med (Praha). 1990; 36 (1–4): 13–5.

41. Campbell, Jordana. "The many faces of Crohn's Disease: Latest concepts in etiology". Open Journal of Internal Medicine. 2012; 02 (02): 107–115.

42. Canavan C, Abrams KR, Mayberry J; et al. "Meta-analysis: Colorectal and small bowel cancer risk in patients with Crohn's disease". Alimentary Pharmacology and Therapeutics. 2006; 23 (8): 1097–104.

43. Carucci LR, Levine MS; Levine. "Radiographic imaging of inflammatory bowel disease". Gastroenterology Clinics of North America. 2002; 31(1): 93–117, ix.

44. Casanova JL, Abel L. "Revisiting Crohn's disease as a primary immunodeficiency of macrophages.". The Journal of experimental medicine. 2009; 206(9): 1839–43.

45. Catassi C, Rätsch IM, Gandolfi L, et al. "Why is coeliac disease endemic in the people of the Sahara?". Lancet. 1999; 354 (9179): 647–8.

46. Catassi, Carlo . "Where Is Celiac Disease Coming From and Why?".Journal of Pediatric Gastroenterology & Nutrition. 2005; 40(3): 279–282.

47. Cenac N, Andrews CN, Holzhausen M, et al. "Role for protease activity in visceral pain in irritable bowel syndrome". J. Clin. Invest. 2007; 117 (3): 636–47.

48. Cenac N, Coelho AM, Nguyen C, et al. "Induction of Intestinal Inflammation in Mouse by Activation of Proteinase-Activated Receptor-2". Am. J. Pathol. 2002; 161(5): 1903–15.

49. Chamberlin W, Borody, TJ Campbell J. "Primary treatment of Crohn's disease: combined antibiotics taking center stage." Expert review of clinical immunology. 2011; 7(6): 751–60.

50. Chamouard P, Richert Z, Meyer N, et al. "Diagnostic Value of C-Reactive Protein for Predicting Activity Level of Crohn's Disease". Clinical Gastroenterology and Hepatology. 2006; 4(7): 882–7.

51. Chen H, Ruan YC, Xu WM, Chen J, et al. "Regulation of male fertility by CFTR and implications in male infertility". Human Reproduction Update. 2012; 18(6): 703–713.

52. Cheng, K; Ashby, D; Smyth, RL. "Ursodeoxycholic acid for cystic fibrosis-related liver disease.". The Cochrane database of systematic reviews. 2014; 12: CD000222.

53. Chermesh, I.; Azriel, A.; Alter-Koltunoff, et al. "Crohn's disease and SLC11A1 promoter polymorphism.". Dig Dis Sci. 2007; 52 (7): 1632–5.

54. Cho JH, Brant SR. "Recent Insights into the Genetics of Inflammatory Bowel Disease". Gastroenterology. 2011; 140(6): 1704–12.

55. Clevers H. "Inflammatory Bowel Disease, Stress, and the Endoplasmic Reticulum". New England Journal of Medicine. 2009; 360 (7): 726–27.

56. Clinical trial number NCT00803205 for "Study of Ataluren (PTC124™) in Cystic Fibrosis" at ClinicalTrials.gov

57. Cobrin GM, Abreu MT. "Defects in mucosal immunity leading to Crohn's disease". Immunol. Rev. 2005; 206(1): 277–95.

58. Cohn JA, Friedman KJ, Noone PG, et al. "Relation between mutations of the cystic fibrosis gene and idiopathic pancreatitis". N. Engl. J. Med. 1998; 339 (10): 653–8.

59. Colombo C, Russo MC, Zazzeron L, Romano G (July 2006). "Liver disease in cystic fibrosis". J. Pediatr. Gastroenterol. Nutr. 43 (Suppl 1): S49–55.

60. Comalada M, Peppelenbosch MP (September 2006). "Impaired innate immunity in Crohn's disease". Trends Mol Med 12 (9): 397–9.

61. Conwell LS, Chang AB (2012). Conwell, Louise S, ed. "Bisphosphonates for osteoporosis in people with cystic fibrosis". Cochrane Database Syst Rev 4 (4): CD002010.

62. Corazza GR, Villanacci V (1 June 2005). "Coeliac disease". J. Clin. Pathol. 58 (6): 573–74.

63. Corazza GR, Villanacci V, Zambelli C, Milione M, Luinetti O, Vindigni C, Chioda C, Albarello L, Bartolini D, Donato F (2007). "Comparison of the interobserver reproducibility with different histologic criteria used in celiac disease". Clin. Gastroenterol. Hepatol. 5 (7): 838–43.

64. Corfield AP, Cooper MJ, Williamson RC, Mayer AD, McMahon MJ, Dickson AP, Shearer MG, Imrie CW (1985). "Prediction of severity in acute pancreatitis: prospective comparison of three prognostic indices". Lancet 2 (8452): 403–7.

65. Crawford JM. "The Gastrointestinal tract, Chapter 17". In Cotran RS, Kumar V, Robbins SL. Robbins Pathologic Basis of Disease: 5th Edition. W.B. Saunders and Company, Philadelphia, 1994.

66. Cullen DJ, Hawkey GM, Greenwood DC, et al. (1997). "Peptic ulcer bleeding in the elderly: relative roles of Helicobacter pylori and non-steroidal anti-inflammatory drugs". Gut 41 (4): 459–62.

67. Cunningham-Rundles C (September 2001). "Physiology of IgA and IgA deficiency". J. Clin. Immunol. 21 (5): 303–9.

68. Cuthbert AP, Fisher SA, Mirza MM, King K, Hampe J, Croucher PJ, Mascheretti S, Sanderson J, Forbes A, Mansfield J, Schreiber S, Lewis CM, Mathew CG (2002). "The contribution of NOD2 gene mutations to the risk and site of disease in inflammatory bowel disease". Gastroenterology 122 (4): 867–74.

69. Cuthbert AW, Halstead J, Ratcliff R, Colledge WH, Evans MJ (January 1995). "The genetic advantage hypothesis in cystic fibrosis heterozygotes: a murine study". J. Physiol. (Lond.) 482 (Pt 2): 449–54.

70. Danese S, Semeraro S, Papa A, Roberto I, Scaldaferri F, Fedeli G, Gasbarrini G, Gasbarrini A (2005). "Extraintestinal manifestations in inflammatory bowel disease". World Journal of Gastroenterology 11 (46): 7227–36.

71. Darfeuille-Michaud A, Boudeau J, Bulois P, Neut C, Glasser AL, Barnich N, Bringer MA, Swidsinski A, Beaugerie L, Colombel JF (2004). "High prevalence of Adherent-invasive Escherichia coli associated with ileal mucosa in Crohn's disease". Gastroenterology 127 (2): 412–21.

72. David A. Warrell (2005). Oxford textbook of medicine: Sections 18-33. Oxford University Press. pp. 511–. ISBN 978-0-19-856978-7.

73. Davies JC, Alton EW, Bush A (December 2007). "Cystic fibrosis". BMJ 335 (7632): 1255–9.

74. Davis LB, Champion SJ, Fair SO, Baker VL, Garber AM (April 2010). "A cost-benefit analysis of preimplantation genetic diagnosis for carrier couples of cystic fibrosis". Fertil. Sterol. 93 (6): 1793–804.

75. De Lisle RC (September 2009). "Pass the bicarb: the importance of HCO3- for mucin release". J. Clin. Invest. 119 (9): 2535–7.

76. Del Pinto, Rita; Pietropaoli, Davide; Chandar, Apoorva K.; Ferri, Claudio; Cominelli, Fabio (2015-08-12). "Association Between Inflammatory Bowel Disease and Vitamin D Deficiency: A Systematic Review and Meta-analysis". Inflammatory Bowel Diseases 21: 2708–17.

77. Dessein R, Chamaillard M, Danese S (2008). "Innate Immunity in Crohn^s Disease". Journal of Clinical Gastroenterology 42: S144–7.

78. Dewar D, Pereira SP, Ciclitira PJ (2004). "The pathogenesis of coeliac disease". Int J Biochem Cell Biol 36 (1): 17–24.

79. Di Sabatino A, Corazza GR (April 2009). "Coeliac disease". Lancet 373 (9673): 1480–93. van Heel DA, West J (2006). "Recent advances in coeliac disease". Gut 55 (7): 1037–46.

80. Di Sant'Agnese PA, Darling RC, Perera GA, Shea E (November 1953). "Abnormal electrolyte composition of sweat in cystic fibrosis of the pancreas; clinical significance and relationship to the disease". Pediatrics 12 (5): 549–63.

81. Dicke WK (1950). Coeliakie: een onderzoek naar de nadelige invloed van sommige graansoorten op de lijder aan coeliaki.e., PhD thesis (in Dutch). Utrecht, the Netherlands: University of Utrecht.

82. Diegelmann, J.; Czamara, D.; Le Bras, E.; Zimmermann, E.; Olszak, T.; Bedynek, A.; Göke, B.; Franke, A.; et al. (2013). "Intestinal DMBT1 expression is modulated by Crohn's disease-associated IL23R variants and by a DMBT1 variant which influences binding of the transcription factors CREB1 and ATF-2.". PLOS ONE 8 (11): e77773.

83. Dieterich W, Ehnis T, Bauer M, Donner P, Volta U, Riecken EO, Schuppan D (1997). "Identification of tissue transglutaminase as the autoantigen of celiac disease". Nat Med 3 (7): 797–801.

84. Dietz HC (August 2010). "New therapeutic approaches to Mendelian disorders". N. Engl. J. Med. 363 (9): 852–63.

85. Dixon PM, Roulston ME, Nolan DJ; Roulston; Nolan (1993). "The small bowel enema: A ten years review". Clinical Radiology 47 (1): 46–8.

86. Dotan I (2007). "Serologic markers in inflammatory bowel disease: tools for better diagnosis and disease stratification". Expert Rev Gastroenterol Hepatol 1 (2): 265–74.

87. Drake, Richard L.; Vogl, Wayne; Tibbitts, Adam W.M. Mitchell; illustrations by Richard; Richardson, Paul (2005). Gray's anatomy for students. Philadelphia: Elsevier/Churchill Livingstone. p. 273. ISBN 978-0-8089-2306-0.

88. Dubinsky MC, Fleshner PP (2003). "Treatment of Crohn's disease of inflammatory, stenotic, and fistulizing phenotypes". Current Treatment Options in Gastroenterology 6 (3): 183–200.

89. E Medicine Health , Jerry R. Balentine, DO, FACEP , Melissa Conrad Stöppler, MD, Chief Medical Editor

90. Eddleman KA, Malone FD, Sullivan L, Dukes K, Berkowitz RL, Kharbutli Y, Porter TF, Luthy DA, Comstock CH, Saade GR, Klugman S, Dugoff L, Craigo SD, Timor-Tritsch I.E., Carr SR, Wolfe HM, D'Alton ME (November 2006). "Pregnancy loss rates after midtrimester amniocentesis". Obstet Gynecol 108 (5): 1067–72.

91. Eggermont E, De Boeck K (October 1991). "Small-intestinal abnormalities in cystic fibrosis patients". Eur. J. Pediatr. 150 (12): 824–8.

92. Ekbom A, Helmick C, Zack M, Adami HO; Helmick; Zack; Adami (1990). "Increased risk of large-bowel cancer in Crohn's disease with colonic involvement". Lancet 336 (8711): 357–9.

93. Elias S, Annas GJ, Simpson JL (April 1991). "Carrier screening for cystic fibrosis: implications for obstetric and gynecologic practice". Am. J. Obstet. Gynecol. 164 (4): 1077–83.

94. Elliott, David E.; Weinstock, Joel V. (2012). "Where are we on worms?". Current Opinion in Gastroenterology 28 (6): 551–556.

95. Escott-Stump, Sylvia (2008). Nutrition and Diagnosis-Related Care, 7th edition. Baltimore, MD: Lippincott Williams & Wilkins. pp. 1020 (pp 431). ISBN 978-1-60831-017-3.

96. Evans JP, Steinhart AH, Cohen Z, McLeod RS; Steinhart; Cohen; McLeod (2003). "Home Total Parenteral Nutrition an Alternative to Early Surgery for Complicated Inflammatory Bowel Disease". Journal of Gastrointestinal Surgery 7(4): 562–6.

97. Fanconi, G.; Uehlinger, E.; Knauer, C. (1936). "Das coeliakie-syndrom bei angeborener zysticher pankreasfibromatose und bronchiektasien". Wien. Med. Wschr 86: 753–6.

98. Farrell P, Joffe S, Foley L, Canny GJ, Mayne P, Rosenberg M (September 2007). "Diagnosis of cystic fibrosis in the Republic of Ireland: epidemiology and costs". Ir Med J 100 (8): 557–60.

99. Fasano A (2009). "Celiac Disease Insights: Clues to Solving Autoimmunity". Scientific American (August): 49–57.

100. Fasano, A; Catassi, C (Dec 20, 2012). "Clinical practice. Celiac disease.". The New England Journal of Medicine 367 (25): 2419–26.

101. Feller M, Huwiler K, Schoepfer A, Shang A, Furrer H, Egger M (2010). "Long-term antibiotic treatment for Crohn's disease: systematic review and meta-analysis of placebo-controlled trials". Clin. Infect. Dis. 50 (4): 473–80.

102. Ferguson A, Hutton MM, Maxwell JD, Murray D (1970). "Adult coeliac disease in hyposplenic patients". Lancet 1 (7639): 163–4.

103. Ferguson R, Basu MK, Asquith P, Cooke WT (1976). "Jejunal mucosal abnormalities in patients with recurrent aphthous ulceration". Br Med J 1 (6000): 11–13.

104. Ferrante M, Henckaerts L, Joossens M, Pierik M, Joossens S, Dotan N, Norman GL, Altstock RT, Van Steen K, Rutgeerts P, Van Assche G, Vermeire S; Henckaerts; Joossens; Pierik; Joossens; Dotan; Norman; Altstock; Van Steen; Rutgeerts; Van Assche; Vermeire, S (2007). "New serological markers in inflammatory bowel disease are associated with complicated disease behaviour". Gut 56 (10): 1394–403.

105. Fink, G (February 2011). "Stress controversies: post-traumatic stress disorder, hippocampal volume, gastroduodenal ulceration*.". Journal of neuroendocrinology 23 (2): 107–17.

106. Fitzgerald JE, Gupta S, Masterson S, Sigurdsson HH (April 2012). "Laparostomy management using the ABThera™ open abdomen negative pressure therapy system in a grade IV open abdomen secondary to acute pancreatitis". Int Wound J 10 (2): 138–144.

107. Fix OK, Soto JA, Andrews CW, Farraye FA (2004). "Gastroduodenal Crohn's disease". Gastrointestinal Endoscopy 60 (6): 985.

108. Fleckenstein B, Molberg Ø, Qiao SW, Schmid DG, von der Mülbe F, Elgstøen K, Jung G, Sollid LM (2002). "Gliadin T cell epitope selection by tissue transglutaminase in celiac disease. Role of enzyme specificity and pH influence on the transamidation versus deamidation process". J Biol Chem 277 (37): 34109–34116.

109. Flume PA, Mogayzel Jr PJ, Robinson KA, et al. (March 2010). "Cystic Fibrosis Pulmonary Guidelines: Pulmonary Complications: Hemoptysis and Pneumothorax". Am J Respir Crit Care Med 182 (3): 298–306.

110. Forbes A, Kalantzis T (2005). "Crohn's disease: The cold chain hypothesis". International Journal of Colorectal Disease 21 (5): 399–401.

111. Fox, James; Timothy Wang (January 2007). "Inflammation, Atrophy, and Gastric Cancer". Journal Of Clinical Investigation. review 117 (1): 60–69.

112. Franco LP, Camargos PA, Becker HM, Guimarães RE (December 2009). "Nasal endoscopic evaluation of children and adolescents with cystic fibrosis". Braz J Otorhinolaryngol 75 (6): 806–13.

113. Freeman HJ (December 2009). "Adult Celiac Disease and its Malignant Complications" (PDF). Gut and Liver 3 (4): 237–46.

114. Freudenheim, Milt (2009-12-22). "Tool in Cystic Fibrosis Fight: A Registry". New York Times. pp. D1. Retrieved 2009-12-21.

115. Fridell JA, Vianna R, Kwo PY, Howenstine M, Sannuti A, Molleston JP, Pescovitz MD, Tector AJ (October 2005). "Simultaneous liver and pancreas transplantation in patients with cystic fibrosis". Transplant. Proc. 37 (8): 3567–9.

116. Fries, WS; Nazario, B (2007-05-16). "Crohn's Disease: 54 Tips to Help You Manage". WebMD. Retrieved 2008-02-14.

117. Gabriel SE, Brigman KN, Koller BH, Boucher RC, Stutts MJ (October 1994). "Cystic fibrosis heterozygote resistance to cholera toxin in the cystic fibrosis mouse model". Science 266 (5182): 107–9.

118. Gallagher, Eimear (2009). Gluten-free Food Science and Technology. Published by John Wiley and Sons,. p. 320. ISBN 978-1-4051-5915-9.

119. Gasche C, Scholmerich J, Brynskov J, D'Haens G, Hanauer SB, Irvine EJ, Jewell DP, Rachmilewitz D, Sachar DB, Sandborn WJ, Sutherland LR (2007). "A simple classification of Crohn's disease: Report of the Working Party for the World Congresses of Gastroenterology, Vienna 1998". Inflammatory Bowel Diseases 6 (1): 8–15.

120. GBD 2013 Mortality and Causes of Death, Collaborators (17 December 2014). "Global, regional, and national age-sex specific all-cause and cause-specific mortality for 240 causes of death, 1990-2013: a systematic analysis for the Global Burden of Disease Study 2013." Lancet 385: 117–71.

121. GBD 2013 Mortality and Causes of Death, Collaborators (17 December 2014). "Global, regional, and national age-sex specific all-cause and cause-specific mortality for 240 causes of death, 1990-2013: a systematic analysis for the Global Burden of Disease Study 2013." Lancet.

122. Gerasimidis K, McGrogan P, Edwards CA (August 2011). "The aetiology and impact of malnutrition in paediatric inflammatory bowel disease". Journal of Human Nutrition and Dietetics 24 (4): 313–26.

123. Gilljam M, Antoniou M, Shin J, Dupuis A, Corey M, Tullis DE (July 2000). "Pregnancy in cystic fibrosis. Fetal and maternal outcome". Chest 118 (1): 85–91.

124. Girón RM, Domingo D, Buendía B, Antón E, Ruiz-Velasco LM, Ancochea J (October 2005). "Nontuberculous mycobacteria in patients with cystic fibrosis". Arch. Bronconeumol. (in Spanish) 41 (10): 560–5.

125. Glubb DM, Gearry RB, Barclay ML, et al. (2011). "NOD2 and ATG16L1 polymorphisms affect monocyte responses in Crohn's disease". World Journal of Gastroenterology 17 (23): 2829–37.

126. Goddard AF, James MW, McIntyre AS, Scott BB; James; McIntyre; Scott; British Society of Gastroenterology (2011). "Guidelines for the management of iron deficiency anaemia". Gut 60 (10): 1309–1316.

127. Goddard CJ, Gillett HR (November 2006). "Complications of coeliac disease: are all patients at risk?". Postgrad Med J 82 (973): 705–12.

128. Goering, Richard (20 May 2014). MIMS Medical Microbiology. Philadelphia: Elsevier. pp. 32, 64, 294, 133–4, 208, 303–4, 502. ISBN 978-0-3230-4475-2.

129. Goh J, O'Morain CA; O'Morain (2003). "Nutrition and adult inflammatory bowel disease". Alimentary Pharmacology and Therapeutics 17 (3): 307–20.

130. Gray, Henry (1918). Gray's Anatomy. Philadelphia: Lea & Febiger.

131. Green PH, Cellier C (2007). "Celiac disease". N. Engl. J. Med. 357 (17): 1731–43.

132. Greenstein AJ, Janowitz HD, Sachar DB (September 1976). "The extra-intestinal complications of Crohn's disease and ulcerative colitis: a study of 700 patients". Medicine (Baltimore) 55 (5): 401–12.

133. Guandalini, S; Assiri, A (March 2014). "Celiac disease: a review.". JAMA pediatrics 168 (3): 272–8.

134. Gujral N, Freeman HJ, Thomson AB (November 2012). "Celiac disease: prevalence, diagnosis, pathogenesis and treatment." (PDF). World Journal of Gastroenterology 18 (42): 6036–59.

135. Haas SV (1924). "The value of the banana in the treatment of coeliac disease". Am J Dis Child 24 (4): 421–37.

136. Hadithi M, von Blomberg BM, Crusius JB, Bloemena E, Kostense PJ, Meijer JW, Mulder CJ, Stehouwer CD, Peña AS (2007). "Accuracy of serologic tests and HLA-DQ typing for diagnosing celiac disease". Ann. Intern. Med. 147 (5): 294–302. doi:10.7326/0003-4819-147-5-200709040-00003. PMID 17785484.

137. Hamosh A, FitzSimmons SC, Macek M, Knowles MR, Rosenstein BJ, Cutting GR (February 1998). "Comparison of the clinical manifestations of cystic fibrosis in black and white patients". J. Pediatr. 132 (2): 255–9.

138. Hansen CR, Pressler T, Koch C, Høiby N (March 2005). "Long-term azitromycin treatment of cystic fibrosis patients with chronic Pseudomonas aeruginosa infection; an observational cohort study". J. Cyst. Fibros. 4 (1): 35–40.

139. Hara AK, Leighton JA, Heigh RI, Sharma VK, Silva AC, De Petris G, Hentz JG, Fleischer DE (2005). "Crohn Disease of the Small Bowel: Preliminary Comparison among CT Enterography, Capsule Endoscopy, Small-Bowel Follow-through, and Ileoscopy". Radiology 238 (1): 128–34.

140. Hardin DS (August 2004). "GH improves growth and clinical status in children with cystic fibrosis – a review of published studies". Eur. J. Endocrinol. 151 (Suppl 1): S81–5.

141. Hardin DS, Rice J, Ahn C, Ferkol T, Howenstine M, Spears S, Prestidge C, Seilheimer DK, Shepherd R (March 2005). "Growth hormone treatment enhances nutrition and growth in children with cystic fibrosis receiving enteral nutrition". J. Pediatr. 146 (3): 324–8.

142. Harrison's Principles of Internal Medicine. p. Chapter 370 Approach to the Patient with Pancreatic Disease. ISBN 978-0-07-1802161.

143. Häuser W, Gold J, Stein J, Caspary WF, Stallmach A (July 2006). "Health-related quality of life in adult coeliac disease in Germany: results of a national survey". Eur J Gastroenterol Hepatol 18 (7): 747–54.

144. Haworth CS, Selby PL, Webb AK, Dodd ME, Musson H, McL Niven R, Economou G, Horrocks AW, Freemont AJ, Mawer EB, Adams JE (November 1999). "Low bone mineral density in adults with cystic fibrosis". Thorax 54 (11): 961–7.

145. HCP: Pill Cam, Capsule Endoscopy, Esophageal Endoscopy

146. Hegarty M, Macdonald J, Watter P, Wilson C (July 2009). "Quality of life in young people with cystic fibrosis: effects of hospitalization, age and gender, and differences in parent/child perceptions". Child Care Health Dev 35 (4): 462–8.

147. Helander HF, Fändriks L. Surface area of the digestive tract – revisited. Scand J Gastroenterol 49: 681-9, 2014.

148. Helander HF, Fändriks L., "Surface area of the digestive tract – revisited", Scand J Gastroenterol 49: 681-9, 2014.

149. Henckaerts L, Figueroa C, Vermeire S, Sans M (May 2008). "The role of genetics in inflammatory bowel disease". Curr Drug Targets 9 (5): 361–8.

150. Hill ID (April 2005). "What are the sensitivity and specificity of serologic tests for celiac disease? Do sensitivity and specificity vary in different populations?" (PDF). Gastroenterology 128 (4 Suppl 1): S25–32.

151. Hill ID, Dirks MH, Liptak GS, et al. (2005). "Guideline for the diagnosis and treatment of celiac disease in children: recommendations of the North American Society for Pediatric Gastroenterology, Hepatology and Nutrition". J. Pediatr. Gastroenterol. Nutr. (North American Society for Pediatric Gastroenterology) 40 (1): 1–19.

152. Hischenhuber C, Crevel R, Jarry B, Mäki M, Moneret-Vautrin DA, Romano A, Troncone R, Ward R (March 2006). "Review article: safe amounts of gluten for patients with wheat allergy or coeliac disease". Aliment. Pharmacol. Ther. 23 (5): 559–75.

153. Hodson, Margaret; Geddes, Duncan; Bush, Andrew, eds. (2012). Cystic fibrosis (3rd ed.). London: Hodder Arnold. p. 3. ISBN 978-1-4441-1369-3.

154. Hofmann AF (1967). "The syndrome of ileal disease and the broken enterohepatic circulation: cholerhetic enteropathy.". Gastroenterology 52 (4): 752–7.

155. Högenauer C, Santa Ana CA, Porter JL, Millard M, Gelfand A, Rosenblatt RL, Prestidge CB, Fordtran JS (December 2000). "Active intestinal chloride secretion in human carriers of cystic fibrosis mutations: an evaluation of the hypothesis that heterozygotes have subnormal active intestinal chloride secretion". Am. J. Hum. Genet. 67 (6): 1422–7.

156. Høiby N (June 1995). "Isolation and treatment of cystic fibrosis patients with lung infections caused by Pseudomonas (Burkholderia) cepacia and multiresistant Pseudomonas aeruginosa". Neth J Med 46 (6): 280–87.

157. Hopper AD, Cross SS, Hurlstone DP, McAlindon ME, Lobo AJ, Hadjivassiliou M, Sloan ME, Dixon S, Sanders DS (2007). "Pre-endoscopy serological testing for coeliac disease: evaluation of a clinical decision tool". The BMJ 334 (7596): 729.

158. Hou, Jason K; Abraham, Bincy; El-Serag, Hashem (April 2011). "Dietary Intake and Risk of Developing Inflammatory Bowel Disease: A Systematic Review of the Literature" (PDF) Am. J Gastroenterology 106: 563–573.

159. Houlston RS, Ford D (1996). "Genetics of coeliac disease". QJM 89 (10): 737–43.

160. http://www.plos.org/media/press/2012/PLoS_%20HMP_Collection_Manuscript_Summaries.pdf

161. Hugot JP, Alberti C, Berrebi D, Bingen E, Cézard JP (2003). "Crohn's disease: the cold chain hypothesis". Lancet 362 (9400): 2012–5.

162. Hultén, K.; Almashhrawi, A.; El-Zaatari, FA.; Graham, DY. (Mar 2000). "Antibacterial therapy for Crohn's disease: a review emphasizing therapy directed against mycobacteria". Dig Dis Sci 45 (3): 445–56.

163. Huth MM, Zink KA, Van Horn NR (2005). "The effects of massage therapy in improving outcomes for youth with cystic fibrosis: an evidence review". Pediatr Nurs 31 (4): 328–32.

164. Hytönen M, Patjas M, Vento SI, Kauppi P, Malmberg H, Ylikoski J, Kere J (December 2001). "Cystic fibrosis gene mutations deltaF508 and 394delTT in patients with chronic sinusitis in Finland". Acta Otolaryngol. 121 (8): 945–7.

165. Inflamm Bowel Dis Volume 13, Number 12, December 2007

166. Israeli E, Grotto I, Gilburd B, Balicer RD, Goldin E, Wiik A, Shoenfeld Y; Grotto; Gilburd; Balicer; Goldin; Wiik; Shoenfeld (2005). "Anti-Saccharomyces cerevisiae and antineutrophil cytoplasmic antibodies as predictors of inflammatory bowel disease". Gut 54 (9): 1232–6.

167. Izzo AA, Coutts AA; Coutts (2005). "Cannabinoids and the digestive tract". Handbook of Experimental Pharmacology. Handbook of Experimental Pharmacology 168 (168): 573–98.

168. Johnson CD, Hosking S (1991). "National statistics for diet, alcohol consumption, and chronic pancreatitis in England and Wales, 1960–88". Gut 32 (11): 1401–5.

169. Jones AM, Govan JR, Doherty CJ, Dodd ME, Isalska BJ, Stanbridge TN, Webb AK (June 2003). "Identification of airborne dissemination of epidemic multiresistant strains of Pseudomonas aeruginosa at a CF centre during a cross infection outbreak". Thorax 58 (6): 525–27.

170. Joos S, Brinkhaus B, Maluche C, Maupai N, Kohnen R, Kraehmer N, Hahn E.G., Schuppan D; Brinkhaus; Maluche; Maupai; Kohnen; Kraehmer; Hahn; Schuppan (2004). "Acupuncture and moxibustion in the treatment of active Crohn's disease: a randomized controlled study". Digestion 69 (3): 131–9.

171. Jores RD, Frau F, Cucca F, Grazia Clemente M, Orrù S, Rais M, De Virgiliis S, Congia M (2007). "HLA-DQB1*0201 homozygosis predisposes to severe intestinal damage in celiac disease". Scand. J. Gastroenterol. 42 (1): 48–53.

172. Jostins L, Ripke S, Weersma RK; et al. (2012). "Host-microbe interactions have shaped the genetic architecture of inflammatory bowel disease". Nature 491 (7422): 119–24.

173. Kagnoff MF, Paterson YJ, Kumar PJ, Kasarda DD, Carbone FR, Unsworth DJ, Austin RK (1987). "Evidence for the role of a human intestinal adenovirus in the pathogenesis of coeliac disease". Gut 28 (8): 995–1001.

174. Kaila B, Orr K, Bernstein CN; Orr; Bernstein (2005). "The anti-Saccharomyces cerevisiae antibody assay in a province-wide practice: accurate in identifying cases of Crohn's disease and predicting inflammatory disease". The Canadian Journal of Gastroenterology 19 (12): 717–21. PMID 16341311. Retrieved 2006-07-02.

175. Kapoor, Vinay Kumar (13 Jul 2011). Gest, Thomas R., ed. "Large Intestine Anatomy". Medscape.

176. Karell K, Louka AS, Moodie SJ, Ascher H, Clot F, Greco L, Ciclitira PJ, Sollid LM, Partanen J (2003). "HLA types in celiac disease patients not carrying the DQA1*05-DQB1*02 (DQ2) heterodimer: results from the European Genetics Cluster on Celiac Disease". Hum. Immunol. 64 (4): 469–77.

177. Kaser A, Lee AH, Franke A, Glickman JN, Zeissig S, Tilg H, Nieuwenhuis EE, Higgins DE, Schreiber S, Glimcher LH, Blumberg RS (5 September 2008). "XBP1 links ER stress to intestinal inflammation and confers genetic risk for human inflammatory bowel disease". Cell 134 (5): 743–56.

178. Kato, Ikuko; Abraham M. Y. Nomura; Grant N. Stemmermann; Po-Huang Chyou (1992). "A Prospective Study of Gastric and Duodenal Ulcer and Its Relation to Smoking, Alcohol, and Diet". American Journal of Epidemiology 135 (5): 521–530.

179. Kaukinen K, Peräaho M, Collin P, Partanen J, Woolley N, Kaartinen T, Nuutinen T, Halttunen T, Mäki M, Korponay-Szabo I (2005). "Small-bowel mucosal tranglutaminase 2-specific IgA deposits in coeliac disease without villous atrophy: A Prospective and radmonized clinical study". Scand J Gastroenterology 40 (5): 564–572.

180. Kaur G, Sarkar N, Bhatnagar S, Kumar S, Rapthap CC, Bhan MK, Mehra NK (2002). "Pediatric celiac disease in India is associated with multiple DR3-DQ2 haplotypes". Hum. Immunol. 63 (8): 677–82.

181. Kellerman D, Rossi Mospan A, Engels J, Schaberg A, Gorden J, Smiley L (2008). "Denufosol: a review of studies with inhaled P2Y(2) agonists that led to Phase 3". Pulmonary Pharmacology and Therapeutics 21 (4): 600–7.

182. Kere J, Savilahti E, Norio R, Estivill X, de la Chapelle A (September 1990). "Cystic fibrosis mutation delta F508 in Finland: other mutations predominate". Hum. Genet. 85 (4): 413–5.

183. Khoshoo V, Udall JN (February 1994). "Meconium ileus equivalent in children and adults". Am. J. Gastroenterol. 89 (2): 153–7.

184. Kim C, Quarsten H, Bergseng E, Khosla C, Sollid L (2004). "Structural basis for HLA-DQ2-mediated presentation of gluten epitopes in celiac disease". Proc Natl Acad Sci USA 101 (12): 4175–9.

185. Kim SK. Small intestine transit time in the normal small bowel study. American Journal of Roentgenology 1968; 104(3): 522-524.

186. Kirsner JB (1988). "Historical aspects of inflammatory bowel disease". J. Clin. Gastroenterol. 10 (3): 286–97.

187. Koning F, Schuppan D, Cerf-Bensussan N, Sollid LM (Jun 2005). "Pathomechanisms in celiac disease". Best practice & research. Clinical gastroenterology 19 (3): 373–387.

188. Korponay-Szabó IR, Dahlbom I, Laurila K, Koskinen S, Woolley N, Partanen J, Kovács JB, Mäki M, Hansson T (2003). "Elevation of IgG antibodies against tissue transglutaminase as a diagnostic tool for coeliac disease in selective IgA deficiency". Gut 52 (11): 1567–71.

189. Kulczycki LL, Shwachman H (August 1958). "Studies in cystic fibrosis of the pancreas; occurrence of rectal prolapse". N. Engl. J. Med. 259 (9): 409–12.

190. Kumar, Vinay; Abbas, Abul K.; Fausto, Nelson (July 30, 2004). "The Gastrointestinal Tract". Robbins and Cotran: Pathologic Basis of Disease (7th ed.). Philadelphia, Pennsylvania: Elsevier Saunders. p. 847. ISBN 0-7216-0187-1.

191. Kunjathaya P, Ramaswami PK, Krishnamurthy AN, Bhat N (2013). "Acute necrotizing pancreatitis associated with vildagliptin". JOP : Journal of the pancreas 14 (1): 81–84.

192. Kupper C (2005). "Dietary guidelines and implementation for celiac disease". Gastroenterology 128 (4 Suppl 1): S121–7.

193. Kurata Ph.D., M.P.H., John H.; Nogawa, Aki N. M.S. (Jan 1997). "Meta-analysis of Risk Factors for Peptic Ulcer: Nonsteroidal Antiinflammatory Drugs, Helicobacter pylori, and Smoking". Journal of Clinical Gastroenterology 24 (1): 2–17.

194. Kuver R, Lee SP (April 2006). "Hypertonic saline for cystic fibrosis". N. Engl. J. Med. 354 (17): 1848–51; author reply 1848–51.

195. Lalande JD, Behr MA (2010). "Mycobacteria in Crohn's disease: How innate immune deficiency may result in chronic inflammation". Expert review of clinical immunology 6 (4): 633–41.

196. Lammers KM, Lu R, Brownley J, Lu B, Gerard C, Thomas K, Rallabhandi P, Shea-Donohue T, Tamiz A, Alkan S, Netzel-Arnett S, Antalis T, Vogel SN, Fasano A (2008). "Gliadin induces an increase in intestinal permeability and zonulin release by binding to the chemokine receptor CXCR3". Gastroenterology 135 (1): 194–204.e3.

197. Lankisch, PG; Apte, M; Banks, PA (20 January 2015). "Acute pancreatitis.". Lancet 386: 85–96. Yadav, D; Lowenfels, AB (June 2013). "The epidemiology of pancreatitis and pancreatic cancer.". Gastroenterology 144 (6): 1252–61.

198. Lawrence W. Tierney, Stephen J. McPhee. Medicine. McGraw-Hill. ISBN 0-07-144441-6.

199. Layrisse Z, Guedez Y, Domínguez E, Paz N, Montagnani S, Matos M, Herrera F, Ogando V, Balbas O, Rodríguez-Larralde A (2001). "Extended HLA haplotypes in a Carib Amerindian population: the Yucpa of the Perija Range". Hum Immunol 62 (9): 992–1000.

200. Lebwohl, B; Ludvigsson, JF; Green, PH (5 October 2015). "Celiac disease and non-celiac gluten sensitivity". BMJ (Clinical research ed.) 351: h4347.

201. Leeds JS, Hopper AD, Sanders DS (2008). "Coeliac disease". Br Med Bull 88 (1): 157–70.

202. Lesko SM, Kaufman DW, Rosenberg L, Helmrich SP, Miller DR, Stolley PD, Shapiro S (1985). "Evidence for an increased risk of Crohn's disease in oral contraceptive users". Gastroenterology 89 (5): 1046–9.

203. Li JY, Yu T, Chen GC, Yuan YH, Zhong W, Zhao LN, Chen QK. (Jun 6, 2013). "Enteral Nutrition within 48 Hours of Admission Improves Clinical Outcomes of Acute Pancreatitis by Reducing Complications: A Meta-Analysis.". PLoS One. 8 (6): e64926.

204. Lichtarowicz, A.M.; Mayberry, J.F. (August 1, 1988). "Antoni Lésniowski and his contribution to regional enteritis (Crohn's disease)". Journal of the Royal Society of Medicine 81 (8): 468–470.

205. Lieberman J (July 1968). "Dornase aerosol effect on sputum viscosity in cases of cystic fibrosis". JAMA 205 (5): 312–3.

206. Lionetti, Elena; Castellaneta, Stefania; Francavilla, Ruggiero; Pulvirenti, Alfredo; et al. (2014). "Introduction of Gluten, HLA Status, and the Risk of Celiac Disease in Children". New England Journal of Medicine (comparative study) 371 (14): 1295–1303. "The Gluten Connection". Health Canada. Retrieved 1 October 2013.

207. Lomer MC (August 2011). "Dietary and nutritional considerations for inflammatory bowel disease". The Proceedings of the Nutrition Society 70 (3): 329–35.

208. Lomer MC, Hutchinson C, Volkert S, Greenfield SM, Catterall A, Thompson RP, Powell JJ (December 2004). "Dietary sources of inorganic microparticles and their intake in healthy subjects and patients with Crohn's disease". Br. J. Nutr. 92 (6): 947–55.

209. Londei M, Ciacci C, Ricciardelli I, Vacca L, Quaratino S, Maiuri L (2005). "Gliadin as a stimulator of innate responses in celiac disease". Mol Immunol 42 (8): 913–918.

210. Longmore, Murray (2014). Oxford handbook of Clinical Medicine. Oxford University Press. p. 280. ISBN 9780199609628.

211. Longmore, Murray; Ian Wilkinson; Tom Turmezei; Chee Kay Cheung (2007). Oxford Handbook of Clinicial Medicine (7th ed.). Oxford University Press. pp. 266–7. ISBN 0-19-856837-1.

212. Losowsky MS (2008). "A history of coeliac disease". Dig Dis 26 (2): 112–20.

213. Lower Gastrointestinal Tract at the US National Library of Medicine Medical Subject Headings (MeSH)

214. Macdonald WC, Dobbins WO, Rubin CE (1965). "Studies of the familial nature of celiac sprue using biopsy of the small intestine". N Engl J Med 272 (9): 448–56.

215. Mackalski BA, Bernstein CN; Bernstein (2005). "New diagnostic imaging tools for inflammatory bowel disease". Gut 55 (5): 733–41.

216. MacKenzi.e., T; Gifford, AH; Sabadosa, KA; Quinton, HB; Knapp, EA; Goss, CH; Marshall, BC (Aug 19, 2014). "Longevity of patients with cystic fibrosis in 2000 to 2010 and beyond: survival analysis of the cystic fibrosis foundation patient registry.". Annals of internal medicine 161 (4): 233–41.

217. Mahadeva U, Martin JP, Patel NK, Price AB (July 2002). "Granulomatous ulcerative colitis: a re-appraisal of the mucosal granuloma in the distinction of Crohn's disease from ulcerative colitis". Histopathology 41 (1): 50–5.

218. Makker K, Agarwal A, Sharma R (April 2009). "Oxidative stress & male infertility" (PDF). Indian J. Med. Res. 129 (4): 357–67.

219. Maldonado M, Martínez A, Alobid I, Mullol J (December 2004). "The antrochoanal polyp". Rhinology 42 (4): 178–82.

220. Malfroot A, Dab I. "New insights on gastro-esophageal reflux in cystic fibrosis by longitudinal follow up". Arch. Dis. Child. 1991; 66 (11): 1339–45.

221. Marieb and Hoehn, (2014) Human Antomy and Physiology, Chapter 22: The Respiratory System, pg 906, Pearson Education

222. Marks DJ, Harbord MW, MacAllister R, et al. "Defective acute inflammation in Crohn's disease: a clinical investigation". Lancet. 2006; 367 (9511): 668–78.

223. Marks DJ, Rahman FZ, Sewell GW, Segal AW (2010). "Crohn's disease: An immune deficiency state". Clinical reviews in allergy and immunology 38 (1): 20–31.

224. Marks DJ, Segal AW (January 2008). "Innate immunity in inflammatory bowel disease: a disease hypothesis". J Pathol. 214 (2): 260–6.

225. Marks J, Shuster S, Watson AJ (1966). "Small-bowel changes in dermatitis herpetiformis". Lancet 2 (7476): 1280–2.

226. Marks SC, Kissner DG (1997). "Management of sinusitis in adult cystic fibrosis". Am J Rhinol 11 (1): 11–4.

227. Marsh MN. "Gluten, major histocompatibility complex, and the small intestine. A molecular and immunobiologic approach to the spectrum of gluten sensitivity ('celiac sprue')". Gastroenterology. 1992; 102 (1): 330–54.

228. Marshall B.J. "Unidentified curved bacillus on gastric epithelium in active chronic gastritis". Lancet. 1983; 1 (8336): 1273–75.

229. Marshall B.J., Warren J.R. (1984). "Unidentified curved bacilli in the stomach patients with gastritis and peptic ulceration". Lancet 1 (8390): 1311–15.

230. Martin, David F.; Captain Elizabeth Montgomery, et al. "Campylobacter pylori, NSAIDS, and Smoking: Risk Factors for Peptic Ulcer Disease". American Journal of Gastroenterology. 2008; 84 (10): 1268–72.

231. Massa F, Monory K; Monory (2007). "Endocannabinoids and the gastrointestinal tract". Journal of Endocrinological Investigation 29 ((Suppl)): 47–57.

232. Massa F, Storr M, Lutz B; Storr; Lutz. "The endocannabinoid system in the physiology and pathophysiology of the gastrointestinal tract". Journal of Molecular Medicine. 2005; 83 (12): 944–54.

233. Massi.e., J; Delatycki, MB (December 2013). "Cystic fibrosis carrier screening.". Paediatric respiratory reviews 14 (4): 270–5.

234. Matveyenko AV, Dry S, Cox HI, Moshtaghian A, Gurlo T, Galasso R, Butler AE, Butler PC (July 2009). "Beneficial endocrine but adverse exocrine effects of sitagliptin in the human islet amyloid polypeptide transgenic rat model of type 2 diabetes: interactions with metformin". Diabetes 58 (7): 1604–15.

235. McCallum TJ, Milunsky JM, Cunningham DL, Harris DH, Maher TA, Oates RD (October 2000). "Fertility in men with cystic fibrosis: an update on current surgical practices and outcomes". Chest 118 (4): 1059–62.

236. McCoy KS, Quittner AL, Oermann CM, Gibson RL, Retsch-Bogart GZ, Montgomery AB (November 2008). "Inhaled aztreonam lysine for chronic airway Pseudomonas aeruginosa in cystic fibrosis". Am. J. Respir. Crit. Care Med. 178 (9): 921–8.

237. MedlinePlus Encyclopedia Small bowel bacterial overgrowth

238. Mee AS, Burke M, Vallon AG, Newman J, Cotton PB (1985). "Small bowel biopsy for malabsorption: comparison of the diagnostic adequacy of endoscopic forceps and capsule biopsy specimens". The BMJ 291 (6498): 769–72.

239. Michalski JP, McCombs CC, Arai T, Elston RC, Cao T, McCarthy CF, Stevens FM (1996). "HLA-DR, DQ genotypes of celiac disease patients and healthy subjects from the West of Ireland". Tissue Antigens 47 (2): 127–33.

240. Mishra A, Greaves R, Massie J. "The relevance of sweat testing for the diagnosis of cystic fibrosis in the genomic era.". The Clinical biochemist. Reviews / Australian Association of Clinical Biochemists. 2005; 26 (4): 135–53.

241. Mitchell, Richard Sheppard; Kumar, Vinay; Robbins, Stanley L.; Abbas, Abul K.; Fausto, Nelson (2007). Robbins basic pathology. Saunders/Elsevier. ISBN 1-4160-2973-7.

242. Modiano G, Ciminelli BM, Pignatti PF (March 2007). "Cystic fibrosis and lactase persistence: a possible correlation". Eur. J. Hum. Genet. 15 (3): 255–9.

243. Moran A, Dunitz J, Nathan B, et al. "Cystic fibrosis-related diabetes: current trends in prevalence, incidence, and mortality". Diabetes Care. 2009; 32 (9): 1626–31.

244. Moran A, Pyzdrowski KL, Weinreb J, Kahn BB, Smith SA, Adams KS, Seaquist ER (August 1994). "Insulin sensitivity in cystic fibrosis". Diabetes 43 (8): 1020–6.

245. Moran F, Bradley JM, Piper AJ (2009). Moran, Fidelma, ed. "Non-invasive ventilation for cystic fibrosis". Cochrane Database Syst Rev (1): CD002769.

246. Mowat AM (2003). "Coeliac disease – a meeting point for genetics, immunology, and protein chemistry". Lancet 361 (9365): 1290–1292.

247. Mowat C, Cole A, Windsor A, et al. "Guidelines for the management of inflammatory bowel disease in adults". Gut. 2011; 60(5): 571–607.

248. Mpofu CM, Campbell BJ, Subramanian S, et al. "Microbial Mannan Inhibits Bacterial Killing by Macrophages: A Possible Pathogenic Mechanism for Crohn's Disease". Gastroenterology. 2007; 133 (5): 1487–98.

249. Muddana V, Whitcomb DC, Papachristou GI. "Current management and novel insights in acute pancreatitis". Expert Rev Gastroenterol Hepatol. 2009; 3 (4): 435–44.

250. Muniraj, T; Aslanian, HR; Farrell, J; Jamidar, PA (December 2014). "Chronic pancreatitis, a comprehensive review and update. Part I: epidemiology, etiology, risk factors, genetics, pathophysiology, and clinical features.". Disease-a-month : DM 60 (12): 530–50.

251. Munoz A, Katerndahl DA (July 2000). "Diagnosis and management of acute pancreatitis". Am Fam Physician 62 (1): 164–74.

252. Murphy, Kenneth (20 May 2014). Janeway's Immunobiology. New York: Garland Science, Taylor and Francis Group, LLC. pp. 389–398. ISBN 978-0-8153-4243-4.

253. Naftali, T; Mechulam, R; Lev, LB; Konikoff, FM (2014). "Cannabis for inflammatory bowel disease.". Digestive diseases (Basel, Switzerland) 32 (4): 468–74.

254. Nakagome, S.; Mano, S.; Kozlowski, L.; Bujnicki, JM.; Shibata, H.; Fukumaki, Y.; Kidd, JR.; Kidd, KK.; et al. (Jun 2012). "Crohn's disease risk alleles on the NOD2 locus have been maintained by natural selection on standing variation.". Mol Biol Evol 29 (6): 1569–85.

255. Nandiwada SL, Tebo AE. "Testing for antireticulin antibodies in patients with celiac disease is obsolete: a review of recommendations for serologic screening and the literature". Clin. Vaccine Immunol. 2013; 20 (4): 447–51.

256. Naser SA, Collins MT. "Debate on the lack of evidence of Mycobacterium avium subsp. paratuberculosis in Crohn's disease". Inflamm. Bowel Dis. 2005; 11 (12): 1123.

257. Naser SA, Sagramsingh SR, Naser AS, and Naser ST (June 2014). "Mycobacterium avium subspecies paratuberculosis causes Crohn's disease in some inflammatory bowel disease patients". World J Gastroenterol. 20 (23): 7403–7415.

258. National Institute for Health and Clinical Excellence. Clinical guideline 61: Irritable bowel syndrome. London, 2008.

259. Nazareth, D; Walshaw, M (October 2013). "Coming of age in cystic fibrosis - transition from paediatric to adult care.". Clinical medicine (London, England) 13 (5): 482–6.

260. Nicolas ME, Krause PK, Gibson LE, Murray JA (August 2003). "Dermatitis herpetiformis". Int. J. Dermatol. 42 (8): 588–600.

261. NIDDK (July 2008). "Pancreatitis". National Digestive Diseases Information Clearinghouse. U.S. National Institute of Diabetes and Digestive and Kidney Diseases. 08–1596.

262. Niveloni S, Fiorini A, Dezi R, Pedreira S, Smecuol E, Vazquez H, Cabanne A, Boerr LA, Valero J, Kogan Z, Mauriño E, Bai JC (1998). "Usefulness of videoduodenoscopy and vital dye staining as indicators of mucosal atrophy of celiac disease: assessment of interobserver agreement". Gastrointestinal Endoscopy 47 (3): 223–29.

263. Noel RA, Braun DK, Patterson RE, Bloomgren GL (May 2009). "Increased risk of acute pancreatitis and biliary disease observed in patients with type 2 diabetes: a retrospective cohort study". Diabetes Care 32 (5): 834–8.

264. Norris JM, Barriga K, Hoffenberg EJ, Taki I, Miao D, Haas JE, Emery LM, Sokol RJ, Erlich HA, Eisenbarth GS, Rewers M (2005). "Risk of celiac disease autoimmunity and timing of gluten introduction in the diet of infants at increased risk of disease". JAMA 293 (19): 2343–2351.

265. Oberhuber G, Granditsch G, Vogelsang H (October 1999). "The histopathology of coeliac disease: time for a standardized report scheme for pathologists". Eur. J. Gastroenterol. Hepatol. 11 (10): 1185–94.

266. Ogura Y, Bonen DK, Inohara N, Nicolae DL, Chen FF, Ramos R, Britton H, Moran T, Karaliuskas R, Duerr RH, Achkar JP, Brant SR, Bayless TM, Kirschner BS, Hanauer SB, Nuñez G, Cho JH (2001). "A frameshift mutation in NOD2 associated with susceptibility to Crohn's disease". Nature 411 (6837): 603–6.

267. O'Keefe SJ (1996). "Nutrition and gastrointestinal disease". Scand. J. Gastroenterol. Suppl. 220: 52–9.

268. O'Malley CA (May 2009). "Infection control in cystic fibrosis: cohorting, cross-contamination, and the respiratory therapist" (PDF). Respir Care 54 (5): 641–57.

269. Onady GM, Stolfi A (2005). Onady, Gary M, ed. "Insulin and oral agents for managing cystic fibrosis-related diabetes". Cochrane Database Syst Rev (3): CD004730.

270. Ong, T; Ramsey, BW (15 September 2015). "Update in Cystic Fibrosis 2014.". American journal of respiratory and critical care medicine 192 (6): 669–75.

271. Online 'Mendelian Inheritance in Man' (OMIM) CYSTIC FIBROSIS; CF -219700

272. |access-date= requires |url= (help)O'Sullivan, BP; Freedman, SD (30 May 2009). "Cystic fibrosis.". Lancet 373 (9678): 1891–904..

273. Ozuner G, Fazio VW, Lavery IC, Milsom JW, Strong SA; Fazio; Lavery; Milsom; Strong (1996). "Reoperative rates for Crohn's disease following strictureplasty. Long-term analysis". Dis. Colon Rectum 39 (11): 1199–203.

274. Pages 152-156 (Section: Inflammatory bowel disease(IBD)) in: Elizabeth D Agabegi; Agabegi, Steven S. (2008). Step-Up to Medicine (Step-Up Series). Hagerstwon, MD: Lippincott Williams & Wilkins. ISBN 0-7817-7153-6.

275. Pai VB, Nahata MC (October 2001). "Efficacy and safety of aerosolized tobramycin in cystic fibrosis". Pediatr. Pulmonol. 32 (4): 314–27.

276. Pankhurst CL, Philpott-Howard J (April 1996). "The environmental risk factors associated with medical and dental equipment in the transmission of Burkholderia (Pseudomonas) cepacia in cystic fibrosis patients". J. Hosp. Infect. 32 (4): 249–55.

277. Papachristou GI, Muddana V, Yadav D, et al. "Comparison of BISAP, Ranson's, APACHE-II, and CTSI scores in predicting organ failure, complications, and mortality in acute pancreatitis.". Am J Gastroenterol. 2010; 105(2): 435–41.

278. Papp M, Altorjay I, Dotan N, Palatka K, Foldi I, Tumpek J, Sipka S, Udvardy M, Dinya T, Lakatos L, Kovacs A, Molnar T, Tulassay Z, Miheller P, Norman GL, Szamosi T, Papp J, Lakatos PL; Altorjay; Dotan; Palatka; Foldi; Tumpek; Sipka; Udvardy; Dinya; Lakatos; Kovacs; Molnar; Tulassay; Miheller; Norman; Szamosi; Papp; Hungarian Ibd Study; Lakatos (2008). "New serological markers for inflammatory bowel disease are associated with earlier age at onset, complicated disease behavior, risk for surgery, and NOD2/CARD15 genotype in a Hungarian IBD cohort". The American Journal of Gastroenterology 103 (3): 665–81.

279. Parenti DM, Steinberg W, Kang P (November 1996). "Infectious causes of acute pancreatitis". Pancreas 13 (4): 356–71.

280. Parham, Peter (20 May 2014). The Immune System. New York: Garland Science Taylor and Francis Group LLC. p. 494. ISBN 978-0-8153-4146-8.

281. Paulley JW (1954). "Observation on the aetiology of idiopathic steatorrhoea; jejunal and lymph-node biopsies". Br Med J 2 (4900): 1318–21. doi:10.1136/bmj.2.4900.1318. PMC 2080246. PMID 13209109.

282. Pegues DA, Carson LA, Tablan OC, FitzSimmons SC, Roman SB, Miller JM, Jarvis WR (May 1994). "Acquisition of Pseudomonas cepacia at summer camps for patients with cystic fibrosis. Summer Camp Study Group". J. Pediatr. 124 (5 Pt 1): 694–702.

283. Phillipson GT, Petrucco OM, Matthews CD (February 2000). "Congenital bilateral absence of the vas deferens, cystic fibrosis mutation analysis and intracytoplasmic sperm injection". Hum. Reprod. 15 (2): 431–5.

284. Pier GB, Grout M, Zaidi T, Meluleni G, Mueschenborn SS, Banting G, Ratcliff R, Evans MJ, Colledge WH (May 1998). "Salmonella typhi uses CFTR to enter intestinal epithelial cells". Nature 393 (6680): 79–82.

285. Pietzak MM (2014). "Dietary supplements in celiac disease". In Rampertab SD, Mullin GE. Celiac disease. pp. 137–59. ISBN 978-1-4614-8559-9.

286. Pihet M, Carrere J, Cimon B, Chabasse D, Delhaes L, Symoens F, Bouchara JP (June 2009). "Occurrence and relevance of filamentous fungi in respiratory secretions of patients with cystic fibrosis—a review". Med Mycol. 47 (4): 387–97.

287. Pitts-Tucker TJ, Miller MG, Littlewood JM (June 1986). "Finger clubbing in cystic fibrosis". Arch. Dis. Child. 61 (6): 576–9.

288. Pommerville, Jeffrey (2014). Fundamentals of microbiology. Burlington, MA: Jones and Bartlett Learning. ISBN 9781449688615.

289. Poolman EM, Galvani AP (February 2007). "Evaluating candidate agents of selective pressure for cystic fibrosis". Journal of the Royal Society, Interface 4 (12): 91–8.

290. Powell JJ, Thoree V, Pele LC (October 2007). "Dietary microparticles and their impact on tolerance and immune responsiveness of the gastrointestinal tract". Br. J. Nutr. 98 Suppl 1: S59–63.

291. Prescott NJ, Fisher SA, Franke A, Hampe J, Onnie CM, Soars D, Bagnall R, Mirza MM, Sanderson J, Forbes A, Mansfield JC, Lewis CM, Schreiber S, Mathew CG (2007). "A nonsynonymous SNP in ATG16L1 predisposes to ileal Crohn's disease and is independent of CARD15 and IBD5". Gastroenterology 132 (5): 1665–71.

292. Prescott, NJ.; Dominy, KM.; Kubo, M.; Lewis, CM.; Fisher, SA.; Redon, R.; Huang, N.; Stranger, BE.; et al. (May 2010). "Independent and population-specific association of risk variants at the IRGM locus with Crohn's disease.". Hum Mol Genet 19 (9): 1828–39.

293. Presutti RJ, Cangemi JR, Cassidy HD, Hill DA (2007). "Celiac disease". Am Fam Physician 76 (12): 1795–802.

294. Pseudomonas cepacia at summer camps for persons with cystic fibrosis. MMWR Morb. Mortal. Wkly. Rep. 42 (23): 456–9. June 1993.

295. Qiao SW, Bergseng E, Molberg Ø, et al. (August 2004). "Antigen presentation to celiac lesion-derived T cells of a 33-mer gliadin peptide naturally formed by gastrointestinal digestion". J. Immunol. 173 (3): 1757–62.

296. Quinton PM (June 2007). "Cystic fibrosis: lessons from the sweat gland". Physiology (Bethesda) 22 (3): 212–25.

297. Rajesh A, Maglinte DD; Maglinte (2006). "Multislice CT enteroclysis: technique and clinical applications". Clinical Radiology 61 (1): 31–9.

298. Ramalho AS, Beck S, Meyer M, et al. "Five percent of normal cystic fibrosis transmembrane conductance regulator mRNA ameliorates the severity of pulmonary disease in cystic fibrosis". Am. J. Respir. Cell Mol. Biol. 2002; 27(5): 619–27.

299. Ramsey B, Richardson MA. "Impact of sinusitis in cystic fibrosis". J. Allergy Clin. Immunol. 1992; 90(3 Pt 2): 547–52.

300. Rapaka RR, Kolls JK. "Pathogenesis of allergic bronchopulmonary aspergillosis in cystic fibrosis: current understanding and future directions". Med Mycol. 2009; 47 (Suppl 1): S331–7.

301. Ratjen F, Döring G. "Cystic fibrosis". Lancet. 2003; 361 (9358): 681–9..

302. Ratjen FA. "Cystic fibrosis: pathogenesis and future treatment strategies" (PDF). Respir Care. 2009; 54(5): 595–605.

303. Reaves J, Wallace G . "Unexplained bruising: weighing the pros and cons of possible causes". Consultant for Pediatricians. 2010; 9: 201–2.

304. Reddy D, Siegel CA, Sands BE, Kane S . "Possible association between isotretinoin and inflammatory bowel disease". The American journal of gastroenterology. 2006; 101(7): 1569–73.

305. Redondo-Cerezo E, Sánchez-Capilla AD, De La Torre-Rubio P, De Teresa J. "Wireless capsule endoscopy: Perspectives beyond gastrointestinal bleeding". World J. Gastroenterol. 2014; 20(42): 15664–73.

306. Reniers DE, Howard JM. "Isotretinoin-induced inflammatory bowel disease in an adolescent". Annals of Pharmacotherapy. 2001; 35(10): 1214–6.

307. Rewers M. "Epidemiology of celiac disease: what are the prevalence, incidence, and progression of celiac disease?" (PDF). Gastroenterology. 2005; 128(4 Suppl 1): S47–51.

308. Rhodes, M. "Intestinal transplant for Crohn's disease". Everyday Health. Retrieved. 2006; 2009-03-22.

309. Richard Coico, Geoffrey Sunshine, Eli Benjamini. Immunology: a short course. 2003; New York: Wiley-Liss. ISBN 0-471-22689-0.

310. Riordan JR, Rommens JM, Kerem B, et al. "Identification of the cystic fibrosis gene: cloning and characterization of complementary DNA". Science. 1989; 245(4922): 1066–73.

311. Rommens JM, Iannuzzi MC, Kerem B, et al. "Identification of the cystic fibrosis gene: chromosome walking and jumping". Science. 1989; 245 (4922): 1059–65.

312. Rosenfeld M, Davis R, FitzSimmons S, et al. "Gender gap in cystic fibrosis mortality". Am. J. Epidemiol. 1997; 145 (9): 794–803.

313. Rosenstein BJ, Cutting GR. "The diagnosis of cystic fibrosis: a consensus statement. Cystic Fibrosis Foundation Consensus Panel". J. Pediatr. 1998; 132(4): 589–95.

314. Rosenstein BJ, Zeitlin PL. "Cystic fibrosis". Lancet. 1998; 351 (9098): 277–82.

315. Ross LF. "Newborn screening for cystic fibrosis: a lesson in public health disparities". The Journal of Pediatrics. 2008; 153(3): 308–13.

316. Rowe SM, Miller S, Sorscher EJ. "Cystic fibrosis". The New England Journal of Medicine. 2005; 352 (19): 1992–2001.

317. Russell, Peter (2011). Biology: the dynamic science. (2nd ed.). Belmont, CA: Brooks/Cole, Cengage Learning. p. 304. ISBN 978-0-538-49372-7.

318. Rutgeerts P, Geboes K, Vantrappen G, Beyls J, Kerremans R, Hiele M; Geboes; Vantrappen; Beyls; Kerremans; Hiele (October 1990). "Predictability of the postoperative course of Crohn's disease". Gastroenterology 99 (4): 956–63.

319. Saiman L (2004). "Microbiology of early CF lung disease". Paediatric Respiratory Reviews 5 (Suppl A): S367–69.

320. Salih, Barik; M Fatih Abasiyanik; Nizamettin Bayyurt; Ersan Sander (June 2007). "H pylori infection and other risk factors associated with peptic ulcers in Turkish patients: A retrospective study". World Journal of Gastroenterology 13 (23): 3245–8.

321. Salim AF, Phillips AD, Farthing MJ (1990). "Pathogenesis of gut virus infection". Baillieres Clin Gastroenterol 4 (3): 593–607.

322. Salmi TT, Collin P, Korponay-Szabó IR, Laurila K, Partanen J, Huhtala H, Király R, Lorand L, Reunala T, Mäki M, Kaukinen K (2006). "Endomysial antibody-negative coeliac disease: clinical characteristics and intestinal autoantibody deposits". Gut 55 (12): 1746–53.

323. Sandborn WJ, Colombel JF, Enns R, et al. "Natalizumab Induction and Maintenance Therapy for Crohn's Disease". New England Journal of Medicine. 2005; 353 (18): 1912–25.

324. Sasaki M, Sitaraman SV, Babbin BA, et al. "Invasive Escherichia coli are a feature of Crohn's disease". Laboratory investigation; a journal of technical methods and pathology. 2007; 87(10): 1042–54.

325. Satsangi J, Jewell DP, Bell JI; et al. "The genetics of inflammatory bowel disease". Gut. 1997; 40 (5): 572–4.

326. Sblattero D, Berti I, Trevisiol C, et al. "Human recombinant tissue transglutaminase ELISA: an innovative diagnostic assay for celiac disease". Am. J. Gastroenterol. 2000; 95(5): 1253–57.

327. Scheinfeld NS, Teplitz E, McClain SA. "Crohn's disease and lichen nitidus: a case report and comparison of common histopathologic features". Inflammatory Bowel Diseases. 2001; 7(4): 314–8.

328. Schuppan D, Junker Y, Barisani D. "Celiac disease: from pathogenesis to novel therapies". Gastroenterology. 2009; 137(6): 1912–33.

329. Schwank G, Koo BK, Sasselli V, et al. "Functional repair of CFTR by CRISPR/Cas9 in intestinal stem cell organoids of cystic fibrosis patients". Cell Stem Cell. 2013; 13 (6): 653–8.

330. Scribano, ML; Prantera, C. "Use of antibiotics in the treatment of Crohn's disease.". World journal of gastroenterology : WJG. 2013; 19(5): 648–53.

331. Section "Antibiotics and Ulcerative Colitis" in: Prantera C, et al. "Antibiotics and probiotics in inflammatory bowel disease: why, when, and how". Curr. Opin. Gastroenterol. 2009; 25(4): 329–33.

332. Seow CH, Stempak JM, Xu W, et al. "Novel anti-glycan antibodies related to inflammatory bowel disease diagnosis and phenotype". Am J Gastroenterol. 2009; 104(6): 1426–34.

333. Shan L, Qiao SW, Arentz-Hansen H, et al. "Identification and analysis of multivalent proteolytically resistant peptides from gluten: implications for celiac sprue". J. Proteome Res. 2005; 4(5): 1732–41.

334. Shanahan, Fergus (1 January 2002). "Crohn's disease". The Lancet. 2002; 359(9300): 62–69.

335. Shepherd NA. "Granulomas in the diagnosis of intestinal Crohn's disease: a myth exploded?". Histopathology. 2002; 41(2): 166–8.

336. Shoda R, Matsueda K, Yamato S, et al. "Epidemiologic analysis of Crohn disease in Japan: increased dietary intake of n-6 polyunsaturated fatty acids and animal protein relates to the increased incidence of Crohn disease in Japan". The American journal of clinical nutrition. 1996; 63 (5): 741–5.

337. Short DB, Trotter KW, Reczek D, et al. "An apical PDZ protein anchors the cystic fibrosis transmembrane conductance regulator to the cytoskeleton". J. Biol. Chem. 1998; 273(31): 19797–801.

338. Skovbjerg H, Norén O, Anthonsen D, et al. "Gliadin is a good substrate of several transglutaminases: possible implication in the pathogenesis of coeliac disease". Scand J Gastroenterol. 2002; 37(7): 812–7.

339. Smart HL, Mayberry JF, Atkinson M; et al. "Alternative medicine consultations and remedies in patients with the irritable bowel syndrome". Gut. 1986; 27(7): 826–8.

340. Smith, Emma; Murray Longmore; Wilkinson, Ian; et al. Oxford handbook of clinical medicine. 7th edtion 2007. Oxford [Oxfordshire]: Oxford University Press. p. 584. ISBN 0-19-856837-1.

341. Snowden FM. "Emerging and reemerging diseases: a historical perspective". Immunol. Rev. 2008; 225 (1): 9–26.

342. Stefanelli T, Malesci A, Repici A, et al. "New Insights into Inflammatory Bowel Disease Pathophysiology: Paving the Way for Novel Therapeutic Targets". Current Drug Targets. 2008; 9(5): 413–8.

343. Stene LC, Honeyman MC, Hoffenberg EJ, et al. "Rotavirus infection frequency and risk of celiac disease autoimmunity in early childhood: a longitudinal study". Am J Gastroenterol. 2006; 101 (10): 2333–40.

344. Stern RC. "The diagnosis of cystic fibrosis". N. Engl. J. Med. 1997; 336(7): 487–91.

345. Subramanian S, Roberts CL, Hart CA, et al. "Replication of Colonic Crohn's Disease Mucosal Escherichia coli Isolates within Macrophages and Their Susceptibility to Antibiotics". Antimicrobial Agents and Chemotherapy. 2007; 52(2): 427–34.

346. Suman S, Williams EJ, Thomas PW, et al. "Is the risk of adult coeliac disease causally related to cigarette exposure?". Eur J Gastroenterol Hepatol. 2003; 15(9): 995–1000.

347. Tabor A, Philip J, Madsen M, et al. "Randomised controlled trial of genetic amniocentesis in 4606 low-risk women". Lancet. 19886; 1 (8493): 1287–93.

348. Tan KH, Mulheran M, Knox AJ, et al. "Aminoglycoside prescribing and surveillance in cystic fibrosis". Am. J. Respir. Crit. Care Med. 2003; 167(6): 819–23.

349. Tan, WC.; Allan, RN. "Diffuse jejunoileitis of Crohn's disease.". Gut. 1993; 34(10): 1374–8.

350. Tate S, Elborn S. "Progress towards gene therapy for cystic fibrosis". Expert Opin Drug Deliv. 2005; 2(2): 269–80.

351. Taylor BA, Williams GT, Hughes LE, et al. "The histology of anal skin tags in Crohn's disease: An aid to confirmation of the diagnosis". International Journal of Colorectal Disease. 1989; 4(3): 197–9.

352. Tersigni C, Castellani R, de Waure C, et al. "Celiac disease and reproductive disorders: meta-analysis of epidemiologic associations and potential pathogenic mechanisms". Human Reproduction Update. 2014; 20 (4): 582–593.

353. Thrash B, Patel M, Shah KR, et al. "Cutaneous manifestations of gastrointestinal disease: part II". Journal of the American Academy of Dermatology. 2013; 68 (2): 211 e1–33.

354. Tobias, Edward. Essential Medical Genetics. 2011. John Wiley & Sons. p. 312. ISBN 1-118-29370-3.

355. Tresca, AJ (2007-01-12). "Resection Surgery for Crohn's Disease". About.com. Retrieved. 2008-02-14.

356. Triester SL, Leighton JA, Leontiadis GI, et al. "A meta-analysis of the yield of capsule endoscopy compared to other diagnostic modalities in patients with non-stricturing small bowel Crohn's disease". The American Journal of Gastroenterology. 2006; 101(5): 954–64.

357. Trikudanathan G, Venkatesh PG, Navaneethan U. "Diagnosis and therapeutic management of extra-intestinal manifestations of inflammatory bowel disease". Drugs. 2012; 72 (18): 2333–49.

358. Tümmler B, Koopmann U, Grothues D, et al. "Nosocomial acquisition of Pseudomonas aeruginosa by cystic fibrosis patients". J. Clin. Microbiol. 1991; 29(6): 1265–7.

359. Tysk C, Lindberg E, Järnerot G, et al. "Ulcerative colitis and Crohn's disease in an unselected population of monozygotic and dizygotic twins. A study of heritability and the influence of smoking". Gut. 1988; 29(7): 990–6.

360. Uday C Ghoshal, Vikas Sengar, and Deepakshi Srivastava. Colonic Transit Study Technique and Interpretation: Can These Be Uniform Globally in Different Populations With Non-uniform Colon Transit Time? J Neurogastroenterol Motil. 2012; 18(2): 227–228.

361. Van der Schans C, Prasad A, Main E. Van Der Schans, Cees P, ed. "Chest physiotherapy compared to no chest physiotherapy for cystic fibrosis". Cochrane Database Syst Rev. 2000; (2): CD001401.

362. Van der Windt DA, Jellema P, Mulder CJ, et al. "Diagnostic testing for celiac disease among patients with abdominal symptoms: a systematic review". JAMA. 2010; 303 (17): 1738–46.

363. Vandemergel X, Decaux G. "[Review on hypertrophic osteoarthropathy and digital clubbing]". Revue Médicale de Bruxelles (in French). 2003; 24(2): 88–94.

364. Verkman AS, Song Y, Thiagarajah JR. Role of airway surface liquid and submucosal glands in cystic fibrosis lung disease. Am J Physiol Cell Physiol. 2003; 284(1):C2–C15

365. Verma N, Bush A, Buchdahl R. "Is there still a gender gap in cystic fibrosis?". Chest. 2005; 128 (4): 2824–34.

366. Wainwright, CE. "Ivacaftor for patients with cystic fibrosis.". Expert review of respiratory medicine. 2005; 8(5): 533–8.

367. Walcher, Dwain N. and Kretchmer, Norman. Food, nutrition, and evolution: food as an environmental factor in the genesis of human variability. Papers presented at the International Congress of the International Organization for the Study of Human Development, Masson Pub. USA. 1981; pp. 179–199. ISBN 0-89352-158-2.

368. Wang, AY; Peura, DA. "The prevalence and incidence of Helicobacter pylori-associated peptic ulcer disease and upper gastrointestinal bleeding throughout the world.". Gastrointestinal endoscopy clinics of North America. 2011; 21(4): 613–35.

369. Weinstock, Joel V.; Elliott, David E. "Translatability of helminth therapy in inflammatory bowel diseases". International Journal for Parasitology. 2013; 43 (3–4): 245–51.

370. Wennberg C, Kucinskas V. "Low frequency of the delta F508 mutation in Finno-Ugrian and Baltic populations". Hum. Hered. 1994; 44(3): 169–71.

371. Westerman EM, Le Brun PP, Touw DJ, et al. "Effect of nebulized colistin sulphate and colistin sulphomethate on lung function in patients with cystic fibrosis: a pilot study". J. Cyst. Fibros. 2004; 3(1): 23–8.

372. Whiting, P; Al, M; Burgers, L; et al. "Ivacaftor for the treatment of patients with cystic fibrosis and the G551D mutation: a systematic review and cost-effectiveness analysis.". Health technology assessment (Winchester, England). 2014; 18 (18): 1–106.

373. Wier LM, Steiner CA, Owens PL. "Surgeries in Hospital-Owned Outpatient Facilities, 2012". 2015; HCUP Statistical Brief #188. Rockville, MD: Agency for Healthcare Research and Quality.

374. Williams SG, Westaby D, Tanner MS, et al. "Liver and biliary problems in cystic fibrosis". Br. Med. Bull. 1992; 48(4): 877–92.

375. Williams, N. "Footprint fears for new TB threat". Current Biology. 2006; 16(19): R821.

376. Wilschanski M, Yahav Y, Yaacov Y, et al. "Gentamicin-induced correction of CFTR function in patients with cystic fibrosis and CFTR stop mutations". N. Engl. J. Med. 2003; 349(15): 1433–41.

377. Wiuf C. "Do delta F508 heterozygotes have a selective advantage?". Genet. Res. 2001; 78(1): 41–7.

378. Wong RC, Steele RH, Reeves GE, et al. "Antibody and genetic testing in coeliac disease". Pathology. 2003; 35(4): 285–304.

379. Yamada T, Alpers DH; et al. Textbook of gastroenterology. 5th edtion 2009; Chichester, West Sussex: Blackwell Pub. pp. 2774–2784. ISBN 978-1-4051-6911-0.

380. Yamamoto T, Bamba T, Umegae S, et al. "The impact of early endoscopic lesions on the clinical course of patients following ileocolonic resection for Crohn's disease: A 5-year prospective cohort study". United European Gastroenterol. 2013; J 1(4): 294–8.

381. Yamamoto-Furusho JK, Korzenik JR. "Crohn's disease: Innate immunodeficiency?". World Journal of Gastroenterology. 2006; 12(42): 6751–5.

382. Yeomans, ND. "The ulcer sleuths: The search for the cause of peptic ulcers.". Journal of gastroenterology and hepatology. 26 Suppl. 2011; 1: 35–41.

383. Zadik Y, Drucker S, Pallmon S. "Migratory stomatitis (ectopic geographic tongue) on the floor of the mouth". Journal of the American Academy of Dermatology. 2011; 65 (2): 459–60.

384. Zanoni G, Navone R, Lunardi C, et al. "In celiac disease, a subset of autoantibodies against transglutaminase binds toll-like receptor 4 and induces activation of monocytes". PLoS Med. 2006; 3(9): e358..

385. Zhernakova A, Elbers CC, Ferwerda B, et al. "Evolutionary and functional analysis of celiac risk loci reveals SH2B3 as a protective factor against bacterial infection". American Journal of Human Genetics. 2010; 86 (6): 970–7.

386. Zipser RD, Farid M, Baisch D, et al. "Physician awareness of celiac disease: a need for further education". J Gen Intern Med. 2005; 20 (7): 644–6.

387. Zirbes J, Milla CE. "Cystic fibrosis related diabetes". Paediatr Respir Rev. 2009; 10 (3): 118–23; quiz 123.

388. Zisman TL, Rubin DT; Rubin. "Colorectal cancer and dysplasia in inflammatory bowel disease". World Journal of Gastroenterology. 2008; 14(17): 2662–9.

7

The Hypothalamus and Pituitary Gland

INTRODUCTION

Pituitary, also known as hypophysis, is a small gland suspended from the brain by the hypophyseal stem. It is located in a cavity of the sphenoid bone called 'turkish saddle'. Pituitary is composed of two lobes—anterior lobe or adenohypophysis and posterior lobe or neuro-hypophysis. Although, closely related anatomically, they are embryologically and functionally quite distinct. The anterior pituitary comprises primarily glandular tissue, while the posterior pituitary is of neural origin. The pituitary gland is situated at the base of the brain, in close relation to the hypothalamus (Fig. 7.1), which has an essential role in the regulation of pituitary function.

ANTERIOR PITUITARY HORMONES

The cells of the anterior lobe which accounts for 80% of the pituitary gland's weight and the back posterior lobe synthesize and release several hormones necessary for normal growth and development and also stimulate the activity of several target glands.

Growth Hormone

Growth hormone (GH) which regulates growth and physical development and has important effects on body shape by stimulating muscle formation and reducing fat tissue. GH stimulates somatic growth and regulates metabolism. Growth hormone-releasing hormone (GHRH) is the major stimulator and somatostatin is the major inhibitor of the synthesis and release of GH. GH controls synthesis of insulin-like growth factor 1 (IGF-1, also called somatomedin-C), which largely controls growth. Although, IGF-1 is produced by many tissues, the liver is the major source. A variant of IGF-1 occurs in

muscle, where it plays a role in enhancing muscle strength. It is less under control of GH than is the liver variant.

The metabolic effects of GH are biphasic. GH initially exerts insulin-like effects, increasing glucose uptake in muscle and fat, stimulating amino acid uptake and protein synthesis in liver and muscle, and inhibiting lipolysis in adipose tissue. Several hours later, more profound anti-insulin-like metabolic effects occur. They include inhibition of glucose uptake and use, causing blood glucose and lipolysis to increase, which increases plasma free fatty acids. GH levels increase during fasting, maintaining blood glucose levels and mobilizing fat as

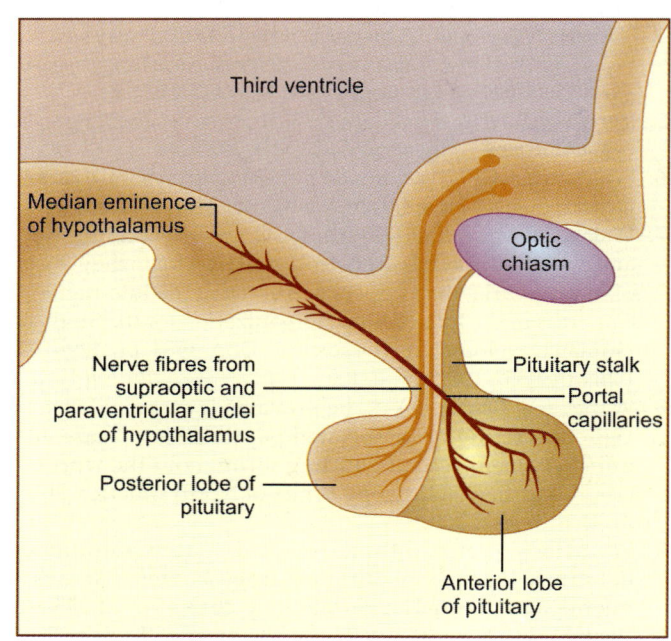

Fig. 7.1: Diagrammatic sagittal section through part of the brain to show the anatomical structures

an alternative metabolic fuel. Production of GH decreases with aging. Ghrelin, a hormone produced in the fundus of the stomach, promotes GH release from the pituitary, increases food intake, and improves memory.

Thyroid-stimulating Hormone

Thyroid-stimulating hormone (TSH) which regulates the structure and function of the thyroid gland and stimulates synthesis and release of thyroid hormones. TSH synthesis and release are stimulated by the hypothalamic hormone thyrotropin-releasing hormone (TRH) and suppressed (by negative feedback) by circulating thyroid hormones.

Thyroid-stimulating hormone (hyrotrophin) is a glycoprotein (molecular weight 28 kDa) composed of an α- and a β-subunit; the amino acid composition of the α-subunit is common to TSH, the pituitary gonadotrophins and human chorionic gonadotrophin (hCG), but the β-subunit is unique to TSH.

The normal plasma concentration of TSH in health is approximately 0.3–5.0 mU/L, but the lower value in particular is dependent on the assay used. TSH binds to specific receptors on thyroid cells, and in doing so stimulates the synthesis and secretion of thyroid hormones. Secretion of TSH is stimulated by the hypothalamic tripeptide TSH-releasing (or thyrotrophin-releasing) hormone (TRH) and this effect, and probably the release of TRH itself, is inhibited by high circulating concentrations of thyroid hormones.

Thus, thyroid hormone secretion is regulated by a negative feedback system; if plasma concentrations of thyroid hormones decrease, TSH secretion increases, stimulating thyroid hormone synthesis; if they increase, TSH secretion is suppressed. In primary hypothyroidism, TSH secretion is increased; in hyperthyroidism it is decreased. TSH deficiency can cause hypothyroidism, but hyperthyroidism due to TSH-secreting tumors is rare.

Adrenocorticotropic Hormone

Adrenocorticotropic hormone (ACTH) also called corticotropin, is a polypeptide (molecular weight 4500 Da), comprising a single chain of 39 amino acids. Its biological function, which is to stimulate adrenal glucocorticoid (but not mineralocorticoid) secretion, is dependent on the N-terminal 24 amino acids. ACTH is a fragment of a much larger precursor, pro-opiomelanocortin (POMC, molecular weight 31 kDa) (Fig. 7.2), which is the precursor not only of ACTH, but also of β-lipotrophin, itself the precursor of endogenous opioid peptides (endorphins). The control of the release of β-lipotrophin and the endorphins has not been fully elucidated, but ACTH release is controlled by a hypothalamic peptide, corticotropin-releasing hormone (CRH). ACTH secretion is pulsatile and also shows diurnal variation, the plasma concentration being

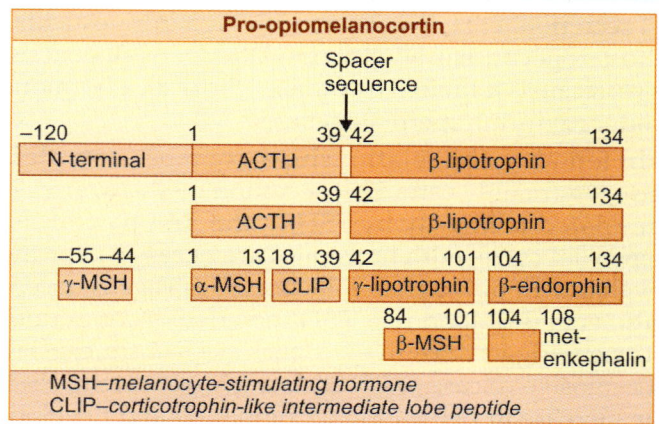

Fig. 7.2: ACTH is derived by proteolysis of a precursor, pro-opiomelanocortin lipotropin

highest at approximately 08:00 h and lowest at midnight. Secretion is greatly increased by stress and is inhibited by cortisol. Thus cortisol secretion by the adrenal cortex is controlled by negative feedback, but this and the circadian variation can be overcome by the effects of stress. The normal value for plasma ACTH concentration at 09:00 h is <50 ng/L.

Increased secretion of ACTH by the pituitary is seen with pituitary tumors (Cushing's disease) and in primary adrenal failure (Addison's disease). The hormone may also be secreted ectopically by non-pituitary tumors. Excessive ACTH synthesis is associated with increased pigmentation, owing to the melanocyte-stimulating action of ACTH and other POMC-derived peptides. Decreased secretion of ACTH may be an isolated phenomenon, but is more commonly associated with generalized pituitary failure.

GONADOTROPHINS

Follicle-stimulating hormone (FSH) and luteinizing hormone (LH) are both glycoproteins having a molecular weight of approximately 30 kDa, and consist of two subunits: the α-subunits are unique to each hormone, but the amino acid sequence of the α-subunits is the same, as it also is in those of both TSH and hCG.

The synthesis and release of both hormones are stimulated by the hypothalamic decapeptide, gonadotrophin-releasing hormone (GnRH), these effects being modulated by circulating gonadal steroids. GnRH is secreted episodically, resulting in pulsatile secretion of gonadotrophins with peaks in plasma concentration occurring at approximately 90-minute intervals. In males, LH stimulates testosterone secretion by Leydig cells in the testes—both testosterone and estradiol, derived from the Leydig cells themselves and from the metabolism of testosterone, feedback to block the action of GnRH on

LH secretion. FSH, in concert with high intratesticular testosterone concentrations, stimulates spermatogenesis; its secretion is inhibited by inhibin (Fig. 7.3), a hormone produced during spermatogenesis.

In females, the relationships are more complex. Estrogen (mainly estradiol) secretion by the ovaries is stimulated primarily by FSH in the first part of the menstrual cycle; both hormones are necessary for the development of Graafian follicles. As estrogen concentrations in the blood rise, FSH secretion declines until estrogens trigger a positive feedback mechanism, causing an explosive release of LH and, to a lesser extent, FSH. The increase in LH stimulates ovulation and development of the corpus luteum, but rising concentrations of estrogens and progesterone then inhibit FSH and LH secretion; inhibin from the ovaries also appears to inhibit FSH secretion. If conception does not occur, declining concentrations of estrogens and progesterone from the regressing corpus luteum trigger menstruation and the release of LH and FSH, initiating the maturation of further follicles in a new cycle (Fig. 7.4). Before puberty, plasma concentrations of LH and FSH are very low and unresponsive to exogenous GnRH. With the approach of puberty, FSH secretion increases before that of LH.

Increased concentrations of gonadotrophins are seen in ovarian failure in females, whether pathological or after the natural menopause. High concentrations of FSH are seen in azoospermic men, and LH is increased if testosterone secretion is decreased.

Gonadotrophin-secreting tumors (secreting either LH or FSH) of the pituitary are rare. Decreased gonadotrophin secretion, leading to secondary gonadal failure, is more common. It can either be an isolated phenomenon, due to hypothalamic dysfunction, or occur with generalized pituitary failure.

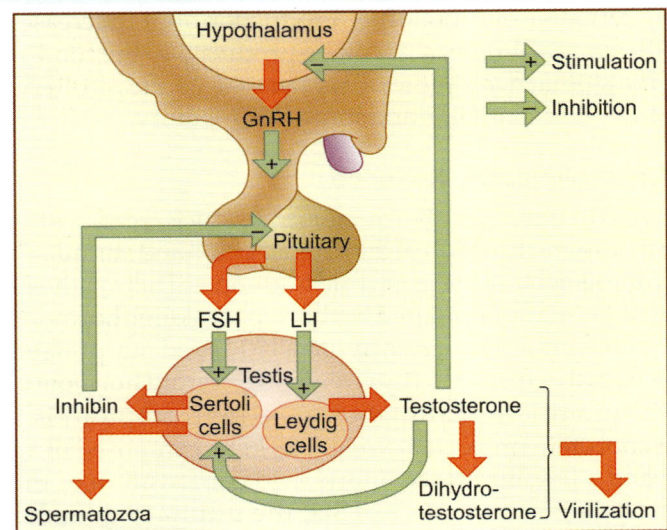

Fig. 7.3: Control of testicular function by pituitary gonadotrophins

Prolactin

Prolactin is a 199 amino acid polypeptide hormone, which circulates in monomeric and various polymeric forms. Its principal physiological action is to initiate and sustain lactation. It also has a role in breast development in females; at high concentrations, it inhibits the synthesis and release of gonadotrophin-releasing hormone from the hypothalamus, and thus gonadotrophins from the pituitary, inhibiting ovulation in females and spermatogenesis in males. Prolactin secretion is controlled by the hypothalamus through the release of dopamine, which normally exerts a tonic inhibition. There is no known specific hypothalamic prolactin-releasing hormone in humans. Although, both TRH and vasoactive intestinal polypeptide (VIP) stimulate prolactin secretion, it is not thought that this is physiologically important. The principal physiological

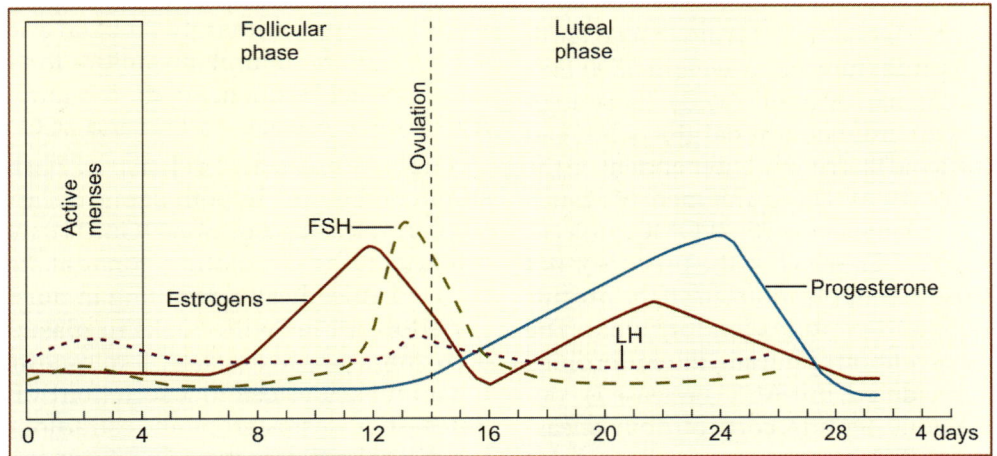

Fig. 7.4: Changes in the plasma concentration of pituitary gonadotrophins during the menstrual cycle

stimuli to prolactin secretion are pregnancy and suckling. Increased prolactin secretion occurs with prolactin-secreting tumors and is also frequently seen with other pituitary tumors, if they obstruct blood flow from the hypothalamus and thus the dopamine-dependent inhibition of prolactin secretion. In the absence of dopamine, prolactin secretion is autonomous.

The secretion of prolactin is pulsatile, increases during sleep, after meals, after exercise and with stress (both physical and psychological), and, in females, is dependent on estrogen status, making it difficult to define a precise upper limit for plasma prolactin concentration in normal men and females, although 500 mU/L is often regarded as the upper reference value in non-pregnant females and 300 mU/L in men. There is no useful lower reference value for plasma prolactin concentration. Its secretion increases during pregnancy but concentrations fall to normal within approximately 7 days after birth if a woman does not breast feed. With breast-feeding, concentrations start to decline after about 3 months, even if breast-feeding is continued beyond this time. Hyperprolactinemia may cause galactorrhea (production and spontaneous flow of breast milk) and disruptions in the normal menstrual period in females and hypogonadism, infertility and erectile dysfunction in men. Prolactin deficiency is uncommon but does occur, e.g. with pituitary infarction; its principal manifestation is failure of lactation.

Other Hormones

The anterior lobe also produces several other hormones. These include POMC, (which gives rise to ACTH), α-and β-melanocyte-stimulating hormone (MSH), β-lipotropin (β-LPH), the enkephalins, and the endorphins. POMC and MSH can cause hyperpigmentation of the skin and are only significant clinically in disorders in which ACTH levels are markedly elevated (e.g. Addison's disease, Nelson's syndrome). The function of β-LPH is unknown. Enkephalins and endorphins are endogenous opioids that bind to and activate opioid receptors throughout the CNS.

DISORDERS OF ANTERIOR PITUITARY FUNCTION

Hypopituitarism

Refers to endocrine deficiency syndromes due to partial or complete loss of anterior lobe pituitary function. Various clinical features occur depending on the specific hormones that are deficient. Diagnosis involves imaging tests and measurement of pituitary hormone levels basally and after various provocative stimuli. Treatment depends on cause but generally includes removal of any tumor and administration of replacement hormones.

Hypopituitarism is divided into primary—caused by disorders that affect the pituitary gland and secondary—caused by disorders of the hypothalamus (Table 7.1).

Table 7.1	Causes of hypopituitarism
Cause	**Examples**
Causes primarily affecting the pituitary gland (primary hypopituitarism)	
Pituitary tumors	Adenoma, craniopharyngioma
Infarction or Ischemic necrosis	Hemorrhagic infarction (pituitary apoplexy)
	Shock, especially postpartum (Sheehan syndrome), or in diabetes mellitus or sickle cell anemia
	Vascular thrombosis or aneurysm, especially of the internal carotid artery
Inflammatory processes	Meningitis (tubercular, other bacterial, fungal, malarial)
	Pituitary abscess, sarcoidosis
Infiltrative disorders	Hemochromatosis
	Langerhans cell histiocytosis (Hand-Schüller-Christian disease)
Idiopathic isolated or multiple pituitary hormone deficiencies	—
Iatrogenic	Irradiation, surgical extirpation
Autoimmune dysfunction	Lymphocytic hypophysitis
Causes primarily affecting the hypothalamus (secondary hypopituitarism)	
Hypothalamic tumors	Craniopharyngioma, ependymoma, meningioma, metastatic tumor, pinealoma
Inflammatory processes	Sarcoidosis
Neurohormone deficiencies of the hypothalamus	Isolated, multiple
Iatrogenic	Surgical transection of the pituitary stalk
Trauma	Basal skull fracture

Symptoms and Signs

Relate to the underlying disorder and to the specific pituitary hormones that are deficient or absent. Onset is usually insidious and may not be recognized by the patient; occasionally, onset is sudden or dramatic.

Most commonly, GH is lost first, then gonadotropins, and finally TSH and ACTH. Vasopressin deficiency is rare in primary pituitary disorders, but is common with lesions of the pituitary stalk and hypothalamus. Function of all target glands decreases when all hormones are deficient (panhypopituitarism).

Lack of LH and FSH in children leads to delayed puberty. Premenopausal females develop amenorrhea, reduced libido, regression of secondary sexual characteristics, and infertility. Men develop erectile dysfunction, testicular atrophy, reduced libido, regression of secondary sexual characteristics, and decreased spermatogenesis with consequent infertility.

Growth hormone deficiency may contribute to decreased energy but is usually asymptomatic and clinically undetectable in adults. Suggestions that GH deficiency accelerates atherosclerosis are unproved. TSH deficiency leads to hypothyroidism, with such symptoms as facial puffiness, hoarse voice, bradycardia, and cold intolerance. ACTH deficiency results in hypoadrenalism with attendant fatigue, hypotension, and intolerance to stress and infection. ACTH deficiency does not result in the hyperpigmentation, a characteristic of primary adrenal failure.

Hypothalamic lesions, which can result in hypopituitarism, can also disturb the centers that control appetite, causing a syndrome resembling anorexia nervosa, or sometimes hyperphagia with massive obesity.

Sheehan syndrome, which affects postpartum females, is pituitary necrosis due to hypovolemia and shock occurring in the immediate peripartum period. Lactation does not start after childbirth, and the patient may complain of fatigue and loss of pubic and axillary hair.

Pituitary apoplexy is a symptom complex caused by hemorrhagic infarction of either a normal pituitary gland or, more commonly, a pituitary tumor. Acute symptoms include severe headache, stiff neck, fever, visual field defects, and oculomotor palsies. The resulting edema may compress the hypothalamus, resulting in somnolence or coma. Varying degrees of hypopituitarism may develop suddenly, and the patient may present with vascular collapse because of deficient ACTH and cortisol. The CSF often contains blood, and MRI documents hemorrhage.

Treatment

Adults of ≤50 years deficient in GH are treated with GH doses of 0.002–0.012 mg/kg SC once a day. Benefits of treatment include improved energy and quality of life, increased body muscle mass, and decreased body fat mass. Suggestions, that GH replacement can prevent an acceleration of atherosclerosis induced by GH deficiency are unproved.

In pituitary apoplexy, immediate surgery is warranted if visual field disturbances or oculomotor palsies develop suddenly or if somnolence progresses to coma because of hypothalamic compression. Although management with high-dose corticosteroids and general support may suffice in a few cases, transsphenoidal decompression of the tumor should generally be undertaken promptly.

Surgery and radiation therapy may be followed by the loss of other pituitary hormone functions. Irradiated patients may lose endocrine function slowly over years. Therefore, post-treatment hormonal status should be evaluated frequently, preferably at 3 and 6 months and yearly thereafter for at least 10 years and preferably up to 15 years after radiation therapy. Such evaluation should include at least assessment of thyroid and adrenal function. Patients may also develop visual difficulties related to fibrosis of the optic chiasm. Sellar imaging and visual field assessment should be done at least every 2 years initially for about 10 years, particularly if residual tumor tissue is present.

ANOREXIA NERVOSA

Anorexia nervosa, a disorder characterized by self-imposed starvation as a result of a preoccupation with (and impaired perception of) body size, may clinically resemble hypopituitarism. Amenorrhea, due to decreased gonadotrophin secretion, is common to both conditions. However, pubic and axillary hair, which may be lost in hypopituitarism, is normal in anorexia nervosa, and there may even be additional (lanugo) hair on the body. The weight loss of anorexia nervosa is usually severe in comparison with that which typically occurs in hypopituitarism. Plasma cortisol and GH concentrations tend to be elevated in anorexia nervosa.

Pituitary Tumors

Pituitary tumors may be purely destructive but are often functional, producing excessive quantities of a hormone. Even tumors that appear to be non-functional may secrete small (clinically insignificant) quantities of the glycoprotein pituitary hormones or just the α-subunit. Non-functional tumors usually present over the age of

60 years. The order of frequency with which hormone secretion occurs in patients with pituitary tumors is prolactin (about 25% of all tumors), GH, ACTH, with gonadotrophins or TSH being very rare. Any pituitary tumor may give rise to clinical features due to the destruction of normal pituitary tissue (i.e. hypopituitarism) and of intracranial space-occupying lesions such as headache, vomiting, and papilloedema. Visual field defects may develop when an upward growing tumor impinges on the optic chiasm and occasionally a patient's sight may be threatened.

Growth Hormone Excess

Acromegaly and gigantism are syndromes of excessive secretion of GH (hypersomatotropism) that are nearly always due to a pituitary adenoma. Before closure of the epiphyses, the result is gigantism. Later, the result is acromegaly, which causes distinctive facial and other features. Diagnosis is clinical and by skull and hand X-rays and measurement of growth hormone levels. Treatment involves removal or destruction of the responsible adenoma.

Many GH-secreting adenomas contain a mutant form of the G_s protein, which is a stimulatory regulator of adenylate cyclase. Cells with the mutant form of G_s protein, secrete GH even in the absence of growth hormone-releasing hormone. A few cases of ectopic GHRH-producing tumors, especially of the pancreas and lung, also.

ACROMEGALY

Symptoms and Signs

In acromegaly, GH hypersecretion usually starts between the 20s and 40s. When GH hypersecretion begins after epiphyseal closure, the earliest clinical manifestations are coarsening of the facial features and soft-tissue swelling of the hands and feet. Appearance changes, and larger rings, gloves, and shoes are needed. Photographs of the patient are important in delineating the course of the disease.

In adults with acromegaly, coarse body hair increases and the skin thickens and frequently darkens. The size and function of sebaceous and sweat glands increase, such that patients frequently complain of excessive perspiration and offensive body odor. Overgrowth of the mandible leads to protrusion of the jaw (prognathism) and malocclusion of teeth. Cartilaginous proliferation of the larynx leads to a deep, husky voice. The tongue is frequently enlarged and furrowed. In long-standing acromegaly, costal cartilage growth leads to a barrel chest. Articular cartilaginous proliferation occurs early in

response to GH excess, with the articular cartilage possibly undergoing necrosis and erosion. Joint symptoms are common, and crippling degenerative arthritis may occur.

Peripheral neuropathies occur commonly because of compression of nerves by adjacent fibrous tissue and endoneural fibrous proliferation. Headaches are common because of the pituitary tumor. Bitemporal hemianopia may develop if suprasellar extension compresses the optic chiasm. The heart, liver, kidneys, spleen, thyroid gland, parathyroid glands, and pancreas are larger than normal. Cardiac disease (e.g. coronary artery disease, cardiomegaly, sometimes cardiomyopathy) occurs in perhaps one-third of patients, with a doubling in the risk of death from cardiac disease. Hypertension occurs in up to one-third of patients. The risk of cancer, particularly of the gastrointestinal (GI) tract, increases 2-fold to 3-fold. GH increases tubular reabsorption of phosphate and leads to mild hyperphosphatemia. Impaired glucose tolerance occurs in nearly half the patients with acromegaly and in gigantism, but clinically significant diabetes mellitus occurs in only about 10% of patients.

Galactorrhea occurs in some females with acromegaly, usually in association with hyperprolactinemia. However, galactorrhea may occur with GH excess alone, because GH itself stimulates lactation. Decreased gonadotropin secretion often occurs with GH-secreting tumors. About one-third of men with acromegaly develop erectile dysfunction, and nearly all females develop menstrual irregularities or amenorrhea.

Treatment

Ablative Therapy

Ablative therapy with surgery or radiation is generally indicated. Trans-sphenoidal resection is preferred, but choices vary at different institutions. Stereotactic supervoltage radiation, delivering about 5000 cGy to the pituitary, is used, but GH levels may not fall to normal for several years. Treatment with accelerated protons (heavy particle radiation) permits delivery of larger doses of radiation (equivalent to 10,000 cGy) to the pituitary; such therapy poses higher risk of cranial nerve and hypothalamic damage and is available only in a few centers. Development of hypopituitarism several years after irradiation is common. Because radiation damage is cumulative, proton beam therapy should *not* be used after conventional γ-irradiation. A combined approach with both surgery and radiation therapy is indicated for patients with progressive extrasellar involvement by a pituitary tumor and for patients whose entire tumor cannot be resected, which is often the case.

Surgical removal of the tumor is likely to have been curative, if GH levels measured after a glucose load and IGF-1 levels reach normal values. If one or both values are abnormal, further therapy is usually needed. If GH excess is poorly controlled, hypertension, heart failure, and a doubling in the death rate occur. If GH levels are <5 ng/mL, however, mortality does not increase.

Drug Therapy

In general, drug therapy is indicated if surgery and radiation therapy are contraindicated, if they have not been curative, or if radiation therapy is being given time to work. In such instances, a somatostatin analog, octreotide, is given at 0.05–0.15 mg sc q 8 to 12 h; it suppresses GH secretion effectively. Longer-acting somatostatin analogs, such as mannitol-modified release octreotide (octreotide LAR) given 10–30 mg IM q 4 to 6 weeks and lanreotide given 30 mg IM q 10 to 14 days, are more convenient. Bromocriptine mesylate (1.25–5 mg by mouth twice a day) may effectively lower GH levels in a small percentage of patients, but is less effective than somatostatin analogs.

Pegvisomant, a GH receptor blocker, has been shown to reduce the effects of GH and lower IGF-1 levels in people with acromegaly, without apparent increase in pituitary tumor size. This drug may find a place in treating patients who are partially or totally unresponsive to somatostatin analogs.

PITUITARY GIGANTISM

This rare condition occurs if GH hypersecretion begins in childhood, before closure of the epiphyses. Skeletal growth velocity and ultimate stature are increased, but little bony deformity occurs. However, soft-tissue swelling occurs, and the peripheral nerves are enlarged. Delayed puberty or hypogonadotropic hypogonadism is also frequently present, resulting in a eunuchoid habitus.

Hyperprolactinemia and Galactorrhea

Galactorrhea is a common endocrine abnormality which is characterized by the inappropriate production and secretion of milk, with its associated hyperprolactinemia, is an extremely common clinical entity. It is often accompanied by menstrual disturbance and infertility and may herald the presence of pituitary tumors, which can produce considerable morbidity and rarely mortality.

Etiology

Hyperprolactinemia is associated with numerous types of pathology (Table 7.2), the four most common causes of hyperprolactinemia are central dopamine metabolism disturbance (functional hyperprolactinemia), prolactinomas, hypothyroidism, and drug ingestion. Patients with hypothyroidism deserve special comment. These

Table 7.2	Causes of hyperprolactinemia
Cause	Example
Physiologic	Nipple stimulation in females
	Pregnancy
	Postpartum period
	Stress
	Food ingestion
	Sexual intercourse in some females
	Sleep
	Hypoglycemia
	Early infancy (up to 3 months)
Hypothalamic disorders	Hypothalamic tumors
	Nontumerous hypothalamic infiltration: Sarcoidosis, TB, Langerhans cell histiocytosis (Hand-Schüller-Chrisitan disease)
	Postencephalitis
	Idiopathic galactorrhea (presumed abnormality in dopamine secretion)
	Head trauma
Pituitary disorders	Prolactin-secreting pituitary tumors
	Tumors causing pituitary stalk compression
	Surgical pituitary stalk section and other stalk lesions
	Empty sella syndrome
Other endocrine disorders	Acromegaly
	Cushing's disease
	Primary hypothyroidism
Disorders of other systems	Chronic renal failure
	Liver disease
	Ectopic production of prolactin: Bronchogenic carcinoma (not squamous cell; mostly small cell undifferentiated)
	Hypernephroma
Chest wall lesions	Surgical scars, trauma, tumors, herpes zoster
Pharmacologic	Antihypertensive drugs: Resperine, α-methyldopa, labetalol, atenolol, verapamil, clonidine
	H2-antagonists (e.g. ranitidine)
	Oral contraceptives and estrogens
	Opioids
	Psychoactive drugs, e.g. phenothiazines, tricyclic and some other antidepressants, butyrphenones (haloperidol), benzamides (metoclopramide, sulpiride)
	Thyrotropin-releasing hormone

patients present with compensated primary hypothyroidism and may demonstrate a normal thyroxine level with markedly elevated TSH levels. They often have pituitary enlargement mimicking an adenoma and may have visual impairment. It is necessary to evaluate thyroid function in all patients before considering neurosurgical exploration.

Symptoms and Signs

The primary symptom of galactorrhea is the discharge of milky fluid from one or both breasts. Females with galactorrhea commonly also have amenorrhea or oligomenorrhea. Females with galactorrhea and amenorrhea may also have symptoms and signs of estrogen deficiency, including dyspareunia, due to inhibition of pulsatile luteinizing hormone and follicle-stimulating hormone release by high prolactin levels. However, estrogen production may be normal, and signs of androgen excess have been observed in some females with hyperprolactinemia. Hyperprolactinemia may occur with other menstrual cycle disturbances besides amenorrhea, including infrequent ovulation and corpus luteum dysfunction.

Males with prolactin-secreting pituitary tumors typically have headaches or visual difficulties. About two-thirds of affected males have loss of libido and erectile dysfunction.

Treatment

The treatment of microprolactinomas is controversial. Asymptomatic patients who have prolactin levels < 100 ng/mL and normal CT or MRI results or who have only microadenomas can probably be observed; serum prolactin often normalizes within years. Patients with hyperprolactinemia should be monitored with quarterly measurement of prolactin levels and undergo sellar CT or MRI annually for at least an additional 2 years. The frequency of sellar imaging can then be reduced if prolactin levels do not increase.

In Females

Indications for treatment include, desire for pregnancy, amenorrhea or significant oligomenorrhea (because of the risk of osteoporosis) hirsutism and low libido.

In Males

Galactorrhea itself is rarely troublesome enough to require treatment; indications for treatment include hypogonadism (because of the risk of osteoporosis), erectile dysfunction and low libido.

The initial treatment is usually a dopamine agonist, such as bromocriptine 1.25–5 mg by mouth twice a day or the longer-acting cabergoline 0.25–1.0 mg by mouth once a week or twice a week, which lower prolactin levels. Cabergoline is the treatment of choice because it appears to be more easily tolerated and more potent than bromocriptine. Females trying to become pregnant should switch to bromocriptine at least 1 month before planned conception and stop bromocriptine use at the time of a positive pregnancy test result; long-term safety data are better established for bromocriptine than for cabergoline, although evidence for the safety of cabergoline is increasing. Exogenous estrogen can be given to females with a microadenoma who are clinically hypoestrogenic or have low estradiol levels. Exogenous estrogen is unlikely to cause tumor expansion. Quinagolide, a nonergot-derived dopamine agonist, is also an option for hyperprolactinemia. It is started at 25 µg by mouth once a day and titrated over 7 days up to the usual maintenance dose of 75 µg once a day (maximum dose 600 µg once a day).

Patients with macroadenomas generally should be treated with dopamine agonists or surgically, but only after thorough testing of pituitary function and evaluation for radiation therapy. Dopamine agonists are usually the initial treatment of choice and usually shrink a prolactin-secreting tumor, but will not shrink a non-functioning tumor causing pituitary stalk compression, although prolactin levels will decrease. If prolactin levels fall and symptoms and signs of compression by the tumor abate, no other therapy may be necessary. However, typically, larger, nonfunctioning lesions need additional treatment, usually surgery. Surgery or radiation therapy may be easier to do or yield better results after tumor shrinkage induced by a dopamine agonist. Although, dopamine agonist treatment usually needs to be continued long-term, prolactin-secreting tumors sometimes remit, either spontaneously or perhaps aided by the drug therapy. Sometimes, therefore, dopamine agonists can be stopped without a recurrence of the tumor or a rise in prolactin levels; remission is more likely with microadenomas than macroadenomas. Remission is also more likely after pregnancy.

High doses of dopamine agonists, particularly cabergoline and pergolide, are thought to have caused valvular heart disease in some patients with Parkinson disease. It is not clear whether the lower doses of dopamine agonists used for hyperprolactinemia similarly increase the risk of valvular heart disease, but the possibility should be discussed with patients, and echocardiographic surveillance should be considered. The risk may be less with bromocriptine or quinagolide.

Radiation therapy should be used only in patients with progressive disease who do not respond to other forms of therapy. With irradiation, hypopituitarism often develops several years after therapy. Monitoring endocrine function and sellar imaging are indicated yearly for life.

CUSHING'S DISEASE

Cushing's disease, in which increased secretion of cortisol by the adrenal cortex is secondary to increased secretion of ACTH by the anterior pituitary, is discussed in

Chapter 8. Patients who have been treated in the past for Cushing's disease by adrenalectomy alone may later develop hyperpigmentation and the clinical features of a large pituitary tumor (Nelson's syndrome). The pigmentation is due to the melanocyte-stimulating activity of ACTH and its precursors. Nelson's syndrome is uncommon in patients in whom treatment for Cushing's disease has included pituitary surgery or irradiation in addition to adrenalectomy.

Nelson's syndrome

Nelson's syndrome occurs when the pituitary gland continues to expand after bilateral adrenalectomy, causing a marked increase in the secretion of ACTH and its precursors, resulting in severe hyperpigmentation. It occurs in ≥50% of patients who undergo adrenalectomy. The risk is probably reduced if the patient undergoes pituitary radiation therapy. Although, irradiation may arrest continued pituitary growth, many patients also require hypophysectomy. The indications for hypophysectomy are the same as for any pituitary tumor; an increase in size such that the tumor encroaches on surrounding structures, causing visual field defects, pressure on the hypothalamus, or other complications. Routine irradiation is often done after hypophysectomy if it was not done previously, especially when a tumor is clearly present. Radiation therapy may be delayed if there is no obvious lesion. Radiosurgery or focused radiation therapy, can be given in a single fraction when standard external beam radiation therapy has already been done, as long as the lesion is at a reasonable distance from the optic nerve and chiasm.

Other Conditions Related to Pituitary Tumors

Tumors that secrete TSH or gonadotrophins are rare. The finding of a high plasma concentration of α-subunits may provide a clue to their presence. Approximately 30% of pituitary tumors, usually chromophobe adenomas, are non-functioning. They can present with features of hypopituitarism because of the physical presence of the tumor, and are occasionally diagnosed incidentally from a skull radiograph taken for some other purpose.

Even apparently non-functioning tumors may secrete small but clinically insignificant quantities of hormones. Some secrete only the α-subunit of the glycoprotein hormones, and measurement of plasma α-subunit concentration may be useful in assessing the success of treatment in such cases.

Asymptomatic pituitary tumors may be discovered incidentally (incidentalomas). If pituitary function is demonstrably normal and there are no mass effects, no intervention is required.

MEASUREMENT OF ANTERIOR PITUITARY HORMONES

Measurements of pituitary hormone concentrations are required in both suspected hypofunction and hyperfunction (the latter is usually the result of a pituitary tumor, and is often accompanied by partial hypofunction). The investigation of suspected pituitary hypofunction should begin with measurement of pituitary and target organ hormones in a blood sample taken at 09:00 h. TSH deficiency will be apparent from a low total or free thyroxine concentration without the elevation of TSH characteristic of primary hypothyroidism. Plasma TSH concentration may be normal or low in hypopituitarism; it is rarely undetectable.

In males, a normal plasma testosterone concentration indicates normal LH secretion. In hypopituitarism, plasma testosterone concentration is low, and LH and FSH concentrations are normal or low. In premenopausal females, amenorrhea with a low plasma estradiol concentration and normal or low gonadotrophins suggests hypothalamic or pituitary dysfunction. A clomiphene test may help to distinguish between these. A normal ovulatory plasma progesterone concentration indicates the integrity of the hypothalamo-pituitary–ovarian axis without the need for further testing; a history of regular, normal menstrual cycles also effectively excludes gonadotrophin deficiency. In normal postmenopausal women, plasma gonadotrophin concentrations are grossly elevated; in hypopituitarism, they are normal or low.

Tests involving the administration of TRH and GnRH followed by measurement of TSH and gonadotrophins have traditionally been used in the investigation of pituitary disease, often combined with the insulin hypoglycemia test (IHT, see below). However, the use of these tests has been criticized on the grounds that the responses to these releasing hormones only reflect the readily releasable pituitary pools of the hormones concerned and do not assess the physiological integrity of the pituitary. Normal responses can occur in spite of other evidence of pituitary hypofunction. The response to the releasing hormones is often delayed in patients with hypothalamic, as opposed to pituitary dysfunction, but such delayed responses can also occur in pituitary disease. In practice, the releasing hormone tests often add little to what can be deduced from clinical observation and the results of basal hormone measurements.

Because GH is secreted sporadically, it may be undetectable in the plasma of normal individuals. Thus, while a concentration of >20 mU/L in a single sample excludes significant deficiency, a low concentration is not necessarily indicative of deficiency. Growth hormone secretion can be assessed using the IHT; a peak plasma concentration <20 mU/L after adequate hypoglycemia (blood glucose concentration <2.2 mmol/L) is reliable evidence of GH deficiency.

Because the IHT is potentially hazardous, various other tests of GH secretion have been devised, involving the administration of, e.g. GHRH, glucagon, arginine, yeast extract or l-DOPA. Although the relevance of these pharmacological stimuli to the physiological secretion of GH is questionable. GH concentrations >20 mU/L are usually regarded as excluding GH deficiency, but lesser responses are not conclusive evidence of deficiency. Vigorous exercise also stimulates GH secretion, but even with standardized protocols an apparently subnormal response may not indicate GH deficiency. More reliable information may be provided by the measurement of GH secretion during sleep, by means of frequent blood sampling through an indwelling cannula, but there are obvious practical drawbacks to this procedure.

Measurements of IGF-1 are increasingly being used together with GH stimulation tests in the investigation of suspected GH deficiency. A low plasma concentration of IGF-1, together with an impaired or absent GH response to stimulation, confirms GH deficiency. Some patients who appear clinically to have GH deficiency have normal or elevated plasma GH concentrations, but because of a receptor or intracellular signaling defect, are resistant to its action. This syndrome is known as Laron dwarfism; patients have low plasma IGF-1 concentrations. It should be noted that, while plasma IGF-1 concentrations are much more stable than those of GH, they vary with age and nutritional status; measured values should always be assessed with reference to age- and sex-matched reference values. The IGFs are carried in the plasma bound to IGF-binding proteins (IGFBPs), and measurement of IGFBP-3 may be a better marker of growth hormone deficiency in children.

The integrity of the hypothalamo-pituitary-adrenal axis can also be tested using the IHT. A rise in plasma cortisol concentration to at least 550 nmol/L after adequate hypoglycemia indicates a normal axis. It has been shown that if the basal (09:00 h) plasma cortisol concentration is <100 nmol/L, the cortisol response to hypoglycemia is never normal, whereas it invariably is normal if the basal concentration is >400 nmol/L. A formal IHT may therefore not be necessary in patients whose basal plasma cortisol concentrations are outside the range 100–400 nmol/L. The short ACTH stimulation test (tetracosactide or synacthen test), used primarily in the investigation of adrenal failure, has also been advocated as a test for ACTH deficiency. This may seem illogical, but the rationale is that ACTH deficiency causes adrenal atrophy and thus decreases adrenal responsiveness to ACTH. A good correlation between the results of the IHT and short ACTH stimulation tests has been demonstrated: a plasma cortisol concentration >550 nmol/L 30 minutes after the administration of synthetic ACTH (250 µg, IV) excludes ACTH deficiency. Experience with the low dose (1 µg) tetracosactide test in this context is presently limited, but it may be less sensitive in identifying partial failure of ACTH secretion.

Prolactin secretion is increased by stress but, in practice, the measurement of prolactin in an IHT adds nothing to the information provided by a single basal measurement.

INSULIN HYPOGLYCEMIA TEST

In this test, the stress of insulin-induced hypoglycemia is used to assess the secretion of GH and ACTH by the pituitary (in practice, cortisol is usually measured for the reasons explained above and because the assay of ACTH is technically more demanding). The test is potentially hazardous because of the possible sequelae of hypoglycemia. A doctor should always be present when the test is performed. It is contraindicated in patients with a history of fits or ischemic heart disease and it should not be performed in patients whose 09:00 hours serum cortisol concentration is low. In children, it should only be performed in specialized units. Concentrated dextrose solution must be available for immediate administration should severe hypoglycemia develop. Giving glucose because of severe symptomatic hypoglycemia does not invalidate the results of the test. The stress needs only to be very brief to be effective. It is important that documented hypoglycemia is obtained, as if it does not occur a lack of response might be due to the inadequacy of the stimulus rather than to pituitary failure. If hypoglycemia does not develop, a further dose of insulin must be given. The test can be combined with releasing hormone tests, although, as discussed, the results of these tests often provide little additional useful information.

It may be preferable to give the insulin by continuous intravenous infusion. The rate can be adjusted until hypoglycemia develops, whereupon the infusion is stopped. This is a more certain and safer way of producing hypoglycemia than giving a single bolus of insulin. When the induction of hypoglycemia is contraindicated, glucagon can be used to stimulate cortisol and GH secretion instead of insulin.

Imaging the Pituitary

Once a pituitary disorder has been diagnosed on the basis of the clinical findings and laboratory investigations, imaging techniques are used to provide essential anatomical information. Computerized tomography (CT) allows visualization of the bony structures in the vicinity of the pituitary, but magnetic resonance imaging (MRI) is superior for imaging the soft tissues. Formal assessment and documentation of the visual fields is also essential, because pituitary tumors can extend to damage the optic pathways.

The Posterior Lobe of the Pituitary Hormones

Antidiuretic hormone (ADH) (also called vasopressin or arginine vasopressin) and oxytocin, both hormones are released in response to neural impulses and have half-lives of about 10 minutes.

Antidiuretic Hormone

It acts primarily to promote water conservation by the kidney by increasing the permeability of the distal tubular epithelium to water. At high concentrations, ADH also causes vasoconstriction. Like aldosterone, ADH plays an important role in maintaining fluid homeostasis and vascular and cellular hydration. The main stimulus for ADH release is increased osmotic pressure of water in the body, which is sensed by osmoreceptors in the hypothalamus. The other major stimulus is volume depletion, which is sensed by baroreceptors in the left atrium, pulmonary veins, carotid sinus, and aortic arch, and then transmitted to the CNS through the vagus and glossopharyngeal nerves. Other stimulants for ADH release include pain, stress, emesis, hypoxia, exercise, hypoglycemia, cholinergic agonists, β-blockers, angiotensin, and prostaglandins. Inhibitors of ADH release include alcohol, β-blockers, and glucocorticoids.

A lack of ADH causes central diabetes insipidus and the inability of the kidneys to respond normally to ADH causes nephrogenic diabetes insipidus. Removal of the pituitary gland usually does not result in permanent diabetes insipidus because some of the remaining hypothalamic neurons produce small amounts of ADH. Copeptin is coproduced with ADH in the posterior pituitary. Measuring it may be useful in distinguishing the cause of hyponatremia.

Oxytocin

Oxytocin has two major targets—the myoepithelial cells of the breast, which surround the alveoli of the mammary gland, and the smooth muscle cells of the uterus. Suckling stimulates the production of oxytocin, which causes the myoepithelial cells to contract. This contraction causes milk to move from the alveoli to large sinuses for ejection (i.e. the milk letdown reflex of nursing mothers). Oxytocin stimulates contraction of uterine smooth muscle cells, and uterine sensitivity to oxytocin increases throughout pregnancy. However, plasma levels do not increase sharply during parturition, and the role of oxytocin in the initiation of labor is unclear. There is no recognized stimulus for oxytocin release in men, although men have extremely low levels.

DISORDERS OF POSTERIOR PITUITARY GLAND

Diabetes Insipidus

Diabetes insipidus (DI) is a condition that results from insufficient production of the ADH, a hormone that helps the kidneys and body conserve the correct amount of water. Normally, the antidiuretic hormone controls the kidneys' output of urine. It is secreted by the hypothalamus (a small gland located at the base of the brain) and stored in the pituitary gland and then released into the bloodstream. ADH is secreted to decrease the amount of urine output so that dehydration does not occur. Diabetes insipidus, however, causes excessive production of much diluted urine and excessive thirst. The disease is categorized into groups:

- **Central diabetes insipidus (CDI):** Insufficient production or secretion of ADH; can be a result of damage to the pituitary gland caused by head injuries, genetic disorders, tumors, surgery, and other diseases.
- **Nephrogenic diabetes insipidus (NDI):** Lack of kidney response to normal levels of ADH: can be caused by drugs or chronic disorders, such as kidney failure, sickle cell disease, or polycystic kidney disease.

Pathophysiology

The posterior lobe of the pituitary is the primary site of vasopressin storage and release, but ADH is synthesized within the hypothalamus. Newly synthesized hormone can still be released into the circulation as long as the hypothalamic nuclei and part of the neurohypophyseal tract are intact. Only about 10% of neurosecretory neurons must remain intact to avoid CDI. The pathology of CDI thus always involves the supraoptic and paraventricular nuclei of the hypothalamus or a major portion of the pituitary stalk.

CDI may be complete (absence of vasopressin) or partial (insufficient amounts of vasopressin). CDI may be primary, in which there is a marked decrease in the hypothalamic nuclei of the neurohypophyseal system.

Etiology

Primary CDI

Genetic abnormalities of the vasopressin gene on chromosome 20 are responsible for autosomal dominant forms of primary CDI, but many cases are idiopathic.

Secondary CDI

Central diabetes incipidus may also be secondary (acquired), caused by various lesions, including hypophysectomy, cranial injuries (particularly basal skull fractures), suprasellar and intrasellar tumors (primary or metastatic), Langerhans cell histiocytosis (Hand-Schüller-Christian disease), lymphocytic hypophysitis, granulomas (sarcoidosis or TB), vascular lesions (aneurysm, thrombosis), and infections (encephalitis, meningitis).

Symptoms and Signs

Onset may be insidious or abrupt, occurring at any age. The only symptoms in primary CDI are polydipsia and polyuria. In secondary CDI, symptoms and signs of the associated lesions are also present. Enormous quantities of fluid may be ingested, and large volumes (3–30 L/day) of very dilute urine (specific gravity usually <1.005 and osmolality <200 mOsm/L) are excreted. Nocturia almost always occurs. Dehydration and hypovolemia may develop rapidly if urinary losses are not continuously replaced.

Diagnosis

CDI must be differentiated from other causes of polyuria, particularly psychogenic polydipsia (Table 7.3) and NDI. All tests for CDI (and for NDI) are based on the principle that increasing the plasma osmolality in normal people will lead to decreased excretion of urine with increased osmolality.

The water deprivation test is the simplest and most reliable method for diagnosing CDI, but should be done only while the patient is under constant supervision. Serious dehydration may result. Additionally, if psychogenic polydipsia is suspected, the patient must be observed to prevent surreptitious drinking. The test is started in the morning by weighing the patient, obtaining venous blood to determine electrolyte concentrations and osmolality, and measuring urinary osmolality. Voided urine is collected hourly, and its specific gravity or, preferably, osmolality is measured. Dehydration is continued until orthostatic hypotension and postural tachycardia appear, ≥5% of the initial body weight has been lost, or the urinary concentration does not increase >0.001 specific gravity or >30 mOsm/L in sequentially voided specimens. Serum electrolytes and osmolality are again determined, and 5 units of aqueous vasopressin are injected sc. Urine for specific gravity or osmolality measurement is collected one final time 60 minutes postinjection, and the test is terminated.

A normal response produces maximum urine osmolality after dehydration (often >1.020 specific gravity or >700 mOsm/L), exceeding the plasma osmolality; osmolality does not increase more than an additional 5% after injection of vasopressin. Patients with CDI are generally unable to concentrate urine to greater than the plasma osmolality, but are able to increase their urine osmolality by >50% after vasopressin administration. Patients with partial CDI are often able to concentrate urine to above the plasma osmolality but show a rise in urine osmolality of >9% after vasopressin administration. Patients with NDI are unable to concentrate urine to greater than the plasma osmolality and show no additional response to vasopressin administration.

Measurement of circulating vasopressin is the most direct method of diagnosing CDI; levels at the end of the water deprivation test (before the vasopressin injection) are low in CDI and appropriately elevated in NDI. However, vasopressin levels are difficult to measure, and the test is not routinely available. In addition, water deprivation is so accurate that direct measurement of vasopressin is unnecessary. Plasma vasopressin levels are diagnostic after either dehydration or infusion of hypertonic saline.

Table 7.3	Common causes of polyuria	
Mechanism	**Example**	
Vasopressin-sensitive polyuria		
Decreased synthesis of vasopressin	Primary diabetes insipidus, hereditary (usually autosomal dominant)	
	Primary diabetes insipidus, hereditary associated with diabetes mellitus, optic nerve atrophy, nerve deafness, and atonia of bladder and ureters	
	Acquired (secondary) diabetes insipidus (causes outlined in text)	
Decreased release of vasopressin	Psychogenic polydipsia (dipsogenic diabetes insipidus)	
Vasopressin-resistant polyuria		
Renal resistance to vasopressin	Congenital nephrogenic diabetes insipidus (usually X-linked recessive trait)	
	Acquired nephrogenic diabetes insipidus: Chronic kidney disease, systemic or metabolic disease (e.g. myeloma, amyloidosis, hypercalcemic or hypokalemic nephropathy, sickle cell disease), certain drugs (e.g. lithium, demeclocycline)	
Osmotic diuresis	Hyperglycemia (in diabetes mellitus)	
	Poorly resorbed solutes (mannitol, sorbitol, urea)	

PSYCHOGENIC POLYDIPSIA

Psychogenic polydipsia may present a difficult problem in differential diagnosis. Patients may ingest and excrete up to 6 L of fluid/day and are often emotionally disturbed. Unlike patients with CDI and NDI, they usually do not have nocturia, nor does their thirst wake them at night. Continued ingestion of large volumes of water in this situation can lead to life-threatening hyponatremia.

Patients with acute psychogenic water drinking are able to concentrate their urine during water deprivation. However, because chronic water intake diminishes medullary tonicity in the kidney, patients with long-standing polydipsia are not able to concentrate their urine to maximal levels during water deprivation, a response similar to that of patients with partial CDI. However, unlike CDI, patients with psychogenic polydipsia show no response to exogenous vasopressin after water deprivation. This response resembles NDI, except that basal vasopressin levels are low compared with the elevated levels present in NDI. After prolonged restriction of fluid intake to ≥2 L/day, normal concentrating ability returns within several weeks.

Treatment

CDI can be treated with hormone replacement and treatment of any correctable cause. In the absence of approzpriate management, permanent renal damage can result.

Desmopressin, a synthetic analog of vasopressin with minimal vasoconstrictive properties, has prolonged antidiuretic activity lasting for 12–24 hours in most patients and may be administered intranasally, SC, IV, or orally. Desmopressin is the preparation of choice for both adults and children and is available as an intranasal solution in two forms. A dropper bottle with a calibrated nasal catheter has the advantage of delivering incremental doses from 5–20 µg, but is awkward to use. A spray bottle that delivers 10 µg of desmopressin in 0.1 mL of fluid is easier to use but delivers a fixed quantity. For each patient, the duration of action of a given dose must be established, because variation among individuals is great. The duration of action can be established by following timed urine volumes and osmolality. The nightly dose is the lowest dose required to prevent nocturia. The morning and evening doses should be adjusted separately. The usual dosage range in adults is 10–40 µg, with most adults requiring 10 µg bid. For children age 3 months to 12 years, the usual dosage range is 2.5–10 µg twice a day.

Over dosage can lead to fluid retention and decreased plasma osmolality, possibly resulting in seizures in small children. In such instances, furosemide can be given to induce diuresis. Headache may be a troublesome adverse effect but generally disappears if the dosage is reduced. Infrequently, desmopressin causes a slight increase in BP. Absorption from the nasal mucosa may be erratic, especially when upper respiratory infection (URI) or allergic rhinitis occurs. When intranasal delivery of desmopressin is inappropriate, it may be administered sc using about one-tenth of the intranasal dose. Desmopressin may be used IV if a rapid effect is necessary (e.g. for hypovolemia). With oral desmopressin, dose equivalence with the intranasal formulation is unpredictable, so individual dose titration is needed. The initial dose is 0.1 mg by mouth 3 times a day, and the maintenance dose is usually 0.1–0.2 mg 3 times a day.

BIBLIOGRAPHY

1. "Adrenal Insufficiency and Addison's Disease". National Endocrine and Metabolic Diseases Information Service. Retrieved 26 November 2010.
2. Baltimore: Lippincott Williams & Wilkins,1999: 189–98.
3. Belanoff; et al. (2001). "Corticosteroids and cognition". J Psychiatric Research 35 (3): 127–145.
4. Biller BM. Hyperprolactinemia. Int J FertilWomens Med 1999; 44: 74–7.
5. Boron, Walter F.; Boulpaep, Emile L. (2009). Medical Physiology (2nd ed.). Philadelphia: Saunders Elsevier. pp. 1016–1017. ISBN 978-1-4160-3115-4.
6. Buckman M, Peake G. Untitled response to: Kemmann E. Incidence of galactorrhea.JAMA1976; 236:2747.
7. Clark, M., Kumar, P. Kumar and Clark's Clinical Medicine. 7th Ed.
8. Crowley RK, Sherlock M, Agha A, Smith D, Thompson CJ (2007). "Clinical insights into adipsic diabetes insipidus: a large case series". Clin. Endocrinol. (Oxf) 66 (4): 475–82.
9. Davajan V, Kletzky O, March CM, Roy S, Mishell DR. The significance of galactorrhea in patients with normal menses, oligomenorrhea, and secondary amenorrhea. Am J Obstet Gynecol 1978;130:894-904.
10. Dunn NR, Freemantle SN, Pearce GL, Mann RD. Galactorrhoea with moclobemide. Lancet 1998;351:802.
11. Edge DS, Segatore M. Assessment and management of galactorrhea. Nurse Pract 1993; 18:35-6, 38, 43–4.
12. Egberts AC, Meyboom RH, De Koning FH, Bakker A, Leufkens HG. Non-puerperal lactation associated with antidepressant drug use. Br J ClinPharmacol 1997;44:277-81.
13. Elizabeth D Agabegi; Agabegi, Steven S. (2008). Step-Up to Medicine (Step-Up Series). Hagerstwon, MD: Lippincott Williams and Wilkins. ISBN 0-7817-7153-6.
14. Faubion WA, Nader S. Spinal cord surgery and galactorrhea: a case report. Am J Obstet Gynecol1997;177:465-6.
15. Fetrow CW, Avila JR. Professional's handbook of complementary & alternative medicines. Springhouse, Pa.: Springhouse, 1999:82-3, 248–9.
16. Finch CK, Kelley KW, Williams RB (April 2003). "Treatment of lithium-induced diabetes insipidus with amiloride". Pharmacotherapy 23 (4): 546–50.

17. Fujiwara TM, Bichet DG (2005). "Molecular Biology of Hereditary Diabetes Insipidus". Journal of the American Society of Nephrology 16 (10): 2836–2846.

18. Fujiweira, TM. , Morgan, K. 1995. Molecular Biology of Diabetes Insipidus. Annu. Rev. Med. 46:331-43.

19. Ganella, Despina E.; Allen, Nicholas B.; Simmons, Julian G.; Schwartz, Orli; Kim, Jee Hyun; Sheeber, Lisa; Whittle, Sarah. "Early life stress alters pituitary growth during adolescence—A longitudinal study". Psychoneuroendocrinology 53: 185–194.

20. Gibo H, Hokama M, Kyoshima K, Kobayashi S (1993). "[Arteries to the pituitary]". Nippon Rinsho 51 (10): 2550–4.

21. Guven K, Kelestimur F. Hyperprolactinemia and galactorrhea with standard-dose famotidine therapy [Letter]. Ann Pharmacother 1995;29:788.

22. Guyton, A., Hall, J. Textbook of Medical Physiology. 11th Ed.

23. James, William; Berger, Timothy; Elston, Dirk (2005). Andrews' Diseases of the Skin: Clinical Dermatology. (10th ed.). Saunders. ISBN 0-7216-2921-0.

24. Kalelioglu I, KubatUzum A, Yildirim A, Ozkan T, Gungor F, Has R (2007). "Transient gestational diabetes insipidus diagnosed in successive pregnancies: review of pathophysiology, diagnosis, treatment, and management of delivery". Pituitary 10 (1): 87–93.

25. Katsuren E, Ishikawa S, Honda K, Saito T. Galactorrhoea and amenorrhoea due to an intraduralneurinoma originating from a thoracic intercostal nerve radicle. ClinEndocrinol [Oxf] 1997;46: 631–6.

26. Katznelson L, Klibanski A. Hyperprolactinemia: physiology and clinical approach. In: Krisht AF, TindallGT,eds. Pituitary disorders: comprehensive management.

27. Kleinberg DL, Noel GL, Frantz AG. Galactorrhea: a study of 235 cases, including 48 with pituitary tumors. N Engl J Med 1977; 296: 589–99.

28. Knepel W, Homolka L, Vlaskovska M, Nutto D. (1984). Stimulation of adrenocorticotropin/beta-endorphin release by synthetic ovine corticotropin-releasing factor in vitro. Enhancement by various vasopressin analogs. Neuroendocrinology. 38(5): 344–50.

29. Kumar, V., Abbas, A., Fausto, N., Aster, J. Robbins and Cotrans Pathologic Basis of Disease. 8th Ed.

30. Labeur M, Arzt E, Stalla GK, Páez-Pereda M. New perspectives in the treatment of Cushing's syndrome. Current Drug Targets-Immune, Endocrine and Metabolic Disorders. 2004; 4: 335–342.

31. Lado-Abeal, J; Rodriguez-Arnao, J; Newell-Price, JD; Perry, LA; Grossman, AB; Besser, GM; Trainer, PJ (September 1998). "Menstrual abnormalities in women with Cushing's disease are correlated with hypercortisolemia rather than raised circulating androgen levels." (PDF). The Journal of Clinical Endocrinology and Metabolism 83 (9): 3083–8.

32. Laureti S, Casucci G, Santeusanio F, Angeletti G, Aubourg P, Brunetti P (1996). "X-linked adrenoleukodystrophy is a frequent cause of idiopathic Addison's disease in young adult male patient". The Journal of Clinical Endocrinology and Metabolism 81 (2): 470–474.

33. Lee ST. Hyperprolactinemia, galactorrhea, and atenolol [Letter]. Ann Intern Med 1992;116:522.

34. Lin D, Loughlin K. Diagnosis and management of surgical adrenal diseases. Urology. 2005;66:476-483.

35. Livingstone, C., Rampes, H. 2006. Lithium: a review of its metabolic adverse effects. J Psychopharmacol. 20:347-355.

36. Loffing J (November 2004). "Paradoxical antidiuretic effect of thiazides in diabetes insipidus: another piece in the puzzle". J. Am. Soc. Nephrol. 15 (11): 2948–50.

37. Longmore, M., Wilkinson, I., Davidson, E., Foulkes, A., Mafi, A. Oxford Handbook of Clinical Medicine 8th Ed.

38. Madlon-Kay DJ. 'Witch's milk.' Galactorrhea in the newborn. Am J Dis Child 1986;140:252-3.

39. Mancall, Elliott L.; Brock, David G., eds. (2011). "Cranial Fossae". Gray's Clinical Anatomy. Elsevier Health Sciences. pp. 154. ISBN 9781437735802.

40. Melmed, Shlomo (2011). The Pituitary - (Third Edition). San Diego, CA 92101-4495, USA: Academic Press is an imprint of Elsevier. pp. 23–25. ISBN 978-0-12-380926-1.

41. Michels A, Michels N (1 Apr 2014). "Addison disease: early detection and treatment principles". Am Fam Physician 89 (7): 563–8.

42. Molitch ME. Management of prolactinomas during pregnancy. J Reprod Med 1999;44:1121-6.

43. Molitch ME. Medical treatment of prolactinomas. Endocrinol Metab Clin North Am 1999;28:143-69.

44. Newell-Price J, Bertagna X, Grossman A, Nieman L. Cushing's syndrome. The Lancet. 2006;367:1605-1617.

45. Nieman L, Ilias I. Evaluation and treatment of Cushing's syndrome. The American Journal of Medicine. 2005;118: 1340–1346.

46. Perkins RM, Yuan CM, Welch PG (March 2006). "Dipsogenic diabetes insipidus: report of a novel treatment strategy and literature review". Clin. Exp. Nephrol. 10 (1): 63–7.

47. Physicians' desk reference: companion guide. Montvale, N.J.: Medical Economics, 2000:1293,1315, 1337.

48. Pocock, Gillian (2006). Human Physiology (Third ed.). Oxford University Press. p. 193. ISBN 978-0-19-856878-0.

49. Quinkler M, Dahlqvist P, Husebye ES, Kämpe O (Jan 2015). "A European Emergency Card for adrenal insufficiency can save lives". Eur J Intern Med 26 (1): 75–6.

50. Romer, Alfred Sherwood; Parsons, Thomas S. (1977). The Vertebrate Body. Philadelphia, PA: Holt-Saunders International. pp. 549–550. ISBN 0-03-910284-X.

51. Rothenberg RE, LaRaja RD, Pryce E, Mueller SC. Breast cancer and idiopathic galactorrhea. J Med Assoc Ga 1990;79: 363–5.

52. Sanfilippo JS. Implications of not treating hyperprolactinemia. J Reprod Med 1999; 449(12 suppl):1111-5.

53. ShlomoMelmed (3 December 2010). The pituitary. Academic Press. p. 40. ISBN 978-0-12-380926-1.

54. Siminoski, K; Goss, P; Drucker, DJ (1989). "The Cushing syndrome induced by medroxyprogesterone acetate". Annals of internal medicine 111 (9): 758–60.

55. Sinha A, Ball S, Jenkins A, Hale J, Cheetham T (2011). "Objective assessment of thirst recovery in patients with adipsic diabetes insipidus". Pituitary 14 (4): 307–11.

56. Smith D, McKenna K, Moore K, et al. "Baroregulation of vasopressin release in adipsic diabetes insipidus". J. Clin. Endocrinol. Metab. 2002; 87(10): 4564–8.

57. Steffensen, C; Bak, AM; Rubeck, KZ; Jørgensen, JO (2010). "Epidemiology of Cushing's syndrome.". Neuroendocrinology. 92 Suppl 1: 1–5.

58. Stuart M, ed. The Encyclopedia of herbs and herbalism. New York: Grosset and Dunlap, 1979:176,191, 239, 276–7.

59. Tietz textbook of clinical chemistry and molecular biology 5fifth edition, Philadelphia, W.B Saunders company (2012).

60. Tolis G, Somma M, Van Campenhout J, Friesen H. Prolactin secretion in sixty-five patients with galactorrhea. Am J Obstet Gynecol 1974; 118:91-101.

61. Turner, H., Wass, J., Oxford Handbook of Endocrinology and Diabetes

62. Turton DB, Shakir KM. Galactorrhea caused by esophagitis. Am J ObstetGynecol 1995; 173:1629-30.

63. Verhelst J, Abs R, Maiter D, Van den Bruel A, Vandeweghe M, Velkeniers B, et al. Cabergoline in the treatment of hyperprolactinemia: a study in 455 patients. J Clin Endocrinol Metab 1999; 84:2518-22.

64. Wells, M. J.; Wells, J. (1969). "Pituitary Analogue in the Octopus". Nature 222 (5190): 293–294.

65. William Marshall, MártaLapsley, Stephen K Bangert. Elsevier.com: Clinical Chemistry, 7th Edition; ISBN-9780723437031. (2012).

66. Windgassen K, Wesselmann U, Schulze Monking H. Galactorrhea and hyperprolactinemia in schizophrenic patients on neuroleptics: frequency and etiology. Neuropsychobiology 1996;33: 142–6.

67. Yarkony GM, Novick AK, Roth EJ, KirschnerKL,Rayner S, Betts HB. Galactorrhea: a complication ofspinal cord injury. Arch Phys Med Rehabil 1992;73: 878–80.

68. Yazigi RA, Quintero CH, Salameh WA. Prolactin disorders. FertilSteril 1997;67: 215–25.

69. Yudófsky, Stuart C.; Robert E. Hales (2007). The American Psychiatric Publishing Textbook of Neuropsychiatry and Behavioral Neurosciences (5th ed.). American Psychiatric Pub, Inc. ISBN 1-58562-239-7.

8

The Adrenal Glands

INTRODUCTION

The adrenal glands have two functionally distinct parts, each weighs approximately 4 g and sits in close proximity to a kidney. The cortex forms about 90% of its mass, the remaining core being the adrenal medulla. In the adult, it can be divided morphologically and functionally into three layers (the glomerulosa, fasciculata, and reticularis) (Fig. 8.1). Each layer has a distinct

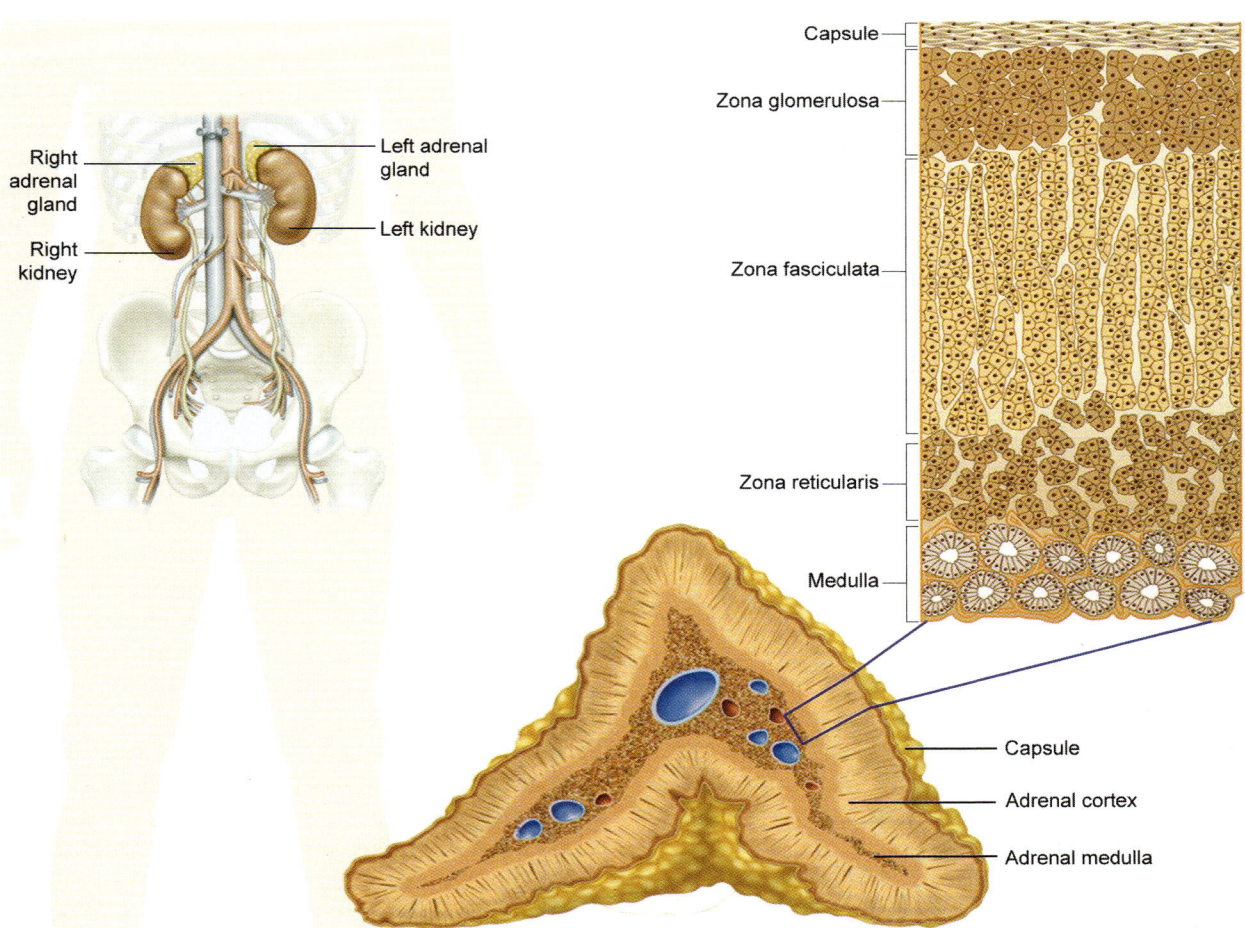

Fig. 8.1: The human adrenal gland

histological appearance and secretes different steroid hormones.

Glucocorticoids, of which the most important is cortisol, are secreted in response to adrenocorticotropic hormone (ACTH), which is itself secreted by the pituitary in response to the hypothalamic corticotropin releasing hormone (CRH). Cortisol exerts negative feedback control on ACTH release through inhibiting the action of CRH; it also inhibits CRH secretion. Glucocorticoids have many actions (Table 8.1), and are particularly important in mediating the body's response to stress. Corticosterone, a precursor of aldosterone, is a weak glucocorticoid (30% of the activity of cortisol).

The most important mineralocorticoid is aldosterone. This is secreted in response to angiotensin II, produced as a result of the activation of the renin–angiotensin system by a decrease in renal blood flow and other indicators of decreased extracellular fluid (ECF) volume (Fig. 8.2). Secretion of aldosterone is also directly stimulated by hyperkalemia. The main action of aldosterone is to stimulate the reabsorption of sodium and the excretion of potassium and hydrogen ions in the distal convoluted tubules of the kidneys; its effect on sodium results in its having a central role in the determination of the ECF volume. ACTH does not have a major physiological role in aldosterone secretion, although it has a role in its synthesis through stimulating cholesterol desmolase, the first step in the biosynthetic pathway of the adrenal steroids. Curiously, the secretion of aldosterone by adrenal tumors is affected by ACTH. 11-Deoxycorticosterone and corticosterone also have mineralocorticoid activity. Cortisol has as high affinity for mineralocorticoid receptors, as does aldosterone, and its concentration in the blood is considerably higher, but renal tubular cells contain 11β-hydroxysteroid dehydrogenase, which converts cortisol to cortisone. The latter has low affinity for mineralocorticoid receptors, thus allowing these to respond primarily to aldosterone and not be overwhelmed by cortisol.

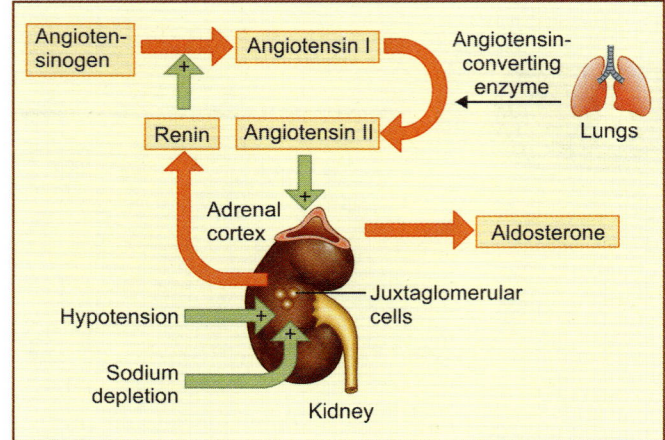

Fig. 8.2: Stimulation of aldosterone secretion through activation of the renin–angiotensin system. Renin, released into the plasma from the juxtaglomerular cells of the kidney in response to various stimuli, catalyzes the formation of angiotensin I from angiotensinogen, an α_2-globulin. Angiotensin I is metabolized to an octapeptide, angiotensin II, by angiotensin-converting enzyme during its passage through the lungs. Angiotensin II stimulates the release of aldosterone from the adrenal cortex; it is a powerful pressor agent and also stimulates thirst and the secretion of vasopressin

The adrenal cortex is also a source of androgens, including dehydroepiandrosterone (DHEA), DHEA sulphate (DHEAS) and androstenedione. These stimulate libido and the development of pubic and axillary hair in females, but are weak androgens in comparison with testosterone, and have only a minor physiological function in males. The clinical effects of excessive adrenal androgens can be a prominent feature of adrenal disorders in females.

ADRENAL STEROID HORMONE BIOSYNTHESIS

Corticosteroid biosynthesis has been well characterized, and is presented in simplified form in Fig. 8.3. Cholesterol, the precursor to all steroid biosynthetic pathways, is converted to a variety of steroid molecules in a series of reactions catalyzed by several cytochrome enzymes. While some cholesterol can be synthesized within the adrenal cortex, the vast majority of cholesterol used in steroid biosynthesis is taken up from a pool of circulating cholesterol bound to low-density lipoproteins in the plasma. After synthesis, corticosteroids are rapidly secreted. Because corticosteroids are not stored in the adrenal cortex, the rate of steroid synthesis is essentially equal to the rate of secretion from the adrenal gland. An awareness of these pathways is important for the understanding of congenital adrenal hyperplasia, a group of conditions each caused by a lack of one of these enzymes.

Table 8.1	Principal physiological functions of glucocorticoids

Increase protein catabolism

Increase hepatic glycogen synthesis

Increase hepatic gluconeogenesis

Inhibit ACTH secretion

Sensitize arterioles to action of norepinephrine (maintenance of blood pressure)

Permissive effect on water excretion

Inhibit the inflammatory and immune response

Inhibit bone formation through inhibition of type 1 collagen synthesis

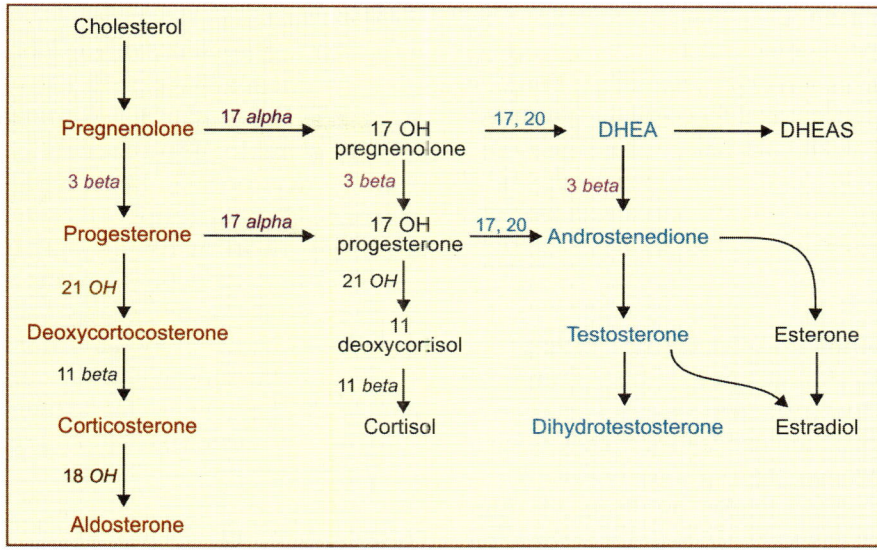

Fig. 8.3: Principal pathways for adrenal steroid hormone synthesis steps

Measurement of Adrenal Steroid Hormones

Adrenal steroid hormones can all be measured by immunoassays, although some cross-reactivity occurs between some steroids in some assays (e.g. between 11-deoxycortisol and cortisol). The plasma concentrations of steroid hormones can fluctuate for various reasons and the results of single estimations must be interpreted with caution.

The measurement of urinary cortisol excretion is valuable in investigations of Cushing's syndrome. **Urinary 'steroid profiling'**, in which steroids are separated and quantified by gas–liquid chromatography, often combined with mass spectrometry, is particularly valuable in the investigation of suspected congenital adrenal hyperplasia; it may also be helpful in the investigation of suspected adrenal carcinoma.

Cortisol

Some 95% of cortisol in the blood is bound to protein, principally to the cortisol-binding globulin, transcortin. Free cortisol concentration, and thus the amount of cortisol that can be excreted unchanged in the urine, is very low. Transcortin is almost fully saturated at normal cortisol concentrations. Because of this, if cortisol production increases, the concentration present in the plasma in the free form, and thus the amount that is excreted, increases to a disproportionately greater extent than the total. For this reason, measurement of the 24 hours urinary excretion of cortisol, provided that an accurate urine collection can be made, is a sensitive way of detecting increased, but not decreased, secretion of the hormone.

Plasma cortisol concentrations show a diurnal variation, being highest in the morning and lowest at night (Fig. 8.4). Blood for cortisol measurement should usually be drawn between 08:00 hour and 09:00 hour; however, samples can be taken at 23:00 hour to detect loss of the diurnal variation, an early feature of adrenal hyperfunction (Cushing's syndrome). Random measurements are rarely of any value in the diagnosis of adrenal disease, except that a high concentration in a sick patient may reasonably be taken to exclude adrenal failure.

Cortisol is secreted in response to stress, mediated through ACTH, and thus stress must be kept to a minimum if results are to be interpreted correctly. Investigations of adrenal hypofunction or hyperfunction

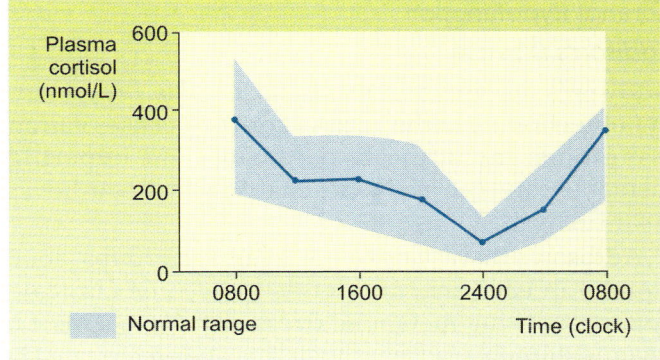

Fig. 8.4: Diurnal variation in plasma cortisol concentration. Plasma cortisol concentrations are at their highest shortly after waking and then decline throughout the day to reach a nadir in the late evening. Because of this variation, it is important that blood samples are taken at times that coincide either with the peak or the trough, random samples being of little value. The graph shows mean values and the range in a sample of healthy people

often involve measurement of cortisol after attempting to stimulate or suppress its secretion.

When interpreting plasma cortisol results, it should be remembered that the synthetic glucocorticoid prednisolone may cross-react with cortisol in immunoassays for the hormone. Cross-reaction does not occur with dexamethasone, nor with spironolactone, an aldosterone antagonist used as a diuretic.

Aldosterone

Renin is secreted by the juxtaglomerular cells of the kidneys in response to changes in plasma volume. An increase in renin normally produces an increase in aldosterone through angiotensin intermediates. Renin's physiological effects are manifested mainly through its changes on aldosterone production; therefore, it is often helpful to measure the plasma renin activity at the same time as the concentration of aldosterone, to establish whether aldosterone secretion is autonomous or under normal control. Calculation of the plasma **aldosterone–renin ratio** in a random blood sample is a useful screening test for excessive aldosterone secretion; this is excluded by a low value. Plasma aldosterone concentration varies with posture; the use of samples taken from patients while they are recumbent or ambulant is discussed further in connection with the investigation of excessive secretion of aldosterone.

Androgens

Measurements of adrenal androgens are of value in the diagnosis and management of congenital adrenal hyperplasia and in the investigation of virilization in women.

DISORDERS OF THE ADRENAL CORTEX
Adrenal Hypofunction
Addison's Disease

Addison's disease is an insidious, usually progressive hypofunctioning of the adrenal cortex. It causes various symptoms, including hypotension and hyperpigmentation, and can lead to adrenal crisis with cardiovascular collapse.

Addison's disease develops in all age groups, about equally in each sex, and tends to become clinically apparent during metabolic stress or trauma. Onset of severe symptoms (adrenal crisis) may be precipitated by acute infection (a common cause, especially with septicemia). Other causes include trauma, surgery, and Na loss from excessive sweating. Even with treatment, Addison's disease may cause a slight increase in mortality. It is not clear whether this increase is due to mistreated adrenal crises or long-term complications of inadvertent over-replacement.

Etiology

About 70% of cases are due to idiopathic atrophy of the adrenal cortex, probably caused by autoimmune processes. The remainder result from destruction of the adrenal gland by granuloma (e.g. TB, histoplasmosis), tumor, amyloidosis, hemorrhage, or inflammatory necrosis. Hypoadrenocorticism can also result from administration of drugs that block corticosteroid synthesis (e.g. ketoconazole, the anestheticetomidate). Addison's disease may coexist with diabetes mellitus or hypothyroidism in polyglandular deficiency syndrome. In children, the most common cause of primary adrenal insufficiency is congenital adrenal hyperplasia (CAH), but other genetic disorders are being increasingly recognized as causes.

Pathophysiology

Disease results from both mineralocorticoids and glucocorticoids deficiency as a result of either destruction of the three layers of the adrenal cortex (the glomerulosa, fasciculata, and reticularis) and disruption of hormone synthesis.

Mineralocorticoid Deficiency

Because mineralocorticoids stimulate Na reabsorption and K excretion, deficiency results in increased excretion of Na and decreased excretion of K, chiefly in urine but also in sweat, saliva, and the gastrointestinal (GI) tract. A low serum concentration of Na and a high concentration of K result. Urinary salt and water loss cause severe dehydration, plasma hypertonicity, acidosis, decreased circulatory volume, hypotension, and, eventually, circulatory collapse. However, when adrenal insufficiency is caused by inadequate ACTH production, electrolyte levels are often normal or only mildly deranged.

Glucocorticoid Deficiency

It contributes to hypotension and causes severe insulin sensitivity and disturbances in carbohydrate, fat, and protein metabolism. In the absence of cortisol, insufficient carbohydrate is formed from protein, hypoglycemia and decreased liver glycogen result. Weakness follows, due in part to deficient neuromuscular function. Resistance to infection, trauma, and other stress is decreased. Myocardial weakness and dehydration reduce cardiac output, and circulatory failure can occur. Decreased blood cortisol results in increased pituitary ACTH production and increased blood β-lipotropin, which has melanocyte-stimulating activity and, together with ACTH, causes the hyperpigmentation of skin and mucous membranes characteristic of Addison's disease. Thus, adrenal insufficiency secondary to pituitary failure does not cause hyperpigmentation.

Symptoms and Signs

Weakness, fatigue, and orthostatic hypotension are early symptoms and signs. Hyperpigmentation (Fig. 8.5) is characterized by diffuse tanning of exposed and, to a lesser extent, unexposed portions of the body, especially on pressure points (bony prominences), skin folds, scars, and extensor surfaces. Black freckles are common on the forehead, face, neck, and shoulders. Bluish black discolorations of the areolae and mucous membranes of the lips, mouth, rectum, and vagina occur. Anorexia, nausea, vomiting, and diarrhea often occur. Decreased tolerance to cold, with hypometabolism, may be noted. Dizziness and syncope may occur. The gradual onset and nonspecific nature of early symptoms often lead to an incorrect initial diagnosis of neurosis. Weight loss, dehydration, and hypotension are characteristic of the later stages of Addison's disease.

ADRENAL CRISIS

Adrenal crisis is a life-threatening emergency, which usually manifests with nausea, vomiting, abdominal pain, and shock. Patients may be previously undiagnosed or have chronic primary adrenal insufficiency (AI), with no or inadequate glucocorticoid replacement. Abdominal tenderness and fever are common findings, and adrenal crisis may manifest as an acute abdomen. In these cases, surgical exploration without glucocorticoid coverage can be lethal. The major hormonal factor precipitating adrenal crisis is mineralocorticoid deficiency. Therefore, adrenal crisis rarely occurs with secondary adrenal insufficiency.

Treatment of adrenal crisis should not be delayed. Diagnostic workup in a patient with no history of AI should include a plasma sample for cortisol and ACTH level determination, immediately followed by an IV bolus of hydrocortisone, 100 mg, and adequate fluid replacement (normal saline). Hydrocortisone should be

continued, 50 mg every 8 hours, while awaiting laboratory results.

Diagnosis

The diagnosis of adrenocortical insufficiency rests on the assessment of the functional capacity of the adrenal cortex to synthesize cortisol. This is accomplished primarily by use of the rapid ACTH stimulation test (corrosion, cosyntropin, tetracosactide, or synacthen).

ACTH, through complex mechanisms, activates cholesterol esterase enzymes and leads to the release of free cholesterol from cholesterol esters. It also activates the 20, 22-desmolase enzyme, which catalyzes the rate-limiting step in adrenal steroidogenesis and increases the NADPH (nicotinamide adenine dinucleotide phosphate) levels necessary for the various hydroxylation steps in steroidogenesis.

Within 15–30 minutes of ACTH infusion, the normal adrenal cortex releases 2–5 times its basal plasma cortisol output. Although, ACTH stimulation is not normally the major stimulus for aldosterone production, it increases aldosterone production to peak levels within 30 minutes. This response, however, is affected by dietary sodium intake. An increase in the plasma cortisol and aldosterone levels above basal levels after ACTH injection reflects the functional integrity of the adrenal cortex.

Performing the Rapid Adrenocorticotropic Hormone Test

A plasma cortisol concentration of <50 nmol/L in a blood sample drawn at 09:00 hour is effectively diagnostic of adrenal failure (unless a patient is being treated with synthetic corticosteroids), while a concentration of >550 nmol/L excludes the diagnosis. However, in the majority of patients with adrenal failure, whether primary or secondary, the plasma cortisol concentration lies between these extremes, and an ACTH stimulation test must be performed to establish the diagnosis. The normal response to a single dose of soluble ACTH (tetracosactide or synacthen) ('short synacthen test') (Fig. 8.5). If the response is in any way abnormal, the patient should be assumed to have adrenal failure. In both primary and secondary adrenal failure, the response in the short ACTH stimulation test is absent or blunted. This should be regarded as a screening test for adrenal failure. The distinction between primary and secondary adrenal failure can usually be made on the basis of measurement of the plasma ACTH concentration at 09:00 hour; high values (a result of decreased negative feedback by cortisol) are typical of primary adrenal failure; low, or low–normal values, are typical of secondary adrenal failure. Alternatively, a long ACTH stimulation test can be performed (Fig. 8.6). There are various protocols for this investigation. Typically, a single dose of depot ACTH

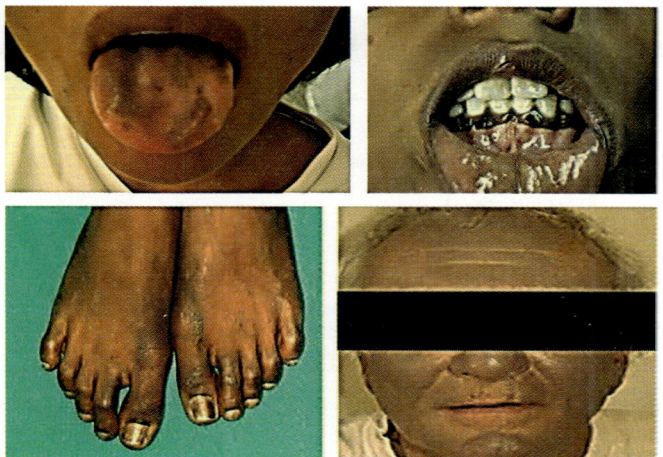

Fig. 8.5: Classic hyperpigmentation as seen in Addison's disease

(1 mg IM), which has a longer duration of action, is given and plasma cortisol is measured after 6 and 24 hours. A failure to increase is typical of primary adrenal failure, whereas in secondary adrenal failure there is usually an increase at 6 hours and a further increase after 24 hours. If no increase occurs, but secondary adrenal failure remains a possibility, depot ACTH can be given over 3 days; a failure of cortisol to increase over this time excludes the diagnosis.

Although, ideally, these tests should be done before starting treatment, when a severely ill patient is judged clinically to have adrenal failure treatment should not be delayed. A blood sample can be taken immediately for later cortisol measurement. Treatment can then be commenced with a synthetic glucocorticoid that does not cross-react with cortisol in the laboratory assay (e.g. dexamethasone) and an ACTH stimulation test perfor-med as soon as is convenient. The results will not be vitiated by the treatment if only a short time elapses before the test is done. Patients presenting acutely with adrenal failure require intravenous hydrocortisone and fluid replacement with 0.9% sodium chloride. Plasma potassium and glucose concentrations should be monito-red and intravenous glucose provided if necessary.

Once primary adrenal failure has been diagnosed, the cause should be sought, e.g. by measuring anti-adrenal antibodies (present in 90% of patients with autoimmune disease) and looking for evidence of tuberculosis.

Other Laboratory Tests

- Comprehensive metabolic panel
  - The most prominent findings are hyponatremia, hyperkalemia, and a mild non-anion-gap metabolic acidosis due to the loss of the sodium-retaining and potassium and hydrogen ion-secreting action of aldosterone.
  - Urinary and sweat sodium also may be elevated.
  - The most consistent finding is elevated blood urea nitrogen (BUN) and creatinine due to the hypo-volemia, a decreased glomerular filtration rate, and a decreased renal plasma flow.
  - Hypercalcemia, the cause of which is not well understood, may be present in a small percentage of patients. However, hypocalcemia could occur in patients with Addison's disease accompanied by idiopathic hypoparathyroidism.
  - Hypoglycemia may be present in fasted patients, or it may occur spontaneously. It is caused by the increased peripheral utilization of glucose and increased insulin sensitivity. It is more prominent in children and in patients with secondary adreno-cortical insufficiency.
  - Liver function tests may reveal a glucocorticoid-responsive liver dysfunction.
- Complete blood cell count
  - Complete blood cell count (CBC) count may reveal a normocytic normochromic anemia, which, upon initial presentation, may be masked by dehydration and hemoconcentration. Relative lymphocytosis and eosinophilia may be present.
  - All of these findings are responsive to glucocorticoid replacement.
- Thyroid-stimulating hormone
  - Increased thyroid-stimulating hormone (TSH), with or without low thyroxine, with or without associated thyroid autoantibodies, and with or without symptoms of hypothyroidism, may occur in patients with Addison's disease and in patients with secondary adrenocortical insufficiency due to isolated ACTH deficiency. These findings may be slowly reversible with cortisol replacement.

ACTH stimulation tests	
Short test	**Long test**
Procedure Take blood sample at 09:00 h for measurement of cortisol Inject 250 µg ACTH IM or IV Take further blood samples after 30 minutes and 60 minutes for cortisol measurement **Normal results** Plasma cortisol after ACTH increment of 200 nmol/L with peak of >550 nmol/L	**Procedure** 09:00 h: Take blood for measurement of cortisol 1 mg depot ACTH IM 15:00 h: Take blood for cortisol measurement 09:00 h (next day): Take blood for cortisol measurement **Results** Primary adrenal insufficiency: No increase in cortisol Secondary adrenal insufficiency: Increase in cortisol at 6 hours with further increase at 24 hours; total increment >200 nmol/L

Fig. 8.6: ACTH stimulation tests (also known as tetracosactide or synacthen tests; synacthen is synthetic ACTH) for the diagnosis of adrenal failure. It is important to note that blood should be taken for ACTH assay before giving ACTH. It is not necessary to withhold any treatment until after the tests have been completed, provided that the drug being used does not cross-react with cortisol, as exogenous steroids do not affect the response of the adrenal gland to ACTH in the short term

- In the setting of both adrenocortical insufficiency and hypothyroidism that requires treatment, corticosteroids should be given before thyroid hormone replacement to avoid precipitating an acute adrenal crisis.

■ *Autoantibody testing:* Thyroid autoantibodies, specifically antithyroglobulin (anti-TG) and antimicrosomal or antithyroid peroxidase (anti-TPO) antibodies, and/or adrenal autoantibodies may be present.

■ *Prolactin testing:*

- Modest hyperprolactinemia has been reported in cases of Addison' disease and also in secondary adrenocortical insufficiency. It is responsive to glucocorticoid replacement.

- The cause of the hyperprolactinemia is thought to be the hyperresponsiveness of the lactotroph to thyrotropin-releasing hormone (TRH) in the absence of the steroid-induced or steroid-enhanced hypothalamic dopaminergic tone.

Treatment

Normally, cortisol is secreted maximally in the early morning and minimally at night. Thus, hydrocortisone (identical to cortisol) is given in 2 or 3 divided doses with a typical total daily dose of 15–30 mg. One regimen gives half the total in the morning, and the remaining half split between lunchtime and early evening (e.g. 10 mg, 5 mg, and 5 mg). Others give two-thirds in the morning and one-third in the evening. Doses immediately before retiring should generally be avoided because they may cause insomnia. Alternatively, prednisone 5 mg by mouth in the morning and 2.5 mg by mouth in the evening may be used. Additionally, fludrocortisone 0.1–0.2 mg by mouth once a day is recommended to replace aldosterone. The easiest way to adjust the dosage is to ensure that the renin level is within the normal range. Normal hydration and absence of orthostatic hypotension are evidence of adequate replacement therapy. In some patients, fludrocortisone causes hypertension, which is treated by reducing the dosage or starting a nondiuretic antihypertensive. Some clinicians tend to give too little fludrocortisone in an effort to avoid use of antihypertensives.

Intercurrent illnesses (e.g. infections) are potentially serious and should be vigorously treated; the patient's hydrocortisone dose should be doubled during the illness. If nausea and vomiting preclude oral therapy, parenteral therapy is necessary. Patients should be instructed when to take supplemental prednisone or hydrocortisone and taught to self-administer parenteral hydrocortisone for urgent situations. A preloaded syringe with 100 mg hydrocortisone should be available to the patient. A bracelet or wallet card giving the diagnosis and corticosteroid dose may help in case of adrenal crisis that renders the patient unable to communicate. When salt loss is severe, as in very hot climates, the dose of fludrocortisone may need to be increased.

In coexisting diabetes mellitus and Addison's disease, the hydrocortisone dose usually should not be >30 mg/day; otherwise, insulin requirements are increased.

ADRENAL HYPERFUNCTION

In Cushing's syndrome, there is overproduction primarily of glucocorticoids, although mineralocorticoid and androgen production may also be excessive. In Conn's syndrome, mineralocorticoids alone are produced in excess.

Cushing's Syndrome

Cushing's syndrome is used to describe a condition resulting from long-term exposure to excessive glucocorticoids. The syndrome is most commonly caused by the therapeutic administration of exogenous glucocorticoids. The term 'Cushing's disease' is reserved for Cushing's syndrome that is caused by excessive secretion of ACTH by a pituitary tumor, usually an adenoma.

Cushing's disease is responsible for roughly two-thirds of the cases of endogenous Cushing's syndrome. The remainder of the endogenous cases are caused by ectopic ACTH-secreting tumors and primary adrenal neoplasms. Cushing's disease occurs most frequently in women of reproductive age, but it can affect males and females of any age.

The pituitary tumors in Cushing's disease are usually microadenomas, which, by definition, are 10 mm or less in diameter. Micro-adenomas generally do not cause symptoms by local mass effect. These tumors are most often discovered when clinical manifestations of hypercortisolism resulting from hypersecretion of ACTH prompt an appropriate diagnostic work-up. Occasionally, microadenomas are found incidentally during imaging performed for other reasons.

Macroadenomas are uncommon in patients with Cushing's disease. These tumors cause mass effect when their size exceeds 15 mm in diameter. Suprasellar extension and optic chiasm compression, local bone erosion, cavernous sinus compression and panhypopituitarism may occur as a macroadenoma enlarges.

A common effect of elevated ACTH levels (whatever the source) is bilateral adrenocortical hyperplasia, which may be diffuse or nodular. Rarely, micronodular or macronodular ACTH-independent adrenal hyperplasia can be the cause of Cushing's syndrome.

Etiology

The condition may also be due to your body's own overproduction of cortisol (endogenous Cushing's syndrome). This may occur from excess production by one or both adrenal glands, or overproduction of the adrenocorticotropic hormone, which normally regulates cortisol production. In these cases, Cushing syndrome may be related to:

- Pituitary gland tumor (pituitary adenoma); A noncancerous (benign) tumor of the pituitary gland, located at the base of the brain, secretes an excess amount of ACTH, which in turn stimulates the adrenal glands to make more cortisol. When this form of the syndrome develops, it's called Cushing' disease. It occurs much more often in women and is the most common form of endogenous Cushing's syndrome.
- A primary adrenal gland disease; in some people, the cause of Cushing's syndrome is excess cortisol secretion that doesn't depend on stimulation from ACTH and is associated with disorders of the adrenal glands. The most common of these disorders is a noncancerous tumor of the adrenal cortex, called an adrenal adenoma. Cancerous tumors of the adrenal cortex (adrenocortical carcinomas) are rare, but they can cause Cushing's syndrome as well. Occasionally, benign, nodular enlargement of both adrenal glands can result in Cushing's syndrome.
- An ectopic ACTH-secreting tumor; rarely when a tumor develops in an organ that normally does not produce ACTH, the tumor will begin to secrete this hormone in excess, resulting in Cushing's syndrome. These tumors, which can be noncancerous (benign) or cancerous (malignant), are usually found in the lungs, pancreas, thyroid, or thymus gland (Fig. 8.7).
- Familial Cushing's syndrome; rarely people inherit a tendency to develop tumors on one or more of their endocrine glands, affecting cortisol levels and causing Cushing's syndrome.

Symptoms and Signs

Clinical manifestations include moon facies with a plethoric appearance, truncal obesity with prominent supraclavicular and dorsal cervical fat pads (buffalo hump), and, usually, very slender distal extremities and fingers. Muscle wasting and weakness are present. The skin is thin and atrophic, with poor wound healing and easy bruising. Purple striae may appear on the abdomen (Fig. 8.8). Hypertension, renal calculi, osteoporosis, glucose intolerance, reduced resistance to infection, and mental disturbances are common. Cessation of linear growth is characteristic in children. Females usually have menstrual irregularities. In females with adrenal tumors, increased production of androgens may lead to hypertrichosis, temporal balding, and other signs of virilism.

Cushing's syndrome

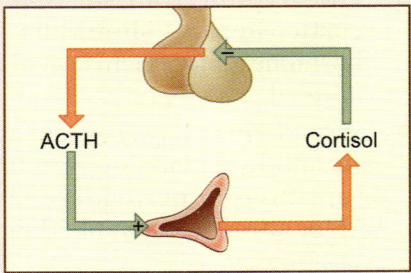

(A) Normal
Production of cortisol by adrenal cortex stimulated by ACTH
Cortisol exerts a negative feedback effect on release of ACTH by pituitary

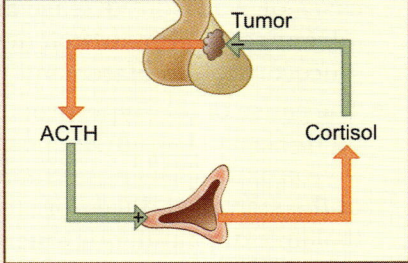

(B) Cushing's disease
ACTH secretion increased
Pituitary insensitive to feedback by normal levels of cortisol
Higher levels of cortisol required to produce negative feedback effect on ACTH secretion

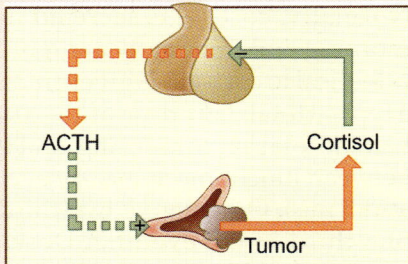

(C) Adrenal tumors
Autonomous cortisol production
High circulating cortisol inhibits ACTH secretion

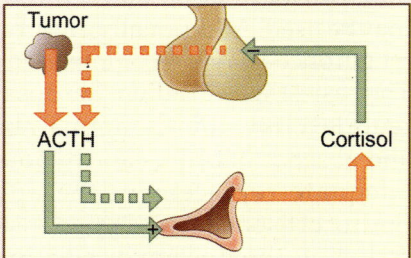

(D) Ectopic ACTH secretion
High level of ACTH secreted by tumor stimulates excessive cortisol production
Inhibition of secretion of ACTH by pituitary

Fig. 8.7: Pituitary–adrenal relationships in Cushing's syndrome. In Cushing's disease, the pituitary usually remains susceptible to feedback by glucocorticoids, but is apparently less sensitive than normal (A) (i.e. a higher concentration of cortisol is necessary to suppress ACTH (B). In Cushing's syndrome caused by adrenal tumors, whether adenomas or carcinomas, and also in ectopic ACTH secretion, there is usually no response to dexamethasone, even at the higher dose, as pituitary ACTH secretion is already suppressed by the high plasma cortisol concentrations (C). This patient's plasma ACTH is raised; with adrenal tumors, feedback of cortisol to the pituitary suppresses ACTH, while with ectopic ACTH secretion, ACTH concentrations are often (but not always) very high (D)

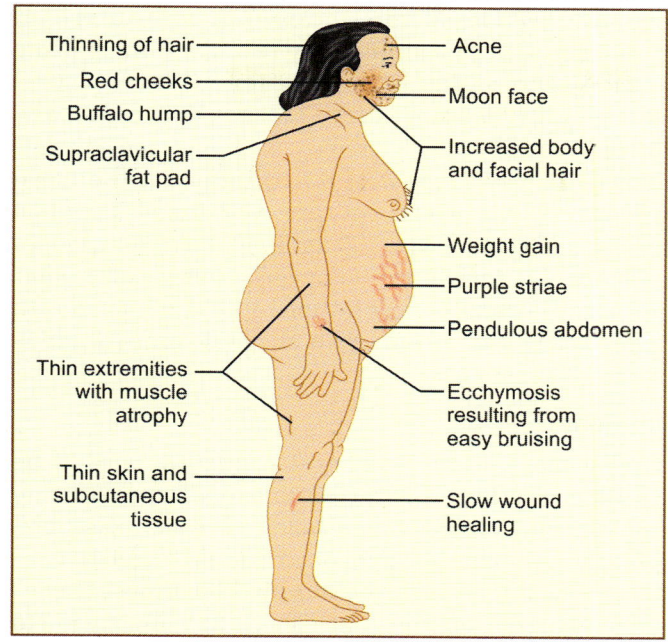

Fig. 8.8: Cushing's syndrome symptoms and signs

Labels (top to bottom, left side): Thinning of hair, Red cheeks, Buffalo hump, Supraclavicular fat pad, Thin extremities with muscle atrophy, Thin skin and subcutaneous tissue

Labels (right side): Acne, Moon face, Increased body and facial hair, Weight gain, Purple striae, Pendulous abdomen, Ecchymosis resulting from easy bruising, Slow wound healing

Diagnosis

There are two diagnostic steps in the investigation of a patient with suspected Cushing's syndrome; the demonstration of increased cortisol secretion and the elucidation of the cause. It is common to see patients who look Cushingoid but it is much less common that Cushing's syndrome is the cause. It is, therefore, often useful to carry out preliminary tests on an outpatient basis, aimed at excluding those patients who do not have adrenal disease and identifying those who may, and who thus merit further investigation. Tests used for this purpose (Fig. 8.9) are the measurement of 24 hours urinary cortisol excretion and the overnight or low-dose dexamethasone suppression test. Isolated measurements of plasma cortisol concentration are of no value. They are often normal during the day in patients with Cushing's syndrome.

Normal 24 hours urinary cortisol excretion is <300 nmol. Increased excretion is characteristic of Cushing's syndrome, but specificity is poor; increased excretion can also occur in pseudo-Cushing's and severe obesity. Sensitivity is also poor but can be improved by making several urine collections (although this may be unacceptable to patients). If the urine collection is incomplete, the true excretion will be underestimated. This problem may be obviated by expressing the results as a ratio to the urinary creatinine excretion.

Dexamethasone is a synthetic glucocorticoid that binds to cortisol receptors in the pituitary and suppresses ACTH release (and thus the secretion of cortisol by the adrenals) in normal individuals. In the overnight test, 1 mg is given at night and blood is drawn for measurement of cortisol at 09:00 hours the next morning. In normal individuals, this should be <50 nmol/L. A failure of suppression is characteristic of Cushing's syndrome, but is not specific as it may also be seen in pseudo-Cushing's syndrome and as a result of stress. Fewer false positives occur if dexamethasone is given at a dose of 0.5 mg 6-hourly for 48 hours, with cortisol being measured on the morning after the last dose. False negatives virtually never occur with either protocol but are a possibility in patients taking drugs, such as phenytoin or carbamazepine, that increase the hepatic metabolism of dexamethasone. It is important that, if urinary cortisol excretion is to be measured, the period of collection does not include the time when dexamethasone is being given (Fig. 8.10).

The insulin hypoglycemia test, also used in the investigation of pituitary function, can be helpful in the diagnosis of Cushing's syndrome, as the normal increase

Screening tests for Cushing's syndrome	
Test	**Normal result**
24, hour urinary cortisol excretion	<300 nmol/24 h
Overnight/48 h low-dose dexamethasone suppression test	Plasma cortisol <50 nmol/L at 09:00 h

Fig. 8.9: Screening tests for Cushing's syndrome. The values for cortisol concentration used for diagnosis may vary slightly between laboratories. Cushing's syndrome is excluded by normal results in these tests.

Typical results of adrenal function tests in Cushing's syndrome					
Condition	**Basal cortisol (nmol/L)**	**Dexamethasone suppression test**		**CRH Test**	**Plasma ACTH ACTH (ng/L)**
		Low dose	High dose		
Cushing's disease	↑ (<1000)	no suppression	suppression	response	↑ (<200)
Adrenal tumor	↑ (variable)	no suppression	no suppression	no response	↓
ctopic ACTH secretion	Greatly ↑ (>1000)	no suppression	no suppression	no response	Greatly ↑ (<200)

Fig. 8.10: Typical results of adrenal function tests in Cushing's syndrome. With ectopic ACTH secretion by carcinoid tumors, the results of these tests may be identical to those seen in Cushing's disease, as the tumor may have glucocorticoid receptors that will respond to dexamethasone

in plasma cortisol concentration that occurs in response to hypoglycemia is abolished even in mild Cushing's syndrome, while in patients with pseudo-Cushing's a normal response occurs.

Loss of diurnal variation of cortisol secretion is an early feature of Cushing's syndrome, and the diagnosis is excluded if the plasma cortisol concentration at 23:00 hours or 24:00 hours is normal (<100 nmol/L). As the patient must be resting and not stressed, plasma cortisol measurement at night is not a practical outpatient procedure. It necessitates hospital admission, itself a stressful event, with the result that false positive results are common. However, if care is taken to minimize stress (ideally blood is taken from the sleeping patient through a previously inserted cannula after 2 or 3 days in hospital), a raised value does indicate pathological overproduction of cortisol. However, the results of salivary cortisol measurements have been shown to give results that are nearly as reliable as those of plasma cortisol, and saliva can be collected by the patient at home.

Cyclical Cushing's syndrome, in which the hypersecretion of cortisol varies with time; sometimes over several years; is uncommon, but well recognized, and can pose a considerable diagnostic.

Once increased cortisol secretion has been documented, measurements of plasma ACTH are used to determine how to investigate the patient further. Low concentrations suggest an adrenal cause (requiring adrenal imaging), and very high concentrations, ectopic secretion of ACTH. However, concentrations may be only slightly elevated in patients with pituitary-dependent Cushing's, and grossly elevated concentrations do not always occur with ectopic secretion of ACTH. Further biochemical investigations used to elucidate the cause of Cushing's syndrome include the high-dose dexamethasone suppression test and the corticotropin-releasing hormone test. The former involves giving 2 mg dexamethasone 6-hourly for 48 hours; plasma cortisol concentration is measured at 09:00 h on the morning following the last dose. In Cushing's disease, the cortisol concentration characteristically decreases to <50% of the pretreatment value. Failure of suppression suggests ectopic ACTH secretion or an adrenal tumor. Exceptions to these typical results occur frequently. Many patients with ectopic ACTH secretion have a characteristic clinical presentation, with weight loss, severe muscle weakness, pigmentation, hypertension, hypokalemic alkalosis and diabetes, but without the classic somatic manifestations of Cushing's disease. In other cases, however (particularly when due to carcinoid tumors), ectopic ACTH secretion may produce a clinical syndrome that is clinically and biochemically identical to Cushing's disease. Imaging techniques, e.g. chest X-ray and pituitary and abdominal computerized tomography (CT) scanning, may reveal a tumor, while selective venous blood sampling for ACTH measurement, to locate the source of ACTH secretion, can also be helpful.

The CRH test can be useful to differentiate between Cushing's disease and ectopic ACTH secretion. In Cushing's disease, CRH (100 µg, IV) typically increases plasma ACTH concentration by 50% over baseline after 60 min, and cortisol concentration by 20%, whereas with ectopic ACTH secretion or an adrenal tumor there is typically no response.

Treatment

Initially, the patient's general condition should be supported by high protein intake and appropriate administration of K. If clinical manifestations are severe, it may be reasonable to block corticosteroid secretion with metyrapone 250 mg to 1 g by mouth three times a day or ketoconazole 400 mg by mouth once a day, increasing to a maximum of 400 mg 3 times a day. Ketoconazole is slower in onset, sometimes hepatotoxic, and its current availability is uncertain.

Pituitary tumors that produce excessive ACTH are removed surgically or extirpated with radiation therapy. If no tumor is shown on imaging but a pituitary source is likely, total hypophysectomy may be attempted, particularly in older patients. Younger patients usually receive supervoltage irradiation of the pituitary, delivering 45 Gy. Improvement usually occurs in <1 year. However, in children, irradiation may reduce secretion of growth hormone and occasionally cause precocious puberty. In special centers, heavy particle beam irradiation, providing about 100 Gy, is often successful, as is a single focused beam of radiation therapy given as a single dose (radiosurgery). Response to irradiation occasionally requires several years, but response is more rapid in children.

Studies suggest that mild cases of persistent or recurrent disease may benefit from the somatostatin analog pasireotide. However, hyperglycemia is a significant adverse effect. The dopamine agonist cabergoline may also occasionally be useful.

Bilateral adrenalectomy is reserved for patients with pituitary hyperadrenocorticism who do not respond to both pituitary exploration (with possible adenomectomy) and irradiation. Adrenalectomy requires life-long corticosteroid replacement.

Adrenocortical tumors are removed surgically. Patients must receive cortisol during the surgical and postoperative periods because their nontumorous adrenal cortex will be atrophic and suppressed. Benign adenomas can be removed laparoscopically. With multinodular adrenal hyperplasia, bilateral adrenalectomy may be necessary. Even after a presumed total adrenalectomy, functional regrowth occurs in a few patients.

Ectopic ACTH syndrome is treated by removing the nonpituitary tumor that is producing the ACTH. However, in some cases, the tumor is disseminated and cannot be excised. Adrenal inhibitors, such as metyrapone 500 mg by mouth 3 times a day (and up to a total of 6 g a day) or mitotane 0.5 g by mouth once a day, increasing to a maximum of 3–4 g a day, usually control severe metabolic disturbances (e.g. hypokalemia). When mitotane is used, large doses of hydrocortisone or dexamethasone may be needed. Measures of cortisol production may be unreliable, and severe hypercholesterolemia may develop. Ketoconazole 400–1200 mg by mouth once a day also blocks corticosteroid synthesis, although it may cause liver toxicity and can cause addisonian symptoms. Alternatively, the corticosteroid receptors can be blocked with mifepristone. Mifepristone increases serum cortisol but blocks effects of the corticosteroid. Sometimes ACTH-secreting tumors respond to long-acting somatostatin analogs, although administration for >2 years requires close follow-up, because mild gastritis, gallstones, cholangitis, and malabsorption may develop.

CONN'S SYNDROME

A disorder caused by excessive aldosterone secretion by a benign tumor of one of the adrenal glands. Aldosterone is the most potent mineralocorticoid produced by the adrenals. It causes Na retention and K loss. In the kidneys, aldosterone causes transfer of Na from the lumen of the distal tubule into the tubular cells in exchange for K and hydrogen. The same effect occurs in salivary glands, sweat glands, cells of the intestinal mucosa, and in exchanges between intracellular fluids (ICFs) and ECFs.

Aldosterone secretion is regulated by the renin-angiotensin system and, to a lesser extent, by ACTH. Renin, a proteolytic enzyme, is stored in the juxtaglomerular cells of the kidneys. Reduction in blood volume and flow in the afferent renal arterioles induces secretion of renin. Renin transforms angiotensinogen from the liver to angiotensin I, which is transformed by angiotensin-converting enzyme (ACE) to angiotensin II. Angiotensin II causes secretion of aldosterone and, to a much lesser extent, secretion of cortisol and deoxycorticosterone; it also has pressor activity. Na and water retention resulting from increased aldosterone secretion increases the blood volume and reduces renin secretion.

Primary aldosteronism is caused by an adenoma, usually unilateral, of the glomerulosa cells of the adrenal cortex or, more rarely, by adrenal carcinoma or hyperplasia. Adenomas are extremely rare in children, but the syndrome sometimes occurs in childhood adrenal carcinoma or hyperplasia. In adrenal hyperplasia, which is more common among older men, both adrenals are overactive, and no adenoma is present. The clinical picture can also occur with congenital adrenal hyperplasia from deficiency of 11 β-hydroxylase and the dominantly inherited dexamethasone-suppressible hyperaldosteronism. Hyperplasia as a cause of hyperaldosteronism may be more common than previously recognized but remains an infrequent cause in the presence of hypokalemia.

Symptoms and Signs

Hypernatremia, hypervolemia, and a hypokalemic alkalosis may occur, causing episodic weakness, paresthesias, transient paralysis, and tetany. Diastolic hypertension and hypokalemic nephropathy with polyuria and polydipsia are common. In many cases, the only manifestation is mild to moderate hypertension. Edema is uncommon.

Diagnosis

There should be three stages to the diagnosis of aldosteronism, i.e. screening, diagnosis, and establishment of the cause. Screening involves measuring aldosterone and plasma renin activity in the same sample. The activity of the renin–aldosterone axis is affected by several drugs; although, it has been suggested that the aldosterone–renin ratio is unaffected by hypotensive medication, it can be increased by β-blockers (which decrease renin secretion) and by spironolactone. Hypokalemia should be corrected before measuring the ratio, as it reduces aldosterone secretion. There is, however, no need to standardize posture. The interpretation of results is indicated in Fig. 8.11, this is a sensitive test and can detect early disease in which aldosterone secretion is only slightly increased, but sufficiently to suppress renin production. Unless the results are clearly normal or abnormal, confirmation or exclusion of the diagnosis is most simply made by

Screening for Conn's syndrome using the plasma aldosterone–renin activity ratio		
Ratio	**Interpretation**	**Action**
<800	Diagnosis excluded	Seek other causes
>1000, <2000	Diagnosis possible	Confirmatory tests
>2000	Diagnosis very likely	Establish cause

Fig. 8.11: Screening for Conn's syndrome using the plasma aldosterone–renin activity ratio, assuming that aldosterone is measured in pmol/L and renin activity in pmol/mL/h. Some laboratories now measure renin mass rather than activity, in which case the units for renin and the cut-off values for the ratio will be different

performing a saline infusion test. This involves the infusion of 1.25 L of 0.9% saline over a period of 2 hours; if plasma aldosterone concentration remains >240 pmol/L, the diagnosis is confirmed. Sodium loading increases the amount of sodium reaching the distal renal tubules and should inhibit aldosterone secretion. Caution is required, particularly in the elderly, because of a small risk of provoking cardiac failure. A more elaborate procedure, regarded by some as the definitive investigation, involves a combination of sodium loading and the administration of fludrocortisone over a period of 4 days. There is a risk of provoking profound hypokalemia, and potassium replacement may be required. However, this test requires admission to hospital, whereas the saline infusion test can be done as an outpatient. Because many antihypertensive drugs, e.g. β-blockers and angiotensin-converting enzyme inhibitors, can affect the secretion of aldosterone, it may be necessary to modify a patient's treatment before performing either of these investigations. α-Adrenergic antagonists can usually be given, but the advice of the laboratory should be sought concerning this.

Treatment

Tumors should be removed laparoscopically. After removal of an adenoma, serum K normalizes and BP decreases in all patients; complete normalization of the BP without the need for hypotensive therapy occurs in 50–70% of patients.

Among patients with adrenal hyperplasia, 70% remain hypertensive after bilateral adrenalectomy; thus, surgery is not recommended. Hyperaldosteronism in these patients can usually be controlled by a selective aldosterone blocker, such as spironolactone, starting with 50 mg by mouth once a day and increasing over 1–3 months to a maintenance dose, usually around 100 mg once a day; or by amiloride 5–10 mg by mouth once a day or another K-sparing diuretic. The more specific drug eplerenone 50 mg by mouth once a day to 200 mg by mouth twice a day may be used because, unlike spironolactone, it does not block the androgen receptor; it is the drug of choice for long-term treatment in men. About half of patients with hyperplasia need additional antihypertensive treatment.

CONGENITAL ADRENAL HYPERPLASIA

The term 'congenital adrenal hyperplasia' (CAH) encompasses a group of **inherited metabolic disorders** of adrenal steroid hormone biosynthesis. Their clinical features depend on the position of the defective enzyme in the synthetic pathway, which determines the pattern of hormones and precursors that is produced (see Fig. 8.3).

21-hydroxylase deficiency CAH, accounts for around 90% of all cases of CAH. It is caused by mutation in the gene CYP21; 6p21. The second most common type is due to deficiency of **11β-hydroxylase,** it is caused by mutation in the gene CYP11B1; 8q21 (Fig. 8.12). In these forms, precursors proximal to the enzyme block accumulate and are shunted into adrenal androgens. The consequent excess androgen secretion causes varying degrees of virilization in external genitals of affected female fetuses; no defects are discernible in external genitals of male fetuses.

In some less common forms affecting enzymes other than 21-hydroxylase and 11β-hydroxylase, the enzyme block impairs androgen synthesis [dehydroepiandrosterone (DHEA) or androstenedione]. As a result, virilization of male fetuses is inadequate, but no defect is discernible in female fetuses.

Congenital Adrenal Hyperplasia Caused by 21-hydroxylase Deficiency

21-hydroxylase deficiency causes 90% of all cases of CAH. Disease severity depends on the specific CYP21A2 mutation and degree of enzyme deficiency. The deficiency completely or partially blocks conversion of 17-hydroxyprogesterone to 11-deoxycortisol, a precursor of cortisol, and conversion of progesterone to deoxycorticosterone, a precursor of aldosterone. Because cortisol synthesis is decreased, ACTH levels increase, which stimulates the adrenal cortex, causing accumulation of cortisol precursors (e.g. 17-hydroxyprogesterone) and excessive production of the adrenal androgens DHEA and androstenedione. Aldosterone deficiency can lead to salt wasting, hyponatremia and hyperkalemia.

Classic 21-hydroxylase Deficiency

Classic 21-hydroxylase deficiency can be divided into 2 forms:

The **salt-wasting form** is the most severe and accounts for 70% of classic 21-hydroxylase deficiency cases; there is complete deficiency of enzyme activity that leads to

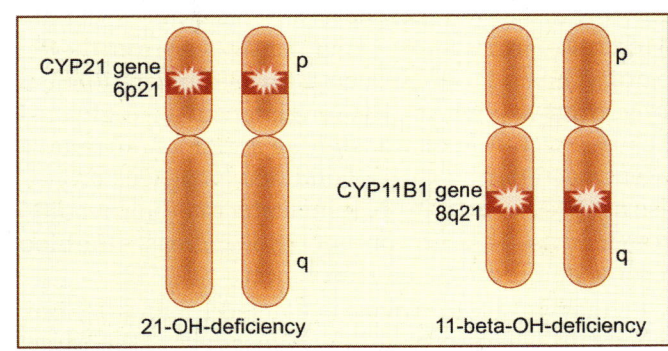

Fig. 8.12: Congenital adrenal hyperplasia classification

very low levels of cortisol and aldosterone. Because minimal aldosterone is secreted, salt is lost, leading to hyponatremia, hyperkalemia, and increased plasma renin activity.

In the **simple virilizing form,** cortisol synthesis is impaired, leading to increased androgen activity, but there is sufficient enzyme activity to maintain normal, or only slightly decreased, aldosterone production.

Nonclassic 21-hydroxylase Deficiency

Nonclassic 21-hydroxylase deficiency is more common than classic 21-hydroxylase deficiency. Incidence ranges from 1/1000–1/2000 live births in white populations (0.1–0.2% prevalence) to 1–2% in certain ethnic groups (e.g. Ashkenazi Jews). Nonclassic 21-hydroxylase deficiency causes a less severe form of the disorder in which there is 20–50% of 21-hydroxylase activity (compared to 0–5% activity in classic 21-hydroxylase deficiency). Salt wasting is absent because aldosterone and cortisol levels are normal, however, adrenal androgen levels are slightly elevated, resulting in mild androgen excess in childhood or adulthood.

Symptoms and Signs

The salt-wasting form causes hyponatremia (sometimes severe), hyperkalemia, and hypotension as well as virilization. If undiagnosed and untreated, this form can lead to life-threatening adrenal crisis, with vomiting, diarrhea, hypoglycemia, hypovolemia, and shock.

With either form of classic 21-hydroxylase deficiency, female neonates have ambiguous external genitals, with clitoral enlargement, fusion of the labia majora, and a urogenital sinus rather than distinct urethral and vaginal openings (Fig. 8.13). Male infants typically have normal genital development, which can delay the diagnosis of the salt-wasting form; affected boys are often identified only through routine newborn screening. Unless detected by newborn screening, boys with the simple virilized form may not be diagnosed for several years, when they develop signs of androgen excess. Signs of androgen excess may include early appearance of pubic hair and increase in growth velocity in both sexes, clitoral enlargement in girls, and penile enlargement and earlier deepening of voice in boys.

Children with nonclassic 21-hydroxylase deficiency do not have symptoms at birth and usually do not present until childhood or adolescence. Affected females may have early pubic hair development, advanced bone age, hirsutism, oligomenorrhea, and/or acne; these symptoms may resemble the manifestations of polycystic ovary syndrome. Affected males may have early pubic hair development, growth acceleration, and advanced bone age.

In affected females, especially those with the salt-wasting form, reproductive function may be impaired as they reach adulthood; they may have labial fusion and anovulatory cycles or amenorrhea. Some males with the salt-wasting form are fertile as adults, but others may develop testicular adrenal rest tumors (benign intratesticular masses composed of adrenal tissue that hypertrophies under chronic ACTH stimulation), Leydig cell dysfunction, decreased testosterone, and impaired spermatogenesis. Most affected males with the non–salt-wasting form, even if untreated, are fertile, but in some, spermatogenesis is impaired.

Diagnosis

Routine newborn screening typically includes measuring serum levels of 17-hydroxyprogesterone. If levels are elevated, the diagnosis is confirmed by identifying low blood levels of cortisol and by identifying high blood levels of DHEA, androstenedione, and testosterone. Rarely, the diagnosis is uncertain, and levels of these hormones must be measured before and 60 minutes after ACTH is given (ACTH or cosyntropin stimulation test). In patients who develop symptoms later, ACTH stimulation testing may help, but genotyping may be required.

Children with the salt-wasting form have hyponatremia and hyperkalemia; low levels of deoxycorticosterone, corticosterone, and aldosterone; and high levels of renin.

Prenatal screening and diagnosis (and experimental treatment) are possible; CYP21 genes are analyzed if risk is high (e.g. the fetus has an affected sibling with the genetic defect). Carrier status (heterozygosity) can be determined in children and adults.

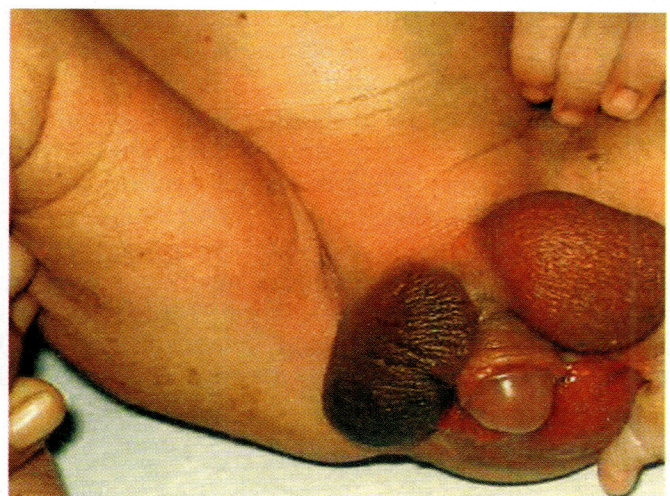

Fig. 8.13: Ambiguous external genital of CAH female neonate

Treatment

For **adrenal crisis** in infants, urgent therapy with IV fluids is needed. Stress doses of hydrocortisone ($100\,mg/m^2/day$) are given by continuous IV infusion to prevent adrenal crisis if the salt-wasting form is suspected; the dose is reduced over several weeks to a more physiologic replacement dose.

Maintenance treatment is corticosteroids as replacement for deficient steroids (typically, oral hydrocortisone $3.5–5\,mg/m^2$ 3 times a day, with total daily dose typically $\leq 20\,mg/m^2$). Postpubertal adolescents and adults may be treated with prednisone 5–7.5 mg by mouth once a day or 2.5–3.75 mg twice a day, or dexamethasone 0.25–0.5 mg once a day or 0.125–0.25 mg twice a day. Cortisone acetate $18–36\,mg/m^2$ IM q 3 days may be used in infants when oral therapy is unreliable.

Response to therapy is monitored in infants every 3 months and in children aged >12 months every 3 to 4 months. Overtreatment with a corticosteroid results in iatrogenic Cushing's syndrome, causing obesity, subnormal growth, and delayed skeletal maturation. Undertreatment results in inability to suppress ACTH with consequent hyperandrogenism, causing virilization and supranormal growth velocity in children and, eventually, premature termination of growth and short stature. Monitoring involves measuring serum 17-hydroxyprogesterone and androstenedione as well as assessing growth velocity and skeletal maturation each year.

Maintenance treatment for the salt-wasting form, in addition to corticosteroids, is mineralocorticoid replacement for restoration of Na and K homeostasis. Oral fludrocortisone (usually 0.1 mg once a day, range 0.05–0.3 mg) is given if salt loss occurs. Infants often require supplemental oral salt for about 1 year. close monitoring during therapy is critical.

Affected female infants may require surgical reconstruction with reduction clitoroplasty and construction of a vaginal opening. Often, further surgery is required during adulthood. With appropriate care and attention to psychosexual issues, a normal sex life and fertility may be expected.

For prenatal treatment, a corticosteroid (usually dexamethasone) is given to the mother to suppress fetal pituitary secretion of ACTH and thus reduce or prevent masculinization of affected female fetuses. Treatment, which is experimental, must begin in the first several weeks of gestation.

Treatment of nonclassic 21-hydroxylase deficiency depends on symptoms. If asymptomatic, no treatment is required. If symptomatic, corticosteroid treatment is similar to classic 21-hydroxylase deficiency, but lower doses are often effective. Mineralocorticoid replacement is not needed.

Congenital Adrenal Hyperplasia Caused by 11β-hydroxylase Deficiency

11β-hydroxylase deficiency causes about 5–8% of all cases of congenital adrenal hyperplasia, conversion of 11-deoxycortisol to cortisol and deoxycorticosterone to corticosterone is partially blocked, leading to

- Increased levels of ACTH
- Accumulation of 11-deoxycortisol (which has limited biological activity) and deoxycorticosterone (which has mineralocorticoid activity)
- Overproduction of adrenal androgens (DHEA, androstenedione, and testosterone)

Symptoms and Signs

Female neonates may present with genital ambiguity, including clitoral enlargement, labial fusion, and a urogenital sinus. Male neonates usually appear normal, but some present with penile enlargement. Some children present later, with sexual precocity or, in females, menstrual irregularities and hirsutism. Salt retention with hypernatremia, hypertension, and hypokalemic alkalosis may result from increased mineralocorticoid activity due to increased deoxycorticosterone levels.

Diagnosis

Prenatal diagnosis is not available. Diagnosis in neonates is established by increased plasma levels of 11-deoxycortisol and adrenal androgens (DHEA, androstenedione, and testosterone). Plasma renin activity is often suppressed because of increased mineralocorticoid activity; this test may be useful in older children but is less reliable in neonates. If the diagnosis is uncertain, levels of 11-deoxycortisol and adrenal androgens are measured before and 60 minutes after ACTH stimulation. In affected adolescents, basal plasma levels may be normal, so ACTH stimulation is recommended.

Hypertension occurs in about two-thirds of patients with CYP11B1 deficiency, and distinguishes it from CYP21A2-deficiency, which causes hypotension. Because both CYP11B1 deficiency and CYP21A2 deficiency can cause increased levels of 17-hydroxyprogesterone, which is measured during routine newborn screening, patients with mild to moderately increased levels of 17-hydroxyprogesterone should have 11-deoxycortisol levels measured. Hypokalemia may occur but not in all patients.

Treatment

Treatment is cortisol replacement, typically with hydrocortisone $3.5–5\,mg/m^2$ 3 times a day, with total daily dose typically ≤ 20 mg/m^2, which prevents further virilization and ameliorates hypertension by reducing levels of 11-deoxycortisol, deoxycorticosterone, and adrenal androgens that are stimulated by ACTH. Unlike CYP21A2 deficiency, mineralocorticoid replacement is not required, because Na and K homeostasis is maintained from mineralocorticoid effects of deoxycorticosterone.

Response to treatment should be monitored, typically by measuring serum 11-deoxycortisol and adrenal androgens and by assessing growth velocity and skeletal maturation. BP should be monitored closely in patients who presented with hypertension. Antihypertensives, such as K-sparing diuretics or Ca channel blockers, may be required.

Affected female infants may require surgical reconstruction with reduction clitoroplasty and construction of a vaginal opening. Often, further surgery is required in adulthood, but with appropriate care and attention to psychosexual issues, a normal sex life and fertility may be expected.

DISORDERS OF THE ADRENAL MEDULLA

The main interest in the adrenal medulla for clinical biochemistry relates to pheochromocytoma. These are tumors that secrete catecholamines, the normal secretory product of the organ, and which are a rare (approximately 0.5% of all cases), but treatable, cause of hypertension. Approximately 10% of pheochromocytoma are found in extramedullary tissue that shares the same embryological origin (i.e. chromaffin tissue derived from neuroectoderm). Catecholamines can also be produced by tumors of embryologically related tissue, e.g. the carotid bodies, and by neuroblastomas, which are rare tumors occurring only in infants and young children and usually presenting as a rapidly enlarging abdominal mass.

PHEOCHROMOCYTOMA

The catecholamines secreted include norepinephrine, epinephrine, dopamine and dopa in varying proportions. About 90% of pheochromocytomas are in the adrenal medulla, but they may also be located in other tissues derived from neural crest cells.

Pheochromocytomas in the adrenal medulla occur equally in both sexes, are bilateral in 10% of cases (20% in children), and are malignant in <10%. Of extra-adrenal tumors, 30% are malignant. Although, pheochromocytomas occur at any age, peak incidence is between the 20s and 40s. About 25–30% are now thought to be due to germline mutations.

Pheochromocytomas vary in size but average 5–6 cm in diameter. They weigh 50–200 g, but tumors weighing several kilograms have been reported. Rarely, they are large enough to be palpated or cause symptoms due to pressure or obstruction. Regardless of the histologic appearance, the tumor is considered benign if it has not invaded the capsule and no metastases are found, although exceptions occur. In general, larger tumors are more likely to be malignant.

Pheochromocytomas may be part of the syndrome of familial multiple endocrine neoplasia (MEN) types 2A and 2B, in which other endocrine tumors (parathyroid or medullary carcinoma of the thyroid) coexist or develop subsequently. Pheochromocytoma develops in 1% of patients with neurofibromatosis (von Recklinghausen disease) and may occur with hemangioblastomas and renal cell carcinoma, as in von Hippel-Lindau disease. Familial pheochromocytomas and carotid body tumors may be due to mutations of the enzyme succinate dehydrogenase as well as of the genes responsible for other more recently described signaling molecules.

Symptoms and Signs

Hypertension, which is paroxysmal in 45% of patients, is prominent. About 1/1000 hypertensive patients has a pheochromocytoma. Common symptoms and signs are tachycardia, diaphoresis, postural hypotension, tachypnea, cold and clammy skin, severe headache, angina, palpitations, nausea, vomiting, epigastric pain, visual disturbances, dyspnea, paresthesias, constipation, and a sense of impending doom. Paroxysmal attacks may be provoked by palpation of the tumor, postural changes, abdominal compression or massage, induction of anesthesia, emotional trauma, unopposed β-blockade (which paradoxically increases BP by blocking β-mediated vasodilation), or micturition (if the tumor is in the bladder). In elderly patients, severe weight loss with persistent hypertension is suggestive of pheochromocytoma.

Physical examination, except for the presence of hypertension, is usually normal unless done during a paroxysmal attack. Retinopathy and cardiomegaly are often less severe than might be expected for the degree of hypertension, but a specific catecholamine cardiomyopathy can occur.

Diagnosis

Pheochromocytoma is suspected in patients with typical symptoms or particularly sudden, severe, or intermittent unexplained hypertension. Diagnosis involves demonstrating high levels of catecholamine products in the serum or urine.

Blood Tests

Plasma free metanephrine is up to 99% sensitive. This test has superior sensitivity to measurement of circulating epinephrine and norepinephrine because plasma metanephrines are elevated continuously, unlike epinephrine and norepinephrine , which are secreted intermittently

Urine Tests

Urinary metanephrine is less specific than plasma free metanephrine, but sensitivity is about 95%. Two or 3 normal results while the patient is hypertensive render the diagnosis extremely unlikely. Measurement of urinary norepinephrine and epinephrine is nearly as accurate. The principal urinary metabolic products of epinephrine and norepinephrine are the metanephrines vanillylmandelic acid (VMA) and homovanillic acid (HVA). Healthy people excrete only very small amounts of these substances. Normal values for 24 hours are as Table 8.2.

In pheochromocytoma, increased urinary excretion of epinephrine and norepinephrine and their metabolic products is intermittent. Elevated excretion of these compounds may also occur in other disorders (e.g. neuroblastoma, coma, dehydration, sleep apnea) or extreme stress; in patients being treated with rauwolfia alkaloids, methyldopa, or catecholamines; or after ingestion of foods containing large quantities of vanilla (especially if renal insufficiency is present).

Other Tests

Blood volume is constricted and may falsely elevate Hb and hematocrit (Hct) levels. Hyperglycemia, glycosuria, or overt diabetes mellitus may be present, with elevated fasting levels of plasma free fatty acid and glycerol. Plasma insulin level is inappropriately low for the plasma glucose. After removal of the pheochromocytoma, hypoglycemia may occur, especially in patients treated with oral antihyperglycemics.

Provocative tests with histamine or tyramine are hazardous and should not be used. Glucagon 0.5 to 1 mg injected rapidly IV provokes a rise in BP of >35/25 mm Hg within 2 minutes in normotensive patients with Pheochromocytoma but is now generally unnecessary. Phentolamine mesylate must be available to terminate any hypertensive crisis.

Screening Tests

Screening tests are preferred to provocative tests. The general approach is to measure plasma metanephrines,

Table 8.2	Normal values epinephrine and norepinephrine, VMA and HVA
Free epinephrine and norepinephrine <582 nmol	
Total metanephrine <7.1 µmol	
VMA <50 µmol	
HVA <82.4 µmol	

24 hours urinary catecholamines, or their metabolites as a screening test and to avoid provocative tests. In patients with elevated plasma catecholamines, a suppression test using oral clonidine or IV pentolinium can be used but is rarely necessary.

IMAGING TESTS TO LOCALIZE TUMORS

Imaging tests to localize tumors are usually done in patients with abnormal screening results. Tests should include CT and MRI of the chest and abdomen with and without contrast. With isotonic contrast media, no adrenoceptor blockade is necessary. Fluorodeoxyglucose-positron emission tomography (FDG-PET) has also been used successfully.

Repeated sampling of plasma catecholamine concentrations during catheterization of the vena cava with sampling at different locations, including the adrenal veins, can help localize the tumor; there will be a step up in norepinephrine level in a vein draining the tumor. Adrenal vein norepinephrine–epinephrine ratios may help in the hunt for a small adrenal source.

Radiopharmaceuticals with nuclear imaging techniques can also help localize pheochromocytomas.

Treatment

Surgical removal is the treatment of choice. The operation is usually delayed until hypertension is controlled by a combination of α-blockers and β-blockers (usually phenoxybenzamine 20–40 mg by mouth 3 times a day and propranolol 20–40 mg by mouth 3 times a day). β-blockers should not be used until adequate α-blockade has been achieved. Some β-blockers, such as doxazosin, may be equally effective but better tolerated.

The most effective and safest preoperative α-blockade is phenoxybenzamine 0.5 mg/kg IV in 0.9% saline over 2 hours on each of the 3 days before the operation. Nitroprusside can be infused for hypertensive crises preoperatively or intraoperatively. When bilateral tumors are documented or suspected (as in a patient with MEN), sufficient hydrocortisone (100 mg IV twice a day) given before and during surgery avoids acute glucocorticoid insufficiency due to bilateral adrenalectomy.

Most pheochromocytomas can be removed laparoscopically. BP must be continuously monitored via an intra-arterial catheter procedure, and volume status is closely monitored. Anesthesia should be induced with a nonarrhythmogenic drug (e.g. a thiobarbiturate) and continued with enflurane. During surgery, paroxysms of hypertension should be controlled with injections of phentolamine 1–5 mg IV or nitroprusside infusion (2–4 µg/kg/min), and tachyarrhythmias should be controlled with propranolol 0.5–2 mg IV. If a muscle relaxant is needed, drugs that do not release histamine are preferred. Atropine should not be used preoperatively.

Preoperative blood transfusion (1–2 units) may be given before the tumor is removed in anticipation of blood loss. If BP has been well controlled before surgery, a diet high in salt is recommended to increase blood volume. An infusion of norepinephrine 4–12 mg/L in a dextrose-containing solution should be started if hypotension develops. Some patients whose hypotension responds poorly to levarterenol may benefit from hydrocortisone 100 mg IV, but adequate fluid replacement is usually all that is required.

Malignant metastatic pheochromocytoma should be treated with α-blockers and β-blockers. The tumor may be indolent and survival longlasting. However, even with rapid tumor growth, BP can be controlled. Iobenguane-metaiodobenzylguanidine (I-MIBG) can help relieve symptoms in patients with residual disease. Radiation therapy may reduce bone pain. Chemotherapy is rarely effective, but the most common regimen tried is the combination of cyclophosphamide, vincristine, and dacarbazine. Recent data have shown some promising results with the chemotherapy agent temozolomide.

BIBLIOGRAPHY

1. Acton S, Rigotti A, Landschulz KT, et al. Identification of scavenger receptor SR-BI as a high density lipoprotein receptor. Science 1996; 271:518.
2. Addison T. On the Constitutional and Local Effects of Disease of the Supra-renal Capsules. London, UK: Samuel Highley; 1855.
3. Babu K, Murthy KR, Babu N, et al. Triple A syndrome with ophthalmic manifestations in two siblings. Indian J Ophthalmol. 2007 Jul-Aug. 55(4): 304–6.
4. Babu PS, Bavers DL, Beuschlein F, et al. Interaction between Dax-1 and steroidogenic factor-1 in vivo: increased adrenal responsiveness to ACTH in the absence of Dax-1. Endocrinology 2002; 143:665.
5. Baker BY, Lin L, Kim CJ, et al. Nonclassic congenital lipoid adrenal hyperplasia: a new disorder of the steroidogenic acute regulatory protein with very late presentation and normal male genitalia. J ClinEndocrinolMetab. 2006 Dec. 91(12): 4781–5.
6. Barnett AH, Donald RA, Espiner EA. High concentrations of thyroid-stimulating hormone in untreated glucocorticoid deficiency: indication of primary hypothyroidism?. Br Med J (Clin Res Ed). 1982 Jul 17. 285(6336): 172–3.
7. Barnett AH, Espiner EA, Donald RA. Patients presenting with Addison's disease need not be pigmented.Postgrad Med J. 1982 Nov. 58(685): 690–2.
8. Bergthorsdottir R, Leonsson-Zachrisson M, Oden A, et al. Premature mortality in patients with Addison's disease: a population-based study. J ClinEndocrinolMetab. 2006 Dec. 91(12):4849–53.
9. Bethune JE. The diagnosis and treatment of adrenal insufficiency. In: De Groot LJ, ed. Endocrinology. 2nd ed. Philadelphia, Pa: WB Saunders; 1989. Vol 2: 1647–59.
10. Bethune JE. The Adrenal cortex: a scope monograph. Kalamazoo, Mich: Upjohn Co; 1974.
11. Betterle C, Lazzarotto F, Spadaccino AC, et al. Celiac disease in North Italian patients with autoimmune Addison's disease. Eur J Endocrinol. 2006 Feb. 154(2): 275–9.
12. Biagi F, Campanella J, Soriani A, et al. Prevalence of coeliac disease in Italian patients affected by Addison's disease. Scand J Gastroenterol. 2006 Mar. 41(3): 302–5.
13. Biason-Lauber A, Schoenle EJ. Apparently normal ovarian differentiation in a prepubertal girl with transcriptionally inactive steroidogenic factor 1 (NR5A1/SF-1) and adrenocortical insufficiency. Am J Hum Genet 2000; 67:1563.
14. Bolté, E, Coudert, S, Lefebvre, Y. Steroid production from plasma cholesterol. II. In vivo conversion of plasma cholesterol to ovarian progesterone and adrenal C19 and C21 steroids in humans. J Clin Endocrinol Metab 1967; 38:394.
15. Borkowski AJ, Levin S, Delcroix C, et al. Blood cholesterol and hydrocortisone production in man: quantitative aspects of the utilization of circulating cholesterol by the adrenals at rest and under adrenocorticotropin stimulation. J Clin Invest 1967; 46:797.
16. Boulpaep, Emile L.; Boron, Walter F. (2003). Medical physiology: a cellular and molecular approach. Philadelphia: Saunders. p. 1065. ISBN 0-7216-3256-4.
17. Burke CW. Adrenocortical insufficiency. Clin Endocrinol Metab. 1985 Nov. 14(4):947-76.
18. Cao G, Zhao L, Stangl H, et al. Developmental and hormonal regulation of murine scavenger receptor, class B, type 1. Mol Endocrinol 1999; 13:1460.
19. Charmandari E, Nicolaides NC, Chrousos GP. Adrenal insufficiency. Lancet. 2014 Jun 21. 383 (9935): 2152–67.
20. Christiansen JJ, Djurhuus CB, Gravholt CH, et al. Effects of cortisol on carbohydrate, lipid, and protein metabolism: studies of acute cortisol withdrawal in adrenocortical failure. J Clin Endocrinol Metab. 2007 Sep. 92(9): 3553–9.
21. Chu JW, Kimura T. Studies on adrenal steroid hydroxylases. Molecular and catalytic properties of adrenodoxin reductase (a flavoprotein). J Biol Chem 1973; 248:2089.
22. Chua SC, Szabo P, Vitek A, et al. Cloning of cDNA encoding steroid 11 beta-hydroxylase (P450c11). Proc Natl Acad Sci U S A 1987; 84:7193.
23. Chung BC, Matteson KJ, Voutilainen R, et al. Human cholesterol side-chain cleavage enzyme, P450scc: cDNA cloning, assignment of the gene to chromosome 15, and expression in the placenta. ProcNatlAcadSci U S A 1986; 83:8962.
24. Clark AJ, Metherell LA, Cheetham ME, Huebner A. Inherited ACTH insensitivity illuminates the mechanisms of ACTH action. Trends Endocrinol Metab 2005; 16:451.
25. Clark BJ, Ranganathan V, Combs R. Steroidogenic acute regulatory protein expression is dependent upon post-translational effects of cAMP-dependent protein kinase A. Mol Cell Endocrinol 2001; 173:183.
26. Coco G, Dal Pra C, Presotto F, et al. Estimated risk for developing autoimmune Addison's disease in patients with

adrenal cortex autoantibodies. J Clin Endocrinol Metab. 2006 May. 91(5): 1637–45.

27. Cone RD, Mountjoy KG. Molecular genetics of the ACTH and melanocyte-stimulating hormone receptors. Trends Endocrinol Metab 1993; 4:242.

28. Cotesta, D; Caliumi, C; Alò, P; Petramala, L; Reale, MG; Masciangelo, R; Signore, A; Cianci, R; et al. (2005). "High plasma levels of human chromogranin A and adrenomedullin in patients with pheochromocytoma". Tumori 91(1): 53–8. PMID 15850005.

29. Dackis CA, Gurpegui M, Pottash AL, et al. Methadone induced hypoadrenalism. Lancet. 1982 Nov 20. 2(8308):1167.

30. Debono M, Ross RJ. Doses and steroids to be used in primary and central hypoadrenalism. Ann Endocrinol (Paris). 2007 Sep. 68(4): 265–7.

31. Demers LM, Whitley RJ. Function of the adrenal cortex: protocol for the rapid ACTH test. In: Burtis CA, Ashwood ER, eds. Tietz Textbook of Clinical Chemistry. 3rd ed. Philadelphia, Pa: WB Saunders; 1999. Vol 43: 1530–60.

32. Dias RP, Chan LF, Metherell LA, et al. Isolated Addison's disease is unlikely to be caused by mutations in MC2R, MRAP or STAR, three genes responsible for familial glucocorticoid deficiency. Eur J Endocrinol. 2010 Feb. 162(2): 357–9.

33. Dickerman Z, Grant DR, Faiman C, Winter JS. Intraadrenal steroid concentrations in man: zonal differences and developmental changes. J Clin Endocrinol Metab 1984; 59:1031.

34. Dickstein G, Shechner C, Nicholson WE, et al. Adreno-corticotropin stimulation test: effects of basal cortisol level, time of day, and suggested new sensitive low dose test. J Clin Endocrinol Metab. 1991 Apr. 72(4): 773–8.

35. Diouf, B.; FaryKa, E. H.; Calender, A.; Giraud, S.; Diop, T. M. (2000). "Association of medullary sponge kidney disease and multiple endocrine neoplasia type IIA due to RET gene mutation: is there a causal relationship?". Nephrology Dialysis Transplantation 15(12): 2062–3. doi:10.1093/ndt/15.12.2062.

36. Dluhy RG, Himathongkam T, Greenfield M. Rapid ACTH test with plasma aldosterone levels. Improved diagnostic discrimination. Ann Intern Med. 1974 Jun. 80(6): 693–6.

37. Donckier JE, Lacrosse M, Michel L. Bilateral adrenal lymphoma with Addison's disease : a surgical pitfall. Acta Chir Belg. 2007 Mar-Apr. 107(2): 219–21.

38. Eisenbarth GS, Wilson PW, Ward F, et al. The polyglandular failure syndrome: disease inheritance, HLA type, and immune function. Ann Intern Med. 1979 Oct. 91(4): 528–33.

39. Elansary EH, Earis JE. Rifampicin and adrenal crisis. Br Med J (Clin Res Ed). 1983 Jun 11. 286(6381): 1861–2.

40. Elfstrom P, Montgomery SM, Kampe O, et al. Risk of primary adrenal insufficiency in patients with celiac disease. J Clin Endocrinol Metab. 2007 Sep. 92(9): 3595–8.

41. Endoh A, Kristiansen SB, Casson PR, et al. The zona reticularis is the site of biosynthesis of dehydroepiandrosterone and dehydroepiandrosterone sulfate in the adult human adrenal cortex resulting from its low expression of 3 beta-hydroxysteroid dehydrogenase. J Clin Endocrinol Metab 1996; 81:3558.

42. Faust JR, Goldstein JL, Brown MS. Receptor-mediated uptake of low density lipoprotein and utilization of its cholesterol for steroid synthesis in cultured mouse adrenal cells. J BiolChem 1977; 252:4861.

43. Gharib H, Hodgson SF, Gastineau CF, et al. Reversible hypothyroidism in Addison's disease. Lancet. 1972 Oct 7. 2(7780): 734–6.

44. Giannini, A. James; Black, Henry R.; Goettsche, Roger L. (1978). Psychiatric, Psychogenic and Somatopsychic Disorders Handbook. Garden City, NY: Medical Examination. pp. 213–4. ISBN 0-87488-596-5.

45. Glasgow BJ, Steinsapir KD, Anders K, et al. Adrenal pathology in the acquired immune deficiency syndrome. Am J Clin Pathol. 1985 Nov. 84(5): 594–7.

46. Goldstein JL, Anderson RG, Brown MS. Coated pits, coated vesicles, and receptor-mediated endocytosis. Nature 1979; 279:679.

47. Gombos Z, Hermann R, Kiviniemi M, et al. Analysis of extended human leukocyte antigen haplotype association with Addison's disease in three populations. Eur J Endocrinol. 2007 Dec. 157(6): 757–61.

48. Gordon WH, Dluhy RG. Diseases of the adrenal cortex. In: Fauci A, Brunwald E, Martin JB, et al, eds. Harrison's Principles of Internal Medicine. 14th ed. New York, NY: μgraw-Hill; 1998. Vol 332: 2035–54.

49. Greene LA, Tischler AS; Tischler (1976). "Establishment of a noradrenergic clonal line of rat adrenal pheochromocytoma cells which respond to nerve growth factor". Proc. Natl. Acad. Sci. U.S.A 73 (7): 2424–8.

50. Greene LW, Cole W, Greene JB, et al. Adrenal insufficiency as a complication of the acquired immunodeficiency syndrome. Ann Intern Med. 1984 Oct. 101(4): 497–8.

51. Guo YK, Yang ZG, Li Y, et al. Addison's disease due to adrenal tuberculosis: contrast-enhanced CT features and clinical duration correlation. Eur J Radiol. 2007 Apr. 62(1):126-31.

52. Gwynne JT, Strauss JF 3rd. The role of lipoproteins in steroidogenesis and cholesterol metabolism in steroidogenic glands. Endocr Rev 1982; 3:299.

53. Hamrahian AH, Oseni TS, Arafah BM. Measurements of serum free cortisol in critically ill patients. N Engl J Med. 2004 Apr 15. 350(16): 1629–38.

54. Hemminki K, Li X, Sundquist J, et al. Subsequent autoimmune or related disease in asthma patients: clustering of diseases or medical care?. Ann Epidemiol. 2010 Mar. 20(3): 217–22.

55. Husebye E, Lovas K. Pathogenesis of primary adrenal insufficiency. Best Pract Res Clin Endocrinol Metab. 2009 Apr. 23(2): 147–57.

56. Husebye ES, Bratland E, Bredholt G, et al. The substrate-binding domain of 21-hydroxylase, the main autoantigen in autoimmune Addison's disease, is an immunodominant T cell epitope. Endocrinology. 2006 May. 147(5): 2411–6.

57. Illingworth DR, Kenny TA, Orwoll ES. Adrenal function in heterozygous and homozygous hypobetalipoproteinemia. J Clin Endocrinol Metab 1982; 54:27.

58. Illingworth DR, Lees AM, Lees RS. Adrenal cortical function in homozygous familial hypercholesterolemia. Metabolism 1983; 32:1045.

59. Imachi H, Murao K, Sato M, et al. CD36 LIMPII analogous-1, a human homolog of the rodent scavenger receptor B1, provides the cholesterol ester for steroidogenesis in adrenocortical cells. Metabolism 1999; 48:627.

60. Jaroszewski, D. E.; Tessier, D. J.; Schlinkert, R. T.; Grant, C. S.; Thompson, G. B.; Van Heerden, J. A.; Farley, D. R.; Smith, S. L.; Hinder, R. A. (2003). "Laparoscopic Adrenalectomy for Pheochromocytoma". Mayo Clinic Proceedings 78 (12): 1501–4.

61. John ME, John MC, Simpson ER, Waterman MR. Regulation of cytochrome P-45011 beta gene expression by adrenocorticotropin. J Biol Chem 1985; 260:5760.

62. Kaplan NM. The adrenal glands. In: Griffin JE, Ojeda S, eds. Textbook of Endocrine Physiology. 3rd ed. Oxford, UK: Oxford University Press; 1996. 284–313.

63. Kasperlik-Zaluska AA, Migdalska B, Czarnocka B, Drac-Kaniewska J, Niegowska E, Czech W. Association of Addison's disease with autoimmune disorders—a long-term observation of 180 patients. Postgrad Med J. 1991 Nov. 67(793): 984–7.

64. Kimura T, Suzuki K. Components of the electron transport system in adrenal steroid hydroxylase. Isolation and properties of non-heme iron protein (adrenodoxin). J BiolChem 1967; 242:485.

65. Kominami S, Hara H, Ogishima T, Takemori S. Interaction between cytochrome P-450 (P-450C21) and NADPH-cytochrome P-450 reductase from adrenocortical microsomes in a reconstituted system. J BiolChem 1984; 259:2991.

66. Kominami S, Ochi H, Kobayashi Y, Takemori S. Studies on the steroid hydroxylation system in adrenal cortex microsomes. Purification and characterization of cytochrome P-450 specific for steroid C-21 hydroxylation. J Biol Chem 1980; 255:3386.

67. Kramer RE, Anderson CM, Peterson JA, et al. Adrenodoxin biosynthesis by bovine adrenal cells in monolayer culture. Induction by adrenocorticotropin. J BiolChem 1982; 257:14921.

68. Kramer RE, Simpson ER, Waterman MR. Induction of 11 beta-hydroxylase by corticotropin in primary cultures of bovine adrenocortical cells. J BiolChem 1983; 258:3000.

69. Kyriazopoulou V, Parparousi O, Vagenakis AG. Rifampicin-induced adrenal crisis in addisonian patients receiving corticosteroid replacement therapy. J ClinEndocrinolMetab. 1984 Dec. 59(6):1204–6.

70. Kyriazopoulou V. Glucocorticoid replacement therapy in patients with Addison's disease. Expert OpinPharmacother. 2007 Apr. 8(6): 725–9.

71. Lever E.G., McKerron CG. Auto-immune Addison's disease associated with hyperprolactinaemia. ClinEndocrinol (Oxf). 1984 Oct. 21(4): 451–7.

72. Likhari T, Magzoub S, Griffiths MJ, et al. Screening for Addison's disease in patients with type 1 diabetes mellitus and recurrent hypoglycaemia. Postgrad Med J. 2007 Jun. 83(980): 420–1.

73. Lin D, Sugawara T, Strauss JF 3rd, et al. Role of steroidogenic acute regulatory protein in adrenal and gonadal steroidogenesis. Science 1995; 267:1828.

74. Lindholm J, Kehlet H. Re-evaluation of the clinical value of the 30 min ACTH test in assessing the hypothalamic-pituitary-adrenocortical function. ClinEndocrinol (Oxf). 1987 Jan. 26(1): 53–9.

75. Lopez D, Shea-Eaton W, Sanchez MD, McLean MP. DAX-1 represses the high-density lipoprotein receptor through interaction with positive regulators sterol regulatory element-binding protein-1a and steroidogenic factor-1. Endocrinology 2001; 142:5097.

76. Lovas K, Gjesdal CG, Christensen M, et al. Glucocorticoid replacement therapy and pharmacogenetics in Addison's disease: effects on bone. Eur J Endocrinol. 2009 Jun. 160(6): 993–1002.

77. Lovas K, Husebye ES. Continuous subcutaneous hydrocortisone infusion in Addison's disease. Eur J Endocrinol. 2007 Jul. 157(1): 109–12.

78. Lovas K, Thorsen TE, Husebye ES. Saliva cortisol measurement: simple and reliable assessment of the glucocorticoid replacement therapy in Addison's disease. J Endocrinol Invest. 2006 Sep. 29(8): 727–31.

79. Ma ES, Yang ZG, Li Y, et al. Tuberculous Addison's disease: morphological and quantitative evaluation with multi-detector-row CT. Eur J Radiol. 2007 Jun. 62(3): 352–8.

80. Magitta NF, Boe Wolff AS, Johansson S, et al. A coding polymorphism in NALP1 confers risk for autoimmune Addison's disease and type 1 diabetes. Genes Immun. 2008 Oct 23.

81. Marx C, Bornstein SR, Wolkersdörfer GW, et al. Relevance of major histocompatibility complex class II expression as a hallmark for the cellular differentiation in the human adrenal cortex. J ClinEndocrinolMetab 1997; 82:3136.

82. Mason AS, Meade TW, Lee JA, et al. Epidemiological and clinical picture of Addison's disease. Lancet. 1968 Oct 5. 2(7571): 744–7.

83. May ME, Carey RM. Rapid adrenocorticotropic hormone test in practice. Retrospective review. Am J Med. 1985 Dec. 79(6): 679–84.

84. McBrien DJ. Steatorrhea in Addison's disease. Lancet. 1963. Vol I:25-6.

85. Meakin JW, Nelson DH, Thorn GW. Addison's disease in two brothers. J Clin Endocrinol Metab. 1959 Jun. 19(6):726-31.

86. Membreno L, Irony I, Dere W, et al. Adrenocortical function in acquired immunodeficiency syndrome. J Clin Endocrinol Metab. 1987 Sep. 65(3): 482–7.

87. Migeon CJ, Kenny EM, Kowarski A, et al. The syndrome of congenital adrenocortical unresponsiveness to ACTH. Report of six cases. Pediatr Res. 1968 Nov. 2(6): 501–13.

88. Miller WL. Molecular biology of steroid hormone synthesis. Endocr Rev 1988; 9:295.

89. Mukherjee S, Newby E, Harvey JN. Adrenomyeloneuropathy in patients with 'Addison's disease': genetic case analysis. J R Soc Med. 2006 May. 99(5): 245–9.

90. Mukhopadhya A, Danda S, Huebner A, et al. Mutations of the AAAS gene in an Indian family with Allgrove's syndrome. World J Gastroenterol. 2006 Aug 7. 12(29): 4764–6.

91. Murao K, Terpstra V, Green SR, et al. Characterization of CLA-1, a human homologue of rodent scavenger receptor BI,

as a receptor for high density lipoprotein and apoptotic thymocytes. J BiolChem 1997; 272:17551.

92. Nieman LK, Chanco Turner ML. Addison's disease. Clin Dermatol. 2006 Jul-Aug. 24(4): 276–80.

93. Norbiato G, Galli M, Righini V, et al. The syndrome of acquired glucocorticoid resistance in HIV infection. Baillieres Clin Endocrinol Metab. 1994 Oct. 8(4): 777–87.

94. Novoselova TV, Jackson D, Campbell DC, et al. Melanocortin receptor accessory proteins in adrenal gland physiology and beyond. J Endocrinol 2013; 217:R1.

95. Oelkers W, Diederich S, Bahr V. Diagnosis and therapy surveillance in Addison's disease: rapid adrenocorticotropin (ACTH) test and measurement of plasma ACTH, renin activity, and aldosterone. J Clin Endocrinol Metab. 1992 Jul. 75(1): 259–64.

96. Pacack, K. (2007). "Preoperative management of the pheochromocytoma patient." J Clin Endocrinol Metab. 92 (11): 4069–79.

97. Papadopoulos V, Baraldi M, Guilarte TR, et al. Translocator protein (18kDa): new nomenclature for the peripheral-type benzodiazepine receptor based on its structure and molecular function. Trends Pharmacol Sci 2006; 27:402.

98. Papadopoulos V, Miller WL. Role of mitochondria in steroidogenesis. Best Pract Res Clin Endocrinol Metab 2012; 26:771.

99. Penhoat A, Lebrethon MC, Bégeot M, Saez JM. Regulation of ACTH receptor mRNA and binding sites by ACTH and angiotensin II in cultured human and bovine adrenal fasciculata cells. Endocr Res 1995; 21:157.

100. Penning TM. Molecular endocrinology of hydroxysteroid dehydrogenases. Endocr Rev 1997; 18:281.

101. Plump AS, Erickson SK, Weng W, et al. Apolipoprotein A-I is required for cholesteryl ester accumulation in steroidogenic cells and for normal adrenal steroid production. J Clin Invest 1996; 97:2660.

102. Pombo M, Devesa J, Taborda A, et al. Glucocorticoid deficiency with achalasia of the cardia and lack of lacrimation. Clin Endocrinol (Oxf). 1985 Sep. 23(3): 237–43.

103. Reisch N, Arlt W. Fine tuning for quality of life: 21st century approach to treatment of Addison's disease. Endocrinol Metab Clin North Am. 2009 Jun. 38(2): 407–18, ix-x.

104. Rigotti A, Trigatti BL, Penman M, et al. A targeted mutation in the murine gene encoding the high density lipoprotein (HDL) receptor scavenger receptor class B type I reveals its key role in HDL metabolism. ProcNatlAcadSci U S A 1997; 94:12610.

105. Rose LI, Williams GH, Jagger PI, et al. The 48-hour adrenocorticotropin infusion test for adrenocortical insufficiency. Ann Intern Med. 1970 Jul. 73(1): 49–54.

106. Roycroft M, Fichna M, Mc Donald D, et al. The tryptophan 620 allele of the lymphoid tyrosine phosphatase (PTPN22 gene) predisposes to autoimmune Addison's disease. ClinEndocrinol (Oxf). 2008.

107. Sekiguchi Y, Hara Y, Matsuoka H, et al. Sibling cases of Addison's disease caused by DAX-1 gene mutations. Intern Med. 2007. 46(1): 35–9.

108. Simpson ER, Waterman MR. Regulation of the synthesis of steroidogenic enzymes in adrenal cortical cells by ACTH. Annu Rev Physiol 1988; 50:427.

109. Sloper JC. The pathology of the adrenals, thymus and certain other endocrine glands in Addison's disease: an analysis of 37 necropsies. Proc R Soc Med. 1955 Aug. 48(8): 625–8.

110. Smith D, McKenna K, Moore K, Tormey W, Finucane J, Phillips J, Baylis P, Thompson CJ (2002). "Baroregulation of vasopressin release in adipsic diabetes insipidus". J. Clin. Endocrinol. Metab. 87 (10): 4564–8.

111. Steffensen, C; Bak, AM; Rubeck, KZ; Jørgensen, JO (2010). "Epidemiology of Cushing's syndrome.". Neuroendocrinology. 92 Suppl 1: 1–5.

112. Stocco DM, Clark BJ. Regulation of the acute production of steroids in steroidogenic cells. Endocr Rev 1996; 17:221.

113. Stuart M, ed. The Encyclopedia of herbs and herbalism. New York: Grosset and Dunlap, 1979: 176, 191, 239, 276–7.

114. Sugawara T, Saito M, Fujimoto S. Sp1 and SF-1 interact and cooperate in the regulation of human steroidogenic acute regulatory protein gene expression. Endocrinology 2000; 141:2895.

115. Sweeney, Ann T; Griffing, George T (August 2, 2011). "Pheochromocytoma". eMedicine.

116. Symington T, ed. Functional Pathology of the Adrenal Gland. Edinburgh, Scotland: Churchill Livingstone; 1969.

117. Taymans SE, Pack S, Pak E, et al. Human CYP11B2 (aldosterone synthase) maps to chromosome 8q24.3. J Clin Endocrinol Metab 1998; 83:1033.

118. Tietz textbook of clinical chemistry and molecular biology 5fifth edition, Philadelphia, W.B Saunders company (2012).

119. Tolis G, Somma M, Van Campenhout J, Friesen H. Prolactin secretion in sixty-five patients with galactorrhea. Am J Obstet Gynecol 1974;118:91-101.

120. Torrejon S, Webb SM, Rodriguez-Espinosa J, et al. Long-lasting subclinical Addison's disease. Exp Clin Endocrinol Diabetes. 2007 Sep. 115(8): 530–2.

121. Trzeciak WH, Simpson ER, Scallen TJ, et al. Studies on the synthesis of sterol carrier protein-2 in rat adrenocortical cells in monolayer culture. Regulation by ACTH and dibutyryl cyclic 3',5'-AMP. J Biol Chem 1987; 262:3713.

122. Turner, H., Wass, J., Oxford Handbook of Endocrinology and Diabetes

123. Turton DB, Shakir KM. Galactorrhea caused by esophagitis. Am J Obstet Gynecol 1995; 173: 1629–30.

124. Van Dellen RG, Purnell DC. Hyperkalemic paralysis in Addison's disease. Mayo Clin Proc. 1969 Dec. 44(12): 904–14.

125. Verhelst J, Abs R, Maiter D, Van den Bruel A, Vandeweghe M, Velkeniers B, et al. Cabergoline in the treatment of hyperprolactinemia: a study in 455 patients. J Clin Endocrinol Metab 1999; 84: 2518–22.

126. Walter M, McDonald CG, Paty BW, et al. Prevalence of autoimmune diseases in islet transplant candidates with severe hypoglycaemia and glycaemiclability: previously undiagnosed coeliac and autoimmune thyroid disease is identified by screening. Diabet Med. 2007 Feb. 24(2): 161–5.

127. Wang XL, Bassett M, Zhang Y, et al. Transcriptional regulation of human 11beta-hydroxylase (hCYP11B1). Endocrinology 2000; 141:3587.

128. Waterhouse R. A case of suprarenal apoplexy. Lancet. 1911. Vol 3:577-8.

129. Waterman MR. A rising StAR: an essential role in cholesterol transport. Science 1995; 267:1780.

130. Wells, M. J.; Wells, J. (1969). "Pituitary Analogue in the Octopus". Nature 222 (5190): 293–294.

131. White K, Arlt W. Adrenal crisis in treated Addison's disease: a predictable but under-managed event. Eur J Endocrinol. 2010 Jan. 162(1): 115–20.

132. White PC, Chaplin DD, Weis JH, et al. Two steroid 21-hydroxylase genes are located in the murine S region. Nature 1984; 312:465.

133. White PC, Curnow KM, Pascoe L. Disorders of steroid 11 beta-hydroxylase isozymes. Endocr Rev 1994; 15:421.

134. White PC, New MI, Dupont B. HLA-linked congenital adrenal hyperplasia results from a defective gene encoding a cytochrome P-450 specific for steroid 21-hydroxylation ProcNatlAcadSci U S A 1984; 81:7505.

135. White PC, Speiser PW. Congenital adrenal hyperplasia due to 21-hydroxylase deficiency. Endocr Rev 2000; 21:245.

136. White PC. Disorders of aldosterone biosynthesis and action. N Engl J Med 1994; 331:250.

137. William Marshall, MártaLapsley, Stephen K Bangert. Elsevier.com: Clinical Chemistry, 7th Edition; ISBN-9780723437031. (2012).

138. Windgassen K, Wesselmann U, Schulze Monking H. Galactorrhea and hyperprolactinemia in schizophrenic patients on neuroleptics: frequency and etiology. Neuropsychobiology 1996;33: 142–6.

139. Wolff AS, Erichsen MM, Meager A, et al. Autoimmune polyendocrine syndrome type 1 in Norway: phenotypic variation, autoantibodies, and novel mutations in the autoimmune regulator gene. J ClinEndocrinolMetab. 2007 Feb. 92(2): 595–603.

140. Wolff AS, Myhr KM, Vedeler CA, et al. Fc-gamma receptor polymorphisms are not associated with autoimmune Addison's disease. Scand J Immunol. 2007 Jun. 65(6): 555–8.

141. Wolkersdörfer GW, Lohmann T, Marx C, et al. Lymphocytes stimulate dehydroepiandrosterone production through direct cellular contact with adrenal zona reticularis cells: a novel mechanism of immune-endocrine interaction. J Clin Endocrinol Metab 1999; 84:4220.

142. Wood JB, Frankland AW, James VH, et al. A rapid test of adrenocortical function. Lancet. 1965 Jan 30. 191: 243–5.

143. Yanase T, Simpson ER, Waterman MR. 17 alpha-hydroxylase/17, 20-lyase deficiency: from clinical investigation to molecular definition. Endocr Rev 1991; 12:91.

144. Yarkony GM, Novick AK, Roth EJ, KirschnerKL,Rayner S, Betts HB. Galactorrhea: a complication ofspinal cord injury. Arch Phys Med Rehabil 1992; 73: 878–80.

145. Yazigi RA, Quintero CH, Salameh WA. Prolactin disorders. Fertil Steril 1997; 67: 215–25.

146. Yudofsky, Stuart C.; Robert E. Hales (2007). The American Psychiatric Publishing Textbook of Neuropsychiatry and Behavioral Neurosciences (5th ed.). American Psychiatric Pub, Inc. ISBN 1-58562-239-7.

9

The Thyroid Gland

INTRODUCTION

The thyroid gland is a butterfly-shaped organ and is composed of two cone-like lobes or wings, lobus dexter (right lobe) and lobus sinister (left lobe), connected via the isthmus. The organ is situated on the anterior side of the neck, lying against and around the larynx and trachea, reaching posteriorly the esophagus and carotid sheath (Fig. 9.1). It starts cranially at the oblique line on the thyroid cartilage (just below the laryngeal prominence, or 'Adam's Apple'), and extends inferiorly to approximately the fifth or sixth tracheal ring. It is difficult to demarcate the gland's upper and lower border with vertebral levels because it moves in position in relation to these structures during swallowing.

The thyroid gland secretes three hormones, i.e. thyroxine (T4) and triiodothyronine (T3), both of which are iodinated derivatives of tyrosine (Fig. 9.2), and calcitonin, a polypeptide hormone. T4 and T3 are produced by the follicular cells but calcitonin is secreted by the C cells, which are of separate embryological origin. Calcitonin is functionally unrelated to the other thyroid hormones. It has a minor role in calcium homoeostasis and disorders of its secretion are rare. Thyroid disorders in which there is either oversecretion or undersecretion of T4 and T3 are, however, common.

Thyroxine synthesis and release are stimulated by the pituitary trophic hormone, thyroid-stimulating hormone (TSH). The secretion of TSH is controlled by negative

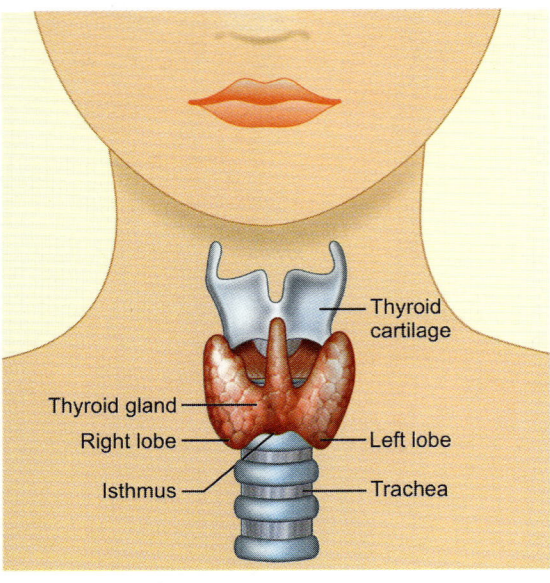

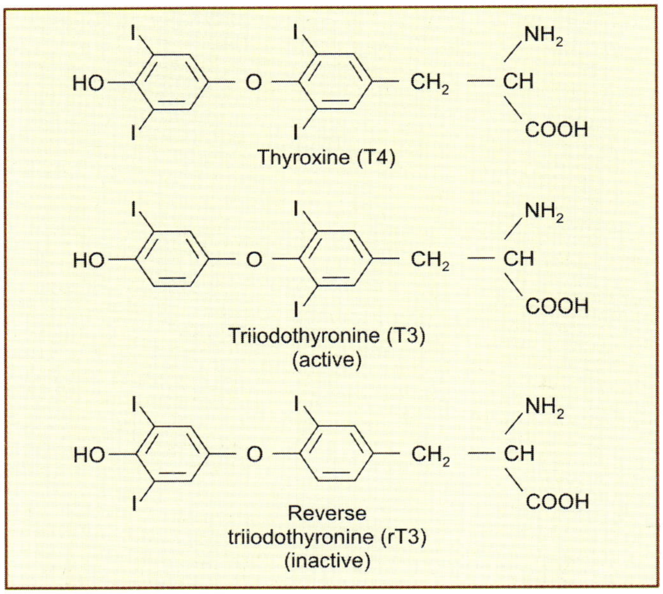

Fig. 9.1: The thyroid gland

Fig. 9.2: Chemical structure of the thyroid hormones, T4 and T3, and the inactive metabolite of T4 and rT3

feedback by the thyroid hormones, which modulate the response of the pituitary to the hypothalamic hormone, thyrotrophin-releasing hormone (TRH; Fig. 9.3). This feedback is mediated primarily by T3 produced by the action of iodothyronine deiodinase on T4 in the thyrotroph cells of the anterior pituitary. Glucocorticoids, dopamine, and somatostatin inhibit TSH secretion. The physiological significance of this is not known, but it may be relevant to the disturbances of thyroid hormones that can occur in non-thyroidal illness. The feedback mechanisms result in the maintenance of steady plasma concentrations of thyroid hormones.

The **major product of the thyroid gland** is T4. Ten times less T3 is produced (the proportion may be greater in thyroid disease), most (approximately 80%) T3 being derived from T4 by deiodination in peripheral tissues, particularly the liver, kidneys, and muscle, catalyzed by selenium-containing iodothyronine deiodinases. T3 is 3–4 times more potent than T4. In tissues, most of the effect of T4 results from this conversion to T3, so that T4 itself is essentially a prohormone. Deiodination can also produce reverse triiodothyronine (rT3; Fig. 9.2), which is physiologically inactive. It is produced instead of T3 in starvation and many non-thyroidal illnesses, and the formation of either the active or inactive metabolite of T4 appears to play an important part in the control of energy metabolism.

SYNTHESIS OF THYROID HORMONES

The first step in the synthesis of thyroid hormones is the organification of iodine. Iodide is taken up, converted to

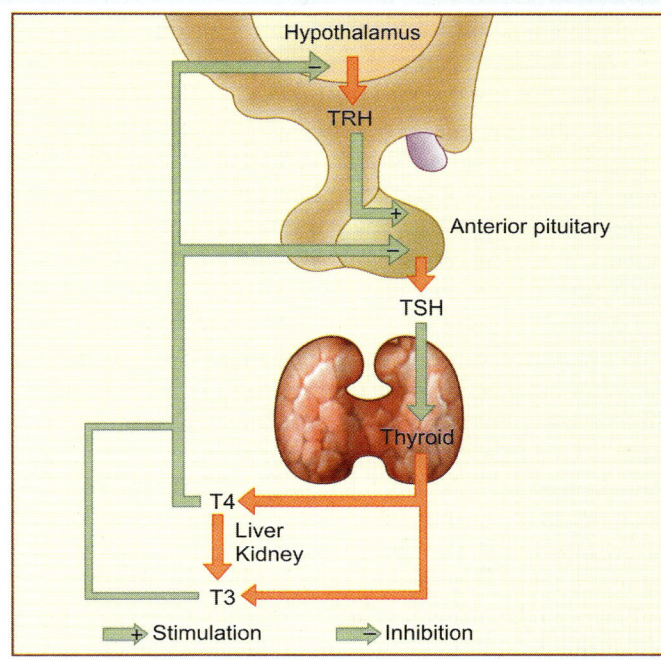

Fig. 9.3: Control of thyroid hormone secretion. TSH is released from the pituitary in response to the hypothalamic hormone, TRH, and stimulates the synthesis and release of thyroid hormones. TSH release is inhibited by thyroid hormones, which decrease the sensitivity of the pituitary to TRH. They may also inhibit TRH release by the hypothalamus

iodine, and then condensed onto tyrosine residues which reside along the polypeptide backbone of a protein molecule called thyroglobulin (Fig. 9.4). This reaction results in either a monoiodotyrosine (MIT) or diiodotyrosine (DIT) being incorporated into thyroglobulin. This

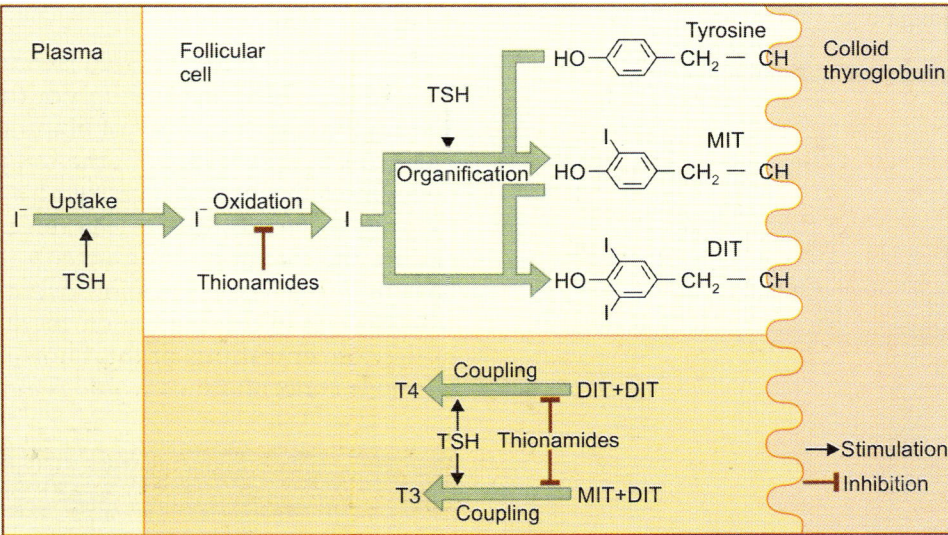

Fig. 9.4: Biosynthesis of the thyroid hormones. The iodination and condensation reactions involve tyrosine residues that are an integral part of the thyroglobulin polypeptide. The thyroid hormones remain protein bound until they are released from the cell. Iodide is actively absorbed into thyroid cells and oxidized to iodine, which is immediately incorporated into tyrosine residues to form monoiodotyrosine (MIT) and diiodotyrosine (DIT). These undergo coupling to form T3 and T4. Anti-thyroid thionamide drugs, such as carbimazole, act by inhibiting the oxidation of iodide and the coupling reaction

newly formed iodothyroglobulin forms one of the most important constituents of the colloid material, present in the follicle of the thyroid unit.

The other synthetic reaction that is closely linked to organification is a coupling reaction, where iodotyrosine molecules are coupled together. If two diiodotyrosine molecules couple together, the result is the formation of T4. If a diiodotyrosine and a monoiodotyrosine molecules are coupled together, the result is the formation of T3.

From the perspective of the formation of thyroid hormone, the major coupling reaction is the diiodotyrosine coupling to produce T4. Although, T3 is biologically more active than T4, the major production of T3 actually occurs outside of the thyroid gland. The majority of T3 is produced by peripheral conversion from T4 in a deiodination reaction involving a specific enzyme which removes one iodine from the outer ring of T4.

Thyroglobulin is stored within the thyroid gland in colloid follicles. These are accumulations of thyroglobulin-containing colloid surrounded by thyroid follicular cells. Release of thyroid hormones (stimulated by TSH) involves pinocytosis of colloid by follicular cells, fusion with lysosomes to form phagocytic vacuoles, and proteolysis (Fig. 9.5). Thyroid hormones are thence released into the bloodstream. Proteolysis also results in the liberation of MIT and DIT; these are usually degraded within thyroid follicular cells and their iodine is retained and reutilized. A small amount of thyroglobulin also reaches the bloodstream.

Thyroid Hormones in Blood

The **normal plasma concentrations of T4 and T3** are 60–150 nmol/L and 1.0–2.9 nmol/L, respectively. Both hormones are extensively protein bound; some 99.98% of T4 and 99.66% of T3 are bound, principally to a specific thyroxine-binding globulin (TBG) and, to a lesser extent, to prealbumin and albumin. TBG is approximately one-third saturated at normal concentrations of thyroid hormones (Fig. 9.6). It is generally accepted that only the free, non-protein-bound, thyroid hormones are physiologically active. Although, the total T4 (tT4) concentration is normally 50 times that of T3, the different extents to which these hormones are bound to protein mean that the free T4 (fT4) concentration is only 2–3 times that of free T3 (fT3) (typical reference ranges are 9–26 pmol/L for fT4 and 3.0–9.0 pmol/L for fT3).

The precise physiological function of TBG is unknown; individuals who have a genetically determined deficiency of the protein show no clinical abnormality. It has, however, been suggested that the extensive binding of thyroid hormones to TBG provides a buffer that maintains the free hormone concentrations constant in the face of any tendency to change. Protein binding also reduces the amount of thyroid hormones that would otherwise be lost by glomerular filtration and subsequent renal excretion.

Total (free + bound) thyroid hormone concentrations in plasma are dependent not only on thyroid function but, also on the concentrations of binding proteins. If these were to increase (Fig. 9.7), the temporary fall in free hormone concentration caused by increased protein binding would stimulate TSH release and this would restore the free hormone concentrations to normal; if binding protein concentrations were to fall, the reverse would occur. In either situation, there would be a change in the concentrations of total hormones, but the free hormone concentrations would remain normal.

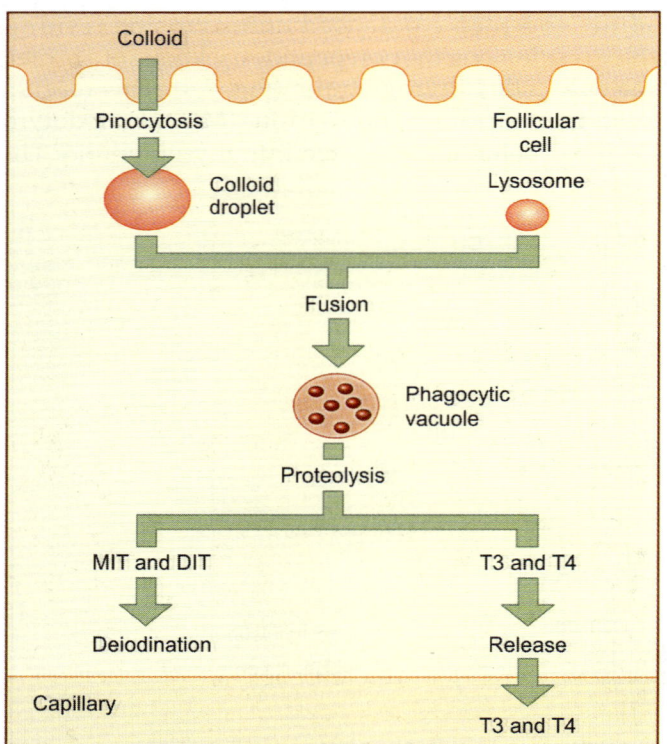

Fig. 9.5: Secretion of the thyroid hormones. Colloid is taken up into follicular cells by pinocytosis and undergoes lysosomal proteolysis, resulting in the release of thyroid hormones

Plasma concentration		Extent of protein	Half-life
Total (nmol/L)	Free (pmol/L)	binding (%)	(days)
T4 60–150	9.0–26.0	99.98	6–7
T3 1.0–2.9	3.0–9.0	99.66	1–1.5

Fig. 9.6: Thyroid hormones in blood. Each laboratory should determine its own reference range for plasma concentrations

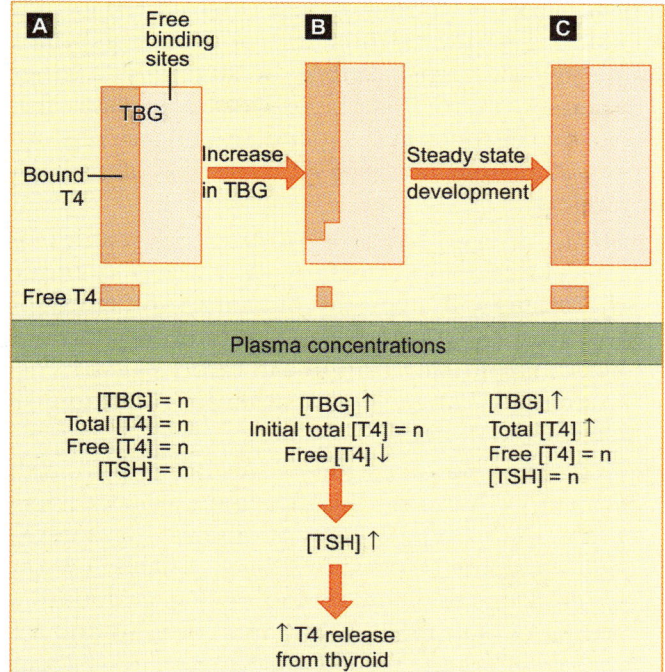

Fig. 9.7: Effect of an increase in TBG concentration on plasma T4 concentration. (A) In the initial steady state, TBG is one-third saturated with T4. (B) TBG concentration increases, causing more T4 to be bound, thus reducing the fT4 concentration. This stimulates TSH secretion, which leads to an increase in the release of T4 from the thyroid. (C) T4 becomes redistributed between the bound and the free states, leading to a new steady state with the same fT4 concentration but an increased tT4

This is a matter of considerable practical importance, as changes in the concentrations of the binding proteins occur in many circumstances (Table 9.1), causing changes in total hormone concentrations, but not necessarily in those of the free (physiologically available) hormones. Furthermore, certain drugs, e.g. salicylates and phenytoin, displace thyroid hormones from their binding

Table 9.1	Causes of abnormal plasma TBG concentrations
Increase	
Genetic	
Pregnancy	
Estrogens, including estrogen containing oral contraceptives	
Decease	
Genetic	
Protein losing states, e.g. nephrotic syndrome	
Malnutrition	
Malabsorption	
Cushing's syndrome	
High-dose corticosteroids	
Severe illness	
Androgens	

proteins, thus reducing total, but not free, hormone concentrations, once a new steady state is attained. If an attempt is made to assess thyroid status in a patient who is not in a steady state, the results may be bizarre and misleading.

Only small amounts of T4 and T3 are excreted by the kidneys owing to the extensive protein binding. The major route of thyroid hormone degradation is by deiodination and metabolism in tissues, but they are also conjugated in the liver and excreted in bile.

Disorders of the Thyroid

The metabolic manifestations of thyroid disease relate to either excessive or inadequate production of thyroid hormones (hyperthyroidism and hypothyroidism, respectively). The clinical syndrome that results from hyperthyroidism is thyrotoxicosis. The term 'myxedema' is often used to describe the entire clinical syndrome of hypothyroidism but strictly refers specifically to the dryness of the skin, coarsening of the features and subcutaneous swelling characteristic of severe hypothyroidism. Patients with thyroid disease may present with a thyroid swelling or goiter. Investigation may reveal hypothyroidism or (more frequently) hyperthyroidism, but there may be no functional abnormality. A goiter can be the presenting feature of thyroid cancer.

HYPERTHYROIDISM

Hyperthyroidism can be classified on the basis of thyroid radioactive iodine uptake and the presence or absence of circulating thyroid stimulators.

Etiology

Hyperthyroidism may result from increased synthesis and secretion of thyroid hormones T4 and T3 from the thyroid, caused by thyroid stimulators in the blood or by autonomous thyroid hyperfunction. It can also result from excessive release of thyroid hormone from the thyroid without increased synthesis. Such release is commonly caused by the destructive changes of various types of thyroiditis. Various clinical syndromes also cause hyperthyroidism.

Graves' disease (toxic diffuse goiter), the most common cause of hyperthyroidism, is characterized by hyperthyroidism and one or more of the following: goiter, exophthalmos, and infiltrative dermopathy. Graves' disease is caused by an autoantibody against the thyroid receptor for TSH; unlike most autoantibodies, which are inhibitory, this autoantibody is stimulatory, thus causing continuous synthesis and secretion of excess T4 and T3. Graves' disease (like Hashimoto thyroiditis), sometimes occurs with other autoimmune disorders, including type 1 diabetes mellitus, vitiligo, premature graying of hair, pernicious anemia, connective tissue disorders, and polyglandular deficiency syndrome. Heredity increases risk of Graves' disease, although the genes involved are still unknown. The pathogenesis of infiltrative ophthalmopathy (responsible for the exophthalmos in Graves' disease) is poorly understood but may result from immunoglobulins directed to the TSH receptors in the orbital fibroblasts and fat that result in release of proinflammatory cytokines, inflammation, and accumulation of glycosaminoglycans. Ophthalmopathy may also occur before the onset of hyperthyroidism or as late as 20 years afterward and frequently worsens or abates independently of the clinical course of hyperthyroidism. Typical ophthalmopathy in the presence of normal thyroid function is called euthyroid Graves' disease.

Inappropriate TSH secretion is a rare cause. Patients with hyperthyroidism have essentially undetectable TSH except for those with a TSH-secreting anterior pituitary adenoma or pituitary resistance to thyroid hormone. TSH levels are high, and the TSH produced in both disorders is biologically more active than normal TSH. An increase in the α-subunit of TSH in the blood (helpful in differential diagnosis) occurs in patients with a TSH-secreting pituitary adenoma.

Molar pregnancy, choriocarcinoma, and hyperemesis gravidarum produce high levels of serum human chorionic gonadotropin (HCG), a weak thyroid stimulator. Levels of HCG are highest during the first trimester of pregnancy and result in the decrease in serum TSH and mild increase in serum fT4 sometimes observed at that time. The increased thyroid stimulation may be caused by increased levels of partially desialated HCG, an hCG variant that appears to be a more potent thyroid stimulator than more sialated hCG. Hyperthyroidism in molar pregnancy, choriocarcinoma, and hyperemesis gravidarum is transient; normal thyroid function resumes when the molar pregnancy is evacuated, the choriocarcinoma is appropriately treated, or the hyperemesis gravidarum abates.

Nonautoimmune autosomal dominant hyperthyroidism manifests during infancy. It results from mutations in the TSH receptor gene that produce continuous thyroid stimulation.

Multinodular goiter (Plummer's disease) sometimes results from TSH receptor gene mutations causing continuous thyroid activation. Patients with toxic nodular goiter have none of the autoimmune manifestations or circulating antibodies observed in patients with Graves' disease. Also, in contrast to Graves' disease, toxic solitary and multinodular goiters usually do not remit.

Inflammatory thyroid disease (thyroiditis) includes subacute granulomatous thyroiditis, Hashimoto thyroiditis, and silent lymphocytic thyroiditis, a variant of Hashimoto thyroiditis. Hyperthyroidism results from destructive changes in the gland and release of stored hormone, not from increased synthesis. Hypothyroidism may follow.

- **Drug-induced hyperthyroidism** can result from amiodarone and interferon-a, which may induce thyroiditis with hyperthyroidism and other thyroid disorders. Although more commonly causing hypothyroidism, lithium can rarely cause hyperthyroidism. Patients receiving these drugs should be closely monitored.

- **Excess iodine ingestion** causes hyperthyroidism with a low thyroid radioactive iodine uptake. It most often occurs in patients with underlying nontoxic nodular goiter (especially elderly patients) who are given drugs that contain iodine (e.g. amiodarone, iodine-containing expectorants) or who undergo radiologic studies using iodine-rich contrast agents. The etiology may be that the excess iodine provides substrate for functionally autonomous (i.e. not under TSH regulation) areas of the thyroid to produce hormone. Hyperthyroidism usually persists as long as excess iodine remains in the circulation.

- **Metastatic thyroid cancer** is a possible cause. Overproduction of thyroid hormone occurs rarely from functioning metastatic follicular carcinoma, especially in pulmonary metastases.

Pathophysiology

In hyperthyroidism, serum T3 usually increases more than does T4, probably because of increased secretion of T3 as well as conversion of T4 to T3 in peripheral tissues. In some patients, only T3 is elevated (T3 toxicosis). T3 toxicosis may occur in any of the usual disorders that cause hyperthyroidism, including Graves' disease, multinodular goiter, and the autonomously functioning solitary thyroid nodule. If T3 toxicosis is untreated, the patient usually also develops laboratory abnormalities typical of hyperthyroidism (i.e. elevated T4 and ^{123}I uptake). The various forms of thyroiditis commonly have a hyperthyroid phase followed by a hypothyroid phase.

Symptoms and Signs

Most symptoms and signs are the same regardless of the cause. Exceptions include infiltrative ophthalmopathy and dermopathy, which occur only in Graves' disease (Fig. 9.8).

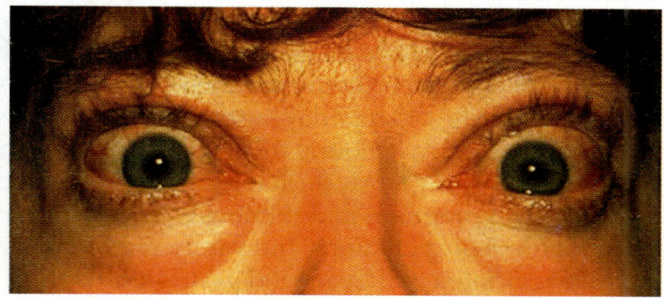

Fig. 9.8: Patient with active thyroid-associated ophthalmopathy

The clinical presentation may be dramatic or subtle. A goiter or nodule may be present. Many common symptoms of hyperthyroidism are similar to those of adrenergic excess, such as nervousness, palpitations, hyperactivity, increased sweating, heat hypersensitivity, fatigue, increased appetite, weight loss, insomnia, weakness, and frequent bowel movements (occasionally diarrhea). Hypomenorrhea may be present. Signs may include warm, moist skin, tremor, tachycardia, widened pulse pressure, atrial fibrillation, and palpitations.

Elderly patients, particularly those with toxic nodular goiter, may present atypically (apathetic or masked hyperthyroidism) with symptoms more akin to depression or dementia. Most do not have exophthalmos or tremor. Atrial fibrillation, syncope, altered sensorium, heart failure, and weakness are more likely. Symptoms and signs may involve only a single organ system.

Eye signs include stare, eyelid lag, eyelid retraction, and mild conjunctival injection and are largely due to excessive adrenergic stimulation. They usually remit with successful treatment. Infiltrative ophthalmopathy, a more serious development, is specific to Graves' disease and can occur years before or after hyperthyroidism. It is characterized by orbital pain, lacrimation, irritation, photophobia, increased retro-orbital tissue, exophthalmos, and lymphocytic infiltration of the extraocular muscles, causing ocular muscle weakness that frequently leads to double vision.

Infiltrative dermopathy, also called pretibial myxedema (a confusing term, because myxedema suggests hypothyroidism), is characterized by nonpitting infiltration by proteinaceous ground substance, usually in the pretibial area. It rarely occurs in the absence of Graves' ophthalmopathy. The lesion is often pruritic and erythematous in its early stages and subsequently becomes brawny. Infiltrative dermopathy may appear years before or after hyperthyroidism.

THYROID STORM

Thyroid storm is an acute form of hyperthyroidism that results from untreated or inadequately treated severe hyperthyroidism. It is rare, occurring in patients with Graves' disease or toxic multinodular goiter (a solitary toxic nodule is a less common cause and generally causes less severe manifestations). It may be precipitated by infection, trauma, surgery, embolism, diabetic keto-acidosis, or preeclampsia. Thyroid storm causes abrupt florid symptoms of hyperthyroidism with one or more of the following: fever, marked weakness and muscle wasting, extreme restlessness with wide emotional swings, confusion, psychosis, coma, nausea, vomiting, diarrhea, and hepatomegaly with mild jaundice. The patient may present with cardiovascular collapse and shock. Thyroid storm is a life-threatening emergency requiring prompt treatment.

Diagnosis

Diagnosis is based on history, physical examination, and thyroid function tests. Serum TSH measurement is the best test because TSH is suppressed in hyperthyroid patients except in the rare instance when the etiology is a TSH-secreting pituitary adenoma or pituitary resistance to the normal inhibition by thyroid hormone. Screening selected populations for TSH level is warranted. FT4 is increased in hyperthyroidism. However, T4 can be falsely normal in true hyperthyroidism in patients with a severe systemic illness (similar to the falsely low levels that occur in euthyroid sick syndrome) and in T3 toxicosis. If fT4 level is normal and TSH is low in a patient with subtle symptoms and signs of hyperthyroidism, then serum T3 should be measured to detect T3 toxicosis; an elevated level confirms that diagnosis.

The cause can often be diagnosed clinically (e.g. exposure to a drug, the presence of signs specific to Graves' disease). If not, radioactive iodine uptake by the thyroid may be measured by using [123] I. When hyperthyroidism is due to hormone overproduction, radioactive iodine uptake by the thyroid is usually elevated. When hyperthyroidism is due to thyroiditis, iodine ingestion, or ectopic hormone production, radioactive iodine uptake is low.

TSH receptor antibodies can be measured to detect Graves' disease, but measurement is rarely necessary except during the third trimester of pregnancy to assess the risk of neonatal Graves' disease; TSH receptor antibodies readily cross the placenta to stimulate the fetal thyroid. Most patients with Graves' disease have circulating antithyroid peroxidase antibodies, and fewer have antithyroglobulin antibodies.

Inappropriate TSH secretion is uncommon. The diagnosis is confirmed when hyperthyroidism occurs with elevated circulating fT4 and T3 concentrations and normal or elevated serum TSH.

If thyrotoxicosis factitia is suspected, serum thyroglobulin can be measured; it is usually low or low-normal; unlike in all other causes of hyperthyroidism.

Treatment

Methimazole and Propylthiouracil

These antithyroid drugs block thyroid peroxidase, decreasing the organification of iodide, and impair the coupling reaction. Propylthiouracil in high doses also inhibits the peripheral conversion of T4_T3. About 20–50% of patients with Graves' disease remain in remission after a 1- to 2-years course of either drug. The return to normal or a marked decrease in gland size, the restoration of a normal serum TSH level, and less severe hyperthyroidism before therapy are good prognostic signs of long-term remission. The concomitant use of antithyroid drug therapy and L-thyroxine does not improve the remission rate in patients with Graves' disease. Because toxic nodular goiter rarely goes into remission, antithyroid drug therapy is given only in preparation for surgical treatment or ^{131}I therapy.

Because of severe hepatic failure in some patients <40, especially children, propylthiouracil is now recommended only in special situations, (e.g. in the first trimester of pregnancy, in thyroid storm). Methimazole is the preferred drug. The usual starting dosage of methimazole is 5–20 mg by mouth 3 times a day and of propylthiouracil 100–150 mg by mouth every 8 hours. When T4 and T3 levels normalize, the dosage is decreased to the lowest effective amount, usually methimazole 5 to 15 mg once a day or propylthiouracil 50 mg 3 times a day. Usually, control is achieved in 2 to 3 months. More rapid control can be achieved by increasing the dosage of propylthiouracil to 150–200 mg every 8 hours. Such dosages or higher ones (up to 400 mg every 8 hours) are generally reserved for severely ill patients, including those with thyroid storm; to block the conversion of T4 to T3, maintenance doses of methimazole can be continued for one or many years depending on the clinical circumstances. Carbimazole, which is used widely in Europe, is rapidly converted to methimazole. The usual starting dose is similar to that of methimazole; maintenance dosage is 5–20 mg by mouth once a day, 2.5–10 mg bid, or 1.7–6.7 mg 3 times a day.

Adverse effects include rash, allergic reactions, abnormal liver function (including hepatic failure with propylthiouracil), and in about 0.1% of patients, reversible agranulocytosis. Patients allergic to one drug can be switched to the other, but cross-sensitivity may occur. If agranulocytosis occurs, the patient cannot be switched to the other drug; other therapy (e.g. radioiodine, surgery) should be used.

Each drug has advantages and disadvantages. Methimazole need only be given once a day, which improves adherence. Furthermore, when methimazole is used in dosages of <40 mg/day, agranulocytosis is less common; with propylthiouracil, agranulocytosis may occur at any dosage. Methimazole has been used successfully in pregnant and nursing women without fetal or infant complications, but rarely methimazole has been associated with scalp and gastrointestinal (GI) defects in neonates and with a rare embryopathy. Because of these complications, propylthiouracil is used in the first trimester of pregnancy. Propylthiouracil is preferred for the treatment of thyroid storm, because the dosages used (800–1200 mg/day) partially block the peripheral conversion of T4 to T3.

The combination of high-dose propylthiouracil and dexamethasone, also a potent inhibitor of T4 to T3 conversion, can relieve symptoms of severe hyperthyroidism and restore the serum T3 level to normal within a week.

β-Blockers

Symptoms and signs of hyperthyroidism due to adrenergic stimulation may respond to β-blockers; propranolol has had the greatest use, but atenolol or metoprolol may be preferable.

Other manifestations typically do not respond.

- *Manifestations typically responding to β-blockers:* Tachycardia, tremor, mental symptoms, eyelid lag; occasionally heat intolerance and sweating, diarrhea, proximal myopathy
- *Manifestations typically not responding to β-blockers:* O_2 consumption, exophthalmos, goiter, bruit, circulating thyroxine levels, weight loss

Propranolol is indicated in thyroid storm. It rapidly decreases heart rate, usually within 2–3 hours when given orally and within minutes when given IV. Esmolol may be used in the ICU, because it requires careful titration and monitoring. Propranolol is also indicated for tachycardia with hyperthyroidism, especially in elderly patients, because antithyroid drugs usually take several weeks to become fully effective. Ca channel blockers may control tachyarrhythmias in patients in whom β-blockers are contraindicated.

Iodine

Iodine in pharmacologic doses inhibits the release of T3 and T4 within hours and inhibits the organification of iodine, a transitory effect lasting from a few days to a week, after which inhibition usually ceases. Iodine is used for emergency management of thyroid storm, for hyperthyroid patients undergoing emergency nonthyroid surgery, and (because it also decreases the vascularity of the thyroid) for preoperative preparation of hyperthyroid patients undergoing subtotal thyroidectomy. Iodine generally is not used for routine treatment of hyperthyroidism. The usual dosage is 2–3 drops (100–150 mg) of a saturated K iodide solution by mouth 3 times a day or 4 times a day or 0.5–1 g Na iodide in 1 L 0.9% saline solution given IV slowly every 12 hours.

Complications of iodine therapy include inflammation of the salivary glands, conjunctivitis, and rash.

Radioactive Sodium Iodine (^{131}I, Radioiodine)

Radioiodine (^{131}I) is the most common treatment for hyperthyroidism. Radioiodine is often recommended as the treatment of choice for Graves' disease and toxic nodular goiter in all patients, including children. Dosage of ^{131}I is difficult to adjust because the response of the gland cannot be predicted; some physicians give a standard dose of 8–15 mCi. Others adjust the dose based on estimated thyroid size and the 24-h uptake to provide a dose of 80–120 mCi/g thyroid tissue.

When sufficient ^{131}I is given to cause euthyroidism, about 25–50% of patients become hypothyroid 1 years later, and the incidence continues to increase yearly. Thus, most patients eventually become hypothyroid. However, if smaller doses are used, incidence of recurrence is higher. Larger doses, such as 10–15 mCi, often cause hypothyroidism within 6 months.

Radioactive iodine is not used during lactation because it can enter breast milk and cause hypothyroidism in the infant. It is not used during pregnancy because it crosses the placenta and can cause severe fetal hypothyroidism. There is no proof that radioiodine increases the incidence of tumors, leukemia, thyroid cancer, or birth defects in children born to previously hyperthyroid women who become pregnant later in life.

Surgery

Surgery is indicated for patients with Graves' disease whose hyperthyroidism has recurred after courses of antithyroid drugs and who refuse ^{131}I therapy, patients who cannot tolerate antithyroid drugs, patients with very large goiters, and in some younger patients with toxic adenoma and multinodular goiter. Surgery may be done in elderly patients with giant nodular goiters.

Surgery usually restores normal function. Postoperative recurrences vary between 2% and 16%; risk of hypothyroidism is directly related to the extent of surgery. Vocal cord paralysis and hypoparathyroidism are uncommon complications. Saturated solution of K iodide 3 drops (about 100–150 mg) by mouth 3 times a day should be given for 10 days before surgery to reduce the vascularity of the gland. Methimazole must also be given, because the patient should be euthyroid before iodide is given. Dexamethasone can be added to rapidly restore euthyroidism. Surgical procedures are more difficult in patients who previously underwent thyroidectomy or radioiodine therapy.

HYPOTHYROIDISM

Hypothyroidism can occur at any age, but is particularly common among the elderly. It occurs in close to 10% of women and 6% of men >65. Although, typically easy to diagnose in younger adults, it may be subtle and manifest atypically in the elderly. Hypothyroidism may be primary; caused by disease in the thyroid, or secondary: caused by disease in the hypothalamus or pituitary.

Primary Hypothyroidism

Primary hypothyroidism is due to disease in the thyroid; TSH is increased. The most common cause is autoimmune. It usually results from Hashimoto thyroiditis and is often associated with a firm goiter or, later in the disease process, with a shrunken fibrotic thyroid with little or no function. The second most common cause is post-therapeutic hypothyroidism, especially after radioactive iodine therapy or surgery for hyperthyroidism or goiter. Hypothyroidism during overtreatment with propylthiouracil, methimazole, and iodide abates after therapy is stopped.

Most patients with non-Hashimoto goiters are euthyroid or have hyperthyroidism, but goitrous hypothyroidism may occur in endemic goiter. Iodine deficiency decreases thyroid hormonogenesis. In response, TSH is released, which causes the thyroid to enlarge and trap iodine avidly; thus, goiter results. If iodine deficiency is severe, the patient becomes hypothyroid.

Iodine deficiency can cause congenital hypothyroidism. In severely iodine-deficient regions worldwide, congenital hypothyroidism (previously termed endemic cretinism) is a major cause of intellectual disability.

Rare inherited enzymatic defects can alter the synthesis of thyroid hormone and cause goitrous hypothyroidism.

Hypothyroidism may occur in patients taking lithium, perhaps because lithium inhibits hormone release by the thyroid. Hypothyroidism may also occur in patients taking amiodarone or other iodine-containing drugs, and in patients taking interferon-α. Hypothyroidism can result from radiation therapy for cancer of the larynx or Hodgkin lymphoma (Hodgkin disease). The incidence of permanent hypothyroidism after radiation therapy is high, and thyroid function (through measurement of serum TSH) should be evaluated at 6–12 months intervals.

Secondary Hypothyroidism

Secondary hypothyroidism occurs when the hypothalamus produces insufficient thyrotropin-releasing hormone or the pituitary produces insufficient TSH. Sometimes, deficient TSH secretion due to deficient TRH secretion is termed tertiary hypothyroidism.

Symptoms and Signs

Symptoms may include cold intolerance, constipation, forgetfulness, and personality changes. Modest weight gain is largely the result of fluid retention and decreased metabolism. Paresthesias of the hands and feet are common, often due to carpal-tarsal tunnel syndrome caused by deposition of proteinaceous ground substance in the ligaments around the wrist and ankle. Women with hypothyroidism may develop menorrhagia or secondary amenorrhea.

The facial expression is dull; the voice is hoarse and speech is slow; facial puffiness and periorbital swelling occur due to infiltration with the mucopolysaccharides hyaluronic acid and chondroitin sulfate; eyelids droop because of decreased adrenergic drive; hair is sparse, coarse, and dry; and the skin is coarse, dry, scaly, and thick. The relaxation phase of deep tendon reflexes is slowed. Hypothermia is common. Dementia or frank psychosis (myxedema madness) may occur.

Carotenemia is common, particularly notable on the palms and soles, caused by deposition of carotene in the lipid-rich epidermal layers deposition of proteinaceous ground substance in the tongue may cause macroglossia. A decrease in both thyroid hormone and adrenergic stimulation causes bradycardia. The heart may appear to be enlarged on examination and imaging, partly because of dilation but chiefly because of pericardial effusion. Pleural or abdominal effusions also may be noted. The pericardial and pleural effusions develop slowly and only rarely cause respiratory or hemodynamic distress.

Elderly patients have significantly fewer symptoms than do younger adults, and complaints are often subtle and vague. Many elderly patients with hypothyroidism present with nonspecific geriatric syndromes confusion, anorexia, weight loss, falling, incontinence, and decreased mobility. Musculoskeletal symptoms (especially arthralgias) occur often, but arthritis is rare. Muscular aches and weakness, often mimicking polymyalgia rheumatica or polymyositis, and an elevated CK level may occur. In the elderly, hypothyroidism may mimic dementia or Parkinsonism.

Although secondary hypothyroidism is uncommon, its causes often affect other endocrine organs controlled by the hypothalamic-pituitary axis. In a woman with hypothyroidism, indications of secondary hypothyroidism are a history of amenorrhea rather than menorrhagia and some suggestive differences on physical examination. Secondary hypothyroidism is characterized by skin and hair that are dry but not very coarse, skin depigmentation, only minimal macroglossia, atrophic breasts, and low BP. Also, the heart is small, and serous pericardial effusions do not occur. Hypoglycemia is common because of concomitant adrenal insufficiency or growth hormone deficiency.

Myxedema Coma

Myxedema coma is a life-threatening complication of hypothyroidism, usually occurring in patients with a long history of hypothyroidism. Its characteristics include coma with extreme hypothermia (temperature 24°–32.2°C), areflexia, seizures, and respiratory depression with CO_2 retention. Severe hypothermia may be missed unless low-reading thermometers are used. Rapid diagnosis based on clinical judgment, history, and physical examination is imperative, because death is likely without rapid treatment. Precipitating factors include illness, infection, trauma, drugs that suppress the CNS, and exposure to cold.

Diagnosis

Serum TSH is the most sensitive test, and screening of selected populations is warranted. In primary hypothyroidism, there is no feedback inhibition of the intact pituitary, and serum TSH is always elevated, whereas serum fT4 is low. In secondary hypothyroidism, fT4 and serum TSH are low (sometimes TSH is normal but with decreased bioactivity).

Many patients with primary hypothyroidism have normal circulating levels of triiodothyronine (T3), probably caused by sustained TSH stimulation of the failing thyroid, resulting in preferential synthesis and secretion of biologically active T3. Therefore, serum T3 is not sensitive for hypothyroidism.

Anemia is often present, usually normocytic-normochromic and of unknown etiology, but it may be hypochromic because of menorrhagia and sometimes macrocytic because of associated pernicious anemia or decreased absorption of folate. Serum cholesterol is usually high in primary hypothyroidism, but less so in secondary hypothyroidism.

In addition to primary and secondary hypothyroidism, other conditions may cause decreased levels of tT4, such as serum thyroxine-binding globulin deficiency, some drugs and euthyroid sick syndrome.

Treatment

Various thyroid hormone preparations are available for replacement therapy, including synthetic preparations of T4 (L-thyroxine), T3 (liothyronine), combinations of the 2 synthetic hormones, and desiccated animal thyroid extract. L-thyroxine is preferred; the usual maintenance dose is 75–150 μg by mouth once a day, depending on age, body mass index, and absorption. The starting dose in young or middle-aged patients who are otherwise healthy can be 100 μg or 1.7 μg/kg by mouth once a day.

However, in the elderly and in patients with heart disease, therapy is begun with low doses, usually 25 μg once a day. The dose is adjusted every 6 weeks until maintenance dose is achieved. The maintenance dose may need to be decreased in elderly patients and increased in pregnant women. Dose may also need to be increased if drugs that decrease T4 absorption or increase its biliary excretion are administered concomitantly. The dose used should be the lowest that restores serum TSH levels to the midnormal range (though this criterion cannot be used in patients with secondary hypothyroidism). In secondary hypothyroidism the dose of L-thyroxine should achieve a fT4 in the midnormal range.

Liothyronine should not be used alone for long-term replacement because of its short half-life and the large peaks in serum T3 levels it produces. The administration of standard replacement amounts (25–37.5 μg twice a day) results in rapidly increasing serum T3 within 4 hours due to its almost complete absorption; these levels return to normal by 24 hours additionally, patients receiving liothyronine are chemically hyperthyroid for at least several hours a day, potentially increasing cardiac risks.

Similar patterns of serum T3 occur when mixtures of T3 and T4 are taken by mouth, although peak T3 is lower because less T3 is given. Replacement regimens with synthetic T4 preparations reflect a different pattern in serum T3 response. Increases in serum T3 occur gradually, and normal levels are maintained when adequate doses of T4 are given. Desiccated animal thyroid preparations contain variable amounts of T3 and T4 and should not be prescribed unless the patient is already taking the preparation and has normal serum TSH.

In patients with secondary hypothyroidism, L-thyroxine should not be given until there is evidence of adequate cortisol secretion (or cortisol therapy is given), because L-thyroxine could precipitate adrenal crisis.

Myxedema Coma

Patients require a large initial dose of T4 (300–500 μg IV) or T3 (25–50 μg IV). The IV maintenance dose of T4 is 75–100 μg once a day and of T3, 10–20 μg twice a day until T4 can be given orally. Corticosteroids are also given because the possibility of central hypothyroidism usually cannot be initially ruled out. The patient should not be rewarmed rapidly, which may precipitate hypotension or arrhythmias. Hypoxemia is common, so PaO_2 should be monitored. If ventilation is compromised, immediate mechanical ventilatory assistance is required. The precipitating factor should be rapidly and appropriately treated and fluid replacement given carefully, because hypothyroid patients do not excrete water appropriately. Finally, all drugs should be given cautiously because they are metabolized more slowly than in healthy people.

SUBCLINICAL HYPOTHYROIDISM

Subclinical hypothyroidism is elevated serum TSH in patients with absent or minimal symptoms of hypothyroidism and normal serum levels of fT4.

Subclinical thyroid dysfunction is relatively common; it occurs in more than 15% of elderly women and 10% of elderly men, particularly in those with underlying Hashimoto thyroiditis.

In patients with serum TSH >10 mU/L, there is a high likelihood of progression to overt hypothyroidism with low serum levels of fT4 in the next 10 years. These patients are also more likely to have hypercholesterolemia and atherosclerosis. They should be treated with L-thyroxine, even if they are asymptomatic. For patients with TSH levels between 4.5 mU/L and 10 mU/L, a trial of L-thyroxine is reasonable if symptoms of early hypothyroidism (e.g. fatigue, depression) are present. L-thyroxine therapy is also indicated in pregnant women and in women who plan to become pregnant to avoid deleterious effects of hypothyroidism on the pregnancy and fetal development. Patients should have annual measurement of serum TSH and fT4 to assess progress of the condition if untreated or to adjust the L-thyroxine dosage.

HASHIMOTO THYROIDITIS

Hashimoto thyroiditis is believed to be the most common cause of primary hypothyroidism in North America. It is twice as prevalent among women. Incidence increases with age and in patients with chromosomal disorders, including Down, Turner, and Klinefelter syndromes. A family history of thyroid disorders is common.

Hashimoto thyroiditis, like Graves' disease, is sometimes associated with other autoimmune disorders, including Addison's disease (adrenal insufficiency), type

1 diabetes mellitus, hypoparathyroidism, vitiligo, premature graying of hair, pernicious anemia, connective tissue disorders [e.g. rheumatoid arthritis (RA), systemic lupus erythematosus (SLE), Sjögren syndrome], celiac disease, and Schmidt syndrome (Addison's disease, diabetes, and hypothyroidism secondary to Hashimoto thyroiditis). There may be an increased incidence of thyroid tumors, rarely thyroid lymphoma. Pathologically, there is extensive infiltration of lymphocytes with lymphoid follicles and scarring.

Symptoms and Signs

Patients complain of painless enlargement of the thyroid or fullness in the throat (Fig. 9.9). Examination reveals a non-tender goiter that is smooth or nodular, firm, and more rubbery than the normal thyroid. Many patients present with symptoms of hypothyroidism, but some present with hyperthyroidism.

Diagnosis

Testing consists of measuring T4, TSH, and thyroid autoantibodies. Early in the disease, T4 and TSH levels are normal and there are high levels of thyroid peroxidase antibodies and, less commonly, of antithyroglobulin antibodies. Thyroid radioactive iodine uptake may be increased, perhaps because of defective iodide organification together with a gland that continues to trap iodine. Patients later develop hypothyroidism with decreased T4, decreased thyroid radioactive iodine uptake, and increased TSH. Testing for other autoimmune disorders is warranted only when clinical manifestations are present.

Treatment

Occasionally, hypothyroidism is transient, but most patients require lifelong thyroid hormone replacement, typically L-thyroxine 75–150 µg by mouth once a day.

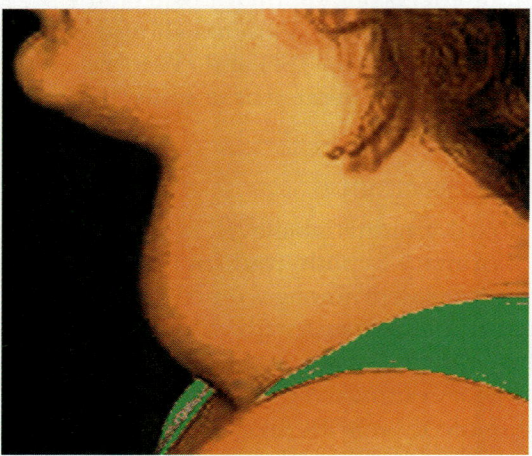

Fig. 9.9: A visibly larger neck, a feeling of fullness in the neck or throat

EUTHYROID SICK SYNDROME

Patients with various acute or chronic nonthyroid disorders may have abnormal thyroid function test results. Such disorders include acute and chronic illness, particularly fasting, starvation, protein-energy undernutrition, major trauma, myocardial infarction (MI), chronic renal failure, diabetic ketoacidosis, anorexia nervosa, cirrhosis, thermal injury, and sepsis.

Decreased triiodothyronine (T3) levels are most common. Patients with more severe or prolonged illness also have decreased thyroxine (T4) levels. Serum reverse T3 (rT3) is increased. Patients are clinically euthyroid and do not have elevated thyroid-stimulating hormone levels.

Pathogenesis is unknown but may include decreased peripheral conversion of T4 to T3, decreased clearance of rT3 generated from T4, and decreased binding of thyroid hormones to thyroxine-binding globulin. Proinflammatory cytokines (e.g. tumor necrosis factor-a, IL-1) may be responsible for some changes.

Interpretation of abnormal thyroid function test results in ill patients is complicated by the effects of various drugs, including the iodine-rich contrast agents and amiodarone, which impairs the peripheral conversion of T4 to T3, and by drugs, such as dopamine and corticosteroids, which decrease pituitary secretion of TSH, resulting in low serum TSH levels and subsequent decreased T4 secretion.

Diagnosis

The best test is measurement of TSH, which in euthyroid sick syndrome is low, normal, or slightly elevated but not as high as it would be in hypothyroidism. Serum rT3 is elevated, although this measurement is rarely done. Serum cortisol is often elevated in euthyroid sick syndrome and low or low-normal in hypothyroidism due to pituitary-hypothalamic disease. Because tests are nonspecific, clinical judgment is required to interpret abnormal thyroid function tests in the acutely or chronically ill patient. Unless thyroid dysfunction is highly suspected.

Treatment

Treatment with thyroid hormone replacement is not appropriate. When the underlying disorder is treated, results of thyroid tests normalize.

SILENT LYMPHOCYTIC THYROIDITIS

The term 'silent' refers to the absence of thyroid tenderness in contrast with subacute thyroiditis, which usually causes thyroid tenderness. Silent lymphocytic thyroiditis causes most cases of postpartum thyroid dysfunction. It occurs in about 5–10% of postpartum women.

Thyroid biopsy reveals lymphocytic infiltration as in Hashimoto thyroiditis but without lymphoid follicles and scarring. Thyroid peroxidase autoantibodies and, less commonly, antithyroglobulin antibodies are almost always positive during pregnancy and the postpartum period in these patients. Thus, this disorder would appear to be a variant of Hashimoto thyroiditis.

Symptoms and Signs

The condition begins in the postpartum period, usually within 12–16 weeks. Silent lymphocytic thyroiditis is characterized by a variable degree of painless thyroid enlargement with a hyperthyroid phase of several weeks, often followed by transient hypothyroidism due to depleted thyroid hormone stores but usually eventual recovery to the euthyroid state (as noted for painful subacute thyroiditis). The hyperthyroid phase is self-limited and may be brief or overlooked. Many women with this disorder are diagnosed when they become hypothyroid, which occasionally is permanent.

Diagnosis

Silent lymphocytic thyroiditis is frequently undiagnosed. Suspicion of the diagnosis generally depends on clinical findings, typically once hypothyroidism has occurred. Eye signs and pretibial myxedema do not occur.

Thyroid function test results vary depending on the phase of illness. Initially, serum T4 and T3 are elevated and TSH is suppressed. In the hypothyroid phase, these findings are reversed. White lood cell (WBC) count and erythrocyte sedimentation rate (ESR) are normal. Needle biopsy provides definitive diagnosis but is usually unnecessary.

Treatment

Because silent lymphocytic thyroiditis lasts only a few months, treatment is conservative, usually requiring only a β-blocker during the hyperthyroid phase. Antithyroid drugs, surgery, and radioiodine therapy are contra-indicated. Thyroid hormone replacement may be required during the hypothyroid phase. Most patients recover normal thyroid function, although some remain permanently hypothyroid. Therefore, thyroid function should be reevaluated after 9–12 months of thyroxine therapy; replacement is stopped for 5 weeks, and TSH is remeasured. This disorder usually recurs after subsequent pregnancies.

SUBACUTE THYROIDITIS

History of an antecedent viral upper respiratory tract infection (URI) is common. Histologic studies show less lymphocytic infiltration of the thyroid than in Hashimoto's thyroiditis or silent thyroiditis, but there is characteristic giant cell infiltration, polymorphonuclear leukocytes (PMNs), and follicular disruption.

Symptoms and Signs

There is pain in the anterior neck and fever of 37.8°–38.3°C. Neck pain characteristically shifts from side-to side and may settle in one area, frequently radiating to the jaw and ears. It is often confused with dental pain, pharyngitis, or otitis and is aggravated by swallowing or turning of the head. Symptoms of hyperthyroidism are common early in the disease because of hormone release from the disrupted follicles. There is more lassitude and prostration than in other thyroid disorders. On physical examination, the thyroid is asymmetrically enlarged, firm, and tender.

Diagnosis

Diagnosis is primarily clinical, based on finding an enlarged, tender thyroid in patients with the appropriate clinical history. Thyroid testing with TSH and at least a fT4 measurement is usually also done. Radioactive iodine uptake should be measured to confirm the diagnosis. When the diagnosis is uncertain, fine-needle aspiration biopsy is useful. Thyroid ultrasonography with color Doppler shows reduced blood flow in contrast with the increased flow of Graves' disease. Laboratory findings early in the disease include an increase in fT4 and T3, a marked decrease in TSH and thyroid radioactive iodine uptake (often 0), and a high ESR. After several weeks, the thyroid is depleted of T4 and T3 stores, and transient hypothyroidism develops accompanied by a decrease in fT4 and T3, a rise in TSH, and recovery of thyroid radioactive iodine uptake. Weakly positive thyroid antibodies may be present. Measurement of fT4, T3, and TSH at 2–4 weeks intervals identifies the stages of the disease.

Treatment

Discomfort is treated with high doses of aspirin or nonsteroidal anti-inflammatory drugs (NSAIDs). In severe and protracted cases, corticosteroids (e.g. prednisone 30–40 mg by mouth once a day, gradually decreasing the dose over 3–4 weeks) eradicate all symptoms within 48 hours.

Bothersome hyperthyroid symptoms may be treated with a short course of a β-blocker. If hypothyroidism is pronounced or persists, thyroid hormone replacement therapy may be required, rarely permanently.

SIMPLE NONTOXIC GOITER (EUTHYROID GOITER)

The most common type of thyroid enlargement, is frequently noted at puberty, during pregnancy, and at menopause. The cause at these times is usually unclear.

Known causes include intrinsic thyroid hormone production defects and, in iodine-deficient countries, ingestion of foods that contain substances that inhibit thyroid hormone synthesis (goitrogens, e.g. cassava, broccoli, cauliflower, and cabbage). Other causes include the use of drugs that can decrease the synthesis of thyroid hormone (e.g. amiodarone or other iodine-containing compounds, lithium).

Iodine deficiency is the most common cause of goiter worldwide (termed endemic goiter). Compensatory small elevations in thyroid-stimulating hormone occur, preventing hypothyroidism, but the TSH stimulation results in goiter formation. Recurrent cycles of stimulation and involution may result in nontoxic nodular goiters. However, the true etiology of most nontoxic goiters in iodine-sufficient areas is unknown.

Symptoms and Signs

The patient may have a history of low iodine intake or over ingestion of food goitrogens, but these phenomena are rare in North America. In the early stages, the goiter is typically soft, symmetric, and smooth. Later, multiple nodules and cysts may develop.

Diagnosis

In the early stages, thyroidal radioactive iodine uptake may be normal or high with normal thyroid scans. Thyroid function tests are usually normal. Thyroid antibodies are measured to rule out Hashimoto's thyroiditis.

In endemic goiter, serum TSH may be slightly elevated, and serum T4 may be low-normal or slightly low, but serum T3 is usually normal or slightly elevated.

Treatment

In iodine-deficient areas, iodine supplementation of salt; oral or IM administration of iodized oil yearly; and iodination of water, crops, or animal fodder eliminates iodine-deficiency goiter. Goitrogens being ingested should be stopped.

In other instances, suppression of the hypothalamic-pituitary axis with thyroid hormone blocks TSH production (and hence stimulation of the thyroid). Full TSH-suppressive doses of L-thyroxine (100–150 µg/day by mouth depending on the serum TSH) are useful in younger patients. L-thyroxine is contraindicated in older patients with nontoxic nodular goiter, because these goiters rarely shrink and may harbor areas of autonomy, so that L-thyroxine therapy can result in hyperthyroidism. Large goiters occasionally require surgery or ^{131}I to shrink the gland enough to prevent interference with respiration or swallowing or to correct cosmetic problems.

THYROID CANCERS

The four general types of thyroid cancer are papillary, follicular, medullary, and anaplastic. Papillary and follicular carcinoma together are called differentiated thyroid cancer because of their histologic resemblance to normal thyroid tissue and because differentiated function (e.g. thyroglobulin secretion) is preserved. Most thyroid cancers manifest as asymptomatic nodules. Rarely, lymph node, lung, or bone metastases cause the presenting symptoms of small thyroid cancers. Diagnosis is often by fine-needle aspiration biopsy, but may involve other tests. Except for anaplastic and metastatic medullary carcinoma, most thyroid cancers are not highly malignant and are seldom fatal. Treatment is surgical removal, usually followed by ablation of residual tissue with radioactive iodine.

Papillary Carcinoma

Papillary carcinoma accounts for 70–80% of all thyroid cancers. The most patients present between ages 30 and 60. The tumor is often more aggressive in elderly patients. Many papillary carcinomas contain follicular elements.

The tumor spreads via lymphatics to regional lymph nodes in one-third of patients and may metastasize to the lungs. Patients <45 years with small tumors confined to the thyroid have an excellent prognosis.

Treatment

Treatment for encapsulated tumors <1.5 cm localized to one lobe is usually near-total thyroidectomy, although some experts recommend only lobectomy and isthmectomy; surgery is almost always curative. Thyroid hormone in thyroid-stimulating hormone—suppressive doses is given to minimize chances of regrowth and cause regression of any microscopic remnants of papillary carcinoma.

Tumors >4 cm or that are diffusely spreading require total or near-total thyroidectomy with postoperative radioiodine ablation of residual thyroid tissue with appropriately large doses of ^{131}I administered, when the patient is hypothyroid or after recombinant TSH injections. Treatment may be repeated every 6–12 months to ablate any remaining thyroid tissue. TSH-suppressive doses of L-thyroxine are given after treatment, and serum thyroglobulin levels help detect recurrent or persistent disease. About 20–30% of patients, mainly older patients, have recurrent or persistent disease.

Follicular Carcinoma

Follicular carcinoma, including the Hürthle cell variant, accounts for about 15% of thyroid cancers. It is more common among older patients and in regions of iodine deficiency. It is more malignant than papillary carcinoma, spreading hematogenously with distant metastases.

Treatment requires near-total thyroidectomy with postoperative radioiodine ablation of residual thyroid tissue as in treatment for papillary carcinoma. Metastases are more responsive to radioiodine therapy than are those of papillary carcinoma. TSH-suppressive doses of L-thyroxine are given after treatment. Serum thyroglobulin should be monitored to detect recurrent or persistent disease.

Medullary Carcinoma

Medullary (solid) carcinoma constitutes about 3% of thyroid cancers and is composed of parafollicular cells (C cells) that produce calcitonin. It may be sporadic (usually unilateral); however, it is often familial, caused by a mutation of the *ret* proto-oncogene. The familial form may occur in isolation or as a component of multiple endocrine neoplasia (MEN) syndromes types 2A and 2B. Although, calcitonin can lower serum Ca and phosphate levels, serum Ca is normal because the high level of calcitonin ultimately down-regulates its receptors. Characteristic amyloid deposits that stain with Congo red are also present.

Metastases spread via the lymphatic system to cervical and mediastinal nodes and sometimes to liver, lungs, and bone.

Symptoms and Signs

Patients typically present with an asymptomatic thyroid nodule, although many cases are now diagnosed during routine screening of affected kindreds with MEN 2A or MEN 2B before a palpable tumor develops.

Medullary carcinoma may have a dramatic bio-chemical presentation when associated with ectopic production of other hormones or peptides (e.g. ACTH, vasoactive intestinal polypeptide, prostaglandins, kallikreins, and serotonin).

Diagnosis

The best test is measurement of serum calcitonin, which is greatly elevated. A challenge with Ca (15 mg/kg IV over 4 hours) provokes excessive secretion of calcitonin. X-rays may show a dense, homogenous, and conglomerate calcification.

All patients with medullary carcinoma should have genetic testing; relatives of those with mutations should have genetic testing and measurement of basal and stimulated calcitonin levels.

Treatment

Total thyroidectomy is indicated even if bilateral involvement is not obvious. Lymph nodes are also dissected. If hyperparathyroidism is present, removal of hyperplastic, or adenomatous parathyroids is required. Pheochromocytoma, if present, is usually bilateral. Pheochromocytomas should be identified and removed before thyroidectomy because of the danger of provoking hypertensive crisis during the operation. Long-term survival is common in patients with medullary carcinoma and MEN 2A; more than two-thirds of affected patients are alive at 10 years. Medullary carcinoma of the sporadic type has a worse prognosis.

Relatives with an elevated calcitonin level without a palpable thyroid abnormality should undergo thyroidectomy because there is a greater chance of cure at this stage. Some experts recommend surgery in relatives who have normal basal and stimulated serum calcitonin levels, but who have the *ret* proto-oncogene mutation.

Anaplastic Carcinoma

Anaplastic carcinoma is an undifferentiated cancer that accounts for about 2% of thyroid cancers. It occurs mostly in elderly patients and slightly more often in women. The tumor is characterized by rapid, painful enlargement. Rapid enlargement of the thyroid may also suggest thyroid lymphoma, particularly if found in association with Hashimoto's thyroiditis.

No effective therapy exists, and the disease is generally fatal. About 80% of patients die within 1 year of diagnosis. In a few patients with smaller tumors, thyroidectomy followed by external beam radiation therapy has been curative. Chemotherapy is mainly experimental.

RADIATION-INDUCED THYROID CANCER

Thyroid tumors develop in people exposed to large amounts of environmental thyroid radiation, as occurs from atomic bomb blasts, nuclear reactor accidents, or incidental thyroid irradiation due to radiation therapy. Tumors may be detected 10 years after exposure, but risk remains increased for 30–40 years. Such tumors are usually benign; however, about 10% are papillary thyroid carcinoma. The tumors are frequently multicentric or diffuse.

Patients who had thyroid irradiation should undergo yearly thyroid palpation, ultrasonography, and measurement of thyroid autoantibodies (to exclude Hashimoto's thyroiditis). A thyroid scan does not always reflect areas of involvement.

If ultrasonography reveals a nodule, fine-needle aspiration biopsy should be done. In the absence of suspicious or malignant lesions, many physicians recommend lifelong TSH-lowering doses of thyroid hormone to suppress thyroid function and thyrotropin secretion and possibly decrease the chance of developing a thyroid tumor.

Surgery is required if fine-needle aspiration biopsy suggests cancer. Near-total or total thyroidectomy is the treatment of choice, to be followed by radioiodine ablation of any residual thyroid tissue if a cancer is found (depending on the size, histology, and invasiveness).

Tests of Thyroid Function

Laboratory tests of thyroid function are required to assist in the diagnosis and monitoring of thyroid disease. Most laboratories offer a standard 'profile' of thyroid function tests (e.g. TSH and fT4), and perform additional tests only if these results are equivocal or the clinical circumstances require it.

Total Thyroxine and Triiodothyronine

Measurement of plasma tT4 concentration was formerly widely used as a test of thyroid function, but this test has the major disadvantage in that it is dependent on binding protein concentration as well as thyroid activity. For example, a slightly elevated plasma tT4 concentration, compatible with mild hyperthyroidism, can occur with normal thyroid function if there is an increase in plasma binding protein concentrations. With the introduction of reliable assays for fT4 there is now little, if any, justification for laboratories continuing to measure tT4 as a test of thyroid function.

Plasma total T3 (tT3) concentration is almost always raised in hyperthyroidism (usually to a proportionately greater extent than tT4, and hence it is the more sensitive test for this condition), but may be normal in hypothyroidism owing to preferential production of T3 in the thyroid and increased peripheral formation from T4. However, tT3 concentrations, like those of tT4, are dependent on the concentration of binding proteins in plasma, and their measurement has been largely superseded by measurements of fT3.

Free Thyroxine and Triiodothyronine

The measurement of free hormone concentrations poses major technical problems because the binding of free hormones in an assay, usually by an antibody, will disturb the equilibrium between bound and free hormone and cause release of hormone from binding proteins. Various techniques have been developed that allow the estimation of fT4 and fT3 concentrations in plasma. Such measurements, in theory, circumvent the problems associated with protein binding, and have rendered obsolete techniques for the indirect assessment of free hormone concentrations, such as the resin uptake test, calculation of the free thyroxine index or measurement of the T4/TBG ratio. However, with gross abnormalities of binding protein concentrations, the results of measurements of free hormones may be misleading owing to technical limitations of the assays.

In **pregnancy**, TBG concentration increases, owing to increased synthesis stimulated by estrogens, and leads to an increase in tT4. The fT4 concentration may rise slightly in early pregnancy, probably as a result of the weak thyroid-stimulating properties of chorionic gonadotrophin, but returns to normal values by 20 weeks; it may fall somewhat in the third trimester, but in most women fT4 remains within the non-pregnant reference range. Measured values should be compared with trimester-specific (and method-specific) reference ranges.

Just as the tT3 concentration can be normal in hypothyroidism (especially in mild cases), so too can the fT3 concentration, and its measurement is of no value in the diagnosis of this condition. FT3 is, however, a sensitive test for hyperthyroidism. In hyperthyroid patients, both fT4 and fT3 are usually elevated (fT3 to a proportionately greater extent), but there are exceptions to this. In a small number of patients with hyperthyroidism, the fT3 concentration is elevated, but fT4 is not (although it is usually high–normal)—a condition called 'T3 toxicosis'. Occasionally, fT4 is elevated, but not fT3. This is usually due to concomitant non-thyroidal illness resulting in decreased conversion of T4 to T3, and the fT3 concentration increases when this illness resolves. Typical results of thyroid function tests in various conditions are shown in Fig. 9.10.

Thyroid-stimulating Hormone

As the release of TSH from the pituitary is controlled through negative feedback by thyroid hormones, measurements of TSH can be used as an index of thyroid function. If primary thyroid disease is suspected and the plasma TSH concentration is normal, it can be safely inferred that the patient is euthyroid. In overt primary hypothyroidism, TSH concentrations are greatly increased, often to 10 or more times the upper limit of normal. Smaller increases are seen in borderline cases, but TSH measurement is more sensitive than T4 under these circumstances; TSH concentrations rise above the reference range before those of T4 fall below it. TSH can also increase transiently during recovery from non-thyroidal illness (see below). Plasma TSH concentrations are suppressed to very low values in hyperthyroidism, but low concentrations can also occur in individuals with subclinical hyperthyroidism and in euthyroid patients with non-thyroidal illness. Indeed, in hospital patients, a low plasma TSH concentration is more often due to non-thyroidal illness than to hyperthyroidism, while a slightly elevated concentration is as frequently due to recovery from such illness as to mild or incipient hypothyroidism.

Plasma fT4			
		High	**Normal**	**Low**

		Plasma fT4: High	**Plasma fT4: Normal**	**Plasma fT4: Low**
Plasma TSH	**High**	TSH-secreting tumor (rare) (fT3↑; TSH may be high–normal)	Borderline/Compensated hypothyroidism	Hypothyroidism (primary) recovery from sick euthyroid state
	Normal	Euthyroid with T4 autoantibodies (uncommon) thyroid hormone resistance	Euthyroid	Sick euthyroid (fT3↓) hypopituitrism (other pituitary hormones↓)
	Low	Hyperthyroidism (fT3↑)	T3 thyrotoxicosis (fT3↑) early in treatment of hyperthyroidism subclinical hyperthyroidism (fT3 N/↑)	Hypopituitarism (other pituitary hormones↓) sick euthyroid (severe) fT3↓

Fig. 9.10: The results of thyroid function tests in various conditions

Clinical biochemistry laboratories undertake large numbers of tests of thyroid function. To simplify their procedures, many adopt the approach of measuring TSH as a first-line test of thyroid function, adding other tests as required, e.g. if the concentration of TSH is found to be outside the euthyroid reference range or if there is a strong suspicion that thyroid dysfunction is secondary to pituitary disease (although, this is far less common than primary thyroid dysfunction). A combination of tests may also be required to assess patients being treated for thyroid disease, particularly in the early stages.

It should be noted that immunometric assays (such as are used for TSH) are subject to interference by naturally occurring heterophilic antibodies against the monoclonal antibodies used in the assay; such interference occurs only infrequently, but can give rise to apparently high results. When the results of assays do not accord with those expected from the patient's clinical condition, it may be prudent to repeat them using an alternative method.

Thyrotrophin-releasing Hormone Test

Plasma TSH is measured immediately before, and 20 and 60 minutes after, giving the patient 200 µg of TRH IV (Fig. 9.11), the normal response is an increase in TSH concentration of 2–20 mU/L in 20 minutes, with reversion towards the basal value at 60 minutes.

This test was formerly mainly used in the assessment of patients in whom other tests of thyroid function gave equivocal results. A normal response excludes thyroid dysfunction. The TSH response to TRH is exaggerated in hypothyroidism, even in borderline cases, while the attenuated (so-called 'flat') response characteristic of frank hyperthyroidism also occurs in incipient or borderline hyperthyroidism.

However, experience with currently available TSH assays has shown that the magnitude of the TSH response to TRH is a function of basal (unstimulated) TSH concentration (e.g. if the TSH is low, there will be no response to TRH). Measuring the TSH response to TRH provides no additional information over that provided by a basal TSH measurement. The TRH test is now mainly used in the investigation of patients with pituitary or hypothalamic disease, to assess the capacity of the pituitary to secrete TSH. TSH secretion is rarely completely lost in pituitary disease, and thus the TSH response to TRH is more usually decreased than absent and may even be normal. In hypothalamic disease, the response is characteristically (although not invariably) delayed, with the plasma TSH concentration at 60 minutes exceeding that at 20 minutes. The TRH test may also be of value in the diagnosis of TSH-secreting tumors.

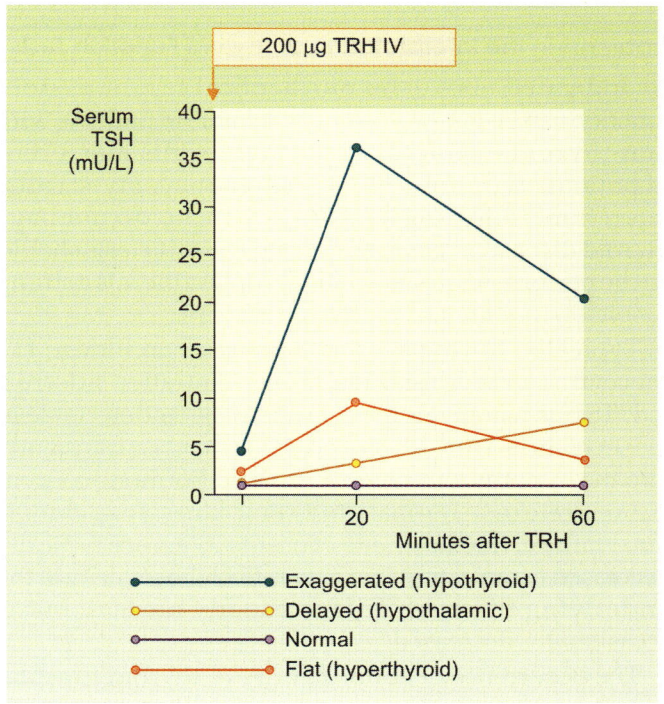

Fig. 9.11: TRH test: 200 µg is given intravenously and serum TSH is measured at 0, 20 and 60 minutes, typical responses are shown

SCREENING FOR THYROID DISEASE

Congenital hypothyroidism (usually due to thyroid agenesis or dysgenesis) is sufficiently serious and common for it to be worthwhile to screen for the condition. Untreated, affected children become cretins, with very low intelligence and impaired growth and motor function. Treatment by replacement of T4 is simple and effective, but this must be started as soon after birth as a reliable diagnosis can be made. The screening method involves measurement of TSH in a capillary blood sample collected on to a Guthrie card at 6–8 days of age. Screening for phenylketonuria and some other inherited conditions is performed at the same time. Maternal thyroxine crosses the placenta and can affect the infant's pituitary–thyroid axis for a short period after birth.

Hypothyroidism and hyperthyroidism, both are common in the elderly (more so the former), with a combined prevalence of approximately 5%. As both the conditions may present insidiously, and atypically, in the elderly, attempts have been made to screen for the conditions in this population. In practice, however, the influence of non-thyroidal illness on the results of thyroid function tests renders this a far from straightforward proposition. Furthermore, while there is evidence that the presence of a slightly raised plasma TSH together with the presence of thyroid autoantibodies indicates an increased risk of future clinical hypothyroidism, people with either one of these abnormalities alone may not be at significant risk.

Problems in the Interpretation of Thyroid Function Tests

As indicated above, no biochemical test of thyroid function can be guaranteed to be reliable in patients with **non-thyroidal illness**. Abnormal results may occur in patients with infections, malignancy, myocardial infarction, following surgery, etc., who do not have thyroid disease. In general, thyroid function tests should not be performed on such patients unless there is a strong suspicion that they have thyroid disease.

Typically, during the acute phase of an illness, fT3 concentration and, less often, fT4 concentration is decreased. TSH is usually normal, but may be undetectable in the severely ill. During recovery, TSH may rise transiently into the hypothyroid range as thyroid hormone concentrations return to normal. In chronic illness, e.g. chronic renal failure, free hormone concentrations are typically decreased (to an extent that may reflect the severity of the underlying disease); TSH is usually normal, but is occasionally decreased.

The occurrence of abnormalities of thyroid function tests in patients with non-thyroidal illness has been termed the 'sick euthyroid syndrome'. Causes include decreased peripheral conversion of T4 to T3; changes in the concentration of binding proteins (to an extent that may reveal technical limitations in the ability of free hormone assays to provide a true measurement of free hormone concentrations); increased plasma concentrations of free fatty acids, which displace thyroid hormones from their binding sites, and non-thyroidal influences on the hypothalamic-pituitary-thyroid axis, e.g. by cortisol, which can inhibit TSH secretion.

Furthermore, many drugs can influence the results of tests of thyroid function. Some examples are given in Fig. 9.12. Amiodarone is particularly noteworthy. This iodine-containing antiarrhythmic can both increase and decrease thyroid hormone synthesis and may occasionally cause clinical thyroid disease more often hypothyroidism in iodine sufficient areas and hyperthyroidism in iodine-deficient areas.

The effects of some drugs on the thyroid	
Drug	**Effect**
Corticosteroids, dopaminergic durgs	Inhibit TSH secretion
Lithium[a], iodine, carbimazole, thiouracils	Inhibit T3 and T4 secretion
Oestrogens, tamoxifen, methadone, heroin	Increase TBG
Corticosteroids, androgens	Decrease TBG
Salicylates, phenytoin	Compete with T4 for binding by TBG
β-antagonists, amiodarone[b]	Inhibit conversion of T4 to T3
Cholestyramine, aluminium hydroxide, sucralfate, ferrous sulphate, calcium salts	Impair absorption of thyroxine
Phenytoin, carbamazepine	Increase hepatic metabolism of T4 (so patients on replacement may need an increased dose

Fig. 9.12: The effects of some drugs on the thyroid. (a) Regular monitoring (6–12-monthly) of thyroid hormone concentration is mandatory for patients treated with lithium, (b) Amiodarone is an iodine-containing anti-arrhythmic drug. It can also both increase and decrease thyroid hormone synthesis and may occasionally cause clinical thyroid disease

BIBLIOGRAPHY

1. Albert DM, Rubenstein RA, Scheie HG: Tumor metastasis to the eye: II. Clinical study in infants and children. Am J Ophthalmol 63:727, 1967
2. Arvan P, Di Jeso B. Thyroglobulin structure, function, and biosynthesis. In: The Thyroid: Fundamental and Clinical Text, 9th, Braverman LE, Utiger RD (Eds), Lippincott Williams and Wilkins, Philadelphia 2005. p.77.
3. Bahn RS, Heufelder AE: Pathogenesis of Graves' ophthalmopathy. N Engl J Med 329:1468, 1993

4. Bartalena L, Marcocci C, Bogazzi F, et al. Use of corticosteroids to prevent progression of Graves' ophthalmopathy after radioiodine therapy for hyperthyroidism. N Engl J Med 321:1349, 1989

5. Bartalena L. Recent achievements in studies on thyroid hormone-binding proteins. Endocr Rev 1990; 11:47.

6. Benvenga S. Thyroid hormone transport proteins and the physiology of hormone binding. In: The Thyroid: Fundamental and Clinical Text, 9th, Braverman LE, Utiger RD (Eds), Lippincott Williams and Wilkins, Philadelphia 2005. p.97.

7. Bianco AC, Kim BW. Deiodinases: implications of the local control of thyroid hormone action. J Clin Invest 2006; 116:2571.

8. Bianco AC, Larsen PR. Intracellular pathways of iodothyronine metabolism. In: The Thyroid: Fundamental and Clinical Text, Braverman LE, Utiger RD (Eds), Lippincott Williams and Wilkins, Philadelphia 2005. p.109.

9. Boucher A, Bernard NF, Zhang ZG, et al. Nature and significance of orbital autoantigens and their corresponding autoantibodies in thyroid-associated ophthalmopathy. Autoimmunity 13:89, 1992

10. Bouzas EA, Mastorakos G, Friedman TC et al. Posterior subcapsular cataract in endogenous Cushing syndrome: an uncommon manifestation. Invest Ophthalmol Vis Sci 34: 3497, 1993

11. Brabant G, Prank K, Hoang-Vu C, et al. Hypothalamic regulation of pulsatile thyrotropin secretion. J Clin Endocrinol Metab 1991; 72:145.

12. Carlsen NL, Schroeder H, Christensen IJ, et al. Signs, symptoms, metastatic spread and metabolic behaviour of neuroblastomas treated in Denmark during the period 1943. Anticancer Res 7:465, 1987

13. Cibis GW, Freeman AI, Pang V, et al. Bilateral choroidal neonatal neuroblastoma. Am J Ophthalmol 109:445, 1990

14. Danforth E Jr, Horton ES, O'Connell M, et al. Dietary-induced alterations in thyroid hormone metabolism during overnutrition. J Clin Invest 1979; 64:1336.

15. Day RM, Carroll FD: Optic nerve involvement associated with thyroid dysfunction. Arch Ophthalmol 67:289, 1962

16. Donaldson SS, Bagshaw MA, Kriss JP: Supervoltage orbital radiotherapy for Graves' ophthalmopathy. J Clin Endocrinol Metab 37:276, 1973

17. Duntas LH. Selenium and the thyroid: a close-knit connection. J Clin Endocrinol Metab 2010; 95:5180

18. Dyess EM, Segerson TP, Liposits Z, et al. Triiodothyronine exerts direct cell-specific regulation of thyrotropin-releasing hormone gene expression in the hypothalamic paraventricular nucleus. Endocrinology 1988; 123:2291.

19. Ebner R: Botulinum toxin type A in upper lid retraction of Graves' ophthalmopathy. J Clin Neuro Ophthalmol 13: 258, 1993.

20. Elston JS, Lee JP, Powell CM, et al. Treatment of strabismus in adults with botulinum toxin A. Br J Ophthalmol 69:718, 1985.

21. Engler D, Burger AG. The deiodination of the iodothyronines and of their derivatives in man. Endocr Rev 1984; 5:151.

22. External beam radiotherapy for differentiated thyroid cancer". Am J Otolaryngol 27 (1): 24–8.

23. Feldon SE, Lee CP, Muramatsu MS, Weiner JM: Quantitative computed tomography of Graves' ophthalmopathy: extraocular muscle and orbital fat in development of optic neuropathy. Arch Ophthalmol 103:213, 1985.

24. Feldon SE, Levin L, Liu SK: Graves' ophthalmopathy: correlation of saccadic eye movements with age, presence of optic neuropathy, and extraocular muscle volume. Arch Ophthalmol 108:1568, 1990.

25. Feldon SE, Muramatsu S, Weiner JM: Clinical classification of Graves' ophthalmopathy: identification of risk factors for optic neuropathy. Arch Ophthalmol 102:1469, 1984.

26. Fells P: Management of dysthyroid eye disease. Br J Ophthalmol 75:245, 1991

27. Fells P: Thyroid-associated eye disease: Clinical management. LanceT338:29, 1991

28. Garrity JA, Fatourechi V, Bergstralh EJ, et al. Results of transantral orbital decompression in 428 patients with severe Graves' ophthalmopathy. Am J Ophthalmol 116: 533, 1993

29. Girod DA, Orcutt JC, Cummings CW: Orbital decompression for preservation of vision in Graves' ophthalmopathy. Arch Otolaryngol Head Neck Surg 119:229, 1993

30. Hallin ES, Feldon SE: Graves' ophthalmopathy: II. Correlation of clinical signs with measures derived from computed tomography. Br J Ophthalmol 72:678, 1988

31. Harnett AN, Doughty D, Hirst A, Plowman PN: Radiotherapy in benign orbital disease: II. Ophthalmic Graves' disease and orbital histiocytosis X. Br J Ophthalmol 72:289, 1988

32. Harrison's Principles of Internal Medicine, 18th edition, pp. 2934

33. Heemstra KA, Soeters MR, Fliers E, et al. Type 2 iodothyronine deiodinase in skeletal muscle: effects of hypothyroidism and fasting. J Clin Endocrinol Metab 2009; 94: 2144.

34. Hegedüs L. Thyroid size determined by ultrasound. Influence of physiological factors and non-thyroidal disease. Dan Med Bull 1990; 37:249.

35. Hennemann G, Docter R, Friesema EC, et al. Plasma membrane transport of thyroid hormones and its role in thyroid hormone metabolism and bioavailability. Endocr Rev 2001; 22:451.

36. Heufelder AE, Dutton CM, Sarkar G, et al. Detection of TSH receptor RNA in cultured fibroblasts from patients with Graves' ophthalmopathy and pretibial dermopathy. Thyroid 3:297, 1993.

37. Hollenberg AN. Regulation of thyrotropin secretion. In: The Thyroid: Fundamental and Clinical Text, 9th, Braverman LE, Utiger RD (Eds), Lippincott Williams and Wilkins, Philadelphia 2005. P. 197.

38. Hosten N, Sander B, Cordes M, et al. Graves' ophthalmopathy: MR imaging of the orbits. Radiology 172:759, 1989

39. Hu MI, Vassilopoulou-Sellin R, Lustig R, Lamont JP. "Thyroid and Parathyroid Cancers" in Pazdur R, Wagman LD, Camphausen KA, Hoskins WJ (Eds) Cancer Management: A Multidisciplinary Approach. 11 ed. 2008.

40. Hudson HL, Levin L, Feldon SE: Graves' exophthalmos unrelated to extraocular muscle enlargement: Superior rectus muscle inflammation may induce venous obstruction. Ophthalmology 98:1495, 1991

41. Jackson IM. Thyrotropin-releasing hormone. N Engl J Med 1982; 306:145.

42. Jacobson DH, Gorman CA: Endocrine ophthalmopathy: current ideas concerning etiology, pathogenesis and treatment. Endocr Rev 5:200, 1984

43. Jain IS, Dinesh K, Mohan K: Ocular and orbital metastasis from systemic malignancies. Indian J Ophthalmol 35:437, 1987

44. Jolin T. Diabetes decreases liver and kidney nuclear 3,5,3'-triiodothyronine receptors in rats. Endocrinology 1987; 120:2144.

45. Jonas JB, Huschle O, Koniszewski G et al: Intraocular pressure in patients with Cushing's disease. Graefes Arch ClinExpOphthalmol 228:407, 1990

46. Just M, Kahaly G, Higer H et al: Graves' ophthalmopathy: role of MR imaging in radiation therapy. Radiology 179: 187, 1991

47. Kaplan MM, Utiger RD. Iodothyronine metabolism in rat liver homogenates. J Clin Invest 1978; 61:459.

48. Kendall-Taylor P, Crombie AL, Stephenson AM et al: Intravenous methylprednisolone in the treatment of Graves' ophthalmopathy. Br Med J 297:1574, 1988

49. Kendler DL, Lippa J, Rootman J: The initial clinical characteristics of Graves' ophthalmopathy vary with age and sex. Arch Ophthalmol 111:197, 1993

50. Knight CL, Hoyt WF, Wilson CB: Syndrome of incipient prechiasmal optic nerve compression: progress toward early diagnosis and surgical management. Arch Ophthalmol 87:1, 1972

51. Kopp P. Thyroid hormone synthesis. In: The Thyroid: Fundamental and Clinical Text, 9th, Braverman LE, Utiger RD (Eds), Lippincott Williams and Wilkins, Philadelphia 2005. p.52.

52. Kumar V, Abbas AK, Fausto N, and Mitchel RN, "Robbins basic Pathology", Saunders, 8th ed., 2007

53. Laitt RD, Hoh B, Wakeley C et al: The value of the short tau inversion recovery sequence in magnetic resonance imaging of thyroid eye disease. Br J Radiology 67:244, 1994

54. Larkin R: Treatment of Graves' ophthalmopathy. Lance T342:941, 1993

55. Larsen PR, Silva JE, Kaplan MM. Relationships between circulating and intracellular thyroid hormones: physiological and clinical implications. Endocr Rev 1981; 2:87.

56. Leboeuf R, Perron P, Carpentier AC, et al. L-T3 preparation for whole-body scintigraphy: a randomized-controlled trial. ClinEndocrinol (Oxf) 2007; 67:839.

57. Ledingham JGG: Secondary hypertension. In Weatherall DJ, Ledingham JGG, Warrell DA (eds): Oxford Textbook of Medicine, p 1382 Oxford, Oxford University Press, 1987

58. Lim VS, Passo C, Murata Y, et al. Reduced triiodothyronine content in liver but not pituitary of the uremic rat model: demonstration of changes compatible with thyroid hormone deficiency in liver only. Endocrinology 1984; 114:280.

59. Liu AH, Juan LY, Yang AH, Chen HS, Lin HD (2006). "Anaplastic thyroid cancer with uncommon long-term survival". J Chin Med Assoc 69 (10): 489–91.

60. Lyons CJ, Rootman J: Orbital decompression for disfiguring exophthalmos in thyroid orbitopathy. Ophthalmology 101:223, 1994

61. Lyons CJ, Vickers SF, Lee JP: Botulinum toxin therapy in dysthyroid strabismus. Eye 4:538, 1990

62. Magner JA. Thyroid-stimulating hormone: biosynthesis, cell biology, and bioactivity. Endocr Rev 1990; 11:354.

63. Maia AL, Kim BW, Huang SA, et al. Type 2 iodothyronine deiodinase is the major source of plasma T3 in euthyroid humans. J Clin Invest 2005; 115:2524.

64. McCord CD: Current trends in orbital decompression. Ophthalmology 92:21, 1985

65. McLenachan J, Davies D: Glaucoma and the thyroid. Br J Ophthalmol 49:441, 1965

66. Mendel CM, Weisiger RA, Jones AL, Cavalieri RR. Thyroid hormone-binding proteins in plasma facilitate uniform distribution of thyroxine within tissues: a perfused rat liver study. Endocrinology 1987; 120:1742.

67. Miller A, Arthurs B, Boucher A et al: Significance of antibodies reactive with a 64 kDa eye muscle membrane antigen in patients with thyroid autoimmunity. Thyroid 2:197, 1992

68. Mitchell WG, Snodgrass SR: Opsoclonus-ataxia due to childhood neural crest tumors: a chronic neurologic syndrome. J Child Neurol 5:153, 1990

69. Molnar I, Balazs C: TSH binding site structures in human eye muscle fractions identified by using covalent-crosslinking. Biomed Pharmacother 46:121, 1992

70. Moreno JC, Klootwijk W, van Toor H, et al. Mutations in the iodotyrosine deiodinase gene and hypothyroidism. N Engl J Med 2008; 358:1811.

71. Moreno JC. Identification of novel genes involved in congenital hypothyroidism using serial analysis of gene expression. Horm Res 2003; 60 Suppl 3:96.

72. Morgan DC, Mason AS: Exophthalmos in Cushing's syndrome. Br Med J 2:481, 1958

73. Mourits MP, Koorneef L, Wiersinga WM et al: Clinical criteria for the assessment of disease activity in Graves' ophthalmopathy: a novel approach. Br J Ophthalmol 73: 639, 1989

74. Musarella MA, Chan HS, DeBoer G, Gallie BL: Ocular involvement in neuroblastoma: prognostic implications. Ophthalmology 91:936, 1984

75. Neigel JM, Rootman J, Belkin RI et al: Dysthyroid optic neuropathy: the crowded orbital apex syndrome. Ophthalmology 95:1515, 1988

76. Nishikawa M, Yoshimura M, Toyoda N et al: Correlation of orbital muscle changes evaluated by magnetic resonance imaging and thyroid-stimulating antibody in patients with Graves' ophthalmopathy. Acta Endocrinol 129:213, 1993

77. Numbers from National Cancer Database in the US, from Page 10 in: F. Grünwald; Biersack, H. J.; GrŸunwald, F. (2005). Thyroid cancer. Berlin: Springer. ISBN 3-540-22309-6.

78. Ohnishi T, Noguchi S, Murakami N et al: Levatorpal pebraesuperioris muscle: MR evaluation of enlargement as a cause of upper eyelid retraction in Graves' disease. Radiology 188:115, 1993

79. Panicker V, Cluett C, Shields B, et al. A common variation in deiodinase 1 gene DIO1 is associated with the relative levels of free thyroxine and triiodothyronine. J Clin Endocrinol Metab 2008; 93:3075.

80. Panicker V, Saravanan P, Vaidya B, et al. Common variation in the DIO2 gene predicts baseline psychological well-being and response to combination thyroxine plus triiodothyronine therapy in hypothyroid patients. J Clin Endocrinol Metab 2009; 94:1623.

81. Pankow BG, Michalak J, Ugee MK. Adult human thyroid weight. Health Phys 1985; 49:1097.

82. Parisi MT, Hattner RS, Matthay KK et al: Optimized diagnostic strategy for neuroblastoma in opsoclonus myoclonus. J Nucl Med 34:1922, 1993

83. Perros P, Crombie AL, Matthews JN, Kendall-Taylor P: Age and gender influence the severity of thyroid-associated ophthalmopathy: a study of 101 patients attending a combined thyroid-eye clinic. ClinEndocrinol (Oxf) 38:367, 1993

84. Perros P, Kendall-Taylor P: Antibodies to orbital tissues in thyroid-associated ophthalmopathy. Acta Endocrinol 126:137, 1992

85. Perros P, Kendall-Taylor P: Biological activity of autoantibodies from patients with thyroid-associated ophthalmopathy: In vitro effects on porcine extraocular myoblasts. Q J Med 84:691, 1992

86. Prummel MF, Mourits MP, Blank L et al: Randomized double-blind trial of prednisone versus radiotherapy in Graves' ophthalmopathy. LanceT342:949, 1993

87. Prummel MF, Wiersinga WM: Smoking and risk of Graves' disease. JAMA 269:479, 1993

88. Rotella CM, Zonefrati R, Toccafondi R et al: Ability of monoclonal antibodies to the thyrotropin receptor to increase collagen synthesis in human fibroblasts: an assay which appears to measure exophthalmogenic immunoglobulins in Graves' sera. J ClinEndocrinolMetab 62:357, 1986

89. Salmi J, Grahne B, Valtonen S, Pelkonen R: Recurrence of chromophobe pituitary adenomas after operation and postoperative radiotherapy. Acta Neurol Scand 66:681, 1982

90. Salvi M, Bernard N, Miller A et al: Prevalence of antibodies reactive with a 64 kDa eye muscle membrane antigen in thyroid-associated ophthalmopathy. Thyroid 1:207, 1991

91. Sawin CT, Hershman JM, Chopra IJ. The comparative effect of T4 and T3 on the TSH response to TRH in young adult men. J Clin Endocrinol Metab 1977; 44:273.

92. Schmidt ED, van der Gaag R, Mourits MP, Koornneef L: Site-dependent distribution of macrophages in normal human extraocular muscles. Invest Ophthalmol Vis Sci 34:2130, 1993

93. Scott WE, Thalacker JA: Diagnosis and treatment of thyroid myopathy. Ophthalmology 88:493, 1981

94. Senelick RC, Van Dyk HJL: Chromophobe adenoma masquerading as corticosteroid-responsive optic neuritis. Am J Ophthalmol 78:485, 1974

95. Shine B, Fells P, Edwards OM, Weetman AP: Association between Graves' ophthalmopathy and smoking. LanceT335:1261, 1990

96. Shupnik MA, Ridgway EC, Chin WW. Molecular biology of thyrotropin. Endocr Rev 1989; 10:459.

97. Silva JE, Leonard JL. Regulation of rat cerebrocortical and adenohypophyseal type II 5'-deiodinase by thyroxine, triiodothyronine, and reverse triiodothyronine. Endocrinology 1985; 116:1627.

98. Slansky HH, Kolbert G, Gartner S: Exophthalmos induced by steroids. Arch Ophthalmol 77:578, 1967

99. Spark RF, Baker R, Bienfang DC, Bergland R: Bromocriptine reduces pituitary tumor size and hypersecretion: requiem for pituitary surgery? JAMA 247:311, 1982

100. Spitzweg C, Heufelder AE, Morris JC. Thyroid iodine transport. Thyroid 2000; 10:321.

101. Stark B, Olivari N: Treatment of exophthalmos by orbital fat removal. ClinPlastSurg 20:285, 1993

102. Tallstedt L, Lundell G, Torring O et al: Occurrence of ophthalmopathy after treatment for Graves' hyperthyroidism: The Thyroid Study Group. N Engl J Med 326:1733, 1992

103. Tietz textbook of clinical chemistry and molecular biology 5fifth edition, Philadelphia, W.B Saunders company (2012).

104. Trobe JD, Glaser JS, Laflamme P: Dysthyroid optic neuropathy: clinical profile and rationale for management. Arch Ophthalmol 96:1199, 1978

105. Trobe JD: Optic nerve involvement in dysthyroidism. Ophthalmology 88:488, 1981

106. Trokel S, Kazim M, Moore S: Orbital fat removal: decompression for Graves' orbitopathy. Ophthalmology 100:674, 1993

107. Van der Heyden JT, Docter R, van Toor H, et al. Effects of caloric deprivation on thyroid hormone tissue uptake and generation of low-T3 syndrome. Am J Physiol 1986; 251:E156.

108. Van Herle AJ, Vassart G, Dumont JE. Control of thyroglobulin synthesis and secretion. (First of two parts). N Engl J Med 1979; 301:239.

109. Vassart G, Dumont JE. The thyrotropin receptor and the regulation of thyrocyte function and growth. Endocr Rev 1992; 13:596.

110. Wall JR, Bernard N, Boucher A et al: Pathogenesis of thyroid-associated ophthalmopathy: an autoimmune disorder of the eye muscle associated with Graves' hyperthyroidism and Hashimoto's thyroiditis. ClinImmunolImmunopathol 68:1, 1993

111. Walsh FB: Papilledema associated with increased intracranial pressure in Addison's disease. Arch Ophthalmol 47:86, 1952

112. Wass JA, Williams J, Charlesworth M et al: Bromocriptine in management of large pituitary tumours. Br Med J 284:1908, 1982

113. Weetman AP, Cohen S, Gatter KC et al: Immunohistochemical analysis of the retrobulbar tissues in Graves' ophthalmopathy. Clin Exp Immunol 75:222, 1989.

114. Weetman AP: Thyroid-associated eye disease: pathophysiology. Lance T338:25, 1991

115. Werner SC: Classification of the eye changes of Graves' disease. Am J Ophthalmol 68:646, 1969

116. Wiersinga WM: Immunosuppressive treatment of Graves' ophthalmopathy. Thyroid 2:229, 1992

117. William Marshall, MártaLapsley, Stephen K Bangert. Elsevier.com: Clinical Chemistry, 7th Edition; ISBN-9780723437031. (2012).

118. Williams TC, Kelijman M, Crelin WC, et al. Differential effects of somatostatin (SRIH) and a SRIH analog, SMS 201-995, on the secretion of growth hormone and thyroid-stimulating hormone in man. J Clin Endocrinol Metab 1988; 66:39.

119. Wilson CB: A decade of pituitary microsurgery: The Herbert Olivecrona lecture. J Neurosurg 64:814, 1984

120. Winsa B, Mandahl A, Karlsson FA: Graves' disease, endocrine ophthalmopathy and smoking. Acta Endocrinol 128: 156, 1993

121. Wu P, Lechan RM, Jackson IM. Identification and characterization of thyrotropin-releasing hormone precursor peptides in rat brain. Endocrinology 1987; 121:108.

122. Yen PM. Genomic and nongenomic actions of thyroid hormones. In: The Thyroid: Fundamental and Clinical Text, 9th, Braverman LE, Utiger RD (Eds), Lippincott Williams and Wilkins, Philadelphia 2005. p.135.

The Gonads

ANDROGENS AND TESTICULAR FUNCTION

The testes are responsible for the synthesis of the male sex hormones (androgens) and the production of spermatozoa. The most important androgen, both in terms of potency and the amount secreted, is testosterone. Other testicular androgens include androstenedione and dehydroepiandrosterone (DHEA). These weaker androgens are also secreted by the adrenal glands, but adrenal androgen secretion does not appear to be physiologically important in the male. In the female, however, it contributes to the development of certain secondary sexual characteristics, in particular the growth of pubic and axillary hair.

Regulation of the Hypothalamic–pituitary–testis Axis

Hypothalamic gonadotropin-releasing hormone (GnRH) regulates the production of the pituitary gonadotropins luteinizing hormone (LH) and follicle stimulating hormone (FSH) (Fig. 10.1). GnRH is released in discrete pulses approximately every 2 hours, resulting in corresponding pulses of LH and FSH. These dynamic hormone pulses account in part for the wide variations in LH and testosterone, even within the same individual. LH acts primarily on the Leydig cell to stimulate testosterone synthesis. The regulatory control of androgen synthesis is mediated by testosterone and estrogen feedback on both the hypothalamus and the pituitary. FSH acts on the Sertoli cell to regulate spermatogenesis and the production of Sertoli products, such as inhibin B, which acts to selectively suppress pituitary FSH. Despite these somewhat distinct Leydig and Sertoli cell-regulated pathways, testis function is integrated at several levels; GnRH regulates both gonadotropins; spermatogenesis requires high levels of testosterone; and

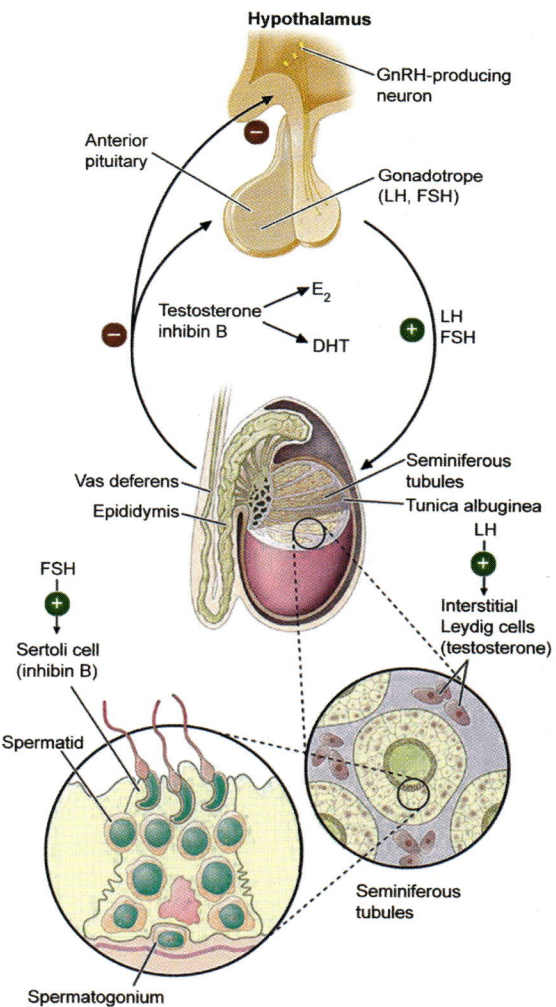

Fig. 10.1: Human pituitary gonadotropin axis, structure of testis, and seminiferous tubule. E$_2$, 17β-estradiol; DHT, dihydrotestosterone; FSH, follicle-stimulating hormones; GnRH, gonadotropin-releasing hormone; LH, luteinizing hormone

numerous paracrine interactions between Leydig and Sertoli cells are necessary for normal testis function.

The Leydig Cell: Androgen Synthesis

Luteinizing hormone (LH) binds to its seven-trans-membrane, G protein–coupled receptor to activate the cyclic adenosine monophosphate (AMP) pathway. Stimulation of the LH receptor induces steroid acute regulatory (StAR) protein, along with several steroidogenic enzymes involved in androgen synthesis. LH receptor mutations cause Leydig cell hypoplasia or agenesis, underscoring the importance of this pathway for Leydig cell development and function. The rate-limiting process in testosterone synthesis is the delivery of cholesterol by the StAR protein to the inner mitochondrial membrane. Peripheral benzodiazepine receptor, a mitochondrial cholesterol-binding protein, is also an acute regulator of Leydig cell steroidogenesis. The five major enzymatic steps involved in testosterone synthesis are summarized in Fig. 10.2. After cholesterol transport into the mitochondrion, the formation of pregnenolone by CYP11A1 (side chain cleavage enzyme) is a limiting enzymatic step. The 17α-hydroxylase and the 17, 20-lyase reactions are catalyzed by a single enzyme, CYP17; post-translational modification (phosphorylation) of this enzyme and the presence of specific enzyme cofactors confer 17, 20-lyase activity selectively in the testis and zona reticularis of the adrenal gland. Testosterone can be converted to the more potent dihydrotestosterone (DHT) by 5α-reductase, or it can be aromatized to estradiol by CYP19 (aromatase). Two isoforms of steroid 5α-reductase, SRD5A1 and SRD5A2, have been described; all known kindreds with 5α-reductase deficiency have had mutations in SRD5A2, the predominant form in the prostate and the skin.

In males, 95% of circulating testosterone is derived from testicular production. Only a small amount of DHT is secreted directly by the testis; most circulating DHT is derived from peripheral conversion of testosterone. Most of the daily production of estradiol in men is derived from aromatase-mediated peripheral conversion of testosterone and androstenedione.

Circulating testosterone is bound to two plasma proteins, i.e. sex hormone-binding globulin (SHBG) and albumin. SHBG binds testosterone with much greater affinity than albumin. Only 0.5–3% of testosterone is unbound. According to the 'free hormone' hypothesis, only the unbound fraction is biologically active; however, albumin-bound hormone dissociates readily in the capillaries and may be bioavailable. SHBG-bound testosterone also may be internalized through endocytic pits by binding to a protein called megalin. SHBG concentrations are decreased by androgens, obesity,

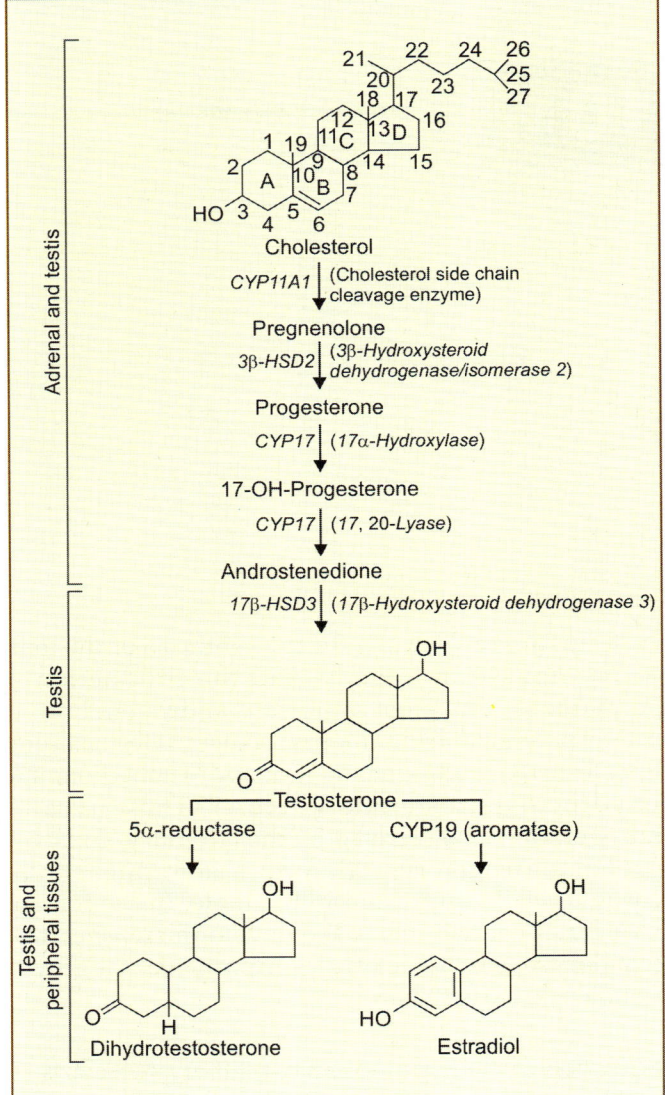

Fig. 10.2: The biochemical pathway in the conversion of 27-carbon sterol cholesterol to androgens and estrogens

diabetes mellitus, insulin, and nephrotic syndrome. Conversely, estrogen administration, hyperthyroidism, many chronic inflammatory illnesses, infections, such as HIV or hepatitis B and C, and aging are associated with high SHBG concentrations.

Testosterone is metabolized predominantly in the liver, although some degradation occurs in peripheral tissues, particularly the prostate and the skin. In the liver, testosterone is converted by a series of enzymatic steps that involve 5α- and 5β-reductases, 3α- and 3β-hydroxysteroid dehydrogenases, and 17β-hydroxysteroid dehydrogenase into androsterone, etiocholanolone, DHT, and 3 α-androstanediol. These compounds undergo glucuronidation or sulfation before being excreted by the kidneys.

Testosterone exerts some of its biologic effects by binding to androgen receptor, either directly or after its conversion to DHT by the steroid 5-α reductase. Testosterone's effects on the skeletal muscle, erythropoiesis, and bone in men do not require its obligatory conversion to DHT. However, the conversion of testosterone to DHT is necessary for the masculinization of the urogenital sinus and genital tubercle. Aromatization of testosterone to estradiol mediates additional effects of testosterone on the bone resorption, epiphyseal closure, sexual desire, vascular endothelium, and fat. DHT can also be converted in some tissues by 3-keto reductase/3β-hydroxysteroid dehydrogenase enzymes to 5α-androstane-3β, 17β-diol, which is a high-affinity ligand and agonist of estrogen receptor β.

The androgen receptor (AR) is structurally related to the nuclear receptors for estrogen, glucocorticoids, and progesterone. The AR is encoded by a gene on the long arm of the X chromosome and has a molecular mass of about 110 kDa. A polymorphic region in the amino terminus of the receptor, which contains a variable number of glutamine repeats, modifies the transcriptional activity of the receptor. The AR protein is distributed in both the cytoplasm and the nucleus. The ligand binding to the AR induces conformational changes that allow the recruitment and assembly of tissue-specific cofactors and causes it to translocate into the nucleus, where it binds to DNA or other transcription factors already bound to DNA. Thus, the AR is a ligand-regulated transcription factor that regulates the expression of androgen-dependent genes in a tissue-specific manner. Some androgen effects may be mediated by nongenomic AR signal transduction pathways. Testosterone binds to AR with half the affinity of DHT. The DHT-AR complex also has greater thermostability and a slower dissociation rate than the testosterone-AR complex. However, the molecular basis for selective testosterone versus DHT actions remains incompletely explained.

The Seminiferous Tubules: Spermatogenesis

The seminiferous tubules are convoluted, closed loops with both ends emptying into the rete testis, a network of progressively larger efferent ducts that ultimately form the epididymis (Fig. 10.1). The seminiferous tubules total about 600 m in length and comprise about two-thirds of testis volume. The walls of the tubules are formed by polarized Sertoli cells that are opposed to peritubular myoid cells. Tight junctions between Sertoli cells create a blood-testis barrier. Germ cells compose the majority of the seminiferous epithelium (~60%) and are intimately embedded within the cytoplasmic extensions of the Sertoli cells, which function as 'nurse cells.' Germ cells progress through characteristic stages of mitotic and meiotic divisions. A pool of type A spermatogonia serve as stem cells capable of self-renewal. Primary spermatocytes are derived from type B spermatogonia and undergo meiosis before progressing to spermatids that undergo spermiogenesis (a differentiation process involving chromatin condensation, acquisition of an acrosome, elongation of cytoplasm, and formation of a tail) and are released from Sertoli cells as mature spermatozoa. The complete differentiation process into mature sperm requires 74 days. Peristaltic-type action by peritubular myoid cells transports sperm into the efferent ducts. The spermatozoa spend an additional 21 days in the epididymis, where they undergo further maturation and capacitation. The normal adult testes produce >100 million sperm per day.

ESTROGENS AND OVARIAN FUNCTION
Estrogens

There are three endogenous nineteen-carbon steroids in humans that have estrogenic activity. The principal ovarian estrogens are 17β-estradiol, which is the primary circulating form, and its metabolite, estrone, which the primary postmenopausal estrogen. During pregnancy the placenta synthesizes estriol. Estrogens coordinate systemic responses during the ovulatory cycle, including regulation of the reproductive tract, pituitary, breasts, and other tissues. Also, some forms of cancer are estrogen-dependent for growth. The hypothalamic-pituitary-ovarian axis and target organs for the actions of estrogens (Fig. 10.3). Estrogens are also responsible for mediating development of secondary sex characteristics when females enter puberty, including progressive maturation of the fallopian tubes, uterus, vagina, and external genitalia. Upon estrogenic stimulation, more fat is deposited in the breast, buttocks, and thighs, leading to the normal adult female habitus.

The following are characteristics promoted by estrogens:

- Breast development by increasing ductal and stromal growth
- Body growth at puberty
- Closure of the epiphyses in the shafts of the long bones
- Synthesis and secretion of prolactin from pituitary lactotrophs
- Proliferation of uterine endometrium and stroma in the absence of progesterone, as occurs in the follicular phase of the menstrual cycle
- Thickening of the vaginal mucosa and thinning of cervical mucus
- Maintenance of bone mass

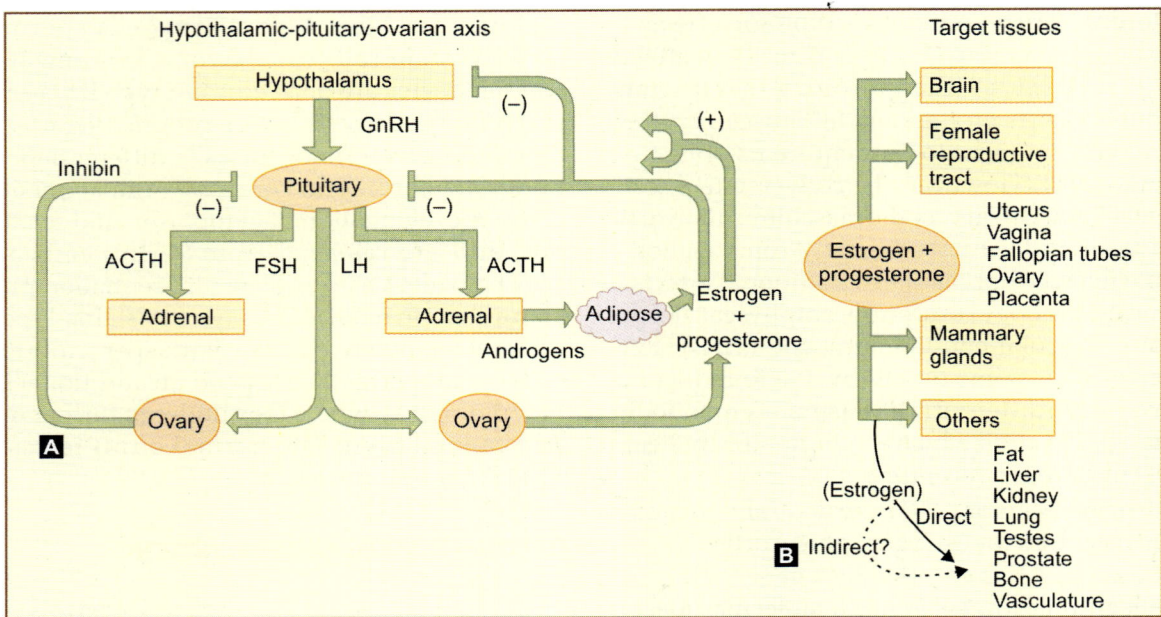

Fig. 10.3: Feedback loops and target tissues. (A) Negative and positive feedback action of estrogens and progesterone on the hypothalamic-pituitary-ovarian axis. (B) Other target tissues for these steroid hormones

- Hepatic production of sex hormone-binding globulin thyroid-binding globulin, blood-clotting factors (VII to X), plasminogen, and high-density lipoprotein (HDL)
- Inhibition of ant thrombin III and low-density lipoprotein (LDL) formation
- Retention of Na^+ and water, occasionally causing edema
- Estrogens may play a direct role in the progression of some endometrial tumors, and lifetime exposure to estrogens is associated with the greatest risk for development of breast cancer. Exposure of the uterus to estrogen without exposure to progesterone is associated with endometrial hyperplasia, episodes of breakthrough bleeding, and an approximate sevenfold increased risk of endometrial cancer.

PROGESTERONE

Estrogen priming is necessary for progesterone receptor (PGR) expression in almost all progesterone-responsive tissues, including the uterus. Progesterone concentrations rise rapidly in the luteal phase of the menstrual cycle, resulting in a modulation of the action of estrogen on the uterus. Progesterone antagonizes estrogen-induced proliferation in the uterus and initiates secretory changes in preparation for embryo implantation. In the absence of pregnancy, plasma progesterone concentrations decrease, resulting in sloughing of the endometrial lining. Progesterone is responsible for causing the increased basal body temperature observed in the luteal phase. Progesterone is important in mammary glandular development and, unlike the uterus, probably stimulates breast cell proliferation. During pregnancy, progesterone can promote maintenance of pregnancy, inhibit uterine contraction, alter carbohydrate metabolism, decrease HDL, increase LDL, and increase Na^+ and water elimination by competitive antagonism of aldosterone interaction with mineralocorticoid receptors. A variety of menstrual cycle disorders are treated with progesterone, estrogen, or both.

BIOSYNTHESIS OF ESTROGENS AND PROGESTERONE

Estrogens and progesterone are produced by steroidogenesis in various tissues. The ovary is the predominant source of these steroids in non-pregnant, premenopausal women. A significant amount of estrogenic activity is also produced by skeletal muscle, liver, and adipose tissue through the conversion of circulating androgens to estrone. Certain brain areas in males and females may also produce estrogens through the action of aromatase on circulating androgens. Small amounts of estradiol can be produced in the male testes.

During the menstrual cycle, the pituitary gonadotropins FSH and LH regulate the synthesis and release of estrogen and progesterone from the ovary. The pulsatile release of hypothalamic gonadotropin-releasing hormone, in turn, regulates FSH and LH synthesis and release. GnRH concentrations are regulated through negative and positive feedback by the steroid hormones. Estrogens and progesterone also act directly on the pituitary gonadotrophin to decrease FSH and LH concentrations. In addition, an ovarian protein, inhibin, negatively affects FSH synthesis. The pathways for the integrated control of hormone regulation are shown in Fig. 10.3.

The ovulatory-menstrual cycle normally spans 25–35 days. The steps in the ovarian and endometrial cycles are shown in Fig. 10.4. The ovarian cycle is divided into the follicular (preovulatory) phase, when ova maturation and estrogen release occurs, ovulation, when follicular rupture leads to ova release, and the postovulatory phase, when the corpus luteum maximally releases progesterone and stimulates growth of the endometrial lining. The follicle is the basic reproductive unit of the ovary and consists of an oocyte surrounded by granulosa cells. At the onset of a menstrual cycle, FSH accelerates maturation of several follicles. Through interactions with its receptor, FSH increases aromatase activity, which stimulates conversion of androgens to estradiol. By days 8–10, FSH decreases, and the dominant follicle becomes more sensitive to circulating gonadotropin because of an increased number of FSH receptors. In the late follicular phase, estradiol levels increase rapidly and initiate a mid-cycle LH surge (16–24 hours before ovulation). Increased LH levels promote follicular production of progesterone, prostaglandin $F_{2\alpha}$, and proteolytic enzymes, and ultimately, follicular rupture and ovulation occur. After ovulation, the granulosa and theca cells become the corpus luteum, which produces and releases progesterone throughout the first half of the luteal phase (10–20 ng/mL). The suppression of FSH and LH release promotes the decline of progesterone and estrogen, luteolysis, initiation of menses, and ultimately a new cycle.

During pregnancy the placenta secretes chorionic gonadotropin into the maternal circulation. The chorionic gonadotropin concentration rises rapidly after implantation and peaks in approximately 6–8 weeks. Chorionic gonadotropin maintains the corpus luteum and stimulates progesterone production, which initially maintains placental implantation and pregnancy. Sometime after the fifth week of pregnancy, the fetal-placental unit becomes the major source of circulating progesterone and estrogens, especially estriol.

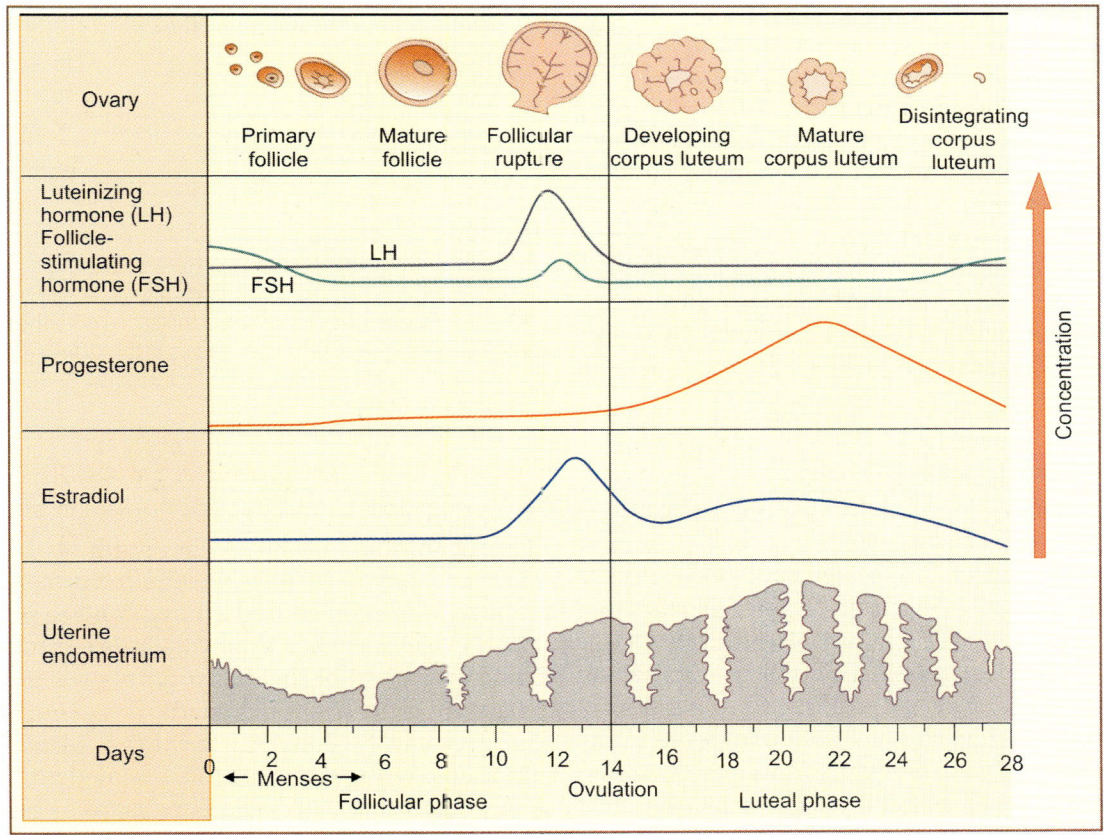

Fig. 10.4: Ovulatory and menstrual cycle. Ovarian and uterine changes that occur with the cyclical hormonal changes during the normal human menstrual cycle. Note the increase in LH, FSH, and estradiol concentrations before ovulation during the follicular phase. Progesterone rises and peaks in the midluteal phase, concomitant with reductions in LH, FSH, and estradiol

As women age, the number of follicles in the ovaries diminish, predominantly as a result of atresia. Eventually, the normal menstrual cycles cease (menopause). Without estrogen and progesterone to suppress the hypothalamic-pituitary axis, FSH, and LH levels increase. Although, adrenal androgens, predominantly androstenedione, can be converted to estrone by peripheral tissues with aromatase activity, circulating estrogen concentrations decrease to extremely low levels. This is associated with symptomology of estrogen deficiency, which can occur rapidly, whereas other symptoms (osteopenia) are delayed. The major acute symptoms include vasomotor instability (hot flashes and sweats) and vaginal atrophy, resulting in discomfort, dyspareunia, and urethral syndrome. Other symptoms, possibly related to decreased estrogen levels, include loss of concentration, loss of libido, weight gain, depression, thinning hair, joint discomfort, and sleep disruption.

TRANSPORT OF HORMONES IN THE BLOOD

Steroid hormones are highly hydrophobic molecules that must be transported by serum proteins to their target tissues. Circulating estrogens are specifically bound by SHBG, and progesterone by corticosteroid-binding globulin (CBG). These are relatively high-affinity, low-capacity interactions compared with those of albumin. The concentration of these binding globulins relative to hormone concentrations determines free hormone concentrations. Free hormone concentrations represents hormone availability to target tissues. The concentrations of the binding globulins are hormonally regulated, and the synthesis of both globulins increase in response to estrogen administration; serum albumin concentrations are unaffected. Synthetic ligands show variable affinities for these serum proteins.

Sex Hormone-binding Globulin

Sex hormone-binding globulin binds both testosterone and estradiol in the plasma, although, it has greater affinity for testosterone. The plasma concentration of SHBG in males is about half that in females. Factors that alter SHBG concentration (Table 10.1) alter the ratio of free testosterone to free estradiol. If SHBG concentration decreases, the ratio of free testosterone to free estradiol increases, although there is an absolute increase in the concentrations of both hormones. If SHBG concentration increases, the ratio decreases. Thus, in either sex, the effect of an increase in SHBG is to increase estrogen-dependent effects, while a decrease in SHBG increases androgen-dependent effects (Fig. 10.5).

Table 10.1	Factors affecting SHBG concentration
Increase	
Estrogens	
Hyperthyroidism	
Liver cirrhosis	
Decrease	
Androgens	
Hypothyroidism	
Glucocorticoids	
Malnutrition and malabsorption	
Protein losing states	
Obesity, particularly in women	

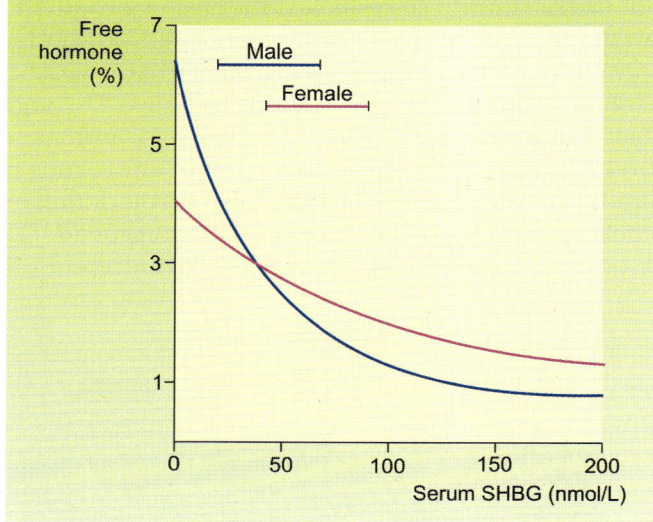

Fig. 10.5: Effect of a change in serum sex hormone-binding globulin (SHBG) concentration on free estradiol (—, magenta) and testosterone (—, blue) concentrations. A decrease in SHBG increases free testosterone concentration more than free estradiol and thus is androgenic; an increase in the concentration of SHBG is anti-androgenic. The normal ranges of SHBG in males and females are shown

DISORDERS OF MALE GONADAL FUNCTION

Delayed puberty and Hypogonadism in Males

It is uncommon for a boy to enter puberty before the age of 9 years. Boys who have not entered puberty by the age of 14 years are considered to have delayed puberty. They often present earlier than this, more often with short stature (a result of the delayed pubertal growth spurt) than with concern about gonadal development. Delayed puberty can be constitutional (i.e. idiopathic, often associated with a family history), related to chronic illness (e.g. coeliac disease, cystic fibrosis) or a consequence of hypogonadism. Delayed puberty should be investigated to diagnose any pathological disorder; constitutional delayed puberty is essentially a diagnosis of exclusion.

The term hypogonadism implies defective spermatogenesis or testosterone production or both. It can be primary (i.e. due to testicular disease) or occur secondarily to pituitary or hypothalamic disease. Primary hypogonadism is sometimes referred to as 'hypergonadotropic hypogonadism' (decreased feedback causes increased gonadotrophin secretion) and secondary hypogonadism as 'hypogonadotropic'.

The hypogonadism is a consequence of decreased gonadotrophin secretion because of either pituitary or hypothalamic disease. Some of the causes are indicated in Table 10.2. Primary hypogonadism can be due to only defective seminiferous tubule function, only defective Leydig cell function, or both. The former leads to infertility through decreased production of spermatozoa,

but masculinization is usually normal. Defective Leydig cell function, on the other hand, results in a failure of testosterone-dependent functions, including spermatogenesis. The effects of decreased testosterone secretion depend on age at the time of onset of the disorder. Secondary sexual characteristics are in part preserved if secretion is lost after puberty.

The basic biochemical characteristics that distinguish between primary and secondary hypogonadism are not always clear-cut. This is partly because most currently available assays for gonadotrophins are insufficiently sensitive to distinguish between low and normal concentrations. The plasma concentration of testosterone shows a circadian rhythm, and the usual recommendation is to measure it at 09:00 hour. Also, the secretion of

Table 10.2	Causes of male hypogonadism

Primary hypogonadism

Klinefelter syndrome. This condition results from a congenital abnormality of the sex chromosomes, X and Y. A male normally has one X and one Y chromosome. In Klinefelter syndrome, two or more X chromosomes are present in addition to one Y chromosome. The Y chromosome contains the genetic material that determines the sex of a child and related development. The extra X chromosome that occurs in Klinefelter syndrome causes abnormal development of the testicles, which in turn results in underproduction of testosterone.

Undescended testicles. Before birth, the testicles develop inside the abdomen and normally move down into their permanent place in the scrotum. Sometimes, one or both of the testicles may not be descended at birth. This condition often corrects itself within the first few years of life without treatment. If not corrected in early childhood, it may lead to malfunction of the testicles and reduced production of testosterone.

Mumps orchitis. If a mumps infection involving the testicles in addition to the salivary glands (mumps orchitis) occurs during adolescence or adulthood, long-term testicular damage may occur. This may affect normal testicular function and testosterone production.

Hemochromatosis. Too much iron in the blood can cause testicular failure or pituitary gland dysfunction affecting testosterone production.

Injury to the testicles. Because they're situated outside the abdomen, the testicles are prone to injury. Damage to normally developed testicles can cause hypogonadism. Damage to one testicle may not impair total testosterone production.

Cancer treatment. Chemotherapy or radiation therapy for the treatment of cancer can interfere with testosterone and sperm production. The effects of both treatments often are temporary, but permanent infertility may occur. Although, many men regain their fertility within a few months after treatment ends, preserving sperm before starting cancer therapy is an option that many men consider.

Secondary hypogonadism

Kallmann syndrome. Abnormal development of the hypothalamus; the area of the brain that controls the secretion of pituitary hormones; can cause hypogonadism. This abnormality is also associated with impaired development of the ability to smell (anosmia) and red-green color blindness.

Pituitary disorders. An abnormality in the pituitary gland can impair the release of hormones from the pituitary gland to the testicles, affecting normal testosterone production. A pituitary tumor or other type of brain tumor located near the pituitary gland may cause testosterone or other hormone deficiencies. Also, the treatment for a brain tumor, such as surgery or radiation therapy, may impair pituitary function and cause hypogonadism.

Inflammatory disease. Certain inflammatory diseases, such as sarcoidosis, histiocytosis and tuberculosis, involve the hypothalamus and pituitary gland and can affect testosterone production, causing hypogonadism.

HIV/AIDS. HIV/AIDS can cause low levels of testosterone by affecting the hypothalamus, the pituitary, and the testes.

Medications. The use of certain drugs, such as opiate pain medications and some hormones, can affect testosterone production.

Obesity. Being significantly overweight at any age may be linked to hypogonadism.

Normal aging. Older men generally have lower testosterone levels than younger men do. As men age, there's a slow and continuous decrease in testosterone production.

Concurrent illness. The reproductive system can temporarily shut down due to the physical stress of an illness or surgery, as well as during significant emotional stress. This is a result of diminished signals from the hypothalamus and usually resolves with successful treatment of the underlying condition.

gonadotrophins and testosterone is pulsatile, and so, ideally, when basal concentrations or the effects of chronic stimulation are to be assessed, measurements should be made on more than one occasion.

Although, biochemical tests are important in establishing that a patient has primary, rather than secondary, gonadal failure, they are less useful in distinguishing between the various causes of primary hypogonadism. In general, seminiferous tubule defects are associated with raised plasma FSH concentrations; Leydig cell defects are associated with raised plasma LH concentrations. HCG, which has an action similar to LH, can be used to test Leydig cell function (Fig. 10. 6). Semen analysis will provide an indication of seminiferous tubule function, and testicular biopsy is valuable in patients with low sperm counts if the cause is not obvious clinically. Careful clinical examination is essential in all cases of gonadal failure.

The treatment of hypogonadism in males should be directed towards the underlying cause wherever possible. Testosterone is given in testosterone deficiency syndromes, but if fertility is required treatment must be with gonadotrophin replacement or, in hypothalamic disorders, pulsatile gonadotropin-releasing hormone administration. Even in constitutional delayed puberty, a course of testosterone can be beneficial, giving a 'kick-start' to puberty, which often continues naturally thereafter. Testosterone replacement should aim to maintain plasma concentrations in the reference range for as long as possible between doses. The actual targets vary with the preparation and only apply once steady state has been reached (after a minimum of four treatments). With implants or injected long-acting testosterone the concentrations should be measured before the next dose is due, with a target range of 10–15 nmol/L; with transdermal patches or gel, 4–6 hours after application, with a target range of 15–20 nmol/L. It is prudent to check liver function tests, prostate-specific antigen (PSA), hematocrit and plasma lipid concentrations at yearly intervals. Because prostate cancer is testosterone dependent, testosterone replacement treatment should be used with caution in older men.

GYNECOMASTIA

Gynecomastia is hypertrophy of breast glandular tissue in males (Fig. 10.7); it must be differentiated from pseudogynecomastia, which is increased breast fat, but no enlargement of breast glandular tissue.

Pathophysiology

During infancy and puberty, enlargement of the male breast is normal (physiologic gynecomastia). Enlargement is usually transient, bilateral, smooth, firm, and symmetrically distributed under the areola; breasts may be tender. Physiologic gynecomastia that develops during puberty usually resolves within about 6 months to 2 years. Similar changes may occur during old age and may be unilateral or bilateral. Most of the enlargement is due to proliferation of stroma, not of breast ducts. The mechanism is usually a decrease in androgen effect or an increase in estrogen effect (e.g. decrease in androgen production, increase in estrogen production, androgen blockade, displacement of estrogen from sex hormone binding globulin, androgen receptor defects). If evaluation reveals no cause for gynecomastia, it is considered idiopathic. The cause may not be found because gynecomastia is physiologic or because there is no longer any evidence of the inciting event.

Etiology

In infants and boys, the most common cause is physiologic gynecomastia, but in men, the most common causes and the common drug causes of gynecomastia are listed in Tables 10.3 and 10.4. Breast cancer, which is uncommon in males, may cause unilateral breast abnormalities, but is rarely confused with gynecomastia.

Human chorionic gonadotrophin test	
Procedure	**Results**
Day 0: 09:00 h; take blood for testosterone; give 5000 U hCG IM	Normal response: Plasma testosterone level increases to above upper limit of reference range
Day 4: 09:00 h; take blood for testosterone	Primary testicular failure: Little or no response
	Secondary testicular failure: Response may be normal

Fig. 10. 6: A protocol for the human chorionic gonadotrophin (HCG) test for primary testicular failure

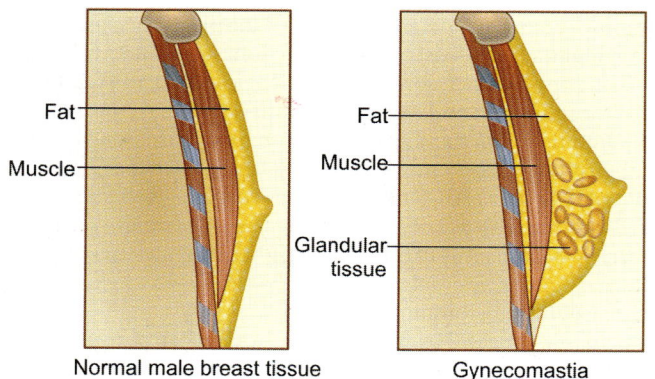

Fig. 10.7: An illustration showing the difference between normal male breast tissue and gynecomastia condition

Table 10.3	Causes of gynecomastia	
Cause	**Suggestive findings**	**Diagnostic approach**
Chronic kidney disease	History of chronic kidney disease	Serum electrolytes, BUN, and creatinine Urinalysis Possibly urine culture and urinary levels of Na, K, and creatinine
Cirrhosis	Often history of liver disease, alcohol use, or both Ascites, spider angiomas, dilated abdominal veins	Routine laboratory testing Sometimes liver biopsy
Feminizing adrenocortical tumor	Palpable mass, testicular atrophy	Imaging (MRI or CT)
Hyperthyroidism	Tremor, heat intolerance, diarrhea, tachycardia, weight loss, goiter, exophthalmos	Thyroid function tests
Hypogonadism	Prepubertal onset: Underdeveloped secondary sexual characteristics Postpubertal onset: Decreased libido, erectile dysfunction, mood changes, decreased muscle and increased fat mass, osteopenia, testicular atrophy, mild cognitive changes	Serum FSH, LH, and testosterone levels
Paraneoplastic ectopic production of human chorionic gonadotropin (hCG)	Possibly signs of primary tumor or symptoms and signs of hypogonadism	Evaluation for suspected primary tumor
Testicular tumors	Testicular mass Possibly symptoms and signs of hypogonadism	Ultrasonography
Feeding after undernutrition	Muscle and fat wasting, hair loss, skin changes, frequent infections, fatigue, signs of vitamin deficiencies (e.g. osteopenia)	Clinical evaluation Selective laboratory testing
Idiopathic gynecomastia	No abnormal findings other than gynecomastia, no symptoms, no apparent cause	Repeat clinical evaluation in 6 months Possibly serum testosterone level

FSH, follicle-stimulating hormone; LH, luteinizing hormone.

Table 10.4	Common drug causes of gynecomastia
Category	**Drugs**
Drugs that inhibit androgen synthesis or activity	Cyproterone (an antiandrogen) Dutasteride and finasteride (5α-reductase inhibitors) Goserelin, histrelin, leuprolide, and triptorelin (LH-RH agonists) Flutamide, bicalutamide, enzalutamide, and nilutamide (antiandrogens used to treat prostate cancer)
Antimicrobials	Efavirenz, ethionamide, isoniazid, ketoconazole, and metronidazole
Antineoplastic drugs	Alkylating drugs, imatinib, methotrexate, and vinca alkaloids
Cardiovascular drugs	ACE inhibitors (e.g. captopril, enalapril), amiodarone, Ca channel blockers (e.g. nifedipine, diltiazem), methyldopa, reserpine, and spironolactone
CNS-acting drugs	Diazepam, haloperidol, methadone, phenothiazines, and tricyclic antidepressants
Antiulcer drugs [†]	Cimetidine, ranitidine, and omeprazole
Hormones	Androgens, anabolic steroids, estrogens, and human growth hormone
Recreational drugs	Amphetamines, ethanol, heroin, and marijuana
OTC herbal drugs	Lavender oil, tea tree oils
Other drugs	Auranofin, diethylpropion, domperidone, metoclopramide, phenytoin penicillamine, sulindac, and theophylline

*Not all drugs that have been associated with gynecomastia have been shown to cause gynecomastia through challenge-rechallenge testing.

[†] Drugs are listed in order of frequency of association.

Signs and Symptoms

History of present illness should help clarify the duration of breast enlargement, whether secondary sexual characteristics are fully developed, the relationship between onset of gynecomastia and puberty, and the symptoms that are cause for concern include, breast tenderness and/or unusual sensitivity/pain, leakage (any type of fluid or secretion), uneven/asymmetrical breasts (one smaller and the other one larger), lump/mass, confirmed calcium deposit or calcified milk and Significant reduction if not total absence of libido.

Diagnosis

Complete examination is done including assessment of vital signs, skin, and general appearance. The neck is examined for goiter. The abdomen is examined for ascites, venous distention, and suspected adrenal masses. Development of secondary sexual characteristics (e.g. the penis, pubic hair, and axillary hair) is assessed. The testes are examined for masses or atrophy.

The breasts are examined while patients are recumbent with their hands behind the head. Examiners bring their thumb and forefinger together from opposite sides of the nipple until they meet. Any nipple discharge is noted. Lumps are assessed and characterized in terms of location, consistency, fixation to underlying tissues, and skin changes. The axilla is examined for lymph node involvement in men who have breast lumps.

Investigations that may help to establish the cause include measurement of plasma testosterone, estradiol, gonadotrophins, HCG, SHBG and prolactin, and tests of renal, liver, thyroid, adrenal and pituitary function. Karyotyping is required to diagnose Klinefelter syndrome, in which an additional X chromosome is present (47XXY). Chest and skull imaging may also be helpful.

With pseudogynecomastia, the examiner feels no resistance between the thumb and forefinger until they meet at the nipple. In contrast, with gynecomastia, a rim of tissue >0.5 cm in diameter surrounds the nipple symmetrically and is similar in consistency to the nipple itself.

Treatment

In most cases, no specific treatment is needed because gynecomastia usually remits spontaneously or disappears after any causative drug (except perhaps anabolic steroids) is stopped or underlying disorder is treated. Some clinicians try tamoxifen 10 mg by mouth twice a day if pain and tenderness are very troublesome in men or adolescents, but this treatment is not always effective. Tamoxifen may also help prevent gynecomastia in men being treated with high-dose antiandrogen (e.g. bicalutamide) therapy for prostate cancer; breast radiation therapy is an alternative. Resolution of gynecomastia is unlikely after 12 months. Thus, after 12 months, if cosmetic appearance is unacceptable, surgical removal of excess breast tissue (e.g. suction lipectomy alone or with cosmetic surgery) may be used.

DISORDERS OF FEMALE GONADAL FUNCTION

Delayed Puberty and Hypogonadism in Females

Few girls enter puberty before about 8 years of age. The great majority of girls will have entered puberty by about 13 years of age. Girls with delayed puberty usually present because of absence of breast development or amenorrhea. Girls with no breast development by the age of 13 or with primary amenorrhea after the age of 15 should be investigated further. As in boys, constitutional delayed puberty is essentially a diagnosis of exclusion. The pathological causes (Table 10.5) can be divided into hypogonadism (hypergonadotropic, i.e. primary ovarian failure; and hypogonadotropic, i.e. secondary to pituitary or hypothalamic disease) or chronic disease (e.g. coeliac disease, and chronic renal failure).

Amenorrhea

Refers to the abnormal cessation of menses. Physiologic amenorrhea exists before puberty, during pregnancy and lactation, and after menopause. However, these physiologic causes are not included in the standard amenorrhea classifications. Amenorrhea can be divided into two major groups based on presentation: primary or secondary amenorrhea.

Primary amenorrhea is the absence of menstruation in a woman who has never menstruated. Because children do not normally menstruate before puberty, the age at which primary amenorrhea is diagnosed depends on the presence or absence of secondary sexual characteristics. In the absence of increased growth or development of secondary sexual characteristics, primary amenorrhea is diagnosed when the patient has no menses by age of 13. In the presence of normal growth and development of secondary sexual characteristics, the diagnosis of primary amenorrhea is reserved for patients who have no menstruation by age of 15.

Table 10.5	Some causes of female hypogonadism
Primary (serum estradiol ↓; FSH and LH ↑)	
Congenital	
Turner's syndrome (45XO), Noonan's syndrome (46XX)	
Acquired	
Chemotherapy and radiotherapy	
Secondary (serum estradiol ↓; FSH and LH ↓ or normal)	
The secondary causes of male hypogonadism	

Secondary amenorrhea refers to cessation of menses after establishment of menstruation for reasons other than pregnancy, lactation, or menopause. By convention, the diagnosis is applied after menses have been absent for a length of time equivalent to at least 3 of the previous menstrual cycle intervals or 6 months.

Pathophysiology

Normally, the hypothalamus generates pulses of gonadotropin-releasing hormone. GnRH stimulates the pituitary to produce gonadotropins FSH and LH, which are released into the bloodstream. Gonadotropins stimulate the ovaries to produce estrogen (mainly estradiol), androgens (mainly testosterone), and progesterone. These hormones do the following:

- **FSH** stimulates tissues around the developing oocytes to convert testosterone to estradiol.
- Estrogen stimulates the endometrium, causing it to proliferate.
- **LH** when it surges during the menstrual cycle, promotes maturation of the dominant oocyte, release of the oocyte, and formation of the corpus luteum, which produces progesterone.
- **Progesterone** changes the endometrium into a secretory structure and prepares it for egg implantation (endometrial decidualization).

If pregnancy does not occur, estrogen and progesterone production decreases, and the endometrium breaks down and is sloughed during menses. Menstruation occurs 14 days after ovulation in typical cycles.

When part of this system malfunctions, ovulatory dysfunction occurs; the cycle of gonadotropin-stimulated-estrogen production and cyclic endometrial changes is disrupted, resulting in anovulatory amenorrhea, and menstrual flow may not occur. Most amenorrhea, particularly secondary amenorrhea, is anovulatory.

However, amenorrhea can occur when ovulation is normal, as occurs when genital anatomic abnormalities prevent normal menstrual flow despite normal hormonal stimulation.

Etiology

Amenorrhea is usually classified as anovulatory and ovulatory, each type has many causes (Tables 10.6 and 10.7, but overall, the most common causes of amenorrhea include:

- Pregnancy (the most common cause in women of reproductive age)
- Constitutional delay of puberty
- Functional hypothalamic anovulation (e.g. due to excessive exercise, eating disorders, or stress)
- Use or abuse of drugs (e.g. oral contraceptives, depo-progesterone, antidepressants, antipsychotics)
- Breastfeeding
- Polycystic ovary syndrome

Contraceptives can cause the endometrium to thin, sometimes resulting in amenorrhea; menses usually begin again about 3 months after stopping oral contraceptives.

Antidepressants and antipsychotics can elevate prolactin, which stimulates the breasts to produce milk and can cause amenorrhea.

Some disorders can cause ovulatory or anovulatory amenorrhea. Congenital anatomic abnormalities cause only primary amenorrhea. All disorders that cause secondary amenorrhea can cause primary amenorrhea.

ANOVULATORY AMENORRHEA

The most common causes involve a disruption of the hypothalamic-pituitary-ovarian axis. The, causes include are listed in Table 10.6. Anovulatory amenorrhea is usually secondary, but may be primary if ovulation never begins (e.g. because of a genetic disorder). If ovulation never begins, puberty and development of secondary sexual characteristics are abnormal. Genetic disorders that confer a Y chromosome increase the risk of ovarian germ cell cancer.

Ovulatory Amenorrhea

The most common causes include; chromosomal abnormalities and congenital anatomic genital abnormalities that obstruct menstrual flow (Table 10.7).

Table 10.6	Causes of anovulatory amenorrhea
Cause	**Examples**
Hypothalamic dysfunction, structural	Genetic disorders (e.g. congenital gonadotropin-releasing hormone deficiency, GnRH receptor gene mutations that result in low FSH and estradiol levels and a high LH level, Prader-Willi syndrome)
	Infiltrative disorders of the hypothalamus (e.g. Langerhans cell granulomatosis, lymphoma, sarcoidosis, TB)
	Irradiation to the hypothalamus
	Traumatic brain injury
	Tumors of the hypothalamus

Contd.

Table 10.6	Causes of anovulatory amenorrhea *(Contd.)*
Cause	**Examples**
Hypothalamic dysfunction, functional	Cachexia
	Chronic disorders, particularly respiratory, GI, hematologic, renal, or hepatic (e.g. Crohn's disease, cystic fibrosis, sickle cell disease, thalassemia major)
	Dieting
	Drug abuse (e.g. of alcohol, cocaine, marijuana, or opioids)
	Eating disorders (e.g. anorexia nervosa, bulimia)
	Exercise, if excessive HIV infection immunodeficiency
	Psychiatric disorders (e.g. stress, depression, obsessive-compulsive disorder, schizophrenia)
	Psychoactive drugs
	Under nutrition
Pituitary dysfunction	Aneurysms of the pituitary
	Hyperprolactinemia*
	Idiopathic hypogonadotropic hypogonadism
	Infiltrative disorders of the pituitary (e.g. hemochromatosis, Langerhans cell granulomatosis, sarcoidosis, TB)
	Isolated gonadotropin deficiency
	Kallmann syndrome (hypogonadotropic hypogonadism with anosmia)
	Postpartum pituitary necrosis (Sheehan syndrome)
	Traumatic brain injury
	Tumors of the brain (e.g. meningioma, craniopharyngioma, gliomas) tumors of the pituitary (e.g. microadenoma)
Ovarian dysfunction	Autoimmune disorders (e.g. autoimmune oophoritis as may occur in myasthenia gravis, thyroiditis, or vitiligo)
	Chemotherapy (e.g. high-dose alkylating drugs)
	Genetic abnormalities, including chromosomal abnormalities (e.g. congenital thymic aplasia, Fragile X syndrome, Turner syndrome [45,X], idiopathic accelerated ovarian follicular atresia)
	Gonadal dysgenesis (incomplete ovarian development, sometimes secondary to genetic disorders)
	Irradiation to the pelvis metabolic disorders (e.g. Addison's disease, diabetes mellitus, galactosemia) viral infections (e.g. mumps)
Other endocrine dysfunction	Androgen insensitivity syndrome (testicular feminization), congenital adrenal virilism (congenital adrenal hyperplasia, e.g. due to 17-hydroxylase deficiency or 17,20-lyase deficiency) or adult-onset adrenal virilism[†]
	Cushing's syndrome[†,‡]
	Drug-induced virilization (e.g. by androgens, antidepressants, danazol, or high-dose progesterone)[†]
	Hyperthyroidism
	Hypothyroidism
	Obesity (which causes excess extraglandular production of estrogen)
	Polycystic ovary syndrome[†]
	True hermaphroditism[†]
	Tumors producing androgens (usually ovarian or adrenal)[†]
	Tumors producing estrogens or tumors producing human chorionic gonadotropin (gestational trophoblastic disease)

*Hyperprolactinemia due to other conditions (e.g. hypothyroidism, use of certain drugs) may also cause amenorrhea.

[†]Females with these disorders may have virilization or ambiguous genitals.

[‡]Virilization may occur in Cushing's syndrome secondary to an adrenal tumor.

Table 10.7	Causes of ovulatory amenorrhea
Cause	**Examples**
Congenital genital abnormalities	Cervical stenosis (rare)
	Imperforate hymen
	Pseudohermaphroditism
	Transverse vaginal septum
	Vaginal or Uterine aplasia (e.g. Müllerian agenesis)
Acquired uterine abnormalities	Asherman syndrome
	Endometrial TB
	Obstructive fibroids and polyps

Obstructive abnormalities are usually accompanied by normal hormonal function. Such obstruction may result in hematocolpos (accumulation of menstrual blood in the vagina), which can cause the vagina to bulge, or in hematometra (accumulation of blood in the uterus), which can cause uterine distention, a mass, or bulging of the cervix. Because ovarian function is normal, external genital organs and other secondary sexual characteristics develop normally. Some congenital disorders (e.g. those accompanied by vaginal aplasia or a vaginal septum) also cause urinary tract and skeletal abnormalities.

Some acquired anatomic abnormalities, such as endometrial scarring after instrumentation for postpartum hemorrhage or infection (Asherman syndrome), cause secondary ovulatory amenorrhea.

Diagnosis

Hormonal causes of amenorrhea requires basal measurements of plasma FSH, LH, and prolactin concentrations. A high FSH concentration is indicative of ovarian failure (and is more sensitive in this respect than LH). If LH, but not FSH, is elevated, and the patient is not pregnant, the most likely diagnosis is polycystic ovary syndrome (PCOS), and pelvic ultrasonography should be performed. If LH and FSH concentrations are normal or low, a pituitary or hypothalamic disorder should be sought, by anatomical studies and dynamic testing of the hypothalamo-pituitary axis in a manner similar to that described for male hypogonadism. As in males, however, the results of such tests do not always distinguish between pituitary and hypothalamic disorders.

If girls have secondary sexual characteristics, a pregnancy test should be done to exclude pregnancy and gestational trophoblastic disease as a cause of amenorrhea. Women of reproductive age should have a pregnancy test after missing one menses.

The approach to primary amenorrhea (Fig. 10.8 evaluation of primary amenorrhea) differs from that to secondary amenorrhea (Fig. 10.9, evaluation of secondary amenorrhea), although no specific general approaches or algorithms are universally accepted.

If patients have primary amenorrhea and normal secondary sexual characteristics, testing should begin with pelvic ultrasonography to check for congenital anatomic genital tract obstruction.

If symptoms or signs suggest a specific disorder, specific tests may be indicated regardless of what an algorithm recommends. For example, patients with abdominal striae, moon facies, a buffalo hump, truncal obesity, and thin extremities should be tested for Cushing's syndrome. Patients with headaches and visual field defects or evidence of pituitary dysfunction require brain MRI.

If clinical evaluation suggests a chronic disease, liver and kidney function tests are done, and ESR is determined.

Often, testing includes measurement of hormone levels; total serum testosterone or dehydroepiandrosterone sulfate (DHEAS) levels are measured only if signs of virilization are present. Certain hormone levels should be remeasured to confirm the results. For example, if serum prolactin is high, it should be remeasured; if serum FSH is high, it should be remeasured monthly at least twice. Amenorrhea with high FSH levels (hypergonadotropic hypogonadism) suggests ovarian dysfunction; amenorrhea with low FSH levels (hypogonadotropic hypogonadism) suggests hypothalamic or pituitary dysfunction.

If patients have secondary amenorrhea without virilization and have normal prolactin and FSH levels and normal thyroid function, a trial of estrogen and a progestogen to try to stimulate withdrawal bleeding can be done (progesterone challenge test).

The progesterone challenge test begins by giving medroxyprogesterone 5–10 mg by mouth once a day or another progestin for 7–10 days.

- If bleeding occurs, amenorrhea is probably not caused by an endometrial lesion (e.g. Asherman syndrome) or outflow tract obstruction, and the cause is probably hypothalamic-pituitary dysfunction, ovarian insufficiency, or estrogen excess.
- If bleeding does not occur, an estrogen (e.g. conjugated equine estrogen 1.25 mg, estradiol 2 mg) once a day is given for 21 days, followed by medroxyprogesterone 10 mg by mouth once a day or another progestin for 7–10 days. If bleeding does not occur after estrogen is given, patients may have an endometrial lesion or outflow tract obstruction. However, bleeding may not occur in patients who do not have these abnormalities (e.g. because the uterus is insensitive to estrogen); thus, the trial using estrogen and progestin may be repeated for confirmation.

However, because this trial takes weeks and results can be inaccurate, diagnosis of some serious disorders may be delayed significantly; thus, brain MRI should be considered before or during the trial.

Mildly elevated levels of testosterone or DHEAS suggest polycystic ovary syndrome, but levels can be elevated in women with hypothalamic or pituitary dysfunction and are sometimes normal in hirsute women with polycystic ovary syndrome. The cause of elevated levels can sometimes be determined by measuring serum LH. In polycystic ovary syndrome, circulating LH levels are often increased, increasing the ratio of LH to FSH.

Treatment

Treatment is directed at the underlying disorder; with such treatment, menses sometimes resume. For example, most abnormalities obstructing the genital outflow tract are surgically repaired.

If a Y chromosome is present, bilateral oophorectomy is recommended because risk of ovarian germ cell cancer is increased.

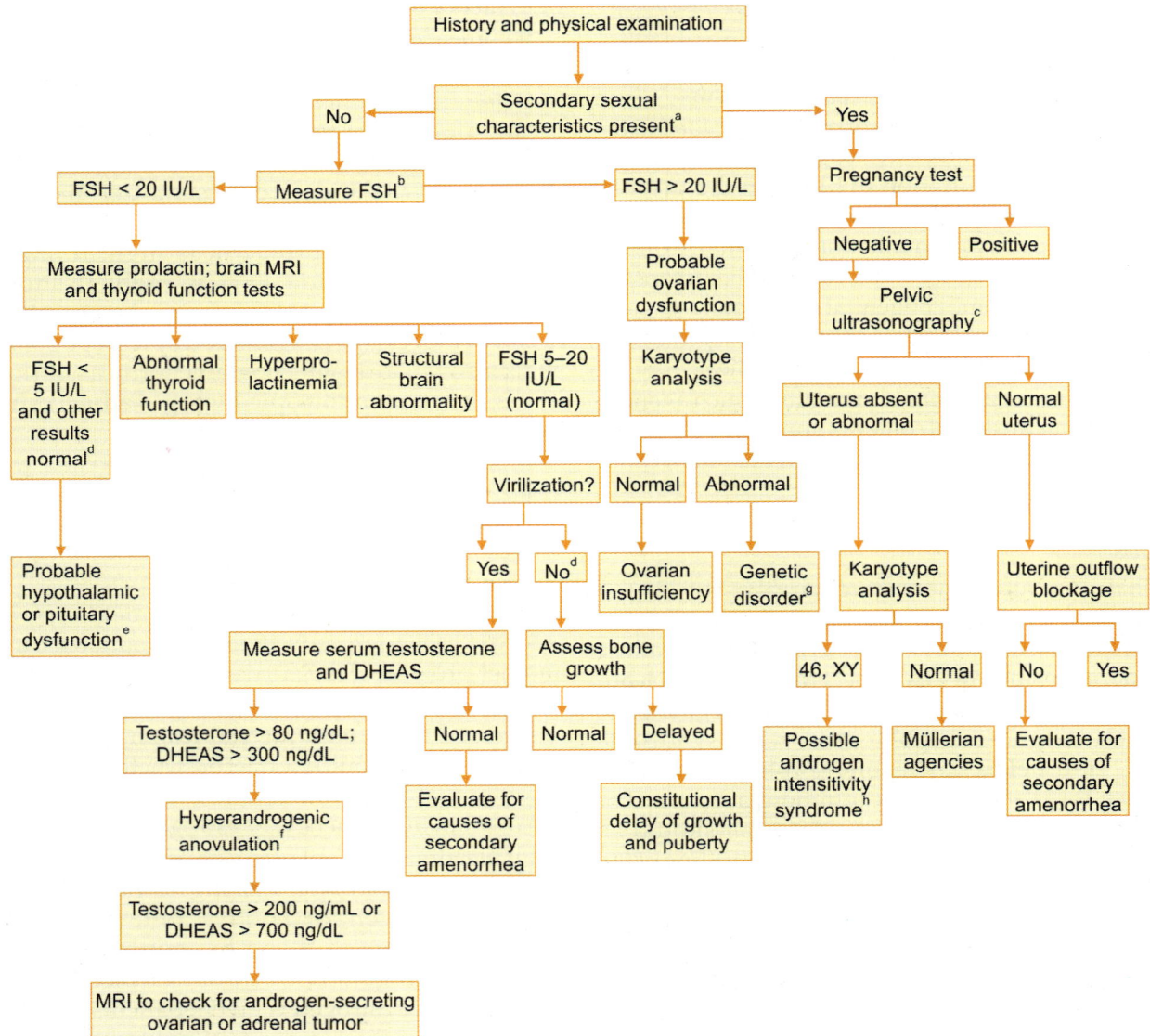

Fig. 10.8: Evaluation of primary amenorrhea, (a) Normal values are; DHEAS: 0.7–0.8 µmol/L, FSH: 5–20 IU/L, LH: 5–40 IU/L, karyotype (female): 46,XX, prolactin: 100 ng/mL and testosterone: 0.7–2.8 nmol/L. (b) some clinicians measure LH levels when they measure FSH levels or when FSH levels are equivocal. (c) If patients have primary amenorrhea and normal secondary sexual characteristics, testing should begin with pelvic ultrasonography to check for congenital anatomic genital tract obstruction. (d) Constitutional delay of growth and puberty is possible. (e) Possible diagnoses include functional hypothalamic chronic anovulation and genetic disorders (e.g. congenital gonadotropin-releasing hormone deficiency, Prader-Willi syndrome). (f) Possible diagnoses include Cushing's syndrome, exogenous androgens, congenital adrenal virilism, and polycystic ovary syndrome. (g) Possible diagnoses include Turner syndrome and disorders characterized by Y chromosome material. (h) Pubic hair may be sparse

pregnancies, can be used to determine whether a fetus is growing normally. The best approach is to compare two serum β-HCG values, obtained 48–72 hours apart and measured by the same laboratory. In a normal single pregnancy, β-HCG levels double about every 1.4–2.1 days during the first 60 days (7.5 weeks), then begin to decrease between 10 weeks and 18 weeks. Regular doubling of the β-HCG level during the first trimester strongly suggests normal growth.

MATERNAL MONITORING

Diabetes

Diabetes during pregnancy increases fetal and maternal morbidity and mortality. Neonates are at risk of respiratory distress, hypoglycemia, hypocalcemia, hyperbilirubinemia, polycythemia, and hyperviscosity. Poor control of preexisting or gestational diabetes during organogenesis (up to about 10 weeks gestation) increases risk of major congenital malformations and spontaneous abortion. Poor control of diabetes later in pregnancy increases risk of fetal macrosomia (usually defined as fetal weight >4000 g or >4500 g at birth), preeclampsia, spontaneous abortion, and shoulder dystocia. However, gestational diabetes can result in fetal macrosomia even if blood glucose is kept nearly normal.

Strict control of diabetes mellitus is vital, for both maternal and fetal health, and entails frequent monitoring of glycated hemoglobin and blood glucose concentrations. Pregnancy can adversely affect maternal glucose homoeostasis; insulin requirements in patients; with type 1 diabetes may increase during pregnancy; patients with type 2 diabetes are usually treated with insulin.

Urine should be tested for proteinuria (and blood pressure measured) at all clinic attendances. The use of urine dipsticks for multiple analytes often means that glucose is checked too; the renal threshold for glucose; is decreased during pregnancy, but if more than a trace of glycosuria is detected, it is advisable to perform a formal test of glucose tolerance. Women with a high risk of gestational diabetes should have a measurement of blood glucose concentration at booking, and all women at 28 weeks. Diabetes diagnosed during pregnancy is termed 'gestational diabetes'. Patients with gestational diabetes are usually treated with insulin during pregnancy, but should have a glucose tolerance test 6 weeks after delivery because glucose tolerance may revert to normal, although even when it does, the woman is at increased risk of developing diabetes in the future.

Preeclampsia

Preeclampsia and eclampsia develop after 20 weeks gestation; up to 25% of cases develop postpartum, most often within the first 4 days, but sometimes up to 6 weeks postpartum.

Untreated preeclampsia usually smolders for a variable time, then suddenly progresses to eclampsia, which occurs in 1/200 patients with preeclampsia. Untreated eclampsia is usually fatal.

Pathophysiology of preeclampsia and eclampsia is poorly understood. Factors may include poorly developed uterine placental spiral arterioles (which decrease uteroplacental blood flow during late pregnancy), a genetic abnormality on chromosome 13, immunologic abnormalities, and placental ischemia or infarction. Lipid peroxidation of cell membranes induced by free radicals may contribute to preeclampsia.

Fetal growth restriction or death may result. Diffuse or multifocal vasospasm can result in maternal ischemia, eventually damaging multiple organs, particularly the brain, kidneys, and liver. Factors that may contribute to vasospasm include decreased prostacyclin (an endothelium-derived vasodilator), increased endothelin (an endothelium-derived vasoconstrictor), and increased soluble Flt-1 (a circulating receptor for vascular endothelial growth factor). Women who have preeclampsia are at risk of abruptio placentae in the current and in future pregnancies, possibly because both the disorders are related to uteroplacental insufficiency.

The coagulation system is activated, possibly secondary to endothelial cell dysfunction, leading to platelet activation. The HELLP syndrome (hemolysis, elevated liver function tests, and low platelet count) develops in 10–20% of women with severe preeclampsia or eclampsia; this incidence is about 100 times that for all pregnancies (1–2/1000). Most pregnant women with this syndrome have hypertension and proteinuria, but some have neither.

Preeclampsia may be asymptomatic or may cause edema or excessive weight gain. Nondependent edema, such as facial or hand swelling (the patient's ring may no longer fit her finger), is more specific than dependent edema. Reflex reactivity may be increased, indicating neuromuscular irritability, which can progress to seizures (eclampsia). Petechiae may develop, as may other signs of coagulopathy.

Severe preeclampsia may cause organ damage; manifestations may include headache, visual disturbances, confusion, and epigastric or right upper quadrant abdominal pain (reflecting hepatic ischemia or capsular distention), nausea, vomiting, dyspnea [reflecting pulmonary edema, acute respiratory distress syndrome (ARDS), or cardiac dysfunction secondary to increased afterload], stroke (rarely), and oliguria (reflecting decreased plasma volume or ischemic acute tubular necrosis).

Diagnosis is suggested by symptoms or presence of hypertension, defined as systolic BP >140 mmHg, diastolic BP >90 mmHg, or both. Except in emergencies, hypertension should be documented in >2 measurements taken at least 4 hours apart. Urine protein excretion is measured in a 24 hours collection. Proteinuria is defined as >300 mg/24 hours. Alternatively, proteinuria is diagnosed based on a protein; creatinine ratio ≥0.3 or a dipstick-reading of 1+ (used only if other quantitative methods are not available). Absence of proteinuria on less accurate tests (e.g. urine dipstick testing, routine urinalysis) does not rule out preeclampsia. At present, there is no way to cure preeclampsia. Sometimes, medication is needed to control blood pressure and prevent convulsions, and the woman may benefit from resting. The only cure is to deliver the baby and the placenta.

Fetal Monitoring

The antenatal diagnosis of inherited metabolic disease in early pregnancy and the use of maternal serum α-fetoprotein measurements to screen for neural tube defects.

Fetal blood can be obtained antenatally by cordocentesis, the aspiration of fetal blood from the umbilical cord under ultrasound control. Analysis of fetal blood for blood gases, hydrogen ion concentration and lactate can aid in the assessment of fetal well-being when non-invasive studies (e.g. ultrasonic determination of umbilical artery blood flow) suggest that the fetus is at risk. Fetal tissue obtained earlier in pregnancy can also be used in the antenatal diagnosis of inherited disease.

Premature babies are at risk of developing respiratory distress due to lack of surfactant. This is a mixture of phospholipids, including lecithin and sphingomyelin, which lowers the surface tension of the alveoli and facilitates the expansion and aeration of the fetal lungs at birth. The concentration of lecithin in amniotic fluid reflects production by fetal lungs. It increases rapidly after 32–34 weeks gestation, corresponding to increasing fetal lung maturity and decreasing risk of development of respiratory distress. Surfactant synthesis can be stimulated by giving corticosteroids to the mother, and this is now routine practice when elective premature delivery is planned for any reason. Natural and synthetic surfactants are available for use in the baby immediately after birth.

Fetal fibronectin is a protein that is involved in attaching the fetal sac to the uterine lining. It is normally present in cervicovaginal secretions up to 22 weeks of gestation, but then disappears until the end of the third trimester. Detection of fetal fibronectin in these secretions during weeks 22–34 in high-risk pregnancies may indicate the possibility of a preterm delivery, although the test is more useful if it is negative, when it is a reliable indicator that preterm delivery will not occur in the next 2 weeks.

During labour, once the cervix is sufficiently dilated, fetal blood hydrogen ion concentration can be measured in capillary samples obtained from the scalp. A concentration of >60 nmol/L (pH <7.22) suggests potentially dangerous fetal hypoxemia. A continuous, direct measurement of fetal PO_2 can be made using a transcutaneous oxygen electrode.

METABOLIC EFFECTS OF ORAL CONTRACEPTIVES

Oral contraceptives contain either a combination of an estrogen and a progestagens or a progestagens alone. In addition to suppressing ovulation, these contraceptives have a number of metabolic effects similar to some of those that occur in normal pregnancy. There has been considerable interest in the effects of oral contraceptives on plasma lipid concentrations, and hence on cardiovascular risk. The precise effects depend on the agents used. In general, combined oral contraceptives tend slightly to lower plasma low-density lipoprotein concentrations and raise high-density lipoprotein concentrations. There is no increase in cardiovascular risk in normotensive women who do not smoke. There is a slightly increased risk of venous thromboembolic disease, but the absolute risk is very low, and lower than that associated with pregnancy. There is no increase in cardiovascular or thromboembolic disease associated with progestagens only contraception.

BIBLIOGRAPHY

1. Adams J, Polson DW, Franks S. Prevalence of polycystic ovaries in women with anovulation and idiopathic hirsutism. Br Med J (Clin Res Ed) 1986; 293:355.
2. Aitken DA, Wallace EM, Crossley JA, Swanston IA, van Pareren Y, van Maarle M, et al. Dimeric inhibin A as a marker for Down's syndrome in early pregnancy. N Engl J Med 1996; 334: 1231–1236.
3. Alexander E. K., Marqusee E., Lawrence J., Jarolim P., Fischer G. A., Larsen P. R. (2004). Timing and magnitude of increases in levothyroxine requirements during pregnancy in women with hypothyroidism. N. Engl. J. Med. 351 241–249 10.
4. Anderson G. D. (2005). Pregnancy-induced changes in pharmacokinetics: a mechanistic-based approach. Clin. Pharmacokinet.
5. Avis NE, Brambilla D, McKinlay SM, Vass K. A longitudinal analysis of the association between menopause and depression. Results from the Massachusetts Women's Health Study. Ann Epidemiol 1994; 4:214.
6. Azziz R, Carmina E, Sawaya ME. Idiopathic hirsutism. Endocr Rev 2000; 21:347.

7. Azziz R, Sanchez LA, Knochenhauer ES, et al. Androgen excess in women: experience with over 1000 consecutive patients. J ClinEndocrinolMetab 2004; 89:453.

8. Bader R. A., Bader M. G., Rose D. J., Braunwald E. (1955). Hemodynamics at rest and during exercise in normal pregnancy as studied by cardiac catheterization. J. Clin. Invest. 34 1524–1536 10.

9. Baldwin G. R., Moorthi D. S., Whelton J. A., MacDonnell K. F. (1977). New lung functions in pregnancy. Am. J. Obstet. Gynecol. 127 235–239.

10. Barnabei VM, Cochrane BB, Aragaki AK, et al. Menopausal symptoms and treatment-related effects of estrogen and progestin in the Women's Health Initiative. ObstetGynecol 2005; 105:1063.

11. Barron W. M., Lindheimer M. D. (1984). Renal sodium and water handling in pregnancy. Obstet. Gynecol. Annu. 13 35–69.

12. Bernard DJ, Chapman SC, Woodruff TK. Mechanisms of inhibin signal transduction. Recent ProgHorm Res 2001; 56: 417–450.

13. Bilezikjian LM, Corrigan AZ, Blount AL, Chen Y, Vale WW. Regulation and actions of Smad7 in the modulation of activin, inhibin, and transforming growth factor-β signaling in anterior pituitary cells. Endocrinology 2001;142: 1065–1072.

14. Black A, Francoeur D, Rowe T, et al. SOGC clinical practice guidelines: Canadian contraception consensus. J Obstet Gynaecol Can 2004; 26:219.

15. Blümel JE, Chedraui P, Baron G, et al. Menopause could be involved in the pathogenesis of muscle and joint aches in mid-aged women. Maturitas 2013; 75:94.

16. Broer SL, Eijkemans MJ, Scheffer GJ, et al. Anti-mullerian hormone predicts menopause: a long-term follow-up study in normoovulatory women. J ClinEndocrinolMetab 2011; 96:2532.

17. Bromberger JT, Assmann SF, Avis NE, et al. Persistent mood symptoms in a multiethnic community cohort of pre- and perimenopausal women. Am J Epidemiol 2003; 158:347.

18. Bromberger JT, Meyer PM, Kravitz HM, et al. Psychologic distress and natural menopause: a multiethnic community study. Am J Public Health 2001; 91:1435.

19. Bromberger JT, Schott LL, Kravitz HM, et al. Longitudinal change in reproductive hormones and depressive symptoms across the menopausal transition: results from the Study of Women's Health Across the Nation (SWAN). Arch Gen Psychiatry 2010; 67:598.

20. Burger HG, Hale GE, Dennerstein L, Robertson DM. Cycle and hormone changes during perimenopause: the key role of ovarian function. Menopause 2008; 15:603.

21. Burger HG. Unpredictable endocrinology of the menopause transition: clinical, diagnostic and management implications. Menopause Int 2011; 17:153.

22. Capeless E. L., Clapp J. F. (1991). When do cardiovascular parameters return to their preconception values? Am. J. Obstet. Gynecol. 165 883–886 10.

23. Cappell M., Garcia A. (1998). Gastric and duodenal ulcers during pregnancy. Gastroenterol. Clin. North Am. 27 169–195.

24. Carbillon L., Uzan M., Uzan S. (2000). Pregnancy, vascular tone, and maternal hemodynamics: a crucial adaptation. Obstet. Gynecol. Surv. 55 574–581.

25. Carmina E, Koyama T, Chang L, et al. Does ethnicity influence the prevalence of adrenal hyperandrogenism and insulin resistance in polycystic ovary syndrome? Am J Obstet Gynecol 1992; 167:1807.

26. Carmina E, Rosato F, Jannì A, et al. Extensive clinical experience: relative prevalence of different androgen excess disorders in 950 women referred because of clinical hyperandrogenism. J Clin Endocrinol Metab 2006; 91:2.

27. Carter B. L., Garnett W. R., Pellock J. M., Stratton M. A., Howell J. R. (1981). Effect of antacids on phenytoin bioavailability. Ther. Drug. Monit. 3 333–340.

28. Chetkowski RJ, DeFazio J, Shamonki I, et al. The incidence of late-onset congenital adrenal hyperplasia due to 21-hydroxylase deficiency among hirsute women. J Clin Endocrinol Metab 1984; 58:595.

29. Chlebowski RT, Cirillo DJ, Eaton CB, et al. Estrogen alone and joint symptoms in the Women's Health Initiative randomized trial. Menopause 2013; 20:600.

30. Clark S. L., Cotton D. B., Lee W., Bishop C., Hill T., Southwick J., et al. (1989). Central hemodynamic assessment of normal term pregnancy. Am. J. Obstet. Gynecol. 161 1439–1442.

31. Clements J. A., Heading R. C., Nimmo W. S., Prescott L. F. (1978). Kinetics of acetaminophen absorption and gastric emptying in man. Clin. Pharmacol. Ther. 24 420–431.

32. Cohen LS, Soares CN, Joffe H. Diagnosis and management of mood disorders during the menopausal transition. Am J Med 2005; 118 Suppl 12B:93.

33. Cohen LS, Soares CN, Vitonis AF, et al. Risk for new onset of depression during the menopausal transition: the Harvard study of moods and cycles. Arch Gen Psychiatry 2006; 63:385.

34. Cutler WB, Garcia CR, McCoy N. Perimenopausal sexuality. Arch Sex Behav 1987; 16:225.

35. Davison J. M., Dunlop W. (1984). Changes in renal hemodynamics and tubular function induced by normal human pregnancy. Semin. Nephrol. 4 198

36. Dawes M., Chowienczyk P. J. (2001). Pharmacokinetics in pregnancy. Best Pract. Res. Clin. Obstet. Gynaecol. 15 819–826.

37. De Haan G., Edelbroek P., Segers J., Engelsman M., Lindhout D., Devile-Notschaele M., et al. (2004).Gestation-induced changes in lamotrigine pharmacokinetics: a monotherapy study. Neurology 63 571–573.

38. De Kretser DM, Meinhardt A, Meehan T, Phillips DJ, O'Bryan MK, Loveland KA. The roles of inhibin and related peptides in gonadal function. Mol Cell Endocrinol2000;161: 43–46.

39. Dennerstein L, Dudley EC, Hopper JL, et al. A prospective population-based study of menopausal symptoms. Obstet Gynecol 2000; 96:351.

40. Deplewski D, Rosenfield RL. Role of hormones in pilosebaceous unit development. Endocr Rev 2000; 21:363.

41. Derby CA, Crawford SL, Pasternak RC, et al. Lipid changes during the menopause transition in relation to age and weight: the Study of Women's Health Across the Nation. Am J Epidemiol 2009; 169:1352.

42. Derksen J, Nagesser SK, Meinders AE, et al. Identification of virilizing adrenal tumors in hirsute women. N Engl J Med 1994; 331:968.

43. DeUgarte CM, Woods KS, Bartolucci AA, Azziz R. Degree of facial and body terminal hair growth in unselected black and white women: toward a populational definition of hirsutism. J Clin Endocrinol Metab 2006; 91:1345.

44. Dewailly D, Vantyghem MC, Lemaire C, et al. Screening heterozygotes for 21-hydroxylase deficiency among hirsute women: lack of utility of the adrenocorticotropin hormone test. Fertil Steril 1988; 50:228.

45. Dugan SA, Powell LH, Kravitz HM, et al. Musculoskeletal pain and menopausal status. Clin J Pain 2006; 22:325.

46. Elkus R., Popovich J. (1992). Respiratory physiology in pregnancy. Clin. Chest Med. 13 555–565.

47. Elting MW, Korsen TJ, Rekers-Mombarg LT, Schoemaker J. Women with polycystic ovary syndrome gain regular menstrual cycles when ageing. Hum Reprod 2000; 15:24.

48. Elting MW, Kwee J, Korsen TJ, et al. Aging women with polycystic ovary syndrome who achieve regular menstrual cycles have a smaller follicle cohort than those who continue to have irregular cycles. Fertil Steril 2003; 79:1154.

49. Escobar-Morreale HF, Serrano-Gotarredona J, García-Robles R, et al. Mild adrenal and ovarian steroidogenic abnormalities in hirsute women without hyperand rogenemia: does idiopathic hirsutism exist? Metabolism 1997; 46:902.

50. Evans W. E., Relling M. V. (1999). Pharmacogenomics: translating functional genomics into rational therapeutics. Science 286 487–491.

51. Ferriman D, Gallwey JD. Clinical assessment of body hair growth in women. J Clin Endocrinol Metab 1961; 21:1440.

52. Florio P, Severi FM, Cobellis L, Danero S, Bome A, Luisi S, et al. Serum activin A and inhibin A. New clinical markers for hydatidiform mole. Cancer 2002; 94:2618-2622.

53. Frederiksen M. C. (2001). Physiologic changes in pregnancy and their effect on drug disposition.Semin. Perinatol. 25 120–123.

54. Freedman RR, Roehrs TA. Sleep disturbance in menopause. Menopause 2007; 14:826.

55. Freeman EW, Grisso JA, Berlin J, et al. Symptom reports from a cohort of African American and white women in the late reproductive years. Menopause 2001; 8:33.

56. Freeman EW, Sammel MD, Gracia CR, et al. Follicular phase hormone levels and menstrual bleeding status in the approach to menopause. Fertil Steril 2005; 83:383.

57. Freeman EW, Sammel MD, Lin H, Nelson DB. Associations of hormones and menopausal status with depressed mood in women with no history of depression. Arch Gen Psychiatry 2006; 63:375.

58. Freeman EW, Sammel MD, Liu L, et al. Hormones and menopausal status as predictors of depression in women in transition to menopause. Arch Gen Psychiatry 2004; 61:62.

59. Friedman CI, Schmidt GE, Kim MH, Powell J. Serum testosterone concentrations in the evaluation of androgen-producing tumors. Am J Obstet Gynecol 1985; 153:44.

60. Glickman SP, Rosenfield RL. Androgen metabolism by isolated hairs from women with idiopathic hirsutism is usually normal. J Invest Dermatol 1984; 82:62.

61. Glinoer D. (1997). The regulation of thyroid function in pregnancy: pathways of endocrine adaptation from physiology to pathology. Endocr. Rev. 18 404–433.

62. Glinoer D. (1999). What happens to the normal thyroid during pregnancy? Thyroid 9 631–635.

63. Gold EB, Colvin A, Avis N, et al. Longitudinal analysis of the association between vasomotor symptoms and race/ethnicity across the menopausal transition: study of women's health across the nation. Am J Public Health 2006; 96:1226.

64. Greendale GA, Derby CA, Maki PM. Perimenopause and cognition. Obstet Gynecol Clin North Am 2011; 38:519.

65. Greendale GA, Ishii S, Huang MH, Karlamangla AS. Predicting the timeline to the final menstrual period: the study of women's health across the nation. J Clin Endocrinol Metab 2013; 98:1483.

66. Groome N. Ultrasensitive two-site assays for inhibin-A and activin-A using monoclonal antibodies raised to synthetic peptides. J Immunol Methods 1991; 145: 65–69.

67. Groome NP, Illingworth PJ, O'Brien M, Cooke I, Ganesan TS, Baird DT, et al. Detection of dimeric inhibin throughout the human menstrual cycle by two-site enzyme immunoassay. ClinEndocrinol (Oxf) 1994; 40: 717–723.

68. Hale GE, Manconi F, Luscombe G, Fraser IS. Quantitative measurements of menstrual blood loss in ovulatory and anovulatory cycles in middle- and late-reproductive age and the menopausal transition. Obstet Gynecol 2010; 115:249.

69. Hall JE. Neuroendocrine physiology of the early and late menopause. EndocrinolMetabClin North Am 2004; 33:637.

70. Harlow SD, Gass M, Hall JE, et al. Executive summary of the Stages of Reproductive Aging Workshop + 10: addressing the unfinished agenda of staging reproductive aging. J Clin Endocrinol Metab 2012; 97:1159.

71. Hatch R, Rosenfield RL, Kim MH, Tredway D. Hirsutism: implications, etiology, and management. Am J Obstet Gynecol 1981; 140:815.

72. Hawkins LA, Chasalow FI, Blethen SL. The role of adrenocorticotropin testing in evaluating girls with premature adrenarche and hirsutism/oligomenorrhea. J Clin Endocrinol Metab 1992; 74:248.

73. Hee J, MacNaughton J, Bangah M, Burger HG. Perimenopausal patterns of gonadotrophins, immunoreactive inhibin, oestradiol and progesterone. Maturitas 1993; 18:9.

74. Hehhgren M. (1996). hemostasis during pregnancy and puerperium. Hemostasis 26 244–247.

75. Hollander LE, Freeman EW, Sammel MD, et al. Sleep quality, estradiol levels, and behavioral factors in late reproductive age women. Obstet Gynecol 2001; 98:391.

76. Hytten F. E., Paintin D. B. (1963). Increase in plasma volume during normal pregnancy. J. Obstet. Gynaecol. Br. Commonw. 70 402–407.

77. Illingworth PJ, Groome NP, Byrd W, Rainey WE, McNeilly AS, Mather JP, et al. Inhibin-B: a likely candidate for the physiologically important form of inhibin in men. J Clin Endocrinol Metab 1996; 81: 1321–1325.

78. Joffe H, Hall JE, Soares CN, et al. Vasomotor symptoms are associated with depression in perimenopausal women seeking primary care. Menopause 2002; 9:392.

79. Juang KD, Wang SJ, Lu SR, et al. Hot flashes are associated with psychological symptoms of anxiety and depression in peri- and post- but not premenopausal women. Maturitas 2005; 52:119.

80. Karrer-Voegeli S, Rey F, Reymond MJ, et al. Androgen dependence of hirsutism, acne, and alopecia in women: retrospective analysis of 228 patients investigated for hyperandrogenism. Medicine (Baltimore) 2009; 88:32.

81. Kato T, Seki K, Matsui H, Sekiya S. Circulating inhibin forms in patients with hydatidiform mole. GynecolObstet Invest 2002; 54: 114–117.

82. Kirschner MA, Samojlik E, Silber D. A comparison of androgen production and clearance in hirsute and obese women. J Steroid Biochem 1983; 19:607.

83. Knight GJ, Palomaki GE, Neveux LM, Haddow JE, Lambert-Messerlian GM. Clinical validation of a new dimeric inhibin-A assay suitable for second trimester Down's syndrome screening. J Med Screen 2001; 8: 2–7.

84. Knight PG, Glister C. Potential local regulatory functions of inhibins, activins and follistatin in the ovary. Reproduction 2001; 121: 503–512.

85. Knochenhauer ES, Key TJ, Kahsar-Miller M, et al. Prevalence of the polycystic ovary syndrome in unselected black and white women of the southeastern United States: a prospective study. J Clin Endocrinol Metab 1998; 83:3078.

86. Koller O. (1982). The clinical significance of hemodilution during pregnancy. Obstet. Gynecol. Surv.37 649–652.

87. Kravitz HM, Ganz PA, Bromberger J, et al. Sleep difficulty in women at midlife: a community survey of sleep and the menopausal transition. Menopause 2003; 10:19.

88. Kronenberg F. Hot flashes: epidemiology and physiology. Ann N Y AcadSci 1990; 592:52.

89. Kuttenn F, Couillin P, Girard F, et al. Late-onset adrenal hyperplasia in hirsutism. N Engl J Med 1985; 313:224.

90. La Marca A, Sighinolfi G, Papaleo E, et al. Prediction of age at menopause from assessment of ovarian reserve may be improved by using body mass index and smoking status. PLoS One 2013; 8:e57005.

91. Labrie F. Intracrinology. Mol Cell Endocrinol 1991; 78:C113.

92. Lambert-Messerlian GM, Hall JE, Sluss PM, et al. Relatively low levels of dimeric inhibin circulate in men and women with polycystic ovarian syndrome using a specific two-site enzyme-linked immunosorbent assay. J Clin Endocrinol Metab 1994;79: 45–50.

93. Lee CG, Carr MC, Murdoch SJ, et al. Adipokines, inflammation, and visceral adiposity across the menopausal transition: a prospective study. J Clin Endocrinol Metab 2009; 94:1104.

94. Letsky E. A. (1995). Erythropoiesis in pregnancy. J. Perinat. Med. 23 39–45.

95. Little B. B. (1999). Pharmacokinetics during pregnancy: evidence-based maternal dose formulation.Obstet. Gynecol. 93 858–868.

96. Lockitch G. (1997). Clinical biochemistry of pregnancy. Crit. Rev. Clin. Lab. Sci. 34 67–139.

97. MacGregor EA. Menstruation, sex hormones, and migraine. Neurol Clin 1997; 15:125.

98. Maki PM, Freeman EW, Greendale GA, et al. Summary of the National Institute on Aging-sponsored conference on depressive symptoms and cognitive complaints in the menopausal transition. Menopause 2010; 17:815.

99. Manson JM, Sammel MD, Freeman EW, Grisso JA. Racial differences in sex hormone levels in women approaching the transition to menopause. FertilSteril 2001; 75:297.

100. Mason AJ, Farnworth PG, Sullivan J. Characterization and determination of the biological activities of noncleavable high molecular weight forms of inhibin A and activin A. Mol Endocrinol 1996;10:1055-1065.

101. Matteri RK, Stanczyk FZ, Gentzschein EE, et al. Androgen sulfate and glucuronide conjugates in nonhirsute and hirsute women with polycystic ovarian syndrome. Am J Obstet Gynecol 1989; 161:1704.

102. Matthews KA, Crawford SL, Chae CU, et al. Are changes in cardiovascular disease risk factors in midlife women due to chronological aging or to the menopausal transition? J Am CollCardiol 2009; 54:2366.

103. Matthews KA, Wing RR, Kuller LH, et al. Influence of the perimenopause on cardiovascular risk factors and symptoms of middle-aged healthy women. Arch Intern Med 1994; 154:2349.

104. Mattison D., Zajicek A. (2006). Gaps in knowledge in treating pregnant women. Gend. Med. 3 169–182.

105. McAuliffe F., Kametas N., Costello J., Rafferty G. F., Greenough A., Nicolaides K. (2002).Respiratory function in singleton and twin pregnancy. BJOG 109 765–768.

106. McKinlay SM, Brambilla DJ, Posner JG. The normal menopause transition. Maturitas 1992; 14:103.

107. McKinlay SM. The normal menopause transition: an overview. Maturitas 1996; 23:137.

108. McManus SS, Levitsky LL, Misra M. Polycystic ovary syndrome: clinical presentation in normal-weight compared with overweight adolescents. EndocrPract 2013; 19:471.

109. Meldrum DR, Abraham GE. Peripheral and ovarian venous concentrations of various steroid hormones in virilizing ovarian tumors. ObstetGynecol 1979; 53:36.

110. Messenger AG. The control of hair growth: an overview. J Invest Dermatol 1993; 101:4S.

111. Miro F, Parker SW, Aspinall LJ, et al. Origins and consequences of the elongation of the human menstrual cycle during the menopausal transition: the FREEDOM Study. J Clin Endocrinol Metab 2004; 89:4910.

112. Mitchell A. A., Hernandez-Diaz S., Louik C., Werler M. M. (2001). Medication use in pregnancy.w Pharmacoepidemiol. Drug Saf. 10 S146.

113. Mohyi D, Tabassi K, Simon J. Differential diagnosis of hot flashes. Maturitas 1997; 27:203.

114. Moltz L, Pickartz H, Sörensen R, et al. Ovarian and adrenal vein steroids in seven patients with androgen-secreting ovarian neoplasms: selective catheterization findings. Fertil Steril 1984; 42:585.

115. Moore A, Magee F, Cunningham S, et al. Adrenal abnormalities in idiopathic hirsutism. Clin Endocrinol (Oxf) 1983; 18:391.

116. National Institutes of Health. National Institutes of Health State-of-the-Science Conference statement: management of menopause-related symptoms. Ann Intern Med 2005; 142:1003.

117. Neer RM, SWAN Investigators. Bone loss across the menopausal transition. Ann N Y Acad Sci 2010; 1192:66.

118. O'Driscoll JB, Mamtora H, Higginson J, et al. A prospective study of the prevalence of clear-cut endocrine disorders and polycystic ovaries in 350 patients presenting with hirsutism or androgenic alopecia. ClinEndocrinol (Oxf) 1994; 41:231.

119. Pacheco L., Costantine M. M, Hankins G. D. V. (2013). "Physiologic changes during pregnancy," inClincal Pharmacology During Pregnancy ed. Mattison D. R., editor. (San Diego: Academic Press ;) 5–14.

120. Parry E., Shields R., Turnbull A. C. (1970). Transit time in the small intestine in pregnancy. J. Obstet. Gynaecol. Br. Commonw. 77 900–901.

121. Paus R, Cotsarelis G. The biology of hair follicles. N Engl J Med 1999; 341:491.

122. Peck T. M., Arias F. (1979). Hematologic changes associated with pregnancy. Clin. Obstet. Gynecol. 22 785–798.

123. Pritchard J. A. (1965). Changes in the blood volume during pregnancy and delivery. Anesthesiology 26 394–399.

124. Randolph JF Jr, Crawford S, Dennerstein L, et al. The value of follicle-stimulating hormone concentration and clinical findings as markers of the late menopausal transition. J Clin Endocrinol Metab 2006; 91:3034.

125. Randolph JF Jr, Sowers M, Bondarenko I, et al. The relationship of longitudinal change in reproductive hormones and vasomotor symptoms during the menopausal transition. J Clin Endocrinol Metab 2005; 90:6106.

126. Randolph JF Jr, Sowers M, Gold EB, et al. Reproductive hormones in the early menopausal transition: relationship to ethnicity, body size, and menopausal status. J Clin Endocrinol Metab 2003; 88:1516.

127. Randolph JF Jr, Zheng H, Sowers MR, et al. Change in follicle-stimulating hormone and estradiol across the menopausal transition: effect of age at the final menstrual period. J Clin Endocrinol Metab 2011; 96:746.

128. Rasmussen P. E., Nielse F. R. (1988). Hydronephrosis during pregnancy: a literature survey. Eur. J. Obstet. Gynaecol. Reprod. Biol. 27 249–259.

129. Robertson D, Burger HG, Sullivan J, Cahir N, Groome N, Poncelet E, et al. Biological and immunological characterization of inhibin forms in human plasma. J Clin Endocrinol Metab 1996; 81: 669–676.

130. Robertson DM, Stephenson T, Pruysers E, Burger HG, McCloud P, Tsigos A, et al. Inhibins/activins as diagnostic markers for ovarian cancer. Mol Cell Endocrinol 2002; 191: 97–103.

131. Robson SC, Hunter S, Boys R J, Dunlop W. (1989). Serial study of factors influencing changes in cardiac output during human pregnancy. Am. J. Physiol. 256 H1060–H1065.

132. Rose MP, Gaines Das RE. International collaborative study by in vitro bioassays and immunoassays of the First International Standard for Inhibin, Human Recombinant. Biologicals 1996; 24: 1–18.

133. Rosenfield RL. Clinical practice. Hirsutism. N Engl J Med 2005; 353:2578.

134. Rubler S., Damani P., Pinto E. (1977). Cardiac size and performance during pregnancy estimated with echocardiography. Am. J. Cardiol. 49 534–540.

135. Samojlik E, Kirschner MA, Silber D, et al. Elevated production and metabolic clearance rates of androgens in morbidly obese women. J Clin Endocrinol Metab 1984; 59:949.

136. Santoro N, Brockwell S, Johnston J, et al. Helping midlife women predict the onset of the final menses: SWAN, the Study of Women's Health Across the Nation. Menopause 2007; 14:415.

137. Sarrel PM. Ovarian hormones and vaginal blood flow: using laser Doppler velocimetry to measure effects in a clinical trial of post-menopausal women. Int J Impot Res 1998; 10 Suppl 2:S91.

138. Schmidt PJ, Haq N, Rubinow DR. A longitudinal evaluation of the relationship between reproductive status and mood in perimenopausal women. Am J Psychiatry 2004; 161:2238.

139. Schou M, Amdisen A, Steenstrup OR (1973). Lithium and pregnancy: hazards to women given lithium during pregnancy and delivery. Br. Med. J. 2 137–138.

140. Schwartz J. B. (2003). The influence of sex on pharmacokinetics. Clin. Pharmacokinet. 42 107–121.

141. Seely E. W., Ecker J. (2011). Chronic hypertension in pregnancy. N. Engl. J. Med. 365 439–446

142. Sherman BM, Korenman SG. Hormonal characteristics of the human menstrual cycle throughout reproductive life. J Clin Invest 1975; 55:699.

143. Soules MR, Sherman S, Parrott E, et al. Executive summary: Stages of Reproductive Aging Workshop (STRAW). Fertil Steril 2001; 76:874.

144. Sternfeld B, Wang H, Quesenberry CP Jr, et al. Physical activity and changes in weight and waist circumference in midlife women: findings from the Study of Women's Health Across the Nation. Am J Epidemiol 2004; 160:912.

145. Su HI, Sammel MD, Freeman EW, et al. Body size affects measures of ovarian reserve in late reproductive age women. Menopause 2008; 15:857.

146. Szoeke CE, Cicuttini F, Guthrie J, Dennerstein L. Self-reported arthritis and the menopause. Climacteric 2005; 8:49.

147. Szoeke CE, Cicuttini FM, Guthrie JR, Dennerstein L. The relationship of reports of aches and joint pains to the menopausal transition: a longitudinal study. Climacteric 2008; 11:55.

148. Taffe JR, Dennerstein L. Menstrual patterns leading to the final menstrual period. Menopause 2002; 9:32.

149. Taylor M. (1961). An experimental study of the influence of the endocrine system on the nasal respiratory mucosa. J. Laryngol. Otol. 75 972–977.

150. Thurston RC, Joffe H. Vasomotor symptoms and menopause: findings from the Study of Women's Health across the Nation. Obstet Gynecol Clin North Am 2011; 38:489.

151. Tsai C, De Leeuw N. K. (1982). Changes in 2,3-diphosphoglycerate during pregnancy and puerperium in normal women and in beta-thalassemia heterozygous women. Am. J. Obstet. Gynecol.142 520–523.

152. Turan O. M., De Paco C., Kametas N., Khaw A., Nicolaides K. H. (2008). Effect of parity on maternal cardiac function during the first trimester of pregnancy. Ultrasound Obstet. Gynecol. 32 849–854.

153. Van Disseldorp J, Faddy MJ, Themmen AP, et al. Relationship of serum antimüllerian hormone concentration to age at menopause. J Clin Endocrinol Metab 2008; 93: 2129.

154. Van Voorhis BJ, Santoro N, Harlow S, et al. The relationship of bleeding patterns to daily reproductive hormones in women approaching menopause. Obstet Gynecol 2008; 112:101.

155. Wald NJ, Huttly WJ, Hackshaw AK. Antenatal screening for Down's syndrome with the quadruple test. Lancet 2003; 361: 835–836.

156. Wald NJ, Kennard A, Hackshaw A, McGuire A. Antenatal screening for Down's syndrome. J Med Screen 1997; 4: 181–246.

157. Welt CK, Arason G, Gudmundsson JA, et al. Defining constant versus variable phenotypic features of women with polycystic ovary syndrome using different ethnic groups and populations. J Clin Endocrinol Metab 2006; 91:4361.

158. Welt CK, McNicholl DJ, Taylor AE, Hall JE. Female reproductive aging is marked by decreased secretion of dimeric inhibin. J Clin Endocrinol Metab 1999; 84:105.

159. Welt CK, McNicholl DJ, Taylor AE, Hall JE. Female reproductive aging is marked by decreased secretion of dimeric inhibin. J Clin Endocrinol Metab 1999; 84: 105–111.

160. Winkel C. A., Milewich L., Parker C. R., Jr., Grizzle W. E., Blevins J. K., Hawkes K. (1980).Conversion of plasma progesterone to desoxycorticosterone in men, non pregnant, and pregnant women, and adrenalectomized subjects. J. Clin. Invest. 66 803–812.

161. Woodard GA, Brooks MM, Barinas-Mitchell E, et al. Lipids, menopause, and early atherosclerosis in sudy of Women's Health Across the Nation Heart women. Menopause 2011; 18:376.

162. Woods NF, Mitchell ES. Sleep symptoms during the menopausal transition and early postmenopause: observations from the Seattle Midlife Women's Health Study. Sleep 2010; 33:539.

163. Woods NF, Mitchell ES. Symptoms during the perimenopause: prevalence, severity, trajectory, and significance in women's lives. Am J Med 2005; 118 Suppl 12B:14.

11

Disorders of Carbohydrate Metabolism

INTRODUCTION

Glucose is a major energy substrate. It typically provides more than half the total energy requirements of a typical 'western' diet and is the only utilizable source of energy for some tissues, e.g. erythrocytes and, in the short term, the central nervous system. Many tissues are capable of oxidizing glucose completely to carbon dioxide; others metabolize it only as far as lactate, which can be converted back into glucose, principally in the liver and also in the kidneys, by gluconeogenesis. Even in tissues capable of completely oxidizing glucose, lactate is produced, if insufficient oxygen is available. The body's sources of glucose are dietary carbohydrate and endogenous production by glycogenolysis (release of glucose stored as glycogen) and gluconeogenesis (glucose synthesis from, e.g. lactate, glycerol, and most amino acids). Glycogen is stored in the liver and skeletal muscle, but only the former contributes to blood glucose.

Blood glucose concentration depends on the relative rates of influx of glucose into the circulation and of its utilization. Its concentration is normally subject to rigorous control, rarely falling below 2.5 mmol/L at any time or rising above 8.0 mmol/L in healthy subjects after a meal or above 5.2 mmol/L after an overnight fast. Following a meal, glucose is stored as glycogen, which is mobilized during fasting. Blood glucose concentration usually falls to pre-meal concentrations within no more than 4 hours after a meal; although the blood glucose concentration falls somewhat if fasting continues, and hepatic glycogen stores are used up after about 24 hours, adaptive changes lead to the attainment of a new steady state. After approximately 72 hours, blood glucose concentration stabilizes and can then remain constant for many days. The principal source of glucose becomes gluconeogenesis, from amino acids and glycerol, while ketones, derived from fat, become the major energy substrate.

The integration of these various processes, and thus the control of blood glucose concentration, is achieved through the concerted action of various hormones; these are insulin (the actions of which tend to lower blood glucose concentration) and the 'counter-regulatory' hormones, namely glucagon, cortisol, catecholamines and growth hormone, which have the opposite effect. Their effects are summarized in Fig. 11.1.

The two most important hormones in glucose homoeostasis are insulin and glucagon.

INSULIN

Insulin is a protein hormone produced by the β-cells of the islets of Langerhans in the pancreas. Insulin was the first protein hormone to be sequenced, the first substance to be measured by radioimmunoassay (RIA), and the first compound produced by recombinant DNA technology for clinical use. It is an anabolic hormone that stimulates the uptake of glucose into fat and muscle, promotes the conversion of glucose to glycogen or fat for storage, inhibits glucose production by the liver, stimulates protein synthesis, and inhibits protein breakdown.

Human insulin consists of 51 amino acids (MW 5808 Da), in two chains (A and B) joined by two disulfide bridges, with a third disulfide bridge within the A chain. The amino acid sequence of human insulin differs slightly from insulin of other species, but the carboxyl terminal region of the B chain (B23 to B26), which appears crucial for the biological actions of insulin, is highly conserved among species. Insulin from most animals is immunologically and biologically similar to human insulin, and in the past, patients were treated with insulin purified from beef or pig pancreas. The most commonly used forms now are recombinant human insulins.

Preproinsulin, a protein of about 100 amino acids (MW 12,000 Da), is formed by ribosomes in the rough endoplasmic reticulum of the pancreatic β-cells (Fig. 11.1). Preproinsulin is not detectable in the circulation under normal conditions, because it is rapidly converted by cleaving enzymes to proinsulin (MW 9000 Da), an 86 amino acid polypeptide.

This is stored in secretory granules in the Golgi complex of the β-cells, where proteolytic cleavage to insulin and connecting peptide (C-peptide) occurs. Cleavage of proinsulin is catalyzed by two Ca^{2+}-regulated endopeptidases–prohormone convertases 1 and 2 (PC1 and PC2). PC1 (sometimes designated PC3) hydrolyzes the molecule on the C-terminal end of Arg-31 and Arg-32 (at the BC junction) to yield split-32,33-proinsulin (Fig. 11.2). PC2 cleaves proinsulin on the C-terminal side of dibasic

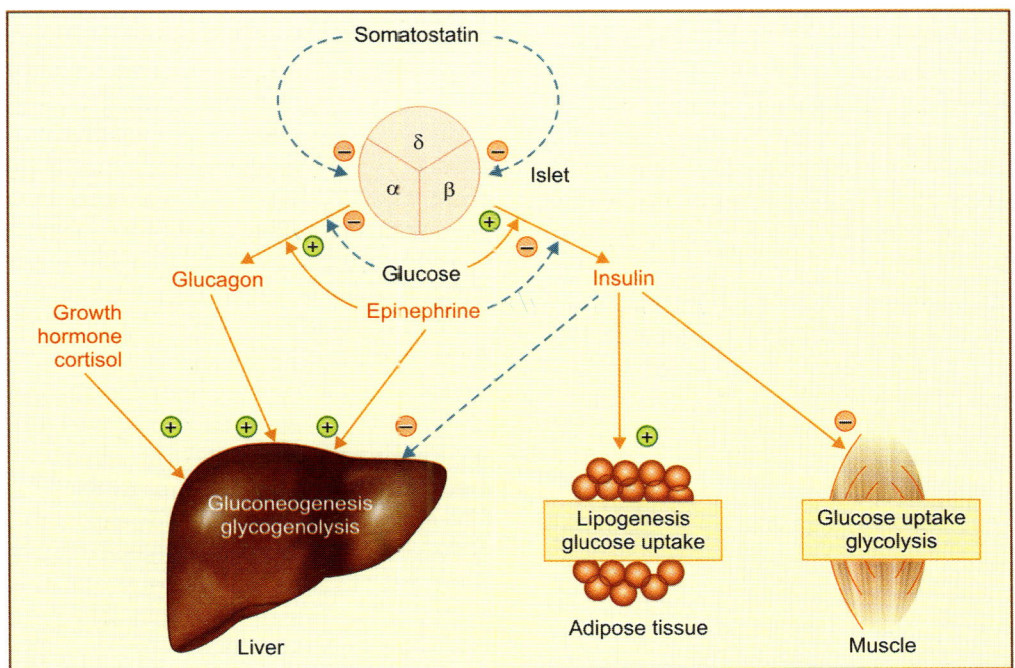

Fig. 11.1: Hormonal regulation of blood glucose. Key: +, stimulation; –, inhibition. Cortisol, growth hormone, and epinephrine antagonize the effects of insulin

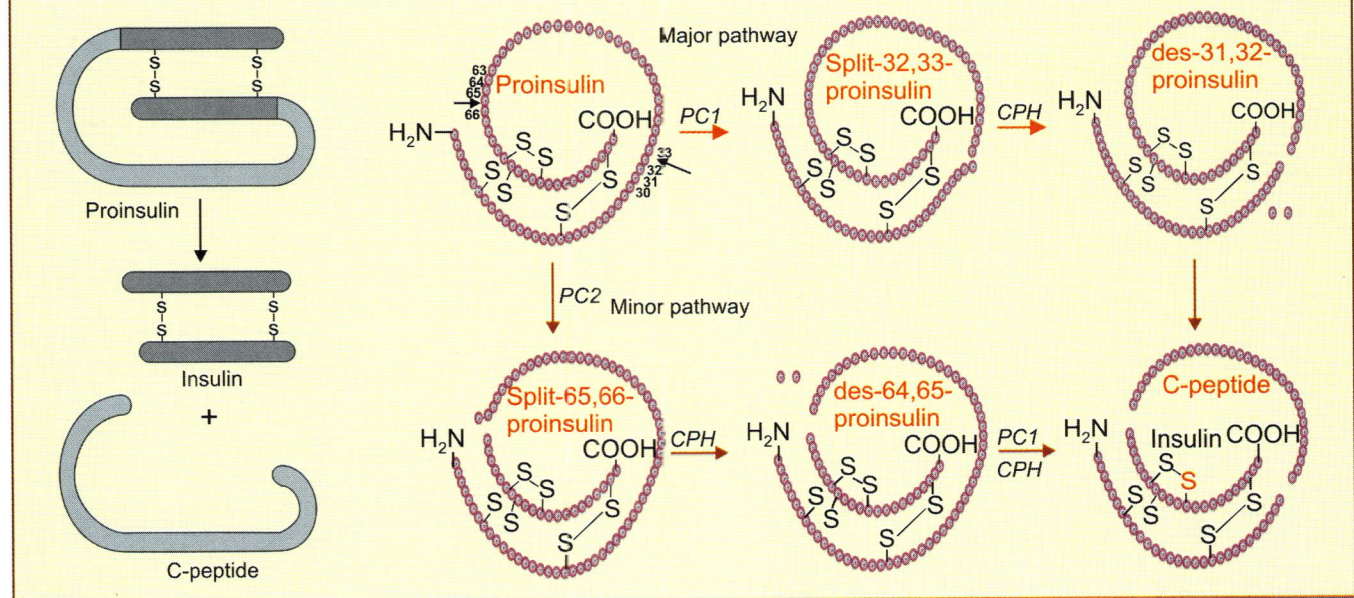

Fig. 11.2: Processing of proinsulin. The enzymes prohormone convertase and 2(PC I and PC2) act on proinsulin to form the appropriate split proinsulins. Carboxypeptidase-H (CPH) removes the two exposed basic amino acid residues (circles)

residues Lys-64 and Arg-65 to generate split-65, 66-proinsulin. Each enzymatic hydrolysis is rapidly followed by the removal of two newly exposed C-terminal basic amino acids by carboxypeptidase-H to produce insulin and C-peptide.

The split proinsulin intermediates are rarely detected in patient samples because of the relatively high quantity of carboxypeptidase-H. This enzyme produces the more commonly observed proinsulin intermediates, des-31, 32-proinsulin and des-64, 65-proinsulin (Fig. 11.3). Most proinsulin processing is sequential. Intact proinsulin is initially hydrolyzed by PC1 or carboxypeptidase-H. The resultant des-31, 32-proinsulin is converted by PC2 and carboxypeptidase-H to insulin and C-peptide. Less than 10% of proinsulin is metabolized via des-(64-65)-proinsulin, which is present in negligible amounts in humans. Des-31, 32-proinsulin is the major proinsulin conversion intermediate.

Glucose regulates biosynthesis of both proinsulin and PC1, but has no effect on PC2 or carboxypeptidase-H. At the cell membrane, insulin and C-peptide are released into the portal circulation in equimolar amounts. In addition, small amounts of proinsulin and intermediate cleavage forms enter the circulation.

Glucose, amino acids, pancreatic and gastrointestinal hormones (e.g. glucagon, gastrin, secretin, pancreozymin, gastrointestinal polypeptide), and some medications (e.g. sulfonylureas, p-adrenergic agonists) stimulate insulin secretion. Insulin release is inhibited by hypoglycemia, somatostatin (produced in the pancreatic δ-cells), and various drugs, e.g. α-adrenergic agonists, β-adrenergic blockers, diazoxide, phenytoin, phenothiazines, nicotinic acid. In healthy individuals, insulin is secreted in a pulsatile fashion, with glucose and insulin the main signals in the feedback loop.

Glucose elicits the release of insulin from the pancreas in two phases. The first phase begins 1–2 minutes after intravenous injection of glucose and ends within 10 minutes. This phase, illustrated by the sharp spike in Fig. 11.3A represents the rapid release of stored insulin. The second phase, beginning at the point, where the first phase ends, depends on continuing insulin synthesis and release and lasts until normoglycemia has been restored, usually within 60–120 minutes. With progressive failure of p-cell function, the first phase insulin response to glucose is lost, but other stimuli, such as glucagon or amino acids may be able to elicit this response. Although, the second-phase insulin response is preserved in most patients with type 2 diabetes mellitus, both the first-phase response (Fig. 11.3B) and normal pulsatile insulin secretion are lost. In contrast, patients with type I diabetes mellitus exhibit minimal or no insulin response (Fig. 11.3C).

On the first pass through the portal circulation, approximately 50% of insulin is extracted by the liver, where it is degraded. Because the amount extracted is variable, plasma insulin concentrations may not accurately reflect the rate of insulin secretion. Additional insulin degradation occurs in the kidneys. Insulin is filtered through the glomeruli, reabsorbed, and degraded in the proximal tubule. The basal insulin secretory rate is about I U (43 µg)/h, with total daily secretion of about 40 U. The half-life of insulin in the circulation is between 4 minutes and 5 minutes.

PROINSULIN

Proinsulin, which has relatively low biological activity (approximately 10% of insulin potency), is the major

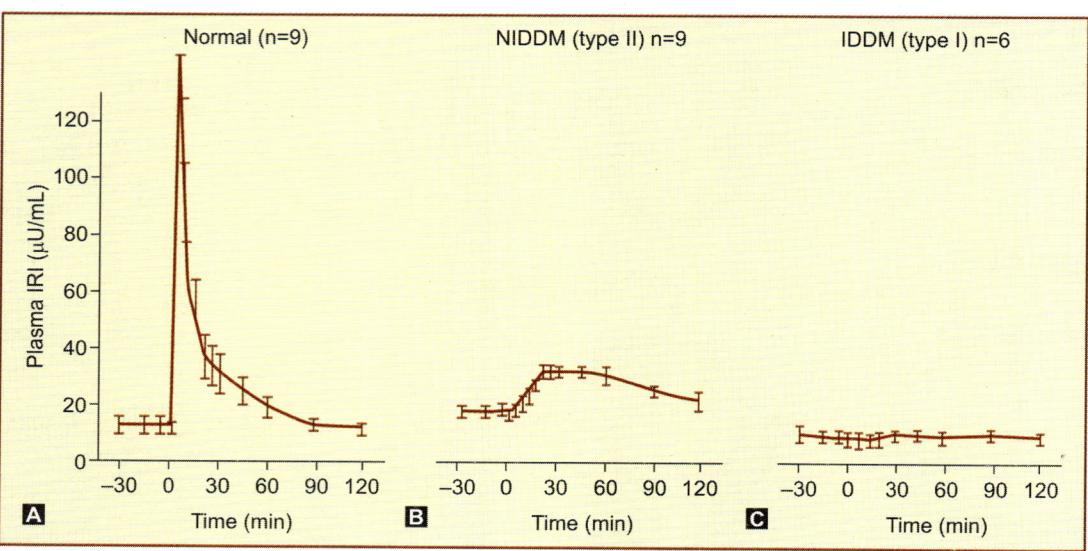

Fig. 11.3: Response of plasma insulin to glucose stimulation. A 20 g glucose pulse is given intravenously at time 0. (A) Healthy subjects. (B) Patients with type 2 diabetes mellitus (NIDDM). (C) Patients with type I diabetes mellitus (100M). IRI, Immunoreactive insulin. Values before time 0 represent baseline

storage form of insulin. Normally, only small amounts (about 3% of the amount of insulin, on a molar basis) of proinsulin enter the circulation. However, the hepatic clearance rate for proinsul in is only 25% of that for insulin, and the half-life of proinsulin is approximately 30 minutes. Therefore, in the fasting state, circulating, proinsulin concentrations are approximately 10–15% of insulin concentrations.

C-Peptide

Proinsulin is cleaved to a 31 amino acid connecting C-peptide (MW 3600 Da) and insulin (Fig. 11.2). C-peptide is devoid of biological activity, but appears necessary to ensure the correct structure of insulin. Although, insulin and C-peptide are secreted into the portal circulationin equimolar amounts, fasting C-peptide concentrations are fivefold to 10-fold higher than those of insulin owing to the longer half-life of C-peptide (approximately 35 minutes). The liver does not extract C-peptide, which is removed from the circulation by the kidneys and degraded, with a fraction excreted unchanged in the urine.

The Mechanism of Insulin Action

Although, the metabolic effects produced by insulin are well known, the molecular mechanism of insulin action remains incompletely understood. It is generally accepted that the initial event is the binding of insulin to specific receptors in the plasma membrane (Fig. 11.4). The human insulin receptor, which is well characterized, is a

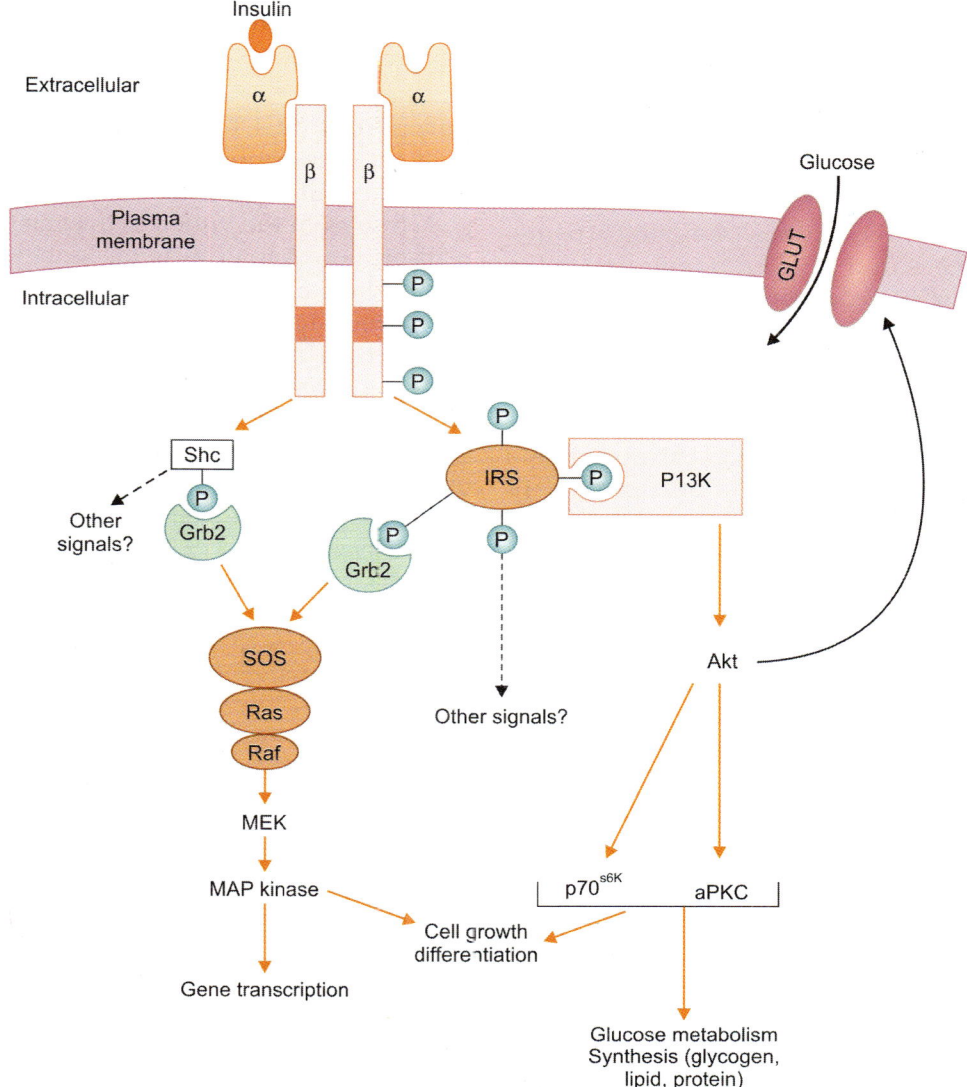

Fig. 11.4: Mechanism of insulin action. Binding of insulin to the extracellular α-subunit of the insulin receptor induces autophosphorylation of the β-subunit of the receptor and phosphorylation of selected intracellular proteins, such as Shc and the insulin-receptor substrate (IRS) family. These latter phosphoproteins interact with other targets, thereby activating phosphorylation cascades, which result in glucose uptake (in adipose tissue and skeletal muscle), glucose metabolism, synthesis (of glycogen, lipid, and proteins), enhanced gene expression, cell growth, and differentiation. A PKC, atypical protein kinase C; p, protein phosphorylation

heterotetramer,comprising two α- and two β-subunits. The α-subunit (MW 135,000 Da) is located on the outer surface of the plasma membrane and contains the site where insulin binds. The β-subunit (MW 95,000 Da) extends intracellularly through the plasma membrane and contains an intrinsic tyrosine kinase. Binding of insulin to the α-subunits induces a conformational change in the receptor, resulting in activation of tyrosine kinase, which catalyzes the phosphorylation of tyrosine residues on several proteins. One of the major substrates for this tyrosine kinase is the receptor itself.

In addition to phosphorylating itself, the insulin receptor catalyzes the tyrosine phosphorylation of various specific intracellular proteins (Fig. 11.4). These include the four members of the family of insulin-receptor substrate (IRS) proteins (termed IRS-I, IRS-2, IRS-3, and IRS-4), Shc, and Gab-I. The phosphorylated tyrosines on these target.

Proteins act as docking sites for selected intracellular signal transducer proteins. Most of these transducer proteins contain one or more Src homology 2 (SH2) domains. The SH2 domain is a sequence of approximately 100 amino acids that recognizes phosphotyrosine. Sequence differences in the SH2 domain dictate the specificity of binding. SH2-containing proteins depicted in (Fig. 11.4), include those labeled phosphatidylinositol 3-kinase (PI3K) and growth factor receptor bound protein 2 (Grb2), both of which mediate downstream signal transduction events. Similar to other growth factors, insulin stimulates the mitogen-activated protein (MAP) kinase cascade via Ras. In addition, phosphatidylinositol 3'-kinase activates atypical protein kinase C (aPKC) via Akt. The latter enzymes regulate glucose transport by modulating translocation of GLUT4 (the insulin-sensitive glucose transporter) to the plasma membrane. Akt also phosphorylates and inactivates GSK-3, thereby enhancing glycogen synthesis.

Some of these events are listed in Fig. 11.4. The pathways are elaborate, and although several components have been identified, there remain considerable gaps in our knowledge and understanding. Recent studies have clarified a fundamental concept that insulin-mediated signaling events are highly redundant. For example, when two key insulin signaling molecules, IRS-l and GLUT4, were knocked out in transgenic mouse experiments, the resulting animals had minor metabolic defects rather than overt diabetes. Similarly, mice with knockout of insulin receptors from skeletal muscle or liver do not develop diabetes.

Glucose Transport

The transport of glucose into cells is modulated by two families of proteins. The sodium-dependent glucose transporters (SGLTs) use the electrochemical sodium gradient to transport glucose against its concentration gradient. SGLTs promote the uptake of glucose and galactose from the lumen of the small bowel and their reabsorption from urine in the kidney (Fig. 11.5).

Members of the second family of glucose carriers are called facilitative glucose transporters (GLUT) (Table 11.1). These transporters are designated GLUTl to GLUT14, based on the order in which they were identified. Eleven have been shown to catalyze sugar transport. They can be divided into three classes, based on sequence similarities and characteristics.

The best characterized are class I. Less is known about those in classes II and III. GLUTl is widely expressed and provides many cells with their basal glucose requirement.

Table 11.1	Facilitative human glucose transporters		
Name	Class	Tissue	Function
GLUTl	I	Wide distribution, especially brain, kidney, colon, and fetal tissues	Basal glucose transport
GLUT2	I	Liver, β-cells of pancreas, small intestine, and kidney	Non-rate limiting glucose transport
GLUT3	I	Wide distribution especially neurons, placenta, and testis	Glucose transport in neurons
GLUT4	I	Skeletal muscle, cardiac muscle, adipose tissue	Insulin stimulated glucose transport
GLUT5	II	Small intestine, kidney, skeletal muscle, brain, and adipose tissue	Transports fructose (not glucose)
GLUT6	III	Brain, spleen, leukocytes	
GLUT7	II	Intestine, testis, prostate	
GLUT8	III	Testis, heart, brain	
GLUT 9	II	Kidney, liver	
GLUT 10	III	Liver, pancreas	
GLUT 11	II	Pancreas, kidney, placenta, skeletal muscle	
GLUTl2	III	Heart, prostate	
HMIT		Brain	Transports myo-inositol (not glucose)
GLUTl4	III	Testis	

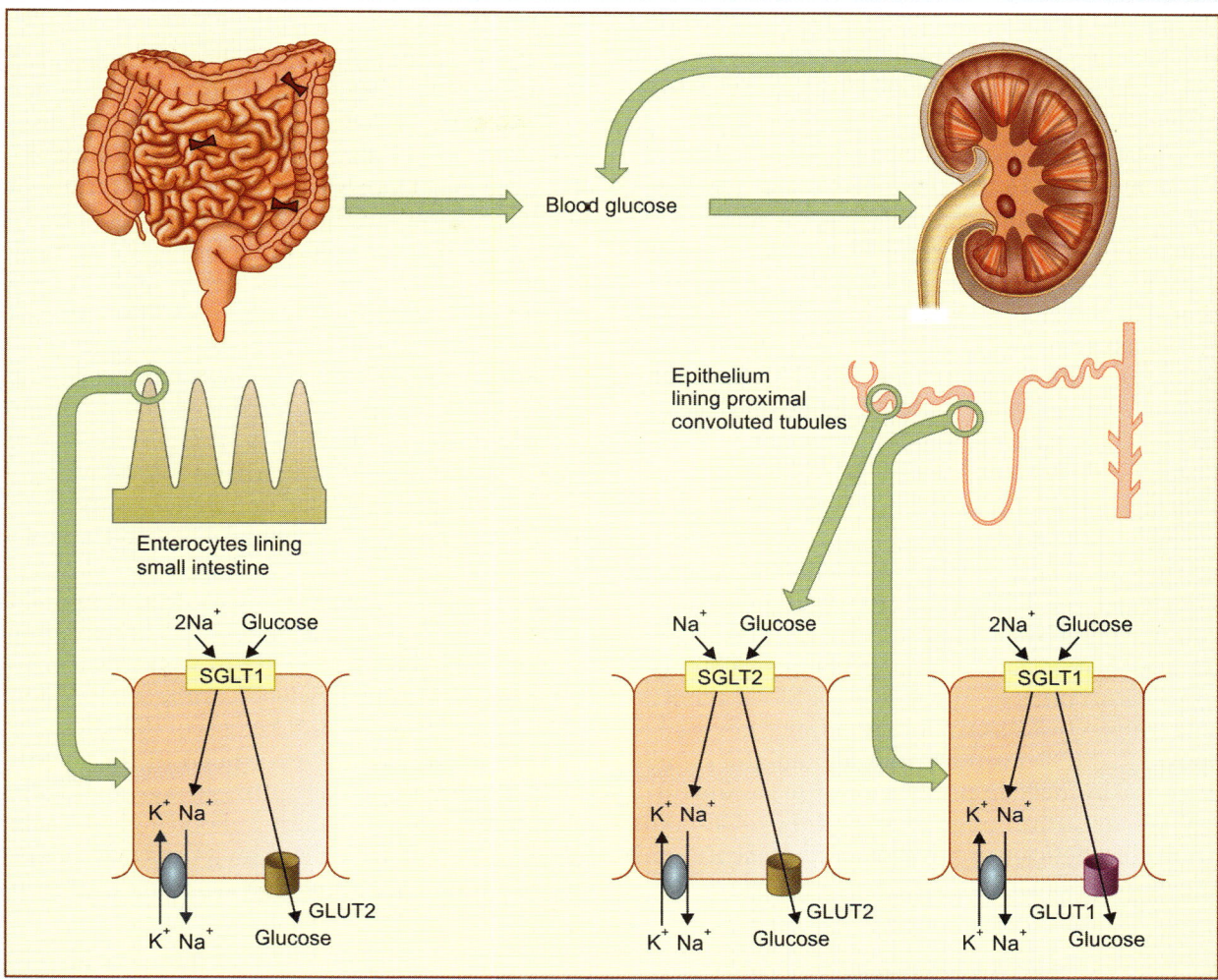

Fig. 11.5: Sodium-dependent glucose transporter (SGLT), use the electrochemical sodium gradient to transport glucose against its concentration gradient

GLUTl in the blood-brain barrier and GLUT3 in neuronal cells provide the constant high concentrations of glucose required by the brain. GLUT2 is expressed in hepatocytes, β-cells of the pancreas, and basolateral membranes of intestinal and renal epithelial cells. It is a low-affinity, high-capacity transport system that allows non-rate-limiting movement of glucose into and out of these cells. GLUT4 catalyzes the rate-limiting step for glucose uptake and metabolism in skeletal muscle, the major organ of glucose consumption. GLUT4 is also present in adipose tissue. When circulating insulin concentrations are low, most of the GLUT4 is localized in intracellular compartments and is inactive. After eating, the pancreas releases insulin, which stimulates the translocation of GLUT4 to the plasma membrane, thereby promoting glucose uptake into skeletal muscle and fat. Insulin-stimulated glucose transport into skeletal muscle is defective in type 2 diabetes mellitus, but the mechanism has not been established.

INSULIN-LIKE GROWTH FACTORS

Insulin-like growth factors 1 and 2 (IGF-1 and IGF-2) are polypeptides structurally related to insulin. These hormones (previously referred to as non-suppressible insulin-like activity or somatomedin) exhibit metabolic and growth promoting effects similar to those of insulin. Accumulating evidence implicates the IGF axis in the development of several common cancers. IGF-1 (previously known as somatomedin-C) is an important mediator of growth hormone action and is one of the major regulators of cell growth and differentiation.

The physiologic role of IGF-2 is not known. Synthesis of IGF-1 depends on growth hormone and occurs predominantly in the liver. In addition, many other cells produce IGF-l that does not enter the circulation but acts locally. Circulating IGF concentrations are approximately 1000-fold higher than insulin concentrations, and the hormone is kept inactive by binding to a family of at least six specific binding proteins. These proteins regulate IGF by protecting the ligands in the circulation and delivering them to their target tissue. In contrast to insulin, which is unbound in the circulation, less than 10% of total serum IGF-1 is free.

The biological actions of IGF are exerted through specific IGF receptors or the insulin receptor. The IGF-1 receptor is closely related to the insulin receptor in structure and biochemical properties. In contrast, the IGF-2 receptor is quite different; it lacks tyrosine kinase activity, and its physiologic relevance is not understood. The IGF-1 receptor has a high affinity for both IGF-1 and IGF-2, but a low affinity for insulin. The IGF-2 receptor has high, low, and no affinity for IGF-2, IGF-1, and insulin, respectively. The insulin receptor binds insulin with high affinity and IGF-1 and IGF-2 with low affinity.

The significance of IGFs in normal carbohydrate metabolism is not known. Exogenous administration produces hypoglycemia, whereas a deficiency of IGF-1 results in dwarfism. IGFs, particularly IGF-2, may be produced in excess by extrapancreatic neoplasms, and patients may have fasting hypoglycemia. The high concentrations of both IGF-2 protein in the blood and IGF-2 messenger RNA (mRNA) in tumor extracts have led to the proposal that IGF-2 is the humoral mediator of non-islet cell tumor-induced hypoglycemia. Measurement of plasma IGF-1 concentration may be useful in evaluating growth hormone deficiency and excess (acromegaly), and in monitoring response to nutritional support.

Glucagon

Glucagon is a 29 amino acid polypeptide secreted by the α-cells of the pancreatic islets; its secretion is decreased by a rise in the blood glucose concentration. In general, its actions oppose those of insulin, the combined effects of insulin and glucagon are shown diagrammatically in Fig. 11.6. Glucagon stimulates the production of glucose in the liver by glycogenolysis and gluconeogenesis. In addition, glucagon enhances ketogenesis in the liver. A minor target organ for glucagon is adipose tissue, where the hormone increases lipolysis. Glucagon secretion is regulated primarily by plasma glucose concentrations, with low and high plasma glucose being stimulatory and inhibitory, respectively. Long-standing diabetes mellitus impairs the glucagon response to hypoglycemia, resulting in an increased incidence of hypoglycemic episodes. Stress, exercise, and amino acids induce glucagon release.

Insulin inhibits glucagon release from the pancreas and decreases glucagon gene expression, thereby attenuating its biosynthesis. Increased glucagon concentrations, secondary to insulin deficiency, are believed to contribute to the hyperglycemia and ketosis of diabetes.

Proglucagon is also produced in the distal gut by L-cells, which process it into glucagon, glucagon-like peptide-1 (GLP-1), and (GLP-2). Food ingestion stimulates release of GLP-1, which acts on β-cells of the pancreas to stimulate insulin gene transcription and potentiate

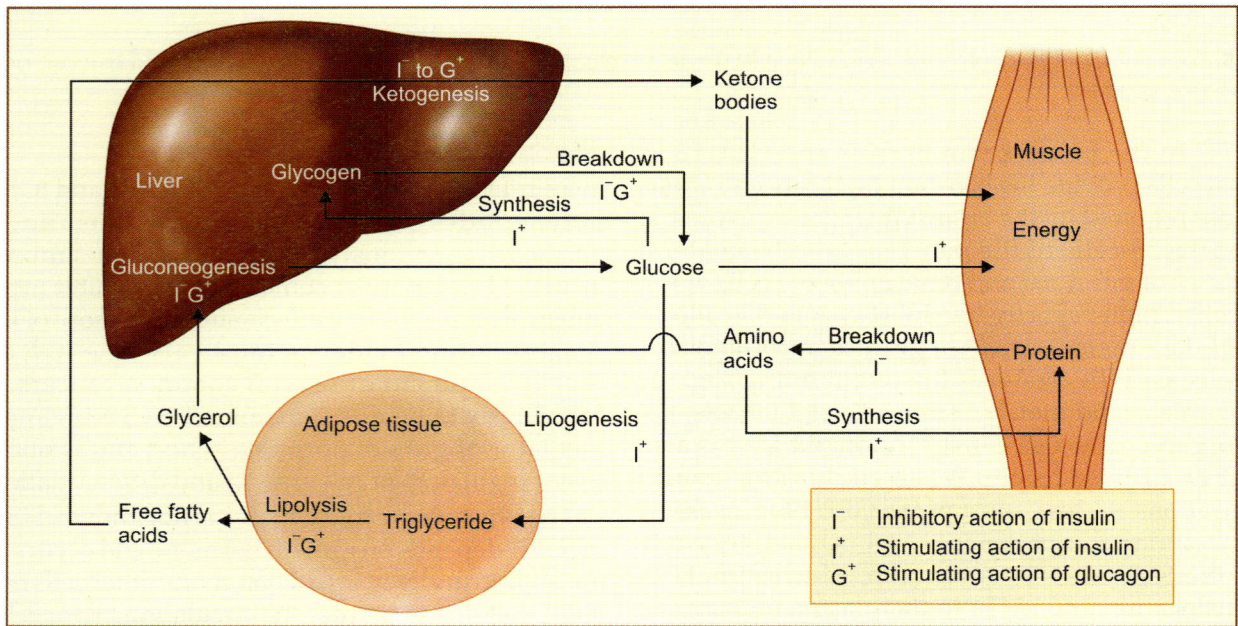

Fig. 11.6: Combined effects of insulin and glucagon on substrate flows between liver, adipose tissue and muscle. When the ratio of the concentrations of insulin to glucagon falls (e.g. during starvation), there is increased hepatic glucose and ketone production and decreased tissue glucose utilization. When the ratio is high (e.g. after a meal), glucose is stored as glycogen and converted into fat

glucose-induced insulin secretion. GLP-l and glucose-dependent insulinotropic polypeptide (GIP) are incretin hormones that are responsible for 70% of postprandial insulin secretion. GLP-l reduces hyperglycemia by regulating insulin and glucagon secretion, thus providing gastric emptying and satiety. For these reasons, GLP-l analogs are generating interest in the treatment of type 2 diabetes, and two (exenatide and liraglutide) have received food and drug administration (FDA) approval.

DISORDERS OF CARBOHYDRATE METABOLISM

Diabetes Mellitus

Diabetes mellitus (DM) is a group of metabolic diseases characterized by hyperglycemia resulting from defects in insulin secretion, insulin action, or both. The chronic hyperglycemia of diabetes is associated with long-term damage, dysfunction, and failure of various organs, especially the eyes, kidneys, nerves, heart, and blood vessels.

There are two main categories of DM—type 1 and type 2, which can be distinguished by a combination of features (Table 11.2). Terms that describe the age of onset (juvenile or adult) or type of treatment (insulin or non-insulin-dependent) are no longer accurate because of overlap in age groups and treatments between disease types.

Impaired glucose regulation is an intermediate, possibly transitional, state between normal glucose metabolism and DM that becomes more common with aging. It is a significant risk factor for DM and may be present for many years before onset of DM. It is associated with an increased risk of cardiovascular disease, but typical diabetic microvascular complications are not very common (microalbuminuria and/or retinopathy develop in 6–10%).

Etiology

Type 1 Diabetes Mellitus

In type 1 DM (previously called juvenile-onset or insulin-dependent), insulin production is absent because of autoimmune pancreatic β-cell destruction possibly triggered by an environmental exposure in genetically susceptible people. Destruction progresses sub-clinically over months or years until β-cell mass decreases to the point that insulin concentrations are no longer adequate to control plasma glucose levels. Type 1 DM generally develops in childhood or adolescence and until recently was the most common form diagnosed before age of 30; however, it can also develop in adults (latent autoimmune diabetes of adulthood, which often initially appears to be type 2 DM). Some cases of type 1 DM, particularly in nonwhite populations, do not appear to be autoimmune in nature and are considered idiopathic. Type 1 accounts for <10% of all cases of DM.

The pathogenesis of the autoimmune β-cell destruction involves incompletely understood interactions between susceptibility genes, autoantigens, and environmental factors.

Susceptibility genes include those within the major histocompatibility complex (MHC), which are present in >90% of patients with type 1 DM and those outside the MHC, which seem to regulate insulin production and processing and confer risk of DM in concert with MHC

Table 11.2	General characteristics of types 1 and 2 diabetes mellitus	
Characteristic	**Type 1**	**Type 2**
Age at onset	Most commonly <30 years	Most commonly >30 years
Associated obesity	Uncommon	Very common
Propensity to ketoacidosis requiring insulin treatment for control	Yes	No
Plasma levels of endogenous insulin	Extremely low to undetectable	Variable; may be low, normal, or elevated depending on degree of insulin resistance and insulin secretory defect
Twin concordance	≤ 50%	>90%
Associated with specific HLA-D antigens	Yes	No
Pancreatic autoantibodies at diagnosis	Yes, but may be absent	No
Islet pathology	Insulitis, selective loss of most β-cells	Smaller, normal-appearing islets; amyloid (amylin) deposition common
Prone to develop diabetic complications (retinopathy, nephropathy, neuropathy, atherosclerotic cardiovascular disease)	Yes	Yes
Hyperglycemia responds to oral antihyperglycemic drugs	No	Yes, initially in many patients

genes. Susceptibility genes are more common among some populations than among others and explain the higher prevalence of type 1 DM in some ethnic groups.

Auto antigens include glutamic acid decarboxylase, insulin, proinsulin, insulinoma-associated protein, zinc transporter ZnT8, and other proteins in β-cells. It is thought that these proteins are exposed or released during normal β-cell turnover or β-cell injury (e.g. due to infection), activating primarily a T-cell mediated immune response resulting in β-cell destruction (insulitis). Glucagon-secreting β-cells remain unharmed. Antibodies to autoantigens, which can be detected in serum, seem to be a response to (not a cause of) β-cell destruction.

Several **viruses** (including coxsackie virus, rubella virus, cytomegalo virus, Epstein–Barr virus, and retroviruses) have been linked to the onset of type 1 DM. Viruses may directly infect and destroy β-cells, or they may cause β-cell destruction indirectly by exposing autoantigens, activating autoreactive lymphocytes, mimicking molecular sequences of autoantigens that stimulate an immune response (molecular mimicry), or other mechanisms.

Diet may also be a factor. Exposure of infants to dairy products (especially cow's milk and the milk protein β-casein), high nitrates in drinking water, and low vitamin D consumption have been linked to increased risk of type 1 DM. Early (<4 months) or late (>7 months) exposure to gluten and cereals increases islet cell auto-antibody production. Mechanisms for these associations are unclear.

Type 2 Diabetes Mellitus

In type 2 DM (previously called adult-onset or non–insulin-dependent), insulin secretion is inadequate because patients have developed resistance to insulin. Hepatic insulin resistance leads to an inability to suppress hepatic glucose production, and peripheral insulin resistance impairs peripheral glucose uptake. This combination gives rise to fasting and postprandial hyperglycemia. Often insulin levels are very high, especially early in the disease. Later in the course of the disease, insulin production may fall, further exacerbating hyperglycemia. The disease generally develops in adults and becomes more common with increasing age; up to one-third of adults > age of 65, have impaired glucose tolerance. In older adults, plasma glucose levels reach higher levels after eating than in younger adults, especially after meals with high carbohydrate loads. Glucose levels also take longer to return to normal, in part because of increased accumulation of visceral and abdominal fat and decreased muscle mass.

Type 2 DM is becoming increasingly common among children as childhood obesity has become epidemic; 40–50% of new-onset DM in children is now type 2. Over 90% of adults with DM have type 2 disease. There are clear genetic determinants, as evidenced by the high prevalence of the disease within ethnic groups and in relatives of people with the disease. Although, several genetic polymorphisms have been identified over the past several years, no single gene responsible for the most common forms of type 2 DM has been identified.

Pathogenesis is complex and incompletely understood. Hyperglycemia develops when insulin secretion can no longer compensate for insulin resistance. Although insulin resistance is characteristic in people with type 2 DM and those at risk of it, evidence also exists for β-cell dysfunction and impaired insulin secretion, including impaired first-phase insulin secretion in response to IV glucose infusion, a loss of normally pulsatile insulin secretion, an increase in proinsulin secretion signaling impaired insulin processing, and an accumulation of islet amyloid polypeptide (a protein normally secreted with insulin). Hyperglycemia itself may impair insulin secretion, because high glucose levels desensitize β-cells, cause β-cell dysfunction (glucose toxicity), or both. These changes typically take years to develop in the presence of insulin resistance.

Obesity and weight gain are important determinants of insulin resistance in type 2 DM. They have some genetic determinants, but also reflect diet, exercise, and life style. An inability to suppress lipolysis in adipose tissue increases plasma levels of free fatty acids (FFAs) that may impair insulin-stimulated glucose transport and muscle glycogen synthase activity. Adipose tissue also appears to function as an endocrine organ, releasing multiple factors (adipocytokines) that favorably (adiponectin) and adversely [tumor necrosis factor-α, interleukin 6 (IL-6), leptin, resistin] influence glucose metabolism. Intra-uterine growth restriction and low birth weight have also been associated with insulin resistance in later life and may reflect adverse prenatal environmental influences on glucose metabolism.

Symptoms and Signs

The most common symptoms of DM are those of hyperglycemia. The mild hyperglycemia of early DM is often asymptomatic; therefore, diagnosis may be delayed for many years. More significant hyperglycemia causes glycosuria and thus an osmotic diuresis, leading to urinary frequency, polyuria, and polydipsia that may progress to orthostatic hypotension and dehydration. Severe dehydration causes weakness, fatigue, and mental status changes. Symptoms may come and go as plasma glucose levels fluctuate. Polyphagia may accompany symptoms of hyperglycemia but is not typically a primary patient concern. Hyperglycemia, can also cause weight loss, nausea and vomiting, and blurred vision, and it may predispose to bacterial or fungal infections.

Patients with type 1 DM typically present with symptomatic hyperglycemia and sometimes with diabetic ketoacidosis (DKA). Some patients experience a long but transient phase of near-normal glucose levels after acute onset of the disease (honeymoon phase) due to partial recovery of insulin secretion.

Patients with type 2 DM may present with symptomatic hyperglycemia but are often asymptomatic, and their condition is detected only during routine testing. In some patients, initial symptoms are those of diabetic complications, suggesting that the disease has been present for some time. In some patients, hyperosmotic coma occurs initially, especially during a period of stress or when glucose metabolism is further impaired by drugs, such as corticosteroids.

COMPLICATIONS

Poorly controlled hyperglycemia lead to multiple, primarily vascular complications that affect small vessels (microvascular), large vessels (macrovascular), or both. The mechanisms by which vascular disease develops include glycosylation of serum and tissue proteins with formation of advanced glycation end products; superoxide production; activation of protein kinase C, a signaling molecule that increases vascular permeability and causes endothelial dysfunction; accelerated hexosamine biosynthetic and polyol pathways leading to sorbitol accumulation within tissues; hypertension and dyslipidemias that commonly accompany DM; arterial microthromboses; and proinflammatory and prothrombotic effects of hyperglycemia and hyperinsulinemia that impair vascular autoregulation. Immune dysfunction is another major complication and develops from the direct effects of hyperglycemia on cellular immunity.

Microvascular disease underlies the three most common and devastating manifestations of DM—retinopathy, nephropathy, and neuropathy. It may also impair skin healing, so that even minor breaks in skin integrity can develop into deeper ulcers and easily become infected, particularly in the lower extremities. Intensive control of plasma glucose can prevent or delay many of these complications, but may not reverse them once established.

Macrovascular disease involves atherosclerosis of large vessels, which can lead to Angina pectoris and myocardial infarction (MI), transient ischemic attacks and strokes and peripheral arterial disease.

Diagnosis

The diagnosis of DM depends on the demonstration of hyperglycemia. In a patient with classic symptoms and signs, this may be inferred from the presence of glycosuria, but glycosuria is not diagnostic of diabetes, even in the presence of classic clinical features. In a patient with such features, a random venous plasma or capillary blood glucose concentration ≥11.1 mmol/L (venous blood glucose ≥10 mmol/L) is diagnostic of diabetes; so, too, is a fasting venous plasma glucose concentration ≥7.0 mmol/L (venous or capillary blood glucose ≥6.1 mmol/L). In the absence of symptoms, any of these limits must be exceeded on more than one occasion for the diagnosis to be made. Even in symptomatic patients, diabetes is unlikely, if a random venous plasma glucose concentration is <5.5 mmol/L (venous or capillary blood glucose <4.4 mmol/L). Individuals who have fasting plasma glucose concentrations that are elevated (≥6.1 mmol/L), but not in the diabetic range have impaired fasting glycaemia. Their response to a glucose load should be tested to determine whether they have diabetes.

These values are those adopted by the World Health Organization (WHO) in 1996, based on the recommendations of an expert committee of the American Diabetic Association (ADA), but more recently (2003) the ADA has suggested that the upper limit of normal for fasting plasma glucose should be 5.6 mmol/L.

The other indications and the protocol for the oral glucose tolerance test (OGTT) are given in Table 11.3, and the interpretation of results in Table 11.4. In the majority of patients suspected of having diabetes, the measurements indicated above will establish the diagnosis, and formal glucose tolerance testing is superfluous; it is only indicated when the diagnosis is in doubt. Note that the diagnostic values are the glucose concentrations fasting and 2 hours after glucose; taking samples at 30 minutes intervals, as used to be recommended, is not required.

The OGTT also defines a category of hyperglycemia termed impaired glucose tolerance (IGT), which does not equate to diabetes, but represents a stage in the natural history of transition from normal glucose tolerance to frank diabetes. IGT is not a clinical entity in itself, but defines a risk category for progression to diabetes. Impaired fasting glycaemia is a further category of abnormal glucose tolerance; some individuals thus classified are found to be diabetic on formal testing; others have IGT. Patients with IGT should be given dietary and lifestyle advice and reviewed regularly. Some will become frankly diabetic; others revert to normal glucose tolerance. All appear to have a similar predisposition to myocardial infarction and stroke as patients with frank

Table 11.3	The oral glucose tolerance test
Indication	**Procedure**
• Equivocal fasting/random blood glucose concentrations	• Patient should eat normal diet, containing at least 250 g carbohydrate per day for 3 days.
• Unexplained glycosuria, particularly in pregnancy	• Fast patient overnight.
• Clinical feature of DM or its complications with normal blood glucose concentrations.	• Take basal blood sample for glucose determination.
• Diagnosis of acromegaly	• Give 75 g glucose in water orally; take further blood same at least 120 minutes for glucose determination.
	• Patient should rest throughout test; smoking not permitted; drinks of water are allowed.

Table 11.4	Diagnostic blood glucose concentrations (mmol/L)			
Diagnosis	**Sample**	**Venous plasma**	**Venous blood**	**Capillary blood**
Normal	Fasting	<6.1	<5.6	<5.6
impaired fasting glycemia	Fasting	≥6.1 and <7.0	≥ 5.6 and <6.1	≥5.6 and <6.1
	2 h post glucose	<7.8	<6.7	<7.8
Impaired glucose tolerance	Fasting	<7.0 and	< 6.1 and	< 6.1 and
	2 h post glucose	≥7.8 and <11.1	≥6.7 and <10.0	≥7.8 and <11.1
Diabetes mellitus	Fasting	≥7.0 or	≥6.1 or	≥6.1 or
	2 h post glucose	≥11.1	≥10.0	≥11.1

diabetes, but they are not at increased risk of microvascular complications.

It should be noted that measurements of blood glucose are no exception to the potential for analytical and biological variation to affect results. Although, precise figures are used as cut-offs for diagnosis, the existence of such variation can result in patients being misclassified if their results are close to cut-off values; this is why a confirmatory measurement is required before diabetes is diagnosed in the absence of clinical features. The results of glucose tolerance tests are additionally affected by factors such as the rate of gastric emptying and, because of the implications of making a diagnosis of diabetes (or of missing it), it may be prudent to repeat an OGTT if the results are at the borderline for diagnosis.

Other Specific Types of Diabetes Mellitus

MODY Diabetes

Maturity-onset diabetes of the young (MODY) is an autosomal dominant inherited group of clinically heterogeneous types of diabetes which are not always insulin dependent. They are characterized by various disorders in the functions of β-cells in the pancreas. MODY is the most frequent form of monogenic diabetes and it is usually diagnosed prior to 25 years old; however, frequently, it is initially interpreted as diabetes type 1 or 2. If gestational diabetes is present, the possibility of MODY diabetes (in approximately 5%) should be considered as well.

The various forms of MODY diabetes have been classified according to their signs and symptoms as well as the respective genes affected by mutations. Today, there are 13 different types, while with a frequency of 83%, MODY type 2 and 3 are the most frequently occurring forms.

MODY type 2 exhibits a persistent, mild hyperglycemia, which usually does not require medical treatment and can be easily treated by adapting the diet. It is caused by mutations in the glucokinase gene (GCK).

MODY type 3 is marked by severe hyperglycemia. The affected patients respond very well to treatment with sulfonylureas or to smallest doses of insulin and show above average frequent episodes of hypoglycemia under treatment. It is caused by mutations in the HNF1A gene, which encodes for the transcription factor hepatocyte nuclear factor 1-α.

The other forms of MODY type 1, 4, and 5 are caused by mutations in the genes of various transcription factors (HNF4A, PDX1, and HNF1B). The signs and symptoms of MODY type 1 are similar to the ones of type 3. The occurring hyperglycemia requires medical intervention. MODY type 4 has been associated with a mild course of the disease due to its mild hyperglycemia. MODY 5 is a rare condition. Besides severe hyperglycemia, the clinical signs and symptoms furthermore include polycystic kidney disease or malformations in the urogenital tract, which allows a clear distinction from other forms.

MODY is diagnosed through sequencing of the suspected gene, and detecting a mutation. However, molecular genetic testing is expensive and not widely available. It is also evident from the description of the various MODY phenotypes that the clinical spectrum is extremely varied and has significant overlap with both common types of diabetes, making it a challenge to identify MODY patients. As a consequence, many patients with MODY remain undiagnosed. A targeted selection of individuals for genetic testing is necessary to improve the yield of diagnosis, particularly in situations where there are limited resources.

GESTATIONAL DIABETES

Gestational diabetes is diabetes or IGT with onset or first recognized during pregnancy. Different authorities recommend different diagnostic criteria, but, in effect, pregnant patients with any degree of glucose intolerance should be managed as if they have diabetes. Pregnancy decreases glucose tolerance, and patients with gestational diabetes may revert to a normal glucose tolerance postpartum.

Measurement of glycated hemoglobin (HbA_{1c}) has recently been recommended by the ADA as a diagnostic test for diabetes, with a cut-off of >48 mmol/mol (>6.5%) (The value at which the risk of retinopathy begins to increase), but this has only been conditionally endorsed by the WHO, and it should be emphasized that normal values do not exclude the diagnosis.

Management

There are many aspects to the management of DM. Education of patients is vital; they will have diabetes for the rest of their lives and must, to a considerable extent, be responsible for their own treatment, albeit with guidance from physicians, nurse specialists, and other health care professionals. The successful management of diabetes requires effective teamwork, with the patient being an active member of the team. Regular follow-up is essential to monitor treatment and detect early signs of complications, particularly retinopathy, which can in many cases be treated successfully, and nephropathy, as treatment may slow its progression.

The aims of treatment are twofold; to alleviate symptoms and prevent the acute metabolic complications of diabetes, and to prevent long-term complications. The first of these objectives is usually attainable with dietary control (essentially, substitution of complex for simple carbohydrates, an increase in dietary fiber and restriction of energy intake when necessary) with or without oral hypoglycemic agents in patients with type 2 DM (at least initially insulin is often required later in the course of the condition), and with diet and insulin in patients with type 1 DM.

The demonstration that intensive glycemic control reduces the risk of microvascular complications in diabetes means that the goal of treatment should be to attempt to maintain the blood glucose concentration within the physiological range. In practice, this may be difficult to achieve, and intensification of treatment increases the risk of episodes of hypoglycemia, particularly in patients treated with insulin. Indeed, some insulin-treated patients prefer to avoid the risk of hypoglycemia by maintaining a level of glycemic control that prevents the development of symptomatic acute hyperglycemia, but is less than optimal in terms of reducing the risk of complications long term.

It is beyond the scope of this book to discuss treatment strategies in detail. In type 1 DM, there is an increasing tendency to use 'basal–bolus' regimens of insulin injections, whereby a long-acting insulin is given at night (to mimic the basal insulin secretion that occurs even during fasting) with boluses of short-acting insulin at meal times. Such regimens can provide plasma insulin concentrations that more closely mimic those seen in non-diabetic individuals. They also allow greater flexibility with regard to meals (timing and content) than the traditional twice daily injections of short- and long-acting insulins. Continuous subcutaneous insulin infusion is also being used, but is demanding for the patient.

In patients with type 2 DM, improved control over that achieved with oral hypoglycemics alone can often be achieved by giving a single injection of a long-acting insulin at night, continuing with the oral agents during the day, but standard insulin regimens may be required for some patients.

Drugs used in the treatment of type 2 DM include metformin, a biguanide, the precise mechanism of action of which is unclear but which appears to increase sensitivity to insulin; sulphonylureas, which enhance insulin secretion; thiazolidinediones (glitazones), activators of the peroxisome proliferator-activated receptor γ (PPARγ), which enhance the actions of insulin; and meglitinides, rapidly (and short) acting insulin secretagogues. More recently, drugs based on the action of incretins have been developed. These are of two types: incretin enhancers and incretin mimetics. The first group (the gliptins) act by inhibiting dipeptidyl peptidase 4 (DPP-4), an enzyme responsible for the rapid degradation of GLP-1. The second group (e.g. exenatide and liraglutide) mimic the action of GLP-1 and are resistant to degradation by DPP-4.

It is sometimes considered that less strict glycemic control may be acceptable in older patients developing type 2 DM on the basis that their life expectancy is such that they are not at significant risk of developing long-term complications. Such patients may not experience acute symptoms of hyperglycemia, even with persisting blood glucose concentrations of the order of 15 mmol/L, and they are not at significant risk of developing ketoacidosis. However, although such a view may sometimes be appropriate, and the targets of treatment should always be assessed on an individual basis, the underlying metabolic abnormality will often have been present for several years before clinical presentation, and indeed patients with type 2 DM sometimes present clinically as a result of complications rather than symptoms of hyperglycemia.

Whatever the treatment, the fluctuations in blood glucose concentration that occur in most diabetic patients are still greater than those that occur in normal subjects.

Monitoring Treatment

The efficacy of treatment in diabetes is monitored clinically, by ensuring that the patient's symptoms are controlled, and by measurement of blood glucose concentration and other objective indicators of glycemic control.

Many patients monitor their own blood glucose concentrations at home using reagent strips and a glucose meter. This may be done more or less frequently as circumstances require; exercise, illness, or a change of diet may alter insulin requirements, and more frequent testing will allow the patient to adjust the dosage accordingly. In type 1 diabetes, currently recommended targets for treatment in adults are preprandial blood glucose concentrations of 4.0–7.0 mmol/L and postprandial concentrations of <9.0 mmol/L. The corresponding figures in children are 4.0–8.0 mmol/L and <10 mmol/L. Urine testing for glucose is now little used; it should not be used to monitor type 1 diabetes. Such testing is only semi-quantitative and is of no value in the detection of hypoglycemia; the urine is virtually free of glucose at normal blood glucose concentrations. Urine glucose excretion also depends on the renal threshold for glucose; if this is low (as, e.g. in renal glycosuria), glucose may be present in the urine at normal blood glucose concentrations. Urine testing for glucose should be used in type 2 diabetes only in patients unable or unwilling to do blood tests, and in older patients in whom control may not need to be so strict, particularly if they are treated with diet alone.

The measurement of glycated hemoglobin provides an important means of monitoring glycemic control over a longer timespan. Hemoglobin undergoes glycation *in vivo* at a rate proportional to the blood glucose concentration; the reaction proceeds through a reversible stage but, once the major stable product (HbA_{1c}) is formed, it persists in that state for the lifetime of the cell. The proportion of hemoglobin in the glycated form thus effectively 'integrates' the blood glucose concentration over the previous 6–8 weeks. HbA_{1c} has, until recently, been expressed as a percentage (of normal hemoglobin), but current recommendations are that it is reported as mmol/mol normal hemoglobin. Normal HbA_{1c} is <42 mmol/mol (<6%); in uncontrolled diabetes, it may exceed 86 mmol/mol (10%). Caution with interpretation is required in patients with decreased red cell life spans, e.g. due to hemolytic anemia. In some of the methods used to measure glycated hemoglobin, hemoglobin variants may cross-react and give falsely high results. The measurement and use of glycated hemoglobin has been complicated by the varying specificity of the different assays that are available (some also measure the minor glycated hemoglobins in addition to HbA_{1c}) and problems with standardization, but these problems have largely been resolved. Although, treatment targets should be set on an individual basis, current recommendations are to aim to achieve and maintain an HbA_{1c} value of no more than 58 mmol/mol (<7.5%) in type 1 diabetes, if this can be attained without unacceptably frequent episodes of hypoglycemia. The general target in type 2 diabetes (reflecting the greater risk of macrovascular disease) is 48 mmol/mol (6.5 %). In practice, however, many patients do not achieve these targets.

As the proportion of glycated hemoglobin reflects the mean blood glucose concentration over the previous few weeks, its measurement is particularly useful whenever there is a discrepancy between the patient's history and blood glucose measurements. For example, it will be high in patients who are generally poorly controlled, but who make a special effort to comply with their treatment before attending a clinic in order to please their doctor by having a normal blood glucose concentration.

Other proteins also undergo glycation. Plasma fructosamine concentration is a measure of the glycation of plasma proteins, particularly albumin, and reflects glycemic control over a shorter span than HbA_{1c}, but is much less widely used than glycated hemoglobin.

Other tests of value in monitoring patients with diabetes include the detection of microalbuminuria (for incipient diabetic nephropathy), measurement of plasma creatinine (in established renal disease) and lipids (because of the risk of atherosclerosis), and urine (or blood) ketones (in patients at risk of ketoacidosis). It should be noted that both autoimmune thyroid disease and coeliac disease have a higher prevalence in patients with type 1 diabetes than in normal individuals.

METABOLIC COMPLICATIONS OF DIABETES

Ketoacidosis

Ketoacidosis may be the presenting feature of type 1 DM, or may develop in a patient known to have diabetes who omits to take his/her insulin or whose insulin dosage becomes inadequate because of an increased requirement, e.g. as a result of infection, trauma or any acute illness such as myocardial infarction. Newly diagnosed patients account for 20–25% of cases. It is rare although not unknown occurrence in patients with type 2 DM.

Pathophysiology

Insulin deficiency causes the body to metabolize triglycerides and amino acids instead of glucose for energy. Serum levels of glycerol and free fatty acids (FFAs) rise because of unrestrained lipolysis, as does alanine because of muscle catabolism. Glycerol and alanine provide substrate for hepatic gluconeogenesis, which is stimulated by the excess of glucagon that accompanies insulin deficiency. Glucagon also stimulates mitochondrial conversion of FFAs into ketones. Insulin normally blocks ketogenesis by inhibiting the transport of FFA derivatives into the mitochondrial matrix, but ketogenesis proceeds in the absence of insulin. The major ketoacids produced, acetoacetic acid and β-hydroxybutyric acid, are strong organic acids that create metabolic acidosis. Acetone derived from the metabolism of acetoacetic acid accumulates in serum and is slowly disposed of by respiration.

Hyperglycemia due to insulin deficiency causes an osmotic diuresis that leads to marked urinary losses of water and electrolytes. Urinary excretion of ketones obligates additional losses of Na and K. Serum Na may fall from natriuresis or rise due to excretion of large volumes of free water. K is also lost in large quantities, sometimes >300 mmol/24 hours. Despite a significant total body deficit of K, initial serum K is typically normal or elevated because of the extracellular migration of K in response to acidosis. K levels generally fall further during treatment as insulin therapy drives K into cells. If serum K is not monitored and replaced as needed, life-threatening hypokalemia may develop.

Symptoms and Signs

Diabetic ketoacidosis signs and symptoms often develop quickly, sometimes within 24 hours. For some, these signs and symptoms may be the first indication of having diabetes. Include excessive thirst, frequent urination, nausea and vomiting, abdominal pain, weakness or fatigue, shortness of breath, fruity-scented breath and confusion. Lethargy and somnolence are symptoms of more severe decompensation. Patients may be hypotensive and tachycardic from dehydration and acidosis. Fever is not a sign of DKA itself and, if present, signifies underlying infection. In the absence of timely treatment, DKA progresses to coma and death. More-specific signs of diabetic ketoacidosis which can be detected through home blood and urine testing kits include; high blood sugar level (hyperglycemia) and high ketone levels in the urine.

Acute cerebral edema, a complication in about 1% of DKA patients, occurs primarily in children and less often in adolescents and young adults. Headache and fluctuating level of consciousness herald this complication in some patients, but respiratory arrest is the initial manifestation in others. The cause is not well understood but may be related to too rapid reductions in serum osmolality or to brain ischemia. It is most likely to occur in children <5 years when DKA is the initial manifestation of DM. Children with the highest blood urea nitrogen (BUN) and lowest $PACO_2$ at presentation appear to be at greatest risk. Delays in correction of hyponatremia and the use of HCO_3 during DKA treatment are additional risk factors.

Diagnosis

In patients suspected of having DKA, serum electrolytes, BUN and creatinine, glucose, ketones, and osmolarity should be measured. Urine should be tested for ketones. Patients who appear significantly ill and those with positive ketones should have arterial blood gas (ABG) measurement. DKA is diagnosed by an arterial pH <7.30 with an anion gap >12 and serum ketones in the presence of hyperglycemia. A presumptive diagnosis can be made when urine glucose and ketones are strongly positive. Urine test strips and some assays for serum ketones may underestimate the degree of ketosis because they detect acetoacetic acid and not β-hydroxybutyric acid, which is usually the predominant keto acid.

Symptoms and signs of a triggering illness should be pursued with appropriate studies (e.g. cultures, imaging studies). Adults should have an ECG to screen for acute MI and to help determine the significance of abnormalities in serum K.

Other laboratory abnormalities include hyponatremia, elevated serum creatinine, and elevated plasma osmolality. Hyperglycemia may cause dilutional hyponatremia, so measured serum Na is corrected by adding 1.6 mmol/L for each 100 mg/dL elevation of serum glucose over 100 mg/dL. To illustrate, for a patient with serum Na of 124 mmol/L and glucose of 600 mg/dL, add [1.6 (600–100)/100] = 8 mmol/L to 124 for a corrected serum Na of 132 mmol/L. As acidosis is corrected, serum K drops. An initial K level <4.5 mmol/L indicates marked

K depletion and requires immediate K supplementation. Serum amylase and lipase are often elevated, even in the absence of pancreatitis (which may be present in alcoholic DKA patients and in those with coexisting hyper-triglyceridemia).

Treatment

The most urgent goals are rapid intravascular volume repletion, correction of hyperglycemia and acidosis, and prevention of hypokalemia. Identification of precipitating factors is also important. Treatment should occur in intensive care settings because clinical and laboratory assessments are initially needed every hour or every other hour with appropriate adjustments in treatment.

Intravascular volume should be restored rapidly to raise BP and ensure glomerular perfusion; once intra-vascular volume is restored, remaining total body water deficits are corrected more slowly, typically over about 24 hours. Initial volume repletion in adults is typically achieved with rapid IV infusion of 1–3 L of 0.9% saline solution, followed by saline infusions at 1 L/h or faster as needed to raise BP, correct hyperglycemia, and keep urine flow adequate. Adults with DKA typically need a minimum of 3 L of saline over the first 5 hours. When BP is stable and urine flow adequate, normal saline is replaced by 0.45% saline. When plasma glucose falls to <11.1 mmol/L, IV fluid should be changed to 5% dextrose in 0.45% saline.

For children, fluid deficits are estimated at 60–100 mL/kg body weight. Maintenance fluids (for ongoing losses) must also be provided. Initial fluid therapy should be 0.9% saline (20 mL/kg) over 1–2 hours, followed by 0.45% saline once BP is stable and urine output adequate. The remaining fluid deficit should be replaced over 36 hours, typically requiring a rate (including maintenance fluids) of about 2–4 mL/kg/h, depending on the degree of dehydration.

Hyperglycemia is corrected by giving regular insulin 0.1 unit/kg IV bolus initially, followed by continuous IV infusion of 0.1 unit/kg/h in 0.9% saline solution. Insulin should be withheld until serum K is ≥3.3 mmol/L. Insulin adsorption onto IV tubing can lead to inconsistent effects, which can be minimized by preflushing the IV tubing with insulin solution. If plasma glucose does not fall by 2.8–4.2 mmol/L in the first hour, insulin doses should be doubled. Children should be given a continuous IV insulin infusion of 0.1 unit/kg/h or higher with or without a bolus.

Ketones should begin to clear within hours if insulin is given in sufficient doses. However, clearance of ketones may appear to lag because of conversion of β-hydroxybutyrate to acetoacetate (which is the 'ketone' measured in most hospital laboratories) as acidosis

resolves. Serum pH and HCO_3 levels should also quickly improve, but restoration of a normal serum HCO_3 level may take 24 hours. Rapid correction of pH by HCO_3 administration may be considered if pH remains <7 after about an hour of initial fluid resuscitation, but HCO_3 is associated with development of acute cerebral edema (primarily in children) and should not be used routinely. If used, only modest pH elevation should be attempted (target pH of about 7.1), with doses of 50–100 mmol over 30–60 minutes, followed by repeat measurement of arterial pH and serum K.

When plasma glucose becomes <11.1 mmol/L in adults, 5% dextrose should be added to IV fluids to reduce the risk of hypoglycemia. Insulin dosage can then be reduced to 0.02–0.05 unit/kg/h, but the continuous IV infusion of regular insulin should be maintained until the anion gap has narrowed and blood and urine are consistently negative for ketones. Insulin replacement may then be switched to regular insulin 5–10 units SC q 4–6 hours. When the patient is stable and able to eat, a typical split-mixed or basal-bolus insulin regimen is begun. IV insulin should be continued for 1–4 hours after the initial dose of SC insulin is given. Children should continue to receive 0.05 unit/kg/h insulin infusion until SC insulin is initiated and pH is >7.3.

Hypokalemia prevention requires replacement of 20–30 mmol K in each liter of IV fluid to keep serum K between 4 mmol/L and 5 mmol/L. If serum K is <3.3 mmol/L, insulin should be withheld and K given at 40 mmol/h until serum K is ≥3.3 mmol/L; if serum K is >5 mmol/L, K supplementation can be withheld. Initially normal or elevated serum K measurements may reflect shifts from intracellular stores in response to acidemia and be lie the true K deficits that almost all DKA patients have. Insulin replacement rapidly shifts K into cells, so levels should be checked hourly or every other hour in the initial stages of treatment. Hypophosphatemia often develops during treatment of DKA, but phosphate repletion is of unclear benefit in most cases. If indicated K phosphate 1–2 mmol/kg of phosphate, can be infused over 6–12 hours. If K phosphate is given, the serum Ca level usually decreases and should be monitored. Treatment of suspected cerebral edema is hyperventilation, corticosteroids, and mannitol, but these measures are often ineffective after the onset of respiratory arrest.

NONKETOTIC HYPERGLYCEMIA

Not all patients with uncontrolled diabetes develop ketoacidosis. In type 2 DM, severe hyperglycemia can develop (blood glucose concentration >50 mmol/L), with extreme dehydration and a very high plasma osmolality, but with no ketosis and minimal acidosis. This complication is often referred to as 'hyperosmolar nonketotic hyperglycemia', but patients with ketoacidosis usually also have increased plasma osmolality, although not to the same extent.

Symptoms and Signs

The primary symptom of nonketotic hyperglycemia is altered consciousness varying from confusion or disorientation to coma, usually as a result of extreme dehydration with or without prerenal azotemia, hyperglycemia, and hyperosmolality. In contrast to DKA, focal or generalized seizures and transient hemiplegia may occur.

Diagnosis

Generally, nonketotic hyperglycemia is initially suspected when a markedly elevated glucose level is found in a fingerstick specimen obtained in the course of a workup of altered mental status. If measurements have not already been obtained, measurement of serum electrolytes, BUN and creatinine, glucose, ketones, and plasma osmolality should be done. Urine should be tested for ketones. Serum K levels are usually normal, but Na may be low or high depending on volume deficits. BUN and serum creatinine levels are markedly increased. Arterial pH is usually >7.3, but occasionally mild metabolic acidosis develops due to lactate accumulation.

The average fluid deficit is 10 L, and acute circulatory collapse is a common cause of death. Widespread thrombosis is a frequent finding on autopsy, and in some cases bleeding may occur as a consequence of disseminated intravascular coagulation. Other complications include aspiration pneumonia, acute renal failure, and acute respiratory distress syndrome.

Treatment

0.9% saline solution 1 L IV over 30 minutes, then at 1 L/h to raise BP and improve circulation and urine output. It can be replaced by 0.45% saline when BP becomes normal and plasma glucose reaches 16.7 mmol/L. The rate of infusion of IV fluids should be adjusted depending on BP, cardiac status, and the balance between fluid input and output.

Insulin is given at 0.1 unit/kg IV bolus followed by a 0.1 unit/kg/h infusion after the first liter of saline has been infused. Hydration alone can sometimes precipitously decrease plasma glucose, so insulin dose may need to be reduced. A too quick reduction in osmolality can lead to cerebral edema. Occasional patients with insulin-resistant type 2 DM with nonketotic hyperglycemia require larger insulin doses. Once plasma glucose reaches 16.7 mmol/L, insulin infusion should be reduced to basal levels (1–2 units/hour) until rehydration is complete and the patient is able to eat. Target plasma glucose is between 13.9 mmol/L to 16.7 mmol/L. Addition of 5% dextrose infusion may occasionally be needed to avoid hypoglycemia. After recovery from the acute episode, patients are usually switched to adjusted doses of SC insulin. Most patients can resume using oral antihyperglycemic drugs once their condition is stable. K replacement is similar to DKA; 40 mmol/h for serum K < 3.3 mmol/L; 20–30 mmol/h for serum K between 3.3 mmol/L and 4.9 mmol/L; and none for serum K ≤ 5 mmol/L.

Lactic Acidosis

Lactic acidosis is an uncommon complication of diabetes. It was formerly chiefly seen in patients treated with phenformin, a biguanide oral hypoglycemic drug, but is now more usually associated with severe systemic illness, e.g. severe shock and pancreatitis.

Diabetic Nephropathy

Diabetic nephropathy is a leading cause of chronic kidney disease; it is characterized by thickening of the glomerular basement membrane, mesangial expansion, and glomerular sclerosis. These changes cause glomerular hypertension and progressive decline in glomerular filtration rate (GFR). Systemic hypertension may accelerate progression. The disease is usually asymptomatic until nephrotic syndrome or renal failure develops.

Diagnosis is by detection of urinary albumin. Once diabetes is diagnosed urinary microalbumin level should be monitored, so that nephropathy can be detected early. Monitoring can be done by measuring the albumin—creatinine ratio on a spot urine specimen or total urinary albumin in a 24 hours collection. A ratio >30 mg/g or an albumin excretion 30–300 mg in 24 hours signifies microalbuminuria and early diabetic nephropathy. A urine dipstick positive for protein signifies albumin excretion >300 mg/day and advanced diabetic nephropathy (or an improperly collected or stored specimen).

Treatment is rigorous glycemic control combined with BP control. An angiotensin-converting enzyme (ACE) inhibitor or an angiotensin II receptor blocker should be used to treat hypertension and, at the earliest sign of microalbuminuria, to prevent progression of renal disease because these drugs lower intraglomerular BP and thus have renoprotective effects. These drugs have not been shown to be beneficial for primary prevention (i.e. in patients who do not have microalbuminuria).

Diabetic Retinopathy

Diabetic retinopathy is the most common cause of adult blindness; it is characterized initially by retinal capillary microaneurysms (background retinopathy) and later by neovascularization (proliferative retinopathy) and macular edema. There are no early symptoms or signs, but focal blurring, vitreous or retinal detachment, and partial or total vision loss eventually develop; rate of progression is highly variable.

Screening and diagnosis is by retinal examination, which should be done regularly (usually annually) in both type 1 and type 2 DM. Early detection and treatment are critical to preventing vision loss. Treatment for all patients includes intensive glycemic and BP control. More advanced proliferative retinopathy may require panretinal laser photocoagulation or more rarely vitrectomy. Vascular endothelial growth factor (VEGF) inhibitors are promising new drugs for macular edema and as adjunctive therapy for proliferative retinopathy.

Diabetic Neuropathy

Diabetic neuropathy is the result of nerve ischemia due to microvascular disease, direct effects of hyperglycemia on neurons, and intracellular metabolic changes that impair nerve function. There are multiple types, including symmetric polyneuropathy (with small- and large-fiber variants), autonomic neuropathy, radiculopathy, cranial neuropathy and mononeuropathy.

Lipoprotein Metabolism in Diabetes Mellitus

Insulin has a major role in the control of fat metabolism, and both type 1 and type 2 DM are associated with abnormalities of plasma lipids. In type 1 DM, at presentation, or if glycemic control deteriorates, marked hypertriglyceridemia (manifest as an increase in very low density lipoprotein (VLDL), and often by chylomicronemia as well) is often present, as a result of decreased activity of lipoprotein lipase (which insulin stimulates) and increased activity of hormone-sensitive lipase (which insulin inhibits), leading to increased flux of free fatty acids from adipose tissue that act as a substrate for hepatic triglyceride synthesis. Both these effects are reversed by insulin treatment. Indeed, the degree of hypertriglyceridemia correlates well with glycemic control. Low density lipoprotein (LDL) concentration can also be increased, and that of high density lipoprotein (HDL) decreased.

In type 2 DM, hypertriglyceridemia is also common, although it is not usually as severe as in uncontrolled type 1 DM, unless there is an additional, genetic, predisposition. It is due mainly to increased hepatic synthesis. The VLDL contains increased triglyceride and cholesteryl esters in relation to the amount of apoprotein and, although LDL cholesterol concentrations are not much increased, the particles tend to be smaller and denser, and are more atherogenic. As in type 1 DM, the HDL concentration is often decreased. In both type 1 and type 2 DM, glycation of apolipoprotein B may enhance the atherogenicity of LDL by reducing its affinity for the LDL receptor, thus leading to increased uptake by macrophage scavenger receptors.

Plasma lipid concentrations usually become normal in patients with well-controlled type 1 DM; HDL concentrations may even become increased. In contrast, the abnormalities seen in type 2 DM may persist despite adequate glycemic control. Because of the greatly increased risk of cardiovascular disease in diabetes, treatment with lipid-lowering drugs should be considered in all patients with diabetes; many experts recommend the same targets for treatment as in patients with established cardiovascular disease, even when there is no clinical evidence of this.

HYPOGLYCEMIA IN DIABETIC PATIENTS

Hypoglycemia is a condition characterized by abnormally low blood glucose levels. Most commonly, symptomatic hypoglycemia is a complication of drug treatment of DM. Oral antihyperglycemics or insulin may be involved.

Symptomatic hypoglycemia unrelated to treatment of DM is relatively rare, in part because the body has extensive counter-regulatory mechanisms to compensate for low blood glucose levels. Glucagon and epinephrine levels surge in response to acute hypoglycemia and appear to be the first line of defense. Cortisol and growth hormone levels also increase acutely and are important in the recovery from prolonged hypoglycemia. The threshold for release of these hormones is usually above that for hypoglycemic symptoms.

Etiology

Insulin-mediated causes include exogenous administration of insulin or an insulin secretagogue and insulin-secreting tumors (insulinomas). A helpful practical classification is based on clinical status; whether hypoglycemia occurs in patients who appear healthy or ill. Within these categories, causes of hypoglycemia can be divided into drug-induced and other causes. Pseudohypoglycemia occurs when processing of blood specimens in untreated test tubes is delayed and cells, such as RBCs and leukocytes (especially if increased, as in leukemia or polycythemia), consume glucose. Factitious hypoglycemia is true hypoglycemia induced by nontherapeutic administration of sulfonylureas or insulin.

Symptoms and Signs

The surge in autonomic activity in response to low plasma glucose causes sweating, nausea, warmth, anxiety, tremulousness, palpitations, and possibly hunger and paresthesias. Insufficient glucose supply to the brain causes headache, blurred or double vision, confusion, difficulty in speaking, seizures, and coma. In controlled settings, autonomic symptoms begin at or beneath a plasma glucose level of about 3.3 mmol/L, whereas CNS symptoms occur at or below a glucose level of about 2.8 mmol/L. However, symptoms suggestive of hypoglycemia are far more common than the condition itself. Most people with glucose levels at these thresholds have no symptoms, and most people with symptoms suggestive of hypoglycemia have normal glucose concentrations.

Diagnosis

In principle, diagnosis requires verification that a low plasma glucose level (<2.8 mmol/L) exists at the time hypoglycemic symptoms occur and that the symptoms are responsive to dextrose administration. If a practitioner is present when symptoms occur, blood should be sent for glucose testing. If glucose is normal, hypoglycemia is ruled out and no further testing is needed. If glucose is abnormally low, serum insulin, C-peptide, and proinsulin measured from the same tube can distinguish insulin-mediated from non-insulin-mediated and factitious from physiologic hypoglycemia and can obviate the need for further testing. Insulin growth factor 2 (IGF-2) levels may help identify non–islet cell (IGF-2 secreting) tumors, which are an unusual cause of hypoglycemia.

In practice, however, it is unusual that practitioners are present when patients experience symptoms suggestive of hypoglycemia. Home glucose meters are unreliable for quantifying hypoglycemia, and there are no clear glycosylated Hb (HbA$_{1c}$) thresholds that distinguish long-term hypoglycemia from normoglycemia. So, the need for more extensive diagnostic testing is based on the probability that an underlying disorder that could cause hypoglycemia exists given a patient's clinical appearance and coexisting illnesses.

A 72-hours fast done in a controlled setting is the standard for diagnosis. Patients drink only noncaloric, noncaffeinated beverages, and plasma glucose is measured at baseline, whenever symptoms occur. Serum insulin, C-peptide, and proinsulin should be measured at times of hypoglycemia to distinguish endogenous from exogenous (factitious) hypoglycemia. The fast is terminated at 72 hours, if the patient has experienced no symptoms and glucose remains normal, sooner if glucose decreases to ≤2.5 mmol/L in the presence of hypoglycemic symptoms. End-of-fast measurements include β-hydroxybutyrate (which should be low in insulinoma), serum sulfonylurea to detect drug-induced hypoglycemia,

and plasma glucose after IV glucagon injection to detect an increase characteristic of insulinoma. Sensitivity, specificity, and predictive values for detecting hypoglycemia by this protocol have not been reported. There is no definitive lower limit of glucose that unequivocally defines pathologic hypoglycemia during a 72 hours fast. Normal women tend to have lower fasting glucose levels than men and may have glucose levels as low as 1.7 mmol/L without symptoms. If symptomatic hypoglycemia has not occurred by 72 hours, the patient should exercise vigorously for about 30 minutes. If hypoglycemia still does not occur, insulinoma is essentially excluded and further testing is generally not indicated.

Treatment

Immediate treatment of hypoglycemia involves provision of glucose. Patients able to eat or drink canned juices, sucrose water, or glucose solutions; eat candy or other foods; or chew on glucose tablets when symptoms occur. Infants and younger children may be given 10% dextrose solution 2–5 mL/kg IV bolus. Adults and older children unable to eat or drink can be given glucagon 0.5 (<20 kg) or 1 mg (≤ 20 kg) SC or IM or 50% dextrose 50–100 mL IV bolus, with or without a continuous infusion of 5–10% dextrose solution sufficient to resolve symptoms. The efficacy of glucagon depends on the size of hepatic glycogen stores; glucagon has little effect on plasma glucose in patients who have been fasting or who are hypoglycemic for long periods.

Underlying disorders causing hypoglycemia must also be treated. Islet cell and non-islet cell tumors must first be localized, then removed by enucleation or partial pancreatectomy; about 6% recur within 10 years. Diazoxide and octreotide can be used to control symptoms while the patient is awaiting surgery or when a patient refuses or is not a candidate for a procedure. Islet cell hypertrophy is most often a diagnosis of exclusion after an islet cell tumor is sought but not identified. Drugs that cause hypoglycemia, including alcohol, must be stopped. Treatment of hereditary and endocrine disorders; hepatic, renal, and heart failure; and sepsis and shock are described elsewhere.

POSTPRANDIAL HYPOGLYCEMIA

In patients who have undergone gastric surgery involving either a gastrointestinal anastomosis or a pyloroplasty, hypoglycemia, developing 90–150 minutes after a meal, particularly a meal rich in sugar, is common. There is rapid passage of glucose into the small intestine and release of hormones that stimulate insulin secretion. The insulin response is excessive and hypoglycemia ensues as glucose absorption from the gut falls off rapidly, rather than slowly as it does when gastric emptying is normal.

Symptoms suggestive of hypoglycemia, following meals may be described by people who have not undergone surgery (essential or idiopathic postprandial hypoglycemia). Although, transient hypoglycemia is common from 90–150 minutes after taking 75 g glucose orally in a glucose tolerance test, it is often asymptomatic and the relevance of hypoglycemia after this artificial stimulus is questionable. It is more relevant to examine the blood glucose response to a standard mixed meal, and this diagnosis should not be made unless a low blood glucose concentration is recorded at a time when the patient is symptomatic, and the symptoms are abolished by giving glucose. Thus defined, idiopathic reactive hypoglycemia is uncommon. Its cause remains uncertain; there is no evidence of any impairment of glucose homoeostasis in these patients.

Alcohol and Reactive Hypoglycemia

Insulin- and drug-induced reactive hypoglycemia are potentiated by alcohol. Alcohol also increases insulin release in response to an oral glucose load, and this may enhance any tendency to postprandial reactive hypoglycemia.

Fasting Hypoglycemia

Insulinoma

Insulinomas are tumors of the insulin-secreting β-cells of the pancreatic islets. Although uncommon, they are an important cause of fasting hypoglycemia. The blood glucose concentration should be measured in any patient who experiences a fit, faint, transient ischemic attack or 'funny turn' in order to exclude hypoglycemia as a cause, although many patients with an insulinoma present with behavioral changes rather than with the classic features of acute hypoglycemia. For this reason, there is often a delay before the diagnosis is considered and appropriate investigations are performed.

Other causes of fasting hypoglycemia are usually obvious clinically and, with the exception of insulin- and sulphonylurea-induced hypoglycemia, and hypoglycemia caused by sepsis, are associated with low plasma insulin concentrations. The presence of an insulin-secreting tumor can be inferred from the presence of an inappropriately high plasma insulin concentration (>20 pmol/L) at a time when the blood glucose concentration is low (<2.2 mmol/L). C-peptide should also be measured. Although, secreted in equimolar amounts with insulin, C-peptide is cleared from the circulation more slowly, so it may be a more reliable marker of endogenous insulin secretion than insulin itself.

A concentration of >100 pmol/L implies continuing endogenous insulin secretion. Measurement of plasma 3-hydroxybutyrate concentration is sometimes recommended. Insulin inhibits lipolysis and hence the production of 3-hydroxybutyrate. High concentrations (>600 μmol/L) occur in hypoglycemia with suppressed insulin secretion (e.g. cortisol deficiency, liver disease). In hyperinsulinemia and tumor-related hypoglycemia, 3-hydroxybutyrate concentrations are usually low. However, they can also be low even when insulin secretion is suppressed, if fat stores are severely depleted.

Ideally, blood should be collected for these measurements while the patient is symptomatic. If this cannot be done, or if symptoms of acute hypoglycemia do not occur, blood samples should be collected after an overnight fast on three consecutive mornings; when this is done, biochemical (although often asymptomatic) hypoglycemia is demonstrable in 90% of patients with an insulinoma. If hypoglycemia does not occur under these circumstances, patients suspected of having an insulinoma can be fasted for longer. Clinical hypoglycemia develops in almost all patients with an insulinoma during a 72-hours fast, and can often be provoked by exercise during this time. Blood samples should be collected every 4–6 hours and during any episode of clinical hypoglycemia; plasma insulin and C-peptide concentrations are measured in any sample in which the blood glucose concentration is low. Although, normal subjects occasionally develop hypoglycemia during such a fast (women more frequently than men), this is asymptomatic and the plasma insulin concentration is low (usually <20 pmol/L).

The 72-hours fast is a time-consuming procedure and, as an alternative, when required, an insulin hypoglycemia test can be performed. Hypoglycemia is induced with insulin (with the usual strict monitoring mandatory for this test) and the plasma C-peptide concentration is measured. C-peptide is not present in insulin produced for therapeutic use. In normal individuals the induction of hypoglycemia suppresses endogenous insulin and C-peptide secretion. In patients with an insulinoma there is continuing C-peptide secretion, implying continuing insulin secretion. Some insulinomas secrete mainly proinsulin, but this is measured as insulin in many insulin assays, and separate measurement of proinsulin is not usually required.

It should be noted that glucose tolerance tests have no role in the investigation of possible insulinomas.

Once hyperinsulinism has been demonstrated (and administration of exogenous insulin excluded as a cause of the hypoglycemia), imaging techniques is used to localize the tumor. The great majority are benign, and surgical resection is then curative. Medical treatment (usually with diazoxide, although somatostatin analogues are also used) can provide relief of symptoms if the tumor cannot be localized and in malignant disease.

Non-pancreatic Neoplasms

Hypoglycemia can also occur in association with non-pancreatic neoplasms, including hepatocellular and adrenal carcinomas, carcinoid tumors and large mesenchymal tumors such as retroperitoneal sarcomas. Patients are usually not ketotic and, except with some carcinoid tumors, plasma insulin concentrations are not increased. It has been suggested that increased glucose uptake by the tumor may be a factor, but this is unlikely ever to be the sole cause. Hepatic glucose output is often reduced, although there is a normal glucogenic response to glucagon. It is probable that most such tumor-related hypoglycemia is related to the secretion of insulin-like growth factors (IGFs). Plasma IGF-1 concentrations are consistently low in such patients, but IGF-2 (particularly in the non-protein-bound form) is often increased, and the IGF-1/IGF-2 ratio decreased. Cytokines, such as tumor necrosis factor (TNFα) have also been implicated.

HEPATIC AND RENAL DISEASE

Although, the liver is central to glucose homoeostasis, its functional reserve is so great that hypoglycemia is a rare feature of hepatic disease. It may occur, however, with the rapid, massive hepatocellular destruction that can follow poisoning with paracetamol and other toxins. The kidneys are the only organs other than the liver capable of gluconeogenesis; they are also responsible for insulin degradation. These facts may in part explain the severe hypoglycemia that is occasionally a feature of end-stage renal disease.

Endocrine Disease

Deficiency of hormones antagonistic to insulin is a recognized, but uncommon cause of hypoglycemia. Lack of cortisol can be due either to primary adrenal failure or secondary to panhypopituitarism; hypoglycemia can be a feature of either condition. Mild hypoglycemia can occur with isolated deficiency of ACTH or growth hormone, but in the latter condition it is never symptomatic.

Rather surprisingly, in view of its role in carbohydrate metabolism, decreased secretion of epinephrine (adrenaline) in patients who have undergone bilateral adrenalectomy and who are maintained on corticoid hormone replacement neither causes hypoglycemia nor interferes with the ability to recover from artificially induced hypoglycemia.

Sepsis

Hypoglycemia sometimes develops in patients with septicemia. It is thought to be a result of the release of cytokines, which may stimulate insulin secretion or have a direct effect on hepatic glucose production. Renal impairment may also be contributory.

HYPOGLYCEMIA IN CHILDHOOD

Neonatal Hypoglycemia

Hypoglycemia may occur transiently in apparently normal babies, but is particularly common in those who have respiratory distress, severe infection, brain damage or who are small-for-dates. Premature and small-for-dates babies are particularly at risk of developing neonatal hypoglycemia, because they are born with low hepatic glycogen stores and are more likely to have feeding problems. Extensive physiological changes occur at birth and, in terms of glucose metabolism, there is a sudden interruption of the maternal glucose supply, so that glycogenolysis must span the period until feeding becomes established. Babies born to mothers with diabetes can have islet cell hyperplasia, which increases the risk of hypoglycemia developing in the immediate postnatal period, although this does not persist thereafter.

Hypoglycemia in Infancy

The inherited metabolic diseases associated with hypoglycemia are particularly likely to present during the first few weeks of life.

Beyond the neonatal period, energy stores are usually sufficient to prevent hypoglycemia during fasting unless there is a defect in homoeostatic mechanisms (e.g. as a result of endocrine disease). In some children, however, starvation often in the setting of an intercurrent illness can lead to hypoglycemia. Insulin secretion is suppressed and ketosis is present. Such children are often thin and sometimes have a history of being small-for-dates. The hypoglycemia is thought to be a result of impaired mobilization of glucogenic precursors (particularly alanine), but no specific defect has been described and there is no defining test for this condition, often called 'idiopathic ketotic hypoglycemia'. Affected children usually lose the tendency to hypoglycemia by the age of 5.

Hyperinsulinism can cause persistent neonatal hypoglycemia. There is often overgrowth of pancreatic ducts and islet cells. This rare condition was formerly known as 'nesidioblastosis', but is now referred to as 'hyperinsulinemic hypoglycemia of infancy'. Many cases have been demonstrated to be the result of genetic mutations, for example in the genes for the sulphonylurea receptor, an ATP-dependent potassium channel in the plasma membrane of islet cells, glucokinase or glutamate dehydrogenase. In infants with glutamate dehydrogenase deficiency, a high protein intake can precipitate the hypoglycemia, which probably explains what was formerly called 'leucine-induced hypoglycemia'. The diagnosis is made on the basis of persistent hypoglycemia without ketosis together with an inappropriate plasma insulin concentration. No tumor is demonstrable. 'Nesidioblastosis' may remit spontaneously in adolescence and should be treated medically (with diazoxide or octreotide), and only surgically, by subtotal pancreatectomy, if medical treatment fails to control the symptoms.

The inherited metabolic diseases associated with hypoglycemia include galactosemia, certain glycogen storage diseases, defects of the β-oxidation of fatty acids, hereditary fructose intolerance, and some organic acidemias and amino acidopathies.

MEASUREMENT OF GLUCOSE CONCENTRATION

Plasma glucose concentration tends to be 10–15% higher than that of whole blood because a given volume of red cells contains less water than the same volume of plasma. The difference is of little significance at normal concentrations, except in making a diagnosis of diabetes. However, when glucose concentration is changing rapidly, there may be a considerable discrepancy because of delayed equilibration of glucose across the red cell membranes.

Many analytical procedures are used to measure blood glucose concentrations. In the past, analyses were often performed with relatively nonspecific methods that could produce falsely increased values. Today, almost all common methods are enzymatic (e.g. hexokinase, glucose oxidase), and older methods, such as photometric or oxidation reduction techniques, are rarely used.

Blood glucose concentrations are now frequently measured using glucose-sensitive reagent strips and a hand-held electronic instrument ('glucose meter'). These instruments are robust and produce reliable results. They are often used to monitor blood glucose concentrations at the bedside in hospitals, and are widely used in the community by patients or their carers to measure blood glucose concentrations at home. Readings obtained from glucose meters should not be relied on for the diagnosis of diabetes; formal laboratory measurement is recommended.

SPECIMEN COLLECTION AND STORAGE

In individuals with a normal hematocrit, fasting whole blood glucose concentration is approximately 10–12% lower than plasma glucose. Although, glucose concentrations in the water phase of red blood cells and plasma are similar (the erythrocyte plasma membrane is freely permeable to glucose), the water content of plasma (93%) is approximately 11% higher than that of whole blood. In most clinical laboratories, plasma or serum is used for most glucose determinations; methods for self-monitoring of glucose use whole blood samples, but may measure the glucose concentration in the plasma phase. Venous plasma is recommended for diagnosis of diabetes. Although, older methods of analysis reported that glucose concentrations in plasma were 5% lower than in serum, study indicated that glucose values measured in serum and plasma are essentially the same. During fasting, capillary blood glucose concentration is slightly higher than that of venous blood. After a glucose load, however, capillary blood glucose concentrations are (20–25%) higher than concurrently drawn venous blood samples. Glycolysis decreases serum glucose by approximately 5–7% in 1 hour in normal uncentrifuged coagulated blood at room temperature. The rate of *in vitro* glycolysis is higher in the presence of leukocytosis or bacterial contamination, but others have observed a slight decrease.

In separated, nonhemolyzed sterile serum, the glucose concentration is generally stable as long as 8 hours at 25°C and up to 72 hours at 4°C; variable stability is observed with longer storage periods. Plasma, removed from the cells after moderate centrifugation, contains leukocytes that also metabolize glucose, although cell-free sterile plasma has no glycolytic activity.

Glycolysis has been found to be inhibited and glucose stabilized for as long as 3 days at room temperature by adding sodium fluoride (NaF) or, less commonly, sodium iodoacetate to the specimen. Fluoride ions prevent glycolysis by inhibiting enolase, an enzyme that requires Mg^{2+}. This inhibition is due to the formation of an ionic complex consisting of Mg^{2+}, inorganic phosphate, and fluoride ions; this complex interferes with the interaction of enzyme and substrate. Fluoride is also a weak anticoagulant, because it binds calcium; however, clotting may occur after several hours. It is therefore advisable to use a combined fluoride-oxalate mixture, such as 2 mg of potassium oxalate ($K_2C_2O_4$) and 2 mg NaF/mL of blood, to prevent late clotting.

Other anticoagulants [e.g. ethylenediaminetetraacetic acid (EDTA), citrate, and heparin] can also be used. Fluoride ions in high concentration inhibit the activity of urease and certain other enzymes; consequently, the specimens are unsuitable for determination of urea in procedures that require urease and for direct assay of some serum enzymes. $K_2C_2O_4$ causes loss of cell water, thereby diluting the plasma. Therefore, samples collected in these tubes should not be used for measurement of analytes other than glucose. Although, fluoride maintains long-term blood glucose stability, the rate of decline in the first hour after sample collection is not altered, and glycolysis may continue for up to 4 hours.

GLYCOSURIA

Although, DM is the commonest cause of glycosuria, it is also seen in patients with a low renal threshold for glucose. This may occur as an isolated and harmless abnormality (renal glycosuria), can develop during pregnancy and is a feature of congenital and acquired generalized disorders of proximal renal tubular function (Fanconi syndrome). The use of reagent sticks containing glucose oxidase are specific for glucose testing, the test strip is impregnated with glucose oxidase, peroxidase, and a chromogen. The reaction is specific for glucose. Ascorbic acid and urates may inhibit the reaction and cause false-negative results. Contamination of urine with hydrogen peroxide or an oxidizing agent, such as bleach may cause a false-positive reaction. Urine glucose may be measure quantitatively using chemical methods (hexokinase method or glucose oxidase method). Uric acid in urine may cause falsely lowered results in glucose oxidase methods, which use hydrogen peroxide and peroxidase indicator reactions. The specimen shall be random or 24 hour specimens may be analyzed. Glucose must be measured promptly or preserved with glacial acetic acid or sodium benzoate.

Glucose in Cerebrospinal Fluid

Glucose concentration in the CSF is frequently measured in patients suspected of having bacterial meningitis, because it is usually decreased as a result of bacterial metabolism. If the CSF is frankly purulent, the measurement of CSF glucose provides no useful additional information. The CSF glucose concentration is normally approximately 65% of the blood glucose concentration, and CSF glucose should always be interpreted in the light of the glucose concentration of a blood sample obtained at the same time.

Glycated Hemoglobin

Glycated hemoglobin (HbA1c), is an indicator of long-term glycemic control. In adults, hemoglobin is a mixture of three forms—Hb A1, Hg A2, and Hb F, with HbA1 predominating. Hemoglobin A1 consists of three sub-forms—HbA1a, HbA1b, and HbA1c, with HbA1c predominating. The term glycated hemoglobin describes a chemically stable conjugate of any of the forms of hemoglobin with glucose. Glycated forms of hemoglobin are formed slowly, non-enzymatically, and irreversibly at a rate that is proportional to the concentration of glucose in the blood. The level of glycated hemoglobin in a blood sample provides a glycemic history of hemoglobin glycation over the life span of the erythrocyte, the cell that contains the hemoglobin.

The average life span of the erythrocyte is 120 days, and glycated hemoglobin describes the average glucose levels in the blood over that life span. Clinically, glycated hemoglobin is used to reflect glycemic control over the previous 90–120 days. Glycated hemoglobin measurements are unaffected by daily variation of glucose from diet and exercise.

Glycated hemoglobin measurements are, however, influenced by conditions that affect the life span of the hemoglobin molecule, such as sickle cell disease and hemolytic disease, which can falsely decrease glycated hemoglobin results.

Glycated hemoglobin may be separated and identified on the basis of charge and structure differences. Methods of analysis include ion-exchange or affinity chromatography, electrophoresis, isoelectric focusing, and immunoassay.

SPECIMEN COLLECTION AND STORAGE

Patients need not be fasting. Venous blood should be collected in tubes containing EDTA, oxalate, or fluoride. Sample stability depends on the assay method used. Whole blood may be stored at 4°C for up to 1 week. Above 4°C, HbA1a+b increases in a time- and temperature-dependent manner, but HbA1c is only slightly affected. Storage of samples at –20°C is not recommended. For most methods, whole blood samples stored at –70°C or colder are stable for at least 18 months. Heparinized samples should be assayed within 2 days and may not be suitable for some methods of analysis (e.g. electrophoresis).

Galactosemia

Galactosemia is a rare disorder of carbohydrate metabolism caused by inherited deficiencies in enzymes that convert galactose to glucose. Three different types of galactosemia have been identified (Fig. 11.7); each of these conditions is caused by mutations in a particular gene and affects different enzymes involved in breaking down galactose.

Classic galactosemia, also known as type I, (galactose-1-phosphate uridyl transferase deficiency; GALT) is the most common and most severe form of the condition. If infants with classic galactosemia are not treated promptly with a low-galactose diet, life-threatening complications appear within a few days after birth. Infants become anorectic and jaundiced within a few days or weeks of consuming breast milk or lactose-containing formula. Vomiting, hepatomegaly, poor growth, lethargy, diarrhea, and septicemia (usually *Escherichia coli*)

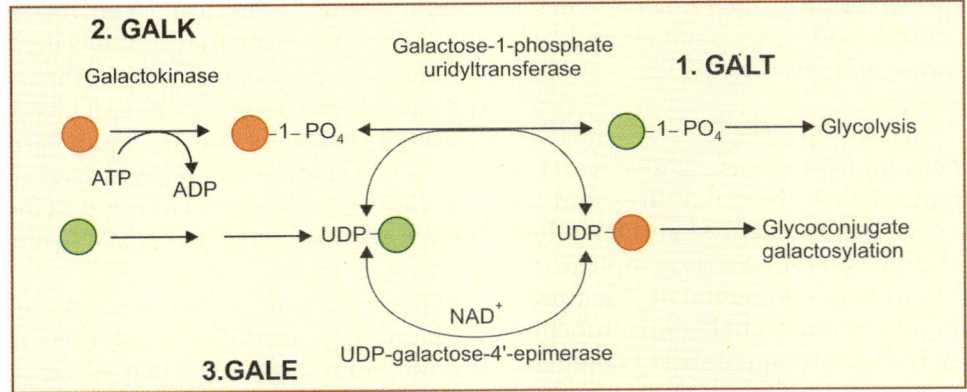

Fig. 11.7: Three different types of galactosemia—galactose 1-phosphate uridyltransferase (GALT) deficiency, galactokinase (GALK) deficiency, and galactose-4'-epimerase (GALE) deficiency

develop, as does renal dysfunction (e.g. proteinuria, aminoaciduria, and Fanconi syndrome), leading to metabolic acidosis and edema. Hemolytic anemia may also occur.

Without treatment, children remain short and develop cognitive, speech, gait, and balance deficits in their teenage years; many also have cataracts, osteomalacia (caused by hypercalciuria), and premature ovarian failure. Patients with the Duarte variant have a much milder phenotype.

Galactosemia type II (galactokinase deficiency; GALK), the patients develop cataracts from production of galactitol, which osmotically damages lens fibers; idiopathic intracranial hypertension (pseudotumor cerebri) is rare.

And galactosemia type III (uridine diphosphate galactose 4-epimerase deficiency; GALE) cause different patterns of signs and symptoms. The benign form is restricted to RBCs and WBCs and causes no clinical abnormalities. The severe form causes a syndrome indistinguishable from classic galactosemia, although sometimes with hearing loss.

GLYCOGEN STORAGE DISORDERS

Glycogen storage diseases (GSDs) is autosomal recessive except for GSD type VIII/IX, which is X-linked. There are many different glycogen storage diseases each is identified by a roman numeral. These diseases are caused by a hereditary lack of one of the enzymes that is essential to the process of forming glucose into glycogen and breaking down glycogen into glucose (Table 11.5). Age of onset, clinical manifestations, and severity vary by type, but symptoms and signs are most commonly those of hypoglycemia and myopathy.

Table 11.5	Glycogen storage diseases		
Disease	**Defective proteins or enzymes**	**Defective gene or genes (chromosomal location)**	**Comments**
GSD I (Von Gierke disease)			Most common type of GSD: Ia (> 80%) Onset: Before 1 year
Type Ia	Glucose-6-phosphatase	G6PC (17q21)*	Clinical features: Before 1 year, severe hypo-
Type Ib	Glucose-6-phosphate translocase	G6PT1 (11q23)*	glycemia, lactic acidosis, and hepatomegaly; later, hepatic adenomas, renomegaly with
Type Ic	Microsomal phosphate or pyrophosphate transporter	G6PT1 (11q23)*	progressive renal insufficiency and hypertension, short stature, hypertriglyceridemia,
Type Id	Microsomal glucose transporter	Probably same as Ic	hyperuricemia, platelet dysfunction with epistaxis, and anemia
			In type Ib, less severe but including neutropenia, neutrophil dysfunction with recurrent infections, and inflammatory bowel disease
			Treatment: Uncooked cornstarch 1.5–2.5 g/kg po q 4–6 h or lactose-free formula with maltodextrin to maintain normoglycemia; nocturnal feedings (important); fructose and galactose restriction; for lactic acidosis, bicarbonate

Contd.

Table 11.5	Glycogen storage diseases *(Contd.)*		
Disease	**Defective proteins or enzymes**	**Defective gene or genes (chromosomal location)**	**Comments**
			0.25–0.5 mmol/kg qid; allopurinol to keep uric acid to <6.4 mg/dL; liver and kidney transplantation (may be successful)
			For type Ib patients with neutropenia, G-CSF
GSD II (Pompe disease)			Onset: Infancy, childhood, or adulthood; residual enzyme activity in child and adult forms
Type IIa	Lysosomal acid α-glucosidase	GAA (17q25)*	Clinical features: In infantile form, cardiomyopathy with heart failure, severe
Type IIb (Danon)	Lysosomal membrane protein-2	LAMP2 (Xq24)*	hypotonia, macroglossia
			In juvenile and adult forms, skeletal myopathy with delayed motor development, progressive peripheral and respiratory muscle weakness
			In type IIb, intellectual disability
			Treatment: None known
			For cardiomyopathy, heart transplantation
GSD III (Forbes disease, Cori disease, limit dextrinosis)			Frequency: IIIa, 85%; IIIb, 15%; IIIc and IIId, rare
			Onset: Infancy or childhood
Types IIIa and IIIb	Debrancher enzyme (amyloglucosidase and oligoglucanotransferase)	AGL (1p21)*	Clinical features: In type IIIa, liver, and muscle involvement with features of type Ia and II
			In type IIIb, only liver involvement plus features of type Ia
Type IIIc	Amyloglucosidase only		In types IIIc and IIId, various features depending
Type IIId	Oligoglucanotransferase only		on tissue affected
			Treatment: Uncooked cornstarch and continuous feeding to maintain normoglycemia, high-protein diet to stimulate gluconeogenesis
GSD IV (Andersen disease)	Branching enzyme	GBE1 (3p12)*	Onset: Early infancy; rarely, the neonatal period, late childhood, or adulthood (manifesting as a variant nonprogressive or a neuromuscular form)
			Clinical features: Hepatomegaly with progressive cirrhosis and hypoglycemia, esophageal varices, and ascites; splenomegaly; failure to thrive
			In neuromuscular forms, hypotonia, and muscle atrophy
			Treatment: None known
			For cirrhosis, liver transplantation, which treats the primary disease as well
GSD V (McArdle disease)	Muscle phosphorylase	PYGM (11q13)*	Onset: Adolescence or early adulthood
			Clinical features: Exercise intolerance due to muscle cramps, rhabdomyolysis
			Treatment: Carbohydrate administration before exercise, high-protein diet
GSD VI (Hers disease)	Liver phosphorylase	PYGL (14q21-q22)*	Frequency: Rare
			Onset: Early childhood
			Clinical features: Benign course with symptoms lessening with aging; growth retardation, hepatomegaly, hypoglycemia, hyperlipidemia, ketosis
			Treatment: None necessary

Contd.

Table 11.5 Glycogen storage diseases *(Contd.)*			
Disease	**Defective proteins or enzymes**	**Defective gene or genes (chromosomal location)**	**Comments**
GSD VII (Tarui disease)	Phosphofructokinase	PFKM (12q13.3)*	Onset: Middle childhood Clinical features: Exercise intolerance due to muscle cramps, rhabdomyolysis, hemolysis Treatment: Nonspecific, avoidance of exercise
GSD VIII/IX		—	Onset: Heterogeneous
Type VIII/IXa:	X-linked phosphorylase kinase	PHKA2 (Xp22)*	Clinical features: Heterogeneous; hepatomegaly, growth retardation, muscle hypotonia, hypercholesterolemia Treatment: Nonspecific
Type IXb	Liver and muscle phosphorylase kinase	PHKB (16q12-q13)*	
Type IXc	Liver phosphorylase kinase	PHKG2 (16p12.1-p11.2)*	
Type IXd	Muscle phosphorylase kinase	PHKA1 (Xq13)*	
GSD O	Glycogen synthase	GYS2 (12p12)*	Onset: Variable but often after cessation of night-time feedings or intercurrent illness Clinical features: Fasting hypoglycemia and ketosis, postprandial lactic acidosis Treatment: Frequent protein-rich meals, uncooked cornstarch at bedtime

*Gene has been identified, and molecular basis has been elucidated.
G-CSF, granulocyte colony-stimulating factor; GSD, glycogen storage disease

Diagnosis of glycogen storage diseases is suspected by history, examination, and detection of glycogen and intermediate metabolites in tissues by MRI or biopsy. Diagnosis is confirmed by significant decrease of enzyme activity in liver (types I, III, VI, and VIII/IX), muscle (types IIb, III, VII, and VIII/IX), skin fibroblasts (types IIa and IV), or RBCs (type VII) or by lack of an increase in venous lactate with forearm activity/ischemia (types V and VII).

Prognosis and treatment of glycogen storage diseases vary by type, but treatment typically includes dietary supplementation with cornstarch to provide a sustained source of glucose for the hepatic forms of GSD and exercise avoidance for the muscle forms.

Defects in glycolysis (rare) may cause syndromes similar to GSDs. Deficiencies of phosphoglycerate kinase, phosphoglycerate mutase, and lactate dehydrogenase mimic the myopathies of GSD types V and VII; deficiencies of glucose transport protein 2 (Fanconi-Bickel syndrome) mimic the hepatopathy of other GSD types (e.g. I, III, IV, VI).

Fructose Metabolism Disorders

Fructose metabolism disorders are a rare autosomal recessive inherited diseases, it can be due to a deficiency of activity of certain enzymes such as, fructose-1-phosphate aldolase, fructokinase, or fructose-1, 6-diphosphatase.

Fructose 1-phosphate aldolase (aldolase B) deficiency is an autosomal recessive causes the clinical syndrome of hereditary fructose intolerance. Infants are healthy until they ingest fructose; fructose 1-phosphate then accumulates, causing hypoglycemia, nausea and vomiting, abdominal pain, sweating, tremors, confusion, lethargy, seizures, and coma. Prolonged ingestion may cause cirrhosis, mental deterioration, and proximal renal tubular acidosis with urinary loss of phosphate and glucose.

Diagnosis of fructose 1-phosphate aldolase deficiency is suggested by symptoms in relation to recent fructose intake and is confirmed by enzyme analysis of liver biopsy tissue or by induction of hypoglycemia by fructose infusion 200 mg/kg IV. Diagnosis and identification of heterozygous carriers of the mutated gene can also be made by direct DNA analysis. Short-term treatment of fructose 1-phosphate aldolase deficiency is glucose for hypoglycemia; long-term treatment is exclusion of dietary fructose, sucrose, and sorbitol. Many patients develop a natural aversion to fructose-containing food. Prognosis is excellent with treatment.

Fructokinase deficiency is an autosomal recessive cause benign elevation of blood and urine fructose levels (benign fructosuria). This condition is asymptomatic and diagnosed accidentally when a non-glucose reducing substance is detected in urine.

Fructose-1,6-biphosphatase deficiency is an autosomal recessive compromises gluconeogenesis and results in fasting hypoglycemia, ketosis, and acidosis. This deficiency can be fatal in neonates. Febrile illness can trigger episodes. Acute treatment of fructose-1, 6-biphosphatase deficiency is oral or IV glucose. Tolerance to fasting generally increases with age.

MUCOPOLYSACCHARIDOSES

Mucopolysaccharidoses (MPS) are inherited deficiencies of enzymes involved in glycosaminogly can break down. Glycosaminoglycans (previously termed mucopolysaccharides) are polysaccharides abundant on cell surfaces and in extracellular matrix and structures. Enzyme deficiencies that prevent glycosaminoglycan breakdown, cause accumulation of glycosaminoglycan fragments in lysosomes and cause extensive bone, soft tissue, and CNS changes. Inheritance is usually autosomal recessive (except for MPS type II). Age at presentation, clinical manifestations, and severity vary by type (Table 11.6).

Common manifestations include coarse facial features, neurodevelopmental delays and regression, joint contractures, organomegaly, stiff hair, progressive respiratory insufficiency (caused by airway obstruction and sleep apnea), cardiac valvular disease, skeletal changes, and cervical vertebral subluxation.

Table 11.6	Mucopolysaccharidoses		
Disease	**Defective proteins or enzymes**	**Defective gene or genes (chromosomal location)**	**Comments**
MPS I-H (Hurler syndrome) MPS I-S (Scheie syndrome) MPS I H/S (Hurler-Scheie syndrome)	α-l-Iduronidase	IDUA (4p16.3)*	Onset: In I-H, first year In I-S, > 5 years In I-H/S, 3–8 years Urine metabolites: Dermatan sulfate, heparin sulfate Clinical features: Corneal clouding, stiff joints, contractures, dysostosis multiplex, coarse facies, coarse hair, macroglossia, organomegaly, intellectual disability with regression, valvular heart disease, hearing and vision impairment, inguinal and umbilical hernia, sleep apnea, hydrocephalus Treatment: Supportive care, enzyme replacement, stem cell or bone marrow transplantation
MPS II (Hunter syndrome)	Iduronate sulfate sulfatase	IDS (Xq28)*	Onset: 2–4 years Urine metabolites: Dermatan sulfate, heparin sulfate Clinical features: Similar to Hurler syndrome but milder and no corneal clouding In mild form, normal intelligence In severe form, progressive intellectual and physical disability, death before age of 15 years Treatment: Supportive care, stem cell or bone marrow transplantation
MPS III (Sanfilippo syndrome) Type III-A Type III-B Type III-C Type III-D	Heparan-S-sulfate sulfamidase N-acetyl-D-glucosaminidase Acetyl-CoA-glucosaminide N-acetyltransferase N-acetyl-glucosaminine-6-sulfate sulfatase	SGSH (17q25.3)* NAGLU (17q21)* (14) GNS (12q14)*	Onset: 2–6 years Urine metabolites: Heparin sulfate Clinical features: Similar to Hurler syndrome but with severe intellectual disability and mild somatic manifestations Treatment: Supportive care

Contd.

Table 11.6	Mucopolysaccharidoses *(Contd.)*		
Disease	**Defective proteins or enzymes**	**Defective gene or genes (chromosomal location)**	**Comments**
MPS IV (Morquio syndrome			Onset: 1–4 years
Type IV-A	Galactosamine-6-sulfate sulfatase	GALNS (16q24.3)*	Urine metabolites: Keratin sulfate; in IV-B, also chondroitin 6-sulfate
Type IV-B	β-Galactosidase	GLB1 (3p21.33*— GM1 gangliosidosis)	Clinical features: Similar to Hurler syndrome but with severe bone changes including odontoid hypoplasia; possibly normal intelligence
			Treatment: Supportive care
			For type IV-A, enzyme replacement therapy with elosulfase alfa
MPS VI (Maroteaux-Lamy syndrome)	*N*-acetyl galactosamine α-4-sulfate sulfatase (arylsulfatase B)	ARSB (5q11-q13)*	Onset: Variable but can be similar to Hurler syndrome
			Urine metabolites: Dermatan sulfate
			Clinical features: Similar to hurler syndrome but normal intelligence
			Treatment: Supportive care
MPS VII (Sly syndrome)	β-Glucuronidase	GUSB (7q21.11)*	Onset: 1–4 years
			Urine metabolites: Dermatan sulfate, heparin sulfate, chondroitin 4-,6-sulfate
			Clinical features: Similar to Hurler syndrome but greater variation in severity
			Treatment: Supportive care, stem cell or bone marrow transplantation
MPS IX (hyaluronidase deficiency)	Hyaluronidase deficiency	HYAL1 (3p21.3-p21.2)*	Onset: 6 months
			Urine metabolites: None
			Clinical features: Bilateral soft-tissue periarticular masses, dysmorphic features, short stature, normal intelligence
			Treatment: Not established

*Gene has been identified, and molecular basis has been elucidated.

Diagnosis of mucopolysaccharidoses is suggested by history, physical examination, and bone abnormalities (e.g. dysostosis multiplex) found during skeletal survey, and elevated total and fractionated urinary glycosaminoglycans. Diagnosis is confirmed by enzyme analysis of cultured fibroblasts (prenatal) or peripheral WBCs (postnatal). (Also see testing for suspected inherited disorders of metabolism.) Additional testing is required to monitor organ-specific changes (e.g. echocardiography for valvular disease, audiometry for hearing changes).

Treatment of MPS type I (Hurler disease) is enzyme replacement with α-l-iduronidase, which effectively halts progression and reverses all non-CNS complications of the disease. Hematopoietic stem cell (HSC) transplantation has also been used. The combination of enzyme replacement and HSC transplantation is under study. For patients with MPS type IV-A (Morquio A syndrome), enzyme replacement with elosulfase alfa may improve functional status, including mobility.

BIBLIOGRAPHY

1. American Diabetes Association: Diagnosis and classification of diabetes mellitus. Diabetes Care, 2006; 29(Suppl 1).

2. American Diabetes Association: Self-monitoring of blood glucose (consensus statement). Diabetes care 1987; 10:93–99.

3. American Society of Health-System Pharmacists (2009-02-01). "Insulin Injection".PubMed Health. National Center for Biotechnology Information, U.S. National Library of Medicine. Retrieved 2012-10-12.

4. Arden C, Trainer A, de la Iglesia N, et al. Cell biology assessment of glucokinase mutations V62M and G72R in pancreatic β-cells: evidence for cellular instability of catalytic activity. Diabetes. 2007;56(7):1773–1782.

5. Atkin SH, et al: Fingerstick glucose determination in shock. Ann Intern Med 1991; 114:1020–1024.

6. Barreau PB, Buttery JI: The effect of the haematocrit value on the determination of glucose levels by reagent strip methods. Med J Aust1987; 147:286–288.

7. Beers M, Berkow R: The Merck Manual of Diagnosis and Therapy, ed 17. Rahway, NJ: Merck & Co., 1999.

8. Bell GI, Pictet RL, Rutter WJ, Cordell B, Tischer E, Goodman HM (March 1980). "Sequence of the human insulin gene". Nature 284 (5751): 26–32.

9. Benziane B, Chibalin AV (2008). "Frontiers: skeletal muscle sodium pump regulation: a translocation paradigm". Am. J. Physiol. Endocrinol. Metab. 295 (3): E553–8.

10. Blundell TL, Cutfield JF, Cutfield SM, Dodson EJ, Dodson GG, Hodgkin DC, Mercola DA, Vijayan M (1971). "Atomic positions in rhombohedral 2-zinc insulin crystals". Nature231 (5304): 506–11.

11. Burke CV, Buettger CW, Davis EA, McClane SJ, Matschinsky FM, Raper SE. Cell-biological assessment of human glucokinase mutants causing maturity-onset diabetes of the young type 2 (MODY-2) or glucokinase-linked hyperinsulinaemia (GK-HI) Biochemical Journal. 1999;342(2):345–352.

12. C. Ronald Kahn; et al. (2005). Joslin's Diabetes Mellitus (14th ed.). Lippincott Williams & Wilkins. ISBN 978-8493531836.

13. Carpenter MW, Coustan DR: Criteria for screening tests for gestational diabetes. Am J ObstetGynecol1982; 144:768–773.

14. Cawston EE, Miller LJ (March 2010). "Therapeutic potential for novel drugs targeting the type 1 cholecystokinin receptor". Br. J. Pharmacol. 159 (5): 1009–21.

15. Chang X, Jorgensen AM, Bardrum P, Led JJ (1997). "Solution structures of the R6 human insulin hexamer,". Biochemistry 36 (31): 9409–22.

16. Chen AV, et al: Effectiveness of sodium fluoride as a preservative of glucose in blood. Clin Chem 1989; 35:315–317.

17. Christesen HBT, Jacobsen BB, Odili S, et al. The second activating glucokinase mutation (A456V): implications for glucose homeostasis and diabetes therapy. Diabetes. 2002;51(4):1240–1246.

18. Christesen HBT, Tribble ND, Molven A, et al. Activating glucokinase (GCK) mutations as a cause of medically responsive congenital hyperinsulinism: prevalence in children and characterisation of a novel GCK mutation. European Journal of Endocrinology. 2008;159(1):27–34.

19. Clark PM: Assays for insulin, proinsulin(s) and C-peptide Ann Clin Biochem1999; 36:

20. Codner E, Rocha A, Deng L, et al. Mild fasting hyperglycemia in children: high rate of glucokinase mutations and some risk of developing type 1 diabetes mellitus. Pediatric Diabetes. 2009; 10(6):382–388.

21. Cohen HT, Spiegel DM: Air-exposed urine dipsticks give false positive results for glucose and false-negative results for blood. Am J Clin Pathol 1991; 96:398–400.

22. Cuesta-Muñoz AL, Huopio H, Otonkoski T, et al. Severe persistent hyperinsulinemic hypoglycemic due to a de novo glucokinase mutation. Diabetes. 2004; 53(8): 2164–2168.

23. Davis B, Mass D, Bishop M: Principles of Clinical Laboratory Utilization and Consultation. Philadelphia: WB Saunders, 1999.

24. Davis EA, Cuesta-Muñoz A, Raoul M, et al. Mutants of glucokinase cause hypoglycaemia- and hyperglycaemia syndromes and their analysis illuminates fundamental quantitative concepts of glucose homeostasis. Diabetologia. 1999; 42 (10):1175–1186.

25. De la Monte SM, Wands JR (February 2005). "Review of insulin and insulin-like growth factor expression, signaling, and malfunction in the central nervous system: relevance to Alzheimer's disease". J. Alzheimers Dis. 7 (1): 45–61.

26. de Souza AM, López JA (2004). "Insulin or insulin-like studies on unicellular organisms: a review.". Braz. arch. biol. technol. 47 (6): 973–981.

27. Diabetes 1964; 13:278.

28. Dokhee TM: An epidemic of childhood diabetes in the United States? Evidence from Allegheny County, Pennsylvania. Pittsburgh Diabetes Epidemiology Research Group. Diabetes Care 1993; 16:1606–1611.

29. Dunn MF (August 2005). "Zinc-ligand interactions modulate assembly and stability of the insulin hexamer — a review". Biometals 18 (4): 295–303.

30. Ellard S, Beards F, Allen LIS, et al. A high prevalence of glucokinase mutations in gestational diabetic subjects selected by clinical criteria. Diabetologia. 2000;43 (2):250–253.

31. Estalella I, Rica I, De Nanclares GP, et al. Mutations in GCK and HNF-1á explain the majority of cases with clinical diagnosis of MODY in Spain. Clinical Endocrinology. 2007;67(4):538–546.

32. Fajans SS, Bell GI, Polonsky KS. Molecular mechanisms and clinical pathophysiology of maturity-onset diabetes of the young. The New England Journal of Medicine. 2001; 345(13):971–980.

33. Fang X, Yu SX, Lu Y, Bast RC, Woodgett JR, Mills GB (October 2000). "Phosphorylation and inactivation of glycogen synthase kinase 3 by protein kinase A". Proc. Natl. Acad. Sci. U.S.A. 97 (22): 11960–5.

34. Froguel P, Vaxillaire M, Sun F, et al. Close linkage of glucokinase locus on chromosome 7p to early-onset non-insulin-dependent diabetes mellitus. Nature. 1992; 356(6365): 162–164.

35. Galán M, Vincent O, Roncero I, et al. Effects of novel maturity-onset diabetes of the young (MODY)-associated mutations on glucokinase activity and protein stability. Biochemical Journal. 2006; 393(1):389–396.

36. Gall MA, et al: Risk factors for development of incipient and overt diabetic nephropathy in patients with non-insulin dependent diabetes mellitus: Prospective, observational study. BMJ 1997; 314:783–788.

37. García-Herrero CM, Galán M, Vincent O, et al. Functional analysis of human glucokinase gene mutations causing MODY2: exploring the regulatory mechanisms of glucokinase activity. Diabetologia. 2007; 50(2):325–333.

38. Gašperíková D, Tribble ND, Staník J, et al. Identification of a novel â-cell glucokinase (GCK) promoter mutation (–71G>C) that modulates GCK gene expression through loss of allele-specific Sp1 binding causing mild fasting hyperglycemia in humans. Diabetes. 2009;58(8):1929–1935.

39. Gerich JE (2002). "Is reduced first-phase insulin release the earliest detectable abnormality in individuals destined to develop type 2 diabetes?". Diabetes (journal) 51(Suppl 1): S117–S121.

40. Gidh-Jain M, Takeda J, Xu LZ, et al. Glucokinase mutations associated with non-insulin-dependent (type 2) diabetes

mellitus have decreased enzymatic activity: implications for structure/function relationships. Proceedings of the National Academy of Sciences of the United States of America. 1993; 90(5): 1932–1936.

41. Gill Carey OJSB, Colclough K, Ellard S, Hattersley AT. Finding a glucokinase mutation alters treatment. Diabetic Medicine. 2007; 24:6–7.

42. Glaser B, Kesavan P, Heyman M, et al. Familial hyper-insulinism caused by an activating glucokinase mutation. The New England Journal of Medicine. 1998;338(4):226–230.

43. Gloyn AL, Tribble ND, van de Bunt M, Barrett A, Johnson PRV. Glucokinase (GCK) and other susceptibility genes for â-cell dysfunction: the candidate approach. Biochemical Society Transactions. 2008;36 (3):306–311.

44. Gloyn AL. Glucokinase (GCK) mutations in hyper- and hypoglycemia: maturity-onset diabetes of the young, permanent neonatal diabetes, and hyperinsulinemia of infancy. Human Mutation. 2003; 22(5):353–362.

45. Goldstein DE, et al: Glycated hemoglobin: Methodologies and clinical applications. Clin Chem 1986; 32:B64–B70.

46. Goldstein DE, et al: Tests of glycemia in diabetes (Technical Review). Diabetes Care 1995; 18:896–909.

47. Gustin N (2005-03-07). "Researchers discover link between insulin and Alzheimer's". EurekAlert!. American Association for the Advancement of Science. Retrieved 2009-01-01.

48. Hattersley AT, Turner RC, Permutt MA, et al. Linkage of type 2 diabetes to the glucokinase gene. The Lancet. 1992; 339 (8805): 1307–1310.

49. Ivanova MI, Sievers SA, Sawaya MR, Wall JS, Eisenberg D (November 2009). "Molecular basis for insulin fibril assembly". Proc. Natl. Acad. Sci. U.S.A. 106 (45): 18990–5.

50. Jang WG, Kim EJ, Park KG, Park YB, Choi HS, Kim HJ, Kim YD, Kim KS, Lee KU, Lee IK (2007). "Glucocorticoid receptor mediated repression of human insulin gene expression is regulated by PGC-1alpha". Biochem. Biophys. Res. Commun. 352 (3): 716–21.

51. Katsoyannis PG, Fukuda K, Tometsko A, Suzuki K, Tilak M (1964). "Insulin Peptides. X. The Synthesis of the B-Chain of Insulin and Its Combination with Natural or Synthetis A-Chin to Generate Insulin Activity". Journal of the American Chemical Society 86 (5): 930–932.

52. Krinsley JS: Effect of an intensive glucose management protocol on the mortality of critically ill adult patients. Mayo Clin Proc 2004; 79: 992–1000.

53. Kung YT, Du YC, Huang WT, Chen CC, Ke LT (November 1965). "Total synthesis of crystalline bovine insulin". Sci. Sin. 14 (11): 1710–6. PMID 5881570.

54. Layden BT, Durai V, Lowe WL Jr (2010). "G-Protein-Coupled Receptors, Pancreatic Islets, and Diabetes". Nature Education 3 (9): 13.

55. LeRoith D, Shiloach J, Heffron R, Rubinovitz C, Tanenbaum R, Roth J (1985). "Insulin-related material in microbes: similarities and differences from mammalian insulins". Can. J. Biochem. Cell Biol. 63 (8): 839–49.

56. Little RR, et al: The National Glycohemoglobin Standardi-zation Program (NGSP): A five-year progress report. ClinChem2001; 47:1985–1992.

57. Lorenzo C, Wagenknecht LE, Rewers MJ, Karter AJ, Bergman RN, Hanley AJ, Haffner SM (2002). "Disposition index, glucose effectiveness, and conversion to type 2 diabetes: the Insulin Resistance Atherosclerosis Study (IRAS)". Diabetes Care 33 (9): 2098–2103.

58. Marglin A, Merrifield RB (1966). "The synthesis of bovine insulin by the solid phase method". J. Am. Chem. Soc. 88 (21): 5051–2.

59. Marotta DE, Anand GR, Anderson TA, et al. Identification and characterization of the ATP-binding site in human pancreatic glucokinase. Archives of Biochemistry and Biophysics. 2005; 436(1):23–31.

60. Matschinsky FM. Regulation of pancreatic â-cell glucokinase: from basics to therapeutics. Diabetes.2002;51(3):S394–S404.

61. McManus EJ, Sakamoto K, Armit LJ, Ronaldson L, Shpiro N, Marquez R, Alessi DR (April 2005). "Role that phosphorylation of GSK3 plays in insulin and Wnt signalling defined by knockin analysis". EMBO J. 24 (8): 1571–83.

62. Melloul D, Marshak S, Cerasi E (2002). "Regulation of insulin gene transcription". Diabetologia 45 (3): 309–26.

63. Menting JG, Whittaker J, Margetts MB, Whittaker LJ, Kong GK, Smith BJ, Watson CJ, Záková L, Kletvíková E, Jiráèek J, Chan SJ, Steiner DF, Dodson GG, Brzozowski AM, Weiss MA, Ward CW, Lawrence MC (2013). "How insulin engages its primary binding site on the insulin receptor". Nature 493 (7431): 241–5.

64. Metzger BE, Coustan DR (eds): Proceedings of the Fourth International Workshop-Conference on Gestational Diabetes Mellitus. Diabetes Care 1998; 21(Suppl 2): B1–B167.

65. Miles Glucometer 3 Blood Glucose Meter 1999 User's Manual. Elkhart, IN: Bayer Inc. Diagnostics Division, 1999.

66. Miller SP, Anand GR, Karschnia EJ, Bell GI, LaPorte DC, Lange AJ. Characterization of glucokinase mutations associated with maturity-onset diabetes of the young type 2 (MODY-2): different glucokinase defects lead to a common phenotype. Diabetes. 1999;48(8):1645–1651.

67. Najjar S (2001). "Insulin Action: Molecular Basis of Diabetes". Encyclopedia of Life Sciences (John Wiley & Sons).

68. Nakaki T, Nakadate T, Kato R (August 1980). "Alpha 2-adrenoceptors modulating insulin release from isolated pancreatic islets". NaunynSchmiedebergs Arch. Pharmacol. 313 (2): 151–3.

69. Njølstad PR, Sagen JV, Bjørkhaug L, et al. Permanent neonatal diabetes caused by glucokinase deficiency: inborn error of the glucose-insulin signaling pathway. Diabetes. 2003; 52(11): 2854–2860.

70. Njølstad PR, Søvik O, Cuesta-Muñoz A, et al. Neonatal diabetes mellitus due to complete glucokinase deficiency. The New England Journal of Medicine. 2001;344(21):1588–1592.

71. O'Sullivan JB, Mahan CM: Criteria for the oral glucose tolerance test in pregnancy.

72. One Touch II Blood Glucose Monitoring System 1992 User's Manual. New Brunswick, NY: Johnson & Johnson, 1992.

73. Osbak KK, Colclough K, Saint-Martin C, et al. Update on mutations in glucokinase (GCK), which cause maturity-onset diabetes of the young, permanent neonatal diabetes, and hyperinsulinemic hypoglycemia.Human Mutation. 2009;30 (11):1512–1526.

74. Pino MF, Kim KA, Shelton KD, et al. Glucokinase thermolability and hepatic regulatory protein binding are essential factors for predicting the blood glucose phenotype of missense mutations. Journal of Biological Chemistry. 2007; 282 (18):13906–13916.

75. Porter JR, Shaw NJ, Barrett TG, Hattersley AT, Ellard S, Gloyn AL. Permanent neonatal diabetes in an Asian infant. Journal of Pediatrics. 2005;146(1):131–133.

76. Ravid M, et al: Long-term renoprotective effect of angiotensin-converting enzyme inhibition in non-insulin-dependent diabetes mellitus: A 7-year follow-up study. Arch Intern Med 1996; 156:286–289.

77. Rhoades, Rodney A.; Bell, David R. (2009). Medical physiology: principles for clinical medicine (3rd ed.). Philadelphia: Lippincott Williams & Wilkins. pp. 644–647. ISBN 978-0-7817-6852-8.

78. Rohlfing CL, et al: Defining the relationship between plasma glucose and HbA1c: Analysis of glucose profiles and HbA1c in the Diabetes Control and Complications Trial. Diabetes Care 2002; 25:275–278.

79. Rubio-Cabezas O, González FD, Aragonés A, Argente J, Campos-Barros A. Permanent neonatal diabetes caused by a homozygous nonsense mutation in the glucokinase gene. Pediatric Diabetes 2008;9(3):245–249.

80. Sacks DS, et al: Guidelines and recommendations for laboratory analyses in the diagnosis and management of diabetes mellitus. Diabetes Care 2002; 25:750–786.

81. Sagen JV, Bjørkhaug L, Molnes J, et al. Diagnostic screening of MODY2/GCK mutations in the Norwegian MODY Registry. Pediatric Diabetes. 2008;9(5):442–449.

82. Sayed S, Langdon DR, Odili S, et al. Extremes of clinical and enzymatic phenotypes in children with hyperinsulinism caused by glucokinase activating mutations. Diabetes. 2009;58(6):1419–1427.

83. Service FJ: Hypoglycemic disorders. N Engl J Med 1995; 332:1144–1152.

84. Sircar S (2007). Medical Physiology. Stuttgart: Thieme Publishing Group. pp. 537–538.ISBN 3-13-144061-9.

85. Sonksen P, Sonksen J (2000). "Insulin: understanding its action in health and disease". Br J Anaesth 85 (1): 69–79. doi:10.1093/bja/85.1.69. PMID 10927996.

86. Steen E, Terry BM, Rivera EJ, Cannon JL, Neely TR, Tavares R, Xu XJ, Wands JR, de la Monte SM (February 2005). "Impaired insulin and insulin-like growth factor expression and signaling mechanisms in Alzheimer's disease—is this type 3 diabetes?". J. Alzheimers Dis. 7 (1): 63–80.

87. Steiner DF, Oyer PE (February 1967). "The biosynthesis of insulin and a probable precursor of insulin by a human islet cell adenoma". Proc. Natl. Acad. Sci. U.S.A. 57 (2): 473–80.

88. Stoffel M, Froguel P, Takeda J, et al. Human glucokinase gene: isolation, characterization, and identification of two missense mutations linked to early-onset non-insulin-dependent (type 2) diabetes mellitus. Proceedings of the National Academy of Sciences of the United States of America. 1992; 89(16): 7698–7702.

89. Stoffel M, Patel P, Lo YMD, et al. Missense glucokinase mutation in maturity-onset diabetes of the young and mutation screening in late-onset diabetes. Nature Genetics. 1992; 2(2):153–156.

90. Takeda J, Gidh-Jain M, Xu LZ, et al. Structure/function studies of human β-cell glucokinase. Enzymatic properties of a sequence polymorphism, mutations associated with diabetes, and other site-directed mutants.Journal of Biological Chemistry. 1993;268(20):15200–15204.

91. The DCCT/EDIC Research Group: Retinopathy and nephropathy in patients with type 1 diabetes four years after a trial of intensive therapy. N Engl J Med 2000; 342:381–389.

92. The Diabetes Control and Complications Trial Research Group: The effect of intensive treatment of diabetes on the development and progression of long-term complications in insulin-dependent diabetes mellitus. N Engl J Med 1993; 329:977–986.

93. The UK Prospective Diabetes Study Group: Effect of intensive blood-glucose control with metformin on complications in overweight patients with type 2 diabetes (UKPDS 34). Lancet 1998; 352:854–865.

94. The UK Prospective Diabetes Study Group: Intensive blood-glucose control with sulphonylureas or insulin compared with conventional treatment and risk of complications in patients with type 2 diabetes (UKPDS 33). Lancet 1998; 352:837–853.

95. Thomas E Creighton (1993). Proteins: Structures and Molecular Properties (2nd ed.). W H Freeman and Company. pp. 81–83. ISBN 0-7167-2317-4.

96. Thomas SH, et al: Accuracy of fingerstick glucose determination in patients receiving CPR. South Med J 1994; 87: 1072–1075.

97. Tietz textbook of clinical chemistry and molecular biology 5fifth edition, Philadelphia, W.B Saunders company (2012).

98. Turkkahraman D, Bircan I, Tribble ND, Akçurin S, Ellard S, Gloyn AL. Permanent neonatal diabetes mellitus caused by a novel homozygous(T168A) glucokinase (GCK) mutation: initial response to oral sulphonylurea therapy. Journal of Pediatrics. 2008;153(1):122–126.

99. Van den Berghe G, et al: Intensive insulin therapy in critically ill patients. N Engl J Med 2001; 345:1359–1367.

100. Weedon MN, Clark VJ, Qian Y, et al. A common haplotype of the glucokinase gene alters fasting glucose and birth weight: association in six studies and population-genetics analyses. American Journal of Human Genetics. 2006;79 (6):991–1001.

101. Weedon MN, Frayling TM, Shields B, et al. Genetic regulation of birth weight and fasting glucose by a common polymorphism in the islet cell promoter of the glucokinase gene. Diabetes. 2005;54 (2):576–581.

102. William Marshall, MártaLapsley, Stephen K Bangert. Elsevier.com: Clinical Chemistry, 7th Edition; ISBN-9780723437031. (2012).

103. Wright, James R.; Yang, Hua; Hyrtsenko, Olga; Xu, Bao-You; Yu, Weiming; Pohajdak, Bill (2014). "A review of piscine islet xenotransplantation using wild-type tilapia donors and the production of transgenic tilapia expressing a "humanized" tilapia insulin".Xenotransplantation 21 (6): 485–495.

104. Young DS, Jackson AJ: Thin-layer chromatography of urinary carbohydrates: A comparative evaluation of procedures. Clin Chem1970; 16:954.

12

Disorders of Bone and Mineral Metabolism

INTRODUCTION

Bone consists of osteoid, a collagenous organic matrix, on which complex inorganic hydrated calcium salts known as hydroxyapatites, are deposited. These have the general formula:

$$Ca_{10}(PO_4)_6(OH)_2$$

Even when growth has ceased, bone remains biologically active. Continuous turnover ('remodeling') occurs with bone resorption (mediated by osteoclasts), being followed by new bone formation (mediated by osteoblasts). At any one time, about 5% of bone mass in adults is subject to remodeling. This process is controlled and coordinated by hormones, growth factors, and cytokines. Bone formation requires osteoid synthesis and adequate calcium and phosphate for the laying down of hydroxyapatite. Alkaline phosphatase, secreted by osteoblasts, is essential to the process, probably acting by releasing phosphate from pyrophosphate. Bone provides an important reservoir of calcium, phosphate and, to a lesser extent, magnesium and sodium.

The main functions of bone are mechanical, protective, and metabolic. Bones are composed of cortical (about 80% of mineral) and trabecular (about 20 % of mineral) bone. The function of cortical bone is primarily mechanical and protective, whereas trabecular bone is metabolically more active. Bone is composed primarily of an extracellular mineralized matrix with a smaller cellular reaction. The organic matrix is primarily type I collagen (about 90%) with lesser amounts of other proteins. The organic matrix is mineralized primarily by the deposition of inorganic calcium and phosphate. Osteoclasts and osteoblasts are the two main types of bone cells. Osteoclasts resorb bone, whereas osteoblasts synthesize new bone.

Turnover or remodeling of bone occurs continuously, enabling the bone to repair damage and adjust strength. Bone remodeling does not occur at random, but instead in discrete packets known as bone remodeling units (Fig. 12.1).

The remodeling cycle includes (1) activation, (2) resorption, (3) reversal, (4) formation, and (5) mineralization

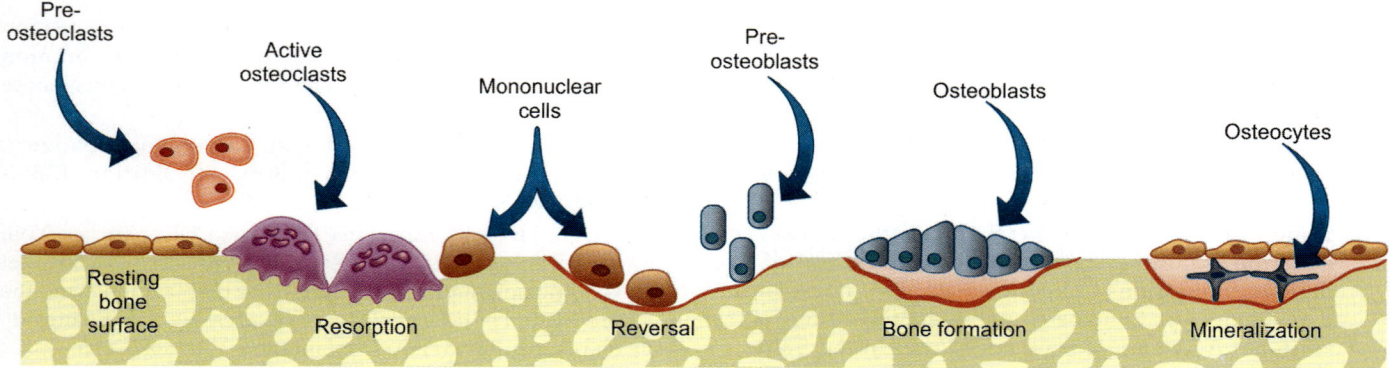

Fig. 12.1: Bone remodeling, bone tissue is removed by osteoclasts, and then new bone tissue is formed by osteoblasts

phases. Circulating osteoclast precursors are recruited, proliferate, and fuse to form osteoclasts. These giant multinucleated cells resorb bone by producing hydrogen ions to mobilize minerals and lysosomal enzymes to digest the organic matrix.

After resorption ceases, a cement line is deposited in the resorption cavity, probably by mononucleated cells. Stromal lining cells differentiate to osteoblasts. Osteoblasts form bone by synthesizing the organic matrix, including type I collagen, and participating in the mineralization of the newly synthesized matrix. An estimated 10–30% of the skeleton is remodeled each year. Bone growth and turnover are influenced by the metabolism of calcium, phosphate, magnesium, and by many hormones, especially parathyroid hormone (PTH), 1,25-dihydroxyvitamin D [1,25(OH)2D], and several cytokines.

Two products of the osteoblast appear to coordinate osteoblast and osteoclast activity. The first, receptor activator of nuclear actor-κB (RANK) ligand, binds to a receptor on osteoclast progenitor cells and increases osteoclast differentiation and activity. The second, osteoprotegerin (OPG), serves as a decoy receptor or RANK ligand. When OPG binds to RANK ligand, the osteoclast-stimulation activity is prevented. The relative ratios of these two molecules determine bone turnover. Bone contains nearly all of the calcium (99%), most of the phosphate (85%), and much of the magnesium (55%) of the body. Their concentrations in plasma depend on the net effect of bone mineral deposition and resorption, intestinal absorption, and renal excretion. PTH and 1,25 [OH] 2D are the principal hormones regulating these processes.

CELL SIGNALING IN BONE

Over the past few years, much new information about control of the bone remodeling cycle has become available. Understanding of signaling pathways has led to the development of potential new therapies. Two key signaling pathways are known as RANK/RANKLI/OPG, and Wnt.

Receptor activator of nuclear factor κB is a membrane protein expressed on the surface of osteoclasts. Its ligand (RANK ligand, or RANKL) is found on the surface of osteoblasts (also on stromal and T cells). Binding of RANK to RANKL activates osteoclasts. Osteoprotegerin is a cytokine [a member of the tumor necrosis factor (TNF) receptor superfamily] and a RANK homolog that can inhibit the production and maturation of osteoclasts by blocking the interaction of RANK with its ligand RANKL. OPG production is stimulated by estrogen, and the

marked decrease in estrogen at menopause diminishes OPG production, leaving the way open for increased activation of osteoclasts and the resultant accelerated bone loss that accompanies menopause. The Wnt signaling pathway is far more complex and is involved in many physiologic systems beyond the skeleton. Key components that have been best studied, thus far with respect to skeletal physiology include the Frizzled family of G protein-coupled receptor proteins, low-density lipoprotein receptor-related protein 5 encoded by the LRP5 gene and associated with high bone mass in affected families, cathepsin K, Dickkopf-related protein 1 (DKKl), and sclerostin.

Bone Remodeling

An estimated 10–30% of the skeleton is remodeled each year, with wide variation among individuals. Bone growth and turnover are influenced by the metabolism of calcium, phosphate, and magnesium and several hormones, the primary ones being parathyroid hormone and 1,25-dihydroxyvitamin D [1,25(OH)2D]. Bone formation and resorption are affected, however, by a large number of other hormones and factors, including thyroid hormones, estrogens, androgens, cortisol, insulin, growth hormone, insulin-like growth factors (IGF-I and IGF-II), transforming growth factor-β (TGF-β), fibroblast growth factor (FGF), and platelet-derived growth factor (PDGF). Numerous cytokines alter bone remodeling primarily by stimulating resorption; these factors include interleukins; macrophage and granulocyte/macrophage colony stimulating factors; and tumor necrosis factor-β (TNF-β). Findings suggest that leptin, which is secreted by adipocytes, can negatively regulate bone formation by osteoblasts.

Exercise is a major factor in maintaining bone mass, and immobilization leads to rapid bone loss. Lack of gravity, as occurs during space flight, results in dramatic bone loss. During childhood and adolescence, bone formation markedly exceeds bone resorption (bone modeling)—a situation that ends with epiphyseal closure at the end of puberty and is followed by a period of consolidation for the next 5–10 years, during which time the bone becomes fully mineralized.

In healthy individuals, resorption and formation remain in balance for the next several decades. At menopause, the decline in estrogen triggers an increase in bone resorption that exceeds the capacity of the formation process and results in a rapid decrease in bone mass. This imbalance continues at an accelerated rate for approximately 5 years before slowing down to a slower rate of loss of bone, termed age-related bone loss. Men do not experience the phase of rapid bone loss unless they develop male hypogonadism, but they do experience age-related loss at a rate similar to that seen in women. The disease resulting from remodeling imbalance is osteoporosis.

Several diseases and medications have adverse effects on bone remodeling and bone balance, in which case the term secondary osteoporosis is used. Systemic skeletal disease is also seen in primary and secondary abnormalities in parathyroid hormone regulation. This latter group includes osteomalacia caused by deficiency of active metabolites of the vitamin D (endocrine system malfunction or metabolic disruption of the vitamin D, as is seen in patients with chronic enal failure or CRF) . Nonsystemic skeletal disease also occurs as in skeletal metastases or Paget disease of bone.

Calcium

Calcium is the fifth most common element in the body and the most prevalent cation; 99% or more of Ca is deposited in bone and the remainder plays a vital role in nerve conduction, muscle contraction, hormone release, and cell signaling. The average adult body contains approximately 25,000 mmol (1 kg), of which 99% is bound in the skeleton. The total calcium content of the extracellular fluid (ECF) is only 22.5 mmol, of which about 9 mmol is in the plasma (Fig. 12.2). Bone is not metabolically inert.

Most of the calcium in bone is stable, but approximately 500 mmol in 24 hours moves between bone and the ECF to support calcium homoeostasis. Approximately 7.5 mmol calcium moves in 24 hours between the stable pool and the ECF in the course of bone remodeling.

In the kidneys, ionized calcium is filtered by the glomeruli (240 mmol per 24 hours). Most of this is reabsorbed in the tubules and normal renal calcium excretion is 2.5–7.5 mmol per 24 hours in males (2.5–6.25 in females). Obligatory renal calcium excretion is approximately 2.5 mmol per 24 hours. Because of the fecal loss, the minimum dietary requirement is about 12.5 mmol in 24 hours (although it is higher during growth, pregnancy, and lactation).

Gastrointestinal secretions contain calcium, some of which is reabsorbed together with dietary calcium. As calcium in the ECF pool is effectively exchanged through the kidneys, gut, and bone about 33 times every 24 hours, a small change in any of these fluxes can have a profound effect on ECF. Ca absorption is controlled by vitamin D while excretion is controlled by parathyroid hormones. However, the distribution from bone to plasma is controlled by both the parathyroid hormones and vitamin D. There is also a constant loss of Ca via the kidneys even if there is none in the diet. This excretion of calcium by the kidneys and its distribution between bone and the rest of the body is primarily controlled by parathyroid hormone.

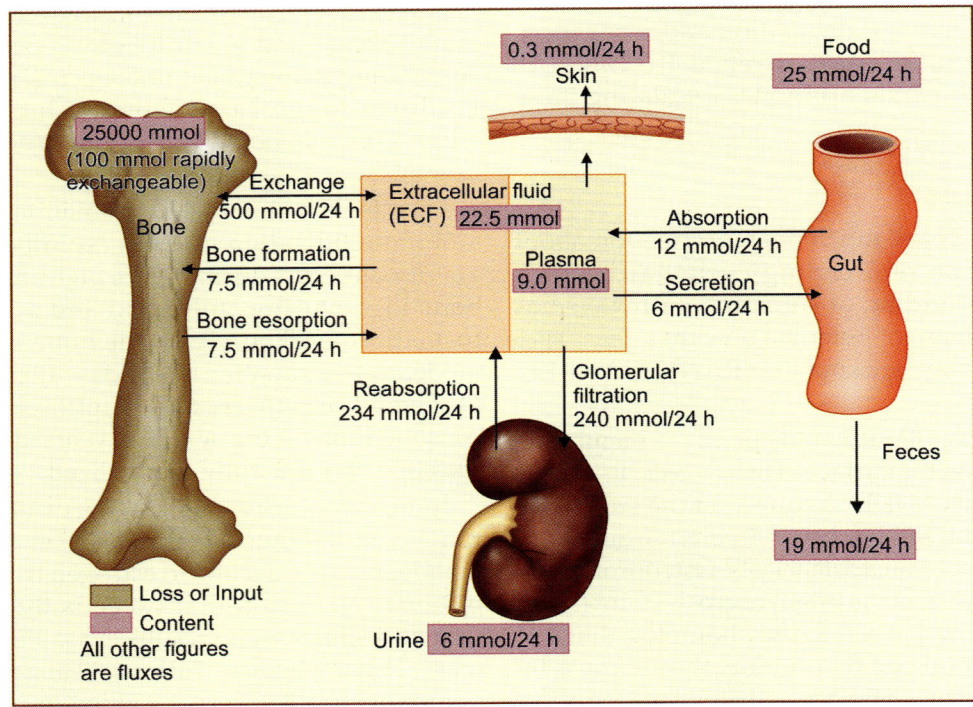

Fig. 12.2: Daily calcium fluxes in the body

Plasma Calcium

In blood, virtually all of the calcium is found in the plasma, which has a mean calcium concentration of (2.38 mmol/L). Calcium exists in three physicochemical states in plasma (Fig. 12.3) bound to protein (mainly albumin), complexed with small diffusible inorganic and organic anions, including bicarbonate, lactate, phosphate, and citrate, and free ions. Only the latter form is physiologically active, and it is the concentration of ionized calcium that is maintained by homoeostatic mechanisms.

The free calcium fraction is the biologically active form. Its concentration in plasma is tightly regulated by the calcium regulating hormones PTH and 1,25(OH)2D. About 80% of protein-bound calcium is associated with albumin, with the remaining 20% associated with globulins. Because calcium binds to negatively charged sites on proteins, its binding is pH dependent. Alkalosis leads to an increase in negative charge and binding and a decrease in free calcium; conversely, acidosis leads to a decrease in negative charge and binding and an increase in free calcium. *In vitro*, for each 0.1 unit change in pH, approximately (0.05 mmol/L) of inverse change occurs in the serum free calcium concentration.

Calcium can be redistributed among the three plasma pools, acutely or chronically, by alterations in the concentrations of protein and small anions, changes in pH, or changes in the quantities of free calcium and total calcium in the serum (Fig. 12.4).

Physiologically, calcium may be classified as intracellular or extracellular. Intracellular calcium has

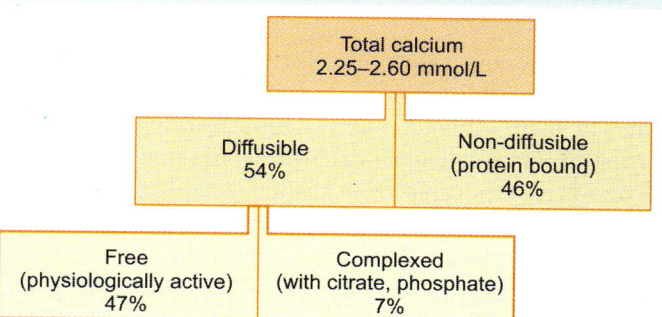

Fig. 12.3: Distribution of calcium in human plasma. Some 80% of the amount bound to protein is bound to albumin, the remainder to γ-globulins

key roles in many important physiologic functions, including muscle contraction, hormone secretion, glycogen metabolism, and cell division. The intracellular concentration of calcium in the cytosol of unstimulated cells is around 0.1 μmol/L, which is less than 1/10,000 of that in extracellular fluid.

Extracellular calcium provides calcium ion for the maintenance of intracellular calcium, bone mineralization, blood coagulation, and plasma membrane potential. Calcium stabilizes the plasma membranes and influences permeability and excitability.

Changes in plasma albumin concentration will affect total calcium concentration independently of the ionized calcium concentration, leading to possible misinterpretation of results in both hypoproteinemic and hyperproteinemic states. Various formulae have been devised to indicate the total calcium concentration to be expected if the albumin concentration were normal.

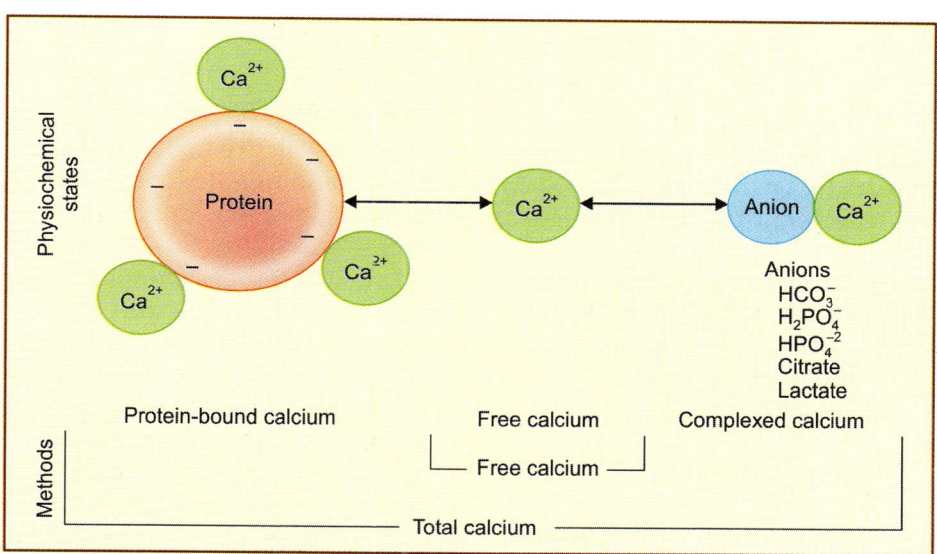

Fig. 12.4: Equilibria and determinations of calcium in serum. Calcium can move between three physiochemical pools—(I) free calcium, (2) protein-bound calcium, and (3) calcium complexed with inorganic and organic anions. Methods for determining total calcium, measure all three pools, whereas methods for determining free calcium, measure only that pool

MEASUREMENT OF CALCIUM

The methods used for quantifying calcium in blood can measure the total concentration of calcium or the free Ca ion. The term ionized calcium, although widely used, is a misnomer because all calcium in plasma or serum is ionized, irrespective of whether or not it is free or is associated with protein or small anions by ionic binding.

Free calcium is the biologically active fraction of blood calcium; it is tightly regulated by PTH and 1,25(OH)2D, and, thus is the best indicator of calcium status. Methods for both total and free calcium are currently in use and have their own sources of error. Free calcium measurements have been recommended because of the consequences of delayed treatment and the cost of working-up patients with misleading total calcium results.

Measurement of Total Calcium

Various methods have been described for total calcium measurement. At present, only photometric, ion selective electrode (ISE), and occasionally atomic absorption spectrophotometry methods are used in clinical laboratories for measuring serum and urine total calcium. ISEs for the measurement of total calcium were introduced more recently than photometric methods. The specimen is acidified to convert protein-bound and complexed calcium to free calcium before calcium is measured by ISE.

Adjusted or Corrected Total Calcium

Various calculations have been used to adjust or correct total calcium or variations in protein concentration. The following equation is often seen in textbooks, but fails to consider the lack of harmonization of albumin and calcium methods, and differences in patient populations:

Adjusted total calcium (mmol/L) = Total calcium (mmol/L) + 0.02 [40 – Albumin (g/L)]

Some factors limiting the ability of total and adjusted calcium to predict free calcium are listed in Table 12.1. When possible, mathematical adjustments or corrections

Table 12.1	Factors altering the distribution of calcium among the protein-bound, complexed, and free pools
Factors altering protein binding of calcium	**Factors altering complex formation**
Altered concentration of albumin or globulins	Citrate
Abnormal proteins	Bicarbonate
Heparin	Lactate
pH	Pyruvate and β-hydroxybutyrate
Free fatty acids	Phosphate
Bilirubin	Sulfate
Drugs	Anion gap
Temperature	

should be replaced by direct determination of free calcium.

SPECIMEN REQUIREMENTS

Serum and heparinized plasma are the preferred specimens. Citrate, oxalate, and ethylenediaminetetraacetic acid (EDTA) anticoagulants should not be used for the spectrophotometric methods, because they interfere by forming complexes with calcium.

Total calcium measurements are little affected by storage, provided that loss of water associated with prolonged refrigerator or freezer storage is prevented (by the use of tightly capped containers designed for such storage), although coprecipitation of calcium with fibrin (e.g. in heparinized plasma) or lipids has been reported with storage or freezing. Plastic and glass may also adsorb calcium from dilute solutions during storage.

Measurement of Free Calcium

Ion selective electrodes are widely used or the rapid measurement offree calcium, electrolytes, and blood gases. Calcium ISEs contain a calcium-selective membrane and an internal reference electrode.

Modern calcium ISEs use liquid membranes containing the ion-selective calcium sensor dissolved in an organic liquid trapped in a polymeric matrix. Neutral carriers are the most commonly used calcium sensors, followed by ion exchangers, such as organophosphate. Temperature affects electrode response and the extent of calcium binding by protein and small anions. Most free calcium analyzers adjust and maintain samples at 37°C, thereby ensuring that results are physiologically relevant or the majority of patients and allowing samples to be chilled before analysis.

Specimen Requirements

Specimens for free calcium measurement must be collected and handled anaerobically and promptly to minimize alterations in pH and free calcium due to the loss of CO_2 and the metabolism of blood cells. Syringes and evacuated tubes should be filled completely and sealed to prevent the loss of CO_2 (increase in pH). Specimens should also be handled to prevent the production of lactic acid (decrease in pH) by erythrocytes or white blood cells during anaerobic metabolism or glycolysis. Unless the specimens can be analyzed or processed promptly, specimens should be (1) collected, (2) transported, and (3) maintained on ice to prevent anaerobic metabolism. Free calcium is measured in (1) heparinized whole blood, (2) heparinized plasma, or (3) serum. For the majority of laboratories in which specimens are analyzed within 30 minutes, heparinized whole blood may be preferable because it reduces processing time and specimen volume requirements and avoids the alteration in pH associated with centrifugation at temperatures other than 37°C. Free calcium is reported to be stable in whole blood specimens or 1 hour at room temperature and or 4 hours at 4°C. If specimens are not promptly analyzed, they should be collected in an ice water slurry to minimize metabolism, but plasma K^+ concentrations may be significantly increased because of the inhibition of Na^+, K^+– ATPase. If analysis is not completed within 1 hour, serum collected in evacuated gel tubes may be the optimal specimen. The tubes should be filled completely. Once centrifuged, specimens are stable or hours at 25°C and or days at 4°C, provided the tube remains sealed. Free calcium has been reported to be less stable in specimens from both acidotic and non-acidotic patients with uremia.

The free calcium concentration and the actual pH o the specimen should be reported on each specimen The pH is use useful in verifying that the specimen has been properly handled. Aerobic handling of specimens and correction of the free calcium to pH 7.4 may be misleading in patients with alkalosis or acidosis and should be avoided.

Hormones Regulating Mineral Metabolism

Parathyroid hormone and 1,25-dihydroxy vitamin D are the primary hormones regulating bone and mineral metabolism. Parathyroid hormone-related peptide (PTHrP) is the principal mediator of humoral hypercalcemia of malignancy, but it also has physiologic functions in fetuses and in women during pregnancy and lactation. Calcitonin probably has only a minor role in calcium homoeostasis.

Parathyroid Hormone

This hormone is a single-chain polypeptide, comprising 84 amino acids; as with many peptide hormones, it is synthesized as a larger precursor, pre-pro-PTH (115 amino acids). Prior to secretion, two amino acid sequences are lost; the removal of a 25 amino acid chain produces pro-PTH, a further six amino acids being removed to form PTH itself. The pre- and pro-sequences are thought to be involved in the intracellular transport of the hormone. The biological activity of PTH resides in the N-terminal 1–34 amino acid sequence of the hormone. PTH is secreted by the parathyroid glands in response to a fall in plasma (ionized) calcium concentration, and secretion is inhibited by hypercalcemia. These effects are mediated by the calcium-sensing receptor (CaSR). 1,25(OH)2D inhibits PTH synthesis. PTH acts on bone and the kidneys, tending to increase the plasma concentration of calcium and reduce that of phosphate (Table. 12.2).

PTH mobilizes calcium from bone; this action is biphasic, a rapid phase involving existing cells (probably osteocytes) and a longer term response dependent on the proliferation of osteoclasts. In the kidneys, PTH increases the fraction of the filtered load that is reabsorbed. However, because increased resorption of bone increases the amount of calcium that is filtered, there is hypercalciuria despite the increased reabsorption. Also in the kidneys, PTH promotes phosphaturia by decreasing the reabsorption of filtered phosphate and stimulates the formation of 1,25(OH)2D, the calcium-regulating hormone derived from vitamin D.

Despite the importance of PTH in the control of phosphate excretion, changes in phosphate concentration do not directly affect secretion of the hormone. Mild hypomagnesaemia stimulates PTH secretion, but more severe hypomagnesaemia reduces it, as the secretion of PTH is magnesium dependent.

Intact PTH has a half-life in the blood of only 3–4 minutes. It is rapidly metabolized in the liver and kidneys, undergoing cleavage in the region of amino acids 33–37 and elsewhere. As a result, various fragments of the hormone are present in the blood as well as the intact hormone; these include an N-terminal fragment, with a similar half-life to that of the intact hormone, a C-terminal fragment (half-life: 2–3 hours) and others (Fig. 12.5). Previously used PTH immunoassays suffered from a lack of specificity for the biologically active moieties; even the now widely used immunometric assays for 'intact PTH' may detect an inactive fragment missing only the N-terminal six amino acids (PTH 7–84) in addition to intact (1–84) PTH; assays that measure only PTH 1–84 ('bioactive PTH') are being introduced, and appear to perform even better.

Table 12.2	Actions of parathyroid hormone	
Target organ	**Action**	**Effect**
Bone	Rapid release of Ca	Increase plasma Ca
	Increase osteoclastic resorption	
Kidney	Increase Ca reabsorption	Increase plasma Ca
	Decrease P reabsorption	Increase plasma P
	Increase 1 α-hydroxylation of 25-dihydroxyvitamin D	Increase Ca and P absorption from gut
	Decrease bicarbonate reabsorption	

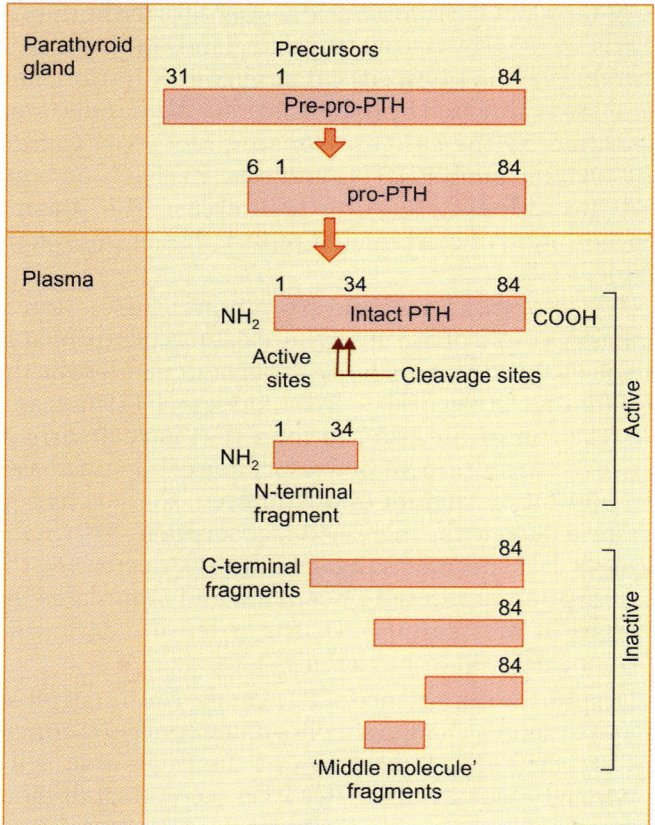

Fig. 12.5: Parathyroid hormone—precursors and cleavage products

MEASUREMENT OF PARATHYROID HORMONE

Two-site or sandwich immunoassays are used to measure intact PTH. These methods require two antibodies capable of simultaneously binding PTH—(1) a solid-phase capture antibody, often directed against the C-terminal region (e.g. amino acid sequences 39–84) and a signal or labeled antibody, often directed against the N-terminal region (e.g. amino acid sequences 1–34). Both antibodies are added in excess to ensure that all PTH is measured. Excess labeled antibody is removed by washing prior to quantification of the labeled antibody attached to the PTH that is captured by the immobilized capture antibody. A problem in most first-generation methods or intact PTH is that N-terminal—truncated fragment(s) cross-react. The degree of overestimation of intact PTH by first-generation intact PTH assays is method-dependent. Overestimation of intact PTH by 50% in patients with chronic renal failure or primary hyperparathyroidism and by 20% in healthy individuals is not unusual. Radioimmunoassays and other competitive immunoassays should not be used because they primarily measure inactive C-terminal fragments or are not sensitive enough to adequately measure intact PTH.

Specimen Requirements

Serum or EDTA plasma is generally preferred. After separation, the serum or plasma should be frozen if the analysis is delayed. Lower concentrations of PTH are observed in serum incubated at room temperature or more than a few hours or held a day or more at 4°C. pH has been reported to be more stable in EDTA plasma.

Vitamin D

Vitamin D is produced endogenously through exposure of skin to sunlight, and is absorbed from foods containing or supplemented with vitamin D. The vitamin is metabolized to its biologically active form, 1,25-dihydroxy vitamin D 1,25(OH)2D, a hormone that regulates calcium and phosphate metabolism. Deficiency of vitamin D results in impaired formation of bone, producing rickets in children and osteomalacia in adults.

Vitamin D and its metabolites may be categorized as cholecalciferols or ergocalciferols (Fig. 12.6). Cholecalciferol (vitamin D3) is the parent compound of the naturally occurring family and is produced in the skin from 7-dehydrocholesterol on exposure to the ultraviolet B portion of sunlight.

Latitude, season, aging, sunscreen use, and skin pigmentation influence production of vitamin D3 by

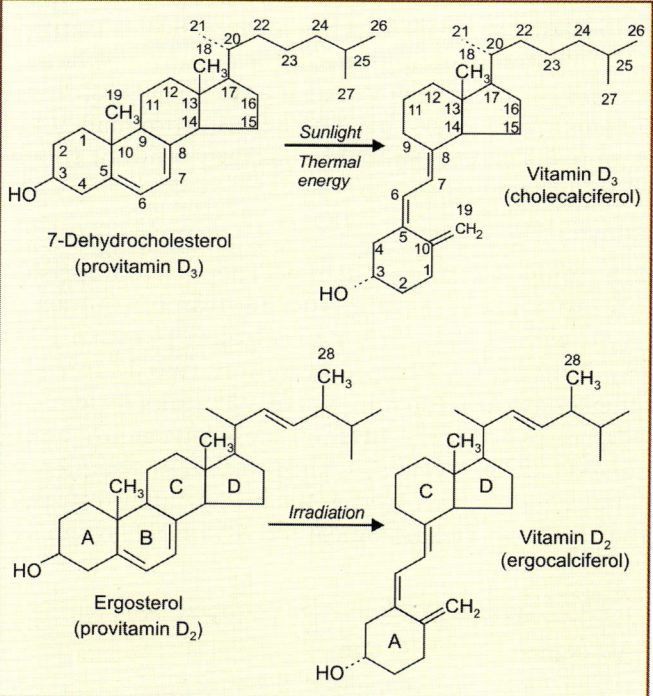

Fig.12.6: Structures of vitamin D3 (cholecalciferol) and vitamin D2 (ergocalciferol) and their precursors. 7-cholecalciferol is produced in the skin from 7-dehydrocholesterol on exposure to sunlight. Ergocalciferol is produced commercially by irradiation of ergosterol

the skin. Vitamin D2 (ergocalciferol), the parent compound of the other family, is manufactured by irradiation of ergosterol produced by yeasts. Vitamin D2 differs from vitamin D3 by the double bond between carbon 22 and carbon 23 and a methyl group on carbon 24. When vitamin D or its metabolites are written without a subscript, both families are included. Only a few foods, primarily fish liver oils, fatty fish, egg yolks, and liver, naturally contain significant amounts of vitamin D. Consequently, before foods were supplemented with vitamin D2 or vitamin D3, most vitamin D in the body was that produced by synthesis in the skin.

Vitamin D2 and vitamin D3 are metabolized to 25-hydroxyvitamin D [25(OH)D] in the liver by vitamin D 25-hydroxylase, a cytochrome P450 enzyme (Fig. 12.7). The concentration of 25(OH)D in serum is approximately 25–162 nmol/L. The half-life of circulating 25(OH)D is 2– 3 weeks and it is biologically inactive in affecting dietary calcium absorption. 25(OH)D2 and 25(OH)D3 are metabolized to 1,25-dihydroxyvitamin D 1,25(OH)2D, the biologically active hormone, by 25(OH)D1α-hydroxylase, a cytochrome P450 enzyme, in kidney and placenta (Fig. 12.7). Normal circulating concentrations are approximately 36–144 pmol/L about 1/1000 that of 25(OH)2D. The half-life of 1,25 (OH) 2D is 4–6 hours.

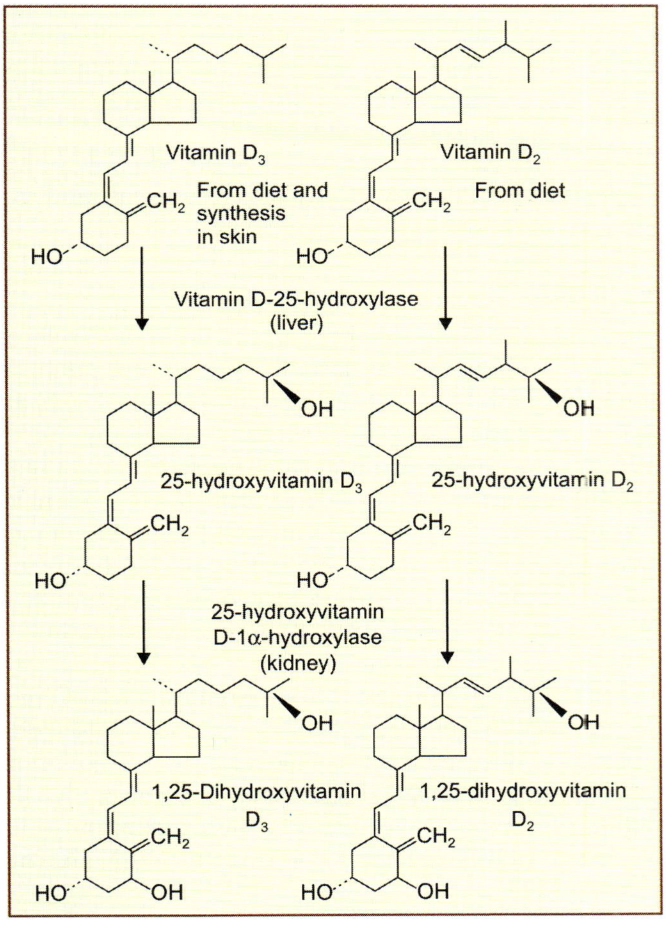

Circulating concentrations of 1,25(OH)2D are tightly regulated, primarily by PTH, phosphate, calcium, and 1,25(OH)2D. PTH and hypophosphatemia increase the synthesis of 1,25(OH)2D by increasing 25(OH)D-1 α-hydroxylase activity, whereas hypocalcemia acts indirectly by stimulating the secretion of PTH. Hypercalcemia, hyperphosphatemia, and 1,25(OH)2D reduce 25(OH)D 1 α-hydroxylase and 1,25(OH)2D. 1,25(OH)2D also induces 25(OH)D 24-hydroxylase, an enzyme producing 24,25-dihydroxy vitamin D [24,25(OH)2D], the most prevalent dihydroxylated vitamin D form in serum. This enzyme is also responsible for inactivating 1,25(OH) vitamin D through the 24-oxidation pathway, leading to formation of calcitroic acid.

In the circulation, vitamin D, 25(OH)D, and 1,25 (OH) 2D are bound to vitamin D-binding protein (DBP), a specific, high-affinity transport protein also known as group-specific component of serum or Gc-globulin. DBP belongs to the albumin and α-fetoprotein gene family. In humans, DBP contains 458 amino acid residues and has a molecular mass of 51,335 Da. DBP is constitutively synthesized by the liver and circulates in great excess (at about 400 mg/L), with less than 5% of the vitamin D binding sites normally occupied. DBP binds vitamin D and its metabolites, particularly the 25-hydroxylated metabolites 25(OH)D, 24,25(OH)2D, and 1,25(OH)2D . Only 0.03% of 25(OH)D and 0.4% of DBP concentrations are increased in pregnancy and with estrogen therapy and are decreased in nephrotic syndrome.

1,25(OH)2D helps to maintain calcium and phosphate in blood through its actions on intestine, bone, kidney, and the parathyroids. In the small intestine, 1,25(OH)2D stimulates calcium absorption, primarily in the duodenum, and phosphate absorption by the jejunum and ileum. Three events serve to absorb calcium from the diet: (1) calcium entry into the brush border cytoplasm (2) diffusion of calcium within the cell fostered by calbindin-D9k, and (3) exit of calcium from the cell across its basolateral membrane by the action of a CaATPase. A diet high in calcium down regulates CaTl and calbindin D expression by down regulating production of 1,25(OH)2D.

At high concentrations, 1,25(OH)2D increases bone resorption by inducing monocytic stem cells in bone marrow to differentiate into osteoclasts and by

Fig. 12.7: Metabolism of vitamin D. Vitamin D2 and vitamin D, are enzymatically hydroxylated to 25-hydroxyvitamin D in the liver and further to 1,25-dihydroxyvitamin D by the kidneys. 1,25-dihydroxy vitamin D2 and 1,25-dihydroxyvitamin D, are the biologically active forms of vitamin D

stimulating osteoblasts to produce cytokines and other factors that influence osteoclast activity. By stimulating osteoblasts, 1,25(OH)2D also increases the circulating concentrations of alkaline phosphatase and osteocalcin. In the kidneys, 1,25(OH)2D inhibits its own synthesis in an ultra-short negative feedback loop and stimulates its own metabolism. 1,25(OH)2D also acts directly on the parathyroids to inhibit the synthesis and secretion of PTH. In addition to a direct transcriptional mechanism, 1,25(OH)2D increases the concentrations of the calcium sensing receptor in the parathyroid gland, thus sensitizing the gland to calcium inhibition.

In target tissues, 1,25(OH)2D exerts its actions by associating with a specific nuclear vitamin D receptor (VDR), analogous to the steroid receptors for androgens, estrogens, and corticosteroids. In addition to the classical vitamin D, effects on calcium metabolism, increasing evidence suggests the role of 1,25(OH)2D in regulation of the immune response and in epithelial differentiation. Inverse relationships have been documented between vitamin D metabolite concentration in blood and the incidence of certain cancers and various other disorders. These findings have led to increased demand for vitamin D testing and have prompted calls for increases in the recommended daily intake of vitamin D. Nevertheless, substantial reductions in the rate of development of various cancers through the use of vitamin D have been difficult to demonstrate in clinical trials.

MEASUREMENT OF VITAMIN D METABOLITES

Specific and sensitive assays have been developed or 25(OH)D and 1,25(OH)2D. The assays or 25(OH)D and 1,25(OH)2D should measure D2 and D3 metabolites equally (with equimolar reactivity), since both D2 and D3 are metabolized to produce biologically active 1,25(OH)2D. Separate measurement of the D2 and D3 forms does not necessarily distinguish between dietary and endogenous sources of vitamin D, as food is supplemented with D2 and D3.

Most assays for 25(OH)D and 1,25(OH)2D require the following steps: (1) deproteinization or extraction, (2) purification, and (3) quantification. Deproteinization or extraction, usually with acetonitrile, frees the metabolites from DBP.

In practice, high performance liquid chromatography (HPLC) and liquid chromatography–mass spectrometry (LC-MS/MS) methods are being more used because of evidence that some immunoassays under estimate the vitamin D2 form of 25(OH)D. HPLC and LC-MS/MS methods measure 25(OH)2D and 25(OH)3D separately. When the sum of the two concentrations is used to determine whether a patient is deficient in vitamin D (or, also, whether a patient has a vitamin D overdose). It is not appropriate to 'treat' an increased or decreased concentration of 25(OH)2D or 25(OH)3D, when the sum of the two concentrations is normal. 1,25(OH)2D circulates at concentrations 1×10^{-3} lower than that of 25(OH)D and at significantly lower concentrations than other dihydroxylated metabolites, greatly complicating its specific determination in serum. The most widely used method requires (1) deproteinization with acetonitrile, (2) oxidation with sodium metaperiodate to eliminate interference from more abundant dihydroxylated metabolites, and (3) purification using a single C18-OH cartridge followed by quantification by radioimmunoassay using a radio iodinated analogue of 1,25(OH)2D. In a newer method, purification of 1,25(OH)2D is carried out with immune capsules containing a gel with immobilized monoclonal anti-1,25(OH)2D antibody, followed then by quantification with an automated chemiluminescent immunoassay.

Specimen Requirements

Serum is typically used in the measurement of vitamin D metabolites. Once separated from the clot, metabolites are relatively stable at both room temperature and 4°C; however, specimens should be frozen if the analysis is delayed. Vitamin D metabolites in serum do not appear to be sensitive to light and do not require special handling in the laboratory.

Calcitonin

Release of calcitonin from the parafollicular or C-cells of the thyroid gland is stimulated by circulating calcium. The hormone has been used pharmacologically as an inhibitor of bone resorption, but the physiologic role of endogenous calcitonin is less certain. No apparent alterations in bone or mineral metabolism are evident in humans with calcitonin deficiency or excess. However, calcitonin measurements have a role in the diagnosis and follow-up of medullary thyroid carcinoma, a malignant tumor of the C-cells, in particular in its familial form.

The C-cells of the thyroid arise from the neural crest and are distributed throughout the gland. These cells belong to amine precursor uptake and decarboxylation (APUD) family, which explains the association of thyroid medullary carcinoma with other tumors, such as multiple endocrine neoplasia type 2A and 2B (MEN2A and MEN2B).

Calcitonin is a 32 amino acid peptide, with a molecular mass of 3418 Da, an N-terminal disulfide bond linking the cysteine residues 1 and 7, and a C-terminal prolineamide (Fig. 12.8). The hormone interacts with a specific G-protein-coupled receptor that is found on fully

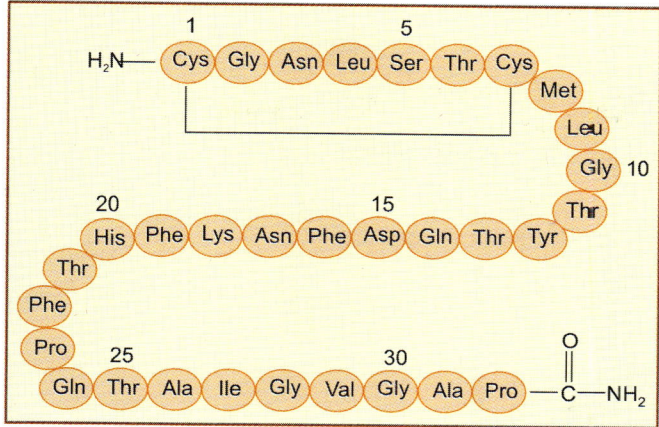

Fig. 12.8: Amino acid sequence of human calcitonin

differentiated osteoclasts. The structures necessary for biological function are the C-terminal portion of the molecule, with its proline-amide residue, the disulfide bond between residues 1 and 7, and the methionine residue at position 8. The amino-terminal amino acids are highly conserved. In humans, salmon calcitonin is 10 times as potent as the human hormone and thus is used pharmacologically, usually as nasal spray. The physiologic regulation of calcitonin secretion is incompletely understood, but the best known secretagogue is the concentration of free calcium in blood. At least in animals, several other peptide hormones (gastrin, cholecystokinin, glucagon, and secretin) can stimulate calcitonin secretion, but their physiologic role in humans is uncertain.

Pharmacologic doses of calcitonin reduce serum calcium and phosphate concentrations primarily by inhibiting osteoclastic bone resorption. Salmon calcitonin has been used to treat Paget disease of bone, osteoporosis, and hypercalcemia due to increased bone resorption. Pharmacologic doses of calcitonin also decrease the renal tubular reabsorption of calcium and phosphate. Calcitonin seems to exert an analgesic effect, which is not necessarily solely explained by its effects on bone.

Higher concentrations of circulating calcitonin can be observed in young children and during pregnancy and lactation, suggesting that the hormone may be important in protecting the skeleton during periods of calcium stress.

In serum, multiple forms of calcitonin can be observed both in healthy individuals and in patients with medullary thyroid carcinoma (MTC) or non-thyroidal malignancies. Much of the immune reactive calcitonin in the circulation is larger than the monomeric hormone. Several reasons for this heterogeneity have been put forward; sulfoxide modification of the monomer, dimerization, glycosylation, presence of biosynthetic precursors of the monomer, and binding to plasma proteins. During the biosynthesis of calcitonin, the original product is a larger precursor form known as procalcitonin. Procalcitonin has attracted attention as a potential infection marker, in relation to the acute-phase response.

CALCIUM AND PHOSPHATE HOMEOSTASIS

The response of the body to a fall in plasma calcium concentration, provided that this is not due to disordered homoeostasis in the first instance, is illustrated in Fig. 12.9. Hypocalcemia stimulates the secretion of PTH, which in turn increases the production of 1,25(OH)2D. There is an increase in the uptake of both calcium and phosphate from the gut, and in their release from bone. PTH is phosphaturic, so the excess phosphate is excreted, but the fractional reabsorption of calcium by the kidney is increased, some of the mobilized calcium is retained and the plasma calcium concentration tends to rise towards normal.

In hypophosphatemia (Fig. 12.10), 1,25(OH)2D secretion is increased but PTH is not. Indeed, any tendency for 1,25(OH)2D to increase the plasma calcium concentration should inhibit PTH secretion. Calcium and phosphate absorption from the gut are stimulated. 1,25(OH)2D has a much smaller effect on renal calcium reabsorption than PTH, with the result that, in the absence of PTH, the excess calcium absorbed from the gut is excreted in the urine. The net outcome is the restoration of the phosphate concentration towards normal, independently of that of calcium.

Phosphate

An adult has about 600 g or approximately 20 mol of phosphorus in inorganic and organic phosphates, of which about 85% is in the skeleton, and the rest is principally in soft tissue.

Plasma contains both inorganic and organic phosphate, but only inorganic phosphate is measured. Inorganic phosphate exists as both monovalent $H_2PO_4^-$ and divalent HPO_4^{-2} phosphate anions. The ratio of $H_2PO_4^-$ to HPO_4^{-2} is pH dependent and varies from approximately 1:1 in acidosis to 1:4 at pH 7.4 and 1:9 in alkalosis. Approximately, 10% of the phosphate in serum is protein-bound; 35% is complexed with sodium, calcium, and magnesium; and the remainder, or 55%, is free. The organic phosphate esters are located primarily within the cellular elements of blood. Inorganic phosphate is a major component of hydroxyapatite in bone; thus, it plays an important role in the structural support of the body and provides phosphate for the extracellular and intracellular pool.

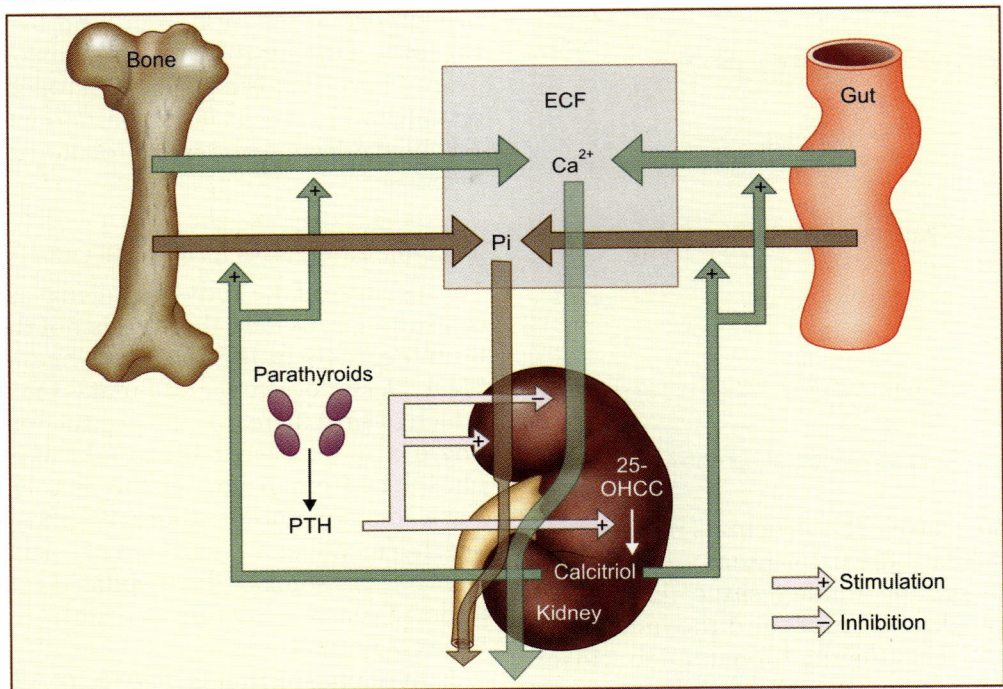

Fig. 12.9: Homoeostatic responses to hypocalcemia. Hypocalcemia stimulates the release of parathyroid hormone (PTH), which in turn stimulates 1,25(OH)2D synthesis. These hormones act together to restore plasma calcium concentration to normal, independently of phosphate concentration. 25-OHCC, 25-hydroxycholecalciferol; ECF, extracellular fluid

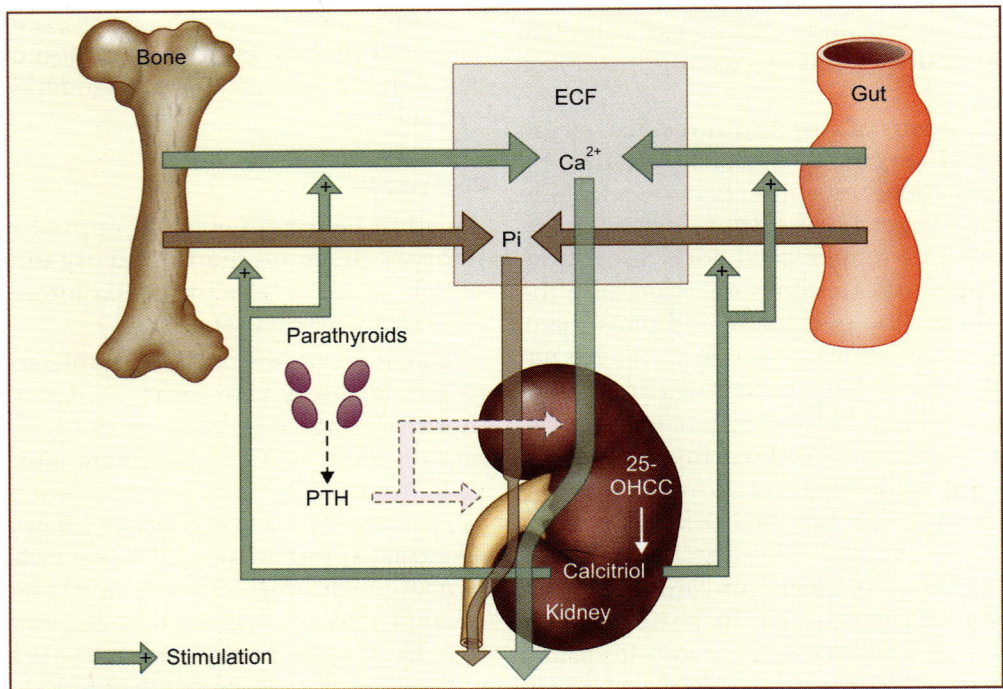

Fig.12.10: Homoeostatic responses in hypophosphatemia. In the absence of parathyroid hormone (PTH) (secretion is not affected by phosphate), an increase in 1,25(OH)2D production due to stimulation of 1α-hydroxylase tends to increase the plasma phosphate independently of calcium concentration

In the soft tissue, most phosphate is cellular. Although, both inorganic and organic phosphates are present in cells, mostly is organic and is incorporated into nucleic acids, phospholipids, phosphoproteins, and high-energy compounds involved in metabolism. ATP and other phosphates, such as creatine phosphate, are involved in many energy-intensive physiologic functions, such as muscle contractility, neurologic function, and electrolyte transport. Phosphate is also an essential element of cyclic nucleotides (such as cyclic AMP) and cofactors, such as nicotinamide-adenine dinucleotide phosphate (NADP). It is important for the activity of several enzymes, including adenylate cyclase, 25-hydroxyvitamin-D 1α-hydroxylase, and those involved in the production of 2,3-diphosphoglycerate, the key compound regulating the oxygen affinity of hemoglobin. Intracellular phosphate therefore is involved in the regulation of intermediary metabolism of proteins, fats, and carbohydrates, and in gene transcription and cell growth. Fibroblast growth factor (FGF)-23 is a key modulator of phosphate homeostasis. FGF-23 increases fractional excretion of phosphate by the kidneys. It also decreases production of the active form of vitamin D, 1,25-dihydoxy vitamin D, by decreasing the activity of the enzyme responsible for its formation (25-hydroxy vitamin D, I-hydroxylase). Both of these key activities lead to decreased serum phosphate. FGF-23 is secreted by bone cells (both osteoblasts and osteoclasts) in response to increased serum phosphate or increased serum 1,25-dihydoxy vitamin D. In chronic kidney disease, FGF-23 increases in a compensatory mechanism to counter increasing serum phosphate. As kidney failure deteriorates further, responsiveness to FGF-23 declines and thus FGF-23 cannot lower serum phosphate.

Measurement of Phosphate

Most methods used to measure serum inorganic phosphate are based on the reaction of phosphate ions with ammonium molybdate to form a phosphomolybdate complex that is then measured by a spectrophotometer.

The colorless phosphomolybdate complex may be measured directly by ultraviolet absorption (340 nm) or reduced to molybdenum blue and measured at 600–700 nm. An acidic pH is necessary for the formation of complexes, but it must be controlled because both complex formation and reduction of molybdate are dependent on pH. A less acidic pH can result in spontaneous reduction of molybdate. The rate of complex formation is also influenced by protein concentration. Solubilizing agents such as Tween 80 are used to prevent protein precipitation.

Measurement of unreduced complexes has several advantages, including simplicity, speed, and reagent stability, and it is the assay that is used in most laboratory analyzers. Disadvantages of the method include greater interference by hemolysis, icterus, and lipemia at 340 nm.

Many reducing agents have been used in producing the blue phosphomolybdate complex, including amino-naphthol-sulfonic acid, stannous chloride, methyl-p-aminophenolsulfate, ferrous ammonium sulfate, ascorbic acid, and N-phenyl-p-phenyldiamine (semidine) HCr. Each of these reagents appears to have some individual advantage, such as increased stability, increased color stability, lower detection limit, or reduced hydrolysis of organic esters. Ferrous sulfate and especially ascorbic acid have often been used for biological specimens containing organic esters, because they cause fewer breakdowns of labile phosphate esters. Aminonaphthol sulfonic acid has been used widely but is unstable, tends to precipitate, and requires careful timing because color continues to increase for several hours. With this reagent, color formation is increased with heating. Stannous chloride provides greater color intensity. Hydrazine has been added to stannous chloride to stabilize the reagent and improve the linearity. Methyl-p-aminophenol sulfate is acid tolerant, allowing for a one-component acid-molybdate reagent. A method using semidine HCL was published as a 'selected method' by the American Association for Clinical Chemistry.

Phosphate concentrations can also be determined by several other procedures, including the vanadate-molybdate and enzymatic methods. Vanadate and molybdate form a yellow complex with phosphate at acid pH, but the method tends to overestimate inorganic phosphate because of hydrolysis of organic esters. Enzymatic methods are rarely used for descriptions.

Specimen Requirements

Serum and heparinized plasma are preferred specimens for the measurement of phosphate. Concentrations of inorganic phosphate are about 0.06–0.10 mmol/L lower in heparinized plasma than in serum. Other anticoagulants such as citrate, oxalate, and EDTA may interfere with formation of the phosphomolybdate complex and thus are not suitable.

The apparent concentration of inorganic phosphate in whole blood specimens may decrease or increase with time, depending on the type of specimen, the storage temperature, and the duration of storage. Phosphate concentrations in plasma or serum are increased by prolonged storage with cells at room temperature or

37°C. Hemolyzed specimens are unacceptable because erythrocytes contain high concentrations of organic phosphate esters, which can be hydrolyzed to inorganic phosphate during storage. Inorganic phosphate increases by 1.29–1.61 mmol/L per day in hemolyzed specimens stored at 4°C, and more rapidly at room temperature or 37°C. Glucose phosphate, creatine phosphate, and other organic phosphates may also be hydrolyzed by assay conditions, resulting in over-estimation of inorganic phosphate concentrations.

Phosphate is considered to be stable in separated serum for days at 4°C and for months when frozen, provided evaporation and lyophilization are prevented.

MAGNESIUM

Magnesium is the fourth most abundant cation in the body and the second most prevalent intracellular cation. The total body magnesium content is about 25 g or approximately 1 mol, of which about 55% resides in the skeleton. One-third of skeletal magnesium is exchangeable and is thought to serve as a reservoir for maintaining the extracellular magnesium concentration. About 45% of magnesium is intracellular.

The concentration of magnesium in cells varies from 1–3 mmol/L. In general, the higher the metabolic activity of a cell, the greater is its magnesium content. Within the cell, most of the magnesium is bound to proteins and negatively charged molecules; 80% of cytosolic magnesium is bound to ATP, and MgATP is the substrate for numerous enzymes. The nucleus, mitochondria, and endoplasmic reticulum contain significant amounts of magnesium. Approximately 0.5–5.0% of the total cellular magnesium is free. Transport of magnesium across the cellular membrane is regulated by a specific magnesium transport system.

Extracellular magnesium accounts for about 1% of the total body magnesium content. About 55% of the magnesium in plasma is free, 30% is associated with proteins (primarily albumin), and 15% is complexed with phosphate, citrate, and other anions. Magnesium is a cofactor for more than 300 enzymes in the body. It is required for formation of substrates of enzymes (e.g. MgATP is a substrate for numerous enzymes that require ATP). In addition, magnesium is an allosteric activator of many enzyme systems. Examples of enzymes that require magnesium for action include adenylate cyclase, Na^+-K^+-adenosine triphosphatase (ATPase), Ca^{2+}-ATPase, phosphofructokinase, and creatine kinase. The guanine nucleotide containing regulatory proteins Gs and Gi require magnesium for activity. Magnesium is important in oxidative phosphorylation, glycolysis, cell replication, nucleotide metabolism, and protein biosynthesis. A decrease in the serum magnesium concentration lowers the threshold of axonal stimulation and increases nerve conduction velocity. Magnesium also influences neurotransmitter release at the neuromuscular junction by competitively inhibiting the entry of calcium into the presynaptic nerve terminal. Reducing the serum magnesium concentration results in increased neuromuscular excitability. Magnesium deficiency can thus result in a variety of metabolic abnormalities and clinical consequences.

Measurement of Total Magnesium

Serum magnesium has been measured by various techniques including photometry, fluorometry, flame emission spectroscopy, and atomic absorption spectrometry (AAS). Today, photometric methods are most commonly used by clinical laboratories; although, AAS is considered the reference method, it is rarely used today.

Measurement of Free (Ionized) Magnesium

Free magnesium is determined in (1) whole blood, (2) plasma, or (3) serum by use of commercially-available instruments using ISEs with neutral carrier ionophores. Current ionophores and electrodes, however, have insufficient selectivity or magnesium over calcium. Free calcium is simultaneously determined and used with the signal from the magnesium electrode to calculate free magnesium concentrations.

Specimen Requirements

Serum and heparinized plasma are the preferred specimens or measuring magnesium. Anticoagulants, such as (1) zinc heparin, (2) lithium-zinc heparin, and (3) some of the newer heparins developed or free calcium determinations should be avoided because they increase magnesium. Other anticoagulants such as (1) citrate, (2) oxalate, and (3) EDTA also should not be used as they form complexes with magnesium. Storage of serum or days at 4°C and or months frozen does not affect measured concentrations of total magnesium, provided evaporation of the specimen is prevented.

Serum or plasma must be separated from the clot or red blood cells as soon as possible to prevent an increase in serum magnesium because of cell leakage. Because erythrocytes contain higher concentrations of magnesium than serum or plasma, hemolyzed specimens are unacceptable.

Disorders of Bone, Calcium, Phosphate, and Magnesium Metabolism

Metabolic Bone Diseases

Metabolic bone disease results from a partial uncoupling or imbalance between bone resorption and formation.

Decreased bone mass, or osteopenia, is more common than abnormal increases in bone mass. The most prevalent metabolic bone diseases are osteoporosis, Paget disease of bone, osteomalacia and rickets and renal osteodystrophy. Osteoporosis, the most prevalent metabolic bone disease in developed countries, is characterized by loss of bone mass, microarchitectural deterioration of bone tissue, and increased risk of fracture. Rickets and osteomalacia, which are more common in the less-developed countries, are characterized by defective mineralization of bone matrix.

Renal osteodystrophy is a complex condition that develops in response to abnormalities of the endocrine and excretory functions of the kidneys. In addition to these three diseases that affect the skeleton in general, two diseases characterized by localized bone involvement are discussed here—paget disease of bone and bone metastases.

Osteoporosis

Osteoporosis is the most prevalent metabolic bone disease associated with increased risk for vertebral, hip, and distal forearm fractures. At the age of 50, women have a lifetime fracture risk (at any of these three sites) of about 40%. Men have a lifetime fracture risk of approximately one-third that of women. Because trabecular bone turns over at 5–7 times the rate of cortical bone, fractures of bones that are predominantly trabecular (vertebra and distal forearm) occur earlier in life.

Pathophysiology

Bone is continually being formed and resorbed. Normally, bone formation and resorption are closely balanced. Osteoblasts (cells that make the organic matrix of bone and then mineralize bone) and osteoclasts (cells that resorb bone) are regulated by parathyroid hormone, calcitonin, estrogen, vitamin D, various cytokines, and other local factors such as prostaglandins.

Peak bone mass in men and women occurs around the age of 30 years old. Men have higher bone mass than women. After achieving peak, bone mass plateaus for about 10 years, during which time bone formation approximately equals bone resorption. After this, bone loss occurs at a rate of about 0.3–0.5% per year. Beginning with menopause, bone loss accelerates in women to about 3–5% per year for about 5–7 years and then the rate of loss decelerates.

Osteoporotic bone loss affects cortical and trabecular (cancellous) bone. Cortical thickness and the number and size of trabeculae decrease, resulting in increased porosity. Trabeculae may be disrupted or entirely absent.

Trabecular bone loss occurs more rapidly than cortical bone loss because trabecular bone is more porous and bone turnover is higher. However, loss of both types contributes to skeletal fragility.

A fragility fracture occurs after less trauma than might be expected to fracture a normal bone. Falls from a standing height or less, including falls out of bed, are typically considered fragility fractures. The most common sites for fragility fractures are the following: distal radius, spine (vertebral compression fractures, the most common osteoporosis-related fracture), femoral neck, greater and trochanter, other sites include the proximal humerus and pelvis.

Classification

Osteoporosis can develop as a primary disorder or secondarily due to some other factor. The sites of fracture are similar in primary and secondary osteoporosis.

Primary Osteoporosis

More than 95% of osteoporosis in women and about 80% in men is primary. Most cases occur in postmenopausal women and older men. Gonadal insufficiency is an important factor in both men and women. Other contributing factors may include decreased Ca intake, low vitamin D levels, certain drugs, and hyperparathyroidism. Some patients have an inadequate intake of Ca during the bone growth, years of adolescence, and thus never achieve peak bone mass.

The major mechanism of bone loss is increased bone resorption, resulting in decreased bone mass and micro architectural deterioration, but sometimes bone formation is impaired. The mechanisms of bone loss may involve the following; local changes in the production of bone-resorbing cytokines, such as increases in cytokines that stimulate bone resorption, impaired formation response during bone remodeling (probably caused by age-related decline in the number and activity of osteoblasts) and other factors such as a decline in local and systemic growth factors.

Fragility fractures rarely occur in children, adolescents, premenopausal women, or men <50 years with normal gonadal function and no detectable secondary cause, even in those with low bone mass. Such uncommon cases are considered idiopathic osteoporosis.

Secondary Osteoporosis

Accounts for <5% of osteoporosis in women and about 20% in men. The causes (Table 12.3) may also further accelerate bone loss and increase fracture risk in patients with primary osteoporosis.

Table 12.3	Causes of secondary osteoporosis

Cancer (e.g. multiple myeloma)

COPD (due to the disorder itself, as well as tobacco use and/or treatment with glucocorticoids)

Chronic kidney disease

Drugs (e.g. glucocorticoids, anticonvulsants, medroxyproge-sterone, aromatase inhibitors, rosiglitazone, pioglitazone, thyroid replacement therapy, heparin, ethanol, tobacco)

Endocrine disease (e.g. glucocorticoid excess, hyperparathyroid-ism, hyperthyroidism, hypogonadism, hyperprolactinemia, diabetes mellitus)

Hypercalciuria

Hypervitaminosis A

Hypophosphatasia

Immobilization

Liver disease

Malabsorption syndromes

Prolonged weightlessness (as occurs in space flight)

RA

COPD, chronic obstructive pulmonary disease
RA, rheumatoid arthritis

Patients with chronic kidney disease may have several reasons for low bone mass, including secondary hyper-parathyroidism, renal osteodystrophy, and adynamic bone.

Symptoms and Signs

Patients with osteoporosis are asymptomatic unless a fracture has occurred. Nonvertebral fractures are typically symptomatic, but about two-thirds of vertebral compression fractures are asymptomatic (although patients may have underlying chronic back pain due to other causes such as osteoarthritis). A vertebral compression fracture that is symptomatic begins with acute onset of pain that usually does not radiate, is aggravated by weight bearing, may be accompanied by point spinal tenderness, and typically begins to subside in 1 week. However, residual pain may last for months or be constant.

Multiple thoracic compression fractures eventually cause dorsal kyphosis, with exaggerated cervical lordosis (Dowager's hump). Abnormal stress on the spinal muscles and ligaments may cause chronic, dull, aching pain, particularly in the lower back. Patients may have shortness of breath due to the reduced intrathoracic volume and/or abdominal discomfort due to the compression of the abdominal cavity as the ribcage approaches the pelvis.

Diagnosis

Bone density should be measured using DXA to screen people at risk and to follow patients with documented low bone density, including those undergoing treatment. Although, low bone density (and the associated increased risk of fracture) can be suggested by plain X-rays, it should be confirmed by a bone density measurement. It is not clear how often DXA should be repeated. For example, it can be done frequently (e.g. every 2–3 years) in women being treated for osteoporosis or who are at high risk, and can be done less frequently, sometimes much less frequently, in women who are at low risk (e.g. T-scores >−2.00 and no risk factors).

Laboratory testing should usually include the following: Ca, Mg, P, 25-hydroxy vitamin D level, alkaline phosphatase, PTH, serum testosterone in men, 24 hour urine for Ca and creatinine (hypercalciuria).

Other tests such as thyroid-stimulating hormone or free thyroxine to check for hyperthyroidism, measurements of urinary free cortisol, and blood counts and other tests to rule out cancer, especially myeloma (e.g. serum and urine protein electrophoresis), should be considered depending on the clinical presentation. Patients with chronic kidney disease can have low bone mass due to hyperparathyroidism, renal osteodystrophy, and adynamic bone, so they may need other tests.

Patients with weight loss should be screened for gastrointestinal (GI) disorders (e.g. malabsorption, celiac disease, inflammatory bowel disease) as well as cancer. Bone biopsy is reserved for unusual cases (e.g. young patients with fragility fractures and no apparent cause, patients with chronic kidney disease who may have other bone disorders, patients with persistently very low vitamin D levels suspected of having osteomalacia).

Treatment

The goals of treatment are to preserve bone mass, prevent fractures, decrease pain, and maintain function. The rate of bone loss can be slowed with drugs. Adequate Ca and vitamin D and physical activity are keys to optimal bone density. All men and women should consume at least 1000 mg of elemental Ca daily. An intake of 1200–1500 mg/day (including dietary consumption) is recommended for postmenopausal women and older men and for periods of increased requirements, such as pubertal growth, pregnancy, and lactation. Ca intake should ideally be from dietary sources, with supplements used if dietary intake is insufficient. Ca supplements are taken most commonly as Ca carbonate or Ca citrate. Ca citrate is better absorbed in patients with achlorhydria, but both are well absorbed when taken with meals. Patients taking proton pump inhibitors or those who have had gastric bypass surgery should take Ca citrate to ensure maximum absorption. Ca should be taken in divided doses of 500–600 mg twice daily or 3 times a day.

Vitamin D supplementation is recommended with 800–1000 IU/day. Patients with vitamin D deficiency may need even higher doses. Supplemental vitamin D is usually given as cholecalciferol, the natural form of vitamin D, although ergocalciferol, the synthetic plant-derived form, is probably also acceptable.

Bisphosphonates are first-line drug therapy. By inhibiting bone resorption, bisphosphonates preserve bone mass and can decrease vertebral and hip fractures by up to 50%. Bone turnover is reduced after 3 months of bisphosphonate therapy and fracture risk reduction is evident as early as 1 year after beginning therapy. DXA scanning, when done serially to monitor response to treatment, need not normally be done at intervals <2 years. Bisphosphonates can be given orally or IV.

Intranasal salmon calcitonin should not regularly be used for treating osteoporosis. Salmon calcitonin may provide short-term analgesia after an acute fracture, such as a painful vertebral fracture, due to an endorphin effect. It has not been shown to reduce fractures.

Estrogen can preserve bone density and prevent fractures. Most effective if started within 4–6 years of meno-pause, estrogen may slow bone loss and possibly reduce fractures even when started much later. Use of estrogen increases the risk of thromboembolism and endometrial cancer and may increase the risk of breast cancer.

Parathyroid hormone, which stimulates new bone formation, is generally indicated in patients who cannot tolerate antiresorptive drugs or have contraindications to their use, who fail to respond (i.e. develop new fractures or lose bone mineral density) to antiresorptive drugs, as well as Ca, vitamin D, and exercise and the one who possibly have severe osteoporosis or multiple vertebral fragility fractures.

PAGET DISEASE OF BONE

Etiology

Several genetic abnormalities, many affecting receptor activator of nuclear factor kappa-B (RANK-NFκB) signaling for osteoclast generation and activity, have been identified. Mutations of the Sequestrum 1 gene related to ubiquitin binding from chromosome 6 are present in about 10% of patients with Paget disease. Appearance of involved bone on electron microscopy suggests a viral infection. Although, a viral cause has not been established, it is hypothesized that in genetically predisposed patients as yet an unidentified virus triggers abnormal osteoclast activity.

Pathophysiology

Any bone can be involved. The bones most commonly affected are, in decreasing order, the pelvis, femur, skull, tibia, vertebrae, clavicle, and humerus.

Bone turnover is accelerated at involved sites. Pagetic lesions are metabolically active and highly vascular. Excessively active osteoclasts are often large and contain many nuclei. Osteoblastic repair is also hyperactive, causing coarsely woven, thickened lamellae, and trabeculae. This abnormal structure weakens the bone, despite bone enlargement and heavy calcification.

Overgrown bone may compress nerves and other structures passing through small foramina. Spinal stenosis or spinal cord compression may develop. Osteoarthritis may develop in joints adjacent to involved bone.

In about 10–15% of patients, increased bone formation and Ca requirement lead to secondary hyperpara-thyroidism; if this need is not matched by an increase in Ca intake, hypocalcemia may occur. Hypercalcemia occasionally develops in patients who are immobile. It also occurs in patients with Paget disease who develop secondary hyperparathyroidism.

Large or numerous lesions may lead to high-output heart failure. Highly vascular bones may bleed excessively during orthopedic surgery.

Symptoms and Signs

There are usually no symptoms for a prolonged period. If symptoms occur, they develop insidiously, with pain, stiffness, fatigue, and bone deformity (Fig. 12.11). Bone pain is aching, deep, and occasionally severe, sometimes worse at night. Pain also may arise from compression neuropathy or osteoarthritis. If the skull is involved, there may be headaches and hearing impairment.

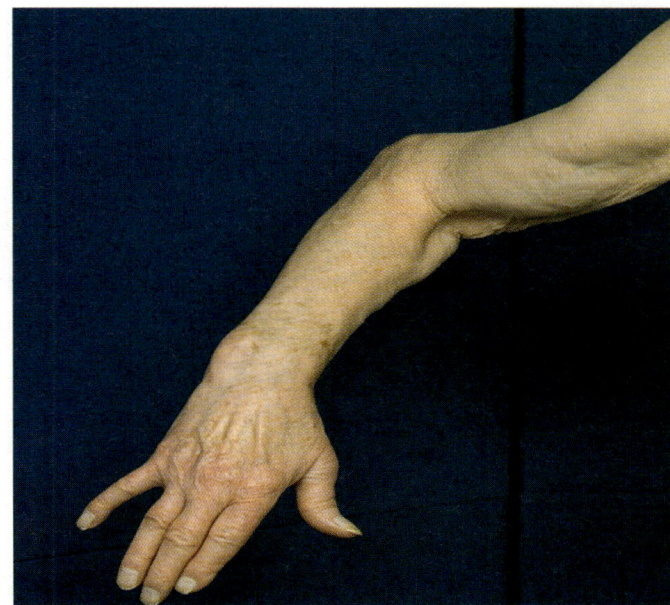

Fig. 12.11: Paget's disease bone deformity

Signs may include skull enlargement bitemporally and frontally (frontal bossing), dilated scalp veins, nerve deafness in one or both ears or vertigo, headaches; angioid streaks in the fundus of the eye, a short kyphotic trunk with simian appearance, hobbling gait, and anterolateral angulation (bowing) of the thigh, leg, or humerus, often with warmth and tenderness. Deformities may develop from bowing of the long bones or osteoarthritis. Pathologic fractures may be the presenting manifestation. Osteosarcoma develops in <1% and is often suggested by increasingly severe pain.

Diagnosis

If Paget disease is suspected, plain X-rays and serum alkaline phosphatase, Ca, and PO_4 levels should be obtained. Confirmation on X-ray is required to establish the diagnosis by findings the following: increased bone sclerosis, abnormal architecture with coarse cortical trabeculation or cortical thickening, bowing, bone enlargement, and may be lateral stress microfractures of the tibia or femur.

Characteristic laboratory findings include elevated serum alkaline phosphatase (increased anabolic activity of bone) but usually normal γ-glutamyl transpeptidase (GGT) and serum PO_4 levels. Serum Ca is usually normal but can increase because of immobilization or hyperparathyroidism or decrease (often transiently) because of increased bone synthesis. If alkaline phosphatase is not elevated or it is unclear whether the increased serum alkaline phosphatase is of bony origin (i.e. if GGT is increased in proportion to alkaline phosphatase), a bone-specific fraction can be measured.

Occasionally, increased catabolic activity of bone, as demonstrated by elevated urine markers of bone collagen turnover (e.g. pyridinoline crosslinks), supplements the findings.

Treatment

Localized, asymptomatic disease requires no treatment. Symptomatic treatment includes a supportive care for symptoms and complications. Orthotics help correct abnormal gait caused by bowed lower extremities. Some patients require orthopedic surgery (e.g. hip or knee replacement, decompression of the spinal cord). Weight bearing should be encouraged, and bed rest should be avoided. Rarely, rapid correction of severe hypercalcemia is necessary, using IV fluids and furosemide.

OSTEOMALACIA AND RICKETS

Osteomalacia and rickets are caused by a mineralization defect that occurs during bone formation, resulting in an increase in osteoid, the unmineralized organic matrix of bone. Defective mineralization produces rickets in children and osteomalacia in adults. Osteomalacia or rickets is usually due to vitamin D deficiency or phosphate depletion. The causes of decreased 25(OH) D and 1,25(OH)2D. Vitamin D deficiency may be secondary to dietary deprivation and/or inadequate exposure to sunlight, vitamin D malabsorption, disorders of vitamin D metabolism, or end-organ resistance to the action of vitamin D. Although, clinical osteomalacia caused by vitamin D deficiency appears to be uncommon, the prevalence of subclinical or mild osteomalacia in the overall population is unknown. Subclinical osteomalacia may coexist with osteoporosis in elderly patients with poor diets and little exposure to sunlight. It has also been shown that mild to moderate vitamin D deficiency may be associated with reduced muscle strength, impaired physical performance, and falls—all factors contributing to osteoporotic fracture. Vitamin D deficiency may develop in patients with malabsorption caused by postgastrectomy syndrome, small bowel disease (e.g. celiac sprue), hepatobiliary disease, or pancreatic insufficiency.

Vitamin D resistance is rare. Vitamin D-dependent rickets type I is an inherited defect in 25(OH)D-1α-hydroxylase that causes impaired formation of 1,25 (OH)2D. The disease is manifested in infancy and can be treated with physiologic doses of 1,25(OH)2D. Vitamin D-dependent rickets type II is an inherited disorder that is characterized by very high serum concentrations of 1,25(OH)2D. This syndrome is caused by resistance to 1,25(OH)2D, secondary to defects in the 1,25(OH)2D receptor.

Osteomalacia and rickets may also occur as the result of phosphate depletion, (also known as hypophosphatemic vitamin D-resistant rickets). This disorder is an X-linked dominant inherited trait characterized by renal phosphate wasting. Tubular phosphate wasting can also occur sporadically in adults and as part of Fanconi syndrome. Certain rare mesenchymal tumors may produce a phosphaturic factor (phosphatonin or FGF-23), resulting in renal phosphate wasting and osteomalacia. In developing countries, dietary calcium deprivation may lead to the clinical picture of rickets, without clear vitamin D or phosphate deficiency. Drugs have also been associated with osteomalacia.

Clinical manifestations of rickets and osteomalacia are a consequence of the defect in mineralization. Rachitic manifestations include bowing of the extremities, short stature, costochondral junction swelling, indentation of the lower ribs, and flattening of the skull. In adults, bone pain is the most common symptom, and stress fractures and frank skeletal fractures may occur. X-rays show classic findings in rickets, such as cupping and fraying of the epiphyseal and diaphyseal ends of the long bone. Pseudofractures are common among adults.

Vitamin D deficiency is diagnosed by measuring serum 25(OH) D. Other laboratory findings in rickets and osteomalacia include increased serum alkaline phosphatase (ALP), with other alterations in bone and mineral metabolism dependent on the cause and severity of the disorder. ALP is usually increased because of increased osteoblastic activity associated with producing unmineralized osteoid. Calcium may be low-normal or low in vitamin D deficiency, depending on the severity of the disease. Phosphate may be normal or low, but falls with the development of secondary hyperparathyroidism. Serum calcium and PTH concentrations are usually normal in renal tubular defects of phosphate transport. Renal phosphate defects can be best assessed through determination of the renal phosphate threshold.

Treatment of rickets and osteomalacia is dictated by the cause of the disorder. Nutritional rickets and osteomalacia are healed by treatment with physiologic doses of vitamin D, whereas higher doses may be required in malabsorption. Adequate dietary intakes of calcium and phosphorus are critical during therapy. Renal phosphate-wasting syndromes require frequent pharmacologic administration of oral phosphorus.

RENAL OSTEODYSTROPHY

Chronic renal failure is associated with a multitude of disorders of bone and mineral metabolism. Renal bone diseases include both high-turnover bone disease (osteitisfibrosa or secondary hyperparathyroidism) and low-turnover bone disease (osteomalacia and adynamic bone disease).

Quantitative histomorphometric analysis of bone biopsies, measurement of bone formation by double tetracycline labeling, and special stains are often necessary for correct diagnosis of patients with osteitis fibrosa, osteomalacia, adynamic bone disease, and mixed bone disease of renal osteodystrophy.

Osteitis fibrosa (hyperparathyroid bone disease) is the most common high-turnover bone disease. This disorder is caused by high concentrations of serum PTH in secondary hyperparathyroidism. Secondary hyperparathyroidism is a consequence of the hypocalcemia associated with hyperphosphatemia and 1,25(OH)2D deficiency. Hyperphosphatemia is a result of the inability of the kidneys to excrete phosphate. 1,25(OH)2D deficiency results from the inability of the kidneys to synthesize 1,25(OH)2D because of decreased renal mass and suppression of 25(OH)D-lα-hydroxylase activity by high concentrations of phosphate. Deficiency of 1,25 (OH)2D leads to reduced intestinal absorption of calcium and reduced inhibition of PTH secretion by 1,25(OH)2D. Skeletal resistance to PTH also contributes to hypocalcemia and secondary hyperparathyroidism.

Low-turnover bone diseases include osteomalacia and adynamic (also known as aplastic) bone disease. Osteomalacia and adynamic bone disease are distinguished by the extent of unmineralized bone matrix or osteoid; osteoid is increased in osteomalacia and normal or low in adynamic bone disease. Osteomalacia in chronic renal failure may reflect vitamin D deficiency caused by decreased renal synthesis of 1,25(OH)2D (osteomalacia and rickets) oraluminum-related disease. In the 1970s and 1980s, aluminumintoxication was a significant contributing factor to the development of osteomalacia and adynamic bone disease.

Aluminum intoxication was commonly caused by aluminum contamination of dialysis water and by therapeutic use of oral aluminum-containing antacids to reduce serum phosphate by binding phosphate and preventing its intestinal absorption. The inability of patients with renal failure to excrete aluminum leads to high concentrations in serum and deposition in bone, inhibiting bone cell function and bone mineralization.

Aluminum-related disease is less common today because of reduced use of aluminum-containing antacids and the use of effective means to decrease the concentrations of aluminum in dialysis water. Other causes of adynamic renal bone disease include calcium supplementation, excessive vitamin D administration, treatment of hyperparathyroidism, advanced age and osteoporosis, diabetes, corticosteroid therapy, and immobilization. Today, oversuppression of parathyroid function (brought about by the use of oral calcium carbonate to control hyperphosphatemia and treatment with vitamin D and dialysate solutions containing high calcium to control hyperparathyroidism) is believed to be the main cause of adynamic renal bone disease.

Amyloid deposition may be noted in bone and in other tissues. It is thought to result from reduced degradation of α2 microglobulin by the kidneys. The amyloid in renal failure is primarily composed of α2 microglobulin. The fraction of patients with amyloidosis increases with the duration of dialysis therapy; 70–80% of patients have clinical features of amyloidosis after 10 or more years of hemodialysis. Amyloidosis may coexist with high-turnover or low-turnover bone disease.

Bone pain is the most common complaint of patients with renal osteodystrophy. The weight-bearing bones are the site of greatest discomfort, with leg and hip pain and back pain being common. If the patient is a growing child, skeletal deformities may result, with bowing of the extremities, kyphoscoliosis, and slipped femoral epiphyses. Extracellular calcification is also commonly found in periarticular areas, in the medial layer of arteries, and in internal organs (lungs, heart muscle, and other tissue).

The central role of serum PTH in guiding therapy requires that the PTH assay used can be relied on to measure only the active hormone. This is not true for any of the assay generations (measurement of PTH), and kidney disease leads to accumulation of inactive PTH fragments well above the concentrations seen in healthy individuals.

Treatment guidelines take this problem into account, but inconsistencies among assays can still lead to situations in which opposite therapeutic decisions could be made for asingle patient, depending on the assay used. Studies are clearly needed to test whether modern biomarkers of bone turnover, when used with measurements of circulating PTH concentrations, could more adequately define the type of osteodystrophy.

Biochemical findings in chronic renal failure include hyperphosphatemia and hypocalcemia. The measured concentration of immune reactive PTH is generally increased, often dramatically, and 1,25(OH)2D is decreased. Serum ALP is increased in patients with hyperparathyroidism or osteomalacia. Because magnesium is cleared by the kidney, modest elevations 0.08–0.16 mmol/L are common, especially in those taking magnesium-containing antacids.

Early management of renal failure calls for dietary restriction of phosphate and administration of phosphate-binding agents. Calcium supplements added to the diet to prevent secondary hyperparathyroidism may also serve as phosphate binders. Administration of 1,25(OH)2D or other active forms of vitamin D enhances intestinal calcium absorption and may act directly on the parathyroid gland to reduce PTH secretion. Ultimately, dialysis or renal transplantation may be necessary.

Disorders of Calcium, Phosphate and Magnesium Metabolism

Hypocalcemia

Low total serum calcium (hypocalcemia) may be due to a reduction in albumin-bound calcium, the free fraction of calcium, or both (Table 12.4). Hypoalbuminemia is the most common cause of apparent hypocalcemia on a standard biochemical profile, particularly in hospitalized patients.

Common clinical conditions associated with low serum albumin include chronic liver disease, nephrotic syndrome, congestive heart failure, malnutrition, and post-surgical volume replacement with saline or colloidal solutions. In these conditions, the concentration of free

Table 12.4	Differential diagnosis of hypocalcemia
Hypoalbuminemia	
Chronic renal failure	
Magnesium deficiency	
Hypoparathyroidism	
Pseudohypoparathyroidism	
Osteomalacia and rickets due to vitamin D deficiency or resistance	
Acute hemorrhagic and edematous pancreatitis, septic shock	
Malignancy, osteoblastic metastases	
Rhabdomyolysis	
Healing phase of bone disease of treated hyperparathyroidism, hyperthyroidism, and hematologic malignancies (hungry bone syndrome)	

calcium typically is maintained in its physiologic reference interval.

Common causes of true hypocalcemia has a number of causes, including, hypoparathyroidism, pseudo-hypoparathyroidism, vitamin D deficiency and dependency and renal disease.

Hypoparathyroidism, is characterized by hypocalcemia and hyperphosphatemia and often causes chronic tetany. Hypoparathyroidism results from deficient parathyroid hormone, which can occur in autoimmune disorders or after the accidental removal of or damage to several parathyroid glands during thyroidectomy. Transient hypoparathyroidism is common after subtotal thyroidectomy, but permanent hypoparathyroidism occurs after <3% of such thyroidectomies done by experienced surgeons. Manifestations of hypocalcemia usually begin about 24–48 hours postoperatively, but may occur after months or years. PTH deficiency is more common after radical thyroidectomy for cancer or as the result of surgery on the parathyroid glands (subtotal or total parathyroidectomy). Risk factors for severe hypocalcemia after subtotal parathyroidectomy include; severe preoperative hypercalcemia, removal of a large adenoma, elevated alkaline phosphatase, and chronic kidney disease.

Idiopathic hypoparathyroidism is an uncommon sporadic or inherited condition in which the parathyroid glands are absent or atrophied. It manifests in childhood. The parathyroid glands are occasionally absent and thymic aplasia and abnormalities of the arteries arising from the brachial arches (DiGeorge syndrome) are present. Other inherited forms include polyglandular autoimmune failure syndrome, autoimmune hypoparathyroidism associated with mucocutaneous candidiasis, and X-linked recessive idiopathic hypoparathyroidism.

Pseudohypoparathyroidism, is an uncommon group of disorders characterized not by hormone deficiency but by target organ resistance to PTH. Complex genetic transmission of these disorders occurs. Patients with type I a pseudohypoparathyroidism (Albright hereditary osteodystrophy) have a mutation in the stimulatory Gs-α1 protein of the adenylyl cyclase complex (GNAS1). The result is failure of normal renal phosphaturic response or increase in urinary cyclic adenosine monophosphate (cAMP) to PTH. Patients are usually hypocalcemic as a result of hyperphosphatemia. Secondary hyperparathyroidism and hyperparathyroid bone disease can occur. Associated abnormalities include short stature, round facies, intellectual disability with calcification of the basal ganglia, shortened metacarpal and metatarsal bones, mild hypothyroidism, and other subtle endocrine abnormalities. Because only the maternal allele for GNAS1 is expressed in the kidneys, patients whose abnormal gene is paternal, although they have many of the somatic features of the disease, do not have hypocalcemia, hyperphosphatemia, or secondary hyperparathyroidism; this condition is sometimes described as pseudohypoparathyroidism. Less is known about type I b pseudohypoparathyroidism. Affected patients have hypocalcemia, hyperphosphatemia, and secondary hyperparathyroidism, but do not have the other associated abnormalities. Type II pseudo-hypoparathyroidism is even less common than type I. In affected patients, exogenous PTH raises the urinary cAMP normally, but does not raise serum Ca or urinary phosphate (PO$_4$). An intracellular resistance to cAMP has been proposed.

Vitamin D deficiency and dependency, may result from inadequate dietary intake or decreased absorption due to hepatobiliary disease or intestinal malabsorption. It can also result from alterations in vitamin D metabolism as occur with certain drugs (e.g. phenytoin, pheno-barbital, rifampin) or decreased formation in the skin due to lack of exposure to sunlight. Aging also decreases skin synthetic capacity. Decreased skin synthesis is an important cause of acquired vitamin D deficiency among people who spend a great deal of time indoors, who live in high northern or southern latitudes, and who wear clothing that covers them completely. Accordingly, subclinical vitamin D deficiency is fairly common, especially during winter months in temperate climates among the elderly. The institutionalized elderly are at particular risk because of decreased skin synthetic capacity, under nutrition, and lack of sun exposure. In fact, most people with deficiency have both decreased skin synthesis and dietary deficiency.

Renal disease, including acquired proximal renal tubular acidosis due to nephrotoxins (e.g. heavy metals) and distal renal tubular acidosis, can cause severe hypocalcemia due to abnormal renal loss of Ca and decreased renal conversion to 1,25(OH)2D. Cadmium, in particular, causes hypocalcemia by injuring proximal tubular cells and interfering with vitamin D conversion. Renal failure can result in hypocalcemia due to dimini-shed formation of 1,25(OH)2D from direct renal cell damage as well as suppression of 1α-hydroxylase by hyperphosphatemia.

Other Causes

- Mg depletion (can cause relative PTH deficiency and end-organ resistance to PTH action, usually when serum Mg concentrations are <0.5 mmol/L; Mg repletion increases PTH concentrations and improves renal Ca conservation).
- Acute pancreatitis (when lipolytic products released from the inflamed pancreas chelate Ca).
- Hypoproteinemia (reduces the protein-bound fraction of serum Ca; hypocalcemia due to diminished protein binding is asymptomatic because ionized Ca is unchanged, this entity has been termed factitious hypocalcemia).
- Hungry bone syndrome (persistent hypocalcemia and hypophosphatemia occurring after surgical or medical correction of moderate to severe hyperparathyroidism in patients in whom serum Ca concentrations had been supported by high bone turnover induced by greatly elevated PTH; hungry bone syndrome has been described after parathyroidectomy, after renal transplantation, and rarely in patients with end-stage renal disease treated with calcimimetics).
- Septic shock (due to suppression of PTH release and decreased conversion of 25(OH)D to 1,25(OH)2D .
- Hyperphosphatemia (causes hypocalcemia by poorly understood mechanisms; patients with renal failure and subsequent PO$_4$ retention are particularly prone)
- Drugs including anticonvulsants (e.g. phenytoin, phenobarbital) and rifampin, which alter vitamin D metabolism, and drugs generally used to treat hypercalcemia. Transfusion of >10 units of citrate-anticoagulated blood and use of radiocontrast agents containing the divalent ion-chelating agent ethylene-diaminetetraacetate, can decrease the concentration of bioavailable ionized Ca while total serum Ca concentrations remain unchanged).
- Infusion of gadolinium (may spuriously lower Ca concentration).

Although, excessive secretion of calcitonin might be expected to cause hypocalcemia, low serum Ca concentrations rarely occur in patients with large amounts of circulating calcitonin due to medullary carcinoma of the thyroid.

Clinically, hypocalcemia most commonly presents with neuromuscular hyper excitability, such as tetany, paresthesia, and seizures. A rapid fall in serum calcium may be associated with hypotension and electro-cardiographic abnormalities. The severity of symptoms is related to the rate of fall in serum calcium concentration. When symptomatic hypocalcemia is considered, the initial laboratory evaluation must include measurement of ionized calcium and is directed toward assessment of renal function and measurement of serum albumin and magnesium concentrations. Serum intact PTH concentrations are low or inappropriately normal in hypoparathyroidism and elevated in pseudohypopara-thyroidism.

Vitamin D deficiency is an uncommon cause of symptomatic hypocalcemia and is characterized by low serum 25(OH)D, high PTH (secondary hyperpara-thyroidism), and high serum alkaline phosphatase. For symptomatic hypocalcemia, calcium may be admini-stered intravenously, and biochemical response to therapy can be monitored by measurement of total serum calcium. If hypocalcemia is secondary to hypopara-thyroidism or pseudohypoparathyroidism, vitamin D and oral calcium supplements are administered.

Activating mutations of the calcium-sensing receptor (CaSR) as a cause of hypocalcemia have been described. Intervention to correct the hypocalcemia may not be needed long term, but in affected neonates) calcium replacement must be provided until genetic confirmation of CaSR status is obtained. Autoimmune destruction of the parathyroid glands may occur in isolation or in combination with other endocrine abnormalities. Post-surgical hypoparathyroidism is uncommon in patients undergoing surgery for primary hyperparathyroidism (PHPT) or secondary hyperparathyroidism (SHPT), but not in patients undergoing extensive neck surgery for treatment of head and neck malignancies. Hypocalcemia in the presence of functional parathyroid glands is a very late manifestation of disease because the interaction of PTH and 1,25(OH)2D will maintain normocalcemia until body stores of 25(OH)D are severely depleted or, in the later stages of chronic renal failure(CRF) 1,25(OH)2D production is inadequate.

Symptoms of hypocalcemia include tingling around the mouth and in the fingers and toes. When more severe, intense, painful spasm of the fingers and toes develops and may be sustained for several minutes. In the most severe cases, life-threatening laryngospasm may occur. These symptoms reflect decreases in the plasma free calcium and may occur despite a normal total calcium concentration when the complexed or protein-bound fraction is increased. For example, this occurs, during massive transfusion (or pheresis) when large quantities of citrated blood are infused rapidly; citrate complexes-calcium, leading to lower free calcium concentration without decreasing the total calcium concentration. An important exception to symptomatic hypocalcemia occurs in CRF when marked acidosis is present. Hypocalcemia triggers muscle contraction, but acidosis hampers muscle contraction. Rapid correction of low serum bicarbonate in patients with CRF without assurance that serum calcium is maintained may trigger muscle spasm.

Hypercalcemia

Hypercalcemia is commonly encountered in clinical practice and results when the influx of calcium into the extracellular fluid compartment from the skeleton, intestine, or kidney is greater than the efflux. For example, when excessive resorption of bone mineral occurs in malignancy, hypercalciuria develops. When the capacity of the kidney to excrete filtered calcium is exceeded, hypercalcemia develops. Hypercalcemia can be caused by increased intestinal absorption (as with rare vitamin D intoxication), increased renal retention (e.g. thiazide diuretics), increased skeletal resorption (e.g. immobiliza-tion), or a combination of mechanisms (as in primary hyperparathyroidism).

The causes of hypercalcemia are listed in Table 12.5. Primary hyperparathyroidism is the most common pathologic cause in outpatients, whereas malignancy is more common in hospitalized patients. Together, these two disorders account for 90–95% of all cases of hypercalcemia.

PHPT is characterized by excessive secretion of PTH that results in hypercalcemia. It is most often due to a solitary adenoma (80–85% of cases), less frequently (about 15%) to hyperplasia involving all glands, and infrequently to parathyroid carcinoma <1 %).

More than 80% of hyper parathyroid patients in developed countries are free of overt symptoms on presentation because of early detection of this disorder through the wide spread use of chemistry panels that include calcium. The most common signs and symptoms of hypercalcemia are nonspecific and are related to the neuromuscular system. They include fatigue, malaise, and weakness with mild hypercalcemia; calcium <3 mmol/L; depression, apathy, and inability to con-centrate may be present at higher calcium concentrations. Hypercalcemia may induce mild nephrogenic diabetes insipidus with thirst, polydipsia, and polyuria. Renal colic caused by kidney stones can result from chronic hypercalcemia and hypercalciuria. Nephrocalcinosis can lead to slowly developing renal failure. Most patients with primary hyperparathyroidism (>60%) are post-menopausal women.

PHPT is diagnosed by laboratory studies. Hyper-calcemia should be documented by measuring total

Table 12.5 Differential diagnosis of hypercalcemia

Primary hyperparathyroidism	Chlorothiazide diuretics
• Adenoma, hyperplasia, carcinoma • Familial • Multiple endocrine neoplasia type 1 with pituitary and pancreatic tumors • Multiple endocrine neoplasia type 2 with medullary thyroid carcinoma and pheochromocytoma	Lithium therapy Milk-alkali syndrome Hyperalimentation regimens Immobilization
Malignancy	**Familial hypocalciuric hypercalcemia**
• With skeletal involvement • Direct tumor erosion of the bone • Local tumor production of bone-resorbing agents • No skeletal involvement (humoral hypercalcemia of malignancy) • Parathyroid hormone-related protein • Growth factor(s) (tumor growth factor, epidermal growth factor, platelet-derived growth factor) • Hematologic malignancy • Cytokines (interleukin-l, tumor necrosis factor, lymphotoxin) • 1,25-dihydroxyvitamin D (lymphoma) • Coexistent primary hyperparathyroidism	Idiopathic hypercalcemia of infancy Loss-of-function mutations in CYP24Al (25-hydroxyvitamin D 24-hydoxylase) Vitamin overdose • Vitamin D • Vitamin A
Other endocrine disorders	**Renal failure**
• Hyperthyroidism • Hypothyroidism • Acromegaly • Acute adrenal insufficiency • Pheochromocytoma	• Chronic renal failure • Acute renal failure-diuretic phase • Post renal transplantation
Granulomatous disease	**Increased serum proteins**
• Sarcoidosis • Tuberculosis • Berylliosis • Coccidioidomycosis	• Hemoconcentration • Hyperglobulinemia due to multiple myeloma

calcium and serum albumin, or by measuring free calcium, on more than one occasion. Measurement of intact PTH (with concomitant measurement of calcium) is the most sensitive and specific test for parathyroid function and is central to the differential diagnosis of hypercalcemia. Serum PTH may not be elevated in some patients, but this should not detract from the diagnosis because, with rare exceptions, non-parathyroid causes of hypercalcemia are associated with suppressed PTH concentrations. Serum 1,25(OH)2D is often in the upper half of the reference interval or is increased in primary hyperparathyroidism, as PTH stimulates its production. By contrast, 1,25(OH)2D (similar to PTH) is low-normal or suppressed in non-parathyroid hypercalcemia, except in sarcoidosis, other granulomatous diseases, and certain lymphomas, in which pathologic tissues contain the 25-hydroxyvitamin D-1α hydroxylase required to produce 1,25(OH)2D.

PTH increases the renal clearance of bicarbonate and phosphate, such that in PHPT a mild hyperchloremic metabolic acidosis may be observed, whereas in non-parathyroid hypercalcemia, a mild hypochloremic metabolic alkalosis may be observed. Although, hypophosphatemia is often seen in PHPT, measurement of serum phosphate is of limited value because hypophosphatemia is also found in hypercalcemic cancer patients.

Symptomatic patients with PHPT should undergo parathyroid surgery. If the patient is asymptomatic, guidelines have been established recommending surgery over monitoring depending on serum calcium concentration, creatinine clearance, urine calcium, bone mineral density, and age. In the 'guidelines for management of asymptomatic primary hyperparathyroidism' from the third international workshop on the topic, serum calcium concentration greater than 0.25 mmol/L above the reference interval was considered an indication for surgical intervention, as was a calculated creatinine clearance less than 60 mL/min. For patients who were to be managed without surgery, annual measurements of serum calcium and creatinine were recommended.

Hypercalcemia occurs in 5–30% of individuals with cancer. Solid tissue malignancies commonly produce parathyroid hormone-related peptide (PTHrP), which is secreted into the circulation and stimulates bone resorption. PTHrP binds to the PTH receptor and is the principal mediator of humoral hypercalcemia of malignancy (HHM). Skeletal metastases from cancer also can produce hypercalcemia, but this is a late manifestation, reflecting a large metastatic burden, and less often presents a diagnostic problem. Cytokines, such as lymphotoxin, interleukin-1, tumor necrosis factor, and PTHrP appear to be important mediators of hypercalcemia in multiple myeloma and other hematologic malignancies.

Some lymphomas associated with acquired immunodeficiency syndrome or human T-lymphotropic virus type 1 (HTLV-1) infection cause hypercalcemia by producing 1,25(OH)2D. It is estimated that less than 5% of patients with hypercalcemic cancer have coexisting primary hyperparathyroidism.

Signs and symptoms of hypercalcemia are more evident in patients with hypercalcemia due to malignancy because the serum calcium increases rapidly and often reaches concentrations higher than those usually seen in PHPT. Lethargy, obtundation, nausea, and vomiting are additional symptoms.

Laboratory test selection is similar to that in suspected hyperparathyroidism, with the addition of PTHrP in some individuals with HHM. However, PTHrP is rarely informative if the PTH is not suppressed. In specific instances (e.g. lymphoma, sarcoidosis), measurement of 1,25(OH)2D may be useful.

Therapies are directed toward treating the malignancy, decreasing the serum calcium concentration by saline diuresis, and decreasing osteoclastic resorption (bisphosphonates, calcitonin, etc.). Corticosteroids are useful in reducing intestinal absorption of calcium in 1,25(OH)3D-mediated hypercalcemia, particularly in granulomatous disease. Familial hypocalciuric hypercalcemia (also called benign familial hypercalcemia) is characterized, as its name implies, by the presence of hypercalcemia and hypocalciuria. It is due to a mutation in the CaSR found in the parathyroids and the kidney tubules.

Very recent studies of four families with idiopathic hypercalcemia of infancy (Table 12.5) have identified a genetic basis for this condition. Sequence analysis of CYP24Al, which encodes 25-hydroxyvitamin D 24-hydroxylase, the key enzyme for degrading the active metabolite of vitamin D3, revealed recessive mutations in the affected children. In addition, CYP24A 1 mutations were identified in a group of infants in whom severe hypercalcemia developed after bolus prophylaxis with vitamin D. Functional characterization revealed a complete loss of function in all CYP24A 1 mutations. The decreased ability to prevent vitamin D actions appears to explain the hypercalcemia seen in the patients.

Primary hyperparathyroidism, is a generalized disorder resulting from excessive secretion of parathyroid hormone by one or more parathyroid glands. It probably is the most common cause of hypercalcemia, particularly among patients who are not hospitalized. Incidence increases with age and is higher in postmenopausal women. It also occurs in high frequency ≥3 decades after neck irradiation. Familial and sporadic forms exist. Familial forms due to parathyroid adenoma occur in patients with other endocrine tumors. Primary hyperparathyroidism causes hypophosphatemia and excessive bone resorption. Although, asymptomatic hypercalcemia is the most frequent presentation, nephrolithiasis is also common, particularly when hypercalciuria occurs due to long-standing hypercalcemia. Histologic examination shows a parathyroid adenoma in about 85% of patients with primary hyperparathyroidism, although it is sometimes difficult to distinguish an adenoma from a normal gland. About 15% of cases are due to hyperplasia of ≥2 glands. Parathyroid cancer occurs in <1% of cases.

Familial hypocalciuric hypercalcemia (FHH), is transmitted as an autosomal dominant trait. Most cases involve an inactivating mutation of the Ca-sensing receptor gene, resulting in higher concentrations of serum Ca being needed to inhibit PTH secretion. Subsequent PTH secretion induces renal phosphate (PO_4) excretion. Persistent hypercalcemia (usually asymptomatic) and often from an early age, normal to slightly elevated concentrations of PTH, hypocalciuria, and hypermagnesemia occur. Renal function is normal, and nephrolithiasis is unusual. However, severe pancreatitis occasionally occurs. This syndrome, which is associated with parathyroid hyperplasia, is not relieved by subtotal parathyroidectomy.

Secondary hyperparathyroidism, occurs most commonly in advanced chronic kidney disease when decreased formation of active vitamin D in the kidneys and other factors lead to hypocalcemia and chronic stimulation of PTH secretion. Hyperphosphatemia that develops in response to chronic kidney disease also contributes. Once established, hypercalcemia or normocalcemia may occur. The sensitivity of the parathyroid to Ca may be diminished because of pronounced glandular hyperplasia and elevation of the Ca set point (i.e. the amount of Ca necessary to reduce secretion of PTH).

Tertiary hyperparathyroidism, results in autonomous hypersecretion of PTH regardless of serum Ca concentration. Tertiary hyperparathyroidism generally occurs in patients with long-standing secondary hyperparathyroidism, as in patients with end-stage renal disease of several years' duration.

Cancer, is a common cause of hypercalcemia, usually in hospitalized patients. Although, there are several mechanisms, elevated serum Ca ultimately occurs as a result of bone resorption. Humoral hypercalcemia of cancer (i.e. hypercalcemia with no or minimal bone metastases) occurs most commonly with squamous cell carcinoma, renal cell carcinoma, breast cancer, prostate cancer, and ovarian cancer. Many cases of humoral hypercalcemia of cancer were formerly attributed to ectopic production of PTH. However, some of these tumors secrete a PTH-related peptide that binds to PTH receptors in both bone and kidney and mimics many of the effects of the hormone, including osteoclastic bone resorption. Hematologic cancers, most often multiple myeloma, but also certain lymphomas and lymphosarcomas, cause hypercalcemia by elaborating a group of cytokines that stimulate osteoclasts to resorb bone, resulting in osteolytic lesions, diffuse osteopenia, or both. Hypercalcemia may result from local elaboration of osteoclast-activating cytokines or prostaglandins, direct bone resorption by the metastatic tumor cells, or both.

Vitamin D toxicity, can be caused by high concentrations of endogenous 1,25(OH)2D. Although, serum concentrations are low in most patients with solid tumors, patients with lymphoma and T-cell leukemia sometimes have elevated concentrations due to dysregulation of the 1α-hydroxylase enzyme present in tumor cells. Exogenous vitamin D in pharmacologic doses causes excessive bone resorption as well as increased intestinal Ca absorption, resulting in hypercalcemia and hypercalciuria.

Immobilization, particularly complete prolonged bed rest in patients can result in hypercalcemia due to accelerated bone resorption. Hypercalcemia develops within days to weeks of onset of bed rest. Reversal of hypercalcemia occurs promptly on resumption of weight bearing. Young adults with several bone fractures and people with Paget disease of bone are particularly prone to hypercalcemia when at bed rest.

Idiopathic infantile hypercalcemia, is an extremely rare sporadic disorder with dysmorphic facial features, cardiovascular abnormalities, Renovascular hypertension, and hypercalcemia. PTH and vitamin D metabolism are normal, but the response of calcitonin to Ca infusion may be abnormal.

Milk-alkali syndrome, excessive amounts of Ca and absorbable alkali are ingested, usually during self-treatment with Ca carbonate antacids for dyspepsia or to prevent osteoporosis, resulting in hypercalcemia, metabolic alkalosis, and renal insufficiency. The availability of effective drugs for peptic ulcer disease and osteoporosis has greatly reduced the incidence of this syndrome.

The most common signs and symptoms of hypercalcemia are nonspecific and are related to the neuromuscular system. They include fatigue, malaise, and weakness with mild hypercalcemia (calcium <3 mmol/L); depression, apathy, and inability to concentrate may be present at higher calcium concentrations. Hypercalcemia may induce mild nephrogenic diabetes insipidus with thirst, polydipsia, and polyuria. Renal colic caused by kidney stones can result from chronic hypercalcemia and hypercalciuria. Nephrocalcinosis can lead to slowly developing renal failure. Most patients with PHPT (>60%) are postmenopausal women. Hypercalcemia should be documented by measuring total calcium and serum albumin, or by measuring free calcium, on more than one occasion. Measurement of intact PTH (with concomitant measurement of calcium) is the most sensitive and specific test for parathyroid function and is central to the differential diagnosis of hypercalcemia. Serum PTH may not be elevated in some patients, but this should not detract from the diagnosis because, with rare exceptions, non-parathyroid causes of hypercalcemia are associated with suppressed PTH concentrations. Serum 1,25(OH)2D is often in the upper half of the reference interval or is increased in primary hyperparathyroidism, as PTH stimulates its production. By contrast, 1,25(OH)2D (similar to PTH) is low-normal or suppressed in non-parathyroid hypercalcemia, except in sarcoidosis, other granulomatous diseases, and certain lymphomas, in which pathologic tissues contain the 25-hydroxyvitamin D-1 alpha hydroxylase required to produce 1,25(OH)3D.

PTH increases the renal clearance of bicarbonate and phosphate, such that in PHPT a mild hyperchloremic metabolic acidosis may be observed, whereas in non-parathyroid hypercalcemia, a mild hypochloremic metabolic alkalosis may be observed. Although, hypophosphatemia is often seen in PHPT, measurement of serum phosphate is of limited value because hypophosphatemia is also found in hypercalcemic cancer patients.

Symptomatic patients with PHPT should undergo parathyroid surgery. If the patient is asymptomatic, guidelines have been established recommending surgery over monitoring depending on serum calcium concentration, creatinine clearance, urine calcium, bone mineral density, and age. In the 'guidelines for management of asymptomatic primary hyperparathyroidism' from the third international workshop on the topic, serum calcium concentration greater than 0.25 mmol/L above the reference interval was considered an indication for surgical intervention, as was a calculated creatinine clearance less than 60 mL/min. For patients who were to be managed without surgery, annual measurements of serum calcium and creatinine were recommended. Hypercalcemia occurs in 5–30% of individuals with cancer. Solid tissue malignancies commonly produce parathyroid hormone-related peptide, which is secreted into the circulation and stimulates bone resorption. PTHrP binds to the PTH receptor and is the principal mediator of humoral hypercalcemia of malignancy. Skeletal metastases from cancer also can produce hypercalcemia, but this is a late manifestation, reflecting a large metastatic burden, and less often presents a diagnostic problem. Cytokines, such as lymphotoxin, interleukin-1, tumor necrosis factor, and PTHrP appear to be important mediators of hypercalcemia in multiple myeloma and other hematologic malignancies.

Some lymphomas associated with acquired immunodeficiency syndrome or human T-lymphotropic virus type 1 (HTLV-1) infection cause hypercalcemia by producing 1,25(OH)2D. It is estimated that less than 5% of patients with hypercalcemic cancer have coexisting primary hyperparathyroidism. Signs and symptoms of hypercalcemia are more evident in patients with hypercalcemia due to malignancy because the serum calcium increases rapidly and often reaches concentrations higher than those usually seen in PHPT. Lethargy, obtundation, nausea, and vomiting are additional symptoms.

Laboratory test selection is similar to that in suspected hyperparathyroidism, with the addition of PTHrP in some individuals with HHM. However, PTHrP is rarely informative if the PTH is not suppressed. In specific instances (e.g. lymphoma, sarcoidosis), measurement of 1,25(OH)2D may be useful.

Therapies are directed toward treating the malignancy, decreasing the serum calcium concentration by saline diuresis, and decreasing osteoclastic resorption (bisphosphonates, calcitonin, etc.). Corticosteroids are useful in reducing intestinal absorption of calcium in 1,25(OH)3D-mediated hypercalcemia, particularly in granulomatous disease.

Familial hypocalciuric hypercalcemia (benign familial hypercalcemia) is characterized, as its name implies, by the presence of hypercalcemia and hypocalciuria. It is due to a mutation in the CaSR found in the parathyroids and the kidney tubules. Very recent studies of four families with idiopathic hypercalcemia of infancy have identified a genetic basis for this condition. A sequence analysis of CYP24A 1, which encodes 25-hydroxyvitamin D 24-hydroxylase, the key enzyme for degrading the active metabolite of vitamin D3, revealed recessive mutations in the affected children. In addition, CYP24A 1 mutations were identified in a group of infants in whom severe hypercalcemia developed after bolus prophylaxis with vitamin D. Functional characterization revealed a complete loss of function in all CYP24A 1 mutations. The decreased ability to prevent vitamin D actions appears to explain the hypercalcemia seen in the patients.

Hypophosphatemia

Defined as the concentration of inorganic phosphate in the serum below the reference interval usually <0.81 mmol/L, is relatively common in hospitalized patients. Hypophosphatemia is not necessarily associated with intracellular phosphate depletion.

Hypophosphatemia may be present when cellular concentrations are normal, and cellular phosphate depletion may exist when serum concentrations are normal or even high.

Hypophosphatemia or phosphate depletion in blood may be caused by—(1) a shift of phosphate from extracellular to intracellular spaces, (2) renal phosphate wasting, (3) decreased intestinal absorption, and (4) loss from intracellular phosphate. A shift of phosphate from extracellular to intracellular fluid is a common cause of hypophosphatemia. A major cause of low serum phosphate is carbohydrate-induced stimulation of insulin secretion, which promotes the transport of glucose and phosphate into insulin-sensitive cells, where phosphate is incorporated into sugar phosphates and ATP. Oral or intravenous carbohydrate and injected insulin decrease serum phosphate. Refeeding of malnourished individuals creates an anabolic state, causing an intracellular shift of phosphate. Respiratory alkalosis leads to an increase in intracellular pH, which activates phosphofructokinase and accelerates glycolysis, causing a shift of phosphate into the cell. Low serum phosphate in these conditions does not indicate a deficiency of phosphate, and hypophosphatemia is self-correcting with stabilization of the patient's condition.

Renal phosphate wasting may also cause hypophosphatemia. Any cause of excessive PTH secretion (primary and secondary hyperparathyroidism) lowers the renal phosphate threshold and may result in hypophosphatemia and phosphate depletion. However, this may not occur if renal failure is the cause of secondary hyperparathyroidism when hyperphosphatemia is more common. The renal phosphate threshold is also lowered in Fanconi syndrome, X-linked hypophosphatemic rickets, and tumor-induced osteomalacia.

Hypophosphatemia and phosphate depletion may result from inadequate intestinal phosphate absorption. Patients taking aluminum- or magnesium-containing antacids may develop hypophosphatemia because these antacids bind phosphate in the intestine, rendering it non-absorbable. The hypophosphatemia observed in patients with malabsorption may be more closely related to their secondary hyperparathyroidism than to malabsorption of phosphate. Because phosphate is abundant in most foods, dietary deprivation is not usually a cause of phosphate depletion in patients with normal intestinal function and an adequate diet.

Intracellular phosphate may be lost in acidosis as a result of catabolism of organic compounds within the cell. Diabetic ketoacidosis is associated initially with high-normal to increased serum phosphate. Treatment of ketosis and acidosis with insulin and intravenous fluids, however, results in a rapid reduction in the serum phosphate concentration. Consequently, patients being treated for diabetic ketoacidosis may have both intra-cellular phosphate depletion and hypophosphatemia.

The clinical manifestations of serum phosphate deple-tion depend on the length and the degree of deficiency. Moderate hypophosphatemia of 0.48–0.77 mmol/L, usually is not associated with clinical signs and symptoms (unless chronic, when osteomalacia or rickets develops).

Plasma concentrations less than 0.48 mmol/L may produce clinical manifestations. Because phosphate is necessary for the formation of ATP, glycolysis, and cellular function are impaired by low intracellular phosphate concentrations.

Muscle weakness, acute respiratory failure, and decreased cardiac output may occur in phosphate depletion.

At very low serum phosphate <0.32 mmol/L, rhabdomyolysis may be seen. Phosphate depletion in erythrocytes decreases erythrocyte 2,3-diphosphogly-cerate, which causes tissue hypoxia as the result of increased affinity of hemoglobin for oxygen. Severe hypophosphatemia (serumphosphate concentration <0.16 mmol/L) may result in hemolysis of the red blood cells. Mental confusion and frank coma may be secondary to low ATP and tissue hypoxia. If hypophosphatemia is chronic, impaired mineralization of bone produces rickets in children and osteomalacia in adults.

Treatment of hypophosphatemia depends on the degree of hypophosphatemia and on the presence of symptoms. Patients with moderate hypophosphatemia often require only treatment of the underlying disorder and, possibly, oral phosphate supplementation. In patients with marked symptoms of hypophosphatemia, particularly if respiratory muscle weakness is present, parenteral administration of phosphate may be indicated.

Hyperphosphatemia

The most common cause of hyperphosphatemia is in ability of the kidneys to excrete phosphate. Hyper-phosphatemia is a major clinical problem in chronic kidney disease. In acute or chronic renal failure, a decrease in glomerular filtration rate (GFR) reduces the renal excretion of phosphate, resulting in hyperphosphatemia. Moderate increase in serum phosphate occur in individuals with low PTH (hypoparathyroidism), PTH resistance (pseudohypoparathyroidism), or acromegaly (increased growth hormone) caused by an increased renal phosphate threshold. Growth hormone is responsible for the increased renal phosphate threshold and the higher phosphate concentrations observed in children. EDTA therapy has also been associated with hyper-phosphatemia. Increased intake and a shift of phosphate from the tissues into the extracellular fluid are also causes of hyperphosphatemia.

Excessive oral, rectal, or intravenous phosphate administration for the treatment of phosphate depletion is a common cause of hyperphosphatemia. Release of phosphate as the result of cell breakdown in cases of rhabdomyolysis, intravascular hemolysis, or chemo-therapy of certain malignancies may cause hyper-phosphatemia. Hyperphosphatemia may also be associated with acidosis, a consequence of the hydrolysis of intracellular organic phosphate-containing com-pounds, with the release of phosphate into the plasma.

The clinical manifestations of hyperphosphatemia depend on its rate of onset. A rapid increase in serum phosphate may be associated with hypocalcemia. Therefore, symptoms may include tetany, seizures, and hypotension. Long-term hyperphosphatemia may be associated with secondary hyperparathyroidism, osteitis fibrosa, and soft tissue calcification of the kidneys, blood vessels, cornea, skin, and periarticular tissue.

Therapy for hyperphosphatemia is directed toward correcting the cause of the increased serum phosphate. In renal failure and in hypoparathyroidism, dietary restriction of phosphate and agents that bind phosphate in the intestine (calcium carbonate and others) are useful in lowering the serum phosphate concentration.

Hypomagnesemia

Hypomagnesemia is common in patients in hospitals. Moderate or severe magnesium deficiency is usually due to loss of magnesium from the gastrointestinal tract or kidneys. Vomiting and nasogastric suction may deplete body stores of magnesium in that upper GI fluids contain approximately 0.5 mmol/L of magnesium. More commonly, magnesium deficiency is associated with losses from the lower intestine. Diarrhea may result in marked losses of magnesium; therefore, acute diarrheal states, regional enteritis, and ulcerative colitis are frequently complicated by magnesium deficiency. Magnesium is most efficiently absorbed from the distal small bowel.

Excessive urinary losses of magnesium from the kidneys are important causes of magnesium deficiency. Clinically important causes include alcohol, diabetes mellitus (osmoticdiuresis), loop diuretics (furosemide), and aminoglycoside antibiotics. Increased sodium excretion (parenteral fluid therapy) and increased calcium excretion (hypercalcemic states) also result in renal magnesium wasting.

Because magnesium deficiency is usually secondary to another disease process or to a therapeutic agent, features of the primary disease process may complicate or mask magnesium deficiency. Neuromuscular hyper-excitability with tetany and seizures may be present. These symptoms and signs may also be due to hypo-calcemia, and magnesium deficiency is a common cause of hypocalcemia. Magnesium deficiency impairs PTH secretion and causes resistance to PTH in the kidneys and bone; it has been linked to osteoporosis in epidemiologic studies and in animal experiments. Deficiency is cardiac arrhythmia. Premature atrial complexes, atrial tachycardia and fibrillation, premature ventricular complexes, ventricular tachycardia, and ventricular fibrillation may be associated with magne-sium deficiency. These effects may be caused in part by the hypokalemia, renal wasting, and intracellular depletion of potassium caused by hypomagnesemia.

Although, extracellular magnesium accounts for only about 1% of total body magnesium, and plasma magnesium concentrations correlate poorly with total body magnesium, determination of serum magnesium is the most widely used test to assess magnesium deficiency. Hypomagnesemia is often transient and is not an indication of magnesium deficiency.

Conversely, intracellular magnesium depletion and magnesium deficiency may exist despite a normal serum magnesium concentration. Consequently, hypocalcemia, hypokalemia, neuromuscular hyperirritability, and cardiac arrhythmias should alert one to the possible presence of magnesium deficiency. Other tests less commonly used include the magnesium loading test (also known as the magnesium tolerance test) and measure-ments of intracellular magnesium (e.g. in red blood cell, lymphocyte, or skeletal muscle). Acute symptomatic magnesium deficiency usually is treated with parenteral magnesium; mild depletion may be treated with oral magnesium.

Hypermagnesemia

Magnesium intoxication is not a frequently encountered clinical problem, although a mild to moderate elevation in the serum magnesium concentration may be noted in as many as 12% of hospital patients. Symptomatic hypermagnesemia is almost always caused by excessive intake, resulting from administration of antacids, enemas, and parenteral fluids containing magnesium. Most of these patients have concomitant renal failure, thereby limiting the ability of the kidneys to excrete excess magnesium. Magnesium used to treat preeclampsia and eclampsia may cause magnesium intoxication in mothers and their neonates.

Depression of the neuromuscular system is the most common manifestation of magnesium intoxication. Deep tendon reflexes disappear at a serum magnesium concentration above 2.06–3.70 mmol/L, whereas depressed respiration and apnea, caused by voluntary muscle paralysis, may occur at serum magnesium concentrations greater than 4.11–4.94 mmol/L. Higher concentrations may result in cardiac arrest. Somnolence, hypotension, nausea, vomiting, and cutaneous flushing may also be seen. Hypermagnesemia induces a decrease in the serum concentration of calcium, presumably because of the inhibition of both PTH secretion and end-organ action of PTH by magnesium.

The possibility of magnesium intoxication should be anticipated in patients receiving magnesium, especially those with renal failure. Replacement therapy should be discontinued in patients with mildly to moderately increased serum magnesium. Higher serum concen-trations are used in the treatment of preeclampsia and eclampsia. Because calcium acutely antagonizes the toxic effects of magnesium, patients with severe magnesium intoxication may be treated with intravenous calcium. If necessary, peritoneal dialysis or hemodialysis against a low-magnesium dialysis bath effectively lowers the serum magnesium concentration.

BIBLIOGRAPHY

1. Abernethy MH, Fowler RT. Micellar improvement of the calmagitecompleximetric measurement of magnesium in plasma. Clin Chern 1982; 28: 520–2.

2. Adami S. Calcitonin. In: Rosen Cj, Compston I.E., Lian IB, eds. Primer on the metabolic bone diseases and disorders of mineral metabolism, 7th edition. Washington, DC: American Society for Bone and Mineral Research, 2008: 250–1.

3. Adams IS, Hewison M. Update in vitamin D. I Clin Endocrinol Metab 2010; 95: 471–8.

4. Ainola M, Valleala H, Nykanen P, Risteli J, Hanemaaijer R, Konttinen YT. Erosive arthritis in a patient with pycnody-sostosis: an experiment of nature. Arthritis Rheum 2008; 58: 3394–401.

5. Almaden Y, Hernandez A, Torregrosa V, Canalejo A, Sabate L, Fernandez Cruz L, et al. High phosphate level directly stimulates parathyroid hormone secretion and synthesis by human parathyroid tissue in vitro. I Am Soc Nephrol 1998; 9: 1845–52.

6. Aloia JF, Talwar SA, Pollack S, Yeh J. A randomized controlled trial of vitamin D3 supplementation in African American women. Arch Intern Med. 2005;165: 1618–1623.

7. Aloia JF, Vaswani A, Yeh JK, Flaster E. Risk for osteoporosis in black women. Calcif Tissue Int.1996; 59: 415–423.

8. Andersen T, McNair P, Fogh-Andersen N, Nielsen TT, Hyldstrup L, Transbol I. Increased parathyroid hormone as a consequence of changed complex binding of plasma calcium in morbid obesity. Metabolism. 1986; 35: 147–151.

9. Anderson He. Sipe IB, Hessle L, Dhanyamraju R, Atti E, Camacho NP, et al. Impaired calcification around matrix vesicles of growth plate and bone in alkaline phosphatase-deficient mice. Am I Pathol 2004;164: 841–7.

10. Anh DJ, Dimai HP, Hall SL, Farley IR. Skeletal alkaline phosphatase activity is primarily released from human osteoblasts in an insoluble form, and the net release is inhibited by calcium and skeletal growth factors. Calcif Tissue Int 1998; 62: 332–40.

11. Atley LM, Mort IS, Lalumiere M, Eyre DR. Proteolysis of human bone collagen by cathepsin K: characterization of the cleavage sites generating by cross-linked N-telopeptide neoepitope. Bone 2000; 26: 241–7.

12. Bailey AI, Knott L. Molecular changes in bone collagen in osteoporosis and osteoarthritis in the elderly. Exp Gerontol 1999; 34: 337–51.

13. Baird GS, Rainey PM, Wener M, Chandler W. Reducing routine ionized calcium measurement. ClinChern 2009; 55: 533–40.

14. Baldwin T, Chernow B. Hypocalcemia in the lCU: coping with the causes and consequences. I Crit Illness 1987; 2: 9–16.

15. Banfi G, Daverio R. In vitro stability of osteocalcin. Clin Chern 1994; 40: 833–4.

16. Barbour HM, Davidson W. Studies on measurement of plasma magnesium: application of the Magon dye method to the "Monarch" centrifugal analyzer. ClinChern 1988; 34: 2103–5.

17. Basuyau IP, Mallet E, Leroy M, Brunelle P. Reference intervals for serum calcitonin in men, women, and children. ClinChern 2004; 50: 1828–30.

18. Beilby I, Randall A, Davis I. Variable citrate interference in arsenazo III dye assays of total calcium in serum. Clin Chern 1990; 36: 824–5.

19. Bell NH, Epstein S, Greene A, Shary J, Oexmann MJ, Shaw S. Evidence for alteration of the vitamin D-endocrine system in obese subjects. J Clin Invest. 1985; 76: 370–373.

20. Bell NH, Epstein S, Shary J, Greene V, Oexmann MJ, Shaw S. Evidence of a probable role for 25-hydroxyvitamin D in the regulation of human calcium metabolism. J Bone Miner Res. 1988; 3: 489–495.

21. Ben Rayana MC, Burnett RW, Covington AK, D'Orazio P, Fogh- Andersen N, lacobs E, et al. IFCC guideline for sampling, measuring and reporting ionized magnesium in plasma. Clin Chern Lab Med 2008; 46: 21–6.

22. Berth M, Delanghe I. Protein precipitation as a possible important pitfall in the clinical chemistry analysis of blood samples containing monoclonal immunoglobulins: 2 case reports and a review of the literature. ActaClinBelg 2004;59:263-73.

23. Bieglmayer C, Vierhapper H, Dudczak R, Niederle B. Measurement of calcitonin by immunoassay analyzers. ClinChern Lab Med 2007; 45:662-6.

24. Bikle D, Adams I, Christakos S. Vitamin D: production metabolism, mechanism of action, and clinical requirements. In: Rosen Cj, Compston I.E., Lian IB, eds. Primer on the metabolic bone diseases and disorders of mineral metabolism, 7th edition. Washington, DC: American Society for Bone and Mineral Research, 2008: 141–9.

25. Bilezikian JP, Khan AA, Potts JT. Guidelines for the management of asymptomatic primary hyperparathyroidism: summary statement from the third international workshop. J EndocrinolMetab 2009;94: 335-9.

26. Bilezikian JP, Rubin MR. Monitoring anabolic treatment. In: Seibel MJ, Robins SP, Bilezikian JP, eds. Dynamics of bone and cartilage metabolism, 2nd edition. San Diego, Calif: Academic Press, 2006: 629–47.

27. Birnbaum J, Van Herle AJ. lmmunoheterogeneity of parathyroid hormone in parathyroid cysts: diagnostic implications. J Endocrinol Invest 1989; 12: 831–6.

28. Blind E, Schmidt-Gayk H, Scharla S, et al. Two-site assay of intact parathyroid hormone in the investigation of primary hyperparathyroidism and other disorders of calcium metabolism compared with a midregion assay. J Clin Endocrinol Metab. 1988; 67: 353–360

29. Blumsohn A, Colwell A, Naylor K, Eastell R. Effect of light and gamma-irradiation on pyridinolines and telopeptides of type I collagen in urine. Clin Chem 1995; 41: 1195–7.

30. Blumsohn A, Hannon RA, Eastell R. Apparent instability of osteocalcin in serum as measured with different commercially available immunoassays. Clin Chem 1995; 41:318 9.

31. Boink AB, Buckley BM, Christiansen TF, Covington AK, Maas AH, Muller-Plathe 0, etaI. IFCC recommendation on sampling, transport and storage for the determination of the concentration of ionized calcium in whole blood, plasma and serum. J Automat Chem 1991; 13: 235–9.

32. Bonde M, Qvist P, Fledelius C, Riis BJ, Christiansen e. Immunoassay for quantifying type I collagen degradation products in urine evaluated. ClinChem 1994; 40: 2022–5.

33. Boudou P, Ibrahim F, Cormier C, Chabas A, Sarfati E, Souberbielle Je. Third- or second-generation parathyroid hormone assays: a remaining debate in the diagnosis of primary hyperparathyroidism. J Clin Endocrinol Metab 2005; 90: 6370–2.

34. Bouillon R, Carmeliet G, Verlinden L, van Etten E, Verstuyf A, Luderer HF, etaI. Vitamin D and human health: lessons from vitamin of receptor null mice. Endocr Rev 2008; 29: 726–76.

35. Bouman AA, Scheffer PG, Ooms ME, Lips P, Netelenbos E. Two bone alkaline phosphatase assays compared with osteocalcin as a marker of bone formation in healthy elderly women. ClinChem 1995; 41: 196–9.

36. Bowers GN Jr, Brassard C, Sena SF. Measurement of ionized calcium in serum with ion-selective electrodes: a mature technology that can meet the daily service needs. ClinChem 1986; 32: 1437–47.

37. Brady JD, Ju J, Robins SP. Isoaspartyl bond formation within N-terminal sequences of collagen type I: implications for their use as markers of collagen degradation. ClinSci (Lond) 1999; 96: 209–15.

38. Brandt J, Krogh TN, Jensen CH, Frederiksen JK, Teisner B. Thermal instability of the trimeric structure of the N-terminal propeptide of human procollagen type I in relation to assay technology. Clin Chem 1999; 45: 47–53.

39. Bringhurst FR. Circulating forms of parathyroid hormone: peeling back the onion. Clin Chem 2003; 49: 1973–5.

40. Brossard JH, Cloutier M, Roy L, Lepage R, Gascon-Barre M, D'Amour P. Accumulation of a non-(1-84) molecular form of parathyroid hormone (PTH) detected by intact PTH assay in renal failure: importance in the interpretation of PTH values. J Clin Endocrinol Metab 1996; 81: 3923–9.

41. Brown EM. Ca'+ -sensing receptor. In: Rosen C), Compston JE, Lian JB, eds. Primer on the metabolic bone diseases and disorders of mineral metabolism, 7th edition. Washington, DC: American Society for Bone and Mineral Research, 2008: 134–41.

42. Brown EM. Calcium receptor and regulation of parathyroid hormone secretion. Rev Endocr Metab Disord 2000; 1: 307–15.

43. Brown IP' Albert C, Nassar BA, Adachi 10, Cole 0, Davison KS, etaI. Bone turnover markers in the management of postmenopausal osteoporosis. ClinBiochem 2009; 42: 929–42.

44. Broyles DL, Nielsen RG, Bussett EM, Lu WD, Mizrahi lA, Nunnelly PA, et aI. Analytical and clinical performance characteristics of Tandem-MP Ostase, a new immunoassay for serum bone alkaline phosphatase. ClinChem 1998; 44: 2139–47.

45. Bucht E, Rong H, Sjoberg HE, Sjostedt U, Granberg B, Tarring 0. Serum calcitonin forms and concentrations in young and elderly healthy females. CalcifTissueInt 1995; 56: 32–7.

46. Buckley BM, Russell LI. The measurement of ionised calcium in blood plasma. Ann ClinBiochem 1988; 25(Pt 5): 447–65.

47. Burnett R'N, Christiansen TF, Covington AK, Fogh-Andersen N, Kulpmann WR, Lewenstam A, et aI. IFCC recommended reference method for the determination of the substance concentration of ionized calcium in undiluted serum, plasma or whole blood. ClinChern Lab Med 2000; 38: 1301–14.

48. Burnett R'N, Covington AK, Fogh-Andersen N, Kiilpman WR, Maas AH, Miiller-Plathe D, et aI. Recommendations on whole blood sampling, transport, and storage for simultaneous determination of pH, blood gases, and electrolytes. International Federation of Clinical Chemistry Scientific Division. lint Fed ClinChern 1994; 6: 115–20.

49. Burtis WI. Parathyroid hormone-related protein: structure, function, and measurement. ClinChern 1992; 38: 2171–83.

50. Cali IP, Bowers GN Ir, Young OS. A referee method for the determination of total calcium in serum. ClinChem 1973; 19: 1208–13.

51. Calvo MS, Eastell R, Offord KP, Bergstralh EI, Burritt MF. Circadian variation in ionized calcium and intact parathyroid hormone: evidence for sex differences in calcium homeostasis. I Clin Endocrinol Metab 1991; 72: 69–76.

52. Calvo MS, Whiting SI. Prevalence of vitamin 0 insufficiency in Canada and the United States: importance to health status and efficacy of current food fortification and dietary supplement use. Nutr Rev 2003; 61: 107–13.

53. Cao Z, Tongate C, Elin RI. Evaluation of AVL988/4 analyzer for measurement of ionized magnesium and ionized calcium. Scand I Clin Lab Invest 2001; 61: 389–94.

54. Cardenas-Rivero N, Chernow B, Stoiko MA, Nussbaum SR, Todres ro. Hypocalcemia in critically ill children. J Pediatr 1989; 114: 946–51.

55. Carmeliet G, Verstuyf A, Maes C, Eelen G, Bouillon R. The vitamin D hormone and its nuclear receptor: mechanisms involved in bone biology. In: Seibel MI, Robins SP, Bilezikian IP, eds. Dynamics of bone and cartilage metabolism, 2nd edition. San Diego, Calif: Academic Press, 2006: 307–25.

56. Carter AB, Howanitz PJ. Intraoperative testing for parathyroid hormone: a comprehensive review of the use of the assay and the relevant literature. Arch Pathol Lab Med 2003; 127: 1424–42.

57. Carter GD, Carter R, Jones J, Berry J. How accurate are assays for 25-hydroxyvitamin D? Data from the International Vitamin D External Quality Assessment Scheme. Clin Chem. 2004; 50: 2195–2197.

58. Carter GO, Carter CR, Gunter E, lones I, lones G, Makin HL, etaI. Measurement of vitamin D metabolites: an international perspective on methodology and clinical interpretation. I Steroid Biochem Mol BioI 2004; 89-90: 467–71.

59. Cecco SA, Hristova EN, Rehak NN, Elin RI. Clinically important intermethod differences for physiologically abnormal ionized magnesium results. Am I ClinPathol 1997; 108: 564–9.

60. Chao TY, Wu YY, lanckila AI. Tartrate-resistant acid phosphatase isoform 5b (TRACP 5b) as a serum maker for cancer with bone metastasis. ClinChimActa 2010; 411: 1553–64.

61. Chapuy MC, Preziosi P, Maamer M, et al. Prevalence of vitamin D insufficiency in an adult normal population. Osteoporos Int. 1997; 7: 439–443.

62. Chapuy MC, Schott AM, Garnero P, Hans D, Delmas PD, Meunier PJ. (EPIDOS Study Group) Healthy elderly French women living at home have secondary hyperparathyroidism and high bone turnover in winter. J Clin Endocrinol Metab. 1996; 81: 1129–1133.

63. Clemens 10, Herrick MV, Singer FR, Eyre DR. Evidence that serum NTx (collagen-type I N-telopeptides) can act as an immunochemical marker of bone resorption. Clin Chern 1997; 43: 2058–63.

64. Clemens TL, Cormier S, Eichinger A, Endlich K, Fiaschi-Taesch N, Fischer E, et aI. Parathyroid hormone-related protein and its receptors: nuclear functions and roles in the renal and cardiovascular systems, the placental trophoblasts and the pancreatic islets. Br I PharmacoI 2001; 134: 1113–36.

65. CloweslA, Hannon RA, Yap TS, Hoyle NR, Blumsohn A, Eastell R. Effect of feeding on bone turnover markers and its impact on biological variability of measurements. Bone 2002; 30: 886–90.

66. Colwell A, Eastell R. The renal clearance of free and conjugated pyridinium cross-links of collagen. I Bone Miner Res 1996;11: 1976–80.

67. Confavreux CB, Levine RL, Karsenty G. A paradigm of integrative physiology, the crosstalk between bone and energy metabolisms. Mol Cell Endocrinol2009;310:21-9.

68. Cooper C, Harvey NC, Dennison EM, van Staa TP. Update on the epidemiology of Paget's disease of bone. I Bone Miner Res 2006; 21(suppI2):P3-8.

69. Corns CM, Ludman C]. Some observations on the nature of the calcium-cresolphthalein complex: one reaction and its relevance to the clinical laboratory. Ann ClinBiochem 1987; 24: 345–51.

70. Cowley DM, Mottram BM, Haling NB, Sinton TJ. Improved linearity of the calcium-cresolphthalein complex one reaction with sodium acetate. ClinChern 1986; 32: 894–5.

71. Crofton PM, Evans N, Taylor MR, Holland Cv. Procollagen type I amino-terminal propeptide: pediatric reference data and relationship with procollagen type I carboxyl-terminal propeptide. ClinChern 2004; 50: 2173–6.

72. Cummings SR, San Martin J, McClung MR, Siris ES, Eastell R, Reid JR, et al. Denosumab for prevention of fractures in postmenopausal women with osteoporosis. N Engl J Med 2009; 361: 756–65.

73. D'Amour P, Brossard JH, Rousseau L, Roy L, Gao P, Cantor T. Amino-terminal form of parathyroid hormone (PTH) with immunologic similarities to hPTH(I -84) is overproduced in primary and secondary hyperparathyroidism. ClinChern 2003; 49: 2037–44.

74. Davidson W, Barbour HM. Determination of urine magnesium using the magon dye method on the "Monarch" centrifugal analyser. Ann Clin Biochem 1990; 27: 595–6.

75. Davis CD. Vitamin D and cancer: current dilemmas and future research needs. Am J Clin Nutr 2008; 88: 565S-9S.

76. Delaisse JM, Andersen TL, Engsig MT, Henriksen K, Troen T, Blavier L. Matrix metalloproteinases (MMP) and cathepsin K contribute differently to osteoclastic activities. Microsc Res Tech 2003; 61: 504–13.

77. Delmas PD, Christiansen C, Mann KG, Price PA. Bone Gla protein (osteocalcin) assay standardization report. J Bone Miner Res 1990; 5: 5–11.

78. Delmas PD. Standardization of bone marker nomenclature. Clin Chern 2001; 47:1497.

79. DeLuca HE Overview of general physiologic features and functions of vitamin D. Am J Clin Nutr 2004; 80: 1689S-96S.

80. Dimeski G, Badrick T, John AS. Ion selective electrodes (lSEs) and interferences-a review. Clin Chim Acta 2010; 411: 309–17.

81. Divieti P, John MR, Juppner H, Bringhurst FR. Human PTH-(7-84) inhibits bone resorption in vitro via actions independent of the type 1 PTH/PTHrP receptor. Endocrinology 2002; 143: 171–6.

82. Donhowe JM, Freier EF, Wong ET, Steffes Mw' Factitious hypophosphatemia related to mannitol therapy. ClinChern 1981; 27: 1765–9.

83. Ducy P, Desbois C, Boyce B, Pinero G, Story B, Dunstan C, et al. Increased bone formation in osteocalcin-deficient mice. Nature 1996; 382: 448–52.

84. Eastell R, Chen P, Saag KG, Burshell AL, Wong M, Warner MR, et al. Bone formation markers in patients with glucocorticoid-induced osteoporosis treated with teriparatide or alendronate. Bone 2010; 46: 929–34.

85. Eknoyan G, Levin A, Levin NW Bone metabolism and disease in chronic kidney disease. Am J Kidney Dis 2003; 42 (suppl): 1–201.

86. Elomaa I, Virkkunen P, Risteli L, Risteli J. Serum concentration of the cross-linked carboxyterminaltelopeptide of type I collagen (lCTP) is a useful prognostic indicator in multiple myeloma. Br J Cancer 1992; 66: 337–41.

87. Endres DB, Morgan CH, Garry PJ, Omdahl JL. Age-related changes in serum immunoreactive parathyroid hormone and its biological action in healthy men and women. J ClinEndocrinolMetab 1987; 65: 724–31.

88. Endres DB, Villanueva R, Sharp CF, Jr, Singer FR. Immunochemiluminometric and immunoradiometric determinations of intact and total immunoreactiveparathyrin: performance in the differential diagnosis of hypercalcemia and hypoparathyroidism. Clin Chem. 1991;37: 162–168.

89. Engelbach M, Gorges R, Forst T, Pfiitzner A, Dawood R, Heerdt S, et al. Improved diagnostic methods in the follow-up of medullary thyroid carcinoma by highly specific calcitonin measurements. J Clin Endocrinol Metab 2000; 85: 1890–4.

90. Eriksen HA, Sharp CA, Robins SP, Sassi ML, Risteli L, Risteli J. Differently cross-linked and uncross-linked carboxy-terminal telopeptides of type I collagen in human mineralised bone. Bone 2004; 34: 720–7.

91. Fall PM, Kennedy D, Smith JA, Seibel MJ, Raisz LG. Comparison of serum and urine assays for biochemical markers of bone resorption in postmenopausal women with and without hormone replacement therapy and in men. OsteoporosInt 2000;11: 481–5.

92. Farley JR, Hall SL, Herring S, Libanati C, Wergedal JE. Reference standards for quantification of skeletal alkaline phosphatase activity in serum by heat inactivation and lectin precipitation. Clin Chern 1993; 39: 1878–84.

93. Favus MJ, Goltzman D. Regulation of calcium and magnesium. In: Rosen CJ, Compston JE, Lian JB, eds. Primer on the metabolic bone diseases and disorders of mineral metabolism, 7th edition. Washington, DC: American Society for Bone and Mineral Research, 2008: 104–8.

94. Fitzpatrick L, Bilezikian JP. Parathyroid hormone: structure, function, and dynamic actions. In: Seibel MJ, Robins SP, Bilezikian JP, eds. Dynamics of bone and cartilage metabolism, 2nd edition. San Diego, Calif: Academic Press, 2006: 273–91.

95. Fledelius C, Johnsen AH, Cloos PA, Bonde M, Qvist P. Characterization of urinary degradation products derived from type I collagen: identification of a beta-isomerized Asp-Gly sequence within the C-terminal telopeptide (alpha 1) region. J Bioi Chern 1997; 272.

96. Flegal KM, Carroll MD, Ogden CL, Johnson CL. Prevalence and trends in obesity among US adults, 1999–2000. JAMA. 2002;288: 1723–1727.

97. Fleisher M, Gladstone M, Crystal D, Schwartz MK. Two whole-blood multi-analyte analyzers evaluated. Clin Chem 1989; 35: 1532–5.

98. Fogh-Andersen N, Bjerrum PJ, Siggaard-Andersen 0. Ionic binding, net charge, and Donnan effect of human serum albumin as a function of pH. Clin Chern 1993; 39:48–52.

99. Foresta C, Strapazzon G, De Toni L, Gianesello L, Calcagno A, Pilon C, et al. Evidence for osteocalcin production by adipose tissue and its role in human metabolism. J Clin Endocrinol Metab 2010; 95: 3502–6.

100. Fraser CG. The application of theoretical goals based on biological variation data in proficiency testing. Arch Pathol Lab Med 1988;112: 404-15.

101. Fraser WD, Robinson J, Lawton R, Durham B, Gallacher SJ, Boyle IT, et al. Clinical and laboratory studies of a new immunoradiometric assay of parathyroid hormone-related protein. ClinChem 1993;39: 414–9.

102. Fritchie K, Zedek D, Grenache DG. The clinical utility of parathyroid hormone-related peptide in the assessment of hypercalcemia. ClinChimActa 2009;402:146-9.

103. Fujita T, Kawakami Y, Kohda S, Takata S, Sunahara Y, Arisue K. Assay of magnesium in serum and urine with use of only one enzyme, isocitrate dehydrogenase (NADP+). ClinChern 1995;41:1302-5.

104. Fukumoto S, Martin TJ. Bone as an endocrine organ. Trends EndocrinolMetab 2009;20:230-6.

105. Gao P, D'Amour P. Evolution of the parathyroid hormone (PTH) assay-importance of circulating PTH immunoheterogeneity and of its regulation. Clin Lab 2005;51: 21–9.

106. Gao P, Scheibel S, D'Amour P, John MR, Rao SD, Schmidt-Gayk H, et al. Development of a novel immunoradiometric assay exclusively for biologically active whole parathyroid hormone 1-84: implications for improvement of accurate assessment of parathyroid function. J Bone Miner Res 2001;16:605-14.

107. Garber CC, Miller RC. Revisions of the 1963 semidine HC1 standard method for inorganic phosphorus. ClinChem 1983;29: 184–8.

108. Garnero P, Borel 0, Byrjalsen I, Ferreras M, Drake FH, McQueney MS, et al. The collagenolytic activity of cathepsin K is unique among mammalian proteinases. J BioiChem 1998;273:32347-52.

109. Garnero P, Borel 0, Delmas PD. Evaluation of a fully automated serum assay for C-terminal cross-linking telopeptide of type I collagen in osteoporosis. Clin Chern 2001; 47: 694–702.

110. Garnero P, Ferreras M, Karsdal MA, Nicamhlaoibh R, Risteli J, Borel D, et al. The type I collagen fragments lCTP and CTX reveal distinct enzymatic pathways of bone collagen degradation. J Bone Miner Res 2003;18: 859–67.

111. Garnero P, Fledelius C, Gineyts E, Serre CM, Vignot E, Delmas PD. Decreased beta-isomerization of the C-terminal telopeptide of type I collagen alpha 1 chain in Paget's disease of bone. J Bone Miner Res 1997;12: 1407–15.

112. Garnero P, Gineyts E, Arbault P, Christiansen C, Delmas PD. Different effects of bisphosphonate and estrogen therapy on free and peptidebound bone cross-link excretion. J Bone Miner Res 1995; 10: 641–9.

113. Garnero P, Grimaux M, Seguin P, Delmas PD. Characterization of immunoreactive forms of human osteocalcin generated in vivo and in vitro. j Bone Miner Res 1994; 9: 255 64.

114. Garnero P, Vergnaud P, Hoyle N. Evaluation of a fully automated serum assay for total N-terminal propeptide of type I collagen in postmenopausal osteoporosis. Clin Chern 2008; 54: 188–96.

115. Gauci C, Moranne 0, Fouqueray B, de la Faille R, Maruani G, Haymannj P, et al. Pitfalls of measuring total blood calcium in patients with CKD. J Am Soc Nephrol 2008;19: 1592–8.

116. GawoskijM, Walsh D. Citrate interference in assays of total calcium in serum. Clin Chern 1989; 35:2140-1.

117. Gelb BD, Shi GP, Chapman HA, DesnickRj. Pycnodysostosis, a lysosomal disease caused by cathepsin K deficiency. Science 1996;273: 1236-8.

118. Glover SJ, Eastell R, McCloskey EV, Rogers A, Garnero P, Lowery J, et al. Rapid and robust response of biochemical markers of bone formation to teriparatide therapy. Bone 2009;45: 1053-8.

119. Glover SJ, Gall M, Schoenborn-Kellenberger 0, Wagener M, Garnero P, Boonen S, et al. Establishing a reference interval for bone turnover markers in 637 healthy, young, premenopausal women from the United Kingdom, France, Belgium, and the United States. j Bone Miner Res 2009;24: 389–97.

120. Goltzman D. Interaction of parathyroid hormone-related peptide with the skeleton. In: Seibel MJ, Robins SP, Bilezikianj P, eds. Dynamics of bone and cartilage metabolism, 2nd edition. San Diego, Calif: Academic Press, 2006: 293–305.

121. Gomez B jr, Ardakani S, Evans Bj, Merrell LD, jenkins OK, Kung VT. Monoclonal antibody assay for free urinary pyridinium cross-links. ClinChern 1996;42: 1168-75.

122. Gomez P, Coca C, Vargas C, Acebillo j, Martinez A. Normal reference-intervals for 20 biochemical variables in healthy infants, children, and adolescents. Clin Chern 1984;30: 407–12.

123. Gonzalez EA, Al Aly Z, Martin Kj. Assessment of bone and joint diseases: renal osteodystrophy. In: Seibel Mj, Robins SP, BilezikianjP, eds. Dynamics of bone and cartilage metabolism, 2nd edition. San Diego, Calif: Academic Press, 2006: 755–65.

124. Goodman WG, jiippner H, SaluskylB, Sherrard OJ. Parathyroid hormone (PTH), PTH-derived peptides, and new PTH assays in renal osteodystrophy. Kidney Int 2003;63: I-II.

125. Gosling P. Analytical reviews in clinical biochemistry: calcium measurement. Ann Clin Biochem 1986; 23: 146–56.

126. Guise TA, Mohammad KS, Clines G, Stebbins E.G., Wong DH, Higgins LS, et al. Basic mechanisms responsible for osteolytic and osteoblastic bone metastases. Clin Cancer Res 2006; 12:6213s-6s.

127. Guise TA. Breaking down bone: new insight into site-specific mechanisms of breast cancer osteolysis mediated by metalloproteinases. Genes Dev 2009; 23: 2117–23.

128. Gundberg CM. Matrix proteins. Osteoporos Int 2003;14 (suppl 5): S37–40.

129. Haddad jG. Plasma vitamin D-binding protein (Gc-globulin): multiple tasks. J Steroid Biochem Mol BioI 1995; 53: 579–82.

130. Halleen 1M, Hentunen TA, Karp M, Kiikonen SM, Pettersson K, Viiiiniinen HK. Characterization of serum tartrate-resistant acid phosphatase and development of a direct two-site immunoassay. j Bone Miner Res 1998;13:683-7.

131. HalleenjM, Alatalo SL, janckila Aj, Woitge HW, Seibel MJ, Viiiiniinen HK. Serum tartrate-resistant acid phosphatase 5b is a specific and sensitive marker of bone resorption. ClinChem 2001;47:597-600.

132. HalleenjM, Alatalo SL, Suominen H, Cheng S, janckila AI, Viiiiniinen HK. Tartrate-resistant acid phosphatase 5b: a novel serum marker of bone resorption. j Bone Miner Res 2000;15:1337-45.

133. Halling Linder C, Narisawa S, Millan jL, Magnusson P. Glycosylation differences contribute to distinct catalytic properties among bone alkaline phosphatase isoforms. Bone 2009;45:987-93.

134. Hannon RA, ClowesjA, Eagleton AC, Al Hadari A, Eastell R, Blumsohn A. Clinical performance of immunoreactive tart rate resistant acid phosphatase isoform 5b as a marker of bone resorption. Bone 2004;34:187-94.

135. Hanson DA, Eyre DR. Molecular site specificity of pyridinoline and pyrrole cross-links in type I collagen of human bone. I BioiChem 1996;271: 26508-16.

136. Hanson DA, Weis MA, Bollen AM, Maslan SL, Singer FR, Eyre DR. A specific immunoassay for monitoring human bone resorption: quanti tat ion of type I collagen cross-linked N-telopeptides in urine. J Bone Miner Res 1992; 7: 1251-8.

137. Harmey 0, Hessle L, Narisawa S, johnson KA, Terkeltaub R, Millan jl.. Concerted regulation of inorganic pyrophosphate and osteopontin by akp2, enpp 1, and ank: an integrated model of the pathogenesis of mineralization disorders. Am j Pathol 2004; 164: 1199-209.

138. Harris EK, Boyd JC. On dividing reference data into subgroups to produce separate reference ranges. Clin Chem. 1990;36: 265–270.

139. Harris EK, Wong ET, Shaw ST., Jr Statistical criteria for separate reference intervals: race and gender groups in creatine kinase. Clin Chem. 1991; 37: 1580–1582.

140. Harvey NC, Dennison EM, Cooper C. Epidemiology of osteoporotic fractures. In: Rosen Cj, Compston I.E., Lian IB, eds. Primer on the metabolic bone diseases and disorders of mineral metabolism, 7th edition. Washington, DC: American Society for Bone and Mineral Research, 2008: 198–203.

141. Haverstick OM, Brill LB 2nd, Scott MG, Bruns DE. Preanalytical variables in measurement of free (ionized) calcium in lithium heparin-containing blood collection tubes. Clin Chim Acta 2009; 403: 102-4.

142. Heaney RP, Horst RL, Cullen OM, Armas LA. Vitamin D3 distribution and status in the body. J Am Coli Nutr 2009; 28: 252–6.

143. Heath H 3rd, EarlljM, Schaaf M, PiechockijT, Li TK. Serum ionized calcium during bed rest in fracture patients and normal men. Metabolism 1972; 21: 633–40.

144. Heider U, Fleissner C, Zavrski I, Kaiser M, Hecht M, Jakob C, et al. Bone markers in multiple myeloma. Eur j Cancer 2006; 42: 1544–53.

145. Henriksen K, Tanko LB, Qvist P, Delmas PO, Christiansen C, Karsdal MA. Assessment of osteoclast number and function: application in the development of new and improved treatment modalities for bone diseases. OsteoporosInt 2007; 18: 681–5.

146. Hermse D, Franzson L, Hoffmann JP, et al. Multicenter evaluation of a new immunoassay for intact PTH measurement on the Elecsys System 2010 and 1010. Clin Lab. 2002; 48(3–4): 131–141.

147. Herrmann M, Seibel Mj. The amino- and carboxy terminal cross linked telopeptides of collagen type I, NTX-l and CTX-I: a comparative review. Clin Chim Acta 2008; 393: 57–75.

148. Hessle L, johnson KA, Anderson HC, Narisawa S, Sali A, GodingjW, et al. Tissue-nonspecific alkaline phosphatase and plasma cell membrane glycoprotein-I are central antagonistic regulators of bone mineralization. Proc Nat! AcadSci USA 2002; 99: 9445–9.

149. Hodsman AB, Bauer DC, Dempster OW, Dian L, Hanley DA, Harris ST, et al. Parathyroid hormone and teriparatide for the treatment of osteoporosis: a review of the evidence and suggested guidelines for its use. Endocr Rev 2005; 26:688-703.

150. Holick MF. The parathyroid hormone D-lema. J Clin Endocrinol Metab. 2003;88: 3499–3500.

151. Inaba M, Nakatsuka K, Imanishi Y, et al. Technical and clinical characterization of the Bio-PTH (1-84) immunochemiluminometric assay and comparison with a second-generation assay for parathyroid hormone.Clin Chem. 2004; 50: 385–390.

152. Intact PTH—Parathyroid Hormone. San Juan Capistrano, CA: Nichols Institute Diagnostics. Catalog No. 60-4446, Item No. 36T-4446: page 6. Rev. C.

153. J Chromatogr B Biomed Sci Appl. D3 and 25- hydroxyvitamin D2 in human plasma with photodiode-array ultraviolet detection. 2001 May 5; 755(1-2):129-35.

154. Lips P, Duong T, Oleksik A, et al. A global study of vitamin D status and parathyroid function in postmenopausal women with osteoporosis: baseline data from the multiple outcomes of raloxifene evaluation clinical trial [erratum in J Clin Endocrinol Metab. 2001;86:3008] J Clin Endocrinol Metab. 2001; 86:1212–1221.

155. Martin KJ, Akhtar I, Gonzalez EA. Parathyroid hormone: new assays, new receptors. Semin Nephrol. 2004; 24:3–9.

156. Sinton TJ, Cowley DM, Bryant SJ. Reference intervals for calcium, phosphate, and alkaline phosphatase as derived on the basis of multichannel-analyzer profiles. Clin Chem. 1986; 32(1 Pt 1):76–79.

157. Souberbielle JC, Cormier C, Kindermans C, et al. Vitamin D status and redefining serum parathyroid hormone reference range in the elderly. J Clin Endocrinol Metab. 2001; 86: 3086–3090.

158. Souberbielle JC, Lawson-Body E, Hammadi B, Sarfati E, Kahan A, Cormier C. The use in clinical practice of parathyroid hormone normative values established in vitamin D-sufficient subjects. J Clin Endocrinol Metab. 2003; 88:3501–3504.

159. Tangpricha V, Pearce EN, Chen TC, Holick MF. Vitamin D insufficiency among free-living healthy young adults. Am J Med. 2002;112:659–662.

160. Tanno Y, Yokoyama K, Nakayama M, et al. IRMA (whole PTH) is a more useful assay for the effect of PTH on bone than the Allegro intact PTH assay in CAPD patients with low bone turnover marker. Nephrol Dial Transplant. 2003;18 (Suppl 3): III97–III98.

161. Tietz textbook of clinical chemistry and molecular biology, 2012. 5fifth edition, Philadelphia, W.B Saunders company.

162. Vieth R, Ladak Y, Walfish PG. Age-related changes in the 25-hydroxyvitamin D versus parathyroid hormone relationship suggest a different reason why older adults require more vitamin D. J Clin Endocrinol Metab. 2003;88:185–191.

163. William Marshall, MártaLapsley, Stephen K Bangert. Elsevier.com: Clinical Chemistry, 2012, 7th Edition; ISBN-9780723437031.

164. Wortsman J, Matsuoka LY, Chen TC, Lu Z, Holick MF. Decreased bioavailability of vitamin D in obesity [erratum in Am J Clin Nutr. 2003;77:1342] Am J Clin Nutr. 2000;72: 690–693.

13

Plasma Proteins

INTRODUCTION

The human body requires 20 amino acids as the building blocks of proteins. Humans make some of these amino acids but must gain the rest, as **essential nutrients**, through the diet. The production of proteins from amino acid building blocks is directed by a template that is produced by the **DNA** of the cell. Therefore, the amino acid sequence of protein is a reflection of the genetic information of the cell. Most enzymes are proteins that are able to catalyze reactions. Through regulation of reactions via enzymes, the genetic information directs the diverse metabolic reactions of the cell. In addition to their function as an energy source and in catalysis, amino acids and proteins are used as transport molecules, structural components of cells and tissues, hormones, clotting agents, and immune agents.

Proteins and amino acids have unique structures (Fig. 13.1) and participate in characteristic chemical reactions. Proteins are polymers consisting of amino acid units. Amino acid units within the protein are joined by peptide bonds. Each amino acid unit contains a unique R group. The amino acid unit on the carboxyl end of the protein contains a free carboxyl group that does not participate in peptide bond formation. The amino acid unit on the amino end of the protein contains a free amino group that does not participate in peptide bond formation.

The carboxyl end may become charged when a hydrogen ion is lost. The amino end may become charged when a hydrogen ion is gained. The peptide bond consists of the covalent linkage of an amino group from one amino acid and a carboxyl group of another amino acid. Proteins are ampholytes, i.e. in aqueous solutions they may have positive and negative charges on the same molecule. This property of proteins is used to separate protein molecules during electrophoresis.

The pH (hydrogen ion concentration) of the solution determines the net charge of the molecule.

At different pH environments, hydrogen ions will be gained or lost from the carboxyl and amino ends and from functional groups of R residues of the amino acids. Since proteins are composed of different amino acids, different proteins will gain or lose hydrogen ions at different pH environments.

Each peptide has a pH at which the net loss and gain of hydrogen ions is equal. This pH is called the pI, or isoelectric point, and is unique for each protein. The pI is unique for each protein because each protein has a unique chemical makeup and structure. In addition to the properties of proteins as ampholytes, proteins also have other representative structural properties. Fibrous proteins usually function as structural components of the body, such as fibrinogen and collagen. Most plasma

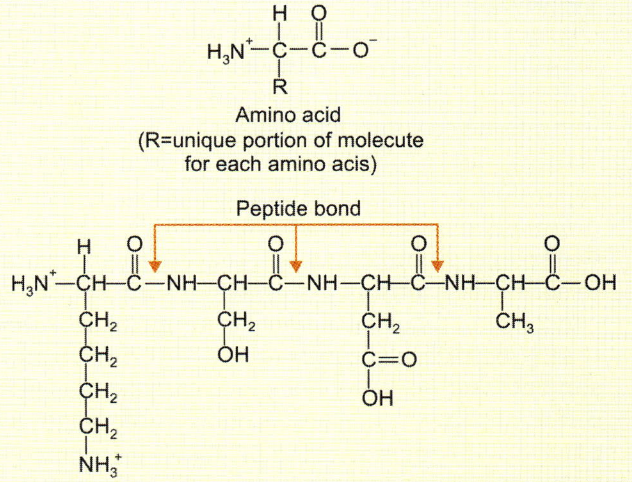

Fig. 13.1: Amino acid and protein structures

proteins and enzymes are globular proteins. Fibrous proteins are insoluble. The structure of fibrous proteins imbues strength to tissue through its linear configuration. Globular proteins play many roles in the body. Globular proteins contain intricate folding sequences. Subgroups within globular proteins interact through non-covalent bonding. Non-covalent interaction is an important character of enzyme proteins.

Proteins may be characterized by the sequence of the amino acids that compose them, the chemical interaction of the components of the protein strand, the regular pattern of folding within the strand, and, finally, the interaction of several protein strands that make up the functional protein. Primary structure refers to the sequence of amino acid units that make up the protein strand. The amino acid sequence is coded from DNA information of the cell in which the protein was created.

Secondary structure refers to the folds of the protein strand. Sections of the protein strand may be folded into regular structures, such as alpha helixes and beta pleats. Tertiary structure refers to folds of sections of the protein. Hydrogen bonds, disulfide bridges, and hydrophobic interactions between functional groups of the protein strand may stabilize tertiary structure. Quaternary structure refers to the association of two or more peptide strands to form one functioning protein.

PHYSICAL PROPERTIES OF PROTEINS

Although, the ionization of individual amino acids may be influenced strongly by neighboring amino acids. Differing physical properties serve as the basis of methods to separate proteins. Some important characteristics include the following:

1. **Differential solubility:** The solubility of proteins is affected by pH, ionic strength, temperature, and the dielectric constant (addition of solvents such as ethanol). Changing solvent pH affects the net charges of a protein; at its pI (net charge zero), a protein in polar solvent usually has its lowest solubility. Changing ionic strength affects the hydration and solubility of proteins. 'Salting-in' and 'salting-out' procedures were early methods for separating and characterizing proteins. Serum was originally divided into albumin, which is soluble in water, and globulins, which require salt to remain in solution. Albumin also stays in solution at high concentrations of salts, such as ammonium sulfate that precipitate globulins. Addition of organic solvents and polyethylene glycol has been used for differential precipitation. Fractional precipitation of plasma with ethanol, using protocols developed by Cohn and coworkers, leads to several Cohn fractions that are enriched in immunoglobulins, a and b-globulins, or albumin (fraction V). Polyethylene glycols induce precipitation by steric exclusion and, therefore, preferentially precipitate large proteins or complexes.

2. **Molecular size:** Separation of small and large molecules can be achieved by dialysis or ultra-filtration. Size exclusion chromatography, ultra-centrifugation, and electrophoresis perform size separations under native conditions, where proteins and peptides are in native globular states or under denaturing conditions. Addition of reducing agents allows separation of disulfide-linked components. Polyacrylamide gel electrophoresis in the presence of the denaturing detergent sodium dodecyl sulfate is a method for estimating the molecular weight of polypeptide chains in proteins.

3. **Molecular mass:** Advances in mass spectrometry allow the determination of masses of peptides and proteins with increasing accuracy. Peptides and proteins can be ionized by matrix-assisted laser desorption/ionization (MALDI) or by electrospray ionization. Highest detection sensitivity and mass accuracy are for peptides, and tandem mass spectrometry can be applied for sequence analysis of peptides. Large proteins with extensive mass heterogeneity due to variable modifications pose challenges related to their high mass and the formation of multiple peaks.

4. **Electrical charge:** Ion-exchange chromatography, isoelectric focusing, and electrophoresis separate peptides and proteins based on charge.

5. **Surface adsorption:** Adsorption of peptides and proteins to particles have been used as the basis for separations. Hydrophobic interaction chromatography and reverse phase chromatography rely on differential hydrophobic interactions of peptides or proteins.

6. **Affinity chromatography:** Specific ligands, antibodies, or other recognition molecules have been used to separate peptides or proteins selectively.

PLASMA PROTEIN CONCENTRATIONS

The characteristic of proteins that has been applied most frequently is their plasma concentration, and the range of plasma concentrations of different proteins measured in clinical assays extends well over 10 logs of concentration. Relative to the highest abundance protein, albumin, concentrations of plasma proteins decrease progressively over several logs of concentration for proteins released from tissues of smaller cell mass, and the ability of endogenous proteins to enter the circulation generally decreases hierarchically: (1) proteins secreted directly into plasma, (2) cell membrane proteins shed into the circulation, (3) secretory proteins in exocrine secretions, (4) high-abundance cytoplasmic proteins, (5) low abundance cytoplasmic proteins, (6) transmembrane proteins, and (7) organellar proteins that must traverse more than one membrane to exit cells. Many proteins serve as useful markers of physiology and disease, as these processes alter the production or release of proteins into plasma.

Changes in plasma concentrations of secretory proteins usually reflect changes in synthetic rates, secretion, or clearance, and plasma concentrations of cytoplasmic and organellar proteins tend to reflect cellular injury and rates of leakage into plasma. In addition to endogenous sources of proteins, multiple exogenous sources of proteins include infectious organisms, dietary sources, and therapeutic interventions.

For diagnostic purposes, clinical laboratories currently assess only a small proportion of the thousands of gene products in the circulation and identify only a small proportion of diversity of post-translational processing. Antibodies and T-cell receptors represent special cases wherein somatic recombination and mutation result in repertoires of millions of sequences and binding specificities. A small portion of this diversity is assessed by serological or functional assay.

Plasma concentrations of proteins depend not only on rates of production and efficiency of entry to the circulation, but also on rates of clearance. Proteins and peptides substantially smaller than albumin are cleared from the circulation by glomerular filtration unless they are bound to larger carriers, such as small apolipoproteins bound to lipoprotein particles or retinol-binding protein bound to prealbumin.

MAJOR PLASMA PROTEINS

Over 100 individual proteins have a physiological function in the plasma. Their principal functions, and some of the proteins, are indicated in Table 13.1. Quantitatively, the single most important protein is albumin. With the exception of fibrinogen, the other proteins are known collectively as globulins. Changes in the concentrations of individual proteins occur in many conditions and their measurement can provide useful diagnostic information. Some plasma proteins are enzymes (e.g. renin, coagulation factors). In addition to these, many primarily intracellular enzymes are detectable in plasma as a result of their loss from cells during normal cell turnover. The measurement of such enzymes provides a sensitive (although, often relatively non-specific) indicator of tissue damage.

Table 13.1	Functions of plasma proteins
Function	**Example**
Transport	Thyroxine-binding globulin (thyroid hormones) apolipoproteins (cholesterol), triglyceride transferrin (iron)
Humoral immunity	Immunoglobulins
Maintenance of oncotic pressure	All proteins, particularly albumin
Enzymes	Renin coagulation factors complement proteins
Protease inhibitors	α1-antitrypsin (acts on proteases)
Buffering	All proteins

The Acute-phase Response

Systemic inflammation in response to infection, tissue injury, or inflammatory disease triggers changes in hepatic production of multiple plasma proteins, as indicated in Table 13.2.

This process, mediated by the action of interleukin-6 (IL-6) and other cytokines has been termed the acute-phase response (APR). It is a nonspecific reaction to

Table 13.2	The acute phase response—changes in plasma protein concentrations
Positive APR	C-reactive protein (extreme)
	Serum amyloid A (extreme)
	α 1 acid glycoprotein
	α 1 antitrypsin
	α 1 anti-chymotrypsin
	Anti-thrombin III
	C3, C4, and C9
	C1 inhibitor
	C4b-binding protein
	Ceruloplasmin
	Factor B
	Ferritin
	Fibrinogen
	Haptoglobin
	Hemopexin
	Lipopolysaccharide-binding protein
	Mannan-binding protein (lectin)
	Plasminogen
	Procalcitonin
Negative APR	Albumin
	Apolipoprotein A-I
	Apolipoprotein B
	α 2 HS glycoprotein
	IGF-I; prealbumin
	Retinol-binding protein
	Thyroxine- binding globulin
	Transferrin

APR, acute-phase response

inflammation, comparable with the increase in temperature or leukocyte count. Studies have suggested that it is possible to therapeutically block the APR with inhibitors of tumor necrosis factor α (TNF-α), which may be beneficial in some cases where products of the APR contribute to inflammation or deposit in tissues as amyloid. In the APR, synthesis of a few proteins, including albumin, transferrin, and prealbumin, is down regulated; such proteins are termed negative acute-phase reactants.

Albumin concentrations fall faster than expected from decreased synthesis; acute response might also reflect increased capillary permeability and redistribution of albumin to extracellular fluids. Production of a number of proteins, including α1-antitrypsin (AAT), α1 acid glycoprotein (AAG), haptoglobin (Hp), ceruloplasmin, C4, C3, and fibrinogen increases several-fold. Production of C-reactive protein (CRP) and serum amyloid A (SAA) increase greatly, and plasma concentrations can increase up to 1000-fold or more in extreme cases. The decrease in apolipoprotein A-I, coupled with increases in serum amyloid A, results in remodeling of high-density lipoproteins (HDLs) from forms with apolipoprotein A-I as the major component to forms with increased amounts of serum amyloid A. These changes in composition of HDL have been related to decreased capacity for reverse cholesterol transport and antioxidant activity, and a general change in function of HDL from anti-inflammatory to proinflammatory.

Procalcitonin is another component measured to assess APRs. Procalcitonin is a polypeptide of 116 amino acids that serves as the precursor for calcitonin in C-cells of the thyroid. In response to inflammation, procalcitonin begins to be synthesized by other tissues, such as liver, kidney, and pancreas, where it is not cleaved into smaller peptide components, and plasma concentrations increase more rapidly than other acute-phase reactants from a very low baseline concentration.

Plasma concentrations of individual acute-phase proteins rise at different rates-first, procalcitonin, CRP, SAA, and Cl1-antichymotrypsin; after the first 12 hours, AAG; after 24–48 hours, AAT, Hp, C4, and fibrinogen; and finally, C3 and ceruloplasmin (Cp). All reach maxima within 2–5 days following an acute insult and then decrease in the same order as their increase.

Measurement of CRP and SAA, which have the greatest change in concentration, can be used to monitor the progress of an inflammatory reaction or its response to treatment. Increased erythrocyte sedimentation rate (ESR) is another indicator of inflammation. Fibrinogen concentrations are considered a major determinant of ESR, so that ESR probably relates to changes in fibrinogen in the acute-phase response. APRs to bacterial infection usually are stronger than those to viral infection, and procalcitonin or other acute-phase reactants sometimes are measured in newborns or in complex adult patients to try to rapidly identify patients with bacterial infection before results from bacterial culture can be obtained. Procalcitonin measurements therefore assist in determining whether antibiotic therapy should be used. Concentrations of procalcitonin are low in infants, and a cutoff of 0.12 ng/mL has been recommended to detect bacterial infection in infants presenting with fever. Concentrations below a higher cutoff of 0.5 ng/mL indicate low risk of sepsis in adult patients in intensive care units. Lipopolysaccharide binding protein is another acute-phase reactant that has been suggested as a useful marker for detecting infection; concentrations of lipopolysaccharide-binding protein are markedly increased in most patients with infectious endocarditis in comparison with noninfectious valvular disease. Qualitative changes in proteins also are seen with the APR, such as altered changes in glycosylation of proteins. Changes in glycosylation of immunoglobulins may have an immunomodulatory effect.

Chronic infection, such as viral hepatitis, yields different changes in the composition of plasma proteins compared with acute infection. Stimulation of lymphocytes to produce antibodies leads initially to increased amounts of IgM and later to increased IgG and IgA antibodies to the infectious agent. Many plasma proteins have been used as indicators of impaired liver function in cirrhotic liver disease, including α2 macroglobulin, apolipoprotein A-I, haptoglobin, vitronectin, and fibronectin, and measures of some of these components have been included in several different multiparameter indices of hepatic fibrosis.

Determination of Total Protein

Plasma normally contains about 6.5–8.5 g/dL protein, and serum about 4% less. Determination of total protein in biological fluids in some respects represents a greater challenge than analysis of a specific protein, because variable protein composition of biological fluids leads to variable carbohydrate composition, charge, and physical characteristics of proteins in the mixture. Many methods of protein measurements respond differentially to different proteins and present problems when applied to specimens of varying protein composition.

Most methods other than the biuret method have not been thoroughly examined for interactions with small peptide components as well as intact proteins, and this may become a significant issue in renal failure with increased accumulation of peptides and small proteins.

Many specific methods have been developed to measure the total protein content of biological fluids, such as, kjeldahl method, biuret method, direct optical methods, dye-binding methods, lowry (folin-ciocalteu) method, refractometry, turbidimetric and nephelometric methods.

Reference Intervals

The total protein concentration of serum obtained from healthy ambulatory adults is 6.3–8.3 g/dL and 6.0–7.8 g/dL for adults at bed rest. Plasma usually contains a protein concentration about 0.3 g/dL higher (unless diluted by a volume of anticoagulant, such as citrate solution) because of the content of fibrinogen and other proteins removed during clotting to form serum.

Hemoconcentration and relative hyperproteinemia, with increased concentrations of all plasma proteins, occur with inadequate water intake or excessive water loss as in severe vomiting, diarrhea, Addison's disease, or diabetic acidosis. Some hemoconcentration also occurs with standing (reduced intravascular volume) or prolonged tourniquet time during blood collection. Hemodilution and relative hypoproteinemia, with decreased concentrations of all plasma proteins, occur with water intoxication or salt retention syndromes, during massive intravenous infusions, and physiologically when cumbent position are is assumed. A recumbent position decreases total protein concentration by 0.3–0.5 g/dL and many individual proteins including albumin by up to 10%. This reflects the redistribution of extracellular fluid from the extravascular space to the intravascular space and therefore dilution of a constant amount of plasma protein in a larger volume. Of the individual serum proteins, albumin is present in such high concentrations that low concentrations of this protein alone may cause hypoproteinemia. Hypoalbuminemia is very common and has many causes. Mild hyperproteinemia may be caused by an increase in the concentration of specific proteins normally present in relatively low concentration as, e.g. in dehydration, with increases in acute-phase reactants, or with increases in polyclonal immunoglobulins as a result of infection. Marked hyperproteinemia may be caused by high concentrations of the monoclonal immunoglobulins produced in paraproteinemias.

SPECIFIC PLASMA PROTEINS

Prealbumin (Transthyretin) and Retinol-binding Protein

Prealbumin and retinol-binding protein (RBP) are non-glycosylated transport proteins. RBP is bound to prealbumin, which was named for its electrophoretic mobility. In 1981, the term transthyretin was proposed for prealbumin to reflect its binding and transport of both thyroid hormones and RBP. Both prealbumin and transthyretin are terms in common use.

Prealbumin (MW 35 kDa) is composed of four identical, non-covalently bound subunits, forming triiodothyronine (T3)- and thyroxine (T4)-binding sites. It binds and transports approximately 10% of both hormones. (Thyroxine-binding globulin transports approximately 70%, and albumin binds approximately 20%). Because of negative cooperativity of thyroid hormone binding, usually only one prealbumin-binding site is occupied. Prealbumin's synthesis is stimulated by glucocorticosteroid hormones, androgens, and many nonsteroidal anti-inflammatory drugs (NSAIDs), including aspirin. Prealbumin is synthesized in the liver and to a lesser extent in the choroid plexus of the brain. Synthesis in the choroid plexus may account for relatively high concentrations of prealbumin in cerebrospinal fluid (CSF).

RBP is a 21-kDa transport protein for all-transretinol, the active form of vitamin A. RBP is synthesized in the liver and in adipose tissue. Minor variants that lack one or two C-terminal residues are observed by mass spectrometry. Studies in the metabolism literature sometimes refer to RBP as retinol-binding protein-4.

Zinc is required for synthesis, and retinol is required for its transportation by the Golgi apparatus. In plasma, RBP occurs mainly as a 1:1 complex with prealbumin, slowing glomerular filtration of RBP. Prealbumin usually has twofold to threefold molar excess over RBP. Uptake of retinol by target cells is followed by dissociation of the prealbumin-RBP complex and clearance of apo-RBP (RBP without retinol) from the circulation by the kidneys. RBP has a half-life of only about 12 hours, but it is extended in renal failure.

Clinical Significance of Prealbumin and RBP

If vitamin A intake is adequate and renal function is normal, concentrations of prealbumin and RBP often rise and fall in parallel.

Adipocytes appear to be a significant site for synthesis of RBP, and its concentrations may increase with obesity or syndromes of insulin resistance.

INCREASED PLASMA CONCENTRATIONS

Serum RBP increases in chronic renal disease, including diabetic nephropathy. Concentrations are increased with corticosteroid or NSAID therapy and in Hodgkin's disease. Interest in RBP has been stimulated by recognition that it is synthesized in adipose tissues, and that excretion from adipose tissue may increase in syndromes of insulin resistance, together with other products of adipocytes, such as leptin, adiponectin, and resistin.

Decreased Plasma Concentrations

Decreased concentrations of prealbumin and RBP are seen primarily in liver disease, protein malnutrition, and the APR. Zinc deficiency results in low serum concentrations of both RBP and vitamin A. Prealbumin concentrations are often used as an indicator of adequacy of protein nutrition because of its relatively short half-life, high proportion of essential amino acids, and small pool size. However, it is a negative APR. Concentrations also fall in cirrhosis of the liver and protein-losing diseases of the gut or kidneys. An acute-phase reactant, such as CRP, should be assayed along with prealbumin if concentrations are to be used to estimate nutritional status. History and physical examination are also important aspects of nutritional assessment.

Laboratory Testing

Prealbumin migrates as a minor component anodal to albumin on routine serum electrophoresis and is not routinely observed by most methods. It is a proportionately greater component of CSF. Prealbumin and RBP usually are measured by immunonephelometric or immunoturbidimetric methods. The adult reference interval for RBP is 3.0–6.0 mg/dL. The RBP concentration at birth is 1.1–3.4 mg/dL and at 6 months increases to 1.8–5.0 mg/dL. The adult reference interval for prealbumin, based on the certified reference material (CRM) 470, is 0.2–0.4 g/L. Concentrations in healthy neonates are approximately half those found in adults; they increase into puberty, with a larger increase noted in boys than girls, and decrease in both sexes after age 50.

Albumin

Albumin represents the largest protein component of human serum that is water soluble, is moderately soluble in concentrated salt solutions, and experiences heat denaturation.

Albumin has an important role in maintaining colloidal oncotic pressure and preventing edema. Since water moves freely through cell membranes and into the intravascular space by osmosis, the high concentration of proteins in intravascular fluid allows movement of water into vessels, and normal blood pressure and cardiac output allow circulation to evenly distribute the fluids. If the concentration of albumin is significantly decreased, fluids accumulate in interstitial spaces and cause edema. Normal protein concentration in blood vessels allows fluid to flow freely from intracellular to interstitial to intravascular spaces. Albumin also serves as a transport molecule for various substances.

Albumin has a non-glycosylated polypeptide chain of 585 amino acids and a calculated molecular weight of 66,438 Da. It has a heart-shaped three dimensional structure stabilized by 17 intrachain S-S bonds. It is a relatively stable protein, resisting denaturation up to higher temperatures than most plasma proteins. Albumin has a high abundance of charged amino acids that contribute to high solubility, and it has a net negative charge of about –12 at neutral pH. Albumin, therefore contributes about 6–10 mmol/L to the anion gap at normal albumin concentrations of 0.5–0.8 mmol/L, and lesser amounts at lower albumin concentrations. At a pH of 8.6 for alkaline electrophoresis, albumin has a net charge of about –25, resulting in high mobility toward the anode. One unpaired cysteine at position 34 occurs partially in reduced form and partially in exchangeable disulfide bonds with small compounds, such as cysteine and homocysteine. The unpaired cysteine has an unusually low pK of <6 and high rates of disulfide exchange. Consequently, it serves as a major plasma carrier of compounds with free sulfhydryls.

Albumin is synthesized by hepatocytes. The synthetic reserve of the liver is substantial; in nephrotic syndrome, albumin synthesis can increase three fold above normal. The synthetic rate is controlled primarily by colloidal osmotic pressure (COP) and secondarily by protein intake. As noted previously, albumin is a negative acute-phase reactant. Catabolism occurs mainly by pinocytosis by multiple tissues, with lysosomal degradation of protein to amino acids. Normally, only small amounts (10–20% of the total catabolized) are lost into the gastrointestinal tract and the glomerular filtrate. Albumin losses by these routes may become substantial, however, in protein-losing enteropathies and glomerular disorders, resulting in nephrotic states. Burn injuries also result in major losses of albumin. The normal plasma half-life of albumin is 15–19 days. Albumin and IgG have several fold longer plasma half-lives than most proteins because of the action of a recycling receptor, the neonatal IgG receptor that recovers these two proteins from pinocytosed fluids.

At high concentrations of albumin, the receptor may be saturated and the half-life of albumin decreased. At low concentrations of albumin, such as in analbuminemia, the half-life of albumin is markedly extended.

Albumin is not essential for humans; rare individuals with analbuminemia have been found. However, the large metabolic expenditure for abundant albumin formation, mechanisms of regulation, and specific recycling mechanisms argue for beneficial functions.

Albumin may serve as a storage form of amino acids that can be delivered to tissues in catabolic states and as an antioxidant, particularly through the action of its free sulfhydryl group. The two most clearly defined functions of albumin are: (1) serving as the major component of colloid osmotic pressure (patients in hypoalbuminemic states, such as nephrotic syndromes, are prone to develop edema; albumin solutions sometimes are administered as a replacement fluid to try to acutely maintain intravascular volume); and (2) serving as a transporter for a diverse range of substances, including fatty acids and other lipids, bilirubin, foreign substances such as drugs, thiol-containing amino acids, tryptophan, calcium, and metals. Some of these substances, such as fatty acids and unconjugated bilirubin, have very low solubility in water in the absence of a carrier molecule; albumin, therefore serves as an important carrier for a variety of hydrophobic metabolic substrates and drugs, assisting with transport to the liver or other sites of metabolism. Albumin has up to six binding sites for free fatty acids. The reference interval of 0.28–0.89 mmol/L for free fatty acids corresponds to a stoichiometry of about one fatty acid per albumin molecule, and this ratio increases in obesity and other states with increased free fatty acids. Purified albumin usually contains bound fatty acids unless special stripping procedures are used.

CLINICAL SIGNIFICANCE OF ALBUMIN

Increased Plasma Concentrations

Increased plasma concentrations occur with dehydration or artifactually from prolonged tourniquet time or specimen evaporation prior to analysis. High albumin concentrations, therefore suggest problems with hydration or specimen handling.

Decreased Plasma Concentrations

Decreased plasma concentrations are associated with decreased survival and poorer outcomes in kidney and cardiovascular disease. Decreased albumin concentrations can result from decreased synthesis, increased metabolic turnover, and increased distribution to extravascular fluids, or losses from glomerular and gastrointestinal disorders, burns, or other wounds. Decreased synthesis occurs with rare genetic variants, acute-phase responses, and liver dysfunction. Hypoalbuminemia leads to decrease in the anion gap. Albumin usually binds half the calcium in the circulation; therefore, decreased albumin concentrations need to be considered in interpretation of total calcium concentrations that may be expressed as values corrected for calcium concentration.

Analbuminemia

Only about 20 families with inherited analbuminemia have been reported. Although affected individuals have plasma albumin concentrations <0.5 g/L (≤1% of normal), symptoms often are absent or consist of mild edema, lipodystrophy, and dyslipidemia. No increased risk for atherosclerosis has been noted. The plasma half-life of infused albumin in affected individuals is prolonged to 50–60 days.

Inflammation

Inflammatory disorders lower albumin by (1) increasing capillary permeability, allowing increased distribution of albumin into the extravascular space; (2) decreasing synthesis in response to inflammatory cytokines, such as IL-6; (3) responding to increased quantities of positive acute-phase reactants that contribute to oncotic pressure; and (4) increasing the catabolism of albumin by cells.

Hepatic Disease

The liver has synthetic capacity to maintain albumin concentrations until parenchymal damage or loss is severe, with loss of more than 50% of function. Mechanisms other than direct loss of function may lead to lower albumin concentrations. Potential mechanisms include nutritional deficiencies, direct inhibition of synthesis by toxins, such as alcohol, and increased distribution of albumin in extravascular spaces.

Urinary Loss/Kidney Disease

Normally, the glomerular filtration barrier efficiently prevents entry into the urinary ultrafiltrate by proteins the size of albumin or larger. Usually, only 1–2 g/day of albumin passes through the glomerular barrier, and 99.9% of albumin in the glomerular ultrafiltrate is taken up by proximal tubules of the kidney and degraded. Only about 10 mg/day of albumin is normally excreted in urine. Small increases and urine albumin excretion to >30 mg/day are indicators of early stages of glomerular or tubular injury. This has been termed microalbuminuria ('micro' refers to excretion of small amounts, not a smaller form, of albumin).

Non-pathologic increases in albumin excretion are observed in some individuals with postural changes, strenuous exercise, and fever. Therefore, urinary albumin should be collected under controlled conditions, and collection repeated if a question arises. First or second voided specimens in the morning may decrease postural effects. Severe glomerular injury and nephrotic syndromes are characterized by excretion of >3.5 g/day. In nephrotic syndrome, the glomerular leakage of proteins is increased but some size selectivity is retained; therefore, very large proteins are still retained. Even though the liver compensates through increased protein synthesis, concentrations of proteins up to about 200 kDa, including albumin, decrease substantially. Concentrations of very large proteins, such as [α2 macroglobulin (AMG)], larger isotypes of Hp (genotypes 2–1 and 2–2), cholinesterase, and apolipoprotein B are increased.

Gastrointestinal Loss

Protein-losing enteropathy may result in losses as great as those seen in the nephrotic syndrome. If protein-losing enteropathy occurs secondary to lymphangiectasis, larger proteins-especially the immunoglobulins may be lost in large quantities. Patients with Menetrier's disease who have gastric protein losses or inflammatory bowel disease of the intestinal tract, such as Crohn's disease with intestinal losses, can develop hypoalbuminemia.

Protein-calorie Malnutrition

Albumin concentrations serve as a means of detecting and monitoring protein-calorie malnutrition, because concentrations vary directly with adequacy of intake. However, the response of albumin to increased or decreased protein ingestion is relatively slow, in part because of its relatively long half-life. Also, effects of acute or chronic inflammation may decrease the correlation of albumin concentration with nutrition.

Burn Injury

Patients with burn injury can experience severe losses of albumin from wounds. Severely decreased plasma albumin concentrations probably relate to combined effects of epithelial losses, accelerated catabolism, and stimulation of the acute-phase response.

Edema and Ascites

Edema and ascites rarely are the result of decreased plasma albumin concentrations per se. Usually, they occur secondary to increased vascular permeability, which permits the loss of albumin into these spaces. Albumin concentrations in these fluids vary from very low to higher than those in plasma, the latter in particular with certain forms of ascites. Increased volumes of extra-vascular fluid may be large enough to contain a sub-stantial portion of total body albumin. In patients with edema or ascites associated with low plasma albumin, effects of albumin infusion are transient because of rapid equilibration with extravascular fluid. In acute hypo-volemic shock, albumin infusion may help to maintain vascular volume, but rapid infusion may result in symptoms of hypocalcemia due to calcium binding by albumin.

LABORATORY TESTING

Plasma and Serum

Most clinical laboratories assay albumin in plasma or serum samples by dye-binding methods, which rely on a shift in the absorption spectrum of dyes, such as bromcresol green (BCG) or purple (BCP) upon albumin binding. The affinity of these dyes is higher for albumin than for other proteins, providing some specificity for albumin.

Bromocresol purple (BCP) generally is slightly more specific for albumin and yields lower values than BCG, particularly for patients with kidney failure. Heparin in collection tubes is reported to affect some dye-binding methods. Dye-binding assays also tend to be less accurate when the serum or plasma protein composition is abnormal. Dye-binding methods have decreased accuracy for patients with cirrhosis, possibly related to oxidize or other modified forms of albumin. Unfortunately, disorders with abnormal plasma protein compositions, such as kidney and liver disease, often present situations in which accurate analysis is most desired. Albumin concentrations are considered an important indicator of adequate nutrition in patients with kidney failure, and guidelines for monitoring patients with kidney failure recommend correcting total calcium values for albumin concentration. Guidelines also recommend nutritional supplementation of patients with kidney failure to maintain serum albumin concentrations of at least 40 g/L by the BCG method. Low albumin concentrations are a strong predictor of unfavorable outcomes for many clinical disorders, including patients on chronic hemodialysis.

Albumin concentrations increasingly are used as a measure of quality of care by physicians or patient care units, so that methods of analysis and accuracy of results are of increasing concern to many medical professionals. Serum albumin also is used as a criterion in the staging of patients with multiple myeloma, with albumin ≥3.5 g/dL necessary for patients to be in stage 1 with best prognosis. Estimation of albumin concentration by serum protein electrophoresis yields discordant values with immunonephelometry and BCG methods for some patients with high paraprotein concentrations. Many ligands of albumin, including drugs and metabolites, bind to albumin, but usually do not affect dye-binding assays of serum or plasma significantly unless their concentrations are very high. Because of their simplicity and low cost, dye-binding assays are likely to remain the predominant means for assaying albumin in serum and plasma. In assessment of albumin in ascitic fluid, dye-binding methods have been noted to give spuriously high results.

Densitometric scans of electrophoretic patterns can determine the percentage of protein made up of albumin. Along with a measure of total protein concentration, albumin concentration can be calculated. Care is needed in calibrating assays and determining ranges of linear responses of staining or absorbance measurements in capillary electrophoresis.

Scanning often offers low precision and linearity, and multiple measurements are combined, generally resulting in measurement with lower accuracy, less precision, and greater potential for interference. Immunoturbidimetry and immunonephelometry offer greater specificity and accuracy of albumin measurement than other methods, along with the higher sensitivity needed for specimens with low albumin concentrations such as urine and CSF.

Reference Intervals of Albumin

Based on the international protein reference, the recommended interim reference interval for albumin in serum of adults 20–60 years of age is 35–52 g/L. Albumin concentrations reach adult concentrations around 20–30 weeks' gestation and remain relatively constant until at least 20 years of age. Concentrations then slowly decrease with age in both sexes. Concentrations are lower in individuals living in the subtropics and tropics, probably because of higher immunoglobulin concentrations secondary to infection. Concentrations are posture dependent, increasing by up to 10–15%, if an individual is standing versus recumbent. This reflects a shift of fluid between intravascular and extravascular spaces; albumin is preferentially retained in the intravascular space. A similar increase in albumin results from prolonged tourniquet time before blood collection.

α1 ACID GLYCOPROTEIN

α1 acid glycoprotein, also known as orosomucoid, was one of the first plasma glycoproteins to be isolated and extensively characterized. AAG is a major constituent of the seromucoid fraction of plasma, which consists of a group of proteins that are 'slimy' because of their high carbohydrate content.

AAG actually consists of two proteins that are products of homologous genes on chromosome. Each of the two gene products has a polypeptide chain of 183 amino acids, but the two differ at about 21 positions. About two-thirds of AAG is the product of the AAG-l (or ORM 1) gene. Both have a molecular mass of 35–40 kDa, of which approximately 45% is carbohydrate (CHO), including approximately 12% sialic acid; 5-N-linked oligosaccharides include a variable mixture of biantennary, triantennary, and tetraantennary structures with terminal sialic acids, resulting in heterogeneity of AAG upon isoelectric focusing. Oligosaccharide structures and charge of AAG change with inflammation, as do many proteins.

AAG is synthesized mainly by hepatocytes, but granulocytes and monocytes may contribute to plasma concentrations in sepsis. Removal of desialylated AAG by hepatic asialoglycoprotein receptors contributes to catabolism. The plasma half-life of intact AAG is approximately 3 days, whereas that of the desialylated protein is only a few minutes.

AAG is a lipocalin, a family of homologous proteins, including RBP, many of which bind lipophilic substances. AAG binds a large number of basic and lipophilic compounds, including progesterone and related steroid hormones. Binding of drugs to AAG increases the total plasma concentration while reducing the proportion of drug that is free and bioactive. Affected drugs include propranolol, quinidine, chlorpromazine, cocaine, imatinib, and benzodiazepines. Because AAG concentrations may change several-fold in acute-phase responses, interpretation of total drug concentrations for some drugs requires measurement of AAG or alternative measurements of free rather than total drug concentrations. Besides its carrier function, AAG has been proposed to serve a variety of functions, including downregulation of the immune response, depression of phagocytosis by neutrophils, inhibition of platelet aggregation, inhibition of mitosis, inhibition of viruses and parasites, and action as a cofactor for lipoprotein lipase; it also acts as a contributor to capillary selectivity.

Clinical Significance of AAG

Various pathologic conditions are associated with increased and decreased concentrations of AAG.

Increased Plasma Concentrations
Acute Phase Response

Plasma AAG concentrations increase up to fourfold in response to inflammation or tissue necrosis, with peak concentrations noted around 3–5 days after the initial insult. As an example, AAG serves as an indicator of the clinical activity of ulcerative colitis.

Hormonal Effects

AAG concentrations are increased by glucocorticoid hormones, either endogenous (e.g. Cushing's syndrome) or exogenous, along with Hp and prealbumin concentrations.

Decreased Plasma Concentrations
Hormonal Effects

Synthesis and plasma AAG concentrations are decreased by estrogens.

Sieving Protein Loss

AAG is slightly smaller than albumin and therefore is lost in the urine in nephrotic syndrome and in gastrointestinal secretions in protein-losing enteropathy.

Laboratory Testing

The major applications of AAG measurement are to monitor APRs and to assess effects on drug binding. Measurement of total drug concentrations may require correction for AAG concentration. Hormonal effects and the APR are similar for AAG and haptoglobin, so that measurement of AAG may assist in interpreting whether changes in haptoglobin are due to *in vivo* hemolysis (which does not affect AAG concentrations).

Although, AAG is one of the proteins of highest concentration in the α1-globulin region on routine serum electrophoresis, it does not stain well with protein stains because of its high carbohydrate content. It can be visualized by using periodic acid-Schiff or other carbohydrate stains. AAG usually is quantified by immunoturbidimetry, immunonephelometry, or radial immunodiffusion (RID).

Reference Intervals for AAG

The proposed interim reference interval for white adolescents and adults is 0.5–8.3 g/L, based on CRM. Concentrations at birth are only 20–30% of this, but approximately adult concentrations are reached by 6–12 months of age.

α1 ANTITRYPSIN

α1 antitrypsin has a single polypeptide chain of 394 amino acid residues with 3 N-linked oligosaccharides, giving a total MW of 51 kDa. It is serpin AI of the serpin superfamily (where A refers to subgroup or clade). It has Met as a reactive site residue at residue 358, helping to define its specificity for inhibition of elastase and its susceptibility to inactivation by oxidation of the methionine side chain.

Serpins are suicide inhibitors of serine proteases, which abortively try to cleave the inhibitor at the reactive site residue but remain covalently linked to the reactive site residue because of a conformational shift of the inhibitor upon cleavage. Serpins usually occur in a 'stressed' conformation, and cleavage leads to a dramatic conformational shift to a 'relaxed' form. AAT and other serpins serve as important models for conformational change in protein function and aggregation.

Most AAT in plasma is synthesized by the hepatocytes, and AAT genotype changes with liver transplantation. AAT is an acute-phase reactant, with hepatic synthesis and plasma concentrations rising up to several-fold. Catabolism occurs by several routes, in addition to usual bulk pinocytosis of plasma proteins; AAT-protease complexes are removed by serpin-enzyme complex receptors [low-density lipoprotein (LDL)-related receptor along with several other serpin enzyme complexes. Proteases complexed with AAT, also may be transferred to AMG; AMG-protease complexes are removed even faster by the liver than are AAT-protease complexes.

AAT can also be removed by asialoglycoprotein receptors, which bind AAT that loses sialic acid. The normal plasma half-life is 6–7 days for the Pi M genotype; Pi S and perhaps other variants have a shorter half-life and secondarily lower plasma concentrations.

AAT covalently binds to the active sites serine proteases, thus blocking their enzymatic activity. Other members of the serpin superfamily include the proteinase inhibitors cxl-antichymotrypsin, cxz-antiplasmin, antithrombin III, heparin cofactor II, and Cl inhibitor, plus angiotensinogen, thyroxine-binding globulin, and other proteins with no apparent inhibitory activity. AAT is one of the 10 most abundant plasma proteins and the most abundant protease inhibitor on a molar basis. AAT inhibits many proteases, but physiologically, one of its most critical actions is inhibiting elastase released from neutrophils. As first established by Laurell, deficiency of AAT is associated with emphysema related to elastin degradation in the lung by neutrophil elastase. Smoking serves as a cofactor in this process by stimulating chronic inflammation and neutrophil infiltration in the lungs, and by promoting inactivation of AA through oxidation of its reactive site metresidue.

Clinical Significance of AAT

Increased plasma concentrations, plasma AAT concentrations are increased in the APR and with estrogens.

Acute Phase Response

In acute inflammatory processes, serum AAT concentrations begin to rise after approximately 24 hours and peak at 3–4 days. Synthesis is stimulated by cytokines, particularly IL-6, and by AAT-elastase complexes taken up via the LDL-related receptor. Cytokines, including IL-6, induce a broader APR. Inflammation of hepatocytes may be associated with increased serum AAT without the other components of the APR.

Estrogens

Synthesis of AAT is stimulated by estrogens; elevated concentrations are seen particularly during late pregnancy and during estrogen therapy.

Decreased Plasma Concentrations

Plasma AAT concentrations are decreased with genetic deficiency, increased turnover, and urinary or gastrointestinal loss.

Genetic Deficiency

More than 75 genetic variants of AAT have been noted, and prevalence of clinical AAT deficiency in the united

States is estimated at 1:3000 to 1:5000. About 10% of individuals express genetic variants of AAT, but clinical disorders usually occur only in individuals expressing variants at both alleles. Severe genetic deficiency of AAT (Pi ZZ or Pi Z null genotypes) increases risk for pulmonary emphysema, and onset of disease is relatively early, with changes beginning in the second to fourth decades of life in 90% of Pi ZZ individuals. Progression of emphysema is highly variable, but age at onset and median age at death are, on average, younger in smokers. Patients with Pi SZ genotype have less risk for lung disease than those with Pi ZZ genotype.

AAT deficiency also is associated with liver disease including neonatal cholestasis or hepatitis, cirrhosis, and hepatocellular carcinoma. About 10% of infants with Pi ZZ or Pi Z null genotype have prolonged obstructive jaundice, 2% progress to liver failure in childhood. Early differentiation of cholestasis from AAT deficiency and biliary atresia can be challenging histologically. Liver disease with AAT variants has a risk for progression to hepatocarcinoma. Hepatic injury in AAT deficiency probably is related to intracellular accumulation of AAT, but many factors may determine disease progression.

Increased Utilization

Low concentrations of AAT are seen in neonatal respiratory distress syndrome, severe neonatal hepatitis, and severe preterminal pancreatic disease. In non-fatal pancreatitis, concentrations increase from the APR, and increased concentrations of complexes with trypsin may indicate diagnosis or prognosis in patients with possible pancreatitis.

Urinary or Gastrointestinal Loss

α1 antitrypsin is similar in size to albumin; therefore, urinary and gastrointestinal losses occur in parallel to those noted with albumin in nephrotic syndromes and protein-losing enteropathies. AAT is normally present in excreted stool, mostly complexed to pancreatic trypsin and elastase. Evaluation of AAT excretion in stool is used as a measure of protein-losing enteropathy.

Laboratory Testing

The global initiative for chronic obstructive lung disease recommends quantitative testing of AAT for patients with chronic obstructive pulmonary disease with family history or onset before age 45. AAT usually is quantified by immunoturbidimetry or immunonephelometry. AAT represents the majority of serum inhibitory activity versus trypsin and elastase and could be assessed by inhibition assays of these enzymes. Leukocyte proteases may be released into serum stored on the clot after blood

drawing, and the proteases may complex with AAT, altering both electrophoretic mobility and immunochemical quantification. Bacterial contamination and release of bacterial proteases can have a similar effect. Serum should be removed from the retracted clot and stored aseptically at 4°C (for up to 3–4 days) or at –70°C (for long-term storage). Phenotyping of AAT usually is performed by isoelectric focusing. For genotyping, the most important types to detect are Z and S, but a large number of other rare alleles are known, and it is important to consider what variants are detected.

AAT usually is the major serum component stained in the α1 globulin band on agarose gel electrophoresis. Decreases in the α1 band suggest a quantitative decrease in AAT or variants with altered mobility. Variants forming dimers with albumin have altered electrophoretic mobility but normal concentrations. The two other highest abundance α1-globulins, AAG, and α-lipoprotein, do not stain well with peptide stains because of their high contents of carbohydrate and lipid, respectively. Five to 8 AAT bands are found on acid gel electrophoresis or isoelectric focusing depending on the genetic phenotype, as shown in Fig. 13.2.

Reference Intervals for AAT

For adults, the recommended consensus reference interval, based on CRM 470, is 0.9–2.0 g/L for individuals with the Pi MM phenotype, with a median of approximately 1.3 g/L. Concentrations are slightly higher in women in childbearing years and in elderly individuals. Concentrations are also higher in patients with inflammatory disorders, malignancy, or trauma, and in women who are pregnant, on estrogen therapy, or taking oral contraceptives. Neonates have higher concentrations, possibly because of maternal estrogen.

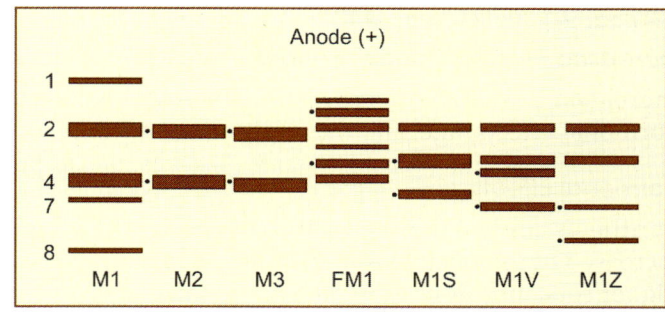

Fig. 13.2: Diagram of common variants of (α1 antitrypsin, as demonstrated by isoelectric focusing. The five major bands are shown for M1, but only the 2 and 4 bands are shown for the other variants (with dots to the left of each). Variants F, S, V, and Z are shown in combination with M1 for the sake of clarity. If cysteine is added to the samples before focusing, the F-2 and F-4 bands shift to the locations of the faint bands

α2 MACROGLOBULIN

α2 macroglobulin (AMG) has four identical subunits with MW of 180 kDa, occurring as a pair of dimers. The dimers are disulfide-linked, whereas the pairs are held together by non-covalent bonds. The dimer is the active unit; one molecule of AMG binds up to two protease molecules.

Each monomer contains a reactive thioester, which is formed internally between cysteine and glutamine side chains at positions 949 and 952 in the peptide chain. The thioester is exposed when a 'bait' region is cleaved by a protease. The thioester reacts to form covalent bonds with the protease, thus immobilizing it, but the active site of proteases is not blocked and retains activity versus low molecular weight substrates. AMG is synthesized primarily by hepatocytes and has a half-life of several days. However, once AMG's thioester is cleaved clearance occurs within minutes via a hepatic receptor. Also, desialylated AMG is removed rapidly by asialoglyco-protein receptors.

AMG is a versatile inhibitor of many proteases, including enzymes in the kinin, complement, coagulation, and fibrinolytic pathways and classes of proteases not inhibited by serpins. In addition, AMG accepts AAT, and AMG-protease complexes are then rapidly removed by receptors. Because of its large size, AMG is restricted primarily to the vascular space. In addition to serving as a protease inhibitor, AMG may serve as a transport molecule for cytokines, growth factors, and zinc. Transport functions may contribute to apparent activity of AMG in modulating immunologic and inflammatory reactions. Oxidation dissociates AMG tetramers into dysfunctional dimers.

Thus, as is the case for AAT and other serpins, inhibitory activity is reduced or eradicated by increased concentrations of oxidants (such as those from cigarette smoke or from neutrophils).

Clinical Significance of AMG

Increased Plasma Concentrations

Increased plasma concentrations of AMG relate to hormonal effects, age, and the nephrotic syndrome.

Hormonal Effects

Synthesis and plasma concentrations of AMG are increased by estrogens; women of child bearing age have higher concentrations than men of the same age.

Age

Synthesis rates in infants and children are up to 3 times adult concentrations. High concentrations of AMG may delay clinical signs and symptoms until after puberty in individuals with anti-thrombin III or Cl inhibitor deficiency.

Nephrotic Syndrome

Hepatic synthesis is increased in the nephrotic syndrome, as is synthesis of most other proteins made by the liver, in attempts to compensate for decreased oncotic pressure. Elevated AMG concentrations may partially compensate physiologically for renal loss of lower molecular weight proteinase inhibitors.

Decreased Plasma Concentrations

Decreased plasma concentrations of AMG result from various genetic conditions, pancreatitis, and prostatic carcinoma. AMG does not change markedly in the acute-phase response. AMG has been measured as one component of some multiparameter indices of hepatic fibrosis.

Laboratory Testing

α2 macroglobulin and Hp together constitute most of the α2-globulin zone on routine clinical serum electrophoresis. In the newborn period and with in vivo hemolysis, AMG alone is the major contributor to this zone. Native and cleaved forms of AMG cannot be distinguished on routine electrophoresis. Higher-resolution separations indicate native AMG migrating slightly cathodal to AMG that has split its thioester. Monoclonal antibodies specific for the two forms indicate that normal plasma contains 0.8–1.9% of AMG in the complexed form.

Reference Intervals for AMG

The interim recommended reference interval for white adults is 1.3–3.0 g/L. Concentrations are approximately twice this in children at a maximum at 2–4 years of age; concentrations in women are 20–30% higher than in men after age 40.

CERULOPLASMIN

Ceruloplasmin (Cp) is an α2-globulin that contains about 95% of serum copper. Each molecule of Cp contains 6–8 copper atoms, most of which are tightly bound. A solution of Cp is blue, and elevated concentrations of Cp may lend plasma a green tint.

Cp has a polypeptide chain with 1046 amino acids and three asparagine-linked oligosaccharides, along with a total carbohydrate content of 8–10%. MW of intact Cp is 132 kDa. Size and charge heterogeneity results from variations in glycosylation, the number of copper atoms, peptide chain variations from alternative DNA splicing, and polymerization. Cp is highly susceptible to proteolysis, leading to earlier reports of more than one peptide chain.

Cp is synthesized primarily by hepatic parenchymal cells, with small amounts from macrophages and lymphocytes. The peptide chain is formed first, then copper is added from an intracellular ATPase (absent in Wilson's disease). Copper appears to be essential for the normal folding of Cp and possibly for normal oligosaccharide attachment. Much of apo-Cp synthesized in the absence of copper or the ATPase is degraded intracellularly; some apo-Cp reaches the circulation, where it has a shortened half-life of a few hours. Consequently, serum Cp is low in Wilson's disease. The normal half-life of Cp is 4–5 days.

Cp is a catalyst for redox reactions in plasma. Cp oxidizes Fe^{2+} to Fe^{3+} (Fig. 13.3), which is important for allowing binding of iron to transferrin. Cp helps control membrane lipid oxidation-probably by direct oxidation of cations, thus preventing their catalysis of lipid peroxidation. In the presence of superoxide, Cp promotes LDL oxidation, which may contribute to atherosclerosis.

Neurologic disorders in hereditary Cp deficiency (aceruloplasminemia) may be due to disordered iron transport in the brain. Cp appears to have a limited role in plasma copper transport to tissues. Albumin and transcuprein appear to be the major copper transport proteins, especially following absorption from the intestinal tract.

Clinical Significance of Cp

Ceruloplasmin is most often measured by immunoassays as a screening test for Wilson's disease. Several factors, including diet, hormone concentrations, and other genetic disorders, may influence plasma concentrations. Immunochemical assays may not distinguish between the active, copper-replete holo-Cp and apo-Cp, which is released into the circulation in most of the disorders

associated with low total Cp concentrations. Functional assays may be helpful to monitor patients on copper-lowering therapy.

Increased Plasma Concentrations

Synthesis of Cp is increased modestly in the APR. This increase occurs relatively slowly, peaking at 4–20 days after a single, acute insult. Synthesis is stimulated markedly by estrogens, with moderate increases seen in women taking estrogen-containing medications, and larger increases noted during pregnancy.

Decreased Plasma Concentrations

Ceruloplasmin concentrations are decreased as a result of various primary and secondary deficiencies.

Genetic Deficiency

Inherited aceruloplasminemia has been reported in several families. Neurodegeneration occurs in these patients associated with iron deposition in the brain. This argues strongly that a major role of Cp is to maintain normal iron transport, particularly in the brain.

Secondary Deficiency

Low plasma Cp concentrations caused by lack of incorporation of Cu^{2+} into the molecule during synthesis are much more common than aceruloplasminemia. Cp deficiency may be due to dietary Cu^{2+} insufficiency (including malabsorption), inability to release Cu^{2+} from the gastrointestinal epithelium into the circulation, or inability to insert Cu^{2+} into the developing Cp molecule. In all cases, apo-Cp (non-copper containing) is still synthesized, but most apo-Cp is catabolized intracellularly, and plasma apo-Cp has a much shorter half-life than Cp. Cp concentrations also may be low in blood loss or in gastrointestinal or renal protein-losing syndromes.

Dietary Cp deficiency is due to nutritional copper deficiency and is associated with neutropenia, thrombocytopenia, low serum iron, and hypochromic, normocytic, or macrocytic anemia unresponsive to iron therapy. The deficiency may be due to inadequate dietary intake, long-term parenteral nutrition without copper supplementation, malabsorption, penicillamine therapy, or combinations of these. Therapy includes dietary changes or copper supplementation, plus treatment of the primary cause of malabsorption if known.

Menkes' Disease

Menkes' disease is an X-linked inherited disorder in which dietary copper is absorbed by gastrointestinal cells that lack an ATPase for copper transfer to plasma. Hence, copper is not available to the liver for incorporation into

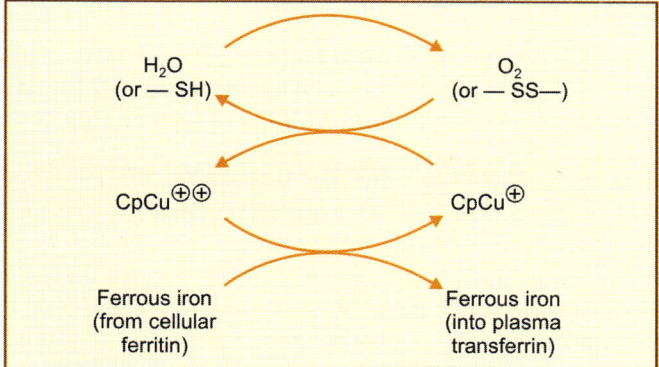

Fig. 13.3: Proposed function of ceruloplasmin copper (CpCu) as an electron recipient from cellular ferrous iron. The resulting oxidation of Fer to the ferric state permits its binding and transport by plasma transferrin. $CpCu^+$ is oxidized (regenerated to CpCu) by reaction with oxygen, oxidized thiol groups, or other oxidizing substances

Cp. Affected infants manifest sparse, brittle, and kinky hair, growth restriction, and neurologic degeneration, with death occurring during the first few years of life if untreated. Subcutaneous injections of copper histidine partially reverse the deleterious effects if started early in life; some residual Menkes' ATPase activity (i.e. incomplete deficiency) may be necessary for this response, however. Patients with deficient gastro-intestinal and blood-brain barrier transport of copper have been described; neurologic symptoms in these patients are not reversed by copper therapy.

Wilson's Disease

Wilson's disease or hepatolenticular degeneration, differs from dietary deficiency and Menkes' disease in that body copper is markedly increased and is deposited in tissue, including the hepatic parenchymal cells, the brain, and the periphery of the iris (resulting in the characteristic Kayser–Fleischer rings). Copper is absorbed and transported to the liver, but the absence of a hepatocellular P type of ATPase encoded on chromosome 13 prevents incorporation of copper into Cp. Symptoms in patients with Wilson's disease usually begin in the second or third decade of life. However, mutations that eliminate gene function may lead to onset of liver disease as early as 3 years of age. The initial clinical presentation may show acute hepatitis or chronic active hepatitis; neurologic signs (e.g. clumsiness, dysarthria, ataxia, tremors); renal indications (e.g. renal tubular acidosis with aminoaciduria); or less commonly, hemolysis secondary to acute release of free copper from tissue. Treatment aims to decrease tissue copper overload through chelation with agents, such as penicillamine or trientene and inhibition of dietary copper intake with supplemental zinc. Most patients with Wilson's disease have low plasma Cp concentrations. A cutoff of 0.2 g/L often has been used, but slight adjustment may be indicated for different populations and assays; an optimal cutoff of 0.14 g/L is recommended from one recent study. However, inflammatory diseases or pregnancy may bring Cp concentrations of affected individuals to above cutoff values. Cp concentrations are slightly reduced in obligate heterozygotes. Low Cp concentrations are also seen in other disorders, as noted earlier. Clinical diagnosis of Wilson's disease therefore, requires the presence of classical signs of the disease, documentation of copper excess, or both. Slit-lamp examination of corneas for Kayser-Fleischer rings, assays of urine copper, and, if these are not diagnostic, liver biopsy for quantitative copper assay may be required for definitive diagnosis. Genetic analysis of the defective ATPase also permits definitive diagnosis in most cases, even in the absence of clinical abnormalities.

Laboratory Considerations for Cp

Cp, usually is measured by immunoturbidimetry or immunonephelometry. It is subject to oxidation and proteolytic degradation during storage that may affect immunoreactivity. This lability may create problems with calibrators, controls, and quality control materials, and with patient samples. Depending on the degree of degradation and the assay method used, apparent concentrations may increase or decrease. Serum or plasma from patient samples should be separated as soon as possible after collection and assayed promptly or stored under proper conditions (up to 3 days at 4°C; longer storage at –70°C). Cp also can be assessed for oxidase activity. Activity assay may serve as a better indicator of functional protein when therapy for copper chelation or other potential sources of copper deficiency is provided.

Reference Intervals for Cp

Ceruloplasmin is undetectable before 20 weeks' gestation. Plasma concentrations gradually rise by term to 25–40% of normal adult concentrations, and by 6 months of age to nearly adult concentrations (Table 13.3).

Serum Cp concentrations reach a maximum at 2 or 3 years of age, then fall slowly until adolescence, when adult concentrations are reached. Concentrations are higher in women during their menstrual years (and longer if estrogen replacement therapy is used). A genetic influence on synthetic rates is apparent; concentrations within families vary less than concentrations among families. Studies have examined the optimal cutoff value for detecting Wilson's disease and suggest a cutoff of 0.14 g/L, but this may require adjustment for local populations. The recommended interim reference interval for all adults of both sexes, based on CRM 470, is 0.2–0.6 g/L.

HAPTOGLOBIN

Haptoglobin (Hp) is an $\alpha 2$ glycoprotein that binds hemoglobin. Hp is synthesized as a single peptide chain by hepatocytes and is cleaved into α and β-chains.

Table 13.3	Plasma ceruloplasmin reference intervals	
Age	**Reference interval (mg/L)**	
Cord (term)	50–330	
Birth to 4 months	150–560	
5–6 months	260–830	
7–36 months	310–900	
4–12 years	250–450	
	Male	Female
13–19 years	150–370	220–500
Adults	220–400	250–600 (no OC)
		270–660 (OC; estrogens)
		300–1200 (pregnane)

The α-chain has some homology to kringle 5 of plasminogen; the α-chain, with 245 amino acid residues plus oligosaccharides, is related to serine proteases. The protein is polymorphic, with two types of α-chain-α^1 and α^2-leading to three Hp genotypes-Hp 1–1, 2–1, and 2–2; that respectively are homozygous for α^1, heterozygous for α^1 and α^2, and homozygous for α^2. Variable numbers of α- and α-chains combine and become covalently linked by disulfides to form Hp. Hp 1–1 consists of four peptide chains $\alpha^1_2 \alpha_2$ with a total MW of 85 kDa. Hp 2–2 consists of multiple forms, including $\alpha^1_2 \beta_2$, $\alpha^1_2\alpha^2\beta_3$, $\alpha^1_2\alpha^2_2\beta_4$, $\alpha^1_2\alpha^2_3\beta_5$, and higher multimers, with MW ranging from 86–300 kDa. Hp 2–2 consists of $\alpha^2_3\beta_3$, $\alpha^2_4\beta_4$, $\alpha^2_5\beta_5$, and higher multimers, ranging from 170–900 kDa.

Hp scavenges hemoglobin in the vascular space. Hemoglobin released by hemolysis dissociates into $\alpha\beta$ dimers at low concentrations, and these dimers of hemoglobin subunits bind to Hp. Each Hp molecule can bind hemoglobin ab dimers, equivalent in number to Hp β-chain binds in the molecule. Hp 1-1 binds hemoglobin with higher affinity than other phenotypes. Hp-hemoglobin complexes are bound by CD 163 receptors and are rapidly removed by reticuloendothelial cells, which degrade proteins and heme and reuse iron and amino acids. This process prevents renal clearance of hemoglobin until Hp-binding capacity is exceeded. Because Hp is degraded after complexing with hemoglobin, its concentration drops severely when intravascular hemolysis occurs. The normal plasma half-life of Hp is about 5.5 days. Hemolysis of specimens after blood collection does not decrease amounts of Hp.

Hp clears hemoglobin from the circulation, thereby preventing iron loss via renal hemoglobin excretion. Hp may have other functions, including antioxidant activity of Hp-hemoglobin complexes, inhibition of cathepsin B release by phagocytes, and bacteriostatic action. Hp synthesis is stimulated by inflammation, but not by hemolysis (and depletion of Hp), suggesting important roles of Hp in inflammatory and immune responses. In chronic hemolytic states, such as sickle cell disease, where haptoglobin is depleted, circulating hemoglobin increases, contributing to vascular disorders, such as pulmonary hypertension by binding nitric oxide.

Clinical Significance of Haptoglobin

Haptoglobin has a capacity to bind only about 1% of the hemoglobin in red cells at usual hematocrits, so intravascular lysis of a small proportion of red cells completely depletes plasma Hp. Once Hp capacity is exceeded, free hemoglobin in the circulation increases.

Free hemoglobin can oxidize to methemoglobin, followed by dissociation of metheme from globin. Metheme binds to hemopexin (high affinity) or albumin (low affinity), keeping it in solution.

Hemopexin-heme complexes are removed by the reticuloendothelial system (as with Hp-hemoglobin complexes, but more slowly), with subsequent intracellular catabolism of the complex and a decrease in the hemopexin concentration in plasma. Hemopexin synthesis is unaffected by other factors (such as estrogen) that decrease Hp synthesis, so low values usually reflect severe or prolonged hemolysis. Similar to Hp, it is a positive (but weak) APR. Disorders with increased red cell breakdown are associated with chronic depletion of Hp and hemopexin. Methemalbumin may be seen when Hp and hemopexin are depleted. Hp depletion may also allow excess hemoglobin $\alpha\beta$ dimers to undergo glomerular filtration. Absorption and catabolism of hemoglobin subunits by the proximal tubules can lead to tubular injury from iron toxicity.

If the absorptive capacity of the proximal tubules is exceeded, overflow proteinuria of hemoglobin into urine occurs. Evaluation of hemoglobinuria tries to distinguish prerenal, renal, and postrenal sources of hemoglobin.

Hp depletion is usually a sensitive biochemical indicator of intravascular hemolysis, followed by hemopexin depletion and finally by the presence of methemalbuminemia, hemoglobinuria, or both. Hp, therefore, is part of the assessment of possible transfusion reactions or other causes of hemolysis. However, Hp concentrations must be considered together with potential sources of protein loss or an APR, which increases Hp.

Increased Plasma Concentrations

Increased concentrations of Hp are seen in the APR and in protein-losing syndromes and are associated with corticosteroid effects.

Acute-phase response; Hp synthesis is increased in the APR 4–6 days after stimulation and takes about 2 weeks to fall to normal after the stimulus is removed.

Protein-losing Syndromes

Most protein-losing syndromes, such as the nephrotic syndromes, compensate by increasing hepatic protein synthesis, including Hp, although Hp 1–1 is relatively small and losses are similar to albumin. Hp 2–1 and 2–2 phenotypes express large forms of Hp that have lower clearance rates, so they are increased in concentration in some protein losing states.

Corticosteroid Effects

Glucocorticoids and androgens increase synthesis and plasma concentrations of Hp. Exogenous steroids, such as dexamethasone, may enhance the response to interleukins rather than directly affecting synthesis.

Decreased Plasma Concentrations

Decreased concentrations of Hp are seen with genetic deficiency, hemolytic disease, ineffective erythropoiesis, estrogens, and hepatocellular disease, and in neonates.

Laboratory Testing

Immunoturbidimetry and immunonephelometry usually are employed for clinical assays. RID requires correction for Hp genotype because of the different molecular sizes and the diffusion of different Hp genotypes. Traditionally, Hp was measured by assaying peroxidase activity after mixing serum with an excess of free hemoglobin, the so-called hemoglobin-binding capacity. On average, 1 mg hemoglobin is bound by 1.5 mg Hp, depending on the genotype.

Reference Intervals for Hp

The recommended reference interval for Hp in serum for adults is 0.3–2.0 g/L. Concentrations are low to absent in the neonatal period and low in women who are pregnant or on exogenous estrogen therapy, including oral contraceptives. For children, the reference interval is approximately 0.2–1.6 g/L.

TRANSFERRIN

Originally named siderophilin, is the principal plasma transport protein for iron (Fe^{3+}). Transferrin (Tf) has a molecular weight of 79.6 kDa, including 5.5% carbohydrate. It is a single polypeptide chain, with two N-linked oligosaccharides and two homologous domains, each with a Fe^{3+}-binding site. It is synthesized mainly in the liver, with lesser amounts in the choroid plexus of the brain. Plasma concentrations are regulated primarily by iron; in iron deficiency, plasma Tf concentrations rise and on successful treatment with iron return to normal. Tf has a usual half-life of 8–10 days. As with albumin, about half of Tf exists in extravascular fluids. Tf reversibly binds two ferric ions and associated anions, usually bicarbonate. The two binding sites for iron have high affinity at physiologic pH, but lower affinity at decreased pH, allowing release of iron in intracellular compartments. Tf has an absorbance maximum at 470 nm related to its iron complex.

Apo transferrin binds iron absorbed from the intestine or released from catabolism of hemoglobin after oxidation of ferrous (Fe^{2+}) to ferric (Fe^{3+}) ions by Cp. Tf is bound by surface receptors for Tf and is internalized into intracellular compartments where Fe^{3+} is released from Tf.

Fe^{3+} is reduced to Fe^{2+} for storage in ferritin or utilization in iron-containing molecules, such as hemoglobin and cytochromes. After delivery of iron, apo-transferrin is recycled back into the circulation.

Clinical Significance of Transferrin

Increased Plasma Concentrations

High concentrations of Tf occur in iron-deficiency anemia, as well as in pregnancy and during estrogen administration. Plasma Tf concentrations assist in evaluating hypochromic microcytic anemia and in monitoring treatment. In iron deficiency, Tf is increased but iron saturation is decreased. On the other hand, in anemia of chronic disease, Tf concentration may be normal or low, but iron saturation is high. In iron overload (e.g. hereditary hemochromatosis, recurrent red cell transfusion), Tf concentration is normal, but saturation (normally 30 to 38%) exceeds 55% and may be as great as 100%. Interpreting serum iron and iron saturation is complicated by large diurnal variation. Serum iron concentration is highest in morning and decreases markedly in the evening. In cases of iron overload, some iron may circulate bound to other proteins such as albumin. Saturation >100% may be observed for toxic overdoses of iron or with administration of parenteral iron preparations.

Decreased Plasma Concentrations

Transferrin is a negative APR; low concentrations occur in inflammation or malignancy. Decreased synthesis occurs with chronic liver disease and malnutrition. Protein loss, as in the nephrotic syndrome or protein-losing enteropathies, also results in low concentrations. In hereditary atransferrinemia, a very low concentration of Tf is accompanied by iron overload and severe hypochromic anemia resistant to iron therapy.

Carbohydrate-deficient Transferrin

Glycosylation of transferrin may be decreased or absent in certain circumstances. Congenital disorders of glycosylation affect glycosylation of many proteins, including Tf, and result in varying multisystem dysfunction, usually with brain involvement. Disorders of glycosylation can be identified by separations of Tf by electrophoresis or isoelectric focusing due to decreased charge from sialic acids.

Laboratory Testing

Transferrin is commonly assayed by immunoturbidimetry and immunonephelometry. It migrates in the PI region on routine serum electrophoresis; genetic variants may have altered mobility. Tf can be estimated from total iron-binding capacity.

Reference Intervals for Transferrin

Serum reference intervals based on CRM 470 as shown in Table 13.4.

β2 MICROGLOBULIN

β2 microglobulin is a small protein that increases in immune activation and in renal failure, because its major clearance mechanism is glomerular filtration.

BMG is a small protein 99 residues in length with MW of 11.8 kDa. It is the non-covalently bound light chain subunit of class I major histocompatibility complex molecules on the surfaces of all nucleated cells. BMG is shed into the blood, particularly by B lymphocytes and some tumor cells. BMG is a non-glycosylated polypeptide chain with one intrachain disulfide-bridge. Its small size allows efficient glomerular filtration, resulting in a plasma half-life of approximately 110 minutes. Minor variants can arise from proteolysis in plasma during renal failure and in urine.

Clinical Significance of BMG

High Plasma Concentrations

High plasma concentrations occur in renal failure, inflammation, and neoplasms, especially those associated with B lymphocytes. Patients with renal failure have a large increase in BMG, because glomerular filtration usually is the primary clearance mechanism. BMG concentrations and efficiency of BMG clearance during dialysis are clinically significant in chronic renal failure, because high plasma concentrations of BMG promote deposition of BMG as amyloid, leading to systemic amyloidosis in many patients on long-term dialysis. In patients with chronic lymphocytic leukemia, high BMG concentrations are a prognostic marker for decreased treatment-free survival and overall survival, although some correction should be made for patients with renal failure.

C-REACTIVE PROTEIN

C-reactive protein consists of five identical, non-glycosylated polypeptide subunits of 23,028 Da non-covalently associated to form a disk-shaped structure with radial symmetry and total mass of 115 kDa. Its pentameric structure leads to the family name pentraxin for CRP and related proteins such as serum amyloid P and pentraxin-3 (PTX3).

CRP binds not only the polysaccharides present in many bacteria, fungi, and protozoal parasites, but in the presence of free calcium ions-phosphorylcholine; phosphatidylcholines, such as lecithin and poly anions, such as nucleic acids. In the absence of calcium ions, CRP also binds polycations such as histones. CRP has a circulating half-life of 18–20 hours.

CRP aids in nonspecific host defense against infectious organisms and breakdown products of cells. CRP complexes activate the classical complement pathway starting at C1q, resulting in phagocytosis via C3b receptors. However, CRP complexes bind factor H, a complement inhibitory factor, greatly reducing the activation of late components (C5–C9) and positive feedback via the alternative pathway (see later section on complement).

C-reactive protein is catabolized when complexes are engulfed by phagocytes. However, whether CRP is catabolized by any other route is not clear. No genetic abnormalities have been reported for circulating CRP.

Clinical Significance of C-reactive Protein

C-reactive protein is one of the strongest acute-phase reactants, with plasma concentrations rising up to 1000-fold after myocardial infarction, stress, trauma, infection, inflammation, surgery, or neoplastic proliferation.

Concentrations >5 to 10 mg/L suggest the presence of an infection or inflammatory process. Concentrations are generally higher in bacterial than viral infection, although concentrations >100 mg/L may be seen in uncomplicated influenza and infectious mononucleosis. The increase with inflammation occurs within 6–12 hours and peaks at about 48 hours. It is generally proportional to tissue damage. Because the increase is nonspecific, however, it cannot be interpreted without other clinical information. Umbilical cord blood normally has low CRP (0.01–0.35 mg/L), but with intrauterine (fetal) bacterial infection, concentrations may be as high as 260 mg/L.

Determination of CRP is clinically useful to screen for organic disease; to assess activity of inflammatory diseases, such as rheumatoid arthritis; to detect intercurrent infections in systemic lupus erythematosus (SLE), in leukemia, or after surgery (secondary rise in plasma concentration); to detect rejection in renal allograft recipients; and to detect neonatal septicemia and meningitis. For unknown reasons, CRP responses vary in some diseases that otherwise are apparently similar. For example, the CRP response in SLE and ulcerative colitis, even when signs and symptoms of inflammation

Table 13.4	Tf serum reference intervals	
Age		**g/L**
Newborn		1.17–2.50
Adults (20–60 years)		2.0–3.6
>60 years		1.6–3.4

are obvious, is slight in contrast to the strong response in rheumatoid arthritis and Crohn's disease.

Risk of Cardiovascular Disease

Epidemiologic studies demonstrate that increased serum CRP concentrations are associated with risk of cardio-vascular disease. Increased concentrations may reflect low-grade, chronic intimal inflammation. The use of CRP for these purposes requires assays with detection limits <0.3 mg/L, that generally are referred to as high-sensitivity CRP assays.

Usually, separate assays are used to assess large increases in CRP with inflammation due to the much higher concentrations that must be measured.

Laboratory Testing

C-reactive protein is normally present in plasma at a concentration <5 mg/L. High concentrations in inflam-matory states are measured with direct immunoturbidi-metric or immunonephelometric assays using antibody to CRP. High-sensitivity assays to measure CRP in healthy subjects often require particle-enhanced (also termed latex-enhanced) immunoturbidimetric or immunonephelometric assays or sandwich-type assay formats. CRP migrates on agarose gel electrophoresis anywhere from the slow-γ to mid-β regions, depending on the calcium ion content of the buffer. Quantities are too small to yield a visibly stained band except in extreme inflammation.

Reference Interval for C-reactive protein

The reference interval for CRP in adults is 0.5 mg/L using less-sensitive assays applied to detection of inflammatory responses.

High-sensitivity assays are needed to measure CRP in healthy individuals and to use CRP as an indicator of cardiovascular risk. A cutoff of 2 mg/L or more was used for increased cardiovascular risk.

COMPLEMENT PROTEINS

The complement system consists of more than 20 proteins, synthesized primarily by the liver. Complement deficiencies are associated with a variety of disease processes, but diagnosis is often overlooked. The complement system has been divided into six groups by function: (1) the classical pathway, which includes Cl, C4, C2, and C3 (in order of activation); (2) the alternative pathway, which includes C3, factors B and D, and properdin; (3) the lectin pathway; (4) the membrane attack complex, which includes C5 through C9, (5) inhibitors and inactivators of the previous pathways, including Cl inhibitor, factors H and I, and C4b-binding protein (C4bp), and (6) cellular regulators and receptors for activated or cell-bound complement factors.

The classical pathway is activated primarily by anti-body–antigen complexes. An antibody-independent or alternative pathway, also termed the properdin pathway, was initially identified through activation of hemolytic activity with cobra venom factor. The alternative path-way is activated by the classical pathway (providing amplification), by bacterial lipopolysaccharides, cellular proteases, or cobra venom factor.

A third pathway, the lectin pathway, is activated by binding of ficolins or mannan-binding protein (MBP; also referred to as mannose-binding protein or lectin, or mannan-binding lectin) to mannose-rich oligosac-charides that are present in the cell walls of many microorganisms. The three types of ficolin and MBP work analogous to C1q in activating two associated protease zymogens: mannan-binding protein associated serine protease-I and -II (MASP-I and MASP-II).

Mannan-binding protein-associated serine protease-II cleaves C4 and C2 analogous to the action of CIs. Activation of pathways generates cascades of protease activation and cleavage products, as outlined in Fig. 13.4.

During activation, many of the complement com-ponents are enzymatically cleaved into two fragments. The larger fragments are designated by a lowercase b, and the smaller ones by a lowercase a. The larger fragments usually contain a binding site for membranes, immune complexes, and protein association, or, in several cases, represent proteases that activate subsequent component(s). Thus, the larger cell-bound fragment of C3 is C3b,

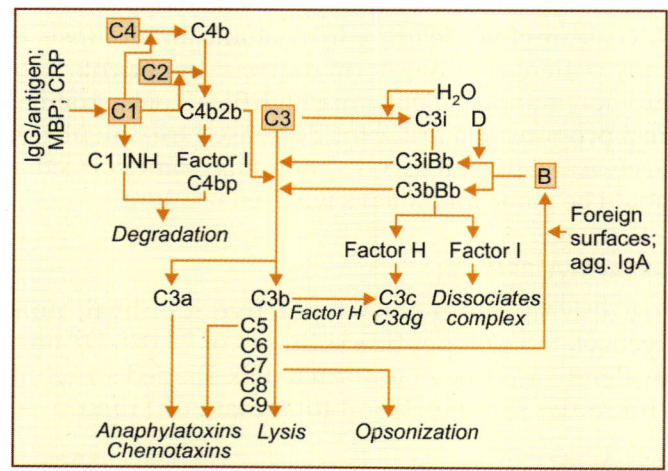

Fig. 13.4: The complement cascades. Activation via the classical pathway is shown on the left and via the alternative pathway on the right. Continuous slow hydrolysis of C3 to C3i is shown at the center top. Direct activation of C3 by neutrophil and plasma proteases also may occur. The control mechanisms are shaded

whereas the small fragment C3a is released to serve as an anaphylatoxic and chemotactic peptide. Inactivated fragments are designated by the letter I (e.g. C3bi). C3i represents C3, in which the thioester essential for activity has degraded. The persisting membrane-bound portion of C3b after inactivation is called C3d, and the major fragment after enzymatic cleavage in solution is called C3c.

Activated complexes often are indicated by a bar over the components. Complement activation results in opsonization or lysis of microorganisms, immune complexes and debris, and immune activation and recruitment of white cells through release of inflammatory mediators. A few of the effector pathways are listed here:

1. Release of bioactive peptides, C3a and C5a in particular, which act as anaphylatoxins and chemotaxins. Anaphylatoxins stimulate the release of histamine from mast cells, contraction of smooth muscles, and increased vascular permeability. Chemotaxins attract neutrophils and macrophages into areas of inflammation.

2. Surface-bound C3b and C4b are opsonins, mediating the binding of microbes or immune complexes to complement receptors on phagocytes, which ingest the particles.

   (Opsonin is derived from a Greek word for 'preparing food for ingestion')

3. Activating the membrane-attack complex through C9 is cytolytic by creating holes in cell membranes. This mechanism appears to be important mainly for control of neisserial infections in human beings, as indicated by genetic deficiencies of C6–C9.

4. C4b and C3b solubilize immune complexes by disrupting lattice formation and directing their removal through opsonization.

5. C3d-kallikrein complexes promote the release of neutrophils from bone marrow.

6. Activation of CIs and C2b can activate the clotting, fibrinolytic, and kinin systems and platelets.

7. Interactions of complement complexes with cellular receptors influence antibody responses.

Through these mechanisms, complement factors are major mediators of inflammatory responses to infection or injury. Increased vascular permeability permits the passage of additional antibody, complement, and phagocytes into extravasculars paces, aiding in the killing and removal of infectious agents and immune complexes. Complement activation by the lectin pathway or CRP binding represents innate responses that may be important in early responses to infection, in immunosuppressed patients, and in infancy before high concentrations of antibody are produced versus a pathogen. After antibodies are produced, complement serves as a further effector mechanism. The high incidence of systemic lupus erythematosus and inflammatory disease in patients with complement deficiencies suggests that complement also has roles in suppressing inflammation, possibly through clearance of immune complexes.

The constant slow ongoing activation of complement factors would lead to accumulation of complement factors on cells, such as red blood cells (RBCs) and would result in their lysis or clearance, if factors were not present on cell surfaces to suppress complement activation and promote removal of C3b and C4b bound to cell surfaces. A few of these factors include decay-accelerating factor or CD55, protectin (CD59), membrane cofactor protein (MCP), and complement receptor 1. Deficiency of these factors can lead to lysis of red cells or other cells. As an example, in the disorder paroxysmal nocturnal hematuria (PNH), amounts of DAF and CD 59 on cell surfaces are decreased by deficiency of enzymes that generate glycosyl-phosphatidylinositol linkages that attach OAF, CD59, and other proteins to cell membranes. Complement regulatory factors on cell surfaces help to prevent destruction of endogenous cells at the same time that foreign cells are destroyed by complement.

The clinical importance of the complement system is demonstrated by the disease associations seen in inherited deficiency of various components, with examples listed in Table 13.5. Deficiencies do not simply increase susceptibility to infectious disease but are also associated with autoimmune disorders, such as SLE and Sjogren's syndrome. Despite the redundancy of multiple

Table 13.5	Clinical disorders associated with inherited deficiencies of complement components	
Component	**Frequency of deficiency**	**Associated disorders**
Ficolins 1-3	Rare?	Recurrent infection
MBP	5%	Infection in infancy; less
MASP	Rare?	Effect on adults
C1q*	Relatively rare	Recurrent infection (e.g.
C1r, CIs	Rare	pneumococcal); inflammation

Contd.

Table 13.5	Clinical disorders associated with inherited deficiencies of complement components *(Contd.)*	
Component	**Frequency of deficiency**	**Associated disorders**
C2	≥0.0003% (homozygous)	SLE, DLE, GNSLE, DLE, infection
		Recurrent infection, vasculitis; SLE, DLE (no antinuclear antibody); half of affected individuals are asymptomatic
C3	Rare	Severe and recurrent bacterial infection, especially with encapsulated, pyogenic bacteria
C4A	13% (heterozygous)	SLE, DLE
C4B	13% (heterozygous)	IgA nephropathy; infection
Combined C4	35% one null; 8–10% 2 nulls; approximately 1% 3 nulls; <0.1 % 4 null alleles	Total deficiency: SLE, GN, DLE (many are anti-ds DNA negative but anti-Ro/SSA positive)
C5–C9	Rare	Severe or recurrent infection
Properdin	Rare	with Neisseria species
Factor D	Rare	X-linked; neisserial infection
Factor H or I	Rare	Recurrent infection
		Hypercatabolism of C3; recurrent bacterial infection; hemolytic-uremic syndrome in factor H deficiency
Cl inhibitor	0.002%	Hereditary angioedema (autosomal dominant)
Decay accelerating Factor (DAF, CD 55)	Rare	Paroxysmal nocturnal hematuria (PNH) related to decreased DAF and CD 59 on cell surfaces

pathways of complement activation, deficiencies in early components of individual pathways are associated with clinical disorders. As an example, genetic deficiency of just one of the three ficolins is associated with recurrent infection. Deficiency of mannan-binding protein may affect about 5% of many populations and is associated with recurrent infection in childhood, before antibodies sreach high concentrations, and in patients with bone marrow transplants. Partial deficiency of C4 also is fairly common. Genetic polymorphism is recognized for a number of components.

Clinical Significance

Increased Plasma Concentrations

C3 concentrations increase with the APR, with biliary obstruction, and with focal glomerulosclerosis.

Acute-phase Response

C3 synthesis is induced by cytokines interleukin-1 (IL-l), IL-6, and TNF-cx. Concentrations rise modestly after trauma or surgery and during inflammatory processes (Table 13.6).

Biliary Obstruction

C3 concentrations increase in biliary obstruction in direct proportion to hyperbilirubinemia.

Focal Glomerulosclerosis

In contrast to nephritic disorders, in which most patients with active disease have low concentrations of C3, about 30% of patients with idiopathic focal glomerulosclerosis have elevated concentrations, which indicate a favorable prognosis.

Table 13.6	Diseases in which estimates of complement factors may be useful for diagnosis
Systemic lupus erythematosus	C4 usually low, C3 sometimes low*
Rheumatoid vasculitis	C3 usually low*
Subacute bacterial endocarditis	Both C3* and C4 low
Shunt nephritis	Both C3* and C4 low
poststreptococcal glomerulonephritis	C3 low,* usually returns to normal in 3 months
Mesangiocapillary glomerulonephritis	C3 low* (persistent), C4 normal
Polymyalgia rheumatica	C3 conversion products found
Mixed cryoglobulinemia	C3 conversion products found
Gram-negative bacteremic shock (early diagnosis)	C3 low,* C4 normal, factor B low
Gram-positive bacteremia	Both C3* and C4 low
Disseminated	C4 very low, C3* normal or increased
Cytomegalovirus infection	*C3 conversion products also present

Decreased Plasma Concentrations

Decreased concentrations of C3 occur with genetic deficiency, increased turnover, and infancy.

Genetic Deficiency

In herited primary deficiency of C3 is associated with a greatly increased risk for infection, particularly with encapsulated bacteria. Deficiency of the inactivators of C3, including factors H and I, results in secondary deficiency of C3 and a similar clinical disorder.

Acquired Deficiency

Any process increasing activation of C3 *in vivo* usually is associated with decreased plasma concentrations; examples are lupus nephritis and severe infection. Turnover is increased and extended by the presence of C3 nephritic factor. In addition to increasing consumption of C3, acute poststreptococcal glomerulonephritis can decrease synthesis for several weeks. Sequential concentrations of C3 can monitor recovery from this disorder. Low C3 concentrations in patients with systemic lupus nephritis suggest risk of active nephritis. Fulminant septicemia, in particular with Neisseria meningitidis, is associated with hypocomplementemia, whether or not shock develops.

Infancy

Concentrations in neonates are approximately two-thirds of adult concentrations, which are reached by approximately 1 year of age.

Laboratory Testing

C3 is usually quantified by immunoturbidimetric or immunonephelometric methods. Because of differences in immunochemical reactivity of C3 and C3c, reference materials should be completely converted to C3c and stabilized, as is the case for the international reference material CRM 470. C3 concentrations measured on fresh samples may be lower than after storage for 8 hours or longer, possibly as the result of conversion of C3 to C3i or C3c. Intact C3 in serum migrates on agarose gel electrophoresis in the $\beta2$ region in the presence of free Ca^{2+}. However, it is a relatively labile protein, with conversion to more anodal forms, C3c and C3dg, on extended storage. Electrophoretic variants, including C3F, may be confused with monoclonal immunoglobulins. Assays for complement activation require plasma samples obtained with precautions to limit activation by plasmin, CIs, and leukocyte proteases. Centrifugation should be performed immediately, and the separated plasma should be frozen at below –40°C.

Reference Intervals for C3

C3 concentrations are low in newborns, then rise and remain relatively constant after the first year of life. The recommended reference interval for adults, based on CRM 470, is 0.9–1.8 g/L. Concentrations are slightly lower in fresh serum (assayed within 8 hours after drawing).

Clinical Significance of C4

Increased Plasma Concentrations

C4 concentrations are modestly increased by the APR.

Decreased Plasma Concentrations

C4 concentrations are low in genetic deficiency, increased turnover, and infancy.

Genetic Deficiency

Complete deficiency of C4 is rare and is strongly associated with autoimmune or collagen vascular disease, particularly SLE, and, in a few cases, with susceptibility for infection. Partial deficiency of C4 is much more common. Isolated deficiency of C4A is markedly increased in patients with SLE as well, but it is not clear whether this results from decreased clearance of immune complexes or from linkage to other genes. Approximately 20% of individuals with deficiency of IgA also have homozygous deficiency of C4A, as do some with combined IgA and IgG subclass deficiencies, suggesting that the gene for a B-cell maturation factor is linked to C4A.

Acquired Deficiency

Concentrations of C4 are more commonly depressed because of consumption; most individuals with SLE and low C4 concentrations do not have genetic deficiency. Other disorders associated with consumption and low concentrations include hereditary angioedema (C1 inhibitor deficiency), autoimmune hemolytic anemia, and autoimmune nephritis.

Infancy

C4 concentrations in newborn infants are approximately 50–75% of adult concentrations.

Laboratory Testing

C4 usually is measured by immunoturbidimetric or immunonephelometric methods. Low concentrations alone cannot differentiate between genetic and acquired deficiency; tests for breakdown products (e.g. C4a des-arginine) or neoantigens may assist in detecting increased turnover. C4 has $\beta1$ elelectrophoretic mobility, similar to that of transferrin, but normally is not visualized because of its low concentration.

Phenotyping of C4 proteins can be performed by electrophoresis of neuraminidase-treated ethylenediaminetetraacetic acid (EDTA) plasma, followed by immunofixation. Hemolytic gel overlay can help identify

C4B bands. DNA genotyping can also determine the types in most cases, but cannot distinguish between synthesizing and non-synthesizing genes. If C4 concentrations are to be used to monitor disease activity in patients with SLE, genotyping or phenotyping of C4 may be indicated.

Reference Intervals for C4

As with C3, concentrations are low in neonates but relatively constant after the first year of life. The recommended interim reference interval for adults, based on CRM 470, is 0.1–0.4 g/L. The baseline plasma concentration of C4 in individuals with one or more null genes is lower.

CYTOKINES

Cytokines are low molecular weight (<80 kDa) peptides secreted by cells involved in inflammation and immunity, which control the activity and growth of these cells. Most of their functions are local, either on nearby cells (paracrine) or on the cells that secrete the peptide (autocrine), but some have remote (endocrine) effects. They show some functional overlap with peptide growth factors, which influence the growth of non-immune cells. The two groups of factors are collectively known as peptide regulatory factors.

Four major classes of cytokines are recognized: (1) interleukins (IL), which are regulators of inflammation; (2) interferons (IF), which are naturally occurring antiviral agents, and in general have an inhibitory effect on cell growth; (3) colony-stimulating factors (CF), which stimulate the growth of macrophages and white blood cells (WBCs); (4) Tumor necrosis factors (TNF), which stimulate the proliferation of many cells, including cytolytic T-cells.

Many cytokines have multiple properties and some cytokine-mediated responses can be brought about by more than one cytokine. Cytokines interact with each other, with the result that the effect of an individual cytokine depends on which other cytokines are present. They are also capable of inducing and inhibiting each other's secretion. More information on these substances can be found in textbooks of immunology.

Cytokines are of considerable importance in the coordination of the immune and inflammatory responses, and in the control of myelopoiesis. Some cytokines are secreted by tumors and can contribute to the effects of those tumors. They can be measured in serum by sensitive and specific assays, although as yet there are no clear clinical indications for doing so in routine practice. Possible applications for cytokine measurements include the early diagnosis of sepsis and graft rejection, for which TNFα and IL-6 show promise.

Growth factors (GF) include epidermal GF, platelet-derived GF, transforming GF and the insulin-like GFs. Secretion of the latter by mesenchymal tumors is a cause of tumor-associated hypoglycemia. Growth factors are now being used therapeutically to stimulate hemopoietic cells following bone marrow grafting for hematological malignancies.

IMMUNOGLOBULINS

The immunoglobulins are a group of plasma proteins that function as antibodies, recognizing and binding foreign antigens. This facilitates the destruction of these antigens by the cellular immune system.

As every immunoglobulin molecule is specific for one antigenic determinant, or epitope, there are vast numbers of different immunoglobulins. All share a similar basic structure (Fig. 13.5), consisting of two identical 'heavy' polypeptide chains and two identical 'light' chains, linked by disulphide bridges. There are five types of heavy chain (γ, α, μ, δ, ε) and two types of light chain (κ, λ), the immunoglobulin class being determined by the type of heavy chain that the molecule contains.

The N-terminal amino acid sequences of both the heavy and light chains show considerable variation between individual immunoglobulin molecules; these form the part of the immunoglobulin molecule responsible for recognition of the antigen (**the antigen binding site**). The amino acid sequence of the rest of the chains varies little within one immunoglobulin class; this constant part of the molecule is concerned with complement activation and interaction with the cellular elements of the immune system. The characteristics and functions of the immunoglobulins are summarized in Table 13.7.

Basic Biochemistry of Immunoglobulins

The major immunoglobulin molecules in humans consist of one or more basic units built of two identical heavy (H) chains and two identical light (L) chains. Each of the four

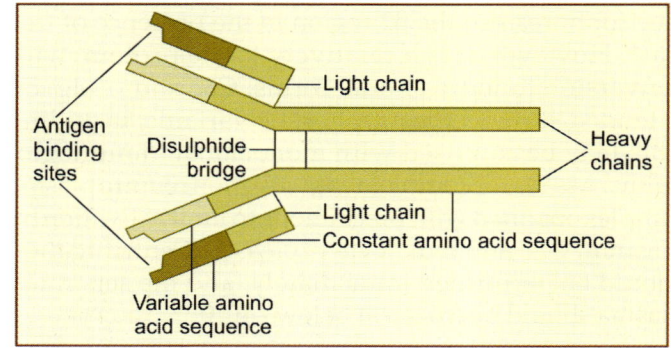

Fig. 13.5: Structure of immunoglobulins. All immunoglobulins have the same basic structure. IgM consists of a pentamer of the basic structure. IgA is secreted as a dimer

Table 13.7	Immunoglobulin characteristics and functions			
Class	Heavy chain	Mean plasma concentration (g/L)	Molecular weight (kDa)	Function
IgG	γ	14.0	146	The major antibody of secondary immune responses
IgA	α	3.5	160	Secreated as a dimer (molecular weight 385 kDa)
				The major antibody in seromucous secretions, e.g. saliva, intestine, bronchial mucus
IgM	μ	1.5	970	A pentamer, confined to the vascular spaces
				The major antibody of the primary immune response
IgD	δ	0.03	184	Present on the surface of B-lymphocytes, involved in antigen recognition
IgE	ε	trace	188	Present on surface of mast cells and basophils
				Probable role in immunity to helminths and associated with immediate hypersensitivity reactions

chains has one variable and one (L chain) or three to four (H chain) constant domains, with the variable region involved in antigen recognition and binding. Extensive diversity in the variable domains is generated by somatic recombination and mutation of the immunoglobulin genes.

Individual plasma cells or clonally expanded cells are committed to synthesis of a single variable domain sequence for heavy and light chains. The amino acid sequences of the variable domains at the N-terminal ends of the four chains form two antigen-binding sites with a high degree of variation in binding specificity, allowing diversity in binding specificity. The constant domains are the same for every immunoglobulin molecule of a given subclass and carrysites for binding to complement receptors and activation of complement.

Immunoglobulins are synthesized by plasma cells, the progeny of B-lymphocyte stem cells in bone marrow (Table 13.8). More mature B-lymphocytes, found mainly in lymph nodes and in blood, develop receptor immunoglobulins on their surface membranes. Recombination of segments of the variable regions of genes by the recombinases RAG 1 and RAG2 helps generate diversity that allows recognition of a wide range of antigens. Upon binding a target antigen, these B lymphocytes proliferate and develop into a clone of plasma cells producing antibody to the target antigen. Somatic mutation of immunoglobulins by activation-induced DNA deaminase leads to further diversity of immunoglobulin variable region and antibody maturation-generally leading to antibodies with higher affinity. B-lymphocytes at first have IgM surface receptors and secrete IgM as the first or 'primary' response to an antigen. Membrane and secreted forms of the antibody arise from differential splicing of the messenger rRNA for heavy chains, which adds a transmembrane segment to the membrane-bound form. Heavy chains of the IgM surface receptor molecules undergo class switching to produce immunoglobulins with γ- or α-heavy chains (IgG or IgA), but the variable regions remain unchanged; as the cells change into plasma cells, second exposure to the same antigen causes a larger secondary or an amnestic response of IgG secretion.

The variable domains contain the antigen-binding regions, and the constant domains of the heavy chains contain sites for complement activation and receptor

Table 13.8	B-lymphocyte lineage and associated malignant neoplasms			
Stages in maturation Surface secreted into and proliferation	Principal site	Surface Receptor	Secreted into blood	Associated Malignant Neoplasms
Stem cell ↓	Bone marrow	None	None	Acute
Early B-lymphocyte antigen ↓	Lymph nodes	IgD	None	lymphoblastic leukemia
Late B-lymphocyte antigen ↓				Lymphoma, chronic lymphocytic leukemia (85%)
Late B-lymphocyte antigen ↓	Lymph nodes	IgM ↓	IgM	Lymphoma, chronic lymphocytic leukemia (15%)
				Waldenstrom's macroglobulinemia
Plasma cell	Lymphatic tissue, bone marrow	IgG, IgA	IgG, IgA	Multiple myeloma

binding. Cleavage of immunoglobulins with pepsin or papain can yield antigen binding fragments (Fab) and constant region fragments (Fe).

Variations in the constant domains of heavy chains (Feregion) result in the classes and subclasses into which immunoglobulins are grouped: IgM, IgG (four subclasses), IgA (two subclasses), IgD, and IgE, respectively, containing heavy chains μ, γ, α, δ and ε.

Light chains, which are produced independently and in slight excess of heavy chains, are of two types—kappa (κ) and lambda (λ)—defined by constant domains with different structures. The heavy-chain genes are located on chromosome 14; K-light chains are encoded by a gene on chromosome 2, whereas the A-chain gene is on chromosome 22. Each plasma cell expresses only one type of light chain, so that each immunoglobulin molecule contains only one type of light chain. The proportions of κ: γ typically are about 2: 1 inimmunoglobulins. Light chains are usually synthesized in excess and secreted as free light chains, but concentrations usually remain low because of rapid glomerular filtration.

Immunoglobulin G

Immunoglobulin G (IgG) accounts for 70–75% of the total immunoglobulins in plasma. Only 35% is found in the plasma space, and 65% is extravascular. IgG consists of two y-heavy and two light chains, linked by disulfides; its molecular weight is approximately 150 kDa, usually including one N-linked oligosaccharide on each heavy chain. The oligosaccharide structure may change in inflammatory states and affect interactions with receptors. On agarose gel electrophoresis, IgG migrates broadly in the γ and slow β regions as a result of its heterogeneity of charge from sequence variation.

Immunoglobulin G has four subclasses: IgG1, IgG2, IgG3, and IgG4. The circulating half-life of IgG1, IgG2, and IgG4 is about 22 days; much longer than most plasma proteins because of recycling from pinocytic vesicles via binding to the neonatal immunoglobulin receptor. IgG3, which does not bind to the receptor, has a half-life of 7 days and IgG2 is weakly complement fixing, and IgG4 does not activate complement. Clustering of multiple IgG molecules is required to activate complement. Both IgG1 and IgG3 bind Fc receptors on phagocytic cells, activate killer monocytes (K-cells), and cross the placenta via receptor-mediated active transport IgG) is the principal IgG to cross the placenta, and neonatal concentrations are similar to maternal concentrations. Neonates have low production of IgG as the result of immaturity of their immune systems, and IgG concentrations fall through infancy as maternally acquired antibody is cleared.

Immunoglobulin M

Immunoglobulin M (IgM) is produced at earlier stages of B-cell development. In the immature immune systems of neonates, IgM is the major immunoglobulin synthesized. In adult serum, it is the third most abundant immunoglobulin, usually accounting for 5–10% of total circulating immunoglobulins. IgM as a membrane receptor molecule is monomeric, but most of the serum IgM is a pentamer, which contains five monomers similar to IgG linked via disulfides to the small J-chain. Plasma cell malignancies may secrete monomeric IgM in addition to, or instead of, pentamers. The high molecular weight of IgM (970 kDa; approximately 10% carbohydrate) prevents its ready passage into extravascular spaces. IgM is not transported across the placenta and therefore is not involved in hemolytic disease of neonates. It activates complement even more efficiently than IgG; binding of one IgM molecule may be adequate to activate complement. In rare hyper IgM syndromes, class switching to IgG and IgA is deficient, shedding light on the process of class switching. Affected patients have deficiency of IgG and IgA and increased susceptibility to infection.

Immunoglobulin A

Approximately 10–15% of serum immunoglobulin is immunoglobulin A (IgA), which contains about 10% carbohydrate, with both N- and O-linked oligosaccharides, has a molecular weight of 160 kDa, and has a half-life of 6 days. In its monomeric form, its structure is similar to that of IgG, but 10–15% of IgA in serum is dimeric, particularly IgA2, which is more resistant to destruction by pathogenic bacteria than IgA1. On electrophoresis, IgA migrates in the β–γ region, anodal to most IgG. IgA is an important component of mucosal immunity. Secretory IgA is found in tears, sweat, saliva, milk, colostrum, and gastrointestinal and bronchial secretions. Secretory IgA has a molecular weight of 380 kDa and consists of two molecules of IgA: a secretory component (70 kDa) and a J-chain (15.6 kDa). It is synthesized mainly by plasma cells in the mucous membranes of the gut and bronchi, and in the ductules of the lactating breast. The secretory component assists with transport of secretory IgA across mucosal epithelium and into secretions. Secretory IgA in colostrum and milk is more abundant than IgG and may aid in protection of neonates from intestinal infection. IgA can activate complement by the alternative pathway (Fig. 13.6), but the exact role of IgA in serum is not clear.

Immunoglobulin D

Immunoglobulin D (IgD) accounts for <1% of serum immunoglobulin. It is monomeric, contains about 12%

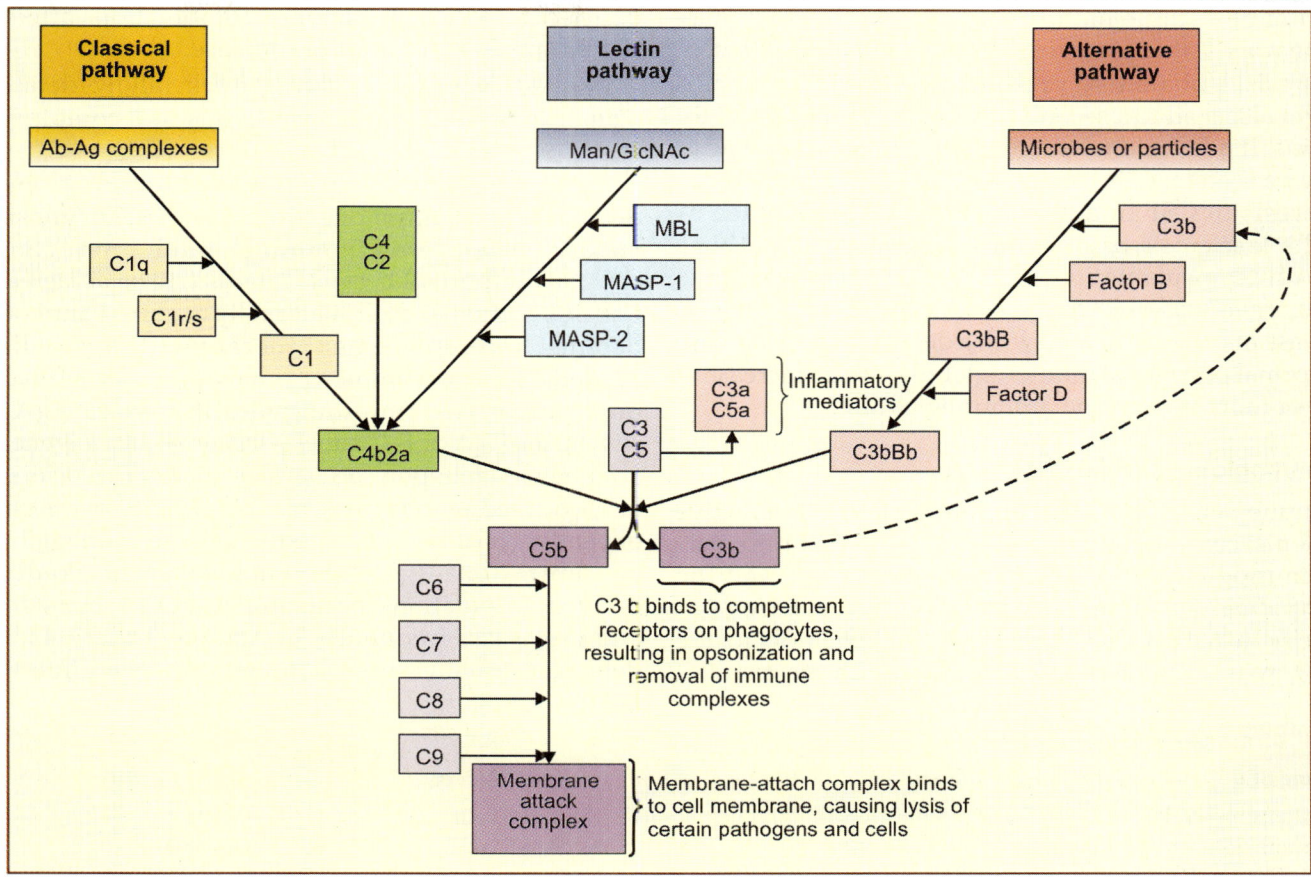

Fig. 13.6: The complement cascades

carbohydrate, and has a molecular weight of 184 kDa. Its structure is similar to that of IgG. Similar to IgM, IgD is a surface receptor for antigen on B-lymphocytes, but its primary function is unknown.

Immunoglobulin E

Immunoglobulin E (IgE) is so rapidly and firmly bound to specific IgE receptors on mast cells that only trace amounts of it are normally present in serum. IgE contains 15% carbohydrate and has a molecular weight of 188 kDa; its quaternary structure is similar to that of IgG. IgE binds to mast cells via sites on its Fc region. When the antigen (allergen) cross-links two of the attached IgE molecules, the mast cell is stimulated to release histamine and other vasoactive amines that increase vascular permeability and smooth muscle contraction, mediating type1 hypersensitivity reactions, such as hay fever, asthma, urticaria, and eczema. Rare regulatory disorders with hyper production of IgE lead to a primary immunodeficiency disorder, Job's syndrome, with eczema, recurrent infection, and markedly increased IgE. IgE molecules specific for particular allergens are analyzed to identify the specificity of allergies. The total serum concentration of IgE may be increased in allergic disorders.

FREE IMMUNOGLOBULIN LIGHT CHAINS

Light chains are usually synthesized in slight excess versus quantities required for intact immunoglobulins. Consequently, small amounts of free light chain, representing only about 0.1% of total immunoglobulin, usually are present in serum or plasma. Amounts in plasma are kept low by renal clearance. Free κ-light chains (23 kDa) are cleared about 3 times faster than free λ-light chains (a disulfide-linked dimer of 46 kDa), which have a half-life of 4–6 hours.

Consequently, even though production of κ-light chains is about twice as great as that of κ-light chains, the plasma concentration of free λ-light chains is usually higher, except in renal failure. Free light chains usually are not functional, but immunoassays specific for free light chains are applied to detect plasma cell disorders.

Clinical Significance

Normally, serum contains a diverse, polyclonal mixture of antibodies with varying amino acid sequences, which represent multiple 'idiotypes' (i.e. the products of many different clones of plasma cells, each producing a specific immunoglobulin molecule). Benign or malignant proliferation of one such clone produces a high concentration of a single monoclonal antibody, which may appear as a sharp, narrow band on protein electrophoresis. Unbalanced production of free light chains might also lead to a second band representing free light chains. If a few clones proliferate, several sharp bands may be seen (e.g. the oligoclonal bands seen in electrophoresis of CSF in demyelinating diseases, such as multiple sclerosis, or in serum following successful bone marrow transplantation, or early during a response to such organisms as *Streptococcus pneumoniae*). Therefore, disease may be associated with a decrease or an increase in normal polyclonal immunoglobulins or an increase in one or more monoclonal immunoglobulins.

Immunoglobulin Deficiency

Immune defense depends on four complex, interactive systems: cell-mediated immunity; humoral antibodies (immunoglobulins); the phagocytic system; and the complement system. 'The last two systems are non-specific in that they have no immunologic memory for the antigen. Immunodeficiency states may be the result of deficiency of a single factor or combinations affecting multiple systems of immune defense.

Analysis of serum or plasma proteins allows detection primarily of deficiencies of antibody and complement systems.

Several genetic disorders with immunoglobulin deficiency are summarized in Table 13.9. Diagnosis of major deficiencies in immunoglobulin production is clinically important because infants will be at increased risk of infection as their maternally acquired antibodies decline, and replacement therapy with IgG will be needed. The most common primary deficiencies involve only one or two immunoglobulin classes (IgA) or subclasses (IgA or IgG subclasses) or ability to generate antibodies versus polysaccharides; such deficiencies may be associated with increased susceptibility to infection, depending on the degree of reduction of immunoglobulin concentrations. IgA deficiency varies markedly in different populations, occurring in about 1: 500 whites, and much less frequently in Asian populations. IgA deficiency usually is not associated with severe infection,

Table 13.9	Genetic disorders with immunoglobulin deficiency		
Name of deficiency syndrome	**Specific abnormality**	**Immune defect**	**Susceptibility**
Severe combined immune deficiency	ADA deficiency	No T or B cells	General
	PNP deficiency	No T or B cells	General
	X-linked scid; Y_c chain deficiency	No T cells	General
	Autosomal scid; DAN repair defect	No T or B cells	General
DiGeorge's syndrome	Thymic aplasia	Variable numbers of T and B cells	General
MHC class I deficiency	TAP mutations	No CD8 T cells	Chronic lung and skin inflammation
MHC class II deficiency	Lack of expression of MHC class II	No CD4 T cells	General
Wiskott-Aldrich syndrome	X-linked; defective; WASP gene	Defective anti-polysaccharide antibody and impaired T cell activation responses	Encapsulated extracellular bacteria
X-linked agammaglobulinemia	Loss of Btk, tyrosine kinase	No B cells	Extracellular bacteria viruses
X-linked hyper-IgM syndrome	Defective CD40 ligand	No isotype switching	Extracellular bacteria *Pneumocystis carinii* *Cryptosporidium parvum*
Common variable immunodeficiency	Unknown; MHC-linked	Defective IgA and IgG production	Extracellular bacteria
Selective IgA	Unknown; MHC-linked	No IgA synthesis	Respiratory infections
Phagocyte deficiencies	Many different	Loss of phagocyte function	Extracellular bacteria and fungi
Complement deficiencies	Many different	Loss of specific complements	Extracellular bacteria especially. *Neisseria* spp
Natural killer (NK) cell defect	Unknown	Loss of NK function	Herpes viruses
X-linked lympho-proliferative	SH2D1A mutant	Inability of control B cell growth	EBV-driven B cell tumors
Ataxia telangiectasia	Gene with Pl 3-kinase homology	T cells reduced	Respiratory infections
Bloom's syndrome	Defective DNA helicase	T cells reduced; reduced anybody levels	Respiratory infections

but the risk of non-severe infection with Giardia or other organisms may be increased. IgA deficiency may lead to false-negative assays for autoantibodies for celiac disease detection, and affected individuals have some risk of anaphylaxis, if they receive blood products containing IgA. Detection of antibodies to IgA serves as an indicator of risk of transfusion reactions. Selective deficiency of IgG subclasses is not rare, but it is unclear whether it is an important risk for infection. Deficiency of IgG2 may be related to poorer responses to polysaccharide antigens and increased risk of infection with encapsulated organisms.

Infants have transient physiologic deficiency of IgG, with a nadir at about 3 months of age; prolonged or severe physiologic deficiency may be associated with increased infection rates, especially with encapsulated bacteria. Concentrations of maternal IgG, transferred across the placenta, rise rapidly in the fetus during the last half of pregnancy but then drop over a few months following birth (Fig. 13.7). Two groups of neonates are at risk for clinically significant IgG deficiency; premature infants, who start with less maternal IgG, and infants with delayed initiation of IgG synthesis. Monitoring of IgG concentrations can identify this problem. Rising IgM and normal salivary IgA concentrations at 6 weeks of age suggest a favorable prognosis.

Contact of the neonate with environmental antigens normally causes B-lymphocytes to begin to multiply and IgM concentrations to start to rise, followed weeks to months later by IgA and IgG.

POLYCLONAL HYPERIMMUNOGLOBULINEMIA

Polyclonal increases in plasma immunoglobulins are the normal response to infection. IgG response predominates in autoimmune responses; IgA in skin, gut, respiratory, and renal infections; and IgM in primary viral infections

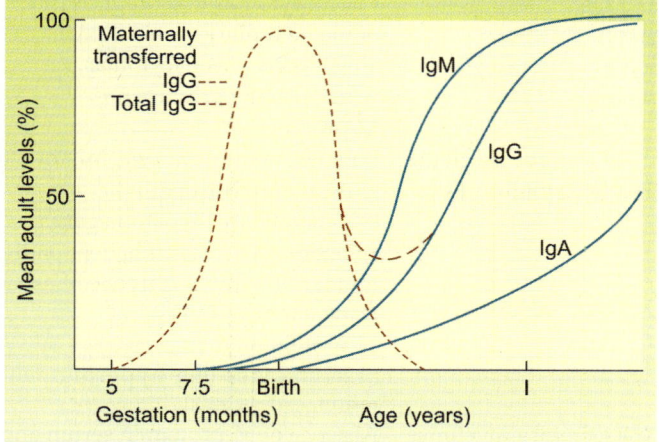

Fig.13.7: Serum immunoglobulin concentrations as percent of mean adult concentrations before birth and for the first year of life

and bloodstream parasites, such as malaria. Chronic bacterial infection may cause increased concentrations of all immunoglobulins.

Selective changes in immunoglobulin concentrations assist in the differential diagnosis of liver disease and of intrauterine infection. In primary biliary cirrhosis, the IgM concentration is greatly increased; in chronic active hepatitis, and sometimes IgM are increased; and in portal cirrhosis, IgA and sometimes IgG are increased. In intrauterine infection, production of IgM by the fetus increases, and the IgM concentration in umbilical cord blood is increased. Measurements of total IgE are used in the management of asthma and other allergic conditions, especially in children. Measurements of allergen-specific IgE assist in identifying allergens that trigger hypersensitivity responses.

Monoclonal Immunoglobulins (Paraproteins)

A single clone of plasma cells produces immunoglobulin molecules with a single defined amino acid sequence. If the clone expands greatly, the concentration of its particular protein in the patient's serum may produce a discrete band on electrophoresis, often referred to as an M-spike or M-protein, which stands out from the diffuse background. These monoclonal immunoglobulins, termed paraproteins, may be polymers, monomers, individual immunoglobulin chains such as free light chains or heavy chains, or fragments of immunoglobulins. About 60% of paraproteins are associated with plasma cell malignancies (multiple myeloma or solitary plasmacy1oma), and approximately 15% are due to over production by B-lymphocytes, mainly in lymph nodes (lymphomas, Waldenstrom's macroglobulinemia, or heavy-chain disease). Up to 25% of paraproteins are benign and have been termed monoclonal gammopathy of undetermined significance (MGUS). The incidence of MGUS increases with age, with 1% incidence for people 50–70 years of age and 3% incidence for people older than 70. Occurrence of MGUS is associated with increased risk of progression to multiple myeloma that should be monitored. Multiple myeloma appears to be preceded consistently by MGUS.

The primary clinical interest in identifying paraproteins is to detect or monitor proliferative disorders of B-cells. However, from the laboratory stand point, paraproteins are also significant as a potentially unpredictable source of interference with many assays. Paraproteins may aggregate or precipitate in a variety of photometric reactions and hematology analyzers. Occasionally, specimens with paraproteins form gels that can plug sample probes of and disable automated analyzers (see discussion of cryoglobulins later).

Many patients with paraproteins have nonspecific presentations, such as anemia or infection. Identification of paraproteins in serum usually is based on serum protein electrophoresis and immunofixation electrophoresis (described in a later section), and urine protein electrophoresis and urine immunofixation electrophoresis are helpful mainly in identifying patients with free immunoglobulin light chains.

Urinary free light chains, as described by Bence Jones in the 1850s, were the first tumor marker. Free light chains, particularly in urine, are often referred to as Bence Jones proteins, although this term was originally used to refer to a subset of free light chains in urine that precipitated and redissolved upon heating. Introduction of capillary electrophoresis and assays for free light chains in serum has led to a variety of approaches for detecting paraproteins. Serum protein electrophoresis together with analysis of free light chains in serum appears to have a diagnostic yield similar to use of immunofixation on serum and urine, except for lower detection of MGUS. Analysis of free light chains tends to detect residual disease or recurrence at lower concentrations than does immunofixation.

Malignancies of B-cells that Commonly Express Paraproteins

Multiple myeloma

Pathophysiology

The M-protein produced by the malignant plasma cells is IgG in about 55% of myeloma patients and IgA in about 20%; of patients producing either IgG or IgA, 40% also have Bence Jones proteinuria, which is free monoclonal κ or λ light chains in the urine. In 15–20% of patients, plasma cells secrete only Bence Jones protein. IgD myeloma accounts for about 1% of cases. Rarely, patients have no M-protein in blood and urine, although a new serum free light chain assay now demonstrates monoclonal light chains in many of these patients.

Diffuse osteoporosis or discrete osteolytic lesions develop, usually in the pelvis, spine, ribs, and skull. Lesions are caused by bone replacement by expanding plasmacytomas or by cytokines that are secreted by malignant plasma cells that activate osteoclasts and suppress osteoblasts. The osteolytic lesions are usually multiple; occasionally, they are solitary intramedullary masses. Increased bone loss may also lead to hypercalcemia. Extraosseous solitary plasmacytomas are unusual, but may occur in any tissue, especially in the upper respiratory tract.

In many patients, renal failure (myeloma kidney) is present at diagnosis or develops during the course of the disorder. Renal failure has many causes, most commonly, it results from deposition of light chains in the distal tubules or hypercalcemia. Patients also often develop anemia usually due to kidney disease or suppression of erythropoiesis by cancer cells, but sometimes also due to iron deficiency.

Susceptibility to bacterial infection may occur in some patients. Viral infections, especially herpes zoster infections, are increasingly occurring as a result of newer treatment modalities, especially use of the proteasome inhibitors bortezomib and carfilzomib. Amyloidosis occurs in 10% of myeloma patients, most often in patients with 2λ-type M-proteins, variant expressions of multiple myeloma occur (Table 13.10)

Symptoms and Signs

Persistent bone pain (especially in the back or thorax), renal failure, and recurring bacterial infections are the most common problems on presentation, but many patients are identified when routine laboratory tests show an elevated total protein level in the blood or show proteinuria. Pathologic fractures are common, and vertebral collapse may lead to spinal cord compression and paraplegia. Symptoms of anemia predominate or may be the sole reason for evaluation in some patients, and a few patients have manifestations of hyperviscosity syndrome. Peripheral neuropathy, carpal tunnel syndrome, abnormal bleeding, and symptoms of hypercalcemia (e.g. polydipsia, dehydration) are common. Patients may also present with renal failure. Lymphadenopathy and hepatosplenomegaly are unusual.

Table 13.10	Variant expressions of multiple myeloma
Form	**Characteristics**
Extramedullary plasmacytoma	Plasmacytomas that occur outside of the medullary system
Solitary plasmacytoma of bone	Single bone plasmacytomas, which usually produce no M-protein
Osteosclerotic myeloma (POEMS syndrome)	Polyneuropathy (chronic inflammatory polyneuropathy)
	Organomegaly (hepatomegaly, splenomegaly, or lymphadenopathy)
	Endocrinopathy (e.g gynecomastia, testicular atrophy)
	M-protein
	Skin changes (e.g hyperpigmentation, excess hair)
Nonsecretory myeloma	Absence of M-protein in serum and urine
	Presence of M-protein in plasma cells

Diagnosis

Multiple myeloma is suspected in patients >40 years with persistent unexplained bone pain, particularly at night or at rest, other typical symptoms, or unexplained laboratory abnormalities, such as elevated blood protein or urinary protein, hypercalcemia, renal insufficiency, or anemia. Laboratory evaluation includes routine blood tests, protein electrophoresis, X-rays, and bone marrow examination.

Routine blood tests include complete blood count (CBC), ESR, and chemistry panel. Anemia is present in 80% of patients, usually normocytic-normochromic anemia with formation of rouleau, which are clusters of 3–12 RBCs that occur in stacks. WBC and platelet counts are usually normal. ESR usually is >100 mm/h; BUN, serum creatinine, LDH, and serum uric acid may be elevated. Anion gap is sometimes low. Hypercalcemia is present at diagnosis in about 10% of patients.

Protein electrophoresis is done on a serum sample and on a urine sample concentrated from a 24-hour collection to quantify the amount of urinary M-protein. Serum electrophoresis identifies M-protein in about 80–90% of patients. The remaining 10–20% are usually patients with only free monoclonal light chains (Bence Jones protein) or IgD. They almost always have M-protein detected by urine protein electrophoresis. Immunofixation electrophoresis can identify the immunoglobulin class of the M-protein (IgG, IgA, or uncommonly IgD, IgM or IgE) and can often detect light-chain protein if serum immunoelectrophoresis is falsely negative; immunofixation electrophoresis is done even when the serum test is negative if multiple myeloma is strongly suspected. Serum free light-chain analysis with delineation of κ and λ ratios helps confirm the diagnosis and can also be used to monitor efficacy of therapy and provide prognostic data. Serum level of β_2-microglobulin is measured if diagnosis is confirmed or very likely and along with serum albumin is used to stage patients as part of the international staging system (Table 13.11).

Table 13.11	International staging system for multiple myeloma	
Stage	**Criteria**	**Median survival (MOS)**
I	β-2 microglobulin <3.5 mcg/mL and Serum albumin ≥3.5 g/dL	62
II	Not stage I or III	44
III	β-2 microglobulin ≥5.5 mcg/mL	29
MOS: Median overall survival		

X-rays include a skeletal survey (i.e. plain X-rays of skull, long bones, spine, pelvis, and ribs). Punched-out lytic lesions or diffuse osteoporosis is present in 80% of cases. Radionuclide bone scans usually are not helpful. MRI can provide more detail and is obtained if specific sites of pain or neurologic symptoms are present. Positron emission tomography–computed tomography (PET-CT) may provide prognostic information and can help determine whether patients have solitary plasmacytoma or multiple myeloma.

Bone marrow aspiration and biopsy are done and reveal sheets or clusters of plasma cells; myeloma is diagnosed when >10% of the cells are of this type. However, bone marrow involvement is patchy; therefore, some samples from patients with myeloma may show <10% plasma cells. Still, the number of plasma cells in bone marrow is rarely normal. Plasma cell morphology does not correlate with the class of immunoglobulin synthesized. Chromosomal studies on bone marrow may reveal specific karyotypic abnormalities in plasma cells associated with differences in survival.

Diagnosis and differentiation from other malignancies (e.g. metastatic carcinoma, lymphoma, leukemia) and monoclonal gammopathy of undetermined significance typically requires multiple criteria:

- Clonal bone marrow plasma cells or plasmacytoma
- M-protein in plasma and/or urine
- Organ impairment (hypercalcemia, renal insufficiency, anemia, or bony lesions)

In patients without serum M protein, myeloma is indicated by Bence Jones proteinuria >300 mg/24 hours or abnormal serum free light chains, osteolytic lesions (without evidence of metastatic cancer or granulomatous disease), and sheets or clusters of plasma cells in the bone marrow.

Prognosis

The disease is progressive and incurable, but median survival has recently improved to >5 years as a result of advances in treatment. Unfavorable prognostic signs at diagnosis are lower serum albumin and higher β2-microglobulin levels. Patients initially presenting with renal failure also do poorly unless kidney function improves with therapy (which typically happens with current treatment options). Certain cytogenetic abnormalities increase risk of poor outcome.

Because multiple myeloma is ultimately fatal, patients are likely to benefit from discussions of end-of-life care that involve their doctors and appropriate family and friends. Points for discussion may include advance directives, the use of feeding tubes, and pain relief.

Treatment

Treatment of myeloma has improved in the past decade, and long-term survival is a reasonable therapeutic target. Therapy involves direct treatment of malignant cells in symptomatic patients or those with myeloma-related organ dysfunction (anemia, renal dysfunction, hypercalcemia, or bone disease). Asymptomatic patients probably do not benefit from treatment, which is usually withheld until symptoms or complications develop. Patients with evidence of lytic lesions or bone loss (osteopenia or osteoporosis) should be treated with monthly infusions of zoledronic acid or pamidronate to reduce the risk of skeletal complications.

Treatment of Malignant Cells

Until recently, conventional chemotherapy consisted only of oral melphalan and prednisone given in cycles of 4–6 weeks with monthly evaluation of response. Recent studies show superior outcome with the addition of either bortezomib or thalidomide. Other chemotherapeutic drugs, including cyclophosphamide, bendamustine, doxorubicin and its newer analog liposomal pegylated doxorubicin also are more effective when combined with an immunomodulatory drug (thalidomide, lenalidomide, or its newer analog pomalidomide) or a proteasome inhibitor (bortezomib, or a newer drug, carfilzomib). Many other patients are effectively treated with bortezomib, corticosteroids, and either thalidomide (or lenalidomide), chemotherapy, or both.

Chemotherapy response is indicated by reduction in bone pain and fatigue, decreases in serum and urine M-protein, increases in RBCs, and improvement in renal function among patients presenting with renal failure.

Autologous peripheral blood stem cell transplantation may be considered for patients who have adequate cardiac, hepatic, pulmonary, and renal function, particularly those whose disease is stable or responsive after several cycles of initial therapy. However, recent studies suggest that the newer treatment options are highly effective and may make transplantation less often necessary. Allogeneic stem cell transplantation after non-myeloablative chemotherapy (e.g. low-dose cyclophosphamide and fludarabine) or low-dose radiation therapy can produce myeloma-free survival of 5–10 years in some patients. However, allogeneic stem cell transplantation with myeloablative or non-myeloablative chemotherapy remains experimental because of the high morbidity and mortality resulting from graft vs host disease.

In relapsed or refractory myeloma, combinations of bortezomib or carfilzomib, and thalidomide, lenalidomide, or pomalidomide, with chemotherapy or corticosteroids may be used. These drugs are usually combined with other effective drugs that the patient has not yet been treated with, although patients with prolonged remissions may respond to retreatment with the same regimen that led to the remission. Patients who fail to respond to a given combination of drugs may respond when another drug in the same class (e.g. proteasome inhibitors, immunomodulatory agents, chemotherapeutic drugs) is substituted.

Maintenance therapy has been tried with nonchemotherapeutic drugs, including interferon alfa, which prolongs remission, but does not improve survival and is associated with significant adverse effects. Following a response to corticosteroid-based regimens, corticosteroids alone are effective as a maintenance treatment. Thalidomide may also be effective as a maintenance treatment, and recent studies show that lenalidomide alone is also an effective maintenance treatment. However, there is some recent concern about secondary malignancy among patients receiving long-term lenalidomide therapy, especially after autologous stem cell transplantation.

Treatment of Complications

In addition to direct treatment of malignant cells, therapy must also be directed at complications, which include anemia, hypercalcemia, renal insufficiency, infections, and skeletal lesions.

Anemia can be treated with recombinant erythropoietin (40,000 units SC once a week) in patients whose anemia is inadequately relieved by chemotherapy. If anemia causes cardiovascular or significant systemic symptoms, packed RBCs are transfused. Plasma exchange is indicated if hyperviscosity develops. Often patients are iron deficient and require intravenous (IV) iron. Patients with anemia should have periodic measurement of serum iron, transferrin, and ferritin levels to monitor iron stores.

Hypercalcemia is treated with vigorous saluresis, IV bisphosphonates after rehydration, and sometimes with calcitonin or prednisone.

Hyperuricemia may occur in some patients with high tumor burden and underlying metabolic problems. However, most patients do not require allopurinol. Allopurinol is indicated for patients with high levels of serum uric acid or high tumor burden and a high risk of tumor lysis syndrome with treatment.

Renal compromise can be ameliorated with adequate hydration. Even patients with prolonged, massive Bence Jones proteinuria (≥ 10–$30\,g/day$) may have intact renal function if they maintain urine output >2000 mL/day. Dehydration combined with high-osmolar IV contrast may precipitate acute oliguric renal failure in patients with Bence Jones proteinuria. Plasma exchange may be effective in some cases.

Infection is more likely during chemotherapy-induced neutropenia. In addition, infections with the herpes zoster virus are occurring more frequently in patients treated with newer antimyeloma drugs especially bortezomib or carfilzomib. Documented bacterial infections should be treated with antibiotics; however, prophylactic use of antibiotics is not routinely recommended. Prophylactic use of antiviral drugs (e.g. acyclovir, valganciclovir, famciclovir) is indicated for patients receiving either bortezomib or carfilzomib. Prophylactic IV immune globulin may reduce the risk of infection but is generally reserved for patients with recurrent infections. Pneumococcal and influenza vaccines are indicated to prevent infection. However, use of live vaccines is not recommended in these immunocompromised patients.

Skeletal lesions require multiple supportive measures. Maintenance of ambulation and supplemental Ca and vitamin D help preserve bone density. Vitamin D levels should be measured at diagnosis and periodically and dosing of vitamin D adjusted accordingly. Analgesics and palliative doses of radiation therapy (18–24 Gy) can relieve bone pain. However, radiation therapy may cause significant toxicity and, because it suppresses bone marrow function, may impair the patient's ability to receive cytotoxic doses of systemic chemotherapy. Most patients, especially those with lytic lesions and generalized osteoporosis or osteopenia, should receive a monthly IV bisphosphonate (either pamidronate or zoledronic acid). Bisphosphonates reduce skeletal complications and lessen bone pain and may have an antitumor effect.

MACROGLOBULINEMIA

Macroglobulinemia is a malignant plasma cell disorder in which B-cells produce excessive amounts of IgM M-proteins. Manifestations may include hyperviscosity, bleeding, recurring infections, and generalized adenopathy. Diagnosis requires bone marrow examination and demonstration of M-protein. Treatment includes plasma exchange as needed for hyperviscosity, and systemic therapy with alkylating drugs, corticosteroids, nucleoside analogs, or monoclonal antibodies.

Macroglobulinemia, an uncommon B-cell cancer, is clinically more similar to a lymphomatous disease than to myeloma and other plasma cell disorders. Cause is unknown. Men are affected more often than women; median age is 65.

After myeloma, macroglobulinemia is the second most common malignant disorder associated with a monoclonal gammopathy. Excessive amounts of IgM M-proteins can also accumulate in other disorders, causing manifestations similar to macroglobulinemia.

Small monoclonal IgM components are present in the sera of about 5% of patients with B-cell non-Hodgkin lymphoma; this circumstance is termed macroglobulinemic lymphoma. Additionally, IgM M-proteins are occasionally present in patients with chronic lymphocytic leukemia or other lymphoproliferative disorders.

Clinical manifestations of macroglobulinemia may be due to the large amount of high molecular weight monoclonal IgM proteins circulating in plasma, but most patients do not develop problems related to high IgM levels. Some of these proteins are antibodies directed toward autologous IgG (rheumatoid factors) or I antigens (cold agglutinins). About 10% are cryoglobulins. Secondary amyloidosis occurs in 5% of patients.

Symptoms and Signs

Most patients are asymptomatic, but many present with anemia or manifestations of hyperviscosity syndrome: fatigue, weakness, skin and mucosal bleeding, visual disturbances, headache, symptoms of peripheral neuropathy, and other changing neurologic manifestations. An increased plasma volume can precipitate heart failure. Cold sensitivity, Raynaud syndrome, or recurring bacterial infections may occur.

Examination may disclose lymphadenopathy, hepatosplenomegaly, and purpura (which rarely can be the first manifestation). Marked engorgement and localized narrowing of retinal veins, which resemble sausage links, suggests hyperviscosity syndrome. Retinal hemorrhages, exudates, microaneurysms, and papilledema occur in late stages.

Diagnosis

Macroglobulinemia is suspected in patients with symptoms of hyperviscosity or other typical symptoms, particularly if anemia is present. However, it is often diagnosed incidentally when protein electrophoresis reveals an M-protein that proves to be IgM by immunofixation. Laboratory evaluation includes tests used to evaluate plasma cell disorders as well as measurement of cryoglobulins, rheumatoid factor, and cold agglutinins; coagulation studies; and direct Coombs test.

Moderate normocytic, normochromic anemia, marked rouleau formation, and a very high ESR are typical. Leukopenia, relative lymphocytosis, and thrombocytopenia occasionally occur. Cryoglobulins, rheumatoid factor, or cold agglutinins may be present. If cold agglutinins are present, the direct Coombs test usually is positive. Various coagulation and platelet function abnormalities may occur. Results of routine blood studies may be spurious if cryoglobulinemia or marked hyperviscosity is present. Normal immunoglobulins are decreased in half of patients.

Immunofixation electrophoresis of concentrated urine frequently shows a monoclonal light chain (usually κ), but gross Bence Jones proteinuria is unusual. Bone marrow studies show a variable increase in plasma cells, lymphocytes, plasmacytoid lymphocytes, and mast cells. Periodic acid-Schiff positive material may be present in lymphoid cells. Lymph node biopsy, done if bone marrow examination is normal, is frequently interpreted as diffuse well-differentiated or plasmacytic lymphocytic lymphoma. Serum viscosity is measured to confirm suspected hyperviscosity and when present is usually >4.0 (normal, 1.4–1.8).

Treatment

The course is variable, with a median survival of 7–10 years. Age >60 years, anemia, and cryoglobulinemia predict shorter survival.

Often, patients require no treatment for many years. If hyperviscosity is present, initial treatment is plasma exchange, which rapidly reverses bleeding as well as neurologic abnormalities. Plasma exchange often needs to be repeated.

Corticosteroids may be effective in reducing tumor load. Treatment with oral alkylating drugs may be indicated for palliation, but bone marrow toxicity can occur. Nucleoside analogs (fludarabine and 2-chloro-deoxyadenosine) produce responses in large numbers of newly diagnosed patients but have been associated with a high risk of myelodysplasia and myeloid leukemia. Rituximab can reduce tumor burden without suppressing normal hematopoiesis. However, during the first several months, IgM levels may increase, requiring plasma exchange. The proteasome inhibitor bortezomib and the immunomodulating agents thalidomide and lenalidomide are also effective in this cancer.

Classification of Plasma Cell Proliferative Disorders

Analysis of paraproteins and other laboratory studies plays an important role in classification and staging of plasma cell proliferative disorders. Evidence of end-organ injury related to paraproteins is provided by hypercalcemia (calcium 2.875 mmol/L), impaired renal function (creatinine >1.95 mg/dL or 172 μmol/L), anemia, and bone lesions.

Monoclonal Gammopathy of Undetermined Significance

Monoclonal gammopathy of undetermined significance (MGUS) is the production of M-protein by noncancerous plasma cells in the absence of other manifestations typical of multiple myeloma. The incidence of MGUS increases with age, from 1% of people aged 25 years to >5% of people >70 years. MGUS may occur in association with

other disorders in which case M-proteins may be antibodies produced in large amounts in response to protracted antigenic stimuli. MGUS usually is asymptomatic, but peripheral neuropathy can occur, and patients are at higher risk of enhanced bone loss and fractures. Although most cases are initially benign, up to 25% (1% per year) progress to myeloma or a related B-cell disorder, such as macroglobulinemia, amyloidosis, or lymphoma.

Diagnosis is usually suspected when M-protein is incidentally detected in blood or urine during a routine examination. On laboratory evaluation, M-protein is present in low levels in serum (<3 g/dL) or urine (<300 mg/24 h). MGUS is differentiated from other plasma cell disorders because M-protein levels remain relatively stable over time and lytic bone lesions, anemia, and renal dysfunction are absent. Because of fracture risk, baseline evaluation with a skeletal survey (i.e. plain X-rays of skull, long bones, spine, pelvis, and ribs) and bone densitometry should be done. Bone marrow shows only mild plasmacytosis (<10% of nucleated cells).

No antineoplastic treatment is recommended. However, recent studies suggest that MGUS patients with associated bone loss (osteopenia or osteoporosis) may benefit from treatment with bisphosphonates. Every 6–12 months, patients should undergo clinical examination and serum and urine protein electrophoresis to evaluate for disease progression.

POEMS Syndrome

POEMS syndrome is a syndrome with polyneuropathy, organomegaly, endocrinopathy, monoclonal protein, and skin changes. Three criteria must be met: (1) presence of a monoclonal plasma cell disorder, (2) peripheral neuropathy, and (3) other related features. A couple of other plasma cell disorders that are not always included with classification lists are light chain deposition disease, in which free light chains are deposited in tissues but lack characteristics of amyloid; and plasma cell leukemia, which is identified by plasma cell counts in peripheral blood >2000 μL and plasma cells >20% of white blood cells.

HEAVY CHAIN DISEASES

Heavy chain diseases are neoplastic plasma cell disorders characterized by overproduction of monoclonal immunoglobulin heavy chains. Symptoms, diagnosis, and treatment vary according to the specific disorder.

Heavy chain diseases are plasma cell disorders that are typically malignant. In most plasma cell disorders, M-proteins are structurally similar to normal antibody molecules. In contrast, in heavy chain diseases, incomplete monoclonal immunoglobulins (true paraproteins) are produced. They consist of only heavy chain components (either α, γ, μ, or δ) without light chains (ε heavy chain disease has not been described). Most heavy chain proteins are fragments of their normal counterparts with internal deletions of variable length; these deletions appear to result from structural mutations. The clinical picture is more like lymphoma than multiple myeloma. Heavy chain diseases are considered in patients with clinical manifestations suggesting lymphoproliferative disorders.

Immunoglobulin A Heavy Chain Disease

Immunoglobulin A heavy chain disease is the most common heavy chain disease and is similar to mediterranean lymphoma (immunoproliferative small intestinal disease). IgA heavy chain disease usually appears between ages 10 and 30 and is geographically concentrated in the Middle East. The cause may be an aberrant immune response to a parasite or other microorganism. Villous atrophy and plasma cell infiltration of the jejunal mucosa are usually present and, sometimes, infiltration of the mesenteric lymph nodes. The peripheral lymph nodes, bone marrow, liver, and spleen usually are not involved. A respiratory tract form of the disease has been reported rarely. Osteolytic lesions do not occur.

Almost all patients present with diffuse abdominal lymphoma and malabsorption. CBC may show anemia, leukopenia, thrombocytopenia, eosinophilia, and circulating atypical lymphocytes or plasma cells. Serum protein electrophoresis is normal in half of cases; often, there is an increased α_2 and β fraction or a decreased γ fraction. Diagnosis requires the detection of a monoclonal α chain on immunofixation electrophoresis. This chain is sometimes found in concentrated urine. If it cannot be found in serum or urine, biopsy is required. The abnormal protein can sometimes be detected in intestinal secretions. The intestinal cellular infiltrate may be pleomorphic and not overtly malignant. Bence Jones proteinuria is absent.

The course is highly variable. Some patients die in 1–2 years, whereas others have remissions that last many years, particularly after treatment with corticosteroids, cytotoxic drugs, and broad-spectrum antibiotics.

Immunoglobulin G Heavy Chain Disease

Immunoglobulin G heavy chain disease is generally similar to an aggressive malignant lymphoma, but is occasionally asymptomatic and benign.

Immunoglobulin G heavy chain disease occurs primarily in elderly men but can occur in children. Associated chronic disorders include rheumatoid arthritis (RA), Sjögren syndrome, SLE, tuberculosis (TB),

myasthenia gravis, hypereosinophilic syndrome, autoimmune hemolytic anemia, and thyroiditis. Reductions in normal immunoglobulin levels occur. Lytic bone lesions are uncommon. Amyloidosis sometimes develops.

Common manifestations include lymphadenopathy and hepatosplenomegaly, fever, and recurring infections. Palatal edema occurs in about one quarter of patients.

The CBC may show anemia, leukopenia, thrombocytopenia, eosinophilia, and circulating atypical lymphocytes or plasma cells. Diagnosis requires demonstration by immunofixation of free monoclonal heavy chain fragments of IgG in serum and urine. Of affected patients, half have monoclonal serum components >1 g/dL (often broad and heterogeneous), and half have proteinuria >1 g/24 h. Although, heavy chain proteins may involve any IgG subclass, the G3 subclass is especially common. Bone marrow or lymph node biopsy, done if other tests are not diagnostic, reveals variable histopathology.

The median survival with aggressive disease is about 1 year. Death usually results from bacterial infection or progressive malignancy. Alkylating agents, vincristine, or corticosteroids, and radiation therapy may yield transient remissions.

Immunoglobulin M Heavy Chain Disease

Immunoglobulin M heavy chain disease, which is rare, produces a clinical picture similar to chronic lymphocytic leukemia or other lymphoproliferative disorders.

Immunoglobulin M heavy chain disease most often affects adults >50 years. Visceral organ involvement (spleen, liver, abdominal lymph nodes) is common, but extensive peripheral lymphadenopathy is not. Pathologic fractures and amyloidosis may occur. Serum protein electrophoresis usually is normal or shows hypogammaglobulinemia. Bence Jones proteinuria (type κ) is present in 10–15% of patients. CBC may show anemia, leukopenia, thrombocytopenia, eosinophilia, and circulating atypical lymphocytes or plasma cells.

Diagnosis usually requires bone marrow examination; vacuolated plasma cells are present in two-thirds of patients and, when present, are virtually pathognomonic. Death can occur in a few months or in many years. The usual cause of death is uncontrollable proliferation of chronic lymphocytic leukemia cells.

Treatment depends on the patient's condition, but may consist of alkylating agents plus corticosteroids or may be similar to treatment of the lymphoproliferative disorder that it most closely resembles.

Cryoglobulinemia and Amyloid Disease

Deposition of monoclonal immunoglobulin light chains or, more rarely, heavy chains in tissues can produce systemic amyloidosis as discussed in a later section of this chapter.

Cryoglobulins are serum proteins or protein complexes that precipitate at temperatures lower than normal core body temperature. Precipitation of cryoglobulins in tissues can result in vasculitis and ischemic injury to peripheral tissues at a lower temperature and tissue loss of fingers, toes, nose, and other sites. Patients need to be kept in a warm environment until treatment can lower cryoglobulin concentrations. Type I cryoglobulins consist of monoclonal immunoglobulins, often IgM. Occasionally, specimens with high paraprotein concentrations will gel, and this can present major problems with plugging sample probes of automated analyzers. Most cryoglobulins consist of immunoglobulin mixed with a monoclonal component (type II) or without a monoclonal component (type III cryoglobulin). Mixed cryoglobulins often present with chronic infection, particularly with hepatitis C. Cryoglobulins require transport and processing of specimens at temperatures near body temperature to prevent loss of the cryoglobulin during serum formation and centrifugation.

For cryoglobulin analysis, serum usually is stored for 7 days under refrigeration. Cryoglobulins precipitated by centrifugation should re-dissolve in saline when warmed to 37°C, whereas cryofibrinogen will not dissolve. Monoclonal immunoglobulins may have unusual solubility characteristics that include not only gelling or precipitating at low temperatures, but also behaving as pyroglobulins (precipitating at 56°C) or precipitating as a result of pH changes. Unusual solubility or physical characteristics may contribute to unpredictable interferences of paraproteins in a variety of photometric assays due to precipitation and turbidity under assay conditions as described in many reports; a recent example describes interference with the biuret assay. Cryoglobulins also are recognized to interfere with automated hematology analyzers.

Laboratory Testing

Immunoglobulins are typically quantified by immunoturbidimetry or immunonephelometry. Immunochemical assays of polyclonal immunoglobulins involve determining the concentration of a mixture of protein molecules having similar constant regions but different variable regions (idiotypes). Reagent antisera and reference immunoglobulin calibrators used in most immunochemical assays have been generated against normal human sera containing a mixture of immunoglobulin subclasses and idiotypes. However, a monoclonal immunoglobulin has only a few of the determinants with which the antiserum usually reacts, and antigen excess may be reached at relatively low concentrations.

If a paraprotein is suspected or previously identified, the assays should be performed at two or more dilutions to check for this; corrected for dilution, the values should agree within approximately 10%. Furthermore, if a new batch of antiserum is introduced, the relationship between paraprotein concentration and the calibration curve is likely to change. For these reasons, many laboratories estimate the concentration of paraproteins by electrophoresis and densitometry.

Reference Intervals

For IgG and IgM in various human adult populations (Table 13.12), differ around the world because of different degrees of antigenic stimulation. IgA concentrations, however, are relatively unaffected by environmental factors. Newborn infants have B lymphocytes with antigen receptors of the IgM type, but do not have significant rates of immunoglobulin synthesis. Essentially all of the IgG in neonates has been transferred across the placenta from the mother.

Measurement of Proteins

Analysis of high-abundance proteins in body fluids depends on a variety of methods for total protein analysis, electrophoretic methods, and specific quantitative immunoassays based on turbidimetry, nephelometry, and radial immunodiffusion. Mass spectrometry is used increasingly for qualitative analysis of high-abundance protein components.

Immunochemical methods nephelometric and turbidimetric methods are performed as equilibrium or rate methods for measuring the amount of light scattering by antigen-antibody complexes. Limits of detection of approximately 10 mg/L are attained with routine nephelometric and turbidimetric methods, adding antibodies in solution. Binding antibodies to particles of latex or other materials enhances light scattering and can lower limits of detection by 10 to 100-fold. Such assays may be described as latex enhanced or as particle-enhanced

Table 13.12	Immunoglobulin reference intervals				
Body fluid	IgG, mg/dL	IgA, mg/dL	IgM, mg/dL	IgD, mg/dL	IgE, mg/dL
Serum newborn (4 days)	700–1480	0–2.2	5–30		
20–60 years	700–1600	70–400	40–230	0–8	0–380
>60 years	600–1560	90–410	30–360		
CSF	0–5.5	0–0.6	0–1.3		

assays. Radial immunodiffusion methods usually are able to detect down to a minimum of 10–20 mg/L.

Nephelometric and turbidimetric assays commonly offer within-run coefficients of variation (CVs) of <5%, except as limits of detection are approached. RID has higher withinrunand run-to-run CVs. Turbidimetric methods can beapplied on most chemistry analyzers capable of performing photometric methods. Nephelometry requires instrumentation capable of measuring light scattering at an angle.

SPECIMEN COLLECTION AND STORAGE FOR IMMUNOASSAY

Test specimens should be nonhemolyzed, cell-free serum, urine, or CSF. CSF specimens may require centrifugation if cells are present. Serum and CSF samples may be stored at 2–8°C for up to 3 days or at –20°C for longer periods. Repeated freezing and thawing of specimens may cause denaturation of some proteins and should be avoided.

Protein Electrophoresis

Electrophoresis is used to separate proteins by charge and thereby to assess protein variants or the concentrations of specific components in serum or other fluids. Electrophoretic techniques commonly performed in clinical laboratories include non-denaturing electrophoresis on cellulose acetate strips or agarose gels, capillary electrophoresis (CE), immunofixation, and 'Western blotting;' Protein separation in one or two dimensions with polyacrylamide gel is a power ful separation technique frequently used for research.

Serum Protein Electrophoresis

Generally, serum rather than plasma is used for electrophoresis of proteins on agarose gels to avoid the fibrinogen band at the β– γ interface, Fig. 13.8 illustrates examples of serum electrophoretic patterns for normal specimens. Analysis usually is performed with low-ionic strength buffers at pH of 8.6. For agarose gels, the usual sample is 3–5 μL, applied evenly across a lane. Much smaller volumes are injected for capillary electrophoresis via electrokinetic or hydrostatic injection. Separation times are typically about 1 hour for agarose gels and a few minutes for capillary electrophoresis. A variety of stains are used to visualize proteins in gels including amido black, Ponceau S, Coomassie brilliant blue, and related dyes. Levels of detection and linearity of protein detection vary with different dyes.

Only a few of the most abundant proteins are visualized, and intensities of bands with protein stains usually relate to the mass of peptide; oligosaccharides and lipids may reduce rather than contribute to band intensities. Therefore, glycoproteins with a high proportion of carbohydrate (e.g. AAG) have lower detec-

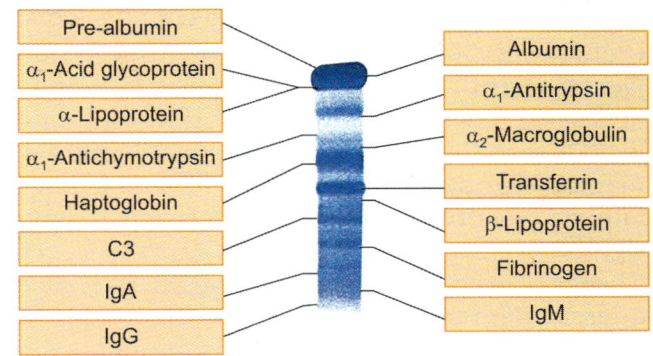

Fig. 13.8: Examples of serum electrophoretic patterns for normal specimens

tion responses than a non-glycosylated protein such as albumin. Quantitative analysis relies on densitometry, which provides relative proportions of different components rather than absolute amounts. Quantitation of individual components relies on calculations based on total protein concentration. Lipophilic stains such as Sudan black are needed to visualize lipoproteins such as HDL (α1 lipoprotein), very-low-density lipoprotein (VLDL) (pre-β region), LDL (β lipoprotein), or chylomicrons (origin). Capillary electrophoresis detects proteins passing through a flow cell by their light absorbance at wavelengths below 220 nm. This offers a more unbiased assessment of protein concentration than staining intensity, as absorbance of proteins in the low ultraviolet region is more consistently related to mass. Small molecules at high concentrations, such as metabolites, radio contrast dyes, or drugs, may also yield absorbance peaks, and this presents problems with analysis of urine specimens.

The major clinical application of serum protein electrophoresis is the detection of monoclonal immunoglobulins (paraproteins) to assist in the diagnosis and monitoring of multiple myeloma and related disorders. Most of the monoclonal immunoglobulins are observed in the β region and γ region, but (especially the IgA class) may migrate more anodally, towards the β region. Quantitation of monoclonal components serves as a means of monitoring disease progression and response to therapy. Identification of paraproteins requires distinction from a variety of other sources of additional bands or pseudoparaproteins by means, such as immunofixation electrophoresis. Incompletely clotted specimens contain fibrinogen. Genetic or post-translational variants of proteins, such as transferrin, haptoglobin, and C3 may migrate in different than usual positions. Large increases in CRP may yield a detectable band in the β or γ region. Increased lysozyme in monocytic leukemia may produce a band in the post-γ-region. Hemoglobin will yield a band in hemolyzed specimens.

Various Other Findings of Potential Clinical Significance

1. Changes in albumin concentration or migration. Decreases in concentration suggest nutritional deficiency, protein losing disorders, APR, or advanced liver disease. Changes in mobility or bisalbuminemia may indicate genetic variants or increased binding of fatty acids or drugs; usually this is not of great clinical significance.

2. Changes in α1 region relate to changes in AAT, and to a lesser degree in AAG or HDL. Decreases are associated with AAT deficiency or protein-losing disorders. Increases are related to inflammation.

3. Changes in α2 region usually relate to changes in HPT and AMG. Migration of HPT varies with genotype. HPT decreases with *in vivo* hemolysis and increases with the APR. AMG and high molecular weight forms of HPT increase in nephrotic syndrome, while most other protein components decrease.

4. Bands in β region are related to transferrin, C3, and LDL. Migration of transferrin may change from the β1 region to β2 region with carbohydrate-deficient transferrin. Transferrin decreases and C3 increases in the APR. Transferrin increases in iron deficiency. LDL may increase in dyslipidemias.

5. An increase between β and γ bands, so-called bridging of β and γ bands, suggests an increase in IgA as seen with cirrhosis, respiratory tract or skin infection, and rheumatoid arthritis.

6. Increases or decrease in the γ region suggest changes inimmunoglobulins. Increases result from chronic infectionor paraproteins. Decreases occur with many immunodeficiency states. Multiple myeloma may suppress general production of immunoglobulins other than from the expanded clone. Therefore, a decrease in the γ-region may suggest the need for additional studies, such as immunofixation electrophoresis to detect paraproteins.

Automated systems for protein electrophoresis are available for large volumes of samples for electrophoresis. An automated system is capable of separating 10–100 samples simultaneously. There are several different automated systems and the number of process steps that are automated varies. Automated steps may include reagent addition, sample application, electrophoresis separation, staining, and detection.

IMMUNOFIXATION ELECTROPHORESIS

An agarose gel electrophoresis first separates the proteins in a serum sample. Antiserum against the protein of interest is spread directly on the gel. The protein of interest precipitates in the gel matrix. After a wash step to remove other proteins, the precipitated protein is stained. This method is qualitative and is used to identify proteins found in multiple myeloma.

Below is the immunofixation electrophoresis (IFE) gel from a serum sample analyzed on IFE agarose gel (Fig. 13.9). After electrophoresis, the precipitated proteins are stained with acid violet. The SP lane represents a routine serum protein electrophoresis of this specimen. On the next three protein separations, antiserum against IgG, IgA, and IgM were applied to the G, A, M lanes respectively. Antiserum to κ light chain was added to the next protein separation and antiserum to κ light chain to the last protein separation.

Capillary Electrophoresis

Capillary electrophoresis of proteins relies on zone electrophoresis in small-bore (10–100 11m), fused silica capillary tubes 20–200 cm in length. Electrokinetic or hydrostatic injection introduces a small amount of protein that is resolved rapidly under high voltage. One of the challenges is to avoid adsorption of proteins to the surface of the capillary. CE is suitable for automation and offers rapid analysis with no need for gel handling or staining. Direct ultraviolet detection offers slightly different specificity than protein staining and offers better reproducibility of quantitation than densitometry. Immunofixation cannot be performed with CE immunosubtraction with specific antisera is used as an alternative procedure to identify paraproteins.

Western Blotting

For Western blotting, proteins separated on a gel are transferred by diffusion or electroblotting onto a membrane made of materials such as nitrocellulose or polyvinylidene fluoride. Proteins bound on the membrane are identified with specific antibodies using labels such as peroxidase, alkaline phosphatase, or chemiluminescent probes.

MASS SPECTROMETRY

Multiple types of mass spectrometry (MS) instrumentation provide qualitative or quantitative information about proteins. An advantage of MS is the ability to analyze a

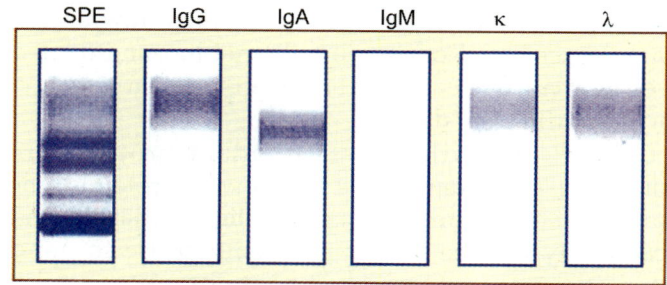

Fig. 13.9: A serum sample analyzed on IFE agarose gel

large number of components in a single analysis, including rapid sequence analysis of peptides. MS, therefore, has been an enabling technology in proteomics, defined as the effort to study the complete set of proteins in an organism or in sub-compartments of an organism such as plasma. Ionization of peptides and proteins has been accomplished by electrospray or matrix assisted laser desorption/ionization sources. Electrospray sources take a solution containing proteins and forma spray of fine droplets with an applied electrical charge.

Solvent is evaporated, generating multiply charged protein ions for mass analysis. In MALDI sources, proteins are deposited on a target surface together with a light-absorbing compound (the matrix) such as dihydroxybenzoic acid. Under a high vacuum, the matrix and proteins are vaporized by pulses of light from a laser; proteins usually are preferentially ionized in a singly charged form. Once proteins are ionized, they can be separated by quadrupoles, iontraps, time-of-flight, and other types of mass analyzers. In general, MS is better suited to analyzing small peptides than proteins, because it provides better resolution, a smaller number of charge states of ions, and better detection sensitivity. It is difficult to quantitatively interpret the absolute magnitude of detector responses in MS, but accurate ratios of similar peptides can be determined. Use of stable.

Isotope-labeled internal standards allows the absolute quantitation of peptides or proteins (based on analysis of proteotypic peptides released by proteolysis). Use of tandem MS with an intermediate fragmentation step between two stages of MS separation offers high sensitivity and specificity for the quantitative analysis of peptides, as it does for most small molecules. Quantitative analysis usually uses selected ion monitoring (also referred to as multiple reaction monitoring for multiple components), which selects particular precursor and product ions for analysis. This form of analysis is performed very efficiently by triple quadrupole MS. Qualitative analysis of peptides, identifying their sequences and post-translational modification, often uses mass spectrometers, such as ion traps that are well suited for scanning all peptide fragments generated by fragmentation. Advantages of using MS for quantitative analysis include the ability to analyze components without developing specific antibodies and the ability to multiplex a large number of measurements. MS can provide information about post-translational modifications that is difficult to assess by immunoassays and chromatographic or electrophoretic techniques. Examples of clinical applications include identification of genetic variants of prealbumin and carbohydrate-deficient transferrin. MS techniques are likely to increasingly serve as reference methods for accurate determination of protein concentrations, such

as recently applied for standardization of hemoglobin Ale measurement and for concentrations of peptides such as insulin and C-peptide. For analysis of bioactive peptides, the ability to distinguish between peptides differing in length by one or two amino acids or by a post-translational modification often is critical. MS is likely to find increased use for clinical laboratory analysis of bioactive peptides and other components of the peptidome.

BIBLIOGRAPHY

1. Amaral S, Hwang W, Fivush B, Neu A, Frankenfield D, Furth S. Serum albumin concentration and risk of mortality and hospitalization in adolescents on hemodialysis. Clin I Am Soc NephroI 2008; 3: 759–67.

2. Anderson NL, Anderson NG, Pearson T\N, Borchers CH, Paulovich AG, Patterson SD, et al. A human proteome detection and quantitation project. Mol Cell Proteomics 2009; 8: 883–6.

3. Anderson NL, Anderson NG. The human plasma proteome: history, character, and diagnostic prospects. Mol Cell Proteomics 2002; I: 845–67.

4. Bachmann-Harildstad G. Diagnostic values of beta-2 transferrin and beta-trace protein as markers for cerebrospinal fluid fistula. Rhinology 2008;46:82-5.

5. Beck FX, Neuhofer W. Response of renal medullary cells to osmotic stress. Contrib NephroI 2005; 148: 21–34.

6. Becker K, Frieling T, Haussinger D. Quantification of fecal alpha I-antitrypsin excretion for assessment of inflammatory bowel diseases. Eur I Med Res 1998;3: 65–70.

7. Becker KL, Snider R, Nylen ES. Procalcitonin assay in systemic inflammation, infection, and sepsis: clinical utility and limitations. Crit Care Med 2008; 36: 941–52.

8. Bergen HR, Zeldenrust SR, Butz ML, Snow DS, Dyck PJ, Dyck IB,et al. Identification of transthyretin variants by sequential proteomic and genomic analysis. Clin Chern 2004; 50: 1544–52.

9. Biffi S, Tamaro G, Bortot B, Zamberlan S, Severini GM, Carrozzi M. Carbohydrate deficient transferrin (CDT) as a biochemical tool for the screening of congenital disorders of glycosylation (CDGs). Clin Biochem 2007; 40: 1431–4.

10. Biou D, Benoist IF, Huong CN, Morel P, Marchand M. Cerebrospinalfluid protein concentrations in children: age-related values in patientswithout disorders of the central nervous system. Clin Chem 2000; 46: 399–403.

11. Blirup- Iensen S, Iohnson AM, Larsen M. IFCC Committee on Plasm Proteins. Protein standardization. V: value transfer. A practicaprotocol for the assignment of serum protein values from a referencmaterial to a target material. Clin Chem Lab Med 2008; 46: 1470–9.

12. Bornhorst lA, Calderon FRO, Procter M, Tang W, Ashwood ER, MaoR. Genotypes and serum concentrations of human alpha-I-antitrypsin "P" protein variants in a clinical population. I Clin Pathol 2007; 60: 1124–8.

13. Brown R, Nelson M, Aklilu E, Kabani D, Yang S, Blayney B, et al. Aevaluation of the Dia Med assays for immunoglobulin A antibodies(anti-IgA) and IgA deficiency. Transfusion 2008; 48: 2057–9.

14. Carrell RW, Lomas DA. Alphal-antitrypsin deficiency-a model for conformational diseases. N Engl I Med 2002; 346: 45–53.

15. Carter K, Worwood M. Haptoglobin: a review of the major allele frequencies worldwide and their association with diseases. Int IHaematoI 2007; 29: 92–110.

16. Chehab FE Obesity and lipodystrophy-where do the circles intersect? Endocrinology 2008;149: 925–34.

17. Chromy V, Svachova B, Novosad L, Jarkovsky J, Sedlak P, Horak P,et al. Albumin based or albumin-linked calibrators cause a positive bias in serum proteins assayed by the Biuret method. Clin Chern Lab Med 2009; 47: 91–101.

18. Coppinger lA, Maguire PB. Insights into the platelet releasate. Curr Pharm Des 2007; 13: 2640–6.

19. Corlin DB, Sen IW, Ladefoged S, Lund GB, Nissen MH, Heegaard NH. Quantification of cleaved beta2-microglobulin in serum from patients undergoing chronic dialysis. Clin Chern 2005; 51: 1177–84.

20. Costacou T, Ferrell RE, Orchard TI. Haptoglobin genotype: a determinant of cardiovascular complication risk in type I diabetes. Diabetes 2008; 57: 1702–6.

21. Craig WY, Ledue TB, Ritchie RE Plasma proteins: clinical utility and interpretation. Scarborough, ME: Foundation for Blood Research, 2001.

22. Dati F, Schumann G, Thomas L, Aguzzi F, Baudner S, Bienvenu I, et al. Consensus of a group of professional societies and diagnostic companies on guidelines for interim reference ranges for 14 proteins in serum based on the standardization against the IFCC/BCR/CAP reference material (CRM 470). Eur I Clin Chern Clin Biochem 1996; 34: 517–20.

23. Delgado I, Pratt G, Phillips N, Briones I, Fegan C, Nomdedeu I, et al. Beta(2)-microglobulin is a better predictor of treatment-free survival in patients with chronic lymphocytic leukemia if adjusted according to glomerular filtration rate. Br I HaematoI 2009;145: 801–5.

24. Denne SC, Poindexter BB. Evidence supporting early nutritional support with parenteral amino acid infusion. Semin Perinatol 2007; 31: 56–60.

25. Devoto G, Gallo F, Marchello C, Racchi 0, Garbini R, Bonassi S,et al. Prealbumin concentrations as a useful tool in the assessment ofmalnutrition in hospitalized patients. Clin Chern 2006; 52: 2281–5.

26. Dimopoulos MA, Gertz MA, Kastritis E, Garcia-Sanz R, Kimby EK,Leblond V, et al. Update on treatment recommendations from theFourth International Workshop on Waldenstrom's macroglobulinemia. J Clin OncoI 2009; 27: 120–6.

27. Dispenzieri A, Kyle R, Merlini G, Miguel JS, Ludwig H, Hajek R, et al.International Myeloma Working Group guidelines for serum free lightchain analysis in multiple myeloma and related disorders. Leukemia 2009; 23: 215–24.

28. Dobson CM. Protein folding and misfolding. Nature 2003; 426: 884–90.

29. Domon B, Aebersold R. Mass spectrometry and protein analysis. Science 2006;312: 212–7.

30. Durandy A, Peron S, Fischer A. Hyper-1gM syndrome. Curr Opin RheumatoI 2006; 18: 369–76.

31. Elango R, Ball RO, Pencharz PB. Amino acid requirements inhumans: with a special emphasis on the metabolic availability ofamino acids. Amino Acids 2009;37: 19–27.

32. Ellington AA, Kullo IJ, Bailey KR, Klee GG. Measurement and qualitycontrol issues in multiplex protein assays: a case study. Clin Chern 2009; 55: 1092–9.

33. Engel H, Bac DJ, Brouwer R, Blijenberg BG, Lindemans J. Diagnosticanalysis of total protein, albumin, white cell count and differential inascitic fluid. Eur J Clin Chern Clin Biochem 1995; 33: 239–42.

34. Erikson N, Benditt EP. Serum amyloid A (ApoSAA) and lipoproteins.Methods Enzymol 1986; 128: 311–20.

35. Felgenhauer K. Protein size and cerebrospinal fluid composition. KlinWochenschr 1974; 52: 1158–64.

36. Ferrante M, Penninckx F, De Hertogh G, Geboes K, D'Hoore A,Noman M, et al. Protein-losing enteropathy in Crohn's disease. ActaGastroenterol Belg 2006; 69: 384–9.

37. Fogh-Andersen N, Bjerrum BJ, Siggaard-Andersen O. Ionic binding,net charge, and Donnan effect of human serum albumin as a functionof pH. Clin Chern 1993; 39: 48–52.

38. Fournier T, Medjoubi NN, Porquet D. Alpha-I-acid glycoprotein. Biochim Biophys Acta 2000;1482: 157–171.

39. Fox PL, Mazumder B, Ehrenwald E, Mukhopadhyay CK. Ceruloplasmin and cardiovascular disease. Free Radic BioI Med 2000; 28: 1735–44.

40. Freeman AF, Domingo DL, Holland SM. Hyper IgE (Job's) syndrome:a primary immunodeficiency with oral manifestations. Oral Dis 2009; 15: 2–7.

41. Fuchs SA, de Sain-van der Velden MG, de Barse MM, Roeconcentrationd MM, Hendriks M, Dorland L, et al. Twomass-spectrometric techniques for quantifying serine enantiomersand glycine in cerebrospinal fluid: potential confounders andage-dependent ranges. Clin Chern 2008; 54: 1443–50.

42. Gabay C, Kushner I. Acute-phase proteins and other systemicresponses to inflammation. N Engl J Med 1999; 340: 448–54.

43. Gladwin MT, Vichinsky E. Pulmonary complications of sickle celldisease. N Engl JMed 2008; 359: 2254–65.

44. Glembotski cc. Endoplasmic reticulum stress in the heart. Circ Res 2007; 101: 975–84.

45. Gornick, 0, Lauc G. Glycosylation of serum proteins in inflammatorydiseases. Dis Markers 2008; 25: 267–78.

46. Gressner OA, Weiskirchen R, Gressner AM. Biomarkers of liverfibrosis: clinical translation of molecular pathogenesis or based onliver-dependent malfunction tests. Clin Chim Acta 2007; 381: 107–13.

47. Hahn BH, Grossman J, Ansell BJ, Skaggs BJ, McMahon M.Altered lipoprotein metabolism in chronic inflammatory states:proinflammatory high-density lipoprotein and acceleratedatherosclerosis is systemic lupus erythematosus and rheumatoidarthritis. Arthritis Res Ther 2008;10:213.

48. Hamilton RG, Franklin Adkinson N. In vitro assays for the diagnosisof 19E-mediated disorders. J Allergy Immunol 2004; 114: 213–25.

49. Hart GW, Housley MP, Slawson C. Cycling of O-linked beta-Nacetylglucosamineon nucleocytoplasmic proteins. Nature 2007; 446: 1017–22.

50. Hay Ww. Strategies for feeding the preterm infant. Neonatology 2008; 94: 245–54.

51. Heffner JE. Discriminating between transudates and exudates. ClinChest Med 2006; 27: 241-52.

52. Henderson JM, Stein SF, Kutner M, Wiles MB, Ansley JD, Rudman D.Analysis of twenty-three plasma proteins in ascites: the depletion offibrinogen and plasminogen. Ann Surg 1980;192:738-42.

53. Hochstrasser M. Origin and function of ubiquitin-like proteins.Nature 2009; 458: 422–9.

54. Hoofnagle AN, Becker JO, Wener MH, Heinecke Jw. Quantification of thyroglobulin, a low-abundance serum protein, by immunoaffinitypeptide enrichment and tandem mass spectrometry. Clin Chern 2008; 54: I 796–804.

55. Hortin GL, Jortani SA, Ritchie Jc' Valdes R, et al. Proteomics:a new diagnostic frontier. Clin Chern 2006; 52: 1218–22.

56. Hortin GL, Meilinger B. Cross-reactivity of amino acids and othercompounds in the Biuret reaction: interference with urinary peptidemeasurements. Clin Chern 2005; 51: 1411–9.

57. Hortin GL, Seam N, Hoehn GT. Bound homocysteine, cysteine, andcysteinylglycine distribution between albumin and globulins. ClinChern 2006; 52: 2258–64.

58. Hortin GL, Sviridov D, Anderson L. High-abundance polypeptides ofthe human plasma proteome comprising the top 4 logs of polypeptideabundance. Clin Chern 2008; 54: 1608–16.

59. Hortin GL, Warshawsky I, Laude-Sharp M. Macromolecular chromogenic substrates for measuring proteinase activity. Clin Chern 2001; 47: 215–22.

60. Hortin GL. Can mass spectrometric protein profiling meet desiredstandards of clinical laboratory practice? Clin Chern 2005; 5 I: 3–5.

61. Hortin GL. The MALDl-TOF mass spectrometric view of the plasmaproteome and peptidome. Clin Chern 2006; 52 1223–37.

62. Horwich TB, Kalantar-Zadeh K, MacLellan RW, Fonarow Gc.Albumin concentrations predict survival in patients with systolic heart failure. Am Heart J 2008;155: 883–9.

63. Hosafci G, Klein 0, Oremek G, Mantele W. Clinical chemistry without reagents? An infrared spectroscopic technique fordetermination of clinically relevant constituents of body fluids. AnalBioanal Chem 2007; 387: 1815–22.

64. Hu S, Loo JA, Wong DT. Human saliva proteome analysis and diseasebiomarker discovery. Expert Rev Proteomics 2007; 4: 531–8.

65. Hutchison CA, Harding S, Hewins P, Mead GP, Townsend J, BradwellAR, et al. Quantitative assessment of serum and urinary free lightchains in patients with chronic kidney disease. Clin J Am Soc Nephrol 2008; 3: 1684–90.

66. Ivandic BT, Spanuth E, Haase D, Lestin HG, Katus HA. Increasedplasma concentrations of soluble CD40 ligand in acute coronarysyndrome depend on in vitro platelet activation. Clin Chern 2007; 53: 1231–4.

67. Jahoor F, Badaloo A, Reid M, Forrester T. Protein metabolism insevere childhood malnutrition. Ann Trop Paediatr 2008; 28: 87–101.

68. Jensen JK, Dolmer K, Gettins PG. Specificity of binding of the lowdensity lipoprotein receptor-related protein (LRP) to differentconformational states of the clade E serpins PAI-1 and PNI. J BioI Chern 2009; 284: 17989–97.

69. Jeschke MG, Finnerty CC, Kulp GA, Przkora R, Micak RP, NerndonDN. Combination of recombinant human growth hormone andpropranolol decreases hypermetabolism and inflammation in severelyburned children. Pediatr Crit Care Med 2008; 9: 209–16.

70. Johnson AM. Amino acids, peptides, and proteins. In: Burtis CA,Ashwood ER, Bruns DE, eds. Tietz textbook of clinical chemistry, 4thedition. Philadelphia: WB Saunders, 2006: 531–95.

71. Joseph J, Handy DE, Loscalzo J. Quo vadis: whither homocysteineresearch? Cardiovasc Toxicol 2009; 9: 53–63.

72. Kaneko Y, Nimmerjahn F, Ravetch jv. Anti-inflammatory activityof immunoglobulin G resulting from Fc sialylation. Science 2006; 313: 670–3.

73. Katzmann jA, Kyle RA, Benson), Larson DR, Snyder MR, Lust jA,et al. Screening panels for detection of monoclonal gammopathies.Clin Chern 2009; 55: 1–6.

74. Keersmaekers T, Claes K, Kuypers DR, de Vlam K, Verschueren P,Westhovens R. Long-term efficacy of infliximab treatment forAA-amyloidosis secondary to chronic inflammatory arthritis. Ann Rheum Dis 2009; 68: 759–61.

75. Kielstein jT, Zoccali C. Asymmetric dimethylarginine: a novel markerof risk and a potential target for therapy in chronic kidney disease. Curr Opin Nephrol Hypertens 2008; 17: 609–15.

76. Kochanek PM, Berger RP, Bayir H, Wagner AK, jenkins LW, Clark RS. Biomarkers of evolving damage in traumatic and ischemic braininjury: diagnosis, prognosis, probing mechanisms, and therapeuticdecision making. Curr Opin Crit Care 2008;14: 135–41.

77. Kolodziej Sj, Klueppelberg HU, Nolasco N, Ehses W, Strickland OK,Stoops jK. Three-dimensional structure of the human plasminalpha2-macroglobulin complex. j Struct BioI 1998; 123: 124–33.

78. Kricka Lj, Master SR, joos TO, Fortina P. Current perspectives inprotein array technology. Ann Clin Biochem 2006; 43: 457–67.

79. Kuhn E, Addona T, Keshishian H, Burgess M, Mani DR, Lee RT, et al.Developing multiplexed assays for troponin 1 and interleukin-33 inplasma by peptide immunoaffinity enrichment and targeted massspectrometry. Clin Chern 2009; 55: 1108–17.

80. Kurpad AV. The requirements of protein and amino acid during acuteand chronic infections. Indian j Med Res 2006; 124: 129–148.

81. Kwong LK, Uryu K, Trojanowski jQ, Lee VM. TDP-43 proteinopathies: neurodegenerative protein misfolding diseaseswithout amyloidosis. Neuro-signals 2008;16: 41–51.

82. Kyle RA, Rajkuma Sv. Criteria for diagnosis, staging, risk stratificationand response assessment of multiple myeloma. Leukemia 2009; 23: 3–9.

83. Kyte j, Doolittle RF. A simple method for displaying the hydropathiccharacter of a protein. j Mol Bioi 1982; 157: 105–132.

84. Labriola B, Wallemacq P, Gulbis B, jadoul M. The impact of theassay for measuring albumin on corrected ("adjusted") calciumconcentrations. Nephrol Dial Transplant 2009; 24: 1834–8.

85. Lam HS, Ng pc. Biochemical markers of neonatal sepsis. Pathology 2008; 40: 141–8.

86. Landgren 0, Kyle RA, Pfeiffer RM, Katzmann jA, Caporaso NE,Hayes RB, et al. Monoclonal gammopathy of undetermined significance (MGUS) consistently precedes multiple myeloma: aprospective study. Blood 2009; 113: 5412–7.

87. Langlois MR, Delanghe JR. Biological and clinical significance ofhaptoglobin polymorphism in humans. Clin Chern 1996; 42: 1589–600.

88. Law RH, Zhang Q, McGowan S, Buckle AM, Silverman GA, Wong W,et al. Anoverview of the serpin superfamily. Genome Bioi 2006; 7:216.

89. Lentine K, Wrone EM. New insights into protein intake and progression of renal disease. Curr Opin Nephrol Hypertens 2004; 13: 333–6.

90. Ling MM, Ricks C, Lea P. Multiplexing molecular diagnostics andimmunoassays using emerging microarray technologies. Expert RevMol Diagn 2007; 7: 87–98.

91. Livrea P, Trojano M, Simone IL, Zimatore GB, Pisicchio L, LogroscinoG, et al. Heterogeneous models for blood-cerebrospinal fluid barrierpermeability to serum proteins in normal and abnormal cerebrospinalfluid/serum protein concentration gradients. J Neurol Sci 1984; 64: 245–58.

92. Lu j, Holmgren A. Selenoproteins. J Bioi Chem 2009; 284: 723–7.

93. Lundblad RL. The evolution from protein chemistry to proteomics: basic science to clinical application. Boca Raton, Fla: CRC Press, 2006.

94. Luque FA, Jaffe SL. Cerebrospinal fluid analysis in multiple sclerosis. Int Rev Neurobiol 2007; 79: 341–56.

95. Madsden E, Gitlin jD. Copper deficiency. Curr Opin Gastroentero 2007; 23: 187–92.

96. Mak CM, Lam CW Diagnosis of Wilson's disease: a comprehensive review. Crit Rev Clin Lab Sci 2008; 45: 263–90.

97. Mak CM, Lam WW, Tam S. Diagnostic accuracy of serumceruloplasmin in Wilson disease: determination of sensitivity andspecificity by ROC curve analysis among ATP7B-genotyped subjects.Clin Chem 2008; 54: 1356–62.

98. Maniaci V, Dauber A, Weiss S, Nylen E, Becker KL, Bachur R.Procalcitonin in young febrile infants for the detection of seriousbacterial infections. Pediatrics 2008; 122:70 1–10.

99. Mantovani A, Garlanda C, Doni A, Bottazzi B. Pentraxins in innateimmunity: from C-reactive protein to the long pentraxin PTX3. j Clin ImmunoI 2008; 28: 1–13.

100. Marklova E, Albahri Z. Screening and diagnosis of congenital disorders of glycosylation. Clin Chim Acta 2007; 385: 6–20.

101. Mathivanan S, Pandey A. Human proteinpedia as a resource forclinical proteomics. Mol Cell Proteomics 2008; 7: 2038–47.

102. Matthews ST, Deutsch DO, Iyer G, Hora N, Pati B, Marsh j, et al.Plasma alpha2-HS glycoprotein concentrations in patients with acutemyocardial infarction quantified by a modified ELISA. Clin ChimActa 2002; 319: 27–34.

103. McCudden CR, Mathews SP, Hainsworth SA, Chapman jF,Hammett-Stabler CA, Willis MS, et al. Performance comparisonof capillary and agarose electrophoresis for the identification and characterization of monoclonal immunoglobulins. Am j Clin Pathol2008;129: 451–8.

104. Meng QH, Krahn j. Lithium heparinized blood-collection tubesgive falsely low albumin results with an automated

105. Miller WG, Bruns DE, Hortin GL, Sandberg S, Aakre KM, McQueenM), et al. Current issues in measurement and reporting of urinaryalbumin excretion. Clin Chem 2009; 55: 24–38.

106. Miller WG, Thienpont LM, Van Uytfanghe K, Clark PM, Lindstedt P,Nilsson G, et al.Toward standardization of insulin immunoassays. Clin Chem 2009; 55: 10 11–8.

107. Miura H, Ozaki N, Sawada M, Isobe K, Ohta T, Nagatsu T. A linkbetween stress and depression: shifts in the balance between thekynurenine and serotonin pathways of tryptophan metabolismand the etiology and pathophysiology of depression. Stroke 2008; 11: 198–209.

108. Mizazaki 0, Yazaki M, Gono T, Kametani F, Tsuchiya A, Matsuda M,et al. AH amyloidosis associated with an immunoglobulin heavychain variable region (VH1) fragment: a case report. Amyloid 2008; 15: 125–8.

109. Moldonado F, Hawkins FJ, Daniels CE, Doerr CH, Decker PA, Ryuj H. Pleural fluid characteristics of chylothorax. Mayo Clin Proc 2009; 84: 129–133.

110. Mora S, Musunuru K, Blumenthal RS. The clinical utility ofhigh-sensitivity C-reactive protein in cardiovascular disease and thepotential implication for JUPITER on current practice guidelines.Clin Chern 2009; 55: 219-28. Ill. Morris CR. Asthma management: reinventing the wheel in sickle celldisease. Am j Hematol 2009; 84: 234–41.

111. Morris SM. Arginine: beyond protein. Am j Clin Nutr 2006; 83: 508S–12S.

112. Mulder C, Verwey NA, van der Flier WM, Bouwman FH, Kok A,van Elk Ej, et al. Amyloid-3(l-42), total tau, and phosphorylated tauas cerebrospinal fluid biomarkers for the diagnosis of Alzheimerdisease. Clin Chern 2010; 56: 248–53.

113. Munthe-Fog B, Hummelshoj T, Honore C, Madsen HO, Permin H,Garred P. Immunodeficiency associated with FCN3 mutation andficolin-3 deficiency. N Engl j Med 2009; 360: 2637–44.

114. Nedelkov 0, Kiernan UA, Niederkofler EE, Tubbs KA, Nelson RW.Investigating diversity in human plasma proteins. Proc Natl Acad Sci USA 2005; 102: 10852–7.

115. Neuberger MS. Antibody diversification by somatic mutation: from Burnet onwards. 1mmunol Cell BioI 2008; 86: 124–32.

116. Norden AGW, Lapsley M, Lee Pj, Pusey CD, Schenman S), Tam FWK,et al. Glomerular protein sieving and implications for renal failure in Fanconi syndrome. Kidney Int 2001; 60: 1885–92.

117. Ridker PM. Clinical application of C-reactive protein for cardiovascular disease detection and prevention. Circulation 2003; 107: 363–9.

118. Ridker PM. C-reactive protein: eighty years from discovery to emergence as a major risk marker for cardiovascular disease. Clin Chern 2009; 55: 209–215.

119. Roopenian DC, Akilesh S. FeRn: the neonatal Fe receptor comes of age. Nat Rev ImmunoI 2007; 7: 715–25.

120. Roth E. Nonnutritive effects of glutamine. J Nutr 2008:138: 2025S–3IS.

121. Runyon BA, Montano AA, Akriviadis EA, Antillon MR, Irving MA, McHutchison JG. The serum-ascites albumin

gradient is superior to the exudate-transudate concept in the differential diagnosis of ascites. Ann Intern Med 1992; 117: 215–20.

122. Saha S, Harrison SH, Shen C, Tang H, Radivojac P, Arnold RJ, et al.HIP2: an online database of human plasma proteins from healthy individuals. BMC Med Genom 2008:1:12.

123. Scheuner D, Kaufman RJ. The unfolded protein response: a pathway that links insulin demand with beta-cell failure and diabetes. Endocr Rev 2008: 29: 317–33.

124. Schiffer E, Mischak H, Vanholder RC. Exploring the uremic toxins using proteomic technologies. Contrib Nephrol 2008: 160: 159–71.

125. Schneider HG, Lam QT. Procalcitonin for the clinical laboratory: are view. Pathology 2007; 39: 383–90.

126. Schreiber G, Aldred AR, Jaworowski A, Nilsson C, Achen MG, Segal ME. Thyroxine transport from blood to brain via transthyretin synthesis in choroid plexus. Am J Physiol 1990; 258:R338.

127. Schrockensnadel K, Wirleitner B, Winkler C, Fuchs D. Monitoring tryptophan metabolism in chronic immune activation. Clin Chim Acta 2006: 364: 82–90.

128. Scott CF, Carrell RW, Glaser CB, Kueppers F, Lewis JH, Colman RW. Alpha-I-antitrypsin Pittsburgh: a potent inhibitor of human plasmafactor XIa, kallikrein, and factor XIIf. J Clin Invest 1986; 77: 631–4.

129. Sharp P. The molecular basis of copper and iron interactions. Proc Nutr Soc 2004: 63: 563–9.

130. Shihabi ZK. Cryoglobulins: an important but neglected clinical test. Ann Clin Lab Sci 2006:36: 395–408.

131. Shimizu A, Nakanishi T, Miyazaki A. Detection and characterization of variant and modified structures of proteins in blood and tissues by mass spectrometry. Mass Spectrom Rev 2006; 25: 686–712.

132. Silverman EK, Sandhaus RA. Alphal-antitrypsin deficiency. N Engl JM Med 2009:360: 2749–57.

133. Sivan SS, Wachtel E, Tsitron E, Sakkee N, van der Ham F, DeGroot J, et al. Collagen turnover in normal and degenerate human intervertebral discs as determined by the racemization of aspartic acid. J Bioi Chern 2008: 283: 8796–801.

134. Sjoholm AG, Jonsson G, Braconier JH, Sturfelt G, Truedsson L. Complement deficiency and disease: an update. Mol Immunol 2006: 43: 78–85.

135. Snozek CLH, Saenger AK, Greipp PR, Bryant SC, Kyle RA, Rajkumar SV, et al. Comparison of bromcresol green and agarose protein electrophoresis for quantitation of serum albumin in multiplemyeloma. Clin Chern 2007:53: 1099–103.

136. Stiehm ER. The four most common pediatric immunodeficiencies. J Immunotoxicol 2008; 5: 227–34.

137. Stoevesandt O, Taussig MJ, He M. Protein microarrays: high throughput tools for proteomics. Expert Rev Proteomics 2009:6: 145–57.

138. Takeda H, Nishise S, Furukawa M, Nagashima R, Shizawa H, Takahashi T. Fecal clearance of alpha I-antitrypsin with lansoprazole can detect protein-losing gastropathy. Dig Dis Sci 1999; 44: 2313–8.

139. Tattersall J. Clearance of beta-2-microglobulin and middle molecules in haemodiafiltration. Contrib NephroI 2007; 158: 201–9.

140. Texel SJ, Xu X, Harris ZL. Ceruloplasmin in neurodegenerative diseases. Biochem Soc Trans 2008: 36: 1277–81.

141. Tichy M, Friedecky B, Budina M, Maisner V, Buchler T, Holeckova M, et ai. Interference of IgM-Iambda paraprotein with biuret-type assay for total serum protein quantification. Clin Chem Lab Med 2009: 47: 235–6.

142. Tietz NW, ed. Clinical guide to laboratory tests, 3rd edition. Philadelphia: WB Saunders, 1995.

143. Tietz textbook of clinical chemistry and molecular biology, 2012. 5fifth edition, Philadelphia, W.B Saunders company.

144. Ueland PM. Homocysteine species as components of plasma redoxthiol status. Clin Chem 1995: 41: 340–2.

145. Unsworth DJ. Complement deficiency and disease. J Clin Pathol 2008; 61: 1013–7.

146. Van Asbeck EC, Hoepelman AIM, Scharringa J, Herpers BL, Verhoef J. Mannose binding lectin plays a crucial role in innate immunity against yeast by enhanced complement activation and enhanced uptake of polymorphonuclear cells. BMC Microbiol 2008: 8:229.

147. Wani MA, Haynes LC, Kim J, et al. Familialhypercatabolic hypoproteinemia caused by deficiency of the neonatal Fc receptor, FcRN, due to a mutant beta2-microglobulingene. PNAS USA 2006; 103: 5084–9.

148. Watanabe A, Matsuzaki S, Moriwaki H, Suzuki K, Nishiguchi S. Problems in serum albumin measurement and clinical significance of albumin microheterogeneity in cirrhotics. Nutrition 2004; 2: 351–7.

149. Whicher IT. BCRIlFCC reference material for plasma proteins (CRM470). Community Bureau of Reference. International Federation of Clinical Chemistry. Clin Biochem 1998; 31:459–65.

150. Whitfield IB, Dy V, Madden PA, et al. Measuring carbohydrate-deficient transferring by direct immunoassay: factors affecting diagnostic sensitivity for excessive alcohol intake. Clin Chern 2008; 54: 1158–65.

151. William Marshall, Márta Lapsley, Stephen K Bangert. Elsevier.com: Clinical Chemistry, 2012, 7th Edition; ISBN-9780723437031.

152. Williams AI, Paulson HI. Polyglutamine neurodegeneration: protein misfoldingrevisited. Trends Neurosci 2008; 31: 521–8.

153. Woof 1M, Mestecky I. Mucosal immunoglobulins. Immunol Rev 2005; 206: 64–82.

154. Xu S, Venge P. Lipocalins as biochemical markers of disease. Biochim Biophys Acta 2000; 1482: 298–307.

155. Zetlerberg H. Update on amyloid-beta homeostasis markers for sporadic Alzheimer's disease. Scand I Clin Lab Invest 2009; 69: 18–21.

156. Zhang XL, Ali MA. Ficolins: structure, function and associated diseases. Adv Exp Med 2008: 632: 105–15.

14

Serum Enzymes

INTRODUCTION

Measurements of enzymes are used in medicine in two major ways. Enzymes are measured in serum and other bodily fluids to detect injury to a tissue that makes up the enzyme. Enzymes are also measured, often within a tissue, to identify abnormalities or absence of the enzyme, which may cause disease.

Most such enzymes are primarily intracellular, being released into the blood when there is damage to cell membranes, but many enzymes, e.g. renin, complement factors and coagulation factors, are actively secreted into the blood, where they fulfil their physiological functions. Highly specific markers have been identified (e.g. cardiac troponin 1, which is found only in cardiac myocytes).

Some enzymes are found predominantly in specialized tissue (e.g. lipase in the pancreas); others, more widely distributed, have tissue-specific isoenzymes or isoforms (e.g. the pancreatic isoenzyme of α-amylase, the bone isoform of alkaline phosphatase) that can be evaluated to enhance tissue and organ specificity.

Small amounts of intracellular enzymes are present in the blood as a result of normal cell turnover. When damage to cells occurs, increased amounts of enzymes will be released and their concentrations in the blood will rise. However, such increases are not always due to tissue damage. Other possible causes include (1) increased cell turnover, (2) cellular proliferation (e.g. neoplasia), (3) increased enzyme synthesis (enzyme induction), (4) obstruction to secretion, and (5) decreased clearance.

Little is known about the mechanisms by which enzymes are removed from the circulation. Small molecules, such as amylase, are filtered by the glomeruli, but most enzymes are probably removed by reticuloendothelial cells. Plasma amylase activity rises in acute kidney injury but, in general, changes in clearance rates are not known to be important as causes of changes in plasma enzyme levels.

The timing of the enzyme's diagnostic window is another important aspect to be considered when these markers are used to evaluate acute injury. According to Noe, the diagnostic window for an injury marker is the interval of time following an episode of injury during which plasma concentrations of the marker are increased, thereby demonstrating the occurrence of injury. Marker substances that rapidly enter the circulation (i.e. early indicators) tend to have diagnostic windows that begin soon after onset of the injury. On the contrary, those biomarkers that are slowly released into the circulation and/or are slowly cleared from the circulation (i.e. late indicators) generally have diagnostic windows that begin later and last long after the time of injury.

DIAGNOSTIC ENZYMOLOGY

In general, clinical laboratorians are principally concerned with changes in activity in the serum or plasma of enzymes that are predominantly intracellular and physiologically present in the blood at low activity concentrations only. Changes in the serum activities of these enzymes are used to infer the location and nature of pathologic changes in tissues of the body. Therefore, an understanding of the factors that affect the rate of release of enzymes from their cells of origin and the rate at which they are cleared from the circulation is necessary to interpret correctly changes in activity that occur with disease.

Factors Affecting Enzyme Concentrations in Plasma or Serum

The measured activity of an enzyme in blood is the result not only of the total amount released from its cells of origin, but also of the rate of enzyme catabolism in the circulation, the escape to the extracellular enzyme pool, and the rate at which it is inactivated or removed.

Leakage of Enzymes from Cells

Enzymes are retained within their cells of origin by the plasma membrane surrounding the cell. The plasma membrane is a metabolically active part of the cell, and its integrity depends on the cell's production of ATP. Any process that impairs ATP production by depriving the cell of oxidizable substrates or by reducing the efficiency of energy production by restricting the access of oxygen (ischemia or anoxia) promotes deterioration of the cell membrane. The earliest sign of impaired energy metabolism is the efflux of potassium with influx of sodium; water thus accumulates within the cell, causing it to swell. The next and most serious stage is the entry of Ca^{2+} which stimulates intracellular enzymes, leading to both cell damage and disruption of the cell membrane.

Finally, free radicals formed during these processes may cause further damage. The membrane becomes leaky; if cellular injury becomes irreversible, the cell will die, although enzyme loss may also occur without the occurrence of irreversible injury. Small molecules are the first to leak from damaged or dying cells, followed by larger molecules, such as enzymes and other proteins. Cytosolic proteins appear early on in the plasma, followed much later by mitochondrial and membrane-bound enzymes. It appears that ATP must decline to below a certain level before substantial enzyme release occurs. Ultimately, the complete content of the necrotic cells is discharged.

Because of very high concentrations of enzymes within the cells, thousands or even tens of thousands times greater than concentrations in extracellular fluid and because extremely small amounts of enzyme can be detected by their catalytic activity, increased enzyme activity in the extracellular fluid or plasma is an extremely sensitive indicator of even minor cellular damage, some causes of which are listed in Table 14.1.

A reduction in the supply of oxygenated blood perfusing any tissue will promote enzyme release, as occurs in myocardial infarction. Cells of the affected region rapidly begin to deteriorate and die, releasing their protein and enzyme contents to the systemic circulation, which accounts for the rapid rise in serum biomarkers, i.e. characteristic of this condition. The liver is also very sensitive to hypoxia, which results from diminished cardiac output (heart failure).

Direct attack on the cell membranes by such agents as viruses or organic chemicals also causes enzyme release, which is particularly important in the case of the liver. Skeletal muscles also contribute enzymes to blood. Again, the cause may be poor perfusion, hypothermia, or direct trauma to the muscles (crush injuries). Infection, inflammation (polymyositis), degenerative changes (dystrophies), drugs, and alcohol (alcoholic myopathy) will cause enzyme leakage from myocytes.

Efflux of Enzymes from Damaged Cells

Once conditions for leakage of enzymes from cells have become established, the speed and extent to which the process is reflected in enzyme changes in the blood depend on several factors.

Table 14.1	Causes of cell damage or death
Category	**Examples**
Hypoxia (an extremely common accompaniment of clinical disease)	Loss of blood supply due to narrowing (atheromatous plaques) or blocking (thrombosis) of artery or vein; ischemic-perfusion injury; inadequate oxygenation due to cardiorespiratory failure; loss of oxygen-carrying capacity, CO poisoning, and anemia
Chemicals and drugs	Environmental pollutants—lead, mercury; drugs-use and abuse; alcohol; tobacco
Physical agents	Trauma; extremes of heat and radiation; electrical energy; toxic chemicals
Microbiological agents	Bacteria, viruses, fungi, protozoa, and helminths
Immune mechanisms	Immune disorders can cause tissue damage by a number of mechanisms: (1) anaphylaxis (causing release of vasoactive amines), (2) cytotoxicity (causing the target cell to be lysed) (3) immune complex disease (leading to release of lysosomal enzymes) (4) Cell-mediated hypersensitivity (leading to cytotoxicity)
Genetic defects	Disorders with polygenic inheritance-diabetes mellitus, gout, Mendelian disorders-X-linked disorders, autosomal dominant and recessive disorders, disorders with variable modes of transmission and inborn errors of metabolism
Nutritional disorders	Protein-calorie malnutrition, vitamin deficiencies, mineral deficiencies; obesity and its consequences

The driving force of enzyme release is the steep concentration gradient that exists between the interior and the exterior of the cells. The rate of escape of enzyme molecules is presumably controlled to some extent by diffusion; therefore, smaller enzyme molecules might be expected to appear in the extracellular fluid earlier than larger ones.

The way in which released enzyme molecules are transferred from the interstitial fluid to the blood varies from one tissue to another; they may pass directly through the capillary wall, or lymphatic transfer may occur. Direct transfer occurs to a large extent in the liver, which is a highly vascular tissue with many permeable capillaries, although evidence suggests that liver enzymes may also be subject to lymphatic transfer.

On the other hand, the capillaries of skeletal muscle are relatively impermeable, and in this tissue it is probable that released enzymes mainly reach the circulatory system by way of drainage from the lymphatic system. Lymph drainage is also important in transporting enzymes released from damaged intestinal, pancreatic, and myocardial cells to the circulation, although, following myocardial infarction, a minor proportion of myocardial enzymes reaches the circulation by direct capillary transfer.

The intracellular location of the leaking enzymes affects the rates at which they appear in the circulation. As would be expected, the most c-indicators of cell damage are the molecules that are present in the soluble fraction of the cell.

Release of structurally bound membrane proteins requires both a leaky cell membrane and a dissociation or degradation, which is a slower process. Enzymes associated with subcellular structures, such as mito-chondria, are less readily released into the circulation and often indicate irreversible cellular injury. This fact has been used in attempts to distinguish reversible leakage, presumed to reflect damage only to the cell membrane, from necrotic lesions, in which intracellular structures are destroyed.

The relation between tissue injury and the appearance of enzymes in the circulation is most clearly seen in myocardial infarction, in which a relatively short episode of damage is followed by rapid transfer of enzymes to the circulatory system. About 24 hours after a myocardial infarction, the pattern of relative activity of various enzymes in the circulatory system closely resembles that in myocardial tissue. These relationships are less clearly recognized in other conditions, such as chronic liver disease, in which enzyme release is a process that continues over a period of time. The pattern of relative enzyme activities in serum in chronic disease may also become distorted by differential rates of removal of enzymes from the circulation and possibly by differential changes in rates of enzyme synthesis in affected tissue.

Release of enzymes from damaged or dying cells and changes in the rate of enzyme production constitute the most important mechanisms by which changes in enzyme activity in the serum or plasma are produced. However, other possibilities exist and appear to account for some changes of diagnostic importance. For example, much of the γ-glutamyl transferase activity of liver cells is located on their exterior surfaces. It is possible that ectoenzymes, such as this may be eluted from the surfaces, especially where detergent action of the blood is increased through accumulation of bile salts. This process does not involve cell damage in the sense of increased membrane permeability, as evidenced by lack of correlation between activities in the serum of γ-glutamyltransferase and the aminotransferases in liver disease of different types.

MUSCLE ENZYMES

Enzymes in this category include creatine kinase, aldolase, and glycogen phosphorylase.

CREATINE KINASE

Creatine kinase (CK) (EC 2.7.3.2; adenosine triphosphate: creatine N-phosphotransferase; CK) is a dimeric enzyme (82 kDa) that catalyzes the reversible phosphorylation of creatine (Cr) by adenosine triphosphate (ATP).

Physiologically, when muscle contracts, ATP is converted to adenosine diphosphate (ADP), and CK catalyzes there phosphorylation of ADP to ATP using creatine phosphate (CrP) as the phosphorylation reservoir.

Optimal pH values for the forward (Cr + ATP to ADP +CrP) and reverse (CrP + ADP to ATP + Cr) reactions are 9.0 and 6.7, respectively. At neutral pH, the formation of ATP is favored; a pH of 9.0 is optimal for the formation of CrP, another high-energy compound. Mg^{2+} is an obligate activating ion that forms complexes with ATP and ADP. The optimal concentration range for Mg^{2+} is narrow, and excess Mg^{2+} is inhibitory. Many metal ions, such as Mn^{2+}, Ca^{2+}, Zn^{2+}, and Cu^{2+}, inhibit enzyme activity, as do iodoacetate and other sulfhydryl-binding reagents. Activity is inhibited by excess ADP and by citrate, fluoride, nitrate, acetate, iodide, bromide, malonate, and L-thyroxine. Urate and cystine are potent inhibitors of the enzyme in serum. Even chloride and sulfate ions inhibit activity, and the concentrations of these ions should be kept low in any enzyme assay system based on the CrP + ADP (reverse) reaction. The enzyme in serum is relatively unstable, activity being lost as a result of sulfhydryl group oxidation at the active site of the enzyme. Activity can be partially restored by incubating the enzyme preparation with sulfhydryl compounds, such as N-acetyl cysteine, dithiothreitol (Cleland reagent), and glutathione. The current agent of choice is N-acetyl cysteine, which has the advantage of being a very soluble substance used at a final concentration of 20 mmol/L in the assay reagent. CK activity is greatest in striated muscle and heart tissue, which contain some 2500 and 550 U/g of protein, respectively.

Other tissues, such as the brain, the gastrointestinal tract, and the urinary bladder, contain significantly less activity, and the liver and erythrocytes are essentially devoid of activity. CK is a dimer composed of two subunits, each with a molecular weight of about 40,000 Da. These subunits (B and M) are the products of loci on chromosomes 14 and 19, respectively. Because the active form of the enzyme is a dimer, only three different pairs of subunits can exist: BB (or CK-1), MB (or CK-2), and MM (or CK-3). The Commission on Biochemical Nomenclature has recommended that isoenzymes be numbered on the basis of their electrophoretic mobility, with the most anodal form receiving the lowest number. Accordingly, the CK isoenzymes are numbered CK-1, CK-2, and CK-3. All three of these isoenzyme species are found in the cytosol of the cell or are associated with myofibrillar structures. However, there exists a fourth form that differs from the others both immunologically and by electrophoretic mobility.

This isoenzyme (CK-Mt) is located between the inner and outer membranes of mitochondria, and it constitutes, in the heart for example, up to 15% of total CK activity. The gene for CK-Mt is located on chromosome 15. CK activity may also be found in macromolecular form the so-called macro-CK. Macro-CK is found, often transiently, in the sera of up to 6% of hospitalized patients, but only a minor proportion of these have increased CK activities in serum. It exists in two forms: types 1 and 2. Type 1 is a complex of CK, typically CK-BB, and an immunoglobulin, often IgG, but other complexes have been described, such as CK-MM with IgA. Macro-CK type 1 is not of pathologic significance, but it can be the cause of elevated CK results, resulting in diagnostic confusion and leading to unnecessary further investigation. Prevalence has been estimated at between 0.8% and 2.3%, but this is dependent on the method used and the population studied. Macro-CK type 2 is oligomeric CK-Mt, with a reported prevalence of between 0.5% and 2.6%. It is found predominantly in adults who are severely ill with malignancy or liver disease, or in children who have notable tissue distress. The appearance of this isoenzyme in serum is usually associated with a poor prognosis. Macro-CK can interfere with the assay of CK-MB by some immunoinhibition methods.

Both M and B subunits have a C-terminal lysine residue, but only the former can be hydrolyzed by the action of carboxypeptidases present in blood. Carboxy peptidases B (EC 3.4.17.2) and N (arginine carboxy-peptidase; EC 3.4.17.3) sequentially hydrolyze the lysine residues from CK-MM to produce two CK-MM isoforms: CK-MM2 (one lysine residue removed) and CK-MM! (Both lysine residues removed). Loss of the positively charged lysine produces a more negatively charged CK molecule with greater anodic mobility at electrophoresis.

Because CK-MB has only one M subunit, the dimer coded by the M and B genes is named CK -MB2 and the lysine hydrolyzed dimer is named CK-MB. The assay of the CK isoforms requires a special technique, such as high-voltage electrophoresis (with gel cooling), high-performance liquid chromatography (HPLC), or immunoassay.

Clinical Significance

Serum CK is increased in nearly all patients when injury, inflammation, or necrosis of skeletal or heart muscle occurs. Elevation of serum CK activity may be the only sign of subclinical neuromuscular disorders. In case series, 30–44% of asymptomatic subjects with persistent hyper CKemia up to fivefold the upper reference limit (URL) have myopathy.

Serum CK activity is greatly elevated in all types of muscular dystrophy. In progressive muscular dystrophy (particularly Duchenne sex-linked muscular dystrophy), enzyme activity in serum is highest in infancy and childhood (7–10 years of age) and may be increased long before the disease is clinically apparent. Serum CK activity characteristically falls as patients get older and as the mass of functioning muscle diminishes with progression of the disease. About 50–80% of asymptomatic female carriers of Duchenne dystrophy show threefold to sixfold increases in CK activity. High values of CK are noted in viral myositis, polymyositis, and similar muscle diseases. However, in neurogenic muscle diseases, such as myasthenia gravis, multiple sclerosis, poliomyelitis, and Parkinsonism, serum enzyme activity is not increased. Very high activity is also encountered in malignant hyperthermia, an inherited life-threatening condition characterized by high fever and brought on by administration of inhalation anesthesia (usually halothane) to the affected individual.

Skeletal muscle that is diseased or damaged (such as by extreme exercise) may contain significant proportions of CK-MB owing to the phenomenon of 'fetal reversion;' in which fetal patterns of protein synthesis reappear. Thus, serum CK-MB isoenzyme may increase in such circumstances. This explanation may also account for the elevated CK-MB values sometimes observed in chronic renal failure (uremic myopathy).

In acute rhabdomyolysis due to crush injury, with severe muscle destruction, serum CK activities exceeding 200 times the URL may be found. If the CK remains below 5000 U/L (about 30 times the URL) during the first 3 days after the insult, the probability of developing acute renal failure appears to be low. Serum CK can also be increased by other direct trauma to muscle, including intramuscular injection and surgical intervention. Finally, a number of drugs when given at pharmacologic doses can increase serum CK activities. The drugs principally responsible are statins, fibrates, antiretrovirals, and angiotensin II receptor antagonists. Varying degrees of myopathy may occur with statin use, ranging from mild myalgic syndrome alone to rhabdomyolysis (0.02%).

Changes in serum CK and its MB isoenzyme following acute myocardial infarction have been the mainstay of diagnosis for many years. However, it is now more advantageous to use more cardiac-specific non-enzymatic markers, such as cardiac troponin I or T. CK-MB determination can still be used with some success to estimate the extent of myocardial necrosis to assist with assessment of infarct prognosis. When peak CK-MB is compared with estimates of infarct size, good correlations can be obtained. A problem with using CK-MB for this purpose is the requirement for frequent sampling to ensure that peak CK-MB values are correctly identified.

Hypothyroidism is a common cause of endocrine myopathy. About 60% of hypothyroid subjects show an average elevation of CK activity fivefold greater than the URL. The major isoenzyme present is CK-MM, suggesting muscular involvement.

During normal childbirth, a sixfold elevation in maternal total serum CK activity occurs. Surgical intervention during labor further increases the activity of CK in serum. CK-BB may be elevated in neonates, particularly in brain-damaged or very low birth weight newborns. The presence of CK-BB in blood, usually at low concentrations, may however represent a physiologic finding in the first days of life.

METHODS FOR DETERMINATION OF CREATINE KINASE ACTIVITY

Numerous photometric, fluorometric, and coupled enzyme methods have been developed for the assay of CK activity, using the forward ($Cr \rightarrow CrP$) or the reverse ($Cr \leftarrow CrP$) reaction. Currently, all commercial assays for total CK are based on the reverse reaction, which proceeds about six times faster than the forward reaction.

$$\text{Creatine phosphate} + ADP \xrightarrow[\text{pH } 6.7]{CK} \text{Creatine} + ADP$$

$$ADP + \text{glucose} \xrightarrow{HK} \text{glucose-6-phosphate} + ADP$$

$$\text{Glucose-6-phosphate} + NADP^{\oplus} \xrightarrow{G6PD} \text{6-phosphoglucorate} + NADPH + H^{\oplus}$$

CK catalyzes the conversion of CrP to Cr with concomitant phosphorylation of ADP to ATP. The ATP produced is measured by hexokinase (HK)/glucose-6-phosphate dehydrogenase (G6PD) coupled reactions that ultimately convert NADP+ to NADPH, which is monitored spectrophotometrically at 340 nm. The assay colleagues optimized by adding N-acetyl cysteine to activate CK, EDTA to bind Ca^{2+} and to increase the stability of the reaction mixture, and adenosine penta-phosphate (ApsA) in addition to AMP to inhibit adenylate kinase (AK). The 8SA reference method based on this previous experience was developed by the International Federation of Clinical Chemistry and Laboratory Medicine (IFCC) for the measurement of CK at 37°C. Specimens for CK analysis include serum and plasma heparin. Anticoagulants other than heparin should not be used in collection tubes because they inhibit CK activity. CK activity in serum is relatively unstable and is rapidly lost during storage. Average stabilities are less than 8 hours at room temperature, 48 hours at 4°C, and 1 month at −20°C. Therefore, the serum specimen should be chilled to 4°C, if the serum is not analyzed immediately, and stored at −80°C, if analysis is delayed for longer than 30 days. It is not necessary to add any thiol agent for storage because the optimized assay formulation containing ethylenediaminetetraacetic acid (EDTA), 2 mmol/L, and N-acetyl cysteine, 20 mmol/L, reactivates CK in serum to the extent of 99% after it has been stored for 1 week at 4°C. A moderate degree of hemolysis is tolerated because erythrocytes contain no CK activity. However, severely hemolyzed specimens are unsatisfactory because enzymes and intermediates (AK, ATP, and G6P) liberated from the erythrocytes may affect the lag phase and side reactions occurring in the assay system.

Reference Intervals

Serum CK activity is subject to a number of physiologic variations. It is influenced by sex, age, race, muscle mass, and physical activity. The distributions of CK activity are notably skewed toward higher values in reference populations. Men have higher values than women, and blacks have higher values than non-blacks. In white subjects, the reference interval was found to be 46–171 U/L for males and 34–145 U/L for females, when measured with an assay traceable to the IFCC 37°C reference procedure. Newborns generally have higher CK activity resulting from skeletal muscle trauma during birth.

Serum CK in infants decreases to the adult reference interval by 6–10 weeks. CK activity in the serum of healthy people is due almost exclusively to CK-MM activity (although, small amounts of CK-MB may be present) and is the result of physiologic turnover of muscle tissue. Exercise and muscle trauma can increase serum CK. Sustained exercise, such as that performed by well-trained long-distance runners, increases the CK-MB content of skeletal muscle, which may produce abnormal serum CK-MB concentrations.

ALDOLASE

Aldolase (EC 4.1.2.13; D-fructose-1, 6-bisdiphosphate D glyceraldehyde-3-phosphate-lyase; ALD) catalyzes the splitting of D-fructose-1, 6-diphosphate to D-glyceraldehyde-3-phosphate (GLAP) and dihydroxy-acetone-phosphate (DAP), an important reaction in the glycolytic breakdown of glucose to lactate.

ALD is a tetramer with subunits determined by three separate gene loci. Only two of these loci, those producing A and B subunits, appear to be active simultaneously in most tissues, so the most common isoenzyme pattern consists of various proportions of the components of a five-member set of isoenzymes, of which two members correspond to the A and B homopolymers. The locus that determines the structure of the C subunit is active in brain tissue, as is the A locus, so this tissue contains ALD A and C, together with the three corresponding hetero-polymers.

Clinical Significance

Serum ALD determinations have been of some clinical interest in primary diseases of skeletal muscle. Some researchers believe that increased ALD activity is useful in distinguishing neuromuscular atrophies from myopathies in combination with the CK/AST ratio. In general, however, measurement of ALD activity in the serum of subjects with suspected muscle disease does not add information to that available more readily from measurement of other enzymes, especially CK. ALD measurement has largely been discontinued within clinical laboratories and is not routinely available.

METHODS FOR MEASUREMENT OF ALDOLASE ACTIVITY

All assay methods are based on the forward ALD-catalyzed reaction. In the analytical approach on which all commonly used procedures and kits are based, the ALD reaction is coupled with two other enzyme reactions. Triosephosphate isomerase (EC 5.3.1.1) is added to ensure rapid conversion of all GLAP to DAP. Glycerol-3-phosphate dehydrogenase (EC 1.1.1.8) is added to reduce DAP to glycerol-3-phosphate, with NADH acting as hydrogen donor. The decrease in NADH concentration is then measured.

ALD activity in serum is quite stable. Activity is unchanged at ambient temperatures for up to 48 hours and at 4°C for several days. Hemolyzed specimens should not be used; plasma is preferred over serum because of the possible release of platelet enzyme during the clotting process.

Reference Intervals

The reference interval for the activity of ALD in adults is 2.5–10 U/L, measured at 37°C. However, a definite sex difference has been noted, with men having higher values. Serum ALD activity in the neonate is fourfold that seen in adult, and in children is twice that in the adult. Adult values are attained by the time the child reaches puberty.

LIVER ENZYMES

Enzymes in this category include alkaline phosphatase, alanine and aspartate aminotransferases, glutamate dehydrogenase, Sf-nucleotidase, γ-glutamyl transferase, and glutathione S-transferase. The alkaline phosphatase, aminotransferases, and γ-glutamyl transferase, are widely used and available on automated analyzers.

The most common alterations in liver enzyme activities encountered in clinical practice is divided into two major pathophysiology subgroups-hepatocellular damage (elevated transaminase and glutamate dehydrogenase activities) and cholestasis (elevated alkaline phosphatase, Sf-nucleotidase, and γ-glutamyl transferase activities); although certain liver diseases may display a mixed biochemical picture.

ALKALINE PHOSPHATASE

Alkaline phosphatase [EC 3.1.3.1; or thophosphoric monoester phosphohydrolase (alkaline optimum); ALP] catalyzes the alkaline hydrolysis of a large variety of naturally occurring and synthetic substrates.

ALP activity is present in most organs of the body and is especially associated with membranes and cell surfaces located in the mucosa of the small intestine and the proximal convoluted tubules of the kidney, in bone (osteoblasts), liver, and placenta. Although the exact metabolic function of the enzyme is not yet understood, it appears that ALP is associated with lipid transport in the intestine and with the calcification process in bone. ALP exists in multiple forms, some of which are true isoenzymes, encoded at separate genetic loci. Bone, liver, and kidney ALP forms share a common primary structure coded for by the same genetic locus, but they differ in carbohydrate content.

Some divalent ions, such as Mg^{2+}, CO^{2+}, and Mn^{2+}, are activators of the enzyme, and Zn^{2+} is a constituent metal ion. The correct ratio of Mg^{2+}/Zn^{2+} ions is necessary to avoid displacement of Mg^{2+} and to attain optimal activity. Phosphate, borate, oxalate, and cyanide ions are inhibitors of ALP activity. Variations in Mg^{2+} and substrate concentrations change the pH optimum. The type of buffer present (except at low concentrations) affects the rate of enzyme activity. Buffers can be classified as inert (carbonate and barbital), inhibiting (glycine and propylamine), or activating [2-amino-2-methyl-1-propanol (AMP), tris (hydroxymethyl) aminomethane (TRIS), and diethanolamine (DEA)].

The ALP activity present in the sera of healthy adults originates mainly in the liver, with most of the rest coming from the skeleton. The respective contributions of these two forms to the total activity are age dependent. Minimal amounts of intestinal ALP may also be present, particularly in the sera of individuals of blood group B or O (i.e. those which are secretors of blood group substances). Because intestinal ALP activity in serum may increase after a meal, ALP should be measured preferentially in fasting sera.

Elevations in serum ALP activity commonly originate from one or both of two sources: liver and bone. Consequently, serum ALP measurements are of particular interest in the investigation of two groups of conditions: hepatobiliary disease and bone disease associated with increased osteoblastic activity (see 'Bone Enzymes' section later in this chapter).

Serum ALP was the first enzyme to be used for the investigation of hepatic disease. The response of the liver to any form of biliary tree obstruction induces the synthesis of ALP by hepatocytes. Some of the newly formed enzyme enters the circulation to increase the enzyme activity in serum. Elevation tends to be more notable (greater than threefold) in extrahepatic obstruction (e.g. by stone, by cancer of the head of the pancreas) than in intrahepatic obstruction and is greater the more complete the obstruction. Serum enzyme activities may reach 10–12 times the upper reference limit and usually return to normal on surgical removal of the obstruction. A similar increase is seen in patients with advanced primary liver cancer or widespread secondary hepatic metastases. Liver diseases that principally affect parenchymal cells, such as infectious hepatitis, typically show only moderately (less than threefold) increased or even normal serum ALP activities. Increases may also be seen as a consequence of a reaction to drug therapy. Intestinal ALP isoenzyme, an asialoglycoprotein normally cleared by the hepatic asialoglycoprotein receptors, is often elevated in patients with liver cirrhosis.

An increase of up to 2–3 times normal is observed in women in the third trimester of pregnancy, with the additional enzyme being of placental origin. Reports have also described a benign familial elevation in serum ALP activity due to increased concentrations of intestinal ALP. Transient, benign increases in serum ALP may be observed in infants and children, with changes often more than 10 times the upper reference limit. Increases in both liver and bone forms are seen. These changes seem to reflect a reduction in the removal of ALP from blood caused by transient modifications of enzyme glycosylation.

A result of the application of techniques of isoenzyme analysis to the characterization of ALP in serum was the discovery that forms of the enzyme essentially identical to the normal placental isoenzyme appear in the sera of some patients with malignant disease. These carcino placental isoenzymes (e.g. Regan isoenzyme) appear to result from de-repression of the placental ALP gene. As described later, the presence of these isoenzymes can be readily detected in serum by their stability at 65°C. Tumors have also been found to produce ALPs that appear to be modified forms of nonplacental isoenzymes (Kasahara isoenzyme).

METHODS FOR DETERMINATION OF ALKALINE PHOSPHATASE ACTIVITY

Numerous methods have been developed for determining ALP activity. In general, methodologic developments have been directed toward increasing the speed and sensitivity of the assay by selecting readily hydrolyzed substrates and phosphate-accepting buffers, and toward the use of continuous-monitoring methods based on 'self-indicating' substrates.

The most popular of the chromogenic or self-indicating substrates for ALP is 4-nitrophenyl phosphate (usually abbreviated 4-NPP, or PNPP from the older name, p-nitrophenylphosphate). This ester is colorless, but the final product is yellow at the pH of the reaction.

The enzyme reaction is continuously monitored by observing the rate of formation of the 4-nitrophenoxide ions. With improvement in reaction conditions, this reaction forms the basis of current recommended and standard methods of ALP assay.

Other self-indicating substrates include phenolphthalein monophosphate, thymolphthalein phosphate, and α-naphthyl phosphate. With the ALP methods discussed, the liberated phosphate group is transferred to water. The rate of phosphatase action is enhanced, however, if certain amino alcohols are used as phosphate-accepting buffers.

Among these activators are compounds, such as AMP, DEA, TRIS, ethylaminoethanol (EAE), and N-methyl-D-glucamine(MEG). Enzyme activity in the presence of optimal concentrations of these buffers is twofold to sixfold greater than in the presence of a non-activating buffer, such as carbonate.

ALP catalyzes the hydrolysis of 4-NPP, forming phosphate and free 4-nitrophenol (4-NP, PNP), which in dilute acid solutions is colorless. Under alkaline conditions, 4-NP is converted to the 4-nitrophenoxide ion, which has a very intense yellow color. The rate of formation of 4-NP by the action of the enzyme on 4-NPP at 37°C is then monitored at 405 nm with a recording spectrophotometer. The (provisional) IFCC recommended method uses 4-NPP as the substrate and AMP as the phosphate-acceptor buffer. It includes Mg^{2+} and Zn^{2+}, optimal concentrations of which are controlled by the addition of Mg^{2+} and Zn^{2+}, and the chelating agent N-hydroxyethyl ethylenediaminetriacetic acid (HEDTA). Although, Zn^{2+} ions are present in a total concentration of 1 mmol/L, most are bound to HEDTA, leaving only a small, experimentally determined optimal concentration of free ions. A similar situation exists for Mg^{2+} ions. Thus, HEDTA acts as a metal ion buffer, maintaining optimal concentrations of both ions.

Serum or heparinized plasma, free of hemolysis, should be used. Complexing anticoagulants, such as citrate, oxalate, and EDTA must be avoided, because they bind cations, such as Mg^{2+} and Zn^{2+}, which are necessary cofactors for ALP activity measurement. Blood transfusion (containing citrate) causes a transient decrease in serum ALP through a similar mechanism. Freshly collected serum samples should be kept at room temperature and assayed as soon as possible but preferably within 4 hours after collection. In sera stored at a refrigerated temperature, ALP activity increases slowly (2% per day). Frozen specimens should be thawed and kept at room temperature for 18–24 hours before measurement to achieve full enzyme reactivation.

ALP activities in serum vary with age (Table 14.2). Children show higher ALP activity than healthy adults as a result of the leakage of bone ALP from osteoblasts during bone growth. Using methods traceable to the IFCC procedure at 37°C, the following reference intervals (central 95-percentiles) have been established.

Methods for Separation and Quantification of Alkaline Phosphatase Isoenzymes

Assays for ALP isoenzymes are needed when (1) the source of an elevated ALP in serum is not obvious and should be clarified; (2) the main clinical question is concerned with detecting the presence of liver or bone involvement; and (3) it is important to ascertain any modifications in the activity of osteoblasts to monitor disease activity and the effects of appropriate therapies in the case of metabolic bone disorders.

Criteria that have been used to differentiate the isoenzymes and other multiple forms of ALP include (1) electrophoretic mobility; (2) stability to denaturation by heat or chemicals; (3) response to the presence of selected inhibitors; (4) affinity for specific lectins; and (5) immunochemical characteristics.

The same electrophoretic techniques are used for the separation of ALP isoenzymes in serum as for separation of serum proteins. After electrophoresis, ALP zones are made visible by incubating the gel in a solution of buffered substrate (e.g. 1-naphthyl phosphate, to which a chromogenic system, usually represented by a diazonium salt, is added; in the case of electrophoresis on cellulose acetate, the strips are covered with an agar gel layer containing the staining system). The liver ALP typically moves most rapidly toward the anode.

Table 14.2	ALP activity reference interval	
Sex	**Age**	**Reference interval**
Males/Females	4–15 years	54–369 U/L
Males	20–50 years	53–128 U/L
	≥60 years	56–116 U/L
Females	20–50 years	42–98 U/L
	≥60 years	53–141 U/L

Bone ALP, which typically gives a more diffuse zone than the liver form, has slightly reduced anodal mobility, although the two zones usually overlap to some extent. Intestinal ALP migrates more slowly than the bone enzyme, whereas the placental isoenzyme commonly appears as a discrete band overlying the diffuse bone fraction. An additional band, which is frequently present in the serum of patients with various hepatic diseases, contains a high molecular weight form of ALP, but is also strongly negatively charged. Therefore, it moves slowly in starch gel or may even fail to enter polyacrylamide gel, but it migrates more anodally than the main liver zone on non-sieving media, such as cellulose acetate.

Investigations of this form have revealed that it corresponds to the main liver form attached to the membrane moiety. Complexes between ALP and immunoglobulins, ormacro-ALP, occur occasionally in serum, giving rise to abnormally migrating bands in the α-globulin zone; however, they do not provide specific diagnostic information in the present state of knowledge.

Two approaches have been proposed to improve the electrophoretic separation between bone and liver ALPs. Both methods exploit differences in the carbohydrate portions of the two forms of ALP. With one, electrophoresis is carried out in the presence of wheat germ lectin, binding the N-acetylglucosamine residues present in different amounts on individual fractions, which retards bone ALP migration more than liver enzyme migration. With the other, serum is treated briefly (i.e. for 15 minutes at 37°C) with neuraminidase to remove a portion of the terminal sialic acid residues. Because the sialic acid residues of bone ALP are more readily attacked than those of liver ALP, the electrophoretic mobility of the bone form is reduced more than that of liver ALP. The improved separation allows quantitative estimates to be made by densitometric scanning (Fig. 14.1). As an alternative to electrophoretic fractionation of ALP, measurement of γ-glutamyl transferase, which is increased in liver disease but not in bone disease, may be a useful rapid tool to distinguish between the two diseases as the explanation for an increased serum ALP.

Overnight incubation of the serum sample with neuraminidase is used to confirm the presence of intestinal ALP.

This treatment reduces the anodal mobility of all ALP isoenzymes except that of intestinal origin, which is neuraminidase resistant because terminal sialic acid residues are not present in the molecule. Because placental ALP is heat stable, incubation of the serum sample at a temperature as high as 65°C for 30 minutes provides a convenient test for the presence of this isoenzyme. Immunologic methods provide the best quantitative measurements of intestinal or placental ALPs.

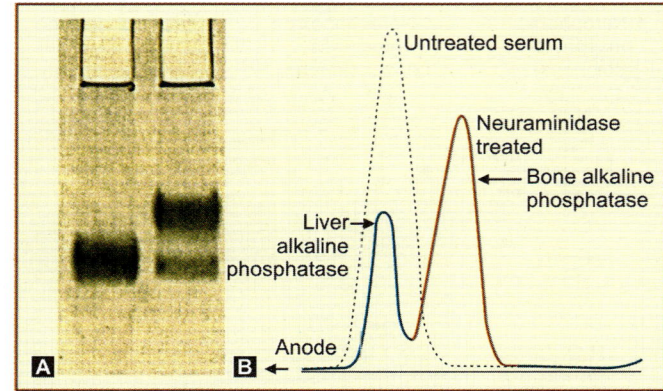

Fig. 14.1: (A) Polyacrylamide-gel electrophoresis of bone and liver alkaline phosphatases in human serum. Left, mixture of two sera containing, respectively, entirely bone phosphatase and entirely liver phosphatase. Right, mixture of the same two sera after each has been treated with neuraminidase for 10 minutes at 37°C. The anodal direction is downward. The more anodal zone is liver phosphatase. (B) Densitometric scans of electrophoretic patterns shown in A. Broken line, scan of mixture of untreated sera; solid line, scan of mixture of sera treated briefly with neuraminidase

Much more difficult is the production of antibodies that selectively react with different products of the tissue nonspecific ALP gene, including liver- and bone-derived isoforms, as these antibodies should recognize specific sugar side-chains instead of a particular amino acid sequence. Until now, no monoclonal antibodies have fully discriminated between liver and bone ALPs. Despite lack of complete specificity, commercially available immunoassays of bone ALP may offer some advantages, but their value has not been convincingly demonstrated, in part because measurements of total ALP provide the required clinical information in many situations

AMINOTRANSFERASES

The aminotransferases constitute a group of enzymes that catalyze the interconversion of amino acids to 2-oxo-acids by transfer of amino groups. Aspartate aminotransferase (EC 2.6.1.1; L-aspartate:2-oxoglutarate aminotransferase; AST) and alanine aminotransferase (EC 2.6.1.2; L-alanine: 2-oxoglutarate aminotransferase; ALT) are examples of aminotransferases that are of clinical interest. The 2-oxoglutarate/L-glutamate couple serves as one amino group acceptor and donor pair in all amino-transfer reactions; the specificity of the individual enzymes derives from the particular amino acid that serves as the other donor of an amino group. Thus, AST catalyzes the as shown on next page.

The reactions are reversible, but the equilibria of the AST and ALT reactions favor formation of aspartate and alanine respectively. Pyridoxal-5′-phosphate (P-5′-P) and its amino analog, pyridoxamine-5′-phosphate, function

$$\underset{\text{L-asparate}}{\overset{\text{COO}^\ominus}{\underset{\text{COO}^\ominus}{|}}\underset{}{\text{H-C-NH}_2}} + \underset{\text{2-oxoglutarate}}{\text{C=O}} \overset{\text{AST, P-5'-P}}{\rightleftharpoons} \underset{\text{Oxaloacetate}}{\text{C=O}} + \underset{\text{L-glutamate}}{\text{H-C-NH}_2}$$

ALT catalyzes the analogous reaction as follows:

$$\underset{\text{L-alanine}}{\text{H-C-NH}_2} + \underset{\text{2-oxoglutarate}}{\text{C=O}} \overset{\text{ALT, P-5'-P}}{\rightleftharpoons} \underset{\text{Pyruvate}}{\text{C=O}} + \underset{\text{L-glutamate}}{\text{H-C-NH}_2}$$

as coenzymes in amino-transfer reactions. The P-5′ -P is bound to the apoenzyme and serves as a true prosthetic group. P-5′-P bound to the apoenzyme accepts the amino group from the first substrate, aspartate or alanine, to form enzyme-bound pyridoxamine-5′-phosphate and the first reaction product, oxaloacetate or pyruvate, respectively. The coenzyme in amino form then transfers its amino group to the second substrate, 2-oxoglutarate, to form the second product, glutamate. P-5′-P is thus regenerated.

Both coenzyme-deficient apoenzymes and holo-enzymes may be present in serum. Therefore, addition of P-5′-P under conditions that allow recombination with the enzymes usually produces an increase in amino-transferase activity. In accordance with the principle that all factors affecting the rate of reaction must be optimized and controlled, the IFCC recommends addition of P-5′-P in aminotransferase methods to ensure that all enzymatic activity is measured. Transaminases are widely distributed throughout the body. AST is found primarily in the heart, liver, skeletal muscle, and kidney, whereas ALT is found primarily in the liver and kidney, with lesser amounts in heart and skeletal muscle. ALT is exclusively cytoplasmic; both mitochondrial and cytoplasmic forms of AST are found in cells. These are genetically distinct isoenzymes with a dimeric structure composed of two identical polypeptide subunits of about 400 amino acid residues.

Clinical Significance

Liver disease is the most important cause of increased transaminase activity in serum. In most types of liver disease, ALT activity is higher than that of AST; exceptions may be seen in alcoholic hepatitis, hepatic cirrhosis, and liver neoplasia. In viral hepatitis and other forms of liver disease associated with acute hepatic necrosis, serum AST and ALT activities are elevated even before the clinical signs and symptoms of disease (such as jaundice) appear. Activities for both enzymes may reach values as high as 100 times the upper reference limit, although 10-fold to 40-fold elevations are most frequently encountered. The most efficient aminotransferase threshold for diagnosing acute liver injury lies at 7 times the upper reference limit (sensitivity and specificity >95%). Peak values of transaminase activity occur between the 7th day and 12th day; activities then gradually decrease, reaching normal levels by the 3rd week to 5th week, if recovery is uneventful.

Peak activities bear no relationship to prognosis and may fall with worsening of the patient's condition. Persistence of increased ALT for longer than 6 months after an episode of acute hepatitis is used to diagnose chronic hepatitis. Most patients with chronic hepatitis have maximum ALT less than 7 times the upper reference limit. ALT may be persistently normal in 15–50% of patients with chronic hepatitis C, but the likelihood of continuously normal ALT decreases with an increasing number of measurements. In patients with acute hepatitis C, ALT should be measured periodically over the next 1–2 years to determine if it becomes and stays normal.

The picture in toxic hepatitis is different from that in infectious hepatitis. In acetaminophen-induced hepatic injury, the transaminase peak is more than 85 times the upper reference limit in 90% of cases—a value rarely seen with acute viral hepatitis. Furthermore, AST and ALT activities typically peak early and fall rapidly.

Nonalcoholic fatty liver disease (NAFLD) is the most common cause of aminotransferase increases other than viral and alcoholic hepatitis. NAFLD includes a spectrum of liver pathology, from simple steatosis to nonalcoholic steatohepatitis (NASH), in which inflammatory changes and focal necrosis may progress to liver fibrosis, cirrhosis, and hepatic failure. NAFLD is now considered to be an additional feature of the 'metabolic syndrome.' Indeed serum aminotransferase elevation in NAFLD is associated with higher body mass index, waist circumference, serum triglycerides, and fasting insulin and lower HDL cholesterol; all features characteristic of this syndrome.

Aminotransferase activities observed in cirrhosis vary with the status of the cirrhotic process and range from the upper reference limit to 4–5 times higher, with an AST/ALT ratio (AAR) greater than 1. This appears to be attributable to a reduction in ALT production in a damaged liver, associated with reduced clearance of AST in advancing liver fibrosis. An AAR 21 has approximate 90% positive predictive value for diagnosing the presence of advanced fibrosis in patients with chronic liver disease. Furthermore, the amount of elevation in the AAR can reflect the grade of fibrosis in these patients.

Twofold to fivefold elevations of both enzymes occur in patients with primary or metastatic carcinoma of the liver, with AST usually being higher than ALT, but activities are often normal in the early stages of malignant infiltration of the liver. Slight or moderate elevations of AST and ALT activities have been observed after administration of various medications, such as non-steroidal anti-inflammatory drugs, antibiotics, antiepileptic drugs, statins, or opiates.

Over-the-counter medications and herbal preparations are also implicated. In patients with increased transaminases, negative viral markers, and a negative history for drugs or alcohol ingestion, the work-up should include less common causes of chronic hepatic injury (e.g. hemochromatosis, Wilson's disease, auto-immune hepatitis, primary biliary cirrhosis, sclerosing cholangitis, celiac disease, α 1-antitrypsin deficiency).

Although serum activities of both AST and ALT become elevated whenever disease processes affect liver cell integrity, ALT is the more liver-specific enzyme. Serum elevations of ALT activity are rarely observed in conditions other than parenchymal liver disease. Moreover, elevations of ALT activity persist longer than do those of AST activity. Thus, the incremental benefit of determination of AST, in addition to ALT, may be limited.

After acute myocardial infarction, increased AST activity appears in serum, as might be expected from the high AST concentration in heart muscle. AST activity is also increased in progressive muscular dystrophy and dermatomyositis, reaching concentrations up to 8 times normal; they are usually normal in other types of muscle disease, especially in those of neurogenic origin. Pulmonary emboli can increase AST to 2–3 times normal, and slight to moderate elevations are noted in acute pancreatitis, crushed muscle injury, and hemolytic disease.

Generally, mitochondrial AST (m-AST) activity in serum shows a marked increase in patients with extensive liver cell degeneration and necrosis. Of particular interest is the usefulness of the ratio between m-AST and total AST activities for diagnosing alcoholic hepatitis. The ratio seems to identify the liver cell 'necrotic type' condition (i.e. slight enzyme increase concomitant with relatively high activities of mitochondrial enzymes) typical of alcoholic hepatitis.

Several authors have described AST linked to immunoglobulins, or macro-AST. Typical findings include a persistent increase in serum AST activity in an asymptomatic subject, with absence of any demonstrable pathology in organs rich in AST. Increased AST activity might reflect decreased clearance of the abnormal complex from plasma. Macro-AST has no known clinical relevance. However, identification is important to avoid unnecessary diagnostic procedures in these subjects. Laboratory procedures for the demonstration of macro-AST include electrophoresis with specific enzyme stain (atypical origin band) and differential precipitation with polyethylene glycol.

METHODS FOR MEASUREMENT OF TRANSAMINASE ACTIVITY

The assay system for measuring transaminase activity contains two amino acids and two oxo-acids. Because no convenient method is available for assaying amino acids, formation or consumption of the oxo-acids is measured. Continuous monitoring methods are commonly used to measure transaminase activity by coupling transaminase reactions to specific dehydrogenase reactions. The oxo-acids formed in the transaminase reaction are measured indirectly by enzymatic reduction to corresponding hydroxy acids, and the accompanying change in NADH concentration is monitored spectrophotometrically. Thus, oxaloacetate, formed in the AST reaction, is reduced to malate in the presence of malate dehydrogenase (MD).

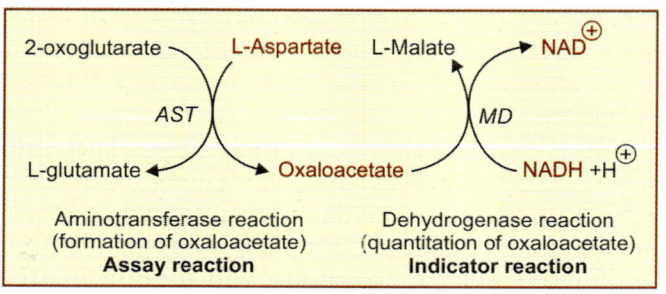

Aminotransferase reaction (formation of oxaloacetate) **Assay reaction**　　Dehydrogenase reaction (quantitation of oxaloacetate) **Indicator reaction**

Pyruvate formed in the ALT reaction is reduced to lactate by lactate dehydrogenase (LD). The substrate, NADH, and an auxiliary enzyme, MD or LD, must be present in sufficient quantity so that the reaction rate is limited only by the amounts of AST and ALT, respectively. As the reactions proceed, NADH is oxidized to NAD^+. The disappearance of NADH is followed by measuring the decrease in absorbance at 340 nm for several minutes, either continuously or at frequent intervals. The change in absorbance per minute (M/min) is proportional to the micromoles of NADH oxidized and in turn to micromoles of substrate transformed per minute. A preliminary incubation period is necessary to ensure that NADH-dependent reduction of endogenous oxo-acids in the sample is completed before 2-oxoglutarate is added to start the transaminase reaction. After a brief lag phase, the change in absorbance (M) is monitored. As already mentioned, supplementation with P-5-P ensures that all transaminase activity of the sample is measured.

Because of the large numbers of AST and ALT activity measurements performed daily in clinical laboratories throughout the world, standardization of transaminase measurements is a priority need for patient care. The reference system approach, based on the concepts of metrologic traceability and the hierarchy of analytical measurement procedures, gives clinical laboratories and the medical community universal means of creating and ensuring the comparability of results. In this system, the IFCC reference measurement procedure forms the highest metrologic level and thereby constitutes the definition of the respective measurable enzyme quantity. Primary IFCC procedures for the measurement of catalytic activity concentrations of AST and ALT at 37°C have been published. Values assigned to the manufacturer's product calibrators and measurement results of lower metrologic levels, including those used in daily routine practice, should be traceable to the top-level reference measurement procedures, thus improving the accuracy and comparability of transaminase results. Its hold be remembered that the concept of the reference system is valid only if the reference procedure and corresponding routine procedures have identical, or at least very similar, specificities for the measured enzyme. Thus, it will not be possible to calibrate procedures for aminotransferases that do not incorporate P-5'-P using a procedure that does, such as the IFCC reference procedure, because the ratio of pre-formed holoenzyme to apoenzyme differs among specimens.

AST activity in serum is stable for up to 48 hours at 4°C. Specimens have to be stored frozen if they are to be kept longer. ALT activity should be assayed on the day of sample collection because activity is lost at room temperature, 4°C, and –25°C. ALT stability is better maintained at –70°C. Hemolyzed specimens should not be used, especially when AST is measured, because of the large amount of this enzyme present in red cells.

Reference Intervals

Using methods traceable to the IFCC reference system, the AST upper reference limit for adults, calculated as the 97.5 percentile of the reference distribution, is 35 U/L, with no significant sex-related differences. Conversely, a clear difference in ALT activities has been noted between adult males and females. Corresponding ALT upper reference limits are 60 U/L and 42 U/L respectively. ALT does not reveal a distinct age dependency during childhood, whereas serum AST activity in neonates and in children younger than 3 years old is twice that in adults. Adult values are attained by the time the child reaches puberty.

GLUTAMATE DEHYDROGENASE

Glutamate dehydrogenase [EC 1.4.1.3; L-glutamate: NAD [oxidoreductase (deaminating) GLD] is a

mitochondrial enzyme found mainly in the liver, heart muscle, and kidneys, but small amounts occur in other tissue, including brain and skeletal muscle tissue, and in leukocytes.

GLD is a zinc-containing enzyme that consists of six polypeptide chains. The smallest active molecule has a molecular weight of about 350,000 Da, but larger polymers are also found. The enzyme catalyzes the removal of hydrogen from L-glutamate to form the corresponding ketimino-acid, which undergoes spontaneous hydrolysis to 2-oxoglutarate.

Although, NAD^+ is the preferred coenzyme, NADP+ also acts as the hydrogen acceptor. GLD is inhibited by metal ions, such as Ag^+ and Hg^+, by several chelating agents, and by L-thyroxine.

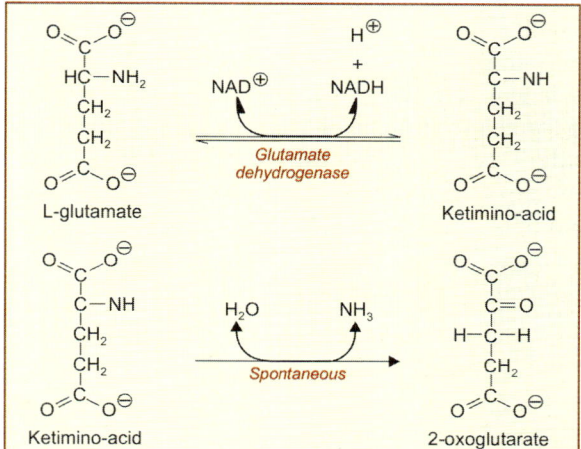

METHODS FOR DETERMINATION OF GLUTAMATE

Dehydrogenase Activity

Continuous-monitoring methods have been developed for determination of GLD using both forward and reverse reactions. The equilibrium favors the formation of glutamate, and higher reaction rates are observed when 2-oxoglutarate is used as a substrate. Serum is added to a solution of NADH, an ammonium salt, and ADP in buffer at pH 7.5, and the reaction is initiated by the addition of the substrate, 2-oxoglutarate. The rate of decrease in absorbance at 340 nm is measured. The German Society for Clinical Chemistry has published optimum reaction conditions for 37°C. Oxamate is incorporated into the reaction mixture because this acid inhibits LD activity, avoiding the critical consumption of NADH by this enzyme in serum. GLD activity in serum is stable at 4°C for 48 hours and at –20°C for several weeks.

Reference Intervals

The GLD upper reference limits are 6 U/L (women) and 8 U/L (men) when a method optimized at 37°C is used.

γ-GLUTAMYL TRANSFERASE

Peptidases are enzymes that catalyze the hydrolytic cleavage of peptides to form amino acids or smaller peptides. They constitute a broad group of enzymes of varied specificity, and some individual enzymes act as amino acid transferases and catalyze the transfer of amino acids from one peptide to another amino acid or peptide. γ-glutamyl transferase (EC2.3.2.2; γ-glutamyl -peptide: amino acid γ-glutamyl transferase; GGT) catalyzes the transfer of the γ-glutamyl group from peptides and compounds to an acceptor. They glutamyl acceptor is the substrate itself, some amino acid or peptide, or even water, in which case simple hydrolysis takes place. The enzyme acts only on peptides or peptide like compounds containing a terminal glutamate residue joined to the remainder of the compound through the terminal (-γ-) carboxyl. Glycylglycine is 5 times more effective as an acceptor than is glycine or the tripeptide (gly-gly-gly), but little is known about the optimal properties of the acceptor cosubstrate. The peptidase transfer reactionis considerably faster than the simple hydrolysis reaction. An example of a reaction catalyzed by the enzyme is shown here.

γ-glutamyl transferase is present (in decreasing order of abundance) in proximal renal tubule, liver, pancreas, and intestine. The enzyme is present in cytoplasm (microsomes), but the larger fraction is located in the cell membrane and may transport amino acids and peptides into the cell across the cell membrane in the form of γ-glutamyl peptides. GGT is critical for the maintenance of adequate intracellular levels of reduced glutathione, a major antioxidant agent,

γ-glutamyl transferase activity in serum comes primarily from liver. The enzyme in serum is heterogeneous with respect to both net molecular charge (e.g. shown by electrophoresis) and size. These forms appear to derive from post-translational modifications of a single type of enzyme molecule rather than resulting from the existence of true isoenzymes. For example, high molecular weight forms may represent the release of cell membrane fragments into the circulation. Despite numerous investigations, clear correlations between patterns of multiple forms and particular diseases cannot be discerned.

Clinical Significance

Even though renal tissue has the highest concentration of GGT, the enzyme present in serum appears to originate primarily from the hepatobiliary system. GGT is a sensitive indicator of the presence of hepatobiliary disease, being elevated in most subjects with liver disease regardless of cause, but its usefulness is limited by lack of specificity. Similar to ALP, it is highest in cases of intrahepatic or posthepatic biliary obstruction, reaching activities some 5–30 times the upper reference limit. High elevations of GGT are also observed inpatients with primary or secondary (metastatic) liver neoplasm.

Moderate elevations (2–5 times normal) occur in infectious hepatitis. Patients with chronic hepatitis C infection and high pretreatment serum GGT are unlikely to have a sustained virologic response to interferon treatment. Small increases in GGT activity are observed in more than 50% of patients with NAFLD, and similar but transient increases are noted in cases of drug intoxication. In acute and chronic pancreatitis and in some pancreatic malignancies (especially if associated with hepatobiliary obstruction), enzyme activity may be 5–15 times the upper reference limit.

Elevated activities of GGT are found in the sera of patients with alcoholic hepatitis and in the majority of sera from people who are heavy drinkers. Increased concentrations of the enzyme are also found in the serum of subjects receiving anticonvulsant drugs, such as phenytoin and phenobarbital. Such an increase in GGT activity in serum may reflect induction of new enzyme activity by the action of the alcohol and drugs and/or their toxic effects on microsomal structures in liver cells.

In acute myocardial infarction, GGT activity is usually normal. If there is a rise, it occurs at about the fourth day, reaches a maximum value in another 4 days, and probably implies liver damage secondary to cardiac insufficiency.

Unlike ALP, GGT is not increased in conditions in which osteoblastic activity is increased.

Recent epidemiologic evidence has shown that serum GGT activity possesses an independent prognostic value for cardiovascular morbidity and mortality. Indeed, experimental work has documented that active enzyme is present in atherosclerotic plaques, and this appears related to the ability of GGT to mediate redox/pro-oxidant reactions at a cellular level.

Methods for Determination of γ-glutamyl Transferase Activity

Early GGT assays used L-γ-glutamyl-p-nitroanilide (GGPNA) as the substrate, with glycylglycine serving as the γ-glutamyl residue acceptor. However, GGPNA has limited solubility in the reaction mixture, and it is therefore difficult to obtain saturating substrate concentrations. The p-nitroaniline produced in the reaction is determined by its yellow color, which is monitored at 405 nm.

Derivatives of GGPNA are also available and have been used in other methods. With these derivatives, various groups have been introduced into the benzene ring to increase solubility in water. The most useful of these substrates is L-γ glutamyl-3-carboxy-4-nitro-anilide, which is readily soluble in water and is split by GGT at a rate comparable with that observed with GGPNA. In the IFCC reference measurement procedure for GGT, L-γ-glutamyl-3-carboxy-4-nitroanilide serves as the substrate, with glycylglycine serving as an acceptor. Buffering is provided by glycylglycine itself. The temperature of the reaction is 37°C, and the wave length of measurement of the reaction product, 5-amino-2-nitrobenzoate, is 410 nm. GGT is a comparatively stable enzyme *in vitro*. Activity is stable for at least 1 month at 4°C and for 1 year at 20°C.

Nonhemolyzed serum is the preferred specimen, but EDTA plasma has also been used. Heparin may produce turbidity in the reaction mixture; citrate, oxalate, and fluoride depress GGT activity by 10–15%.

Reference Intervals

In adults, the upper reference limit for GGT activity in serum is 40 U/L for females and 70 U/L for males, when measured with an assay traceable to the IFCC reference procedure. Reference limits are approximately twofold higher in people of African ancestry. In normal full-term neonates, GGT activity at birth is approximately 6–7 times the adult reference range. The activity then declines, reaching adult values by the age of 5–7 months.

5'-NUCLEOTIDASE

5'-nucleotidase (EC 3.1.3.5; 5'-ribonucleotide phosphohydrolase; NTP) is a phosphatase that acts only on nucleoside-5'-phosphates, such as adenosine-5'-phosphate (adenosine monophosphate, AMP) and adenylic acid, releasing inorganic phosphate.

Clinical Significance

Despite its ubiquitous distribution, serum NTP activities appear to reflect hepatobiliary disease with considerable specificity. NTP is increased threefold to sixfold in those hepatobiliary diseases in which there is interference with the secretion of bile. This may be due to extrahepatic causes (a stone or tumor occluding the bile duct), or it may arise from intrahepatic conditions, such as cholestasis caused by chlorpromazine, malignant infiltration of the liver, or biliary cirrhosis. When parenchymal cell damage is predominant, as in infectious hepatitis, serum NTP activity is only moderately elevated.

The assay of NTP activity has been considered of value as an addition to measurement of nonspecific total ALP in patients with suspected hepatobiliary disease, and abnormal NTP activity is routinely interpreted as evidence of a hepatic origin of increased ALP activity in serum. However, approximately half of individuals in whom liver ALP activity is increased in serum may simultaneously show a normal NTP. On the other hand, increased NTP in the serum of patients with normal liver ALP is very often associated with the presence of liver disease. Thus, the frequent dissociation of the two enzyme activities supports the usefulness of determining both (liver) ALP and NTP to enhance diagnostic efficiency in diseases of the liver.

Methods for Determination of 5'-nucleotidase Activity

The substrates most generally used in measuring the activity of NTP are AMP and inosine-5'-phosphate or inosine mono phosphate) (IMP). However, these substrates are organic phosphate esters and thus can be hydrolyzed to an appreciable degree by other nonspecific (alkaline) phosphatases, even at a pH as low as 7.5, which is the pH assumed optimal for NTP activity. Methods for the estimation of NTP in serum, therefore must incorporate some means for correcting for the hydrolysis of the substrate by the nonspecific phosphatases.

In a commercially available assay, serum NTP catalyzes the hydrolysis of IMP to yield inosine, which is then converted to hypoxanthine by purine-nucleoside phosphorylase (EC 2.4.2.1). Hypoxanthine is oxidized to urate with xanthine oxidase (EC 1.2.3.2). Two moles of hydrogen peroxide are produced for each mole of hypoxanthine liberated and converted to uric acid. The formation rate of hydrogen peroxide is monitored by a spectrophotometer at 510 nm by the oxidation of a chromogenic system. The effect of ALPs on IMP is inhibited by β-glycerophosphate. This material is substrate for ALP but not for NTP, and by forming substrate complexes with the former enzyme, it reduces the proportion of total ALP activity that is directed to the hydrolysis of the NTP substrate, IMP-NTP activity in serum or plasma heparin is stable for at least 4 days at 4°C and 4 months at −20°C.

Reference Interval

The reference interval for NTP activity at 37°C is from 3 to 9 U/L, with no sex-related differences.

PANCREATIC ENZYMES

The most commonly used serum biomarkers for investigation of pancreatic disease, and more specifically acute pancreatitis, are digestive enzymes. Assays of (P-type) amylase, lipase, and trypsin are applied.

AMYLASE

α-Amylase (EC 3.2.1.1; 1,4-α-D glucan glucanohydrolase; AMY) is an enzyme of the hydrolase class that catalyzes the hydrolysis of 1,4-α-glucosidic linkages in polysaccharides.

Both straight-chain (linear) polyglucans, such as amylose, and branched polyglucans, such as amylopectin and glycogen, are hydrolyzed, but at different rates. In the case of amylose, the enzyme splits the chains at alternate α-l,4-hemiacetal (-C-O-C-) links, forming maltose and some residual glucose; maltose, glucose, and a residue of limit dextrins are formed if branched-chain polyglucans are used as substrate. The enzyme does not attack the α-l,6-linkages at the branch points. AMYs are calcium metalloenzymes, with the calcium essential for functional integrity. However, full activity is displayed only in the presence of various anions, such as chloride, bromide, nitrate, cholate, or monohydrogen phosphate with chloride and bromide being the most effective activators. AMY in human serum has a moderately sharp pH optimum at 6.9–7.0.

Amylase normally occurring in human plasma are small molecules with molecular weights varying from 54,000–62,000 Da. The enzyme is thus small enough to pass through the glomeruli of the kidneys, and AMY is the only plasma enzyme normally found in urine. AMY is present in a number of organs and tissues. The greatest concentration is noted in the salivary glands, which secrete a potent AMY (S-type) to initiate hydrolysis of starches while the food is still in the mouth and esophagus. The action of the S-AMY, once referred to as

ptyalin, is terminated by acid in the stomach. In the pancreas, the enzyme (P-type) is synthesized by acinar cells and then is secreted into the intestinal tract by way of the pancreatic duct system. In the intestinal tract, effective action of pancreatic and intestinal AMY is favored by mildly alkaline conditions in the duodenum. Intestinal maltase then further hydrolyzes maltose to glucose. AMY activity is also found in extracts from semen, testes, ovaries, Fallopian tubes, striated muscle, lungs, and adipose tissue. The enzyme is present in colostrum, tears, and milk. Epithelial tumors of lung and ovary may also contain considerable AMY activity. Ascitic and pleural fluids may contain AMY as a result of the presence of a tumor or pancreatitis.

The enzyme present in normal serum and urine is predominantly of pancreatic (P-AMY) and salivary gland (S-AMY) origin. These isoenzymes are products of two closely linked loci on chromosome 1. AMY isoenzymes also undergo post-translational modification of deamidation, glycosylation, and deglycosylation to form a number of isoforms. Indeed, non-enzymic deamidation appears to be the mechanism for 'aging' that occurs when AMY is sequestered (e.g. pancreatic pseudocysts) or subjected to prolonged *in vitro* storage. Although, P-AMY is not glycosylated, S-AMY may exist in both glycosylated and deglycosylated forms; these isoforms can be separated in both serum and urine using isoelectric focusing or electrophoresis. Individuals with isolated P-AMY deficiency, a rare condition, have carbohydrate maldigestion resulting in abdominal distention, flatulence, loose stools, and poor weight gain.

Clinical Significance

Blood AMY activity is physiologically low and constant and greatly increases in acute pancreatitis and salivary gland inflammation. In acute pancreatitis, a rise in serum AMY activity occurs within 5–8 hours of symptom onset; activities typically return to normal by the third or fourth day. A fourfold to sixfold elevation in AMY activity above the upper reference limit is usual, with maximal concentrations attained in 12–72 hours. The magnitude of the elevation of serum enzyme activity is not related to the severity of pancreatic involvement; however, the greater the rise, the greater the probability of acute pancreatitis. A portion of the clearance of AMY from the circulation occurs via renal excretion into the urine, and increased serum activity is reflected in an increase in urinary AMY activity. As compared with serum AMY, urine AMY reaches higher concentrations and persists for longer periods. The clinical specificity of AMY for the diagnosis of acute pancreatitis is low (20–60%, depending on the mix of the patient population studied) because increased values are also found in a number of acute intra-abdominal disorders and in several extrapancreatic conditions (Table 14.3).

Lack of specificity of total AMY measurement has led to interest in the direct measurement of P-AMY instead of total enzyme activity for the differential diagnosis of patients with acute abdominal pain. By applying the best decision limit (an activity equal to threefold the upper reference limit), the clinical specificity of P-AMY for the diagnosis of acute pancreatitis was greater than 90%. Sensitivity in late detection of this condition is also notably improved with P-AMY.

Pancreatic amylase values remain elevated in 80% of patients with uncomplicated pancreatitis 1 week after onset, when only 30% still show increased total AMY activity. This long standing increase in P-AMY activity in serum also makes redundant the traditional measurement of total AMY in urine; a test performed to achieve better diagnostic sensitivity in the late phase of pancreatitis.

Biliary tract diseases, such as cholecystitis, cause up to fourfold elevation in serum P-AMY activity as a result of primary or secondary pancreatic involvement. Various intra-abdominal events can lead to a significant increase in serum P-AMY activities up to a fourfold elevation and sometimes beyond. Such increases may be due to leakage of P-AMY from the intestine into the peritoneal cavity and then into the circulation.

In renal insufficiency, serum AMY activity is increased in proportion to the extent of renal impairment (usually, no more than 5 times the upper reference limit). Hyperamylasemia also occurs in neoplastic disease. Tumors of the lung and serous, and mixed (serous and mucinous) carcinomas of the ovary can produce hyperamylasemia (with an S-type isoenzyme mobility) with elevations as high as 50 times the upper reference limit. The AMY isoenzyme in cases of ruptured ectopic pregnancy is not well characterized. In severe cases presenting late, the increased isoenzyme may be P-AMY (from pancreatic involvement related to peritonitis) despite the fact that S-AMY is present in Fallopian tube. Cases of AMY-producing multiple myeloma have been described.

In 1% of the population, macroamylases are present in sera and may cause hyperamylasemia; these are complexes of ordinary AMY (usually S-type) and IgG or IgA. These macroamylases cannot be filtered through the glomeruli of the kidneys because of their large size (greater than MW 200,000) and are thus retained in the plasma, where their presence may increase AMY activity some twofold to eightfold above the upper reference limit. No clinical symptoms are associated with this disorder, but some cases have been detected during investigation of abdominal pain.

A decrease in serum P-AMY activity (less than the lower reference limit) is highly specific for an exocrine pancreatic insufficiency and can make intubation tests for pancreatic function unnecessary. If, however, P-AMY is normal, reduced pancreatic function cannot be excluded methods for determination of α-amylase activity.

Table 14.3	Causes of hyperamylasemia
Pancreatic disease	Pancreatitis, any cause (P-AMY↑)*
	Pancreatic trauma (P-AMY↑)
Intra-abdominal diseases other than pancreatitis	Biliary tract disease (P-AMY↑)
	Intestinal obstruction (P-AMY↑)
	Mesenteric infarction (P-AMY↑)
	Perforated peptic ulcer (P-AMY↑)
	Gastritis, duodenitis (P-AMY↑)
	Ruptured aortic aneurysm
	Acute appendicitis (perforated)
	Peritonitis
	Trauma
Genitourinary disease	Ectopic, ruptured tubal pregnancy
	Salpingitis (S-AMY↑)
	Ovarian malignancy (S-AMY↑)
	Renal insufficiency (Mixed)
Miscellaneous	Salivary gland lesions (S-AMY↑)
	Acute alcoholic abuse (S-AMY↑)
	Diabetic ketoacidosis (S-AMY↑)
	Macroamylasemia (S-AMY↑ or P-AMY↑)
	Septic shock (S-AMY↑)
	Cardiac surgery (S-AMY↑)
	Tumors (usually S-AMY↑)
	Drugs (usually S-AMY↑)

*Predominant isoenzyme type is shown in parentheses: P-AMY, pancreatic; S-AMY, salivary; Mixed. Either or both isoenzymes may be present.

Methods for Determination of α-Amylase Activity

Historically, saccharogenic, amyloclastic, and chromolytic starch methods were the assays of choice for determining AMY activity. These assays have been completely displaced in favor of ones with well-defined substrates with shorter glucosyl chains. The use of defined AMY substrates and auxiliary and indicator enzymes in the AMY assay has improved the reaction stoichiometry and has led to more controlled and consistent hydrolysis conditions. Substrates used include small oligosaccharides and 4-nitrophenyl (4-NP)-glycoside substrates.

When hydrolyzed by AMY, small oligosaccharide substrates have been found to give better defined products than do starches. For example, both maltopentaose and maltotetraose showed good stability, consistent hydrolysis products, and unambiguous reaction stoichiometry. Several variations of the reaction rate formulation have been devised.

4-Nitrophenyl-glycoside substrates are prepared by bonding 4-NP to the reducing end of a defined oligosaccharide. If the oligosaccharide is maltoheptaose (G7), the substrate is then 4-NPG7. AMY splits this substrate to produce free oligosaccharides (G5, G4, and G3) and 4-NP-G2 (9%), 4-NP-G3 (31%), and 4-NP-G4 (60%). P-AMY hydrolyzes the substrate at a greater rate than does S-AMY in the ratio 1.8:1. G6, G 1, 4-NP-G6, and 4-NP-G5 are not produced in appreciable quantities.

In the original assay, the result of combined hydrolysis by AMY in the specimen and by the reagent α-glucosidase (EC 3.2.1.20; maltase) is that more than 30% of the product is free NP. Free NP is detected by its absorbance at 405 nm α-glucosidase does not react with any oligosaccharide containing more than four glucose molecules in the chain; G4 is hydrolyzed only very slowly. Problems arose with the use of the 4-NP-glycoside assay with regard to the poor stability of the reconstituted assay mixture, because of slow hydrolysis of the 4-NP-glycoside by α-glucosidase. This effect has been reduced by covalently linking a 'blocking' group (i.e. α4,6-ethylidene group) [ethylidene-protected substrate (EPS)] to the non-reducing end of the molecule. The blocked substrate also shows a different and more advantageous hydrolysis pattern. Thus, the ethylidene-4-NP-G7 substrate fragments approximately as 4-NP-G2 (40%), 4-NP-G3 (40%), and 4-NP-G4 (20%). Therefore, liberation of 4-NP is increased; however, the reaction rate is reduced in proportion, so these two effects compensate for each other. A novel-type α-glucosidase is also available (recombinant enzyme AGH-211) that completely hydrolyzes nitrophenylated substrates. As a result, cleavage of one α-glucosidic linkage by AMY results in the release of one molecule of 4-NP.

$$5 \text{ ethylidene-4-NP-G}_7 + 5\,H_2O \xrightarrow{\alpha\text{-amylase}}$$
$$2 \text{ ethylidene-G}_5 + 2\ 4\text{-NP-G}_2 +$$
$$2 \text{ ethylidene-G}_4 + 2\ 4\text{-NP-G}_3 +$$
$$\text{ethylidene-G}_3 + 4\text{-NP-G}_4$$
$$2\ 4\text{-NP-G}_2 + 2\ 4\text{-NP-G}_3 + 10\,H_2O \xrightarrow{\alpha\text{-glucosidase}} 4\ 4\text{-NP} + 10\,G$$

The IFCC has optimized this method at 37°C, recommending it as a reference measurement procedure for AMY. An alternative method based on the 2-chloro-p-nitrophenol (CNP) indicator uses 2-chloro-p-nitrophenyl α-D-maltotrioside (CNP-G3) as a substrate. This assay does not require glucosidases and is considered a 'direct' assay. Its disadvantages have been stated to include its low substrate conversion rate compared with G4, G5, and G7 assays; the variation in molar absorptivity of CNP associated with changes in pH, temperature,

and protein content; and the presence of the activator, potassium thiocyanate, causing allosteric changes to AMY and precluding the use of antibodies for P-AMY determination.

With the exception of heparin, all common anticoagulants inhibit AMY activity because they chelate Ca^{2+}; citrate, EDTA, and oxalate inhibit it by as much as 15%. Therefore, AMY assays should be performed only on serum or heparinized plasma. AMY is quite stable; activity is fully retained during storage for 4 days at room temperature, for 2 weeks at –4°C, for 1 year at –25°C, and for 5 years at –75°C.

Reference Interval

Using the IFCC recommended method at 37°C, the serum reference interval was 31–107 U/L.

LIPASE

Human pancreatic lipase (EC 3.1.1.3; triacylglycerol acylhydrolase; LPS) is a single-chain glycoprotein with a molecular weight of 48,000 Da and an isoelectric point of about 5.8. The LPS gene resides on chromosome 10. LPS concentration in the pancreas is about 5000-fold greater than in other tissues, and the concentration gradient between pancreas and serum is approximately 20,000-fold. For full catalytic activity and greatest specificity, the presence of bile salts and a cofactor called colipase, which is a small molecular weight protein of 10,000 Da secreted by the pancreas, are required. Human LPS can be fully activated in vitro by colipases from other species (e.g. porcine colipase); this property is used in analytical formulations of the LPS assay.

Lipases are defined as enzymes that hydrolyze glycerol esters of long-chain fatty acids. Only ester bonds at carbons 1 and 3 (α-positions) are attacked, and products of the reaction include 2 moles of fatty acids and 1 mole of 2-acylglycerol (β-monoglyceride) per mole of substrate. The latter is resistant to hydrolysis, probably because of steric hindrance, but it can spontaneously isomerize to the α-form (3-acylglycerol).

This isomerization permits the third fatty acid to be split off, but at a much slower rate. A scheme for the steps in complete hydrolysis of a molecule of triglyceride to glycerol and three fatty acids is shown here.

Lipase acts only when the substrate is present in an emulsified form at the interface between water and the substrate. The rate of LPS action depends on the surface area of the dispersed substrate. Bile acids ensure that the surface of the dispersed substrate remains free of other proteins, including lipolytic enzymes, by lining the surface of the insoluble substrate and the aqueous medium. LPS seems to gain access to the substrate surface

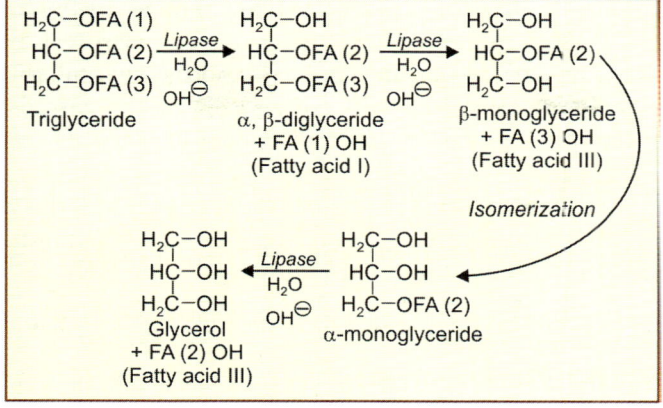

in the following manner. Colipase attaches to a micelle of bile salts, thus forming a colipase-bile salt complex that reconfigures the structure of colipase with exposure of a site with high affinity and high specificity for LPS, which therefore attracts LPS and anchors it to the substrate surface, allowing enzyme action to proceed.

Most LPS activity found in serum derives from the pancreas, but some is secreted by gastric, pulmonary, and intestinal mucosa. LPS is a small enough molecule to be filtered through the glomerulus. It is totally reabsorbed by the renal tubules, and it is not physiologically detected in urine. Evidence suggests that pancreatic LPS may exist in at least two isoforms, although the exact nature of these is unknown. Complete absence of LPS has been reported. Such congenital absence results in fat malabsorption and severe steatorrhea.

Clinical Significance

Lipase measurement of serum is used to diagnose acute pancreatitis. The clinical sensitivity is 80–100% depending on the selected diagnostic cutoff, and the clinical specificity is 80–100% depending on the mix of the patient population studied. After an attack of acute pancreatitis, serum LPS activity increases within 4–8 hours, peaks at about 24 hours, and decreases within 7–14 days. Elevations between 2 times and 50 times the upper reference limit have been reported. The increase in serum LPS activity is not necessarily proportional to the severity of the attack.

Acute pancreatitis is sometimes difficult to diagnose because it must be differentiated from other acute intra-abdominal disorders with similar clinical findings, such as perforated gastric or duodenal ulcer, intestinal obstruction, or mesenteric vascular obstruction. In differential diagnosis, elevation of serum LPS activity to greater than 3 times the upper reference limit, in the absence of renal failure, is a more specific diagnostic finding than increases in serum AMY activity. Furthermore, LPS concentrations remain elevated longer than

those of AMY do, which is another advantage over AMY measurement in patients with delayed presentation (Fig. 14.2). Therefore, it is recommended that LPS should replace AMY as the initial diagnostic test for acute pancreatitis in the emergency department; obtaining both serum AMY and LPS is not warranted.

Obstruction of the pancreatic duct by a calculus or by carcinoma of the pancreas may increase serum LPS activity, depending on the location of the obstruction and the amount of remaining functioning tissue. In patients with a reduced glomerular filtration rate, serum LPS activity is increased.

Thus, care should be exercised in the interpretation of elevated serum LPS values in the presence of renal disease. Finally, investigation of the biliary tract by endoscopic retrograde pancreatography or treatment with opiates (which causes the sphincter of Oddi to contract) may increase serum LPS activity.

METHODS FOR MEASURING LIPASE ACTIVITY

Recently, a synthetic substrate [1,2-O-dilauryl-racgly-cero-3-glutaric acid-(4-methyl-resorufin)-ester] consisting of two glycerol ether bonds and one ester bond has been proposed, and assays based on its use are currently gaining widespread use. LPS hydrolyzes the ester bond in an alkaline medium to an unstable dicarbonic acid ester that spontaneously hydrolyzes to yield glutaric acid and methyl resorufin; this is a bluish-purple chromophore with peak absorption at 580 nm.

The rate of methylresorufin formation is directly proportional to the LPS activity of the sample. The upper reference limit is 38 U/L at 37°C, with no gender- or age-related differences.

Compared with previous LPS spectrophotometric methods, this assay principle is based on a direct reaction and appears to have increased specificity for pancreatic LPS. A newly synthesized thioester (2,3-dibutyrylthio-l-propyloleate) substrate that is believed to be highly selective for pancreatic LPS has also been proposed, but

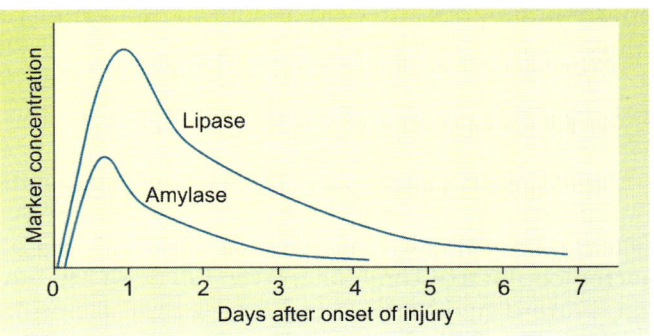

Fig. 14.2: Time-dependent changes in serum amylase and lipase after acute pancreatitis

commercial methods are yet not available to permit its clinical validation. LPS activity in serum is stable at room temperature for 1 week; sera may be stored for 3 weeks in the refrigerator and for several years if frozen.

TRYPSIN

Trypsin (EC 3.4.21.4; no systematic name; TRY) is a pancreas specific serine protease characterized by the presence at the active site of serine and histidine, both of which participate in the catalytic process. TRY hydrolyzes peptide bonds formed by the carboxyl groups of lysine or arginine with other amino acids, although esters and amides involving these amino acids are actually split more rapidly than peptide bonds.

The acinar cells of the human pancreas synthesize two major trypsins (1 and 2) in the form of the inactive proenzymes (or zymogens), trypsinogens-1 and -2. These zymogens are stored in zymogen granules and are secreted into the duodenum under the stimulus of the vagus nerve or the intestinal hormone cholecystokinin-pancreozymin. The two trypsinogens represent approximately 19% of the total protein in pancreatic juice; normally, the pancreas secretes trypsinogen-1 at about twofold to fourfold the concentration of trypsinogen-2, but in pancreatic disease, the ratio of trypsinogen-1 and -2 is reversed. In the intestinal tract, the trypsinogens are converted to the active enzyme TRY by the duodenal enzyme enterokinase or by pre-formed TRY (auto-catalysis). When trypsinogens are converted to active TRY, a small peptide is cleaved from the N-terminal region of trypsinogen [trypsinogen activation peptide (TAP)].

Determinations of urinary TAP may provide information on the severity of acute pancreatitis. TRY-1 is also described as cationic and TRY-2 as anionic because of their differing electrophoretic mobility; the cationic form predominates and is the better documented enzyme. TRY-1 and TRY-2 have molecular weights of 25,800 Da and 22,900 Da and pI values of 4.6–6.5 and greater than 6.5, respectively. TRY-2 differs from TRY-1 in that it rapidly undergoes autolysis at neutral or alkaline pH values, and Ca^{2+} does not stabilize it against autolysis. Because the two trypsins show little immunologic cross-reactivity, a specific immunoassay for each of them is possible.

Materials such as soybeans, lima beans, and egg whites contain natural TRY inhibitors—small polypeptides, such as α1-antitrypsin (α1-protease inhibitor) and α2-macroglobulin that combine irreversibly with TRY and inactivate it by blocking the active center. Similar nondialyzable TRY inhibitors (e.g. pancreatic secretory trypsin inhibitor, PSTI) are present in pancreas, pancreatic juice, serum, and urine. These inhibitors protect plasma and other proteins against hydrolysis by TRY and other proteases if for some reason any appreciable quantity of the enzyme enters the vascular system.

The absence of α1-antitrypsin is associated with an increased tendency toward panlobular emphysema in early life; this example illustrates the effects of uninhibited proteases on organ function.

Clinical Significance

Trypsin-1 (Cationic Trypsin)

In healthy individuals, free trypsinogen-1 is the major form found in serum. After an attack of acute pancreatitis, serum TRY-1 rises in parallel with serum AMY activity to peak values ranging from 2–400 times the upper reference limit.

The distribution of the different forms of TRY-1 appears to be related to the type and severity of acute pancreatitis. Thus, in the mildest form of acute pancreatitis, 80–99% of TRY-1 exists as free trypsinogen-1, with smaller proportions existing as bound TRY-1. In the more severe forms, in which mortality ranges from 20% to more than 50%, the proportion of free trypsinogen-1 may be as low as 30% of the total, with appreciable proportions existing as the α1-antitrypsin- and α2-macroglobulin-bound TRY-1.

Trypsin-1 in serum is elevated in chronic renal failure, as are serum AMY and LPS. Thus, renal failure must be ruled out when elevated concentrations are interpreted. In chronic pancreatitis without steatorrhea, plasma concentrations of TRY-1 do not differ from those found in health; when steatorrhea is present, however, fasting concentrations are extremely low. In the relapsing phase of chronic pancreatitis, plasma TRY may be considerably elevated. In carcinoma of the pancreas, TRY concentrations may be high, normal, or even low.

In comparison with P-AMY and LPS measurements, TRY-1 is a more difficult test to perform, requiring several hours to complete. Because TRY estimation has no distinct role in the routine management of patients with acute pancreatitis, this test is considered of limited clinical value.

Cystic fibrosis is a genetic disorder that primarily affects the lungs and digestive system, resulting in the production of thick mucus that blocks ducts in the pancreas, preventing normal transport of trypsinogen. In this condition, plasma TRY concentrations have been reported to be high in neonates; as the disease progresses, activity falls. Newborn screening is done by the measurement of immunoreactive trypsinogen-1 in dried blood specimens. Infants who have a high TRY concentration on initial testing undergo further assessment via a repeat test 1–3 weeks later, or by analysis of the initial blood spot for specific DNA mutations.

Trypsin-2 (Anionic Trypsin)

Serum trypsinogen-2 increases more than trypsinogen-1 in acute pancreatitis, the concentrations of the former being on average about 10-fold those of the latter. Consequently, larger amounts of trypsinogen-2 are excreted into urine. Urinary trypsinogen-2 measurement has shown high sensitivity and negative predictive value for the diagnosis of acute pancreatitis on admission to the hospital. However, the positive predictive value of this test is low.

As noted earlier, newly formed TRY is inactivated by complexing with α1-antitrypsin. Assays of this serum complex with TRY-2 have shown that this determination could be superior to that of trypsinogen-2 or AMY in acute pancreatitis.

METHODS FOR DETERMINATION OF TRYPSIN

Early studies used catalytic assays, but it was soon recognized that other proteolytic enzymes present in serum could also hydrolyze the same substrates. A major advance has been the development of commercial immunoassays to specifically quantify TRY in blood. In the case of TRY-1, immunoassays detect trypsinogen-I, TRY-1, and the TRY-1-α 1-antitrypsin complex. They do not detect the TRY-1-α 2-macroglobulin complex, for which different assays are necessary. Free TRY-1 is not usually found in serum; it is always complexed. Because no assay standardization is available, reference limits are method dependent.

A rapid (5 minute) urinary trypsinogen-2 test strip is available, which is based on the use of immunochromatography with monoclonal antibodies. The test is considered positive at urinary trypsinogen-2 concentrations greater than 50 μg/L.

ALKALINE PHOSPHATASE (BONE ISOFORM)

Bone, liver, and kidney isoforms of ALP are post-translational modifications of the same gene product and are identified by their unique carbohydrate content. Bone ALP is produced by the osteoblast and has been demonstrated in matrix vesicles deposited as 'buds' derived from the cell's membrane. The enzyme therefore is an excellent indicator of global bone formation activity. Genetic inability to produce tissue-nonspecific ALP, including bone isoform, a rare inherited disorder known as hypophosphatasia, results in severe bone disease and impaired bone growth.

Clinical Significance in Bone Disease

Advantages of using bone ALP concentrations in serum as bone formation markers in clinical practice include low diurnal variability and lack of renal function concerns. Among the bone diseases, the highest concentrations of bone ALP are encountered in Paget's disease (osteitis deformans) as a result of the action of osteoblastic cells as they try to rebuild bone that is being resorbed by uncontrolled activity of osteoclasts. Values from 10–25 times the upper reference limit are not unusual, and in broad terms the increase reflects the extent of disease. In vitamin D deficiency (osteomalacia and rickets), concentrations 2–4 times normal may be observed, and these fall slowly to normal on treatment primary hyperparathyroidism and secondary hyperparathyroidism are associated with slight to moderate elevations of bone ALP in serum, with the existence and degree of elevation reflecting the presence and extent of skeletal involvement. Very high enzyme concentrations are present in patients with osteogenic bone cancer. Bone ALP can be slightly increased in osteoporosis, but osteoporotic individuals are not clearly distinguished from age-matched controls even if, over the entire population, concentrations are inversely correlated with bone mineral density. Transient elevations may be found during healing of bone fractures.

Physiologic bone growth increases bone ALP in serum, and this accounts for the fact that in the sera of growing children, the enzyme concentration is 1.5–7 times that in healthy adult serum, the maximum being reached earlier in girls than in boys.

Methods for Determination of Bone
Alkaline Phosphatase

In general, separation of tissue-nonspecific ALP forms (i.e. bone and liver) is difficult because of structural similarity. At present, bone ALP in serum can be measured by electrophoretic and immunochemical methods (see the section on liver enzymes). Immunoassays for bone ALP, which measure enzyme activity or mass, are commercially available; cross-reactivity with the liver isoform, however, has been established. This general limitation should be borne in mind when test results are interpreted. With the use of immunoassays measuring bone ALP concentrations, the enzyme is said to be stable at −20°C for 2 years.

Reference Intervals

When the electrophoretic procedure is used, the reference interval for bone ALP activity in healthy adults is 10–50 U/L. Mean (SD) bone ALP concentrations, determined by immunoassays in healthy adults, were 13 μg/L.

Miscellaneous Enzymes

Lactate Dehydrogenase

Lactate dehydrogenase (EC 1.1.1.27; L-I actate: NAD$^+$ oxidoreductase; LD) is a hydrogen transfer enzyme that catalyzes the oxidation of L-lactate to pyruvate with the mediation of NAD$^+$ as a hydrogen acceptor.

As indicated, the reaction is reversible, and the reaction equilibrium strongly favors the reduction of pyruvate to lactate (P-7 L)—the 'reverse reaction'. The pH optimum for the lactate-to-pyruvate (L-7 P) reaction is 8.8–9.8, and an assay reaction mixture, optimized for LD-1 at 37°C, contains NAD$^+$, 9 mmol/L, and L-lactate, 80 mmol/L. For the P-7 L assay, at 37°C, the pH optimum is 7.4–7.8, NADH 300 μmol/L, and pyruvate 0.85 mmol/L.

The optimal pH varies with the predominant isoenzymes in the sample and depends on the temperature and on substrate and buffer concentrations. The specificity of the enzyme extends from L-lactate to various related 2-hydroxyacids and 2-oxo-acids. The catalytic oxidation of 2-hydroxybutyrate, the next higher homolog of lactate, to 2-oxobutyrate is referred to as 2-hydroxybutyrate dehydrogenase (HBD) activity. LD does not act on D-lactate, and only NAD$^+$ serves as a coenzyme.

The enzyme has a molecular weight of 134,000 Da and is composed of four peptide chains of two types: M (or A) and H (or B), each under separate genetic control. The structures of LD-M and LD-H are determined by loci on human chromosomes 11 and 12, respectively. The subunit compositions of the five isoenzymes, in order of decreasing anodal mobility in an alkaline medium, are LD-1 (HHHH; H4); LD-2 (HHHM;H3M); LD-3 (HHMM; H2M2); LD-4 (HMMM; HM3); and LD-5 (MMMM; M4). A different, sixth LDH isoenzyme, LD-X (also called LDHd, composed of four X (or C) subunits, is present in postpubertal human testes. A seventh LD, called LD-6, has been identified in the sera of severely ill patients.

Lactate dehydrogenase is inhibited by reagents with reactivity against thiol groups, such as mercuric ions and p-chloromercuribenzoate, the inhibition being reversed by the addition of cysteine or glutathione. Borate and oxalate inhibit by competing with lactate for its binding site on the enzyme; similarly, oxamate competes with pyruvate for its binding site. Both pyruvate and lactate in excess inhibit enzyme activity, although the effect of pyruvate is greater. Inhibition by either substrate is greater for the H form than for the M form, and substrate inhibition decreases with increase in pH. EDTA inhibits the enzyme perhaps by binding Zn^{2+}; however, the postulated activator role for zinc ions is not fully established.

Lactate dehydrogenase activity is present in many cells of the body and is invariably found only in the cytoplasm of the cell. Enzyme concentrations in various tissues are about 1500–5000 times greater than those physiologically found in serum. Therefore, leakage of the enzyme from even a small mass of damaged tissue increases the observed serum activity of LD to a significant extent. Different tissues show different isoenzyme composition. In the heart, kidneys, and erythrocytes, the electrophoretically faster moving isoenzymes LD-1 and LD-2 predominate, whereas in liver and skeletal muscle, the more cathodal LD-4 and LD-5 isoenzymes predominate although skeletal muscle damage may also result in anodic LD patterns. Isoenzymes of intermediate mobility account for the LD activity from many sources (e.g. spleen, lungs, lymphnodes, leukocytes, and platelets).

Clinical Significance

Because of its wide tissue distribution, serum LD elevations occur in a variety of clinical conditions, including myocardial infarction, hepatitis, hemolysis, and disorders of the kidneys, lung, and muscle. Serum LD measurement is, however, relevant only in hematology and oncology.

Hemolytic anemias significantly increase LD concentrations in serum. Marked elevations of LD activity up to 50 times the upper reference limit, have been observed in the megaloblastic anemias. These anemias, usually resulting from the deficiency of folate or vitamin B12, cause the erythrocyte precursor cell to break down in the bone marrow (ineffective erythropoiesis), resulting in the release of large quantities of LD-1 and LD-2 isoenzymes. These elevations rapidly return to normal after appropriate treatment. For monitoring purposes, LD is relevant in predicting disease activity in leukemia, and the survival rate (probability of survival) and duration in Hodgkin's disease and non-Hodgkin's lymphoma.

Patients with malignant disease often show increased LD activity in serum; up to 70% of patients with liver metastases and 20–60% of patients with other non-hepatic metastases (e.g. lymph nodes) have elevated LD activity. Notably elevated LD-1 is observed in germ cell tumors approximately 60% of cases), such as teratoma, seminoma of the testis, and dysgerminoma of the ovary. The percentage of patients with increased LD depended on the stage of the disease. LD appears to be a useful predictor of outcome in patients with testicular non-seminomatous germ cell tumors, melanoma, and small celllung cancer.

Elevations of LD activity (predominant LD-4 and LD-5 isoenzymes) are observed in liver disease, but their routine use in a liver profile appears limited and would not appear to add significantly to the aminotransferase activity investigation.

Macro-LD, usually due to the formation of an auto-antibody-enzyme complex that leads to a persistent increase in the amount of circulating enzyme, has been estimated to occur in <1 in 10,000 people. Documentation of a macro-LD (e.g. by the presence of an abnormally migrating and at electrophoresis) should be established in suspected individuals to avoid additional follow-up investigation or unnecessary treatment.

METHODS FOR DETERMINATION OF LACTATE
Dehydrogenase Activity

Routine methods for quantitation of total LD activity use kinetic spectrophotometry to measure the inter conversion of the coenzyme NAD$^+$ and NADH at 340 nm. The most widely used procedures employ the L → P reaction, because it is claimed that there is less dependence on the NAD$^+$ and lactate concentrations and less contamination of NAD$^+$ with inhibiting products. An L → P reference method, optimized for LD-1, has been developed by the IFCC as a reference procedure for LD at 37°C. Serum is the preferred specimen for measuring LD activity.

Plasma samples may be contaminated with platelets, which contain high concentrations of LD. Serum should be separated from the clot as soon as possible after the specimen has been obtained. Hemolyzed serum must not be used because erythrocytes contain 4000 times more LD activity than does serum. The different isoenzymes vary in their sensitivity to cold, LD-4 and LD-5 being especially labile. Activity of LD-4 and LD-5 is lost if the samples are stored at −20°C. Thus, serum specimens should be stored at room temperature, at which no loss of activity occurs for at least 3 days.

Reference Intervals

The reference interval for LD activity in adult white subjects, determined at 37°C with a procedure traceable to the IFCC reference method, was found to be 125–220 U/L, LD reference limits are higher in children, with a gradual decrease noted over the whole childhood period.

ENZYME ACTIVITY

Enzyme assays usually depend on the measurement of the catalytic activity of the enzyme, rather than the concentration of the enzyme protein itself. As each enzyme molecule can catalyze the reaction of many molecules of substrate, measurement of activity provides great sensitivity. It is, however, important that the conditions of the assay are optimized and standardized to give reliable and reproducible results.

Reference ranges for plasma enzymes are dependent on assay conditions, e.g. temperature, and may also be subject to physiological influences. It is thus important to be aware of both the reference range used by the laboratory providing the assay and the physiological circumstances when interpreting the results of enzyme assays.

DISADVANTAGES OF ENZYME ASSAYS

A major disadvantage in the use of enzymes in the diagnosis of tissue damage is their lack of specificity for a particular tissue or cell type. Many enzymes are common to more than one tissue, with the result that an increase in the plasma activity of a particular enzyme could reflect damage to any one of these tissues. This problem may be obviated to some extent in two ways: first, different tissues may contain (and thus release when they are damaged) two or more enzymes in different proportions; thus alanine and aspartate aminotransferases are both present in cardiac and skeletal muscle and hepatocytes, but there is only a very little alanine aminotransferase in either type of muscle; second, some enzymes exist in different forms (isoforms), colloquially termed **isoenzymes** (although, strictly, the term 'isoenzyme' refers only to a genetically determined isoform). Individual isoforms are often characteristic of a particular tissue; although, they may have similar catalytic activities, they often differ in some other measurable property, such as heat stability or sensitivity to inhibitors.

After a single insult to a tissue, the activity of intra-cellular enzymes in the plasma rises as they are released from the damaged cells, and then falls as the enzymes are cleared. It is thus important to consider the time at which the blood sample is taken in relation to the insult. If taken too soon, there may have been insufficient time for the enzyme to reach the bloodstream, and if too late, it may have been completely cleared. As with all diagnostic techniques, data acquired from measurements of enzymes in plasma must always be assessed in the light of whatever clinical and other information is available, and their limitations borne in mind.

Several enzymes can form complexes with other proteins, most often immunoglobulins, which are cleared from the plasma more slowly than the native forms and are referred to as 'macro' enzymes. The consequence may be a sustained increase in plasma activity, which may cause diagnostic confusion if the possibility is not considered. Macro enzymes are rarely of pathological significance, although occasionally they are associated with paraproteins.

BIBLIOGRAPHY

1. Anderson JL. Lipoprotein-associated phospholipase A, an independentpredictor of coronary artery disease events in primary and secondaryprevention. Am J CardioI 2008; 101 (Suppl): 23F-33F.

2. Apple FS. Wu AHB. Mair J. RavkildeJ. Panteghini M. Tate J. et al. Future biomarkers for detection of ischemia and risk stratification inacute coronary syndrome. Clin Chem 2005; 51: 810–24.

3. Bais R. Edwards JB. Creatine kinase. CRC Crit Rev Clin Lab Sci1982; 16:291-355.

4. Bais R. Phil cox M. Approved recommendation on lFCC methods forthe measurement of catalytic concentration of enzymes. Part 8. IFCC method for lactate dehydrogenase (L-lactate: NAD$^+$ oxidoreductase. EC1.1.1.27). International Federation of Clinical Chemistry (IFCC). Eur J Clin Chem Clin Biochem 1994; 32: 639–55.

5. Beetham R. Biochemical investigation of suspected rhabdomyolysis. Ann Clin Biochem 2000; 37: 581–7.

6. Bertrand A. Buret J. A one-step determination of serum 5′–nucleotidaseusing a centrifugal analyzer. Clin Chim Acta 1982; 119: 275–84.

7. Brancaccio P. Matfulli N. Limongelli FM. Creatine kinase monitoringin sport medicine. Br Med Bull 2007; 81-82: 209–30.

8. Brodrick JW. Geokas MC, Largman Co Fassett M. Johnson JH.Molecular forms of immunoreactive pancreatic cationic trypsin inpancreatitis patient sera. Am J Physiol 1979; 237: E474-80.

9. Broyles DL. Nielsen RG, Bussett EM. Lu WD. Mizrahi IA. Nunnelly PA. et a!. Analytical and clinical performance characteristics ofTandem-MP Ostase. a new immunoassay for serum bone alkalinephosphatase. ClinChem 1998; 44: 2139–47.

10. Cabrera-Abreu JC. Green A. y-GIutamyltransferase: value of itsmeasurement in pediatrics. Ann Clin Biochem 2002; 39: 22–5.

11. Consuegra-Sanchez L. Fredericks S. Kaski Je. Pregnancy-associatedplasma protein-A (PAPP-A) and cardiovascular risk. Atherosclerosis 2009; 203: 346–52.

12. Davidson DF. Watson DJM. Macroenzyme detection by polyethyleneglycol precipitation. Ann ClinBiochem 2003;40: 514–20.

13. Deutsche Gesellschaft fur Klinische Chemie. Proposal of standardmethods for thedetermination of enzyme catalytic concentrations inserum and plasma at 37 0e. III. Glutamate dehydrogenase [L-glutamate:NAD(P)+ oxidoreductase (deaminating). EC 1.4.1.3J. Eur J ClinChemClinBiochem 1992; 30: 493–502.

14. Dolci A, Panteghini M. The exciting story of cardiac biomarkers:from retrospective detection to gold diagnostic standard for acutemyocardial infarction and more. Clin Chim Acta 2006; 369: 179–87.

15. Dufour DR. Lott JA, Nolte FS. Gretch DR. Kotf RS. Seetf LB. Diagnosisand monitoring of hepatic injury. II. Recommendations for use oflaboratory tests in screening, diagnosis. and monitoring. Clin Chem 2000; 46: 2050–68.

16. Emdin M. Pompella A. Paolicchi A. Gamma-glutamyl transferase atherosclerosis. and cardiovascular disease: triggering oxidative stresswithin the plaque. Circulation 2005; 112: 2078–80.

17. Fahie-Wilson MN. Burrows S. Lawson GJ. Gordon T, Wong W.Dasgupta B. Prevalence of increased serum creatine kinase activity dueto macro-creatine kinase and experience of screening programmesindistrict general hospitals. Ann Clin Biochem 2007; 44: 377–83.

18. Foo AY. Amylase measurement-which method? Ann Clin Biochem 1995; 32: 239–43.

19. ForsmarkCEo Baillie J. AGA Institute technical review on acutepancreatitis. Gastroenterology 2007; 132: 2022–44.

20. Frossard JL. Trypsin activation peptide (TAP) in acute pancreatitis:from pathophysiology to clinical usefulness. JOP J Pancreas (Online) 2001; 2:69–77.

21. Goldberg DM. Structural. functional. and clinical aspects ofgammaglutamyltransferase.CRC Crit Rev Clin Lab Sci 1980; 12: 1–58.

22. Hawkins Re. Assessment of the utility of aldolase determination inserum by monitoring patient outcomes. Biochim Clin 2001; 25: 331–5.

23. Hayes PC. BouchierlAD. Beckett GJ. Glutathione S-transferase inhumans in health and disease. Gut 1991; 32: 813–8.

24. Hedstrom J. Sainio V. Kemppainen E. Haapiainen R. Kivilaakso E. Schroder T. et a!. Serum complex of trypsin 2 and u, antitrypsin asdiagnostic and prognostic marker of acute pancreatitis: clinical study inconsecutive patients. Br Med J 1996; 313: 333–7.

25. Heiduk M, Page 1. Kliem C. Abicht K, Klein G. Pediatric referenceintervals determined in ambulatory and hospitalized children andjuveniles. Clin Chim Acta 2009; 406: 156–61.

26. Henriksen K, Tanko LB. Qvist p. Delmas PD. Christiansen C. Karsdal MA. Assessment of osteoclast number and function: application in thedevelopment of new and improved treatment modalities for bonediseases. Osteoporosis Int 2007; 18: 681–5.

27. Hood D. Van Lente F. Estes M. Serum enzyme alterations in chronicmuscle disease: a biopsy-based diagnostic assessment. Am J Clin Pathol 1991; 95: 402–7.

28. Huijgen HJ. Sanders GT. Koster RW, Vreeken J. Bossuyt PM. Theclinical value of lactate dehydrogenase in serum: a quantitative review.Eur J Clin Chem Clin Biochem 1997; 35: 569–75.

29. Ceriotti F. Henny J. Queralt 6 J. Ziyu S. Ozarda Y, Chen B. et al.Common reference intervals for aspartate amino-transferase (AST).alanine aminotransferase (ALT) and γ-glutamyl transferase (GGT) inserum: results from an IFCC multicenter study. ClinChem Lab Med 2010; 48: 1593–60 1.

30. Infusino I. Bonora R. Panteghini M. Traceability in clinical enzymology. Clin Biochem Rev 2007; 28: 155–61.

31. Itkonen O. Koivunen E. Hurme M. Alfthan H, Schroder T. StenmanU-H. Time-resolved immunofluorometric assays

for trypsinogen-1and -2 in serum reveal preferential elevation of trypsinogen-2 inpancreatitis. J Lab Clin Med 1990; 115: 712–8.

32. Iversen KK, Teisner AS. Teisner B. Kliem A. Bay M. Kirk V, et al. Pregnancy-associated plasma protein A in non-cardiac conditions. ClinBiochem 2008;41 :548-53.

33. Junge W. Wortmann W. Wilke B. Waldenstrom J. Kurrle-WeittenhillerA. Finke J. et a!. Development and evaluation of assays for thedetermination of total and pancreatic amylase at 37°C according to theprinciple recommended by the IFCe. ClinBiochem 2001;34:607-15.

34. Kim WR. Flamm SL. Di Bisceglie AM. Bodenheimer He. Serumactivity of alanine aminotransferase (ALT) as an indicator of health anddisease. Hepatology 2008;47:1363-70.

35. Kristensen SR. Mechanisms of cell damage and enzyme release. DanMed Bull 1994;41:423-33.

36. Kristensen SR, Horder M. Principles of diagnostic enzymology. In: Moss DW, Rosalki SB, eds. Enzyme tests in diagnosis. London: EdwardArnold, 1996:7-24.

37. Kruse-arres D, Kaiser C, Hafkenscheid JCM, Hohenwallner W, Stein W, Bohner), et al. Evaluation of a new alpha-amylase assay using4,6-ethylidene- (G7) -1-4- nitrophenyl-(G1) - alpha -D- maltoheptaoside assubstrate.) ClinChemClinBiochem 1989; 27: 103–13.

38. Lessinger M, Ferard G. Plasma pancreatic lipase activity: fromanalytical specificity to clinical efficiency for the diagnosis of acutepancreatitis. Eur Clin Chem Clin Biochem 1994; 32: 377–81.

39. Mair . Tissue release of cardiac markers: from physiology to clinicalapplications. ClinChem Lab Med 1999;37:1077-84.

40. McQueen M. Clinical and analytical considerations in the utilizationof cholinesterase measurements. ClinChimActa 1995; 237: 91–105.

41. Moller-Petersen . Clinical evaluation of cathodic trypsin-likeimmunoreactivity in pancreatic diseases in adults. Scand) Clin LabInvest 1990; 50: 463–77.

42. Moller-Petersen j, Pedersen 0, Thorsgaard-Pedersen N, Nyboe Andersen B. Serumcathodic trypsin-like immunore-activity, pancreaticlipase, and pancreatic isoamylase as diagnostic tests of chronicpancreatitis or pancreatic steator-rhea. Scand) Gastroenterol 1988; 23: 287–96.

43. Morandi L, Angelini C, Prelle A, Pini A, Grassi B, Bernardi G, etal.High plasma creatine kinase: review of the literature and proposal for adiagnostic algorithm. Neurol Sci 2006; 27: 303–11.

44. Mosca A, Bonora R, Ceriotti F, Franzini C, Lando G, Patrosso MC,et al. Assay using succinyldithiocholine as substrate: the method ofchoice for the measurement of cholinesterase catalytic activity inserum to diagnose succinylcholine sensitivity. Clin Chem Lab Med 2003; 41: 317–22.

45. Moss DW. Alkaline phosphatase isoenzymes. Clin Chem 1982; 28: 2007-16.

46. Moss DW. Changes in enzyme expression related to differentiation and regulatory factors: the acid phosphatase of osteoclasts and othermacrophages. ClinChimActa 1992; 209: 131–8.

47. Moss DW. Perspectives in alkaline phosphatase research. Clin Chem 1992; 38: 2486–92.

48. Moss DW. Physicochemical and pathophysiological factors in therelease of membrane-bound alkaline phosphatase from cells. ClinChimActa 1997; 257: 133–40.

49. Moss DW, Edwards RK. Improved electrophoretic resolution of boneand liver alkaline phosphatases resulting from partial digestion with neuraminidase. Clin Chim Acta 1984; 143: 177–82.

50. Moss DW, Raymond FD, Wile DB. Clinical and biological aspects of acid phosphatase. CRC Crit Rev Clin Lab Sci 1995; 32: 431–67.

51. Nicholls S, Hazen SL. Myeloperoxidase and cardiovascular disease. Arterioscler Thromb Vasc Bioi 2005; 25: 1102–11.

52. Noe DA. Tissue injury. In: Noe DA, ed. The logic of laboratorymedicine, 2nd edition. Baltimore: Urban & Schwarzenberg, 2001.

53. Pagani F, Bonora R, Panteghini M. Reference interval for lactatedehydrogenase catalytic activity in serum measured according tothe new IFCC recommendation. ClinChem Lab Med 2003; 41: 970–1.

54. Pagani F, Panteghini M. 5'- Nucleotidase in the detection of increasedactivity of the liver form of alkaline phosphatase in serum. Clin Chem 2001; 47: 2046–8.

55. Paju A, Stenman UH. Biochemistry and clinical role of trypsinogensand pancreatic secretory trypsin inhibitor. Crit Rev Clin Lab Sci 2006; 43: 103–42.

56. Panteghini M. Aspartate aminotransferase isoenzymes. Clin Biochem 1990; 23: 311–9.

57. Panteghini M. Benign inherited hyperphosphatasemia of intestinalorigin: report of two cases and a brief review of the literature. Clin Chem 1991; 37: 1449–52.

58. Panteghini M. Diagnostic application of CK-MB mass determination. Clin Chim Acta 1998; 272: 23–31.

59. Panteghini M. Electrophoretic fractionation of pancreatic lipase. ClinChem 1992;38:1712–6.

60. Panteghini M. Hepatic alkaline phosphatase isoenzyme. I. Biochemicaland pathophysiological aspects. Giorn It ChimClin 1990; 15: 163–71.

61. Panteghini M. Serum isoforms of creatine kinase isoenzymes. Clin Biochem 1988; 21: 211–8.

62. Panteghini M, Bonora R, Pagani F. An alternative approach to theprevention of succinyldicholine-induced apnoea.) Clin Chem Clin Biochem 1988; 26: 85–90.

63. Panteghini M, Bonora R, Pagani F. Automated measurement ofmitochondrial aspartate aminotransferase by selective proteolysis withproteinase K. ClinChem 1993; 39: 2199–200.

64. Panteghini M, Bonora R, Pagani F. Measurement of pancreaticlipase activity in serum by a kinetic colorimetric assay using a newchromogenic substrate. Ann ClinBiochem 2001; 38: 365–70.

65. Panteghini M, Ceriotti F, Pagani F, Secchiero S, Zaninotto M Franzini C; for the Italian Society of Clinical Biochemistry andClinical Molecular Biology (SIBioC) Working Group on Enzymes.Recommendations for the routine use of pancreatic amylasemeasurement instead of total amylase for the diagnosis and monitoringof pancreatic pathology. ClinChem Lab Med 2002; 40: 97–100.

66. Panteghini M, Pagani F. Reference intervals for two bone-derivedenzyme activities in serum: bone isoenzyme of

alkaline phosphatase(ALP) and tartrate-resistant acid phosphatase (TR-ACP). Clin Chem1989; 35: 181–1.

67. Pratt DS, Kaplan MM. Evaluation of abnormal liver-enzyme results inasymptomatic patients. N Engl) Med 2000; 342: 1266–71.

68. Price CPo Multiple forms of human serum alkaline phosphatase:detection and quantitation. Ann ClinBiochem 1993; 30: 355–72.

69. Rauscher E, Gerber M. Pancreatic alpha-amylase assay employingthe synergism of two monoclonal antibodies. Clin Chim Acta 1989; 183: 41–4.

70. Rauscher E, Neumann U, Schaich E, von Bulow S, Wahlefeld AW,Optimized conditions for determining activity concentrationof alpha-amylase in serum, with 1,4-alpha-D-4-nitrophenylmaltoheptaoside as substrate. ClinChem 1985; 31: 14–9.

71. Rees Gw, Trull AK, Doyle S. Evaluation of an enzyme-immunometricassay for serum alpha-glutathione S-transferase. Ann Clin Biochem1995; 32: 575–83.

72. Rosalki SB, Foo AY. Two new methods for separating and quantifyingbone and liver alkaline phosphatase isoenzymes in plasma. Clin Chem 1984; 30: 1182–6.

73. Schindhelm RK, van der Zwan LP, Teerlink T, Scheffer PG.Myeloperoxidase: a useful biomarker for cardiovascular disease riskstratification? Clin Chem 2009; 55:1462–70.

74. Schmidt ES, Schmidt FW, Glutamate dehydrogenase: biochemicaland clinical aspects of an interesting enzyme. ClinChim Acta1988; 43: 43–56.

75. Schumann G, Aoki R, Ferrero CA, Ehlers G, Ferard G, Gella F), et al. IFCC primary reference procedures for the measurement of catalyticactivity concentrations of enzymes at 37°C. Part 8. Referenceprocedure for the measurement of catalytic concentration of α-amylase. ClinChem Lab Med 2006; 44: 1146–55.

76. Schumann G, Bonora R, Ceriotti F, Clerc-Renaud P, Ferrero CA, FerardG, et al. IFCC primary reference procedures for the measurement ofcatalytic activity concentrations of enzymes at 37°C. Part 2. Referenceprocedure for the measurement of catalytic concentration of creatinekinase. Clin Chem Lab Med 2002; 40: 635–42.

77. Schumann G, Bonora R, Ceriotti F, Clerc-Renaud P, Ferrero CA, FerardG, et al. IFCC primary reference procedures for the measurement ofcatalytic activity concentrations of enzymes at 37°C. Part 3. Referenceprocedure for the measurement of catalytic concentration of lactatedehydrogenase. Clin Chem Lab Med 2002; 40: 643–8.

78. Schumann G, Bonora R, Ceriotti F, Clerc-Renaud P, Ferard G, FerreroCA, et al. IFCC primary reference procedures for the measurement ofcatalytic activity concentrations of enzymes at 37°C. Part 6. Referenceprocedure for the measurement of catalytic concentration of γ-glutamyl-transferase. ClinChem Lab Med 2002;40: 734–8.

79. Schumann G, Bonora R, Ceriotti F, Ferard G, Ferrero CA, Franck PFH,et al. IFCC primary reference procedures for the measurement ofcatalytic activity concentrations of enzymes at 37°C. Part 4. Referenceprocedure for the measurement of catalytic concentration of alanineaminotransferase. Clin Chem Lab Med 2002; 40: 718–24.

80. Schumann G, Bonora R, Ceriotti F, Ferard G, Ferrero CA, Franck PFH,et al. IFCC primary reference procedures for the measurement ofcatalytic activity concentrations of enzymes at 37°C. Part 5.Reference procedure for the measurement of catalytic concentrationof aspartate aminotransferase. ClinChem Lab Med 2002; 40: 725–33.

81. Schumann G, Klauke R. New IFCC reference procedures for thedetermination of catalytic activity concentrations of five enzymes inserum: preliminary upper reference limits obtained in hospitalizedsubjects. Clin Chim Acta 2003; 327: 69–79.

82. Shih J, Datwyler SA, Hsu SC, Matias MS, Pacenti DP, Lueders C, et al. Effect of collection tube type and preanalytical handling onmyeloperoxidase concentrations. Clin Chem 2008; 54: 1076–9.

83. Stein P, Rosalki SB, Foo AY, Hjelm M. Transient hyper-phosphatasemiaof infancy and early childhood: clinical and biochemical features of 21cases and literature review. Clin Chem 1987; 33: 313–8.

84. Sunderman FW, The clinical biochemistry of 5'-nucleotidase. Ann Clin Lab Sci 1990; 20: 123–39.

85. Szasz G, Gerhardt W, Gruber W. Creatine kinase in serum. 3. Furtherstudy of adenylate kinase inhibitors. ClinChem 1977; 23: 1888–92.

86. Thompson PO, Clarkson P, KarasRH. Statin-associated myopathy. JAMA 2003; 289: 1681–90.

87. Tietz NW. Support of the diagnosis of pancreatitis by enzymetests-old problems, new techniques. ClinChimActa 1997; 257: 85–98.

88. Tietz NW, Rinker AD, Shaw LM. IFCC methods for the measurementof catalytic concentration of enzymes. Part 5. IFCC method for alkalinephosphatase (orthophosphoric-monoester phosphohydrolase, alkalineoptimum, EC 3.1.3.1). J Clin Chem Clin Biochem 1983; 21: 731–48.

89. Tietz NW, Shuey OF. Lipase in serum-the elusive enzyme: anoverview. Clin Chem 1993; 38: 1000–10.

90. Tietz NW, Shuey OF. Reference intervals for alkaline phosphataseactivity determined by the IFCC and AACC reference methods. Clin Chem 1986; 32: 1593–4.

91. Visnapuu LA, Karlson LK, Dubinsky EH, Szer IS, Hirsch CA. Pediatricreference ranges for serum aldolase. Am J Clin Pathol 1989; 91: 476–7.

92. Von Eyben FE. A systematic review of lactate dehydrogenase isoenzyme 1 and germ cell tumors. Clin Biochem 2001; 34: 441–54.

93. Whitfield JB. Gamma glutamyl transferase. CRC Crit Rev Clin Lab Sci 200 I; 38: 263–355.

94. Whitten RO, Chandler WL, Thomas MGE, Clayson KJ, Fine JS. Surveyof alpha-amylase activity and isoamylases in autopsy tissue. Clin Chem 1988; 34: 1552–5.

95. Wittfooth S, Qin QP, Lund J, Tierala I,Pulkki K, Takalo H, Pettersson K. Immunofluorimetric point-of-care assays for the detection of acutecoronary syndrome-related non-complexed pregnancy-associatedplasma protein A. Clin Chem 2006; 52: 1794–1801.

96. Zalewski A, Macphee C. Role of lipoprotein-associated phospholipase A2 in atherosclerosis: biology, epidemiology, and possible therapeutic target. Arterioscler Thromb Vasc Bioi 2005; 25: 923–31.

15

Lipids, Lipoproteins, and Apolipoproteins

INTRODUCTION

The general term lipid applies to a class of hydrophobic compounds that are soluble in organic solvents and nearly insoluble in water. Chemically, lipids are usually enriched in carbon and hydrogen and after hydrolysis typically yield fatty acids or complex alcohols, which are usually esterified with fatty acids. Some lipids are more complex, containing other chemical groups, such as sialic, phosphoryl, amino, or sulfate groups. The presence of these charged or polar groups makes these lipids amphipathic, which gives them the property of having an affinity for both water and organic solvents; this is an important feature in their ability to form cell membranes. Lipids can been broadly subdivided into five groups based on their chemical structure (Table 15.1).

Table 15.1	Classification of clinically important lipids

Sterol derivatives
Cholesterol and cholesteryl esters
Steroid hormones
Bile acids
Vitamin D
Fatty acids
Short chain (2–4 carbon atoms)
Medium chain (6–10 carbon atoms)
Long chain (12–26 carbon atoms)
Prostaglandins
Glycerol esters
Triglycerides, diglycerides, and monoglycerides
(acyl glycerols)
Phosphoglycerides
Sphingosine derivatives
Sphingomyelin
Glycosphingolipids
Terpenes (isoprene polymers)
Vitamin A, vitamin E, and vitamin K

CHOLESTEROL

Although, every living organism has been found to contain sterols, cholesterol is found almost exclusively in animals, in which it is also the main sterol. Virtually all cells and body fluids contain some cholesterol. Similar to other sterols, cholesterol is a solid alcohol of high molecular weight that possesses a tetracyclic perhydrocyclopentanophenanthrene skeleton. It contains 27 carbon atoms, numbered as shown in Fig. 15.1.

Knowledge of the sterane skeleton structure and numbering system is important not only to clinical laboratorians, but also to practicing clinicians, because

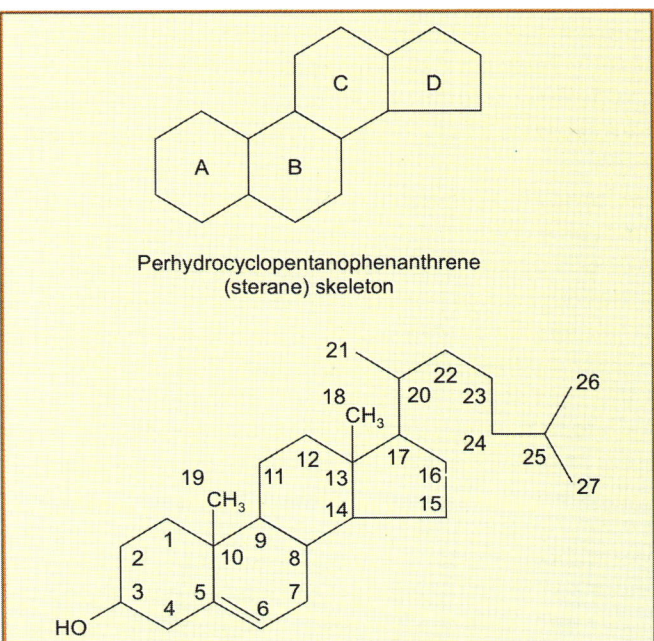

Fig. 15.1: Structure of cholesterol

cholesterol is the starting point in many different metabolic pathways.

These include vitamin D synthesis, steroid hormone synthesis, and bile acid metabolism. Because the enzymes modifying the sterane cholesterol ring or its derivatives are known by their site and type of reaction (e.g. 21-hydroxylase in cortisol synthesis), the diagnosis of many disease states consequently depends on isolating the site of enzyme dysfunction (e.g. 21-hydroxylase deficiency in adrenogenital syndrome).

CHOLESTEROL SYNTHESIS

Although, cholesterol enters the body from the diet, it is also synthesized endogenously by all tissues from acetate. Knowledge of the endogenous cholesterol synthetic pathway has assumed great significance, because drug agents for the treatment of coronary artery disease (CHD) have been sought to suppress or decrease endogenous cholesterol synthesis. The necessity for understanding the fundamental biochemistry of this pathway was originally underscored by the triparanol disaster of 1960. Triparanol is a drug that inhibits the final step in the endogenous cholesterol synthetic pathway; the conversion of desmosterol to cholesterol, but does not inhibit the rate-limiting enzyme of cholesterol synthesis, 3-hydroxy-3-methylglutaryl-CoA (HMG-CoA) reductase (Fig. 15.2). When triparanol was used to treat hypercholesterolemia, the drug caused tissue accumulation of desmosterol, resulting in the development of cataracts, alopecia, and accelerated atherosclerosis.

Many drugs now used to treat CHD selectively suppress the rate-limiting enzyme HMG-CoA reductase, thereby lowering serum cholesterol concentrations significantly without accumulation of water-insoluble intermediates of cholesterol synthesis, such as desmosterol.

Although, essentially all cells have the capacity to synthesize cholesterol from acetyl-CoA, almost 90% of synthesis occurs in the liver and gut; other organs and tissues depend, in part, on cholesterol delivery from the circulation. Cholesterol biosynthesis is best conceptualized as occurring in three stages (Figs 15.2, 15.3, and 15.4). In the first stage, acetyl-CoA, a key metabolic intermediate that can be derived from carbohydrates, amino acids, and fatty acids, forms the six carbon thioester HMG-CoA. In the second stage, HMGCoA is reduced to mevalonate, and then is decarboxylated to form five-carbon isoprene units. These isoprene units are condensed to form first a 10-carbon (geranyl pyrophosphate) and then a 15-carbon intermediate (farnesyl pyrophosphate).

Two of these (CIS) molecules combine to produce the final product of the second stage-squalene, a 30-carbon acyclic hydrocarbon. The second stage is important, because it contains the step involving the microsomal enzyme HMG-CoA reductase, which is the rate-limiting enzyme in cholesterol biosynthesis. The enzyme that forms farnesyl pyrophosphate, geranyl transferase, is an important second site of regulation in cholesterol synthesis. This degree of inhibition still permits the formation of physiologically important intermediate isoprenoids in the absence of cholesterol synthesis. The third and final stage of synthesis occurs in the endoplasmic reticulum, with many of the intermediate products being bound to a specific carrier protein. Squalene, after initial oxidation, undergoes cyclization to form the four-ring, 30-carbon intermediate, lanosterol. In a series of oxidation-decarboxylation reactions, several side-chains are removed from the pentanophenanthrene structure to form the final 27-carbon molecule of cholesterol.

Cholesterol Esterification

Once synthesized, cholesterol is released into the circulation bound to lipoproteins, such as very low-density lipoprotein (VLDL; see later section on lipoprotein metabolism, endogenous pathway), which is one of the primary lipoproteins secreted by the liver. The major apoprotein found in VLDL is apoB-100. It is produced by the same gene as apoB-48, but represents the full-length product of the apoB gene. ApoB-48 is

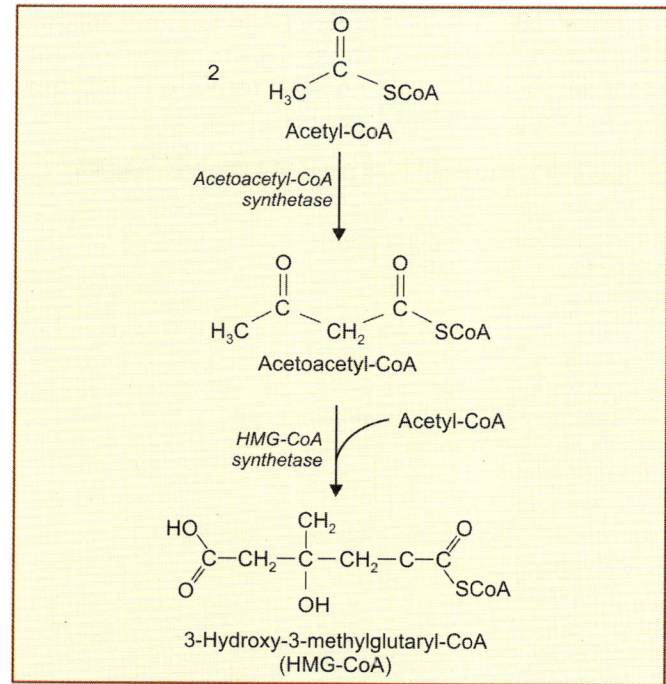

Fig. 15.2: Cholesterol biosynthesis (stage I)

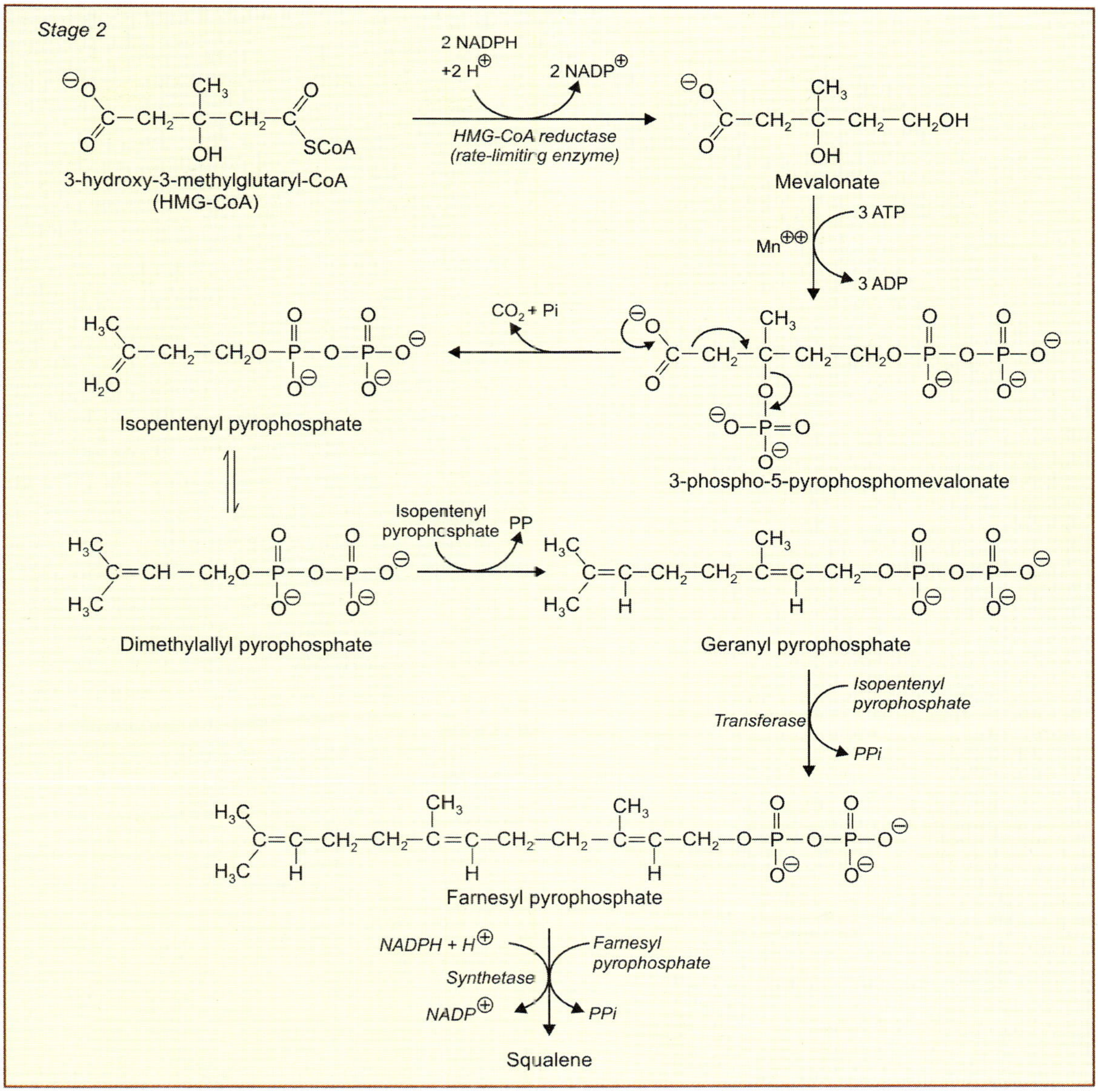

Fig. 15.3: Cholesterol biosynthesis (stage 2)

produced in the intestine by a post-transcriptional editing step, which introduces a stop codon in about the middle of the apoB-100 mRNA transcript, thus resulting in a protein about 48% the length of the full-length apoB 100 protein. The esterification of cholesterol is important, because it serves to enhance the lipid-carrying capacity of the lipoprotein in plasma and prevents intracellular toxicity by free cholesterol. The reaction is catalyzed by lecithin-cholesterol acyltransferase (LCAT) in the plasma and acylcholesterol acyltransferase (ACAT) within the cell. ACAT is an energy requiring enzyme, and the initial reaction (Fig. 15.5) involves activation of a fatty acid with thio coenzyme A (Co-ASH) to form an acyl-CoA, which in turn reacts with cholesterol to form an ester. The LCAT reaction does not require CoASH and results from fatty acid transfer from the second carbon position of phosphatidyl choline (lecithin) to the hydroxyl group on the A-ring of cholesterol (Fig. 15.5). Cholesteryl esters account for about 70% of the total cholesterol in plasma, and LCAT is responsible for the formation of virtually all plasma cholesteryl ester. LCAT is synthesized in the liver and released into the circulation; it primarily resides on lipoproteins and is activated by apoA-I and other apolipoproteins (see later section on apolipoproteins). The esterification of cholesterol by LCAT on the only polar group of cholesterol makes cholesteryl ester more hydrophobic than cholesterol. This causes the cholesterol on the surface of lipoproteins, once esterified,

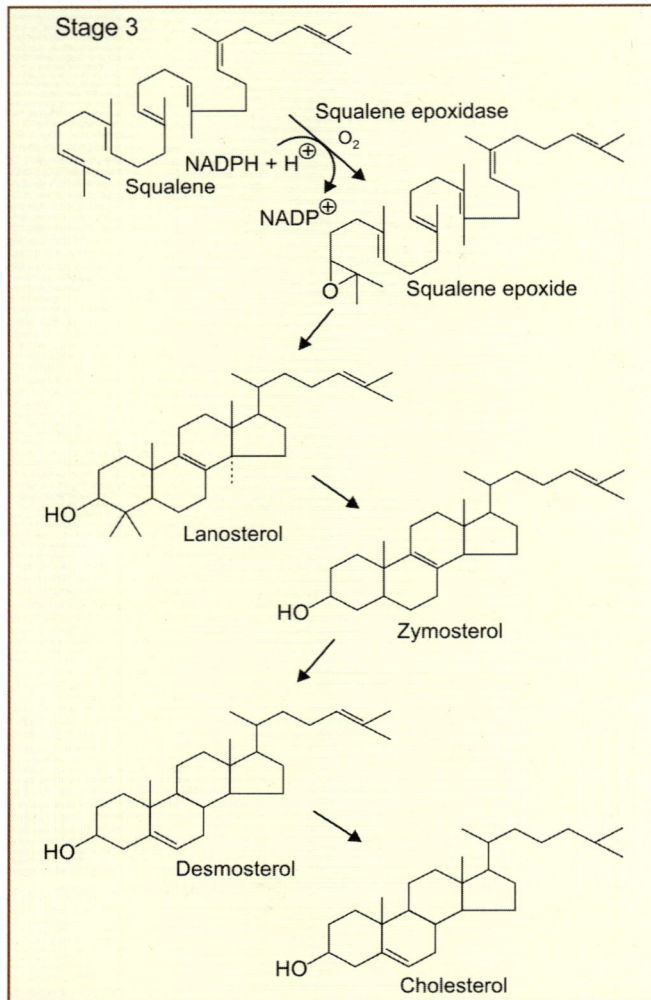

Fig. 15.4: Cholesterol biosynthesis (stage 3)

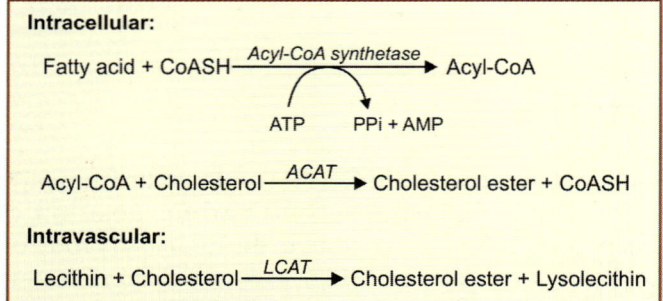

Fig. 15.5: Intracellular and intravascular esterification of cholesterol mediated by ACAT and LCAT, respectively

to partition into the more hydrophobic core of lipo-proteins, where triglycerides are also located.

CHOLESTEROL CATABOLISM

Once a lipoprotein enters the cell, its cholesteryl esters and triglycerides are hydrolyzed by lysosomal acid lipase. Lack or malfunction of this enzyme results in intracellular accumulation of cholesteryl esters and triglycerides, particularly in the liver, and produces a clinical disorder known as cholesteryl ester storage disease, or Wolman's disease.

Cholesterol reaching the liver may be secreted unchanged into bile or metabolized to bile acids or re-secreted on lipoproteins. Approximately, one-third of the daily production of cholesterol, or about 400 mg/day, is converted into bile acids (Fig. 15.6). Conversion of cholesterol to cholic and chenodeoxycholic acids, the major bile acids in humans, involves shortening of the cholesterol side-chain and hydroxylation of the sterol nucleus. The first step, which is also the rate-limiting step, is hydroxylation of the 7-position of the sterol nucleus, catalyzed by the enzyme 7α-hydroxylase (Fig. 15.6).

The bile acids are made more polar after conjugation with glycine or taurine and then are excreted into the bile calculi. After reaching the small intestine, the conjugated bile acids play an active part in cholesterol and fat absorption, as discussed previously. Some of the bile acids are de-conjugated and converted by bacteria in the intestine to secondary bile acids. Cholic acid is converted to deoxycholic acid, and chenodeoxycholic acid is metabolized to lithocholic acid. About 90% of the bile acids, except lithocholic, are reabsorbed in the lower third of the ileum and returned to the liver by the portal vein, which is called the enterohepatic circulation.

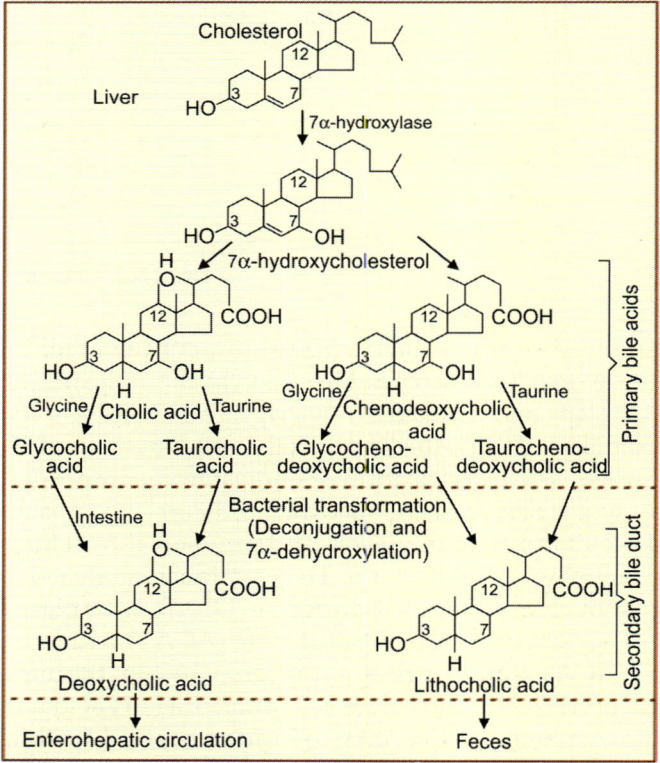

Fig. 15.6: Bile acid synthesis

A significant amount of cholesterol is also excreted directly into the biliary system, where it is solubilized to form mixed micelles with bile acids and phospholipids. If the amount of cholesterol in bile exceeds the capacity of these solubilizing agents, the excess cholesterol can precipitate, forming cholesterol gallstones, which account for about 80% of gallstones in Western societies.

It is important to note that except for the liver and a few endocrine tissues, such as the adrenal gland, most cells cannot further catabolize or modify cholesterol. Because of this and its limited aqueous solubility, cholesterol tends to accumulate in cells or extracellular spaces; this is another feature of cholesterol that contributes to its ability to cause atherosclerosis.

FATTY ACIDS

The fatty acids are one of the simpler molecular forms of lipids. They are generically indicated by the chemical formula RCOOH, where 'R' stands for an alkyl chain. Fatty acid chain lengths vary and are commonly classified according to the number of carbon atoms present. Three somewhat arbitrarily defined groups of fatty acids are those containing 2–4 carbon atoms (short chain), 6–10 carbon atoms (medium chain), and 12–26 carbon atoms (long chain). Those of importance in human nutrition and metabolism' are of the long-chain class containing an even number of carbon atoms.

Fatty acids are further classified according to their degree of saturation. Saturated fatty acids have no double bonds between carbon atoms, monounsaturated fatty acids contain one double bond, and polyunsaturated fatty acids contain more than one double bond (Fig. 15.7). The double bonds in polyunsaturated fatty acids of both animal and plant origin are usually 3 carbon atoms apart. Some fatty acids from marine fish living in deep, cold waters (e.g. salmon), which form oils at room temperature, possess numerous (up to 6) unsaturated bonds and usually are more than 20 carbon atoms long. These fatty acids are prone to oxidation, which occurs at the sites of unsaturation.

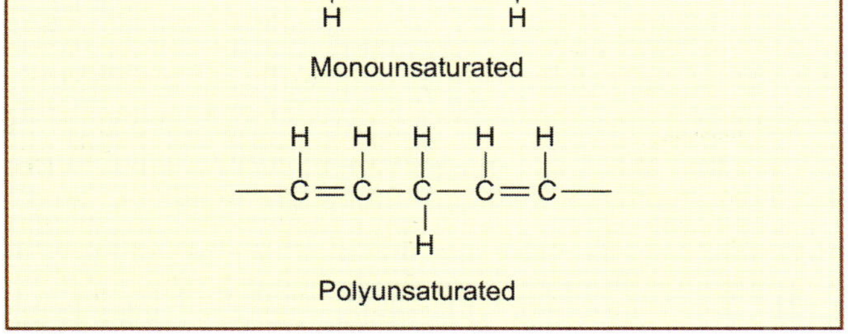

Fatty Acid Catabolism

Long-chain fatty acids are oxidized in the mitochondria and produce energy by a series of reactions that operate in a repetitive manner to shorten the fatty acid chain by two carbon atoms at a time from the carboxy (–COOH) terminal of the molecule through a process known as β oxidation. For example, 1 mole of C16 fatty acid is converted to 8 moles of acetyl-CoA. Acetyl-CoA does not normally accumulate in the cell, but is enzymatically condensed with oxaloacetate, derived largely from carbohydrate metabolism (Fig. 15.8), to yield citrate, which is a major component of the tricarboxylic acid cycle, also called Krebs cycle. The Krebs cycle serves as a common pathway for the final oxidation of nearly all food material, whether derived from carbohydrate, fat, or protein.

It is important to note that the efficiency of the Krebs cycle depends on the availability of sufficient oxaloacetate to serve as an acceptor for acetyl-CoA. Complete oxidation of a single fatty acid molecule produces a relatively large quantity of energy. For example, the complete oxidation of 1 mole of palmitic acid to carbon dioxide and water produces 16 moles of CO_2, 16 moles of H_2O, and 129 moles of adenosine triphosphate, or 2340 calories.

Thus, the standard free energy for oxidation of palmitic acid is 2340 calories, whereas the free energy liberated by hydrolysis of 129 moles of ATP is 940 calories, indicating that the efficiency of energy conservation in fatty acid oxidation is approximately 40% under standard conditions. By means of suitable enzyme reactions, the chemical energy stored in fatty acids can be released for metabolic processes or stored in the form of high-energy compounds, such as ATP. Triglycerides that contain three fatty acid molecules, therefore, are an efficient storage form for metabolic energy. The amount of energy produced by metabolizing 1 mole of palmitic acid (16 carbon atoms) is approximately twice that produced by metabolizing an equivalent amount (2.5 mole) of glucose (6 carbon atoms per molecule). Carbohydrate storage also requires water for hydration; triglyceride storage does not. In addition to their high intrinsic energy content, triglycerides have a low density ≥ 1 g/mL) and, because of their hydrophobic nature and peripheral distribution in the body, provide excellent insulation.

Fig. 15.7: Saturated and unsaturated fatty acids

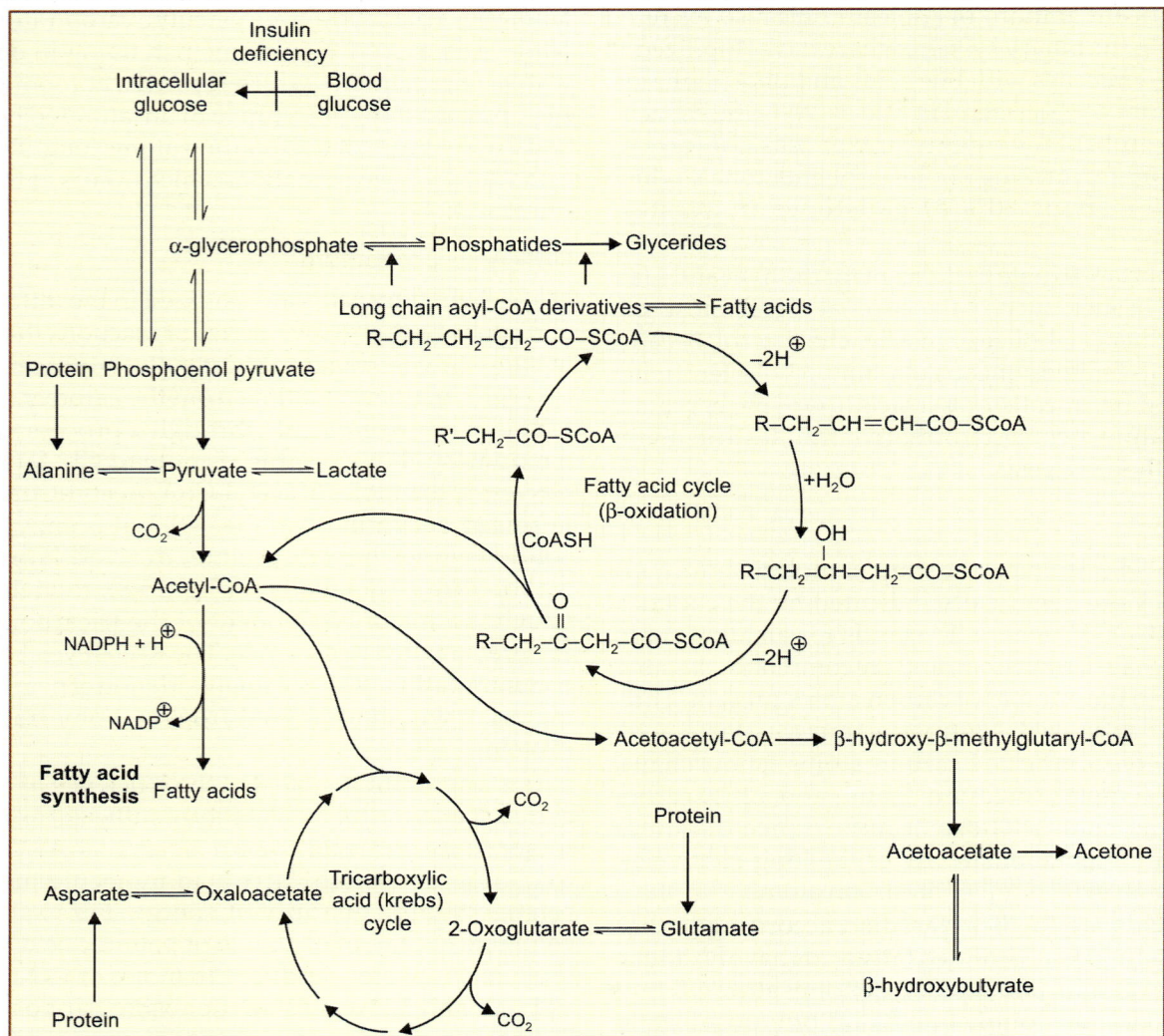

Fig. 15.8: Metabolic relations among intermediates of carbohydrate, fat, and protein metabolism. Note that acetyl-CoA is produced from both carbohydrate and fat. The glucogenic amino acids, derived from protein metabolism, enter glycolytic paths as α-keto acids. Ketogenic amino acids enter as acetyl-CoA

Ketone Formation

During prolonged starvation, or when carbohydrate metabolism is severely impaired, as in uncontrolled diabetes mellitus, the formation of acetyl-CoA exceeds the supply of oxaloacetate. The abundance of acetyl-CoA results from excessive mobilization of fatty acids from adipose tissue and excessive degradation of fatty acids by β-oxidation in the liver. The resulting acetyl-CoA excess is diverted to an alternative pathway in the mitochondria and forms acetoacetic acid, β-hydroxybutyric acid, and acetone—three compounds known collectively as ketone bodies (Fig. 15.9). The presence of ketone bodies is a frequent finding in severe, uncontrolled diabetes mellitus.

As shown in Fig. 15.9, the first product, acetoacetyl-CoA, condenses in the mitochondria with a third

molecule of acetyl-CoA to yield HMG-CoA. This pool of HMG-CoA in the mitochondria is distinct from the pool in the cytosol, which is used for cholesterol biosynthesis. The HMG-CoA produced in the mitochondria is cleaved enzymatically to yield acetoacetate and acetyl-CoA. Some of the acetoacetate formed in liver cells is usually reduced to β-hydroxybutyrate.

Because acetoacetate is unstable, a further portion decomposes to form carbon dioxide and acetone, the third ketone body found in severe, untreated diabetes mellitus. Ketosis, therefore, develops from excessive production of acetyl-CoA because the body attempts to derive necessary energy from stored fat in the absence of an adequate supply of carbohydrate metabolites.

Inadequate incorporation of acetyl-CoA into the Krebs cycle may be further aggravated by inhibition of the

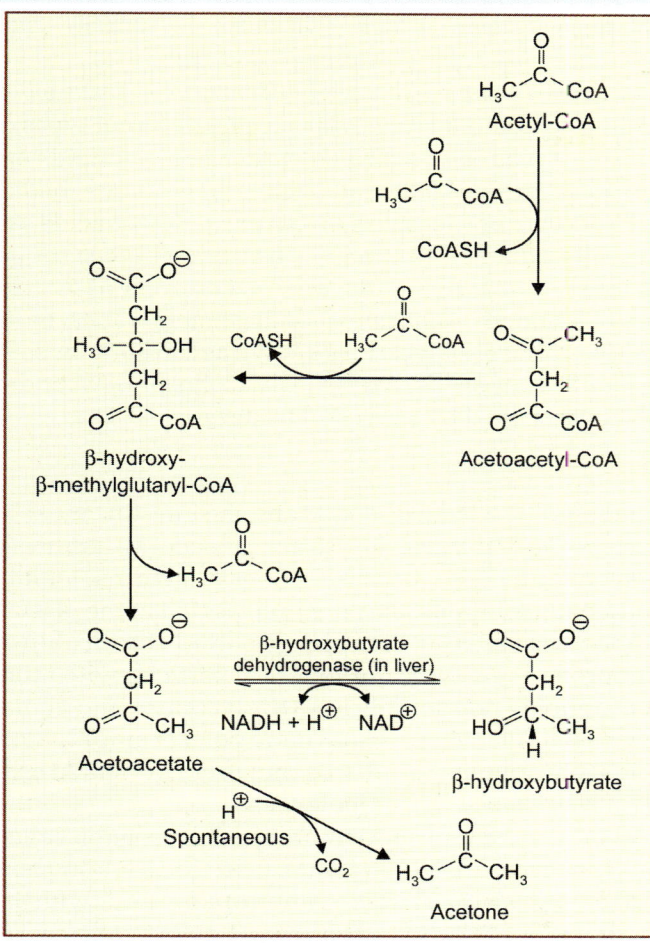

Fig. 15.9: Formation of ketone bodies

interrelationship between carbohydrate, fatty acid, and protein metabolism.

GLYCEROL ESTERS (ACYL GLYCEROLS)

Virtually, all complex lipids contain fatty acids, and in most cases they are covalently linked to an alcohol. One of the most common alcohols found in lipids is glycerol, a three-carbon molecule containing three hydroxyl groups.

The two terminal carbon atoms in the molecule are chemically equivalent and are designated α and α'. The center carbon is labeled β. A common alternative labeling system uses the numeral 1 for the β-carbon, 2 for the α-carbon, and 3 for the α'-carbon.

The class of acyl glycerol (glyceride) is determined by the number of fatty acyl groups present; one fatty acid, mono acyl glycerols (monoglycerides); two fatty acids, dia acyl glycerols (diglycerides); three fatty acids, tri-acyl glycerols (triglycerides). In a mono acyl glycerol, the fatty acid may be linked to any of the three carbon atoms. By convention, the number system is used to indicate the carbon position (e.g. 1-monoglyceride indicates a fatty acid attachment to the α-carbon). This numbering system applies to all acyl glycerols, including the phosphoglycerides, as shown later. Diglycerides may be 1, 2– or 1, 3-diglycerides (Fig. 15.10).

oxaloacetate-generating enzyme system through excess acid-CoA derivatives in the liver. Skeletal muscle and heart (and brain in prolonged fasting) use ketone bodies by resynthesizing their CoA derivatives and subsequently oxidizing them for the production of energy. Although, liver cells are largely responsible for converting fatty acids, they cannot metabolize acetoacetate, because the liver lacks 3-keto acid CoA transferase, the enzyme required for transferring CoA from succinyl-CoA.

The entire process of ketosis is reversed by restoring adequate metabolism of carbohydrate. In starvation, restoration consists of adequate carbohydrate ingestion; in diabetes mellitus, ketosis can be reversed by insulin administration, which permits circulating blood glucose to be taken up by the cells.

With restored concentrations of oxaloacetate, acetyl-CoA can instead enter the Krebs cycle, thus restoring the normal pathway for energy metabolism. Eventually, the release of fatty acids from adipose tissue slows down and is finally reversed. A graphic view of these metabolic reactions is outlined in Fig. 15.8, which shows the

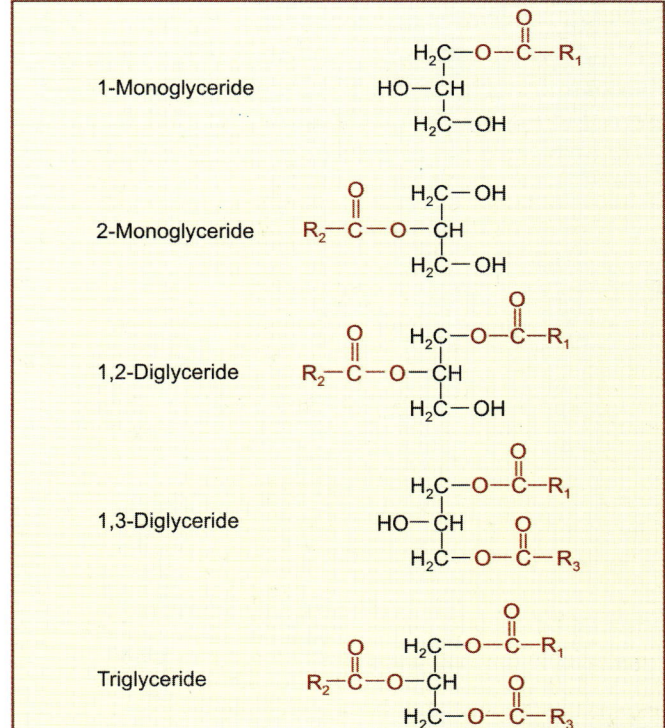

Fig. 15.10: Structure and classification of glycerol esters (acylglycerols). R1 R2, and R3 are fatty acids of varying chain length

Triglycerides are the most prevalent glycerol esters encountered in the body and constitute 95% of tissue storage fat; they are the predominant form of glyceryl ester found in plasma.

Fatty acid residues found in monoglycerides, diglycerides, or triglycerides vary considerably and usually include combinations of the long-chain fatty acids. Triglycerides from plants (e.g. corn, sunflower seed, safflower oils) tend to have large quantities of cis-unsaturated fatty acids, such as C18:2 or linoleic acid, and are liquid at room temperature. Triglycerides from animals, especially ruminants, tend to have C12:0 through C18:0 fatty acid residues (saturated fats) and are solids at room temperature. Rarely, some plant triglycerides, such as coconut oil, are highly saturated and may be solid at room temperature.

Triglycerides are digested in the duodenum and the proximal ileum. Through the action of pancreatic and intestinal lipases and in the presence of bile acids, which activate lipases, they are hydrolyzed to glycerol, monoglycerides, and fatty acids. After absorption, triglycerides are re-synthesized in the intestinal epithelial cells and are combined with cholesterol and apoB-48 to form chylomicrons. Another major class of glycerol esters consists of those containing phosphoric acid at the third α' carbon atom; these esters are called phosphoglycerides (Fig. 15.11). In their simplest form, the A group is an H atom; the molecule is therefore called a dia-acyl phosphoglyceride. Usually, however, the A is an alcohol-derived group, such as choline, serine, inositol, or ethanolamine (Fig. 15.11). If A is choline, the molecule is referred to as phosphatidylcholine; if it is ethanolamine, it will be referred to as phosphatidylethanolamine, etc.

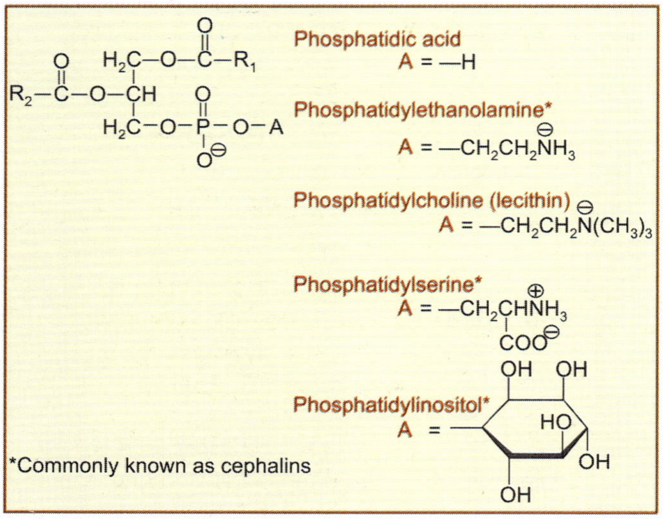

The term lecithin, which is an older designation, is a commonly used term for phosphatidylcholines.

Because of the wide variety of fatty acid residues at positions R1 and R2 (Fig. 15.11), many different types of phospholipids can be formed. These phospholipids are named according to the fatty acid acyl ester attached at C–l and C–2 of the glycerol. Saturated fatty acids are typically attached to the C–l position, whereas (poly) unsaturated fatty acids are often present at the C–2 position. In inner mitochondrial membranes, more complex phosphoglycerides known as cardiolipins scan be found. They are derived from two phosphoglycerides molecules joined by a glycerol bridge.

LIPOPROTEINS

Lipids synthesized in the liver and the intestine must be transported to various tissues to accomplish their metabolic functions. Because of their relative insolubility in aqueous solutions, they are transported in the plasma in macromolecular complexes called lipoproteins. Lipoproteins are typically spherical particles with more hydrophobic nonpolar lipids (triglycerides and cholesteryl esters) in their core, and more polar or amphipathic lipids (phospholipids and free cholesterol) oriented near the surface as a single monolayer.

They also contain one or more specific proteins, called apolipoproteins, which usually are located on their surface (Fig. 15.12). The association of core lipids with the overlying phospholipid, cholesterol, and protein coat is non-covalent, occurring primarily through hydrogen

Fig. 15.11: Structures of phosphoglycerides and common alcohol groups associated with them. R1 and R2 are fatty acid (s) of varying carbon atom lengths

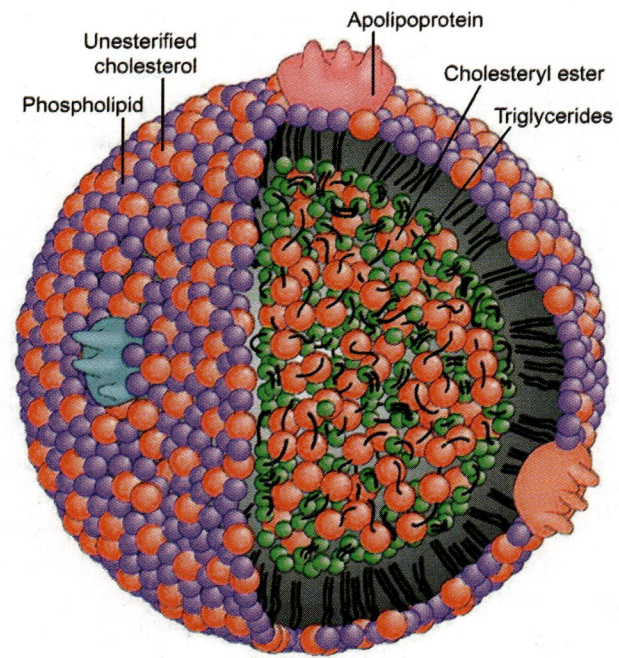

Fig. 15.12: Structure of a typical lipoprotein particle

bonding and van der Waals forces. This binding is lose enough to allow spontaneous exchange of cholesterol, which is more water soluble than the other lipids, among plasma lipoproteins and between cell membranes. The other more hydrophobic lipids require specific transfer proteins to exchange between lipoproteins, such as cholesteryl ester transfer protein (CETP), which exchanges triglycerides and cholesteryl esters between lipoproteins.

Phospholipid transfer protein (PLTP) promotes the transfer of phospholipids between lipoproteins. Lipoproteins have different physical and chemical properties (Table 15.2) because they contain different proportions of lipids and proteins (Table 15.3). Historically, lipoproteins have been categorized on the basis of differences in their hydrated densities, as determined by ultracentrifugation. Categories include (1) chylomicron, (2) VLDL, (3) intermediate density lipoprotein (IDL), (4) low-density lipoprotein (LDL),(5) high-density lipoprotein (HDL), and (6) lipoprotein(a) [Lp(a)]. HDL can be further divided by density into two subpopulations: HDL2 and HDL3. Lp(a) consists of a distinct class of lipoproteins that are structurally related to LDL, because similar to LDL, it contains one apolipoprotein cholesteryl esters.

B-100 per particle and has a similar lipid composition. In contrast to LDL, Lp(a) contains a carbohydrate-rich protein called apo(a), which is covalently bound to apo B-100 through a disulfide linkage. Apo(a) exhibits a significant sequence homology with plasminogen, but unlike plasminogen, Lp(a) is not an active protease. Lp (a) contains a high degree of variation in polypeptide chain length because of a variable number of kringle domains (Fig. 15.13). Apo(a) contains 10 distinct classes

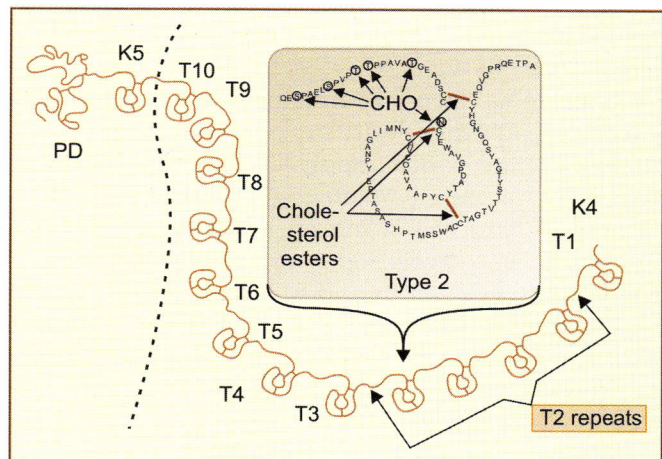

Fig. 15.13: Structure of lipoprotein (a)

Table 15.2	Characteristics of human plasma lipoproteins					
Variable	Chylomicron	VLDL	IDL	LDL	HDL	Lp(a)
Density, g/mL	<0.95	0.95–1.006	1.006–1.019	1.019–1.063	1.063–1.210	1.040–1.130
Electrophoretic mobility	Origin	Pre-β	Between β and pre-β	β	α	Pre-β
Lipid-lipoprotein ratio	99:1	90:10	85:15	80:20	50:50	75:27–64:36
Major lipids	Exogenous triglycerides	Endogenous triglycerides	Endogenous triglycerides, cholesteryl esters	cholesteryl esters	Phospholipids	Cholesteryl esters, Phospholipids
Major proteins	A-I, B-48 C-I, C-II, C-III	B100, C-I C-II, C-III, E	B100, E	B100	A-I, A-II	(a) B100

HDL, High-density lipoprotein; lDL, intermediate-density lipoprotein; LDL, low-density lipoprotein; Lp(a), lipoprotein(a); VLDL, very low-density lipoprotein.

Table 15.3	Chemical composition (%) of normal human plasma lipoproteins				
	Surface components			Core lipids	
	Cholesterol	Phospholipids	Apolipoproteins	Triglycerides	Cholesteryl esters
Chylomicrons	2	7	2	86	3
VLDL	7	18	8	55	12
IDL	9	19	19	23	29
LDL	8	22	22	6	42
HDL2	5	33	40	5	17
HDL3	4	25	55	3	13

*Surface components and core lipids given as percentage of dry mass. HDL, High-density lipoprotein; IDL, intermediate-density lipoprotein; LDL, low-density lipoprotein; VLDL, very low-density lipoprotein.

of kringle 4-like domains that differ from each other in amino acid sequence. Kringle 4 type 1 and kringle 4 types 3–10 are present as a single copy, but kringle 4 type 2 is present in variable numbers of repeats (3 to >40) (Fig. 15.13).

In the fasting state, most plasma triglycerides are present in VLDL. In the postprandial state, chylomicrons appear transiently and contribute significantly to the total plasma triglyceride concentration. LDL normally carries about 70% of total plasma cholesteryl esters but very little triglyceride (Table 15.3). HDL contains about 20–30% of plasma cholesterol.

Lipoproteins can be separated electrophoretically on agarose or on other solid support material, such as cellulose acetate, paper, or polyacrylamide gels. At a pH of 8.6, HDL migrates with the α-globulins, LDL with the β-globulins, and VLDL and Lp(a) between the α- and β-globulins, in the pre-β-globulin region. IDL forms a broad band between β- and pre-β-globulins. Chylomicrons remain at the point of application. This forms the basis for the following common classification of lipoproteins: pre-β-lipoprotein, VLDL; β-lipoprotein, LDL; and β-lipoprotein, HDL.

APOLIPOPROTEINS

Apolipoproteins are the protein components of a lipoprotein. Characteristics and main known functions of the major apolipoproteins are summarized in Table 15.4. Each class of lipoprotein has a variety of Apolipoproteins in differing proportions, with the exception of LDL, which contains only apoB-100. Apo A-I is the major protein in HDL. ApoC-I, C-II, C-III, and E are present in various proportions in all lipoproteins except LDL. Apolipoproteins collectively have three major physiologic functions. They are involved in:

1. Activating important enzymes in the lipoprotein metabolic pathways.

2. Maintaining the structural integrity of the lipoprotein complex.

3. Facilitating uptake of lipoprotein into cells through their recognition by specific cell surface receptors.

Besides these main apolipoproteins, lipoproteins have been found to weakly bind a large number of plasma proteins, but their relevance is not fully understood.

Apolipoprotein A

Together, apolipoprotein A-I and apoA-II constitute about 90% of total HDL protein. The ratio of apoA-I to A-II in HDL is about 3:1. In addition to being an important structural component of HDL, apoA-I is a cofactor for LCAT, the enzyme responsible for forming cholesteryl esters in plasma. Some evidence suggests that apoA-II may inhibit LCAT and activate hepatic triglyceride lipase. ApoA-IV is a component of newly secreted chylomicrons, but it is not a major constituent of chylomicron remnants, VLDL, LDL, and HDL. The primary function of apoA-IV is currently unknown, but it has been shown to activate LCAT in vitro, and available data suggest that it plays a role in the intestinal absorption of lipid.

ApoA-V is a recently described apolipoprotein. It is relatively low in abundance compared with other apolipoproteins and appears to modulate triglyceride concentrations by a mechanism that currently is not well understood. All these proteins, including most of the other apolipoproteins, contain a structural motif called an amphipathic helix. It is an α-helix with approximately half the amino acid residues comprising hydrophobic amino acids, which face toward the neutral lipid core when bound to a lipoprotein particle. The other side of the helix faces outward from the surface of a lipoprotein particle and contains polar or charged amino acids. In general, the binding of amphipathic helices to lipoproteins is relatively weak, thus allowing apolipoproteins to

Table 15.4	Classification and properties of major human plasma apolipoproteins			
Apolipoprotein	Molecular weight, Da	Chromosomal location	Function	Lipoprotein carrier(s)
ApoA-I	29,016	11	Cofactor LCAT	Chylomicron, HDL
ApoA-II	17,414	1	Not known	HDL
ApoA-IV	44,465	11	Activates LCAT	Chylomicron, HDL
ApoB-l00	512,723	2	Secretion of triglyceride from liver binding protein to LDL receptor	VLDL, IDL, LDL
ApoB-48	240,800	2	Secretion of triglyceride from intestine	Chylomicron
ApoC-I	6630	19	Activates LCAT	Chylomicron, VLDL, HDL
ApoC-II	8900	19	Cofactor LPL	Chylomicron, VLDL, HDL
ApoC-III	8800	11	Inhibits apoC-II, activation of LPL	Chylomicron, VLDL, HDL
ApoE	34,145	19	Facilitates uptake of chylomicron remnant and IDL	Chylomicron, VLDL, HDL
Apo(a)	187000–662000	6	Unknown	Lp(a)

exchange between diffident lipoproteins during lipoprotein metabolism.

Apolipoprotein B

Apolipoprotein B exists in two forms: apoB-100 and apo-B-48. ApoB-100, a single polypeptide of more than 4500 amino acids, is the full-length translation product of the apoB gene. In humans, apoB-100 is made in the liver and is secreted into plasma as part of VLDL. Apo B-100 is also the major apolipoprotein of LDL, the end-product of VLDL catabolism. Each VLDL particle contains one molecule of apoB-100. In the fasting state, most of the apoB in plasma is apoB-100. Unlike other Apolipoproteins, however, apoB-100 cannot move from one lipoprotein particle to another, because in addition to amphipathic helices, it has β-sheets—a structural motif with much higher affinity for lipids. It is for this reason that apoB-100 remains with VLDL as it is transformed by lipolysis of its triglycerides and is eventually converted into LDL. ApoB-48 contains 2152 amino acids and is identical to the amino-terminal portion of apoB-100. ApoB-48 results from post-transcriptional modification of internal apoB-100 messenger ribonucleic acid, in which a single base substitution produces a stop codon corresponding to residue 2153 of apoB-100. ApoB-48 is made in the intestine and is the major apo B component of chylomicrons. Both apoB-100 and apoB-48 play important roles in the secretion of VLDL and chylomicrons, respectively.

Apolipoprotein B-100 is recognized by the LDL receptor in hepatic and peripheral tissues; it allows the LDL receptor-mediated internalization of LDL (see later sections on lipoprotein metabolism, endogenous and exogenous pathways).

Apolipoprotein C

Apolipoproteins C-I, C-II, and C-III are associated with all lipoproteins except LDL. ApoC- I, the smallest of the C apolipoproteins, has been reported to activate LCAT *in vitro*, but its *in vivo* function is not clear. Apo-C-II plays an important role in the metabolism of triglyceride-rich lipoprotein (VLDL and chylomicrons) by serving as an activator of lipoprotein lipase (LPL), an enzyme that hydrolyzes lipoprotein triglycerides. Because of differences in sialic acid content, apoC-III exists in at least three polymorphic forms. In contrast to apoC-II, apoC-III decreases lipolysis by the inhibition of LPL.

Apolipoprotein E

Apolipoprotein E is a 34-kDa plasma glycoprotein that is found primarily in chylomicrons, VLDL, HDL, and chylomicron and in VLDL remnants. Removal of apoE-bearing lipoproteins is mediated by several different cellular receptors that recognize a cluster of positively charged amino acids in a specific region of apoE. ApoE plays a central role in the metabolism of chylomicrons and VLDL remnants. It regulates and facilitates lipoprotein uptake in the liver through the interaction of chylomicron remnants with chylomicron remnant receptors, and the binding of VLDL remnants to the LDL receptor, as well as probably proteoglycans.

Three common apoE isoforms, designated E2, E3, and E4, were initially distinguished by isoelectric-focusing electrophoresis. These isoforms have amino acid substitutions at residues 112 and 158. ApoE2 has cysteine residues in both positions, and apoE4 has arginine residues in both positions, whereas apoE3 has cysteine and arginine at positions 112 and 158, respectively. ApoE2 exhibits reduced binding affinity for the band/or E remnant receptor compared with apoE3, which tends to lead to an accumulation of apoE-containing lipoprotein in the circulation, whereas apoE-containing lipoproteins are cleared more rapidly than those containing apoE3. These isoforms are coded for by three alleles of the apoE gene: ε ε2, ε3, and ε4. The ε3 allele is most frequent, although relative proportions of the three alleles vary among populations. These apo E alleles have been shown to contribute significantly to the variability of LDL cholesterol and apoB-100 concentrations within populations.

Individuals with at least one ε2 allele tend to have lower concentrations of apoB-100 and LDL cholesterol than do those who are homozygous for the ε3 allele, whereas individuals with at least one ε4 allele tend to have higher concentrations of these analytes. This most likely occurs because increased hepatic uptake of lipoproteins in the presence of the ε4 allele leads to an increase in hepatic cholesterol and down regulation of the LDL receptor. ApoE4 is also associated with increased cholesterol absorption; in the distant past, this may have offered a selective advantage, but it is a disadvantage with regard to CHD in populations that consume a high-fat diet. Variations at the apoE locus may explain some of the differences observed in plasma lipid and lipoprotein between individual responses to dietary and drug therapy. Finally, the apoE4 allele has been strongly associated with Alzheimer's disease and other neurologic diseases. This association is likely related to the role of apoE in modulating lipid metabolism in the brain, but the exact connection between apoE4 and neurologic diseases is not known.

Lipoprotein Metabolism

The pathways of lipoprotein metabolism are complex and intersect at several points. They include exogenous and endogenous pathways based on whether they carry lipids from dietary or hepatic origin (Figs 15.14 and 15.15).

Also included are the intracellular LDL receptor pathway (Fig. 15.16) and the HDL reverse cholesterol transport pathway (Fig. 15.17).

EXOGENOUS PATHWAY

The primary function of the exogenous pathway is the absorption of dietary lipid and its delivery, particularly triglyceride, to peripheral tissues and the liver. The exogenous pathway begins when nascent chylomicrons are assembled from dietary triglycerides and cholesterol

in the enterocytes and packaged in secretory vesicles in the Golgi apparatus. These particles are transported by exocytosis into the extracellular space and are introduced into the circulation through the lymphatic duct. The lipid content of nascent chylomicrons consists mainly of triglycerides (90% by mass), whereas protein components include apoB-48 and the A apolipoproteins (2% by mass). Shortly after entering the circulation, these particles acquire the C apolipoproteins and apoE from circulating HDL (Fig. 15.14). ApoC-II, now present on the surface of chylomicrons, activates the LPL attached to the luminal surface of endothelial cells; this rapidly hydrolyzes the triglycerides to free fatty acids. The fatty

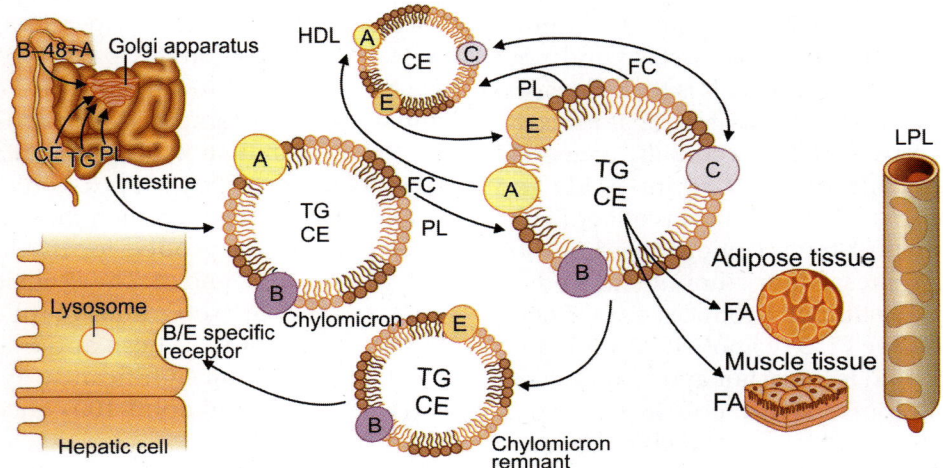

Fig. 15.14: Exogenous lipoprotein metabolism pathway. A—apolipoprotein A-I; B—apolipoprotein B-48; C—apolipoprotein C-II; CE, cholesterol ester; E—apolipoprotein E. FA, fatty acid; FC, free cholesterol; HDL, high-density lipoprotein; LPL, lipoproteinlipase; PL, phospholipid; TG, triglyceride

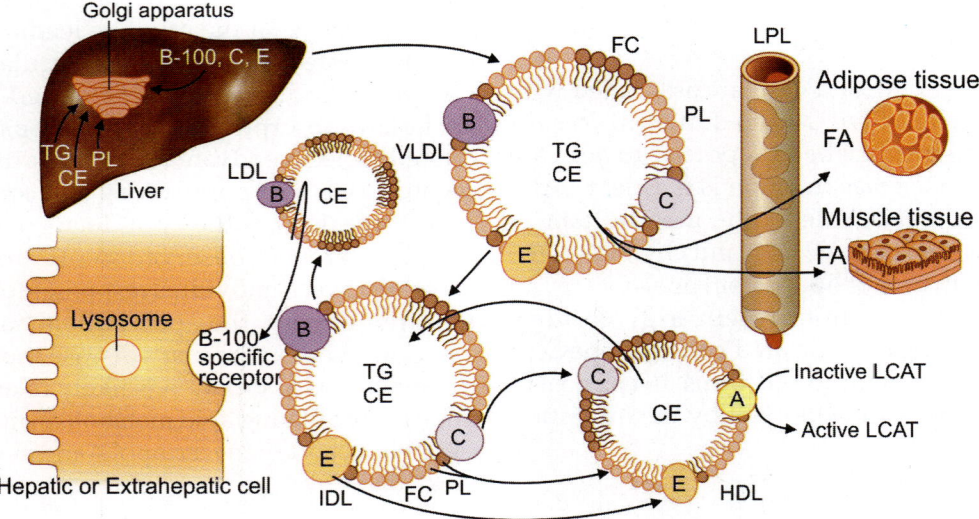

Fig. 15.15: Endogenous lipoprotein metabolism pathway. A—apolipoprotein A-I; B—apolipoprotein B-100; C—apolipoprotein C-II; CE—cholesterol ester; E—apolipoprotein E. FA, fatty acid; FC, free cholesterol; HDL, high-density lipoprotein; IDL, intermediate-density lipoprotein; LCAT, lecithin cholesterol acyl transferase; LDL, ow-density lipoprotein; LPL, lipoprotein lipase; PL, phospholipid; TG, triglyceride; VLDL, very low-density lipoproteins

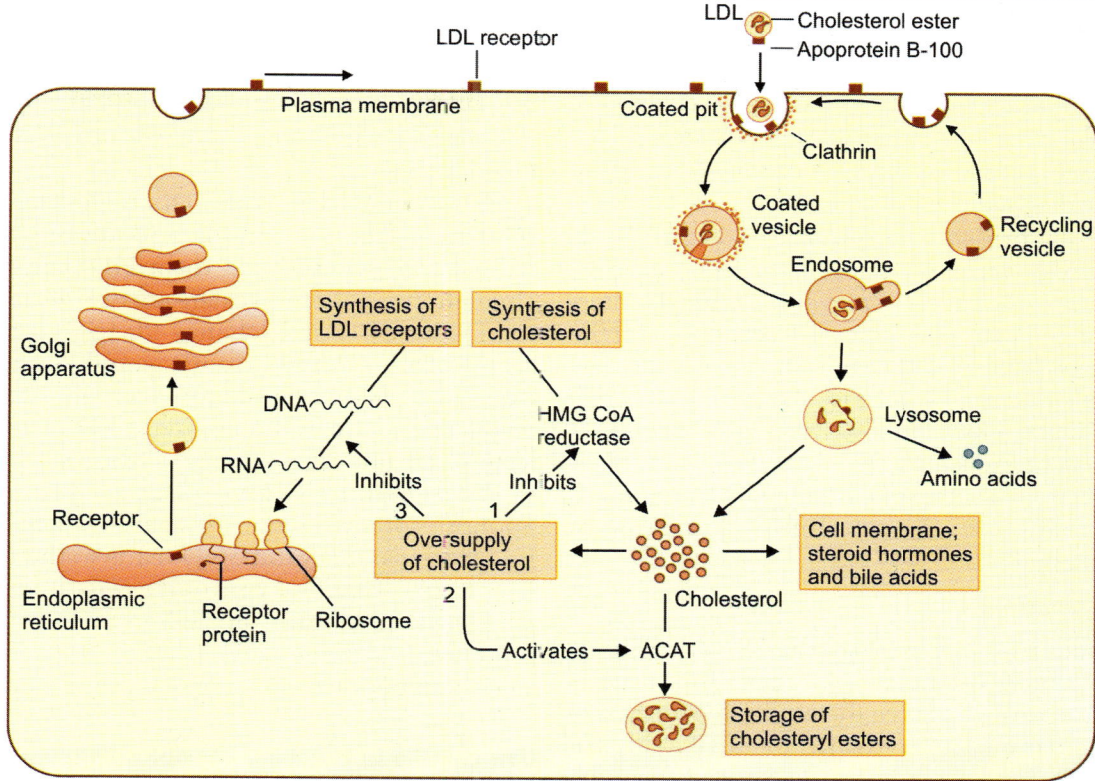

Fig. 15.16: Low-density lipoprotein receptor pathway. ACAT, Acyl-CoA cholesterol acyltransferase; HMG-CoA reductase, 3-hydroxy-3-methylglutaryl coenzyme A reductase; LDL, low-density lipoprotein. Because of the presence of apolipoprotein B-100 on its surface, the LDL particle is recognized by a specific receptor in a coated pit and is taken into the cell in a coated vesicle (top right). Coated vesicles fuse together to form an endosome. The acidic environment of the endosome causes the LDL particle to dissociate from the receptors, which return to the cell surface. LDL particles are taken to a lysosome, where apolipoprotein B-100 is broken down into amino acids and cholesterol ester is converted to free cholesterol for cellular requirements. The cellular cholesterol level is self-regulated. Oversupply of cholesterol will lead to (I) decreased rates of cholesterol synthesis by inhibiting HMG-CoA reductase, (2) increased storage of cholesteryl esters by activating ACAT, and (3) inhibition of manufacture of new LDL receptors by suppressing transcription of the receptor gene into mRNA

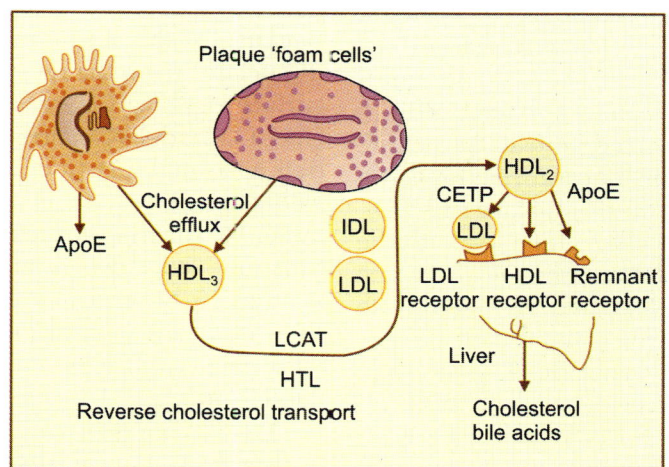

Fig. 15.17: Reverse-cholesterol transport pathway. ABCA I, ATP binding cassette transporter A I; ABCG I, ATP binding cassette transporter GI; apo A-I, apolipoprotein A-I; CETP, cholesteryl ester transfer protein; HDL, high-density lipoprotein; LCA, lecithin cholesterol acyltransferase; LDL, low-density lipoprotein; LDL-R, LDL receptor; SR-BI, scavenger receptor B-1; LDL-R, LDL receptor. After formation in the liver and intestine, nascent discoidal HDL removes cholesterol from peripheral cells by the ABCA I transporter. Additional cholesterol can also be removed from HDL by the ABCG I transporter and by a passive diffusion mechanism. LCAT esterifies the cholesterol content of HDL to prevent it from re-entering the cells. Cholesterol esters are delivered to the liver by the SR-B I receptor or by the LDL-R after transfer to LDL by CETP

acids are associated with albumin and can be taken up by muscle cells as an energy source or into adipose cells for storage. Simultaneously, some of the phospholipids and the apoA apolipoproteins are transferred back to HDL during lipolysis. The newly formed particle, the chylomicron remnant, contains 80–90% of the triglyceride content of the original chylomicron.

Because of the presence of apo B-48 and apoE on its surface, the chylomicron remnant can be recognized by specific hepatic remnant receptors and is quickly internalized within hours by endocytosis. Components of the particle are then hydrolyzed within the lysosomes. The cholesterol released can be used for the synthesis of bile acids, can be incorporated into newly synthesized lipoprotein, or can be stored as cholesteryl ester. Further more, cholesterol from these remnants down regulates HMG-CoA reductase, the rate-limiting enzyme of cholesterol biosynthesis.

ENDOGENOUS PATHWAY

The endogenous pathway involves the delivery of lipids that are packaged in the liver to peripheral cells (Fig. 15.15). Hepatocytes have the ability to synthesize triglycerides from carbohydrates or fatty acids. In addition, when dietary cholesterol acquired from the receptor-mediated uptake of chylomicron remnants is insufficient, hepatocytes can synthesize their own cholesterol by increasing the activity of HMG-CoA reductase. Endogenously made triglycerides and cholesterol are packaged along with apoB-100 into VLDL particles in the endoplasmic reticulum; this involves the microsomal transfer protein. A defective microsomal transfer protein results in the inability to secrete apo B-containing lipoproteins and is referred to as a beta lipoproteinemia. VLDL is a triglyceride-rich particle (55% by mass) that contains apoB-100, apoE, and small quantities of C apolipoproteins on its surface. Additional C apolipoproteins are transferred from HDL to VLDL after it enters the circulation. As in the case of chylomicron metabolism, apoC-I1 present on the surface of VLDL activates LPL on endothelial cells, which leads to the hydrolysis of VLDL triglycerides and the release of free fatty acids. It is important to note, however, that the rate of hydrolysis of VLDL triglyceride is significantly lower than that of chylomicron triglyceride. The average residence time of VLDL triglyceride is 15–60 minutes, compared with 5–10 minutes for chylomicron triglyceride. This difference may be attributed to the fact that VLDL particles are smaller and bind to fewer LPL molecules than do chylomicrons.

During hydrolysis of VLDL triglycerides, C apolipoproteins are transferred back to HDL. VLDL particles are thus converted to VLDL remnants, some of which are taken up by the liver. The rest are converted to smaller, denser particles called IDL. Large IDL particles, which also have several molecules of apoE, bind the hepatic remnant receptors and are removed from the circulation. In humans, about 50% of IDL is removed by hepatocytes.

Surface materials from IDL, including some phospholipids, free cholesterol, and apolipoproteins, are transferred to HDL, or form HDL de novo in the circulation. Cholesteryl esters are transferred from HDL to LDL by CETP in exchange for triglyceride. The net result of the coupled lipolysis and cholesteryl ester exchange reaction is the replacement of much of the triglyceride core of the original VLDL with cholestery lesters. IDL undergoes further hydrolysis, in which most of the remaining triglycerides are removed and all apolipoproteins except B-100 are transferred to other lipoproteins; this ultimately leads to the formation of LDL. Most LDL is eventually returned to the liver by the LDL receptor, but when present in excess, it infiltrates into the vessel wall, where it accumulates. This is a key initiation step in the process of atherosclerosis.

Low-density Lipoprotein Receptor Pathway

The mechanism by which LDL is removed from the circulation is reasonably well understood and primarily occurs via the LDL receptor pathway. Compared with VLDL and chylomicrons.

Low-density lipoprotein has a relatively long residence time in the circulation of about 3 days. Specific receptors present on plasma membranes recognize and bind apoB-100 associated with LDL (Fig. 15.15 and 15.16). LDL particles then are internalized and fuse with endosomes. Because of the acidic milieu of the endosome, LDL dissociates from the receptor, which returns to the cell surface for reuse, whereas LDL migrates to the lysosome. Once LDL is delivered to the lysosome, apoB-100 is degraded into small peptides and amino acids. Cholesteryl esters are also hydrolyzed, with the cholesterol then available for the synthesis of cell membranes, steroid hormone synthesis in endocrine tissues, or bile acid synthesis in hepatocytes. Cells have the ability to regulate their cholesterol content, most likely because of the cytotoxicity of excess cholesterol. Oversupply of free cholesterol.

1. Decreases the rate of endogenous cholesterol synthesis by inhibiting the rate-limiting enzyme HMG-CoA reductase.
2. Increases the formation of cholesteryl esters, which are catalyzed by ACAT.
3. Inhibits the synthesis of new LDL receptors by suppressing transcription of the receptor gene.

Many different intracellular pathways are available for coordinated gene regulation of cholesterol metabolism, but the sterol regulatory element-binding protein (SREBP) transcription factors, which sense intracellular cholesterol concentrations, appear to play the most central role.

Approximately, one-third of LDL is taken up by extrahepatic tissue through scavenger receptors or non-receptor-mediated pinocytosis. Non-receptor-mediated uptake becomes important as plasma LDL concentrations increase, as in familial hypercholesterolemia (FH). Non-receptor-mediated uptake is not saturable and is not regulated.

Scavenger receptors are unregulated and recognize LDL that has been modified in various ways, such as by oxidation. Scavenger receptors are largely found in macrophages; this probably accounts for the accumulation of lipid that occurs in these cells in atherosclerotic plaque. Macrophages that become engorged with cholesteryl esters are called foam cells, and are considered the earliest components of the atherosclerotic lesion.

REVERSE CHOLESTEROL TRANSFER PATHWAY

The reverse cholesterol transport pathway helps the body maintain cholesterol homeostasis by removing excess cholesterol from peripheral cells and delivering it to the liver for excretion. It is mediated mostly by HDL; this in part accounts for the antiatherogenic property of HDL. The pathway begins when HDL is secreted from the liver and intestine as disk-shaped nascent particles that contain phospholipids and apoA-I. Through the extracellular addition of surface components of triglyceride-rich particles, such as phospholipids, cholesterol, and certain apolipoproteins, nascent HDL is converted to spherical particles. Free cholesterol from cell membranes is also transferred to the nascent HDL (Fig. 15.17). This can occur by a passive process called aqueous diffusion, but it can also occur by specific energy, requiring transporters.

The ABCA 1 transporter, which is the defective gene in Tangier disease, promotes the efflux of excess cellular cholesterol and phospholipids to nascent HDL. In contrast, the ABCG 1 transporter and the scavenger receptor class B type I (SR-BI) receptor promote the efflux of cholesterol to more lipid-rich forms of HDL. Once cholesterol is delivered to HDL by whatever mechanism, it is quickly esterified by the action of LCAT in the presence of its cofactor apoA-I. The size of the HDL particle depends strongly on the quantity of accumulated cholesteryl esters and the activity of LCAT. Lysolecithin, a by-product of this reaction (see previous discussion), is removed from circulation after binding with albumin.

HDL cholesteryl esters are delivered to the liver by one of the following mechanisms: (1) cholesteryl esters are selectively taken up from HDL by the SR-BI receptor, and lipid-depleted forms of HDL are returned to the circulation for further transport; (2) cholesteryl esters are transferred from HDL to apoB-100-containing lipoprotein by a process mediated by cholesterol ester transfer protein; they then are taken up by the liver through receptors for the selipoproteins; or (3) HDL can be taken up in toto by holo particle receptors, which possibly recognize apoE. These processes constitute the reverse cholesterol transport mechanism by which cellular and lipoprotein cholesterol is delivered back to the liver for reuse or disposal.

Although, LDL is the major product resulting from the catabolism of VLDL, some conversion of HDL subfractions also occurs during this process. Surface materials from triglyceride-rich particles that have been transferred to the small circulating HDL3 are subsequently esterified by LCAT, as described earlier, to create the larger cholesteryl ester-rich HDL2. It has been shown that in vitro HDL2 is converted back to HDL3 in the presence of hepatic LPL. HDL2 contains twice as many cholesterol molecules per unit of apolipoproteinsas does HDL3.

LIPID DISORDERS

Lipid disorders is an elevation of plasma cholesterol, triglycerides or both, or a low high-density lipoprotein level that contributes to the development of atherosclerosis. Causes may be primary (genetic) or secondary. Diagnosis is by measuring plasma levels of total cholesterol, triglycerides (TGs), and individual lipoproteins. Treatment involves dietary changes, exercise, and lipid-lowering drugs.

DYSLIPIDEMIA (HYPERLIPIDEMIA)

There is no natural cutoff between normal and abnormal lipid levels because lipid measurements are continuous. A linear relation probably exists between lipid levels and cardiovascular risk, so many people with 'normal' cholesterol levels benefit from achieving still lower levels. Consequently, there are no numeric definitions of dyslipidemia; the term is applied to lipid levels for which treatment has proven beneficial. Proof of benefit is strongest for lowering elevated low-density lipoprotein levels. In the overall population, evidence is less strong for a benefit from lowering elevated TG and increasing low high-density lipoprotein levels. HDL levels do not always predict cardiovascular risk. For example, high HDL levels caused by some genetic disorders may not protect against cardiovascular disorders, and low HDL levels caused by some genetic disorders may not increase the risk of cardiovascular disorders. Although, HDL levels predict cardiovascular risk in the overall population, the increased risk may be caused by other factors, such as accompanying lipid and metabolic abnormalities, rather than the HDL level itself.

Classification

Dyslipidemias were traditionally classified by patterns of elevation in lipids and lipoproteins; Fredrickson phenotype (Table 15.5) dyslipidemias as primary or secondary and characterizes them by

- Increases in cholesterol only (pure or isolated hypercholesterolemia)
- Increases in TGs only (pure or isolated hypertriglyceridemia)
- Increases in both cholesterol and TGs (mixed or combined hyperlipidemias)

This system does not take into account specific lipoprotein abnormalities (e.g., low HDL or high LDL) that may contribute to disease despite normal cholesterol and TG levels.

Etiology

Primary (genetic) causes and secondary (lifestyle and other) causes contribute to dyslipidemias in varying degrees. For example, in familial combined hyperlipidemia, expression may occur only in the presence of significant secondary causes.

PRIMARY CAUSES

Primary causes are single or multiple gene mutations that result in either overproduction or defective clearance of TG and LDL cholesterol, or in underproduction or excessive clearance of HDL (Table 15.6). The names of

Table 15.5	Lipoprotein patterns (Fredrickson phenotypes)	
Phenotype	Elevated lipoprotein(s)	Elevated lipids
I	Chylomicrons	TGs
IIa	LDL	Cholesterol
IIb	LDL and VLDL	TGs and cholesterol
III	VLDL and chylomicron remnants	TGs and cholesterol
IV	VLDL	TGs
V	Chylomicrons and VLDL	TGs and cholesterol

LDL, low-density lipoprotein; TGs, triglycerides; VLDL, very-low-density lipoprotein.

Table 15.6	Genetic (primary) dyslipidemias				
Disorder	Genetic defect/ Mechanism	Inheritance	Prevalence	Clinical features	Treatment
Familial hypercholesterolemia	LDL receptor defect Diminished LDL clearance	Codominant or Complex with multiple genes	Present worldwide but increased among French Canadian, Christian Lebanese, and South African populations	—	Diet, lipid-lowering drugs, LDL apheresis (for homozygotes and heterozygotes with severe disease), liver transplantation (for homozygotes)
			Heterozygotes: 1/200–1/500	Tendon xanthomas, arcus cornea, premature CAD (ages 30–50), responsible for about 5% of MIs in people < 60 years TC: (7–13 mmol/L)	
			Homozygotes: 1/1 million (increased among French Canadian, Christian Lebanese, and South African populations)	Planar and tendon xanthomas and tuberous xanthomas, premature CAD (before age 18); TC >13 mmol/L	
Familial defective apoB-100	ApoB (LDL receptor-binding region defect) Diminished LDL clearance	Dominant	1/700	Xanthomas, arcus cornea, premature CAD; TC:7–13 mmol/L	Diet, lipid-lowering drugs

Contd.

Table 15.6 | **Genetic (primary) dyslipidemias** *(Contd.)*

Disorder	Genetic defect/Mechanism	Inheritance	Prevalence	Clinical features	Treatment
PCSK9 gain of function mutations	Increased degradation of LDL receptors	Dominant	Unknown	Similar to familial hypercholesterolemia	Diet, lipid-lowering drugs
Polygenic hypercholesterolemia	Unknown, possibly multiple defects and mechanisms	Variable	Common	Premature CAD; TC: 6.5–9.0 mmol/L	Diet, lipid-lowering drugs
LPL deficiency	Endothelial LPL defect Diminished chylomicron clearance	Recessive	Rare but present worldwide	Failure to thrive (in infants), eruptive xanthomas, hepatosplenomegaly, pancreatitis TG: >8.5 mmol/L	Diet, total fat restriction with fat-soluble vitamin supplementation and medium-chain TG supplementation Gene therapy (approved in European Union)
ApoC-II deficiency	ApoC-II (causing functional LPL deficiency)	Recessive	<1/1 million	Pancreatitis (in some adults), metabolic syndrome (often present) TG: >8.5 mmol/L	Diet, total fat restriction with fat-soluble vitamin supplementation and medium-chain TG supplementation
Familial hypertriglyceridemia	Unknown, possibly multiple defects and mechanisms	Dominant	1/100	Usually no symptoms or findings; occasionally hyperuricemia, sometimes early atherosclerosis TG: 2.3–5.7 mmol/L, possibly higher depending on diet and alcohol use	Diet, weight loss, lipid-lowering drugs
Familial combined hyperlipidemia	Unknown, possibly multiple defects and mechanisms	Dominant	1/50–1/100	Premature CAD, responsible for about 15% of MIs in people <60 years ApoB: Disproportionately elevated TC: 6.5–13.0 mmol/L TG: 2.8–8.5 mmol/L	Diet, weight loss, lipid-lowering drugs
Familial dysbetalipoproteinemia	ApoE (usually ApoE2/E2 homozygotes) Diminished chylomicron and VLDL clearance	Recessive (more common) or dominant (less common)	1/5000 Present worldwide	Xanthomas (especially tuberous and palmar), yellow palmar creases, premature CAD TC: 6.5–13.0 mmol/L) TG: 2.8–5.6 mmol/L	Diet, lipid-lowering drugs
Primary hypoalphalipoproteinemia (familial or non-familial)	Unknown, possibly apo-A-I, C-III, or A-IV	Dominant	About 5%	Premature CAD; HDL: 0.39–0.9 mmol/L	Exercise; HDL-elevating drugs and LDL-lowering drugs
Familial apoA/apoC-III deficiency/mutations	ApoA or apoC-III Increased HDL catabolism	Unknown	Rare	Corneal opacities, xanthomas, premature CAD (in some people) HDL: 0.39–0.8 mmol/L	Nonspecific
Familial LCAT deficiency	LCAT gene	Recessive	Extremely rare	Corneal opacities, anemia, renal failure HDL: <0.26mmol/L	Fat restriction Renal transplantation
Fisheye disease (partial LCAT deficiency)	LCAT gene	Recessive	Extremely rare	Corneal opacities HDL: <0.26 mmol/L	Nonspecific
Tangier disease	ABCA1 gene	Recessive	Rare	Premature CAD (in some people), peripheral neuropathy, hemolytic anemia, corneal opacities, hepatosplenomegaly, orange tonsils HDL: <0.13 mmol/L	Low-fat diet

Contd.

Table 15.6	Genetic (primary) dyslipidemias *(Contd.)*				
Disorder	Genetic defect/ Mechanism	Inheritance	Prevalence	Clinical features	Treatment
Familial HDL deficiency	ABCA1 gene	Dominant	Rare	Premature CAD	Low-fat diet
Hepatic lipase deficiency	Hepatic lipase	Recessive	Extremely rare	Premature CAD	
				TC: 6.5–38.9 mmol/L TG: 10.2–212.4 mmol/L HDL: Variable	Empiric: Diet, lipid-lowering drugs
Cerebrotendinous xanthomatosis	Hepatic mitochondrial 27-hydroxylase defect Blockage of bile acid synthesis and conversion of cholesterol to cholestanol, which accumulates	Recessive	Rare	Cataracts, premature CAD, neuropathy, ataxia	Chenodeoxycholic acid
Sitosterolemia	ABCG5 and ABCG8 genes	Recessive	Rare	Tendon xanthomas, premature CAD	Fat restriction Bile acid sequestrants Ezetimibe
Cholesteryl ester storage disease and Wolman disease	Lysosomal esterase deficiency	Recessive	Rare	Premature CAD Accumulation of cholesteryl esters and TG in lysosomes in the liver, spleen, and lymph nodes Cirrhosis	Possibly statins Enzyme replacement (experimental)

ABCA1, ATP-binding cassette transporter A1; ABCG5 and 8, ATP-binding cassette subfamily G members 5 and 8; Apo, apoprotein; CAD, coronary artery disease; HDL, high-density lipoprotein; LCAT, lecithin-cholesterol acyltransferase; LDL, low-density lipoprotein; LPL, lipoprotein lipase; MI, myocardial infarction; PCSK9, proprotein convertase subtilisin-like/kexin type 9; TC, total cholesterol; TG, triglyceride; VLDL, very-low-density lipoprotein

many primary disorders reflect an old nomenclature in which lipoproteins were detected and distinguished by how they separated into alpha (HDL) and beta (LDL) bands on electrophoretic gels.

SECONDARY CAUSES

Secondary causes contribute too many cases of dyslipidemia in adults. The **most important** secondary cause in developed countries is a sedentary lifestyle with excessive dietary intake of saturated fat, cholesterol, and trans fats.

Trans fats are polyunsaturated or monounsaturated fatty acids to which hydrogen atoms have been added; they are used in many processed foods and are as atherogenic as saturated fat. Other common secondary causes include:

- Diabetes mellitus
- Alcohol overuse
- Chronic kidney disease
- Hypothyroidism
- Primary biliary cirrhosis and other cholestatic liver diseases
- Drugs, such as thiazides, β-blockers, retinoids, highly active antiretroviral agents, cyclosporine, tacrolimus, estrogen and progestins, and glucocorticoids

Secondary causes of low levels of HDL cholesterol include cigarette smoking, anabolic steroids, HIV infection, and nephrotic syndrome.

Diabetes is an especially significant secondary cause because patients tend to have an atherogenic combination of high TGs; high-small, dense LDL fractions; and low HDL (diabetic dyslipidemia, hypertriglyceridemic hyperapoB). Patients with type 2 diabetes are especially at risk. The combination may be a consequence of obesity, poor control of diabetes, or both, which may increase circulating free fatty acids (FFAs), leading to increased hepatic very-low-density lipoprotein production. TG-rich VLDL then transfers TG and cholesterol to LDL and HDL, promoting formation of TG-rich, small, dense LDL and clearance of TG-rich HDL. Diabetic dyslipidemia is often exacerbated by the increased caloric intake and physical inactivity that characterize the lifestyles of some patients with type 2 diabetes. Women with diabetes may be at special risk of cardiac disease from this form.

Symptoms and Signs

Dyslipidemia itself usually causes no symptoms, but can lead to symptomatic vascular disease, including coronary artery disease (CAD), stroke, and peripheral arterial disease. High levels of TGs (>11.3 mmol/L) can cause acute pancreatitis. High levels of LDL can cause arcus cornea and tendinous xanthomas at the Achilles, elbow, and knee tendons and over metacarpophalangeal joints.

Patients with the homozygous form of familial hypercholesterolemia may have the above findings plus planar or tuberous xanthomas. Planar xanthomas (Fig. 15.18) are flat or slightly raised yellowish patches. Tuberous xanthomas (Fig. 15.19) are painless, firm nodules typically located over extensor surfaces of joints. Patients with severe elevations of TGs can have eruptive xanthomas (Fig. 15.20) over the trunk, back, elbows, buttocks, knees, hands, and feet. Patients with the rare

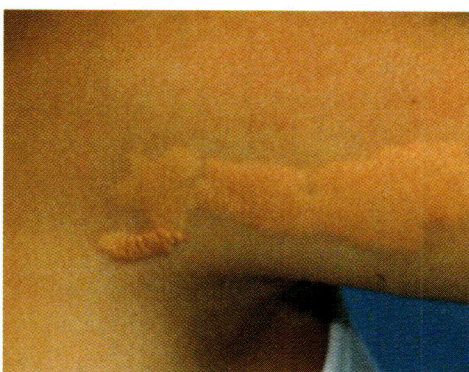

Fig. 15.18: Planar xanthomas are flat or slightly raised yellowish patches

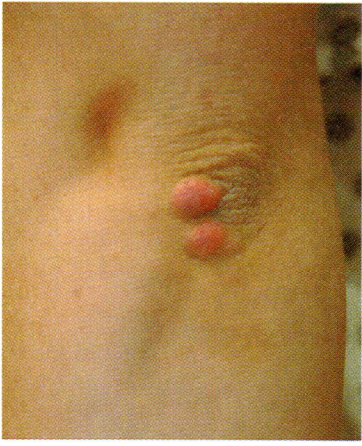

Fig. 15.19: Tuberous xanthomas are painless, firm nodules typically located over extensor surfaces of joints

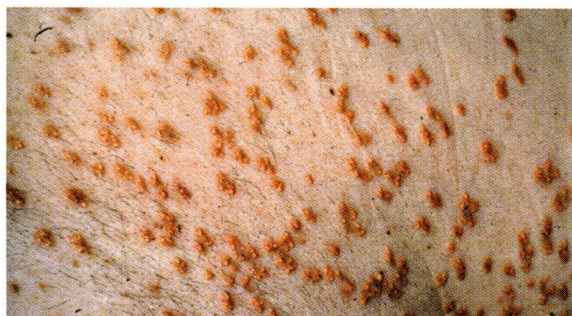

Fig. 15.20: Eruptive xanthoma; patients with severe elevations of TGs can have eruptive xanthomas over the trunk, back, elbows, buttocks, knees, hands, and feet

dys-betalipoproteinemia can have planar and tuberous xanthomas.

Severe hypertriglyceridemia (>22.6 mmol/L) can give retinal arteries and veins a creamy white appearance (lipemia retinalis). Extremely high lipid levels also give a lactescent (milky) appearance to blood plasma. Symptoms can include paresthesias, dypsnea, and confusion.

Diagnosis

Dyslipidemia is suspected in patients with characteristic physical findings or complications of dyslipidemia (e.g. atherosclerotic disease). Primary lipid disorders are suspected when patients have physical signs of dyslipidemia, onset of premature atherosclerotic disease (at <60 years), a family history of atherosclerotic disease, or serum cholesterol >6.2 mmol/L. Dyslipidemia is diagnosed by measuring serum lipids. Routine measurements (lipid profile) include total cholesterol (TC), TGs, HDL cholesterol, and LDL cholesterol.

Screening

Universal screening using a fasting lipid profile (TC, TGs, HDL cholesterol, and calculated LDL cholesterol) should be done in all children between age 9 and 11 (or at age 2 if children have a family history of severe hyperlipidemia or premature CAD). Adults are screened at age 20 years and every 5 years thereafter. Lipid measurement should be accompanied by assessment of other cardiovascular risk factors, defined as

- Diabetes mellitus
- Cigarette use
- Hypertension
- Family history of CAD in a male first-degree relative before age 55 or a female first-degree relative before age 65

A definite age after which patients no longer require screening has not been established, but evidence supports screening of patients into their 80s, especially in the presence of atherosclerotic cardiovascular disease.

Patients with an extensive family history of heart disease should also be screened by measuring Lp(a) levels.

Treatment

The main indication for dyslipidemia treatment is prevention of atherosclerotic cardiovascular disease (ASCVD), including acute coronary syndromes, stroke, transient ischemic attack, or peripheral arterial disease presumed caused by atherosclerosis. Treatment is indicated for all patients with ASCVD (secondary prevention) and for some without (primary prevention).

Treatment of children is controversial; dietary changes may be difficult to implement, and no data suggest that lowering lipid levels in childhood effectively prevents heart disease in adulthood. Moreover, the safety and effectiveness of long-term lipid-lowering treatment are questionable. Children with heterozygous familial hypercholesterolemia should be treated beginning at age 10 years. Children with homozygous familial hypercholesterolemia require diet, medications, and often LDL apheresis to prevent premature death; treatment is begun when diagnosis is made.

Treatment options depend on the specific lipid abnormality, although different lipid abnormalities often coexist. In some patients, a single abnormality may require several therapies; in others, a single treatment may be adequate for several abnormalities. Treatment should always include treatment of hypertension and diabetes, smoking cessation, and in patients with a 10 years risk of MI or death from CAD of ≥20%, low-dose daily aspirin. In general, treatment options for men and women are the same.

Elevated Low-density Lipoprotein Cholesterol Treatment

Treatment options to lower LDL cholesterol in all age groups include lifestyle changes (diet and exercise), drugs, dietary supplements, procedural interventions, and experimental therapies. Many of these options are also effective for treating other lipid abnormalities.

Dietary changes include decreasing intake of saturated fats and cholesterol; increasing the proportion of dietary fiber, and complex carbohydrates; and maintaining ideal body weight. Referral to a dietitian is often useful, especially for older people. Exercise lowers LDL cholesterol in some people and also helps maintain ideal body weight. Dietary changes and exercise should be used whenever feasible, but some guidelines recommend also using drug treatment for certain groups of patients after discussion of the risks and benefits of statin therapy.

For **drug treatment in adults,** the recommended treatment with a statin for four groups of patients, comprised of those with any of the following:
- Clinical ASCVD
- LDL cholesterol ≥4.9 mmol/L
- Age 40–75, with diabetes and LDL cholesterol 1.8–4.9 mmol/L
- Age 40–75, LDL cholesterol 1.8–4.9 mmol/L, and estimated 10-years risk of ASCVD ≥7.5%

Statins are the treatment of choice for LDL cholesterol reduction because they demonstrably reduce cardiovascular morbidity and mortality. Other classes of lipid-lowering drugs are not the first choice because they have not demonstrated equivalent efficacy for decreasing ASCVD. Statin treatment is classified as high, moderate, or low intensity and is given based on treatment group and age (Tables 15.7 A and B). The choice of statin may depend on the patient's co-morbidities, other medications, risk factors for adverse events, statin intolerance, cost, and patient preference. Statins inhibit hydroxymethylglutaryl CoA reductase, a key enzyme in cholesterol synthesis, leading to up-regulation of LDL receptors and increased LDL clearance. They reduce LDL

Table 15.7A	Statins for ASCVD prevention		
Classification	**Effects***	**Recommended for**	**Examples†**
High-intensity	Lowers LDL-C ≥ 50%	For clinical ASCVD, age ≤75 LDL-C ≥ 4.9 mmol/L Diabetes, age 40–75, and 10 years ASCVD risk ≥ 7.5%, age 40–75, 10-years ASCVD risk ≥7.5% Consider additional risk factors	Atorvastatin 40–80 mg Rosuvastatin 20–40 mg
Moderate-intensity	Lowers LDL-C 30 to <50%	Clinical ASCVD, age >75 Diabetes, age 40–75, and 10-years ASCVD risk <7.5% Age 40–75, 10-years ASCVD risk ≥7.5%	Atorvastatin 10–20 mg Fluvastatin XL 80 mg Lovastatin 40 mg Pitavastatin 2–4 mg Pravastatin 40–80 mg Rosuvastatin 5–10 mg Simvastatin 20–40 mg
Low-intensity	Lowers LDL-C < 30%	Patients who cannot tolerate high or moderate intensity treatment	Fluvastatin 20–40 mg Lovastatin 20 mg Pitavastatin 1 mg Pravastatin 10–20 mg

*Individual response may vary.
†All doses oral and once a day.

Table 15.7B	Non-statin lipid-lowering drugs	
Drugs	**Adult doses**	**Comments**
Bile acid sequestrants		Lower LDL-C (primary), slightly increase HDL (secondary), may increase TGs
Cholestyramine	4–8 g by mouth 1–3 times/day with meals	—
Colesevelam	2.4–4.4 g by mouth once/day with a meal	—
Colestipol	5–30 g by mouth once/day with a meal or divided with two or more meals	—
Cholesterol absorption inhibitor		Lowers LDL-C (primary), minimally increases HDL-C
Ezetimibe	10 mg by mouth once/day	—
Drugs for homozygous familial hypercholesteremia		
Lomitapide	5–60 mg by mouth once/day	Risk of hepatotoxicity Increase dose gradually (about every 2 weeks) Measure transaminase levels before increasing dosage
Mipomersen	200 mg sc once/week	Used as an adjunct to diet and other lipid-lowering drugs in patients with familial hypercholesteremia Can cause hepatotoxicity
Fibrates		Lower TGs and VLDL, increase HDL, may increase LDL-C (in patients with high TGs)
Bezafibrate	200 mg by mouth 3 times day or 400 mg by mouth once/day	Decreased dose required in renal insufficiency Not available in US
Ciprofibrate	100–200 mg by mouth once/day	Not available in US
Fenofibrate	34–201 mg by mouth once/day	Decreased dose required in renal insufficiency May be safest fibrate for use with statins
Gemfibrozil	600 mg by mouth bid	Decreased dose required in renal insufficiency
Nicotinic acid (niacin)	Immediate-release: 500 mg twice a day—1000 mg by mouth 3 times day	Increases HDL; lowers TGs (low doses), LDL-C (higher doses), and Lp(a) (secondary) Frequent adverse effects: Flushing, impaired glucose tolerance, increased uric acid
	Extended-release: 500–2000 mg by mouth once/day at bedtime	Aspirin and administration with food minimize flushing
PCSK9 monoclonal antibodies		
Alirocumab	75–150 mg sc q 2 weeks	For patients with familial hypercholesterolemia and for other high-risk patients
Evolocumab	Primary or Mixed dyslipidemia: 140 mg sc q 2 weeks or 420 mg sc once/month* Familial hypercholesterolemia: 420 mg sc once/ month or 420 mg sc q 2 weeks*	For patients with familial hypercholesterolemia and for other high-risk patients
Prescription omega-3 fatty acids		
Omega-3 acid ethyl esters	3–4 g by mouth once/day (4 capsules)	Lower TGs only
Combination products		Combined effects of the 2 drugs
Ezetimibe + Atorvastatin	Ezetimibe 10 mg + atorvastatin 10, 20, 40, 80 mg by mouth once/day	Not recommended as initial therapy. Simvastatin 80 mg should not be used unless patients have already taken it for >1 years without adverse effects
Ezetimibe + Simvastatin	Ezetimibe 10 mg + simvastatin 10, 20, 40, or 80 mg by mouth once/day	
Niacin extended release + Lovastatin	Niacin 500 mg + lovastatin 20 mg by mouth once/day, niacin 2000 mg + lovastatin 40 mg by mouth once/day	
Niacin extended release + Simvastatin	Niacin 500 mg + Simvastatin 20 mg by mouth once/day at bedtime (starting dose) or niacin 750 or 1000 mg + Simvastatin 20 mg by mouth once/day at bedtime	

*Proposed dosages, pending FDA approval.

HDL, high-density lipoprotein; HDL-C, HDL cholesterol; LDL, low-density lipoprotein; LDL-C, LDL cholesterol; Lp(a), lipoprotein (a); TG, triglyceride.

cholesterol by up to 60% and produce small increases in HDL and modest decreases in TGs. Statins also appear to decrease intra-arterial inflammation, systemic inflammation, or both by stimulating production of endothelial nitric oxide and may have other beneficial effects.

Adverse effects are uncommon but include liver enzyme elevations and myositis or rhabdomyolysis. Liver enzyme elevations are uncommon, and serious liver toxicity is extremely rare. Muscle problems occur in up to 10% of patients taking statins and may be dose-dependent in many patients. Muscle symptoms can occur without enzyme elevation. Adverse effects are more common among older patients, patients with several disorders, and patients taking several drugs. In some patients, changing from one statin to another or lowering the dose relieves the problem. Muscle toxicity seems to be most common when some of the statins are used with drugs that inhibit cytochrome P3A4 (e.g. macrolide antibiotics, azole antifungals, and cyclosporine) and with fibrates, especially gemfibrozil. Statins are contraindicated during pregnancy and lactation.

Previous guidelines recommended using specific target LDL cholesterol levels to guide drug treatment. However, evidence suggests that using such targets does not improve ASCVD prevention but does increase risk of adverse effects. Instead, response to therapy is determined by whether LDL cholesterol levels decrease as expected based on therapy intensity (i.e. patients receiving high-intensity therapy should have a ≥50% decrease in LDL cholesterol). If response is less than anticipated, the first intervention is to reinforce the importance of adherence to the drug regimen and lifestyle changes, and assess for drug side effects and secondary causes of hyperlipidemia (e.g. hypothyroidism, nephrotic syndrome).

If response remains less than expected after this, then the statin can be changed or dosage increased. If response continues to be less than expected after patients are on the maximum tolerated intensity of statin therapy, then a non-statin lipid-lowering drug(s) can be added if the ASCVD risk reduction benefit appears to outweigh the potential for adverse effects, particularly for secondary prevention and in patients with genetic dyslipidemias such as familial hypercholesterolemia.

Bile acid sequestrants block intestinal bile acid reabsorption, forcing up-regulation of hepatic LDL receptors to recruit circulating cholesterol for bile synthesis. They are proved to reduce cardiovascular mortality. Bile acid sequestrants are usually used with statins or with nicotinic acid to augment LDL cholesterol reduction and are the drugs of choice for women who are or are planning to become pregnant. Bile acid sequestrants are safe, but their use is limited by adverse effects of bloating, nausea, cramping, and constipation. They may also increase TGs, so their use is contraindicated in patients with hypertriglyceridemia. Cholestyramine and colestipol, but not usually colesevelam, interfere with absorption of other drugs; notably thiazides, beta-blockers, warfarin, digoxin, and thyroxine; an effect that can be decreased by administration at least 4 hour before or 1 hour after other drugs. Bile acid sequestrants should be given with meals to increase their efficacy.

Cholesterol absorption inhibitors, such as ezetimibe, inhibit intestinal absorption of cholesterol and phytosterol. Ezetimibe usually lowers LDL cholesterol by 15–20% and causes small increases in HDL and a mild decrease in TGs. Ezetimibe can be used as monotherapy in patients intolerant to statins or added to statins for patients on maximum doses with persistent LDL cholesterol elevation. Adverse effects are infrequent.

Proprotein convertase subtilisin/kexin type 9 (PCSK9) monoclonal antibodies are available as subcutaneous injections given once or twice per month. These drugs keep PCSK9 from attaching to LDL receptors, leading to improved function of these receptors. LDL cholesterol is lowered by 40–70%. Long-term clinical trials of cardiovascular outcomes are underway.

Dietary supplements that lower LDL cholesterol levels include fiber supplements and commercially available margarines and other products containing plant sterols (sitosterol and campesterol) or stanols. The latter reduce LDL cholesterol by up to 10% without affecting HDL or TGs by competitively displacing cholesterol from intestinal micelles.

Drugs for homozygous familial hypercholesterolemia include mipomersen and lomitapide. Mipomersen is an apoB antisense oligonucleotide that decreases synthesis of apoB in liver cells and decreases levels of LDL, apoB, and Lp(a). It is given by subcutaneous injection and can cause injection site reactions, flu-like symptoms, and increased hepatic fat and liver enzyme elevations. Lomitapide is an inhibitor of microsomal triglyceride transfer protein inhibitor that interferes with the secretion of TG-rich lipoproteins in the liver and intestine. Dose is begun low and gradually titrated up about every 2 weeks. Patients must follow a diet with less than 20% of calories from fat. Lomitapide can cause gastrointestinal (GI) adverse effects (e.g. diarrhea, increased hepatic fat, elevated liver enzymes).

ELEVATED LDL CHOLESTEROL IN CHILDREN

Childhood risk factors besides family history and diabetes include cigarette smoking, hypertension, low HDL cholesterol (<35 mg/dL), obesity, and physical inactivity.

For children, the American Academy of Pediatrics (AAP) recommends dietary treatment for children with LDL cholesterol >2.8 mmol/L. Drug therapy is recommended for children > 8 years and with either of the following:

- Poor response to dietary therapy, LDL cholesterol ≥4.9 mmol/L, and no family history of premature cardiovascular disease
- LDL cholesterol >4.13 mmol/L and a family history of premature cardiovascular disease or ≥2 risk factors for premature cardiovascular disease

Drugs used in children include many of the statins. Children with familial hypercholesterolemia may require a second drug to achieve LDL cholesterol reduction of at least 50%.

Elevated Triglycerides

Although, it is unclear whether elevated TGs independently contribute to cardiovascular disease, they are associated with multiple metabolic abnormalities that contribute to CAD (e.g. diabetes, metabolic syndrome). Consensus is emerging that lowering elevated TGs is beneficial. No target goals exist, but levels <1.7 mmol/L are generally considered desirable. No guidelines specifically address treatment of elevated TGs in children.

The **overall treatment strategy** is to first implement lifestyle changes, including exercise, weight loss, and avoidance of concentrated dietary sugar and alcohol. Intake of 2–4 servings/weeks of marine fish high in omega-3 fatty acids may be effective, but the amount of omega-3 fatty acids is often lower than needed; supplements may be helpful. In patients with diabetes, glucose levels should be tightly controlled. If these measures are ineffective, lipid-lowering drugs should be considered. Patients with very high TGs may need to begin drug therapy at diagnosis to more quickly reduce the risk of acute pancreatitis.

Fibrates reduce TGs by about 50%. They appear to stimulate endothelial LPL, leading to increased fatty acid oxidation in the liver and muscle and decreased hepatic VLDL synthesis. They also increase HDL by up to 20%. Fibrates can cause GI adverse effects, including dyspepsia, abdominal pain, and elevated liver enzymes. They uncommonly cause cholelithiasis. Fibrates may potentiate muscle toxicity when used with statins and potentiate the effects of warfarin.

Statins can be used in patients with TGs <5.65 mmol/L if LDL cholesterol elevations are also present; statins may reduce both LDL cholesterol and TGs through reduction of VLDL. If only TGs are elevated, fibrates are the drug of choice.

Omega-3 fatty acids in high doses [1–6 g/day of eicosapentaenoic acid (EPA) and docosahexaenoic acid (DHA)] can be effective in reducing TGs. The omega-3 fatty acids EPA and DHA are the active ingredients in marine fish oil or omega-3 capsules. Adverse effects include eructation and diarrhea. These effects may be decreased by giving the fish oil capsules with meals in divided doses (e.g. twice or three times a day). Omega-3 fatty acids can be a useful adjunct to other therapies. Prescription omega-3 fatty acid preparations are indicated for triglyceride levels 5.65 mmol/L.

Low High-densiy Lipoprotein

Although, higher HDL levels are associated with lower cardiovascular risk, it is not clear whether treatments to increase HDL cholesterol levels decrease risk of death. Adult treatment panel III (ATP-III) guidelines define low HDL cholesterol as <1.04 mmol/L; the guidelines do not specify an HDL cholesterol target level and recommend interventions to raise HDL cholesterol only after LDL cholesterol targets have been reached. Treatments for LDL cholesterol and TG reduction often increase HDL cholesterol, and the three objectives can sometimes be achieved simultaneously. No guidelines specifically address treatment of low HDL cholesterol in children.

Treatment includes **lifestyle changes** such as an increase in exercise and weight loss. Alcohol raises HDL cholesterol, but is not routinely recommended as a therapy because of its many other adverse effects. Drugs may be successful in raising levels when lifestyle changes alone are insufficient, but it is uncertain whether raising HDL levels reduces mortality.

Nicotinic acid (niacin) is the most effective drug for increasing HDL. Its mechanism of action is unknown, but it appears to both increase HDL production and inhibit HDL clearance; it may also mobilize cholesterol from macrophages. Niacin also decreases TGs and, in doses of 1500–2000 mg/day, reduces LDL cholesterol. Niacin causes flushing, pruritus, and nausea; premedication with low-dose aspirin may prevent these adverse effects. Extended-release preparations cause flushing less often. However, most over-the-counter (OTC) slow-release preparations are not recommended; an exception is polygel controlled-release niacin. Niacin can cause liver enzyme elevations and occasionally liver failure, insulin resistance, and hyperuricemia and gout. It may also increase homocysteine levels. The combination of high doses of niacin with statins may increase the risk of myopathy. In patients with average LDL cholesterol and below-average HDL cholesterol levels, niacin combined with statin treatment may be effective in preventing cardiovascular disorders. In patients treated with statins to lower LDL cholesterol to <1.8 mmol/L, niacin does not appear to have added benefit.

Elevated Lipoprotein (a)

The upper limit of normal for Lp(a) is about 0.8 mmol/L, but values in African Americans run higher. Few data exist to guide the treatment of elevated Lp(a) or to establish treatment efficacy. Niacin is the only drug that directly decreases Lp(a); it can lower Lp(a) by >20% at higher doses. The usual approach in patients with elevated Lp(a) is to lower LDL cholesterol aggressively. LDL apheresis has been used to lower Lp(a) in patients with high Lp(a) levels and progressive vascular disease.

Secondary Causes

Treatment of diabetic dyslipidemia should always involve lifestyle changes and statins to reduce LDL cholesterol. To decrease the risk of pancreatitis, fibrates can be used to decrease TGs when levels are >5.65 mmol/L. Metformin lowers TGs, which may be a reason to choose it over other oral antihyperglycemic drugs when treating diabetes. Some thiazolidinediones (TZDs) increase both HDL cholesterol and LDL cholesterol. Some TZDs also decrease TGs. These antihyperglycemic drugs should not be chosen over lipid-lowering drugs to treat lipid abnormalities in diabetic patients but may be useful adjuncts. Patients with very high TG levels and less than optimally controlled diabetes may have better response to insulin than to oral antihyperglycemic drugs.

Treatment of dyslipidemia in patients with hypothyroidism, renal disease, liver disease, or a combination of these disorders involves treating the underlying disorders primarily and lipid abnormalities secondarily. Abnormal lipid levels in patients with low-normal thyroid function [high-normal thyroid stimulating hormone (TSH) levels] improve with hormone replacement. Reducing the dosage of or stopping drugs that cause lipid abnormalities should be considered.

Monitoring Treatment

Lipid levels should be monitored periodically after starting treatment. No data support specific monitoring intervals, but measuring lipid levels 2–3 months after starting or changing therapies and once or twice yearly after lipid levels are stabilized is common practice.

Despite the low incidence of liver and severe muscle toxicity with statin use (0.5–2% of all users), current recommendations are for baseline measurements of liver and muscle enzyme levels at the beginning of treatment. Routine monitoring of liver enzyme levels is not necessary, and routine measurement of CK is not useful to predict the onset of rhabdomyolysis. Muscle enzyme levels need not be checked regularly unless patients develop myalgias or other muscle symptoms. If statin-induced muscle damage is suspected, statin use is stopped and CK may be measured. When muscle symptoms subside, a lower dose or a different statin can be tried. If symptoms do not subside within 1–2 weeks of stopping the statin, another cause should be sought for the muscle symptoms (e.g. polymyalgia rheumatica).

HYPOLIPIDEMIA

Hypolipidemia is a decrease in plasma lipoprotein caused by primary (genetic) or secondary factors. It is usually asymptomatic and diagnosed incidentally on routine lipid screening. Treatment of secondary hypolipidemia involves treating underlying disorders. Treatment of primary hypolipidemia is often unnecessary, but patients with some genetic disorders require high-dose vitamin E and dietary supplementation of fats and other fat-soluble vitamins.

Etiology

Hypolipidemia is defined as a total cholesterol <3.1 mmol/L or low-density lipoprotein cholesterol <1.3 mmol/L. Secondary causes are far more common than primary causes and include all of the following:

- Hyperthyroidism
- Chronic infections (including hepatitis C infection) and other inflammatory states
- Hematologic and other cancers
- Under nutrition (including that accompanying chronic alcohol use)
- Malabsorption

The unexpected finding of low cholesterol or low LDL cholesterol in a patient not taking a lipid-lowering drug should prompt a diagnostic evaluation, including measurements of aspartate aminotransferase (AST), alanine aminotransferase (ALT), and thyroid-stimulating hormone; a negative evaluation suggests a possible primary cause.

There are three primary disorders in which single or multiple genetic mutations result in underproduction or increased clearance of LDL.

Abetalipoproteinemia (Bassen-Kornzweig Syndrome)

This autosomal recessive condition is caused by mutations in the gene for microsomal triglyceride transfer protein, a protein critical to chylomicron and very-low-density lipoprotein formation. Dietary fat cannot be absorbed, and lipoproteins in both metabolic pathways are virtually absent from serum; TC is typically <1.16 mmol/L, TGs are <0.23 mmol/L, and LDL is undetectable.

The condition is often first noticed in infants with fat malabsorption, steatorrhea, and failure to thrive. Intellectual disability may result. Because vitamin E is distributed to peripheral tissues via VLDL and LDL, most affected people eventually develop severe vitamin E deficiency. Symptoms and signs include visual changes from slow retinal degeneration, sensory neuropathy, posterior column signs, and cerebellar signs of dysmetria, ataxia, and spasticity, which can eventually lead to death. Red blood cell (RBC) acanthocytosis is a distinguishing feature on blood smear. Diagnosis is made by the absence of apoprotein B (apoB) in plasma; intestinal biopsies show lack of microsomal transfer protein.

Treatment is with high doses (100–300 mg/kg once a day) of vitamin E with supplementation of dietary fat and other fat-soluble vitamins. The prognosis is poor.

HYPOBETALIPOPROTEINEMIA

Hypobetalipoproteinemia is an autosomal dominant or co-dominant condition caused by mutations in the gene coding for apoB. Heterozygous patients have truncated apoB, leading to rapid LDL clearance. Heterozygous patients manifest no symptoms or signs except for TC <3.1 mmol/L and LDL cholesterol <2.1 mmol/L. TGs are normal. Homozygous patients have either shorter truncations, leading to lower lipid levels TC <2.1 mmol/L, LDL cholesterol <0.52 mmol/L, or absent apo B synthesis, leading to symptoms and signs of abetalipoproteinemia.

Diagnosis is by finding low levels of LDL cholesterol and apoB; hypobetalipoproteinemia and abetalipoproteinemia are distinguished from one another by family history. People who are heterozygous and people who are homozygous with low but detectable LDL cholesterol require no treatment. Treatment of people who are homozygous with no LDL is the same as for abetalipoproteinemia.

Loss of function mutations of PCSK9 are another cause of low LDL levels. There are no adverse consequences and no treatment.

Chylomicron Retention Disease

Chylomicron retention disease is a very rare autosomal recessive condition caused by an unknown mutation leading to deficient apoB secretion from enterocytes. Chylomicron synthesis is absent, but VLDL synthesis remains intact. Affected infants have fat malabsorption, steatorrhea, and failure to thrive and may develop neurologic disorders similar to those in abetalipoproteinemia. Diagnosis is by intestinal biopsy of patients with low cholesterol levels and absence of postprandial chylomicrons. Treatment is supplementation of fat and fat-soluble vitamins.

ELEVATED HIGH-DENSITY LIPOPROTEIN LOW-DENSITY LIPOPROTEIN LEVEL

Elevated HDL cholesterol levels usually correlate with decreased cardiovascular risk; however, high HDL cholesterol levels caused by some genetic disorders may not protect against cardiovascular disease, probably because of accompanying lipid and metabolic abnormalities.

Primary causes of elevated HDL levels are single or multiple genetic mutations that result in overproduction or decreased clearance of HDL. **Secondary causes** of high HDL cholesterol include all of the following:

- Chronic alcoholism without cirrhosis
- Primary biliary cirrhosis
- Hyperthyroidism
- Drugs (e.g. corticosteroids, insulin, and phenytoin)

The unexpected finding of high HDL cholesterol in patients not taking lipid-lowering drugs should prompt a diagnostic evaluation for a secondary cause with measurements of AST, ALT, and thyroid-stimulating hormone; a negative evaluation suggests a possible primary cause.

Cholesteryl ester transfer protein deficiency is a rare autosomal recessive disorder caused by a CETP gene mutation. CETP facilitates transfer of cholesterol esters from HDL to other lipoproteins, and CETP deficiency affects low-density lipoprotein cholesterol and slows HDL clearance. Affected patients display no symptoms or signs but have HDL cholesterol >3.9 mmol/L. Protection from cardiovascular disorders has not been proved. No treatment is necessary.

Familial hyperalphalipoproteinemia is an autosomal dominant condition caused by various unidentified and known genetic mutations, including those that cause apoprotein A-I overproduction and apoprotein C-III variants. The disorder is usually diagnosed incidentally when plasma HDL cholesterol levels are >2.1 mmol/L. Affected patients have no other symptoms or signs. No treatment is necessary.

Measurement of Lipids, Lipoproteins, and Apolipoproteins

Total cholesterol, TGs, and HDL cholesterol are measured directly. TC and TG values reflect cholesterol and TGs in all circulating lipoproteins, including chylomicrons, VLDL, intermediate-density lipoprotein, LDL, and HDL. TC values can vary by 10% and TGs by up to 25% day-to-day even in the absence of a disorder. TC and HDL cholesterol can be measured in the non-fasting state, but most patients should have all lipids measured while fasting (usually for 12 hours) for maximum accuracy and consistency.

Testing should be postponed until after resolution of acute illness because TG and lipoprotein (a) levels increase and cholesterol levels decrease in inflammatory states. Lipid profiles can vary for about 30 days after an acute myocardial infarction (MI); however, results obtained within 24 hours after MI are usually reliable enough to guide initial lipid-lowering therapy.

LDL cholesterol values are most often calculated as the amount of cholesterol not contained in HDL and VLDL. VLDL is estimated by TG ÷ 5 because the cholesterol concentration in VLDL particles is usually one fifth of the total lipid in the particle. Thus,

LDL cholesterol = Total cholesterol –

$$\text{HDL cholesterol} + \frac{(\text{Triglycerides})}{5}$$

This calculation is valid only when TGs are <4.5 mmol/L and patients are fasting, because eating increases TGs. The calculated LDL cholesterol value incorporates measures of all non-HDL, non-chylomicron cholesterol, including that in IDL and lipoprotein (a).

LDL can also be measured directly using plasma ultracentrifugation, which separates chylomicrons and VLDL fractions from HDL and LDL, and by an immunoassay method. Direct measurement may be useful in some patients with elevated TGs, but these direct measurements are not routinely necessary. The role of apoB testing is under study because values reflect all non-HDL cholesterol (in VLDL, VLDL remnants, IDL, and LDL) and may be more predictive of CAD risk than LDL cholesterol. Non-HDL cholesterol (TC-HDL cholesterol) may also be more predictive of CAD risk than LDL cholesterol.

Other Tests

Patients with premature atherosclerotic cardiovascular disease, cardiovascular disease with normal or near-normal lipid levels, or high LDL levels refractory to drug therapy should probably have Lp (a) levels measured. Lp (a) levels may also be directly measured in patients with borderline high LDL cholesterol levels to determine whether drug therapy is warranted. C-reactive protein may be considered in the same populations. Measurements of LDL particle number or apoprotein B 100 (apoB) may be useful in patients with elevated TGs and the metabolic syndrome. ApoB provides similar information to LDL particle number because there is one apoB molecule for each LDL particle. ApoB measurement includes all atherogenic particles, including remnants and Lp(a).

Total Cholesterol

Testing methods for total cholesterol use cholesterol oxidase reactions along with cholesterol esterase and usually a peroxidase reaction for the 'color' or final determination reaction.

The Reaction

- **Cholesterol esterase**
  Total cholesterol esters → Cholesterol + Free fatty acid
- **Cholesterol oxidase**
  Cholesterol + O_2 → Cholest-3-ene-4-one + H_2O_2
- **Peroxidase**
  $2 H_2O_2$ + 4-aminoantipyrine → $4 H_2O$ + Chromogen

Interference

Remove sample from red cells after blood clots or plasma has been spun down. The peroxidase assay can be susceptible to increases in uric acid, ascorbic acid, bilirubin, hemoglobin, or other reducing substances. Samples should have only the normal amount of these substances present.

The Specimen

Nonhemolyzed serum or plasma, free from clots. The patient need not be fasting if this is the only lipid test requested. However, if total cholesterol is requested as part of a lipid panel, the patient must be fasting for 10–12 hours.

Reference ranges (age-specific)
Male (25–29 year old) 3.37–6.1 mmol/L
Female (25–29 years old) 3.37–5.9 mmol/L
Based on coronary heart disease risk:
Child desirable 4.4 mmol/L
Adult desirable 5.2 mmol/L

Triglyceride

Triglycerides are composed of three fatty acids and a glycerol moiety. Analyzing a serum or plasma sample for triglycerides typically involves four reactions.

The Reaction

- **Lipase (bacterial)**
  Triglycerides → 3 fatty acids + Glycerol
- **Glycerol kinase**
  Glycerol + ATP → Glycerol-3-phosphate + ADP
- **Pyruvate kinase**
  ADP + Phosphoenol pyruvate → ATP + Pyruvate
- **Lactate dehydrogenase**
  NADH + H^+ + Pyruvate → NAD + Lactate

The Specimen

Serum, fasting 10 to 12 hours.
Reference ranges (age-specific)
Male (25–29 years old) 0.51–2.3 mmol/L
Females (25–29 years old) 0.47–1.8 mmol/L

National cholesterol education program risk factors (adult male):

Optimal <1.7 mmol/L
High 1.7–2.2 mmol/L
Hypertriglyceridemic 2.3–5.6 mmol/L
Very high >5.6 mmol/L

Low-density Lipoprotein Cholesterol

Low-density lipoprotein cholesterol (LDL-C) may be calculated or measured directly.

Friedewald Calculation or Derived Beta-quantification

Testing for LDL-C involves a calculation that includes total cholesterol, HDL cholesterol (HDL-C), and triglyceride (TG) values using the formula:

$$LDL\text{-}C = Total\ cholesterol - [HDL\text{-}C + (TG/5)]$$

where TG/5 approximates the VLDL cholesterol concentration in the sample.

Interference

Cannot be used for TG over 4.5 mmol/L.

Specimen

None required for this portion, but 10–12 hours fasting serum specimen for lipid panel.

Reference ranges (age-specific)
Male (25–29 years old) 1.8–4.3 mmol/L
Females (25–29 years old) 1.8–4.2 mmol/L

National cholesterol education program risk factors (adult male):

Optimal <2.6 mmol/L
Near optimal 2.6–3.3 mmol/L
Borderline high 3.4–4.1 mmol/L
High >4.1 mmol/L
Very high >4.9 mmol/L

Direct Measurement of LDL-C

With the advent of homogeneous reagents, LDL-C is now measured using the cholesterol reaction along with reagents that block the contribution of HDL and VLDL to the resulting answer. In the homogeneous LDL assay, detergents block the other two lipoprotein cholesterol products from forming colored chromogens. Only the LDL-C forms a colored chromogen that can be measured spectrophotometrically by automated systems or designated analyzers.

The Specimen

Serum, plasma. The patient need not be fasting if this is the only lipid test requested.
However, if total cholesterol is requested as part of a lipid panel, the patient must be fasting for 10–12 hours.

Reference ranges (age-specific)
Male (25–29 years old) 1.8–4.3 mmol/L
Females (25–29 years old) 1.8–4.2 mmol/L

National cholesterol education program risk factors (adult male):

Optimal <2.6 mmol/L
Near optimal 2.6–3.3 mmol/L
Borderline high 3.4–4.1 mmol/L
High >4.1 mmol/L
Very high >4.9 mmol/L

HDL Cholesterol

Testing for HDL-C using either precipitation methods or homogenous assays.

The Precipitation Reaction

The precipitation methods use either dextran sulfate, polyethylene glycol (PEG), or phosphotungstic acid with magnesium chloride ($MgCl_2$) to precipitate LDL and VLDL lipoproteins from a fasting serum sample, leaving HDL in the supernatant. This HDL supernatant is then assayed for cholesterol. The resulting answer (in mg/dL) represents the amount of HDL in the serum sample. The supernatant is tested for cholesterol concentration.

Interference

Chylomicrons from non-fasting specimens will interfere in these precipitation methods.

The Specimen

Serum, plasma (depending on the precipitating reagent used); 10–12 hours fasting.
Reference ranges (age-specific)
Men (25–29 years old) 0.8–1.6 mmol/L
Women (25–29 years old) 1.0–2.1 mmol/L

National cholesterol education program risk factors (adult male):

Low risk >1.5 mmol/L
High risk <1.0 mmol/L

The Homogeneous Reaction

Homogeneous HDL-C assays do not use precipitation, nor do they require a centrifugation separation step. This improves the yield of HDL recovered from the specimen.

One method uses an antibody to apolipoprotein B-100 to bind LDL and VLDL in the sample. This leaves the HDL-C to react with the second reagent, which contains enzymes and substrate for cholesterol analysis.

In a second method, a synthetic polyanion reagent binds the sites on VLDL and LDL particles, blocking their products from forming cholesterol colored products. The second reagent added has detergent, enzymes, and substrate that react with the HDL-C in the sample. Only the HDL particle cholesterol is allowed to form a colored product and be measured.

The Specimen

Serum, plasma (depends on the method used).
Reference ranges (age-specific)
Men (25–29 years old) 0.8–1.6 mmol/L
Women (25–29 years old) 1.0–2.1mmol/L
National cholesterol education program risk factors (adult male):
Low risk >1.5 mmol/L
High risk <1.0 mmol/L

Apolipoproteins

Apolipoproteins can be measured by antigen-antibody assays in which antibody to a specific apolipoprotein is used to complex with the 'antigen' apoprotein and no other. Enzyme-linked immunosorbent assays (ELISAs) use two antibodies to 'sandwich' the apoprotein of interest.

The Reaction

In the antigen-antibody (Ab) assay, where X = any apoprotein, such as apoprotein A-I:

$$ApoX + Ab \leftrightarrow Ab\text{-}apoX$$
$$Ab\text{-}apoX + Ab2 \text{ complex} \leftrightarrow Ab\text{-}apoX\text{–}Ab2$$

The Specimen

Serum, plasma.

Reference Ranges

Apo A-I 0.94–1.99 g/L
Apo B-100 0.55–1.25 g/L
Other assays use different methods.

BIBLIOGRAPHY

1. Abera AB, Marais AD, Raal FJ, Leisegang F, Jones S, George P, et al. Autosomal recessive hypercholesterolaemia: discrimination of ARH protein and LDLR function in the homozygous FH phenotype. Clin Chim Acta 2007; 378: 33–7.

2. Abuja PM, Esterbauer H. Simulation of lipid peroxidation in low-density lipoprotein by a basic "skeleton" of reactions. Chem Res Toxicol 1995; 8: 753–63.

3. Alaupovic P. Apolipoproteins and lipoproteins. Athero-sclerosis 1971; 13: 141–6.

4. Albers n, Hazzard WR. Immunochemical quantification of human plasma Lp(a) lipoprotein. Lipids 1974; 9: 15–26.

5. Albers n, Marcovina SM. Lipoprotein (a) quantification: comparison of methods and strategies for standardization. Curr Opin Lipidol 1994; 5: 417–21.

6. Albert CM, Ma J, Rifai N, Stampfer MJ, Ridker PM. Prospective study of C-reactive protein, homocysteine, and plasma lipid levels as predictors of sudden cardiac death. Circulation 2002; 105: 2595–9.

7. Albert MA, Danielson E, Rifai N, Ridker PM. Effect of statin therapyon C-reactive protein levels: the pravastatin inflammation/CRP evaluation (PRINCE): a randomized trial and cohort study. JAMA200 I; 286: 64–70.

8. Andersson A, Isaksson A, Brattstrom L, Hultberg B. Homocysteine and other thiols determined in plasma by HPLC and thiol-specificpostcolumnderivatization. Clin Chern 1993; 39: 1590–7.

9. Ariyo AA, Thach C, Tracy R. Lp(a) lipoprotein, vascular disease, and mortality in the elderly. N Engl J Med 2003; 349: 2108–15.

10. Arranz-Pena ML, Tasende-Mata J, Martin-Gil FJ. Com-parisonof two homogeneous assays with a precipitation method and an ultracentrifugation method for the measure-ment of HDL-cholesterol. ClinChern 1998; 44: 2499–505.

11. Assmann G, Eckardstein A, Brewer HB Jr. Familial analphaliproteinemia: Tangier disease. In: Scriver C, BeaudetA,Valle D, Sly W, Childs B, Kinzler K, et aI, eds. The metabolic and molecular bases of inherited diseases. New York: McGraw-Hill, 2001: 2937–81.

12. Assmann G, Herbert PN, Fredrickson DS, Forte T. Isolation and characterization of an abnormal high density lipoprotein in Tangierdisease. J Clin Invest 1977; 60: 242–52.

13. Asztalos BF, Roheim PS, Milani RL, Lefevre M, McNamara JR, Horvath KV, et al. Distribution of ApoA-I-containing HDL subpopulations in patients with coronary heart disease. ArteriosclerThrombVascBioi 2000; 20: 2670–6.

14. Austin MA, Breslow JL, Hennekens CH, Buring JE, Willett WC, Krauss RM. Low-density lipoprotein subclass patterns and risk of myocardial infarction. JAMA 1988; 260: 1917–21.

15. Bachorik PS, Albers n. Precipitation methods for quantifica-tion of lipoproteins. Methods Enzymol 1986; 129: 78–1 00.

16. Bachorik PS, Lovejoy KL, Carroll MD, Johnson CL. Apolipoprotein Band Al distributions in the United States, 1988-1991: results of the National Health and Nutrition Examination Survey 1Il (NHANES [II).ClinChem 1997; 43: 2364–78.

17. Bachorik PS, Rifkind BM, Kwiterovich PO. Lipids and dyslipoproteinemia. In: Henry J, ed. Clinical diagnosis and management by laboratory methods. Philadelphia: WB Saunders, 1996: 208–36.

18. Bachorik PS, Walker R, Brownell KD, et al. Determination of high density lipoprotein-cholesterol in stored human plasma. J Lipid Res 1980; 21: 608–16.

19. Bachorik PS, Walker RE, Virgil DG. High-density-lipoprotein cholesterol in heparin-MnCl2 supernates determined with the Dowenzymic method after precipitation of Mn2+ with HC03-. ClinChem 1984; 30: 839–42.

20. Bachorik PS. Electrophoresis in the determination of plasma lipoprotein patterns. In: Lewis L, OppltJ, eds. CRC handbook of electrophoresis. Boca Raton, Fla: CRC Press, 1980; 7.

21. Balk EM, Lau J, Goudas LC, Jordan HS, Kupelnick B, Kim LU, et al. Effects of statins on non-lipid serum markers associated with cardiovascular disease: a systematic review. Ann Intern Med 2003; 139: 670–82.

22. Bartlett GR. Phosphorus assay in column chromatography. J Bioi Chem 1959; 234: 466–8.

23. Benzaquen LR, Yu H, Rifai N. High sensitivity C-reactive protein: an emerging role in cardiovascular risk assessment. Crit Rev Clin Lab Sci 2002; 39: 459–97.

24. Berenson GS, Wattigney WA, Tracy RE, Newman WP III, Srinivasan SR, Webber LS, et al. Atherosclerosis of the aorta and coronary arteries and cardiovascular risk factors in persons aged 6 to 30 years and studied at necropsy (The Bogalusa Heart Study). Am J Cardiol1992; 70:851-8.

25. Blake GJ, Rifai N, Buring JE, Ridker PM. Blood pressure, C-reactive protein, and risk of future cardiovascular events. Circulation 2003; 108: 2993–9.

26. Blankenhorn DH, Nessim SA, Johnson RL, San marco ME, AzenSP,Cashin-Hemphill L. Beneficial effects of combined colestipol-niacintherapy on coronary atherosclerosis and coronary venous bypass grafts. JAMA 1987; 257: 3233–40.

27. Bookstein L, Gidding SS, Donovan M, Smith FA. Day-to-day variability of serum cholesterol, triglyceride, and high-density lipoprotein cholesterol levels: impact on the assessment of risk according to the National Cholesterol Education Program guidelines. Arch Intern Med 1990; 150: 1653–7.

28. Booth GL, Wang EE. Preventive health care, 2000 update: screening and management of hyper homocysteinemia for the prevention of coronary artery disease events. The Canadian Task Force on Preventive Health Care. CMAJ 2000; 163: 21–9.

29. Breslow JL. Familial disorders of high-density lipoprotein metabolism. In: Scriver C, Beaudet A, Sly W, Valle D, eds. The metabolic and molecular bases of inherited diseases. New York: McGraw-Hill, 1995: 2031–52.

30. Brown G, Albers n, Fisher LD, Schaefer SM, Lin JT, Kaplan C, et al. Regression of coronary artery disease as a result of intensivelipid-lowering therapy in men with high levels of apolipoprotein B.N Engl J Med 1990; 323: 1289–98.

31. Brown MS, Goldstein JL. A receptor-mediated pathway for cholesterol homeostasis. Science 1986; 232: 34–47.

32. Brown MS, Goldstein JL. Lipoprotein metabolism in the macrophage: implications for cholesterol deposition in atherosclerosis. Annu Rev Biochem 1983; 52: 223–61.

33. Brown SA, Hutchinson R, Morrisett J, Boerwinkle E, Davis CE, Gotto AM Jr, et al. Plasma lipid, lipoprotein cholesterol, and apoprotein distributions in selected US communities: the Atherosclerosis Risk in Communities (A RIC) study. Arterioscler Thromb 1993; 13: 1139–58.

34. Brunzell JD, Deeb S. Familial lipoprotein lipase deficiency, apo C-I1 deficiency, and hepatic lipase deficiency. In: Scriver C, Beaudet A, Sly W, Valle D, eds. The metabolic basis of inherited diseases. New York: McGraw-Hill, 2001:2789-819.

35. Burstein M, Legmann P. Lipoprotein precipitation. Monogr Atheroscler 1982; 11: 1–131.

36. Buxtorf JC, Baudet MF, Martin C, Richard JL, lacotot B. Seasonal variations of serum lipids and apoproteins. Ann Nutr Metab 1988; 32: 68–74.

37. Campos H, Blijlevens E, McNamara JR, Ordovas JM. Posner BM, Wilson PW, et al. LDL particle size distribution: results from the Framingham Offspring Study. Arterioscler Thromb 1992; 12: 1410–9.

38. Castelli WP, Doyle JT, Gordon T, Hames CG, Hjortland MC, Hulley SB, et al. HDL cholesterol and other lipids in coronary heart disease: the Cooperative Lipoprotein Phenotyping Study. Circulation 1977; 55: 767–72.

39. Chace DH, Hillman SL, Millington DS, Kahler SG, Adam BW, Levy HL. Rapid diagnosis of homocystinuria and other hypermethioninemias from newborns' blood spots by tandem mass spectrometry. Clin Chem 1996; 42: 349–55.

40. Chae CU, Lee RT, Rifai N, Ridker PM. Blood pressure and inflammation in apparently healthy men. Hypertension 2001; 38: 399–403.

41. Chait A, Albers n, Brunzell JD. Very low density lipoprotein overproduction in genetic forms of hypertriglyceridaemia. Eur J Clin Invest 1980; 10: 17–22.

42. Chen CH, Albers n. Activation of lecithin: cholesterol acyltransferaseby apolipoproteins E-2, E-3, and A-IV isolated from human plasma. Biochim Biophys Acta 1985; 836: 279–85.

43. Christen WG, Ajani UA, Glynn RJ, Hennekens CH. Blood levels of homocysteine and increased risks of cardiovascular disease: causal or casual? Arch Intern Med 2000; 160: 422–34.

44. Chung BH, Segrest JP, Ray MJ, Brunzell JD, Hokanson JE, Krauss RM, et al. Single vertical spin density gradient ultracentrifugation. Methods Enzymol 1986; 128: 181–209.

45. Chung BH, Wilkinson '1', Geer JC, Segrest JP. Preparative and quantitative isolation of plasma lipoproteins: rapid, single discontinuous density gradient ultracentrifugation in a vertical rotor. J Lipid Res 1980; 2 I : 284–9 I.

46. Cohn JS, McNamara JR, Cohn SD, Ordovas JM, Schaefer EJ. Postprandial plasma lipoprotein changes in human subjects of different ages. J Lipid Res 1988; 29: 469–79.

47. Cohn JS, McNamara JR, Schaefer EJ. Lipoprotein cholesterol concentrations in the plasma of human subjects as measured in the fed and fasted states. Clin Chem 1988; 34: 2456–9.

48. Cole TG. Glycerol blanking in triglyceride assays: is it necessary? ClinChem 1990; 36: I267–8.

49. Contois J, McNamara JR, Lammi-Keefe C, Wilson PW, Massov '1', Schaefer EJ. Reference intervals for plasma apolipoprotein A- I determined with a standardized commercial immunoturbidimetric assay: results from the Framingham Offspring Study. ClinChem 1996; 42: 507–14.

50. Contois JH, McConnell JP, Sethi AA, Csako G, Devaraj S, Hoefner DM, et al. Apolipoprotein B and cardiovascular disease risk: position statement from the AACC Lipoproteins and Vascular Diseases Division Working Group on Best Practices. Clin Chem 2009; 55: 407–19.

51. Contois JH, McNamara JR, Lammi-Keefe CJ, Wilson PW, Massov '1',Schaefer EJ. Reference intervals for plasma apolipoprotein Bdetermined with a standardized commercial immunoturbidimetric assay: results from the Framingham Offspring Study. Clin Chem1996; 42: 5 I 5–23.

52. Cooper GR, Smith SJ, Duncan IW, Mather A, Fellows WD, FoleyT,et al. Inter laboratory testing of the transferability of a candidate reference method for total cholesterol in serum. Clin Chem 1986; 32: 92 I–9.

53. Cooper GR, Smith SJ, Wiebe DA, Kuchmak M, Hannon WHO International survey of apolipoproteins A I and B measurements (1983-1984). Clin Chem 1985; 31: 223–8.

54. Cortner JA, Coates PM, Bennett MJ, Cryer DR, Le NA. Familial combined hyperlipidaemia: use of stable isotopes to demonstrate overproduction of very low-density lipoprotein apolipoprotein B by the liver. J Inherit Metab Dis 1991; 14: 915–22.

55. Couderc R, Mahieux F, Bailleul S, Fenelon G, Mary R, Fermanian J. Prevalence of apolipoprotein E phenotypes in ischemic cerebrovascular disease. A case-control study. Stroke 1993; 24: 66 I–4.

56. Curb JD, Abbott RD, Rodriguez BL, Sakkinen P, Popper JS, Yano K,et al. C-reactive protein and the future risk of thromboembolic stroke in healthy men. Circulation 2003; 107: 2016–20.

57. Cushman M, McClure LA, Howard VJ, Jenny NS, Lakoski SG, Howard G. Implications of increased C-reactive protein for cardiovascular risk stratification in black and white men and women in the US. ClinChem 2009; 55: 1627–36.

58. Dallongeville J, Lussier-Cacan S, Davignon J. Modulation of plasma triglyceride levels by apo E phenotype: a meta-analysis. J Lipid Res1992; 33: 447–54.

59. Daniels SR, Greer FR. Lipid screening and cardiovascular health in childhood. Pediatrics 2008; 122: I 98–208.

60. Davignon J, Gregg RE, Sing CF. Apolipoprotein E poly-morphism andatherosclerosis. Arteriosclerosis 1988; 8: I-2 I.

61. deKeijzer MH, Elbers D, Baadenhuijsen H, Demacker PN. Evaluation of five different high-density lipoprotein cholesterol assays: the most precise are not the most accurate. Ann ClinBiochem 1999; 36(Pt 2): 168–75.

62. Deacon AC, Dawson PJ. Enzymic assay of total cholesterol involving chemical or enzymic hydrolysis-a comparison of methods. Clin Chern 1979; 25: 976–84.

63. DeLong DM, Delong ER, Wood PD, Lippel K, Rifkind BM. A comparison of methods for the estimation of plasma Iow- and very low-density lipoprotein cholesterol. The Lipid Research Clinics Prevalence Study. JAMA 1986; 256: 2372-7.

64. Devaraj S, Singh U, Jialal I. The evolving role of C-reactive protein in atherothrombosis. Clin Chern 2009; 55: 229–38.

65. Devaraj S, Xu DY, Jialal I. C-reactive protein increases plasminogen activator inhibitor- I expression and activity in human aortic endothelial cells: implications for the metabolic syndrome and atherothrombosis. Circulation 2003; 107: 398–404.

66. Ducros V, Demuth K, Sauvant MP, Quillard M, Causse E, CanditoM,et al. Methods for homocysteine analysis and biological relevance ofthe results. J Chromatogr B Analyt Technol Biomed Life Sci 2002; 78 I: 207–26.

67. Durrington PN. Lipoprotein (a). Baillieres Clin Endocrinol Metab 1995; 9: 773–95.

68. Ellerbe P, Myers GL, Cooper GR, Hertz HS, Sniegoski LT, Welch MJ,et al. A comparison of results for cholesterol in human serum obtained by the reference method and by the definitive, ethod of the national reference system for cholesterol. Clin Chem 1990; 36: 370–5.

69. Elliot P, Chambers Je, Zhang W, Clarke R, Hopewell JC, PedenJF,et al. Genetic loci associated with C-reactive protein levels and risk of coronary heart disease. JAMA 2009; 302: 37–48.

70. Emi M, Wu LL, Robertson MA, Myers RL, Hegele RA, Williams RR,et al. Genotyping and sequence analysis of apolipoprotein E isoforms. Genomics 1988; 3: 373–9.

71. Enos WF, Holmes RH, Beyer J. Landmark article, July 18, 1953.Coronary disease among United States soldiers killed in action in Korea: preliminary report. JAMA 1986; 256: 2859–62.

72. Ensign W, Hill N, Heward CB. Disparate LDL phenotypic classification among 4 different methods assessing LDL particle characteristics. ClinChem 2006; 52: I 722–7.

73. Esteban-Sahin M, Guimon-Bardesi A, de La Viuda-Unzueta JM,Azcarate-Ania MN, Pascual-Usandizaga P, Amoroto-Del-Rio E.Analytical and clinical evaluation of two homogeneous assays for LDL-cholesterol in hyperlipidemic patients. Clin Chem 2000; 46: Il21–31.

74. Evrovski J, Callaghan M, Cole DE. Determination of homocysteine by HPLC with pulsed integrated ampero-metry. ClinChem 1995; 41: 757–8.

75. Ford ES, Giles WH, Myers GL, Mannino DM. Population distribution of high-sensitivity C-reactive protein among US men: findings from National Health and Nutrition Examination Survey 1999-2000. Clin Chem 2003; 49: 686–90.

76. Forte 'I'M, Shu X, Ryan RO. The ins (cell) and outs (plasma) of apolipoprotein A-V. J Lipid Res 2009; 50(Suppl): SI50-5.

77. Frantzen F, Faaren AL, Alfheim I, Nordhei AK. Enzyme conversion immunoassay for determining total homo-cysteine in plasma orserum. Clin Chem 1998; 44:3 I 1–6.

78. Franzin M, Ferro C, Ceriotti F, Carobene A, Martini R, Guerra E.Optimization of a designed comparison method (DCM) for triglycerides measurement. ClinChem Lab Med 1999; 37:S260.

79. Freedman DS, Srinivasan SR, Shear CL, Franklin FA, Webber LS, Berenson GS. The relation of apolipoproteins A-I and B in children to parental myocardial infarction. N Engl J Med 1986; 315: 721–6.

80. Freeman DJ, Norrie J, Caslake MJ, Gaw A, Ford I, Lowe GD, et al. C-reactive protein is an independent predictor of risk for the development of diabetes in the West of Scotland Coronary Prevention Study. Diabetes 2002; 5 I: I 596–600.

81. Friedewald WT, Levy RI, Fredrickson DS. Estimation of the concentration of low-density lipoprotein cholesterol in plasma, without use of the preparative ultracentrifuge. Clin Chem 1972; I 8: 499–502.

82. Funk CD, FitzGerald GA. COX-2 inhibitors and cardio-vascular risk. J Cardiovasc Pharmacol 2007; 50: 470–9.

83. Garg UC, Zheng ZJ, Folsom AR, Moyer YS, Tsai MY, McGovern P, et al. Short-term and long-term variability of plasma homocysteine measurement. ClinChem 1997; 43: 141–5.

84. Glueck CJ, Mellies MJ, Srivastava L, Knowles HC Jr, FallatRW,Tsang RC, et al. Insulin, obesity, and triglyceride interrelationships in sixteen children with familial hypertriglyceridemia. Pediatr Res 1977; Il: 13–9.

85. Marcovina SM, Albers JJ, Kennedy H, Mei JV, Henderson LO, Hannon WHo International Federation of Clinical Chemistry standardization project for measurements of apolipoproteins A-I and B. IV. Comparability of apolipoprotein B values by use of International Reference Material. ClinChern 1994; 40: 586–92.

86. Marcovina SM, Albers JJ, Scanu AM, et al. Use of a reference material proposed by the International Federation of Clinical Chemistry and Laboratory Medicine to evaluate analytical methods for the determination of plasma lipoprotein(a). Clin Chern 2000; 46: 1956–67.

87. Marcovina SM, Gaur VP, Albers JJ. Biological variability of cholesterol, triglyceride, low- and high-density lipoprotein cholesterol, lipoprotelO(a), and apolipoproteins A-I and B. Clin Chern 1994; 40: 574–8.

88. Marcovina SM, Hobbs HH, Albers JJ. Relation between number of apolipoprotein(a) kringle 4 repeats and mobility of isoforms in agarose gel: basis for a standardized isoform nomenclature. Clin Chern 1996; 42: 436–9.

89. Marcovina SM, Koschinsky ML, Albers JJ, Skarlatos S. Report of the National Heart, Lung, and Blood Institute Workshop on Lipoprotein(a) and Cardiovascular Disease: recent advances and future directions. ClinChern 2003; 49: 1785–96.

90. Marcovina SM, Morrisett JD. Structure and metabolism of lipoprotein (a). Curr Opin Lipidol 1995; 6:136–45.

91. Marcovina SM, Zhang ZH, Gaur VP, Albers JJ. Identification of 34 apolipoprotein(a) isoforms: differential expression of apolipoprotein(a) alleles between American blacks and whites. Biochem Biophys Res Commun 1993; 191: 1192–6.

92. McCabe E. Disorders of glycerol metabolism. In: Scriver C, Beaudet A, Sly W, Valle D, eds. The Metabolic and molecular bases of inherited diseases. New York: McGraw-Hill, 1995: 1631–52.

93. Ridker PM, Hennekens CH, BuringjE, Rifai N. C-reactive protein and other markers of inflammation in the prediction of cardiovascular disease in women. N Engl j Med 2000; 342: 836–43.

94. Ridker PM, Paynter NP, Rifai N, GazianojM, Cook NR. C-reactive protein and parental history improve global cardiovascular risk prediction: the Reynolds Risk Score for men. Circulation 2008; 118: 2243–51.

95. Ridker PM, Rifai N, Clearfield M, et al. Measurement of C-reactive protein for the targeting of statin therapy in the primary prevention of acute coronary events. N Engl j Med 2001; 344: 1959–65.

96. Ridker PM, Rifai N, Pfeffer MA, Sacks F, Braunwald E. Long-term effects of pravastatin on plasma concentration of C-reactive protein. The Cholesterol and Recurrent Events (CARE) Investigators. Circulation 1999; 100: 230–5.

97. Ridker PM, Rifai N, Pfeffer MA, Sacks FM, Moye LA, Goldman S, et al. Inflammation, pravastatin, and the risk of coronary events after myocardial infarction in patients with average cholesterol levels. Cholesterol and Recurrent Events (CARE) Investigators. Circulation 1998; 98: 839–44.

98. Ridker PM, Rifai N, Rose L, BuringjE, Cook NR. Comparison of C-reactive protein and low-density lipoprotein cholesterol levels in the prediction of first cardiovascular events. N Engl J Med 2002; 347: 1557–65.

99. Ridker PM, Stampfer MJ, Rifai N. Novel risk factors for systemic atherosclerosis: a comparison of C-reactive protein, fibrinogen, homocysteine, lipoprotein(a), and standard cholesterol screening as predictors of peripheral arterial disease. JAMA 2001; 285: 2481–5.

100. Rifai N, Heiss G, Doetsch K. Lipoprotein (a) at birth, in blacks and whites. Atherosclerosis 1992; 92: 123–9.

101. Rifai N, Heiss G. Gender and race differences in cord blood lipoprotein. Circulation 1988; 1l: 481.

102. Rifai N, Kwiterovich P Jr. Disorders of lipid and lipoprotein metabolism in children and adolescents. In: Soldin Sj, Rifai N, Hicks JMB, eds. Biochemical bases of inherited disease. Washington, DC: AACC Press, 1995.

103. Rifai N, Neufeld E, Ahlstrom P, Rimm E, D'Angelo L, Hicks jM. Failure of current guidelines for cholesterol screening in urban African-American adolescents. Pediatrics 1996; 98: 383–8.

104. Rifai N, Ridker PM. Population distributions of C-reactive protein in apparently healthy men and women in the United States: implication for clinical interpretation. Clin Chern 2003; 49: 666–9.

105. Rifai N, Silverman LM. Immunoturbidimetric techniques for quantifying apolipoproteins Cll and Clll. Clin Chern 1986; 32: 1969–72.

106. Rifai N. Lipoproteins and apolipoproteins: composition, metabolism, and association with coronary heart disease. Arch Pathol Lab Med 1986; 110: 694–70 1.

107. Roberts WL, Moulton L, Law TC, Farrow G, Cooper-Anderson M, Savory j, et al. Evaluation of nine automated high-sensitivity C-reactive protein methods: implications for clinical and epidemiological applications. Part 2. Clin Chern 2001; 47: 418–25.

108. Rosseneu M, Vercaemst R, Steinberg KK, Cooper GR. Some considerations of methodology and standardization of apolipoprotein B immunoassays. Clin Chern 1983; 29: 427-33.

109. Rousset X, Vaisman B, Amar M, Sethi AA, Remaley AT. Lecithin: cholesterol acyltransferase-from biochemistry to role in cardiovascular disease. Curr Opin Endocrinol Diabetes Obes 2009; 16:163-71.

110. Sandkamp M, Funke H, Schulte H, Kohler E, Assmann G. Lipoprotein(a) is an independent risk factor for myocardial infarction at a young age. Clin Chern 1990; 36: 20–3.

111. Sattar N, Gaw A, Scherbakova 0, Ford I, O'Reilly DS, Haffner SM, et al. Metabolic syndrome with and without C-reactive protein as a predictor of coronary heart disease and diabetes in the West of Scotland Coronary Prevention Study. Circulation 2003; 108: 414–9.

112. Savage DG, Lindenbaum j, Stabler SP, Allen RH. Sensitivity of serum methyl malonic acid and total homocysteine determinations for diagnosing cobalamin and folate deficiencies. Am j Med 1994; 96: 239–46.

113. Schaefer Ej, Blum CB, Levy RI, jenkins LL, Alaupovic P, Foster DM, et al. Metabolism of high-density lipoprotein apolipoproteins in Tangier disease. N Engl j Med 1978; 299: 905–10.

114. Schaefer Ej, Lamon-Fava S, johnson S, OrdovasjM, Schaefer MM, Castelli WP, et al. Effects of gender and menopausal status on the association of apolipoprotein E phenotype with plasma lipoprotein levels: results from the Framingham Offspring Study. ArteriosclerThromb 1994; 14: 1105–13.

115. Schaefer Ej, McNamara JR. Overview of the diagnosis and treatment of lipid disorders. In: Rifai N, Dominiczak M, Warnick GR, eds. Handbook of lipoprotein testing. Washington, DC: AACC Press, 1997.

116. Schaefer Ej. Clinical, biochemical, and genetic features in familial disorders of high density lipoprotein deficiency. Arteriosclerosis 1984; 4: 303–22.

117. Scharnagl H, Nauck M, Wieland H, Marz W. The Friedewald formula underestimates LDL cholesterol at low concentrations. Clin Chern Lab Med 2001; 39: 426–31.

118. Schmitz G, Assmann G, Robenek H, Brennhausen B. Tangier disease: a disorder of intracellular membrane traffic. Proc Natl Acad Sci USA 1985; 82: 6305–9.

119. Schrott HG, Goldstein jL, Hazzard WR, McGoodwin MM, Motulsky AG. Familial hypercholesterolemia in a large kindred: evidence for a monogenic mechanism. Ann Intern Med 1972; 76: 711–20.

120. SegrestjP, Chung BH, Cone jT, Hughes TA. Coronary heart disease risk: assessment by plasma lipoprotein profiles. Ala j Med Sci 1983; 20:76-83.

121. Stary He. The sequence of cell and matrix changes in atheroscleroticlesions of coronary arteries in the first forty years of life. Eur Heart J1990; II(Suppl E):3-19.

122. Steele BW, Koehler DF, Azar MM, Blaszkowski TP, Kuba K, DempseyME. Enzymatic determinations of cholesterol in high-densitylipoproteinfractions prepared by a precipitation technique. ClinChem 1976; 22: 98–10 1.

123. Steinberg D, Witztum JL. Is the oxidative modification hypothesisrelevant to human atherosclerosis? Do the anti-oxidant trialsconducted to date refute the hypothesis? Circulation 2002; 105: 2107–11.

124. Steinberg KK, Cooper GR, Graiser SR, Rosseneu M. Someconsiderations of methodology and standardization of apolipoproteinA-I immunoassays. ClinChem 1983; 29: 415–26.

125. Strong JP, Malcom GT, McMahan CA, Tracy RE, Newman WP III,Herderick EE, et ai. Prevalence and extent of atherosclerosis inadolescents and young adults: implications for prevention from thePathobiological Determinants of Atherosclerosis in Youth Study.JAMA 1999; 281:727-35.

126. Strong JP, McGill HC Jr. The pediatric aspects of atherosclerosis. J Atheroscler Res 1969; 9: 251–65.

127. Stuyt PM, Van't LA. Clinical features of type III hyper-lipoproteinaemia. Neth J Med 1983; 26: 104–11.

128. Sugiuchi H, Irie T, Uji Y, Ueno T, Chaen T, Uekama K, et ai. Homogeneous assay for measuring low-density lipoprotein cholesterolin serum with triblock copolymer and alpha-cyclodextrin sulfate. Clin Chem 1998; 44: 522–31.

129. Sugiuchi H, Uji Y, Obbe H, Irie T, Uekama K, Kayahara N, et ai.Direct measurement of high-density lipoprotein cholesterol in serumwith polyethylene glycol-modified enzymes and sulfated alphacyclodextrin.ClinChem 1995;41: 717–23.

130. Taddei-Peters WC, Butman BT, Jones GR, Venetta TM, Macomber PF, Ransom JH. Quantification of lipoprotein(a) particles containing various apolipoprotein(a) isoforms by a monoclonal anti-apo(a) capture antibody and a polyclonal anti-apolipoprotein B detection antibody sandwich enzyme immunoassay. ClinChem 1993; 39: 1382–9.

131. Takayama M, Itoh S, Nagasaki T, Tanimizu I. A new enzymatic method for determination of serum choline-containing phospholipids. Clin ChimActa 1977; 79: 93–8.

132. Tate JR, Berg K, Couderc R, Dati F, Kostner GM, Marcovina SM, et ai. International Federation of Clinical Chemistry and Laboratory Medicine (IFCC) Standardization Project for the Measurement of Lipoprotein (a). Phase 2. Selection and pro-perties of a proposed secondary reference material for lipoprotein (a). Clin Chem Lab Med 1999; 37: 949–58.

133. Tate JR, Rifai N, Berg K, Couderc R, et al. International Federation of Clinical Chemistry standardization project for the measurement of lipoprotein (a). Phase I. Evaluation of the analytical performance of lipoprotein (a) assay systems and commercial calibrators. Clin Chem 1998; 44: 1629–40.

134. Warnick GR, Spain M, Kloepfer H, et al. Standardization of acommercial (Boehringer Mannheim diagnostics) enzymatic method for cholesterol. ClinChern 1989; 35: 409–13.

135. Webber LS, Srinivasan SR, Wattigney WA, Berenson GS. Tracking of serum lipids and lipoproteins from childhood to adulthood. The Bogalusa Heart Study. Am I Epidemiol 1991; 133: 884–99.

136. Weisgraber KH, Innerarity TL, Mahley RW. Abnormal lipoprotein receptor-binding activity of the human E apoprotein due to cysteine arginine interchange at a single site. I Biol Chern 1982; 257: 2518–21.

137. Weisgraber KH, Newhouse YM, Mahley RW: Apolipoprotein Egenotyping using the polymerase chain reaction and allele-specific oligonucleotide probes. BiochemBiophys Res Commun 1988; 157: 1212–7.

138. Wilder LB, Bachorik PS, Finney CA, et al. The effectof fasting status on the determination of low-density and high-densitylipoprotein cholesterol. Am I Med 1995; 99: 374–7.

139. Wissler RW. New insights into the pathogenesis of atherosclerosis asrevealed by PDAY. Pathobiological Determinants of Atherosclerosis inYouth. Atherosclerosis 1994; 108(Suppl): S3–20.

140. Yamada S, Gotoh T, Nakashima Y, et al. Distribution of serum C-reactive protein and its association withatherosclerotic risk factors in a lapanese population. lichiMedicalSchool Cohort Study. Am I Epidemiol 2001; 153: 1183–90.

141. Yamamoto A, Nakamura M, Hino K, Saito K, Manabe M. Development of a new homogeneous method for serum HDL-C. Clin Chern 2000; 46:A98.

142. Yancey PG, Bortnick AE, Kellner-Weibel G, et al. Importance of different pathways ofcellular cholesterol efflux. Arterioscler Thromb Vasc Bioi 2003; 23: 712–9.

143. Yu HH, Markowitz R, De Ferranti SD, et al. Direct measurement of LDL-C in children:performance of two surfactant-based methods in a general pediatricpopulation. Clin Biochem 2000; 33: 89–95.

144. Zacho I, Tybjaerg-Hansen A, lensen IS, et al. Genetically elevated C-reactive protein andischemic vascular disease. N Engl I Med 2008; 359: 1897–908.

145. Ziccardi P, Nappo F, Giugliano G, et al. Reduction of inflammatory cytokine concentrations andimprovement of endothelial functions in obese women after weightloss over one year. Circulation 2002; 105: 804–9.

146. Zilversmit DB. Atherogenesis: a postprandial phenomenon. Circulation 1979; 60: 473–85.

147. Zwaka TP, Hombach V, Torzewski I. C-reactive protein-mediated lowdensity lipoprotein uptake by macrophages: implications foratherosclerosis. Circulation 2001; 103: 1194–7.

16

Therapeutic Drug Monitoring

INTRODUCTION

The aim of therapeutic drug monitoring (TDM) is to aid the clinician in the choice of drug dosage in order to provide the optimum treatment for the patient and, in particular, to avoid iatrogenic toxicity. It can be based on pharmacogenetic, demographic and clinical information alone (*a priori* TDM), but is normally supplemented with measurement of drug or metabolite concentrations in blood or markers of clinical effect (*a posteriori* TDM). Measurements of drug or metabolite concentrations are only useful where there is a known relationship between the plasma concentration and the clinical effect, no immediate simple clinical or other indication of effectiveness or toxicity and a defined concentration limit above which toxicity is likely. Therapeutic drug monitoring has an established place in enabling optimization of therapy in such cases.

Toxicity may cause organ damage, such as to the liver or kidneys, which further affects the circulating levels of the drug or its by-products. Nephrotoxicity is very common and can lead to acute renal failure. Monitoring the blood level of these drugs is helpful to determine if the dosage amount or interval between doses is appropriate, particularly if the kidneys are failing since elimination of drug is decreased in kidney failure. Subsequent dosage adjustment will be used to maximize drug efficacy while minimizing toxicity. Although, many medications do not cause toxicity when given in the usual doses and therefore don't require TDM, we will focus on general categories and some specific drugs that do.

Patient drug levels are compared to a reference range called the therapeutic range. This range includes a lower value, which is the minimum effective concentration, and an upper value, just below the minimum toxic concentration.

Blood levels of the drug fluctuate, as it is handled by different organ systems within the body. Peak levels depend on how the drug is administered and the body's ability to absorb and distribute the drug.

Trough drug levels depend on the body's ability to metabolize and eliminate the drug. The time frame for a drug concentration to decrease by half is termed the half-life (t1/2). If a drug is given once per t1/2, an equilibrium termed steady state is reached after 4–5 half-lives.

As a rule of thumb, the effectiveness of therapeutic drugs should be monitored by the parameter that is easiest to measure. For example, with certain drugs usefulness may be determined as easing of symptoms. Blood pressure is the best measure of efficacy of furosemide or other blood pressure medication dosage. Periodic measuring of prothrombin time is useful for monitoring warfarin (coumadin) and coagulation management. Tests to monitor the effectiveness of therapeutic drugs should be ordered for the correct time of day, and results should be evaluated carefully.

In a study of hospitalized patients receiving cardio-active medications, 49% of the drug testing was performed for irrational indications and 36% of the drug results were not evaluated correctly. The study concluded that pharmacists should become more involved in monitoring drug assays for interpretation and follow-up.

ROUTES OF DRUG ADMINISTRATION

There are various routes of drug administration. These include but are not limited by mouth (PO), intravenous (IV), intramuscular (IM), on the skin, in the rectum or cheek, and inhalation and epidermal routes. Each route of administration will result in a characteristic concentration versus time that can be depicted graphically. The relationship of drug concentration versus time is termed **pharmacokinetics.** For a drug given intravenously, the gastrointestinal (GI) system is bypassed and the drug is immediately distributed to the bloodstream. The graph of blood concentration of drug versus time illustrated in Fig. 16.1, depicts this immediate absorption. In contrast, a drug taken orally must pass through the GI system before it is absorbed into the bloodstream; Fig. 16.2 depicts the relationship of time versus blood concentration of drug following oral dosage.

Drugs are processed in the body through four main phases. Absorption is the process in which the drug enters the bloodstream from the GI tract with an oral dose, intramuscularly, via skin absorption, or from under the tongue (sublingually).

Drugs taken intravenously enter directly into the bloodstream. Following the absorption phase, distribution occurs. Distribution is the spread of drug via the circulatory system to organs and tissues throughout the body following the absorption phase. Distribution depends on fluid volume and circulation. Drug binding occurs during this stage and, thus, not the entire drug dose becomes available to the tissues. Metabolism begins shortly after distribution and commences the elimination phase. Metabolism is the process in which the parent drug is transformed to a more easily excreted form, such as water insoluble. The metabolite may be pharmacologically active or inactive. Elimination is the process by which drugs are removed from the body by metabolism and excretion processes. Renal excretion is the prime method of eliminating water-soluble drugs and metabolites.

DRUG METABOLISM

Many drugs are metabolized by enzymes working in **first-order (metabolic) kinetics.** As the drug concentration increases, the rate of hepatic metabolism by enzymes increases to keep up with the amount of drug present. In other words, the velocity of drug metabolism by enzymes is proportional to the concentration of the substrate (drug). This type of drug clearance, generally represented by a skewed type of curve, is the typical response with most drugs after administration of only one dose. Patients taking drugs that continue to follow nonlinear kinetics must be monitored by TDM very closely. Some drugs are absorbed by the liver during GI absorptive circulation and metabolized quickly before they have a chance to reach the systemic circulation.

This is termed the 'first-pass effect.' Lidocaine, a cardioactive drug, exhibits first pass metabolism. Therefore, it is retained in circulation longer if it is administered as an intramuscular injection rather than an oral dose.

Some drugs are metabolized by **zero-order kinetics** in which the metabolizing enzyme active sites are fully saturated with drug. The hepatic enzymes metabolize the drug at maximum velocity (Vmax). Therefore, the concentration of the drug does not affect its metabolic rate, which is already at a maximum. **Ethanol**, phenytoin, and salicylates all follow zero-order kinetics at typical or therapeutic levels. The kidneys eliminate water-soluble drugs through glomerular filtration. Only free drugs and water-soluble metabolites can pass through the kidney into the urine for elimination. Other routes of drug elimination are through elimination of bile and feces, especially for lipid-soluble drugs, and through gaseous expiration from the lungs. Due to the role of the kidney in elimination of many drugs, it is also prone to toxicity and possible failure. Effective elimination of drugs requires adequate renal function so, in situations of renal failure, circulating drug levels stay elevated longer than

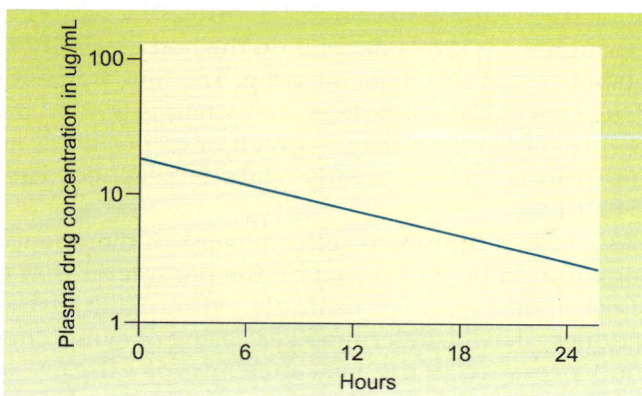

Fig. 16.1: Blood concentration after intravenous dosage

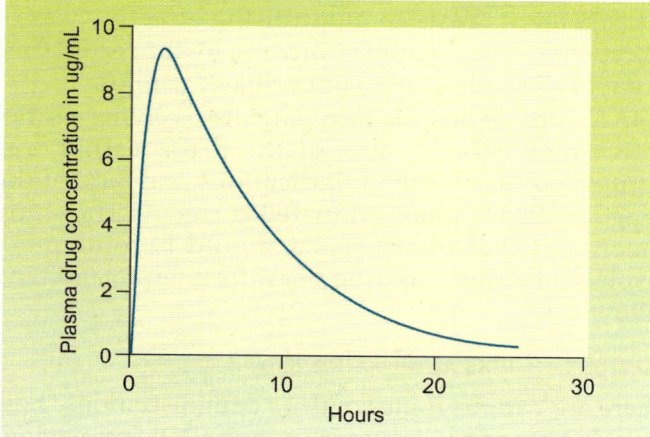

Fig. 16.2: Blood concentration after oral dosage

with normal renal function. Drugs typically measured in TDM are classified into categories. There are seven common categories of drugs monitored by blood levels. These are antibiotics, cardioactive drugs (so-called anti-arrhythmic drugs that control normal heart rhythm), antineoplastics (drugs to control cell growth), medications to control seizures (so called anti-epileptic drugs), bronchodilators (so-called anti-asthmatic drugs), antipsychotics (drugs that control the mind and behavior, including depression), and immunosuppressive agents (drugs that inhibit immunity).

DRUG EXCRETION

Drug excretion (or elimination) is the final removal of drugs from the body. This can occur by numerous routes, including secretion into sweat, breath, and breast milk, incorporation into hair and nails, or even crossing the placenta into the fetal bloodstream. However, by far the most common means of drug elimination is excretion into urine or stool, depending on the water solubility of the compound. The rate of elimination into urine can be estimated using the glomerular filtration rate (e.g. calculated from serum creatinine).

Clearance can also be measured directly for a particular drug. This requires multiple samples from the same patient and is infrequently done, except for therapeutic agents with a narrow window between efficacy and toxicity. An example of this is the alkylating agent busulfan, used in high doses to ablate bone marrow precursor cells prior to hematopoietic stem cell transplant. Given the delicate balance between effective ablation (leading to successful transplant engraftment) and excessive treatment (leading to serious complications, such as veno-occlusive disease of the liver), serial measurements of busulfan are used clinically to assess exposure to the drug and to individualize subsequent doses.

Urine can be a useful matrix for drug testing; it is readily collected in a noninvasive manner, is relatively poor in protein and other analytical interferences, and generally shows higher drug concentrations because of the ability of the kidneys to concentrate compounds filtered from the blood. For these reasons, it is the most common matrix for drugs of abuse testing and other toxicologic applications.

However, it is important to note that the correlation between urine drug concentrations and serum concentrations is poor at best. This is the result of wide variability in several factors that can affect renal drug elimination, including patient hydration status, urine pH, and circadian fluctuations in renal function. Although, it may be possible to normalize urine drug concentrations

somewhat with 24 hours urine samples and correction to a marker of renal function, such as creatinine, in practice urine is rarely used for TDM purposes. In select exceptions, such as assessing patient compliance in pain clinics, samples are obtained frequently, serum concentrations are poorly related to therapeutic efficacy, and risk of drug diversion or misuse is relatively high.

Pharmacokinetic Models

The processes of drug absorption, distribution, metabolism, and elimination are not completely independent steps, but rather occur in an overlapping fashion, often simultaneously, within the body. This is especially true of those agents that are administered serially, as a subsequent dose is typically given before the first dose has been completely eliminated.

Thus, it is necessary to have mathematical means of estimating factors, such as the amount of drug present at a given time, the rate of clearance of a drug from the system, and the overall exposure to a drug for a given dose.

ANTI-EPILEPTIC DRUGS

Many drugs are available for treating seizures (Table 16.1). In general, anti-epileptic drugs prevent or minimize seizures by augmenting inhibitory processes, for example, by enhancing γ-aminobutyric acid (GABA)-mediated neurotransmission or inhibiting excitatory processes (e.g. voltage-gated or ligand-gated ion channels, glutamate-mediated neurotransmission) in the brain. Therefore, it is not surprising that some of these drugs are also used as sedatives; to treat neuropathic pain, migraine headaches, and psychiatric conditions; and to manage addictions.

Anti-epileptic drugs were among the first class of drugs monitored to establish appropriate dosing, in part because both under dosing and overdosing can be manifested by seizure activity, making it difficult to titrate and optimize dose clinically. In addition, therapeutic and toxic effects of early drugs, such as phenobarbital and phenytoin were shown to relate to serum concentrations. TDM provided a vehicle through which noncompliance and drug-drug interactions could be identified. In 1971 a workshop produced an authoritative reference book regarding TDM of anti-epileptic drugs.

Several books and consensus documents evolved from this and subsequent workshops held in locations worldwide. As many laboratories began to develop analytical methods to support TDM of anti-epileptic drugs, it was recognized that substantial variation existed in results among laboratories.

Table 16.1	Pharmacokinetic parameters of anti-epileptic drugs					
Drug	Recommended therapeutic range, mg/L	Meantime to steady state, d	Observed range of half-life in adults, h**	Mean volume of distribution, L/kg	Protein binding %	Important metabolizing enzymes
Carbamazepine	4–12	2–4	8–12	1.4	75	CYP3A4
Clonazepam	0.02–.07	3–10	17–56	3.2	85	CYP3A4
Ethosuximide	40–100	7–10	30–60	0.7	0	CYP3A4
Felbamate	30–60	3–4	14–21	0.8	25	CYP3A4
Gabapentin	2–20	1–2	5–9	0.9	0	NA
Lamotrigine	2.5–15	3–6	20–30	1.2	55	NA
Levetiracetam	12–46	1–2	6–8	0.6	0	NA
Monohydroxy oxcarbazepine (MHD)*	3–35	2–3	8–15	0.8	40	NA
Phenobarbital	10–40	12–24	70–140	0.7	50	CYP2C19
Phenytoin	10–20 (1.0–2.0)	5–17	30–100	0.6	90	CYP2C9, 2CI9
Primidone	5–10	2–4	3–22	0.7	20	CYP2C9, 2CI9
Tiagabine	0.02–0.2	1–2	5–9	1.4	96	CYP3A4
Topiramate	5–20	4–5	20–30	0.7	15	NA
Valproic acid	50–100	2–4	11–20	0.2	90	CYP2C9, 2CI9, 2B6, 2E1, 2A6
Vigabatrin	0.8–36	1–2	5–8	0.8	0	NA
Zonisamide	10–40	9–12	50–70	1.4	50	CYP2CI9, 3A4

*Active metabolite not available as a unique drug.
**Based on average half-life and no interfering medications; NA, not applicable.

Most anti-epileptic therapy is administered long-term, possibly life-long, meaning that dosing requirements will change with age, stage of development, and clinical status. In addition to comparing steady-state concentrations of anti-epileptic drugs versus proposed therapeutic ranges and toxic thresholds, TDM for anti-epileptics is used early in therapy to ensure that steady-state concentrations have been achieved before efficacy is evaluated, particularly for drugs that exhibit nonlinear and/or variable pharmacokinetics.

Therapeutic drug monitoring is useful to identify and manage drug-drug interactions, to manage changes in dose or drug formulation, and to evaluate compliance, particularly when signs of therapeutic failure or toxicity are evident. In general, older anti-epileptic drugs are monitored more frequently than the newer drugs, in part because of the wide availability of automated immunoassays. In general, immunoassay procedures target a single analyte (usually the parent drug) and are fast, inexpensive, and available for a wide variety of analyzers. When immunoassays are not available, or in certain clinical situations wherein higher sensitivity and specificity than can be accomplished through existing immunoassays is required, chromatographic methods are applied to support anti-epileptic TDM. Chromatographic methods are particularly valuable in situations wherein pharmacologically active metabolites are important to monitor with parent drug, when no

commercial methods are available, or when commercial methods are fraught with poor specificity. Another advantage of chromatographic methods is that simultaneous analyses of multiple drugs and active drug metabolites can be accomplished to monitor polypharmacy, but also to improve the efficiency of operations in the laboratory.

Some anti-epileptics are extensively bound to circulating plasma proteins. As with most drugs, only the unbound (free) fraction of drug is able to pass through membranes to exert pharmacologic activity, and many drug-drug interactions occur as a result of competition for protein-binding sites. For patients with unpredictable protein concentrations, or for whom drug-drug interactions are a significant concern, it may be appropriate to provide TDM for the free fraction of drug. For example, if the proportion of drug bound to proteins changes from 95–80%, the amount of active (free) drug in circulation will increase dramatically, while the total drug concentration for that patient may not change. As such, risk of toxicity could be missed and TDM results could be misinterpreted, particularly for pregnant women and elderly persons with poor nutritional status who are managed with multiple medications. Most analytical techniques are designed to measure total drug concentrations and do not distinguish between free and bound drug concentrations. To accommodate TDM of free drug concentrations, protein bound drug can be separated and removed from plasma using physical or chemical techniques. Resulting free drug concentrations can be determined by immunoassays or chromatographic techniques, with calibration and sensitivity designed to accommodate lower concentrations than those observed when total drug concentrations are measured. In theory, measurement of drugs in oral fluid (saliva) could approximate free drug concentrations. Anti-epileptic TDM using saliva is of interest because of the convenience of specimen collection, particularly at the time of a seizure, and for children.

Oral fluid testing is not currently done routinely. However, oral fluid may become an important specimen type of the future. When a standardized method of saliva stimulation is used, a linear relationship between drug concentrations and dose has been observed for some drugs, such as valproic acid, but not for others such as carbamazepine.

Key attributes of TDM support for specific anti-epileptic drugs that are currently in use are provided here, organized along the following historical lines.

1. *Traditional and still widely used:* Anti-epileptic drugs introduced before 1990 and currently in use include carbamazepine, phenytoin, phenobarbital, primidone, clonazepam, diazepam, ethosuximide, fosphenytoin, and valproic acid.

2. *Contemporary:* Anti-epileptic drugs introduced after 1990 and currently in use include felbamate, gabapentin, levetiracetam, lamotrigine, oxcarbazepine, pregabalin, tiagabine, topiramate, vigabatrin, and zonisamide.

3. *Historical and not widely used:* Bromides, methsuximide, ethotoin, and mephobarbital.

CARBAMAZEPINE

Carbamazepine (proprietary name tegretol) is available under other names and in generic form. Similar to phenytoin, carbamazepine modulates the synaptic sodium channel, which prolongs inactivation, reducing the ability of the neuron to respond at high frequency. The physiologic effect of this action is reduction in central synaptic transmission, aiding in control of abnormal neuronal excitability. Carbamazepine is used in the treatment of generalized tonic-clonic, partial, and partial-complex seizures. Carbamazepine also has an anti-diuretic effect, reducing concentrations of antidiuretic hormone, although it is unlikely that this contributes to anti-epileptic activity.

After oral administration, carbamazepine is slowly but erratically absorbed with wide individual formulation-based variability. Approximately 75% of the drug is protein bound.

For this reason, determination of protein-free carbamazepine concentrations for patients with abnormally low or unpredictable concentrations of albumin is sometimes clinically important. The volume of distribution is modest at 1–2 L/kg. The elimination half-life early after the first dose varies from 18–55 hours for adults and from 3–32 hours for children. During maintenance dosing, the half-life is 8–20 hours for adults, 10–14 hours for children, and 30–50 hours in elderly patients. The reduced half-life with long-term therapy is explained somewhat by the induction of CYP3A4.

Because hepatic metabolism is the principal means by which plasma concentration is reduced, any reduction in liver function results in drug accumulation. The active metabolite of carbamazepine is carbamazepine 10, 11 epoxide formed by the action of CYP3A4. This metabolite has been found to accumulate in children and exists in concentrations equivalent to carbamazepine. Monitoring of ratios may be useful for evaluating compliance and drug-drug interactions. Cross reactivity of this metabolite in commercial immunoassays is variable and should be considered when carbamazepine TDM is provided. Because carbamazepine is metabolized by CYP3A4, drugs that induce this enzyme (erythromycin, oxcarbazepine, phenytoin, and St. John's Wort) increase the rate of clearance of carbamazepine. Co-administration of erythromycin, phenytoin, or valproic acid increases the rate of metabolism of carbamazepine, reducing the blood concentration. Itraconazole and grapefruit juice interfere with CYP3A4 activity, increasing carbamazepine concentrations.

The therapeutic concentration range for optimal pharmacologic effect of carbamazepine is 4–12 mg/L. Toxicity associated with excessive carbamazepine may occur at plasma concentrations in excess of 15 mg/L (or free carbamazepine >3 mg/L) and is characterized by symptoms of blurred vision, paresthesia, nystagmus, ataxia, drowsiness, and diplopia. Side effects unrelated to plasma concentration include development of an urticarial rash, which usually disappears on discontinuation of the drug, and hematologic depression (leukopenia, thrombocytopenia, and aplastic anemia).

ETHOSUXIMIDE

Ethosuximide (proprietary name zarontin) is used for the treatment of absence seizures characterized by brief loss of consciousness. Ethosuximide reduces the flow of calcium through T-type calcium channels in the synapse of thalamic neurons. Because thalamic neurons are the main source of 3 Hz spike-wave rhythms in absence seizures, reduction of calcium flow slows the rate of these seizure-inducing pulses. Ethosuximide is a chiral molecule that is used clinically as a racemic mixture.

Ethosuximide is readily absorbed from the gastro-intestinal tract with near complete bioavailability. Several formulations are available, a fact that influences the time to peak concentrations; for example, liquid suspension is absorbed faster than capsules. Peak concentrations also vary with age and occur faster in adults (1–4 hours) than in children (3–7 hours). Ethosuximide is not protein bound, has a volume of distribution (Vd) of 0.7 L/kg, and undergoes extensive metabolism. In children, its half-life is approximately 33 hours, although this may be prolonged to as long as 60 hours in adults. The drug is cleared in a linear fashion, primarily by metabolism mediated by CYP3A4 (hydroxyethyl metabolite) and the glucuronide.

Drug-drug interactions occur primarily as a result of enzyme induction or through CYP3A4. Valproic acid is reported to exert variable effects on ethosuximide concentrations.

The established therapeutic range of ethosuximide is 40–100 mg/L, although it is not uncommon that higher concentrations are required. Toxicity related to an excessive blood concentration of ethosuximide is rare. Symptoms of gastrointestinal distress, lethargy, dizziness, and euphoria may be encountered early in therapy, but patients usually become tolerant to these symptoms.

PHENOBARBITAL

Phenobarbital is a broad-spectrum anti-epileptic drug that was introduced clinically in 1912 under the name luminal. It is now known by a wide variety of proprietary names, is given alone or in combination with many other drugs, and is still used today to manage all but absence seizure types. It is known to reduce synaptic transmission, resulting in decreased excitability of the entire nerve cell, inducing sedation. Phenobarbital potentiates synaptic inhibition through action on the GABA-A receptor by increasing the duration of chloride flow into the synapse. The end result is an increase in seizure threshold with inhibition of the spread of discharges from epileptic foci.

Serum concentrations of phenobarbital are well correlated with dose; however, pharmacokinetics is widely variable.

Absorption of oral phenobarbital is near complete, but the rate of absorption is age dependent, rapid in adults, slow in children. Thus, the time at which peak plasma concentrations are reached ranges from 4 to 10 hours after the dose. Phenobarbital is 40–60% bound to plasma proteins, wherein protein binding is higher in adults than in children.

Children have larger Vd values than adults, although Vd is generally about 0.6–1.0 L/kg. CYP2C19 is the primary hepatic enzyme involved in metabolism, producing an elimination half-life of 70–140 hours; metabolism is also age dependent (children average 70 hours, geriatric patients 100 hours). Phenobarbital is metabolized by CYP2C19 to p-hydroxyphenobarbital, which is largely excreted as the glucuronide. Drug-drug interactions are common. For example, phenobarbital concentrations increase with co-administration of phenytoin, valproic acid, felbamate, and oxcarbazepine. Phenobarbital concentrations decrease with co-administration of other barbiturates, alcohol, rifampin, or carbamazepine. When renal or hepatic function is decreased, patients experience decreased clearance of the drug and a prolonged half-life. Phenobarbital is also recognized to induce hepatic enzymes, which will affect the concentrations of other co-administered medications.

The widely recognized therapeutic range for phenobarbital for adults is between 15 mg/L and 40 mg/L. The predominant side effect observed in adults at blood concentrations greater than 40 mg/L is sedation, although tolerance to this effect develops with long-term therapy. Actual optimal concentrations will vary and may not be realized until tolerance to the sedative effects has occurred. Because of the long elimination half-life of phenobarbital, the blood concentration does not change rapidly. Therefore, blood for TDM can be collected at any time of day, once steady state has been achieved.

PRIMIDONE

Primidone (proprietary name mysoline) is metabolized to phenobarbital. Both compounds have anti-seizure activity. The mechanism of action of this drug is similar to that described for phenobarbital, and the therapeutic effect is due partially to the accumulation of its major metabolite, phenobarbital, created by the action of CYP2C19. A second metabolite of primidone, phenylethylmalonamide (PEMA), created by the action of CYP2C9, also has some anti-epileptic activity.

Primidone is rapidly and nearly completely absorbed after oral administration. Once absorbed, it is not highly protein bound, and it has a half-life of approximately 10 hours; however, because the pharmacokinetics are variable, the half-life may vary from 3–22 hours. Disposition of the drug is known to be affected by drugs that alter CYP2C19 and 2C9 metabolism and by diseases that alter phenobarbital disposition.

Co-administration of acetazolamide with primidone results in decreased gastrointestinal absorption of primidone and subsequent diminished plasma concentrations. Primidone administered in association with phenytoin produces a modest elevation of the phenobarbital-to-primidone ratio because phenytoin competes with the hepatic hydroxylating enzymes associated with the metabolism of phenobarbital.

Co-administration of valproic acid, for the same reasons outlined for phenobarbital, causes a modest increase in both primidone and phenobarbital serum concentrations.

The optimal therapeutic concentration of primidone has been established as 5–10 mg/L. Because phenobarbital is an active metabolite of primidone, concurrent analysis of phenobarbital is required for complete interpretation of results. The previously defined therapeutic range for phenobarbital applies to adequate primidone therapy. Phenobarbital concentrations rise gradually over a period of 1–2 weeks after therapy is initiated. Toxicity due to accumulation of primidone occurs at serum concentrations greater than 15 mg/L and usually is associated with symptoms of sedation, nausea, vomiting, diplopia, dizziness, and ataxia, and a phenobarbital concentration greater than 40 mg/L. In addition to detection of drug-drug interactions, evaluating the ratio of phenobarbital to primidone may assist with detection of noncompliance.

PHENYTOIN

Phenytoin (diphenylhydantoin), most commonly available as dilantin, but also available under other names and in generic form, is used in the treatment of primary or secondary generalized tonic-clonic seizures, partial or complex-partial seizures, and status epilepticus. The drug is not effective for absence seizures. Phenytoin interferes with sodium channel activity by prolonging inactivation, which reduces the ability of the neuron to respond at high frequency. The physiologic effect of this action is reduction in central synaptic transmission, which aids in control of abnormal neuronal excitability.

The pharmacokinetics of phenytoin are complex and unpredictable as the result of variable absorption, high (>90%) protein binding, saturable metabolism, and drug-drug interactions. Absorption of oral phenytoin is slow and sometimes is incomplete. A wide selection of drug preparations contribute to variable and sometimes poor bioavailability, but Vd is 0.6–0.7 L/kg. Phenytoin is not readily soluble in aqueous solutions. When administered by intramuscular injection, most of the dose precipitates at the site of injection and then is slowly absorbed. A prodrug called fosphenytoin (cerebyx) allows intramuscular injection and rapid conversion to and liberation of phenytoin. Monitoring of fosphenytoin is accomplished through the use of routine phenytoin assays. However, specimens collected shortly after administration of fosphenytoin may not accurately reflect active drug concentrations; interpretation of TDM for fosphenytoin should be performed after phenytoin concentrations reach steady state.

Phenytoin is metabolized by hepatic microsomal hydroxylating enzymes CYP2C19 and 2C9. The principal metabolite is 5-(p-hydroxyphenyl)-5-phenylhydantoin, which is excreted principally as a glucuronide. Hepatic metabolism of phenytoin may become saturated within the therapeutic range. Once metabolism is saturated, small dose increments result in large changes in blood concentration; this phenomenon partially explains the wide variation in dose among patients that is required to achieve a therapeutic effect. Because of this saturation phenomenon, first-order kinetics does not apply to phenytoin at plasma concentrations in excess of 5 mg/L (or lower in select patients), and half-life can vary tremendously.

It is noteworthy that some commercially available immunoassays exhibit cross-reactivity for phenytoin metabolites and may generate falsely elevated results. ISS In addition, various drug interactions result in alteration of the disposition of phenytoin. Alcohol, carbamazepine, barbiturates, and rifampin induce CYP2C19 and 2C9; this induction results in increased metabolism of phenytoin, reduced serum concentration of both total and free phenytoin, and reduced pharmacologic effect. Drugs, such as chloramphenicol, cimetidine, disulfiram, isoniazid, omeprazole, and topiramate compete with phenytoin metabolism, resulting in an increase in both total and free phenytoin concentrations and enhancement of the pharmacologic effect. Salicylate, valproic acid, phenyl butazone, sulfisoxazole, and sulfonylureas compete with phenytoin for serum protein-binding sites. The end result is diminished total serum concentration of phenytoin, while the free phenytoin concentration and the pharmacologic effect remain approximately the same.

The optimal therapeutic concentration for seizure control without side effects is 10–20 mg/L. Total phenytoin concentrations greater than 20 mg/L usually do not enhance seizure control and often are associated with nystagmus and ataxia. Total phenytoin plasma concentrations greater than 35 mg/L have been shown to precipitate seizure activity. A side effect of phenytoin not related to plasma concentration is development of gingival hyperplasia.

VALPROIC ACID

Valproic acid (brand names Depakene and Depakote, but also available under other names and in generic form) is used for the treatment of absence seizures. It has also been shown to be useful against tonic-clonic and partial seizures when used in conjunction with other anti-epileptic agents, such as phenobarbital or phenytoin. The drug inhibits the enzyme GABA transaminase, resulting in an increase in the concentration of GABA in the brain. GABA is a potent inhibitor of presynaptic and postsynaptic discharges in the central nervous system.

Valproic acid also modulates the synaptic sodium channel by prolonging inactivation, which reduces the ability of the neuron to respond at high frequency. This action gives it some activity against tonic-clonic seizures.

Valproic acid is rapidly and almost completely absorbed after oral administration and has a very low Vd (0.1–0.5 L/kg). Peak concentrations occur 1–4 hours after an oral dose of conventional tablets and solutions, but they are extended for enteric-coated and sustained-release formulations, as well as when taken with food. Valproic acid is highly protein bound (>90%), but the extent of protein binding decreases with increasing concentration, leading to nonlinear kinetics in some patients. The metabolism of valproic acid is extensive, involving β-oxidation (approximately 30% of dose) and production of several glucuronide conjugates (approximately 40% of dose). The clinical significance of these metabolites is not well understood.

The half-life is shortened from approximately 20 hours with the initial dose to approximately 12 hours as steady state is achieved. The half-life is shorter still in children than in adults, with the exception of neonates with hepatic disease, in whom the half-life becomes prolonged. Relatively poor correlation has been noted between dose and serum concentrations.

Valproic acid modulates the pharmacokinetics of many other anti-epileptic drugs. For example, it inhibits the clearance of phenobarbital and competes with phenytoin for protein-binding sites. The free phenytoin concentration remains approximately the same, but total phenytoin in the plasma is decreased. Other drugs that induce hepatic oxidative enzymes result in increased valproic acid clearance, requiring a higher dose to maintain effective therapeutic concentrations.

The minimum effective therapeutic concentration of valproic acid is 50 mg/L. Concentrations greater than 100 mg/L have been associated with hepatic toxicity and acute toxic encephalopathy. Free concentrations are sometimes clinically useful. Glycine has been observed to accumulate in patients taking valproic acid therapy.

CONTEMPORARY ANTI-EPILEPTICS

Felbamate

Felbamate (felbatol), which was approved for primary or adjunctive therapy of partial seizures, exerts efficacy through several mechanisms, including potentiation of GABA-ergicneurotrans mission and inhibition of glutamate excitation due to interaction with the N-methyl-D-aspartate (NMDA) receptor.

Felbamate is particularly effective in controlling Lennox-Gastaut syndrome. However, its use is limited to those patients who fail other drug treatments, because felbamate carries with it a substantial risk of aplastic anemia and liver failure that is not related to the blood concentrations. Bi-weekly monitoring of complete blood count, serum aminotransferases, and bilirubin is recommended to detect early onset of these side effects.

Felbamate is completely absorbed from the gastro-intestinal tract with peak concentrations observed 2–6 hours after administration. The drug is only 25% bound to plasma proteins and has a volume of distribution less than 1.0 L/kg. It is eliminated by hepatic metabolism (CYP3A4), with its half-life ranging from 14–21 hours. Felbamate saturates metabolism when the concentration exceeds 120 mg/L and is inducible, shifting elimination kinetics from first order to zero order. Half-life is also affected by other drugs and is substantially shorter in children, who may exhibit felbamate clearance 40–65% higher than in adults. The proposed therapeutic range for felbamate is narrow, ranging from 30–60 mg/L. An intermediate metabolite, an atropaldehyde, has been implicated in the idiosyncratic adverse events associated with felbamate.

Gabapentin

Gabapentin (neurontin) is a chemical analog of GABA that promotes the release of GABA. It does not interact directly with the GABA receptor, nor does it inhibit glutamic acid decarboxylase, the enzyme that usually controls cellular concentrations of GABA.

The mechanism of action is somewhat unclear, but is thought to be most related to interactions with voltage-gated calcium channels. A chemically and mechanistically related drug, pregabalin (lyrica) is used primarily for managing neuropathic pain. Gabapentin has proved effective in the treatment of drug-resistant partial seizures, so it is primarily considered adjuvant therapy.

Absorption of oral gabapentin is mediated by the L-amino transport system in the small intestines through a saturable process. Thus, bioavailability is dose dependent. Peak concentrations are observed 2–3 hours after a dose. Absorption is reduced by concomitant use of antacids. Pregabalin does not require active absorption and exhibits far more predictable and linear pharmacokinetics. Gabapentin is less than 10% bound to plasma proteins, and the volume of distribution is 0.65–1.4 L/kg. Gabapentin is not metabolized and does not induce or inhibit metabolic enzymes. The elimination half-life is 5–9 hours, and elimination is proportional to renal clearance. Approximately 30% higher doses are required in children.

The minimum effective concentration of gabapentin is 2 mg/L, and the optimally effective therapeutic serum concentration of gabapentin is reported as between 2– 20 mg/L. Side effects observed in adults at serum concentrations greater than 12 mg/L are somnolence, ataxia, dizziness, and fatigue.

Lamotrigine

Lamotrigine (lamictal) is a broad-spectrum anti-epileptic drug that is widely used. Lamotrigine is thought to act through multiple mechanisms, including blocking sodium and calcium channels to reduce repetitive nerve firings induced by depolarization of spinal cord neurons, and reducing glutamate release. Lamotrigine is completely absorbed from the gastrointestinal tract after oral administration, with peak concentrations occurring at 1–3 hours. A linear relationship between dose and serum concentrations is observed, volume of distribution is 0.9–1.5 L/kg, and binding to plasma proteins is moderate (approximate 55%). Lamotrigine is extensively metabolized and is eliminated primarily as the glucuronide ester. Half-life ranges from 20–30 hours. Autoinduction reduces serum concentrations by approximate 20% within 2 weeks of therapy.

Enzyme-inducing drugs such as phenobarbital, phenytoin, or carbamazepine also result in reduced lamotrigine concentrations. Clearance is greater in children and increases up to 300% in pregnancy.

The proposed therapeutic range for lamotrigine is between 2.5 mg/L and 15 mg/L. Dizziness, ataxia, diplopia, blurred vision, nausea, and vomiting are signs of toxicity that have been reported, although these effects are rare when plasma concentrations are less than 15 mg/L. Lamotrigine is a potent inhibitor of dihydrofolate reductase. Folate concentrations are decreased when this drug is administered. If folate replacement is not implemented, rash and anemia may be experienced when lamotrigine is within the therapeutic range.

Lamotrigine, similar to carbamazepine, has also been associated with the development of severe rash (Stevens-Johnson syndrome) in approximately 1% of patients.

Levetiracetam

Levetiracetam (keppra) is a broad-spectrum anti-epileptic that has been found useful for managing focal and generalized seizures. The primary mechanism of action is unique and appears to be mediated through interactions with synaptic vesicle protein SV2A, which is involved in the release of neurotransmitters from presynaptic terminals. This drug is chiral, and its anti-epileptic activity is highly enantio-selective.

Levetiracetam is 100% bioavailable following an oral dose and reaches maximum concentration in approximately 1 hour. Although absorption is slowed by food, a good correlation between dose and serum concentrations

has been reported. Levetiracetam is less than 10% bound to plasma proteins, has a volume of distribution of 0.5– 0.7 L/kg, and is not extensively metabolized. Renal function and age are the major determinants of elimination kinetics. The possibility of *in vitro* metabolism (after specimen is collected) by blood esterases has been proposed, so plasma should be separated from cells promptly. The half-life ranges from 16–18 hours for newborns and from 6–8 hours in healthy adults. No pharmacokinetic interactions have been noted between levetiracetam and other anti-epileptic drugs.

The minimal effective serum concentration of levetiracetam for seizure control is 3 mg/L, but the effective concentration is not well defined. The pre-dose therapeutic concentration range proposed in a 2008 consensus document is 12–46 mg/L. Toxicity effects known to be associated with levetiracetam use include decreased RBC count and hematocrit, decreased neutrophil count, somnolence, asthenia, and dizziness. These toxicities may be associated with blood concentrations in the therapeutic range.

Oxcarbazepine

Oxcarbazepine (trileptal) is a 10-keto analog of carbamazepine that is useful in managing partial and generalized seizures. Oxcarbazepine is a chiral pro-drug that is metabolized to 10-hydroxy-10, 11-dihydrocarbamazepine, known commonly as monohydroxy carbamazepine (MHD), the metabolite responsible for the therapeutic effect. MHD, similar to carbamazepine, blocks sodium channels; MHD also exhibits inhibitory activity at calcium channels.

Oxcarbazepine is rapidly and completely absorbed, with peak concentrations observed at 1–2 hours; food has no effect on rate or extent of absorption. The half-life of oxcarbazepine is approximately 2 hours. Concentrations of MHD peak at 3–5 hours, protein binding is approximately 40%, and the Vd is less than 1.0 L/kg. Concentrations of the S-enantiomer of MHD are much higher than those of the R-enantiomer because conversion is stereo-selective. The metabolism of MHD is extensive; about 96% of the dose is excreted in the urine as metabolites. Most of the dose is eliminated and recovered as the glucuronide ester of oxcarbazepine or MHD. Metabolism does not involve inducible enzymes, however, so drug-drug interactions are minimal compared with carbamazepine. Because carbamazepine activates the uridine diphosphate glucuronosyl transferase (UGT) enzyme system, patients taking carbamazepine concomitantly with oxcarbazepine have significantly lower MHD concentrations than those not receiving carbamazepine. The elimination half-life for MHD is 8–15 hours. Because MHD is cleared predominantly by the kidney, the dose for patients with creatinine clearance less than 30 mL/min should be half that given to patients with normal renal function. MHD selectively induces CYP3A4 enzymes and may inhibit CYP2C19.

Optimal response is reported when pre-dose MHD concentration is in the range of 3–35 mg/L. Toxicities include hyponatremia, dizziness, somnolence, diplopia, fatigue, nausea, vomiting, ataxia, abnormal vision, abdominal pain, tremor, dyspepsia, and abnormal gait. These toxicities may be transient and may be observed when blood concentrations are in the therapeutic range, although the incidence is highest in patients with serum MHD concentration greater than 30 mg/L. Serum sodium concentration less than 125 mmol/L and decreased thyroxine (T4) have also been seen in patients treated with MHD. To prevent peaks in MHD, it is suggested that dosing be split throughout the day.

Tiagabine

Tiagabine (gabitril) is indicated as adjunctive therapy in adults and children for the treatment of partial seizures. It is frequently administered to patients receiving at least one concomitant anti-epileptic drug. Tiagabine is a nipecotic acid derivative that blocks reuptake of GABA into presynaptic neurons, permitting more GABA to be available for receptor binding on the surface of postsynaptic cells. This drug has been found particularly effective in patients with drug resistant epilepsy associated with glial tumors.

Tiagabine is rapidly and completely absorbed, reaching peak concentration approximately 45 minutes following an oral dose in the fasting state. Administration with food is recommended to reduce fluctuations in plasma concentrations between doses. Pediatric patients reach peak concentration at approximately 2.4 hours. Tiagabine pharmacokinetics is linear over the typical dose range. This drug is highly (approximate 96%) bound to human plasma proteins, mainly to serum albumin and alpha-1-acid glycoprotein (AAG). The volume of distribution is 1.0 L/kg, and it is extensively metabolized, with a major route mediated by CYP3A4. Half-life is approximately 5–9 hours and is extended to 12–16 hours in patients with compromised liver function. Children require higher doses because of accelerated clearance. This drug does not induce or inhibit metabolism of other drugs, but is subject to drug-drug interactions through both protein-binding interactions and enzyme-inducing drugs. For example, co-administration with valproic acid reduces protein binding to 94%, increasing the free fraction of tiagabine by 40%. Naproxen and salicylates are also known to displace tiagabine from protein-binding sites.

A proposed therapeutic range for tiagabine is 20 to 200 saliva µg/L. Serum concentrations greater than 800 µg/L may be associated with adverse effects such as asthenia, ataxia, difficulty concentrating, and depression. Timing of specimen collection is critical for TDM of tiagabine because of the rapid absorption and relatively short half-life.

Topiramate

Topiramate (topamax) is a broad-spectrum anti-epileptic drug that exerts activity through several mechanisms. It has sodium and calcium channel blocking activity, potentiates the activity of GABA, and inhibits glutamate release. Because of this range of activities, topiramate blocks seizure spread rather than raising seizure potential. Topiramate is routinely administered orally, is absorbed rapidly, and peaks at 2–4 hours. Although, time to peak concentration is delayed by food, the peak concentration is not affected, and the relationship between dose and serum concentration is linear. Topiramate minimally bound (approximate 15%) to plasma proteins, and Vi factors is 0.6–0.8 L/kg. Approximately 50% of topiramate is metabolized, with a serum half-life of 20–30 hours in adults, less in children. Topiramate inhibits CYP2C19 and induces CYP3A4, although serum concentrations of other anticonvulsant drugs are not significantly affected by concurrent administration of topiramate.

Enzyme-inducing medications reduce serum topiramate concentrations; serum concentrations are increased by amitriptyline, lithium, and sumatriptan. As with other renally eliminated anticonvulsant drugs, patients with impaired renal function exhibit decreased renal clearance. Most studies have reported a therapeutic range for topiramate of 5–20 mg/L, yet considerable overlap is seen in serum concentrations between responders and non-responders. Concentrations less than 2.0 mg/L indicate that the dose is suboptimal or was administered too infrequently. Adverse side effects (cognitive, emotional, and physical) are related to serum concentrations in some patients.

Vigabatrine

Vigabatrine (flexyx, sabril) is a structural analog of GABA that acts as a suicidal inhibitor of GABA-transaminase, the enzyme responsible for GABA metabolism. This drug is effective for managing infantile spasm associated with tuberous sclerosis and refractory partial epilepsies and is used outside the United States. However, because of irreversible visual field impairment that occurs in approximately one-third of patients, this drug is not widely used within the United States. Because of the mechanism of action, the value of TDM is limited to compliance testing in most cases.

Zonisamide

Zonisamide (proprietary name Zonegran) is a sodium and calcium channel blocker. It binds to the GABA receptor but does not produce a chloride influx. Therefore, zonisamide is a broad-spectrum anti-epileptic. Zonisamide has weak inhibitory activity on carbonic anhydrase, is a free radical scavenger, and promotes dopaminergic and serotonergic neurotransmission, but these actions are not likely to contribute to its anti-epileptic activity.

Peak concentrations of zonisamide are observed 2 to 6 hours after dose administration. Pharmacokinetics becomes nonlinear at high concentrations. As with many other anti-epileptic drugs, children generally require higher doses than adults. It is 50% bound to plasma proteins, but has high affinity for red cell protein components. The Vd is 0.8–1.6 L/kg.

The relatively long half-life (50–70 hours) is shortened considerably (25–35 hours) when enzyme-inducing drugs are also administered. Zonisamide is extensively metabolized, with a primary pathway mediated by CYP2C19 and CYP3A4. Thus, co-administration with CYP-inducing drugs, such as phenobarbital, phenytoin, or carbamazepine results in reduced zonisamide concentration. Zonisamide does not inhibit CYP isozymes, nor does it undergo autoinduction.

The proposed therapeutic range of zonisamide is 10–40 mg/L, but overlap in plasma concentrations between responders and non-responders occurs. Adverse effects on cognition are reported at concentrations that exceed 30 mg/L. Toxicity is likely at concentrations that exceed 70 mg/L.

EPILEPSY

Also called epileptic seizure disorder; is a chronic brain disorder characterized by recurrent (≥2) seizures that are unprovoked (i.e. not related to reversible stressors) and that occur >24 hours apart. A single seizure is not considered an epileptic seizure. Epilepsy is often idiopathic, but various brain disorders, such as malformations, strokes, and tumors, can cause symptomatic epilepsy.

Symptomatic epilepsy is epilepsy due to a known cause (e.g. brain tumor, stroke). The seizures it causes are called symptomatic epileptic seizures. Such seizures are most common among neonates and the elderly.

Cryptogenic epilepsy is epilepsy assumed to be due to a specific cause, but whose specific cause is currently unknown.

Non-epileptic seizures are provoked by a temporary disorder or stressor (e.g. metabolic disorders, CNS infections, cardiovascular disorders, drug toxicity or withdrawal, psychogenic disorders). In children, fever can provoke a seizure (febrile seizures).

Psychogenic non-epileptic seizures (pseudoseizures) are symptoms that simulate seizures in patients with psychiatric disorders but that do not involve an abnormal electrical discharge in the brain.

Etiology

Common causes of seizures (Table 16.2) vary by age of onset. In **reflex epilepsy,** a rare disorder, seizures are triggered predictably by an external stimulus, such as repetitive sounds, flashing lights, video games, music, or even touching certain parts of the body.

In cryptogenic epilepsy and often in refractory epilepsy, a rare but increasingly identified cause is anti-N-methyl-d-aspartate (NMDA) receptor encephalitis, especially in young women. This disorder also causes psychiatric symptoms, a movement disorder, and cerebrospinal fluid (CSF) pleocytosis. Ovarian teratoma occurs in about 60% of women with anti-NMDA receptor encephalitis. Removal of the teratoma (if present) and immunotherapy control the seizures much better than anticonvulsants.

Classification

Seizures are classified as generalized or partial.

Table 16.2	Causes of seizures
Condition	**Examples**
Autoimmune disorders	Cerebral vasculitis, anti-NMDA receptor encephalitis, multiple sclerosis (rarely)
Cerebral edema	Eclampsia, hypertensive encephalopathy
Cerebral ischemia or hypoxia	Cardiac arrhythmias, carbon monoxide toxicity, nonfatal drowning, near suffocation, stroke, vasculitis
Head trauma*	Birth injury, blunt or penetrating injuries
CNS infections	AIDS, brain abscess, falciparum malaria, meningitis, neurocysticercosis, neurosyphilis, rabies, tetanus, toxoplasmosis, viral encephalitis
Congenital or developmental abnormalities	Cortical malformations, genetic disorders (e.g. fifth day fits[†], lipid storage diseases, such as Tay-Sachs disease), neuronal migration disorders (e.g. heterotopias), phenylketonuria

Contd...

Condition	Examples
Drugs and toxins‡	Cause seizures: Camphor, ciprofloxacin, cocaine and other CNS stimulants, cyclosporine, imipenem, lead, pentylenetetrazol, picrotoxin, strychnine, tacrolimus Lower seizure threshold: Aminophylline, antidepressants (particularly tricyclics), sedating antihistamines, antimalarial drugs, some antipsychotics (e.g. clozapine), buspirone, fluoroquinolones, theophylline; when blood levels of phenytoin are very high, a paradoxical increase in seizure frequency
Expanding intracranial lesions	Hemorrhage, hydrocephalus, tumors
Hyperpyrexia	Drug toxicity (e.g. with amphetamines or cocaine), fever, heatstroke
Metabolic disturbances	Commonly, hypocalcemia (e.g. secondary to hypoparathyroidism), hypoglycemia, hyponatremia; less commonly, aminoacidurias, hepatic or uremic encephalopathy, hyperglycemia, hypomagnesemia, hypernatremia; in neonates, vitamin B_6 (pyridoxine) deficiency
Neurocutaneous disorders	Neurofibromatosis, tuberous sclerosis
Pressure-related	Decompression illness, hyperbaric oxygen treatments
Withdrawal syndromes	Alcohol, anesthetics, barbiturates, benzodiazepines

Table 16.2 Causes of seizures (Contd.)

*Post-traumatic seizures occur in 25–75% of patients who have brain contusion, skull fracture, intracranial hemorrhage, prolonged coma, or focal neurologic deficits.

†Fifth day fits (benign neonatal seizures) are tonic-clonic seizures occurring between 4 days and 6 days of age in otherwise healthy infants; one form is inherited.

‡When given in toxic doses, various drugs can cause seizures.

NMDA, N-methyl-d-aspartate.

GENERALIZED SEIZURES

In generalized seizures, the aberrant electrical discharge diffusely involves the entire cortex of both hemispheres from the onset, and consciousness is usually lost. Generalized seizures result most often from metabolic disorders and sometimes from genetic disorders. Generalized seizures include the following:

- Infantile spasms
- Absence seizures
- Tonic-clonic seizures
- Tonic seizures
- Atonic seizures
- Myoclonic seizures (e.g. in juvenile myoclonic epilepsy)

Partial Seizures

In partial seizures, the excess neuronal discharge occurs in one cerebral cortex, and most often results from structural abnormalities. Partial seizures may be simple or complex.

Partial seizures may evolve into a generalized seizure (called secondary generalization), which causes loss of consciousness. Secondary generalization occurs when a partial seizure spreads and activates the entire cerebrum bilaterally. Activation may occur so rapidly that the initial partial seizure is not clinically apparent or is very brief. Partial seizures are called focal seizures, and the following terms are used for subtypes:

- **For simple partial seizures:** Focal seizures without impairment of consciousness or awareness
- **For complex partial seizures:** Focal seizures with impairment of consciousness or awareness
- **For secondarily generalized partial seizures:** Focal seizures evolving to a bilateral or convulsive seizure

Symptoms and Signs

Because epilepsy is caused by abnormal activity in brain cells, seizures can affect any process of the brain coordinates. Seizure symptoms and signs may include: temporary confusion, a staring spell, uncontrollable jerking movements of the arms and legs, loss of consciousness or awareness and psychic symptoms

Symptoms vary depending on the type of seizure. In most cases, a person with epilepsy will tend to have the same type of seizure each time, so the symptoms will be similar from episode to episode.

A **postictal state** often follows generalized seizures; it is characterized by deep sleep, headache, confusion, and muscle soreness; this state lasts from minutes to hours. Sometimes the postictal state includes Todd paralysis (a transient neurologic deficit, usually weakness, of the limb contralateral to the seizure focus).

Most patients appear neurologically normal between seizures, although high doses of the drugs used to treat seizure disorders, particularly anticonvulsants, can reduce alertness. Any progressive mental deterioration is usually related to the neurologic disorder that caused the seizures rather than to the seizures themselves. Occasionally, seizures are unremitting, as in status epilepticus.

Types of Partial Seizures

Simple partial seizures cause motor, sensory, or psychomotor symptoms without loss of consciousness. Specific symptoms reflect the affected area of the brain (Table 16.3). In Jacksonian seizures, focal motor symptoms begin in one hand, then march up the arm (Jacksonian march). Other focal seizures affect the face first, then spread to an arm and sometimes a leg. Some partial motor seizures begin with an arm raising and the head turning toward the raised arm (called fencing posture).

Epilepsia partialis continua, a rare disorder, causes focal motor seizures that usually involve the arm, hand, or one side of the face; seizures recur every few seconds or minutes for days to years at a time. The cause is usually

- *In adults:* A structural lesion (e.g., stroke)
- *In children:* A focal cerebral cortical inflammatory process (e.g. Rasmussen encephalitis), possibly caused by a chronic viral infection or by autoimmune processes

Complex partial seizures are often preceded by an aura. During the seizure, patients may stare. Consciousness is impaired, but patients have some awareness of the environment (e.g. they purposefully withdraw from noxious stimuli). The following may also occur:

- Oral automatisms (involuntary chewing or lip smacking)
- Limb automatisms (e.g. automatic purposeless movements of the hands)
- Utterance of unintelligible sounds without understanding what they say

- Resistance to assistance
- Tonic or dystonic posturing of the extremity contralateral to the seizure focus
- Head and eye deviation, usually in a direction contralateral to the seizure focus
- Bicycling or pedaling movements of the legs if the seizure emanates from the medial frontal or orbitofrontal head regions.

Motor symptoms subside after 1–2 minutes, but confusion and disorientation may continue for another 1 minutes or 2 minutes. Postictal amnesia is common. Patients may lash out if restrained during the seizure or while recovering consciousness if the seizure generalizes. However, unprovoked aggressive behavior is unusual.

Left temporal lobe seizures may cause verbal memory abnormalities; right temporal lobe seizures may cause visual spatial memory abnormalities.

Generalized Seizures

Consciousness is usually lost, and motor function is abnormal from the onset.

Infantile spasms are characterized by sudden flexion and adduction of the arms and forward flexion of the trunk. Seizures last a few seconds and recur many times a day. They occur only in the first 5 years of life, then are replaced by other types of seizures. Developmental defects are usually present.

Typical absence seizures (formerly called petit mal seizures) consist of 10–30-second loss of consciousness with eyelid fluttering; axial muscle tone may or may not be lost. Patients do not fall or convulse; they abruptly stop activity, then just as abruptly resume it, with no postictal symptoms or knowledge that a seizure has occurred. Absence seizures are genetic and occur predominantly in children. Without treatment, such seizures are likely to occur many times a day. Seizures often occur when

Table 16.3	Manifestations of partial seizures by site
Focal manifestation	**Site of dysfunction**
Bilateral tonic posture	Frontal lobe (supplementary motor cortex)
Simple movements (e.g. limb twitching, jacksonian march)	Contralateral frontal lobe
Head and eye deviation with posturing	Supplementary motor cortex
Abnormal taste sensation (dysgeusia)	Insula
Visceral or autonomic abnormalities (e.g. epigastric aura, salivation)	Insular-orbital-frontal cortex
Olfactory hallucinations	Anteromedial temporal lobe
Chewing movements, salivation, speech arrest	Amygdala, opercular region
Complex behavioral automatisms	Temporal lobe
Unusual behavior suggesting a psychiatric cause or sleep disorder	Frontal lobe
Visual hallucinations (formed images)	Posterior temporal lobe or amygdala-hippocampus
Localized sensory disturbances (e.g. tingling or numbness of a limb or half the body)	Parietal lobe (sensory cortex)
Visual hallucinations (unformed images)	Occipital lobe

patients are sitting quietly, can be precipitated by hyperventilation, and rarely occur during exercise. Neurologic and cognitive examination results are usually normal.

Atypical absence seizures usually occur as part of the Lennox-Gastaut syndrome, a severe form of epilepsy that begins before age 4 years. They differ from typical absence seizures as follows:

- They last longer.
- Jerking or automatic movements are more pronounced.
- Loss of awareness is less complete.

Many patients have a history of damage to the nervous system, developmental delay, abnormal neurologic examination results, and other types of seizures. Atypical absence seizures usually continue into adulthood.

Atonic seizures occur most often in children, usually as part of Lennox-Gastaut syndrome. Atonic seizures are characterized by brief, complete loss of muscle tone and consciousness. Children fall or pitch to the ground, risking trauma, particularly head injury.

Tonic seizures occur most often during sleep, usually in children. The cause is usually the Lennox-Gastaut syndrome. Tonic (sustained) contraction of axial muscles may begin abruptly or gradually, then spread to the proximal muscles of the limbs. Tonic seizures usually last 10–15 seconds. In longer tonic seizures, a few, rapid clonic jerks may occur as the tonic phase ends.

Tonic-clonic Seizures

Primarily generalized seizures typically begin with an outcry; they continue with loss of consciousness and falling, followed by tonic contraction, then clonic (rapidly alternating contraction and relaxation) motion of muscles of the extremities, trunk, and head. Urinary and fecal incontinence, tongue biting, and frothing at the mouth sometimes occur. Seizures usually last 1 minute to 2 minutes. There is no aura.

Secondarily generalized tonic-clonic seizures begin with a simple partial or complex partial seizure, then progress to resemble other generalized seizures.

Myoclonic seizures are brief, lightning-like jerks of a limb, several limbs, or the trunk. They may be repetitive, leading to a tonic-clonic seizure. The jerks may be bilateral or unilateral. Unlike other seizures with bilateral motor movements, consciousness is not lost unless the myoclonic seizure progresses into a generalized tonic-clonic seizure.

Juvenile myoclonic epilepsy is an epilepsy syndrome characterized by myoclonic, tonic-clonic, and absence seizures. It typically appears during adolescence. Seizures begin with a few bilateral, synchronous myoclonic jerks, followed in 90% of cases by generalized tonic-clonic seizures. They often occur when patients awaken in the morning, especially after sleep deprivation or alcohol use. Absence seizures may occur in one third of patients.

Febrile seizures occur, by definition, with fever and in the absence of intracranial infection; they are considered a type of provoked seizure. They affect about 4% of children aged 3 months to 5 years. Benign febrile seizures are brief, solitary, and generalized tonic-clonic in appearance. Complicated febrile seizures are focal, last >15 min, or recur ≥2 times in <24 hours. Overall, 2% of patients with febrile seizures develop a subsequent seizure disorder. However, incidence of seizure disorders and risk of recurrent febrile seizures are much greater among children with any of the following:

- Complicated febrile seizures
- Pre-existing neurologic abnormalities
- Onset before age 1 year
- A family history of seizure disorders

Status Epilepticus

Status epilepticus has two forms—convulsive and non-convulsive.

Generalized convulsive status epilepticus involves at least one of the following:

- Tonic-clonic seizure activity lasting >5–10 minutes
- ≥2 seizures between which patients do not fully regain consciousness

The previous definition of >30 minutes duration was revised to encourage more prompt identification and treatment. Untreated generalized seizures lasting >60 minutes may result in permanent brain damage; longer-lasting seizures may be fatal. Heart rate and temperature increase. Generalized convulsive status epilepticus has many causes, including head trauma and rapid withdrawal of anticonvulsants.

Non-convulsive status epilepticus includes complex partial status epilepticus and absence status epilepticus. They often manifest as prolonged episodes of mental status changes. Electroencephalography (EEG) may be required for diagnosis.

Diagnosis

Evaluation must determine whether the event was a seizure vs another cause of obtundation (e.g. a pseudo-seizure, syncope), then identify possible causes or precipitants. Patients with new-onset seizures are evaluated in an emergency department; they can sometimes be discharged after thorough evaluation. Those with a known seizure disorder may be evaluated in a physician's office.

PHYSICAL EXAMINATION

In patients who have lost consciousness, a bitten tongue, incontinence (e.g. urine or feces in clothing), or prolonged confusion after loss of consciousness suggest seizure. In pseudoseizures, generalized muscular activity and lack of response to verbal stimuli may at first glance suggest generalized tonic-clonic seizures. However, pseudoseizures can usually be distinguished from true seizures by clinical characteristics:

- Pseudoseizures often last longer (several minutes or more).
- Postictal confusion tends to be absent.
- Typical tonic phase activity, followed by clonic phase, usually does not occur.
- The progression of muscular activity does not correspond to true seizure patterns [e.g. jerks moving from one side to the other and back (non-physiologic progression), exaggerated pelvic thrusting].
- Intensity may wax and wane.
- Vital signs, including temperature, usually remain normal.
- Patients often actively resist passive eye opening.

Physical examination rarely indicates the cause when seizures are idiopathic but may provide clues when seizures are symptomatic (Table 16.4).

Testing

Testing is done routinely, but normal results do not necessarily exclude a seizure disorder. Thus, the diagnosis may ultimately be clinical. Testing depends on results of the history and neurologic examination.

If patients have a known seizure disorder and examination results are normal or unchanged, little testing is required except for blood anticonvulsant levels. Additional testing is indicated if patients have symptoms or signs of a treatable disorder such as trauma, infection, or a metabolic disorder.

If seizures are new-onset or if examination results are abnormal for the first time, neuroimaging is required. Patients with new-onset seizures or atypical manifestations also require laboratory testing, including blood tests (serum electrolytes, blood urea nitrogen (BUN), creatinine, glucose, Ca, Mg, and P levels), and liver function tests. Other tests may done based on disorders that are suspected clinically:

- *Meningitis or CNS infection with normal neuroimaging results:* Lumbar puncture is required.
- *Unreported use of recreational drugs that can cause or contribute to seizures:* Drug screens may be done, although this practice is controversial because positive results do not indicate causality and test results can be inaccurate.
- *Cryptogenic epilepsy:* Testing for the anti-NMDA receptor antibody should be considered, especially in young women (as many as 26% may test positive); a positive result suggests anti-NMDA receptor encephalitis.

Neuroimaging [typically head computed tomography (CT), but sometimes magnetic resonance imaging (MRI)] is usually done immediately to exclude a mass or hemorrhage. Some experts say that CT can be deferred and possibly avoided in children with typical febrile seizures whose neurologic status rapidly returns to normal.

Follow-up MRI is recommended when CT is negative. It provides better resolution of brain tumors and abscesses and can detect cortical dysplasias, cerebral venous thrombosis, and herpes encephalitis. An epilepsy-protocol MRI of the head uses high-resolution coronal T1 and T2 sequences, which can detect hippocampal atrophy or sclerosis. MRI can detect some common causes of

Table 16.4	Clinical clues to the causes of symptomatic seizures
Finding	**Possible cause**
Fever and stiff neck	Meningitis, subarachnoid hemorrhage, meningoencephalitis
Papilledema	Increased intracranial pressure
Loss of spontaneous venous pulsations (noted during funduscopy)	Increased intracranial pressure (specificity is 80–90%*)
Focal neurologic defects (e.g. asymmetry of reflexes or muscle strength)	Structural abnormality (e.g. tumor, stroke) Postictal paralysis
Generalized neuromuscular irritability (e.g. tremulousness, hyperreflexia)	Drug toxicity (e.g. sympathomimetics), withdrawal syndromes (e.g. of alcohol or sedatives) Certain metabolic disorders (e.g. hypocalcemia, hypomagnesemia)
Skin lesions (e.g. axillary freckling or café-au-lait spots, hypomelanotic skin macules, Shagreen patches)	Neurocutaneous disorders (e.g. neurofibromatosis, tuberous sclerosis)

*Spontaneous venous pulsations are absent in all patients with increased intracranial pressure; these pulsations are also absent in 10–20% of people with normal intracranial pressure, but sometimes only temporarily.

seizures, such as malformations of cortical development in young children and mesial temporal sclerosis, traumatic gliosis, and small tumors in adults.

Electroencephalography is critical in the diagnosis of epileptic seizures, particularly of complex partial or absence status epilepticus, when EEG may be the most definitive indication of a seizure. EEG may detect epileptiform abnormalities (spikes, sharp waves, spike and slow-wave complexes, poly-spike and slow-wave complexes). Epileptiform abnormalities may be bilateral, symmetric, and synchronous in patients with primarily generalized seizures and may be localized in patients with partial seizures. EEG findings may include the following:

- Epileptiform abnormalities in temporal lobe foci between seizures (interictal) in complex partial seizures originating in the temporal lobe
- Interictal bilateral symmetric bursts of 4–7 Hz epileptiform activity in primarily generalized tonic-clonic seizures
- Focal epileptiform discharges in secondarily generalized seizures
- Spikes and slow-wave discharges occurring bilaterally at a rate of 3 per seconds and usually a normal interictal EEG in typical absence seizures
- Slow spike and wave discharges usually at a rate of <2.5/seconds, typically with interictal disorganization of background activity and diffuse slow waves, in atypical absence seizures.
- Bilateral polyspike and wave abnormality at a rate of 4–6 Hz in juvenile myoclonic epilepsy.

However, normal EEG cannot exclude the diagnosis of epileptic seizures, which must be made clinically. EEG is less likely to detect abnormalities if seizures are infrequent. The initial EEG may detect an epileptiform abnormality in only 30–55% of patients with a known epileptic seizure disorder. Serial EEG may detect epileptiform abnormalities in up to 80–90% of such patients. In general, serial EEG with extended recording times and with tests done after sleep deprivation greatly increases the chance of detecting epileptiform abnormalities in patients with epileptic seizures.

Inpatient combined video-EEG monitoring, usually for 2–7 days, records EEG activity and clinical behavior simultaneously. It is the most sensitive EEG testing available and is thus useful in differentiating epileptic from non-epileptic seizures.

If surgical resection of areas of epileptic foci is being considered, advanced imaging tests to identify such areas are available in epilepsy centers. Functional MRI can identify functioning cortex and guide surgical resection.

If EEG and MRI do not clearly identify the epileptic focus, magnetoencephalography with EEG (called magnetic source imaging) may localize the lesion, avoiding the need for invasive intraoperative mapping procedures. Single-photon emission CT (SPECT) during the peri-ictal period may detect increased perfusion in the seizure focus and help localize the area to be surgically removed. Because injection of contrast is required at the time of seizure, patients must be admitted for continuous EEG-video monitoring when SPECT is done during the peri-ictal period.

Neuropsychologic testing may help identify functional deficits before and after surgery and help predict social and psychologic prognosis and capacity for rehabilitation.

Prognosis

With treatment, seizures are eliminated in one-third of patients with epileptic seizures, and frequency of seizures is reduced by >50% in another third. About 60% of patients whose seizures are well-controlled by drugs can eventually stop the drugs and remain seizure-free.

Epileptic seizures are considered resolved when patients have been seizure-free for 10 years and have not taken anticonvulsants for the last 5 years of that time period. Sudden unexplained death in epilepsy (SUDEP) is a rare complication of unknown cause.

ANTIMICROBIAL AGENTS

Antimicrobial agents include a wide range of compounds with very different target organisms, mechanisms of activity, and pharmacokinetics. Efficacy of therapy is dependent on both the drug and the infectious agent, thus TDM for these compounds requires knowledge not only of the pharmacologic and toxicologic characteristics of the drug itself, but also of the nature of the infection it is intended to treat.

Antibacterials

Bacterial susceptibility to antibiotics is commonly measured in terms of the minimum inhibitory concentration (MIC), i.e. the concentration of drug sufficient to inhibit growth of an organism. The MIC varies widely for different strains of the same species, thus cultures must be obtained from each patient to ascertain not only the organism involved, but also its vulnerability to a panel of agents. TDM for antibiotics often involves relating some aspect of the serum concentration of drug [AUC, maximum plasma concentration of the drug (Cmax), or time above a given concentration] to the MIC measured for the specific infectious agent being treated.

AMINOGLYCOSIDES

Aminoglycoside antibiotics inhibit protein synthesis to kill aerobic, gram-negative bacteria. Because oral absorption is poor, aminoglycosides are administered intravenously or by intramuscular injection. Elimination is largely renal, almost entirely as the unchanged parent drug; the presence of kidney dysfunction is therefore a concern with use of these agents and may necessitate adjusting dose or dosing intervals.

Aminoglycosides are associated with the risk of serious toxicity. The most common concentration-related adverse effects are nephrotoxicity (renal tubular necrosis) and potentially irreversible ototoxicity (auditory nerve degeneration) leading to hearing loss. Aminoglycosides include amikacin, gentamicin, and tobramycin, among many others. Several studies have shown that efficacy of these drugs correlates well with the ratio of the Cmax relative to the MIC of the organism; this characteristic is termed concentration dependent killing. Ratios of Cmax and MIC ≥10 are preferred for optimal effect against sensitive bacteria. In contrast, toxicity is best averted when trough concentrations are allowed to decline substantially. This does not adversely affect therapeutic efficacy, because aminoglycosides show a considerable postantibiotic effect, i.e. they continue to enhance bactericidal activity after the drug has been cleared from the body.

A popular dosing strategy for aminoglycosides is extended interval administration, which provides large, less-frequent doses to drive Cmax above the organism MIC with adequate time for substantial drug elimination to minimize toxicity.

Serum concentrations do not reach steady state in extended interval dosing. Peak concentrations should rise well above the MIC (and often above previously published 'toxic' limits for more-frequent administration protocols), but trough concentrations will decline to near-undetectable concentrations. For these reasons, TDM is less routine for extended-interval dosing, although it is still common for patients with renal disease, sepsis, cystic fibrosis, or other conditions necessitating individualized therapy rather than application of population-derived protocols.

If administered more frequently, aminoglycoside TDM samples should be drawn at peak (1 hour post-infusion) and at trough (immediately pre-dose, or at minimum 10–12 hours post-infusion) to monitor both efficacy and risk of toxicity, respectively. In practice, one or both of these samples is often replaced by the use of a nomogram, Bayesian model, or other predictive protocol. However, publications have highlighted the prevalence of suboptimal use of antibiotics, including failure of these predictive models to consistently achieve sufficient concentrations above the MIC, or to allow adequate drug clearance in patients with renal dysfunction or other atypical pharmacokinetic parameters (e.g. elderly, septic patients). Ineffective antibacterial treatment fails to rid patients of infection at the risk of avoidable toxicity; it also enhances the development of antibiotic resistant bacterial strains; thus, TDM-based management of aminoglycoside therapy is recommended to optimize patient outcomes.

GLYCOPEPTIDES

Vancomycin and teicoplanin are glycopeptide antibiotics with activity against antibiotic resistant bacteria, including methicillin-resistant *Staphylococcus aureus* (MRSA). Teicoplanin is generally considered to have minimal toxicity at therapeutic concentrations; it is important to note that early concerns of vancomycin-related nephrotoxicity and ototoxicity were likely due to impurities in early formulations of the drug.

More recent studies evaluating current preparations of vancomycin (>90% pure) show much lower (although not absent) risk for adverse effects, unless administered with other agents capable of damaging hearing or renal function, such as aminoglycosides. TDM of vancomycin has been associated with improved therapy and reduced risk of toxicity; however, until recently, the optimal TDM protocol has remained contested. Recent guidelines suggest that the preferred monitoring parameter for vancomycin is the trough serum concentration, obtained immediately before the fourth dose. For most infections, trough vancomycin concentrations should be maintained above 10 mg/L, depending on the MIC of the pathogen; the target parameter for optimal therapy is an AUC/MIC ratio greater than 400. For more severe infections, such as MRSA endocarditis, more aggressive dosing is required and trough concentrations should be sustained in the range of 15–20 mg/L. Peak vancomycin concentrations do not appear to be helpful in monitoring risk of toxicity. In contrast to vancomycin, teicoplanin efficacy appears to correlate better with the time spent above the MIC [(teicoplanin) > MIC]. TDM of teicoplanin is not routinely necessary. However, in patients with renal dysfunction, atypical pharmacokinetics, or co-medications associated with nephrotoxicity or ototoxicity, frequent TDM of both glycopeptide antibiotics should be considered.

TUBERCULOSIS THERAPY

Management of tuberculosis (TB) typically involves an initial intensive treatment with several agents followed by months of continuation therapy to eliminate residual disease. Most patients respond well to such protocols;

cure rates are high with acceptably low concentrations of adverse effects.

However, certain populations present therapeutic challenges, including those with drug-resistant disease (e.g., isoniazid resistant or multidrug-resistant TB), individuals with comorbidities (e.g. diabetes mellitus, renal failure), and patients with HIV, wherein the disease affects immune response while treatment disrupts the disposition of co-medications.

First-line agents for TB include isoniazid, rifampicin, pyrazinamide, ethambutol, and streptomycin. These compounds are generally effective with minimal toxicity. Second-line therapy involves compounds that are less effectual or are poorly tolerated; second-line agents include cycloserine, p-aminosalicylic acid, and levofloxacin or other fluoroquinolones.

Trough concentrations often are too low to be readily measured, thus peak sampling is preferred. One protocol suggests obtaining a 2-hour sample (close to the serum peak for several primary agents) followed by a 6-hour sample to ascertain delayed absorption, malabsorption, or atypical elimination. Samples should be processed immediately to eliminate issues of drug instability ex vivo (e.g. rifampicin degradation in serum).

Rifampicin and related rifamycin drugs (e.g. rifabutin, rifapentine) are known inducers of most major hepatic phase I enzymes, including CYP2B6, CYP2C8/9/19, CYP2D6, and CYP3A4/5/7. Rifampicin is one of the most potent enzyme inducers characterized to date; thus its use can be a significant concern in patients with co-medications. It also presents a particular concern in patients with HIV, as many anti-retroviral agents inhibit or induce those same enzymes. Resources for TDM in large TB practices are increasing alongside the recognition that TDM is key to manag both drug-drug interactions and multidrug-resistant TB; achieving optimal drug concentrations is essential to successful therapy and preventing the development of other resistant strains.

OTHER ANTIBIOTICS

Analytical methods to detect many other types of antibiotics have been described, but little consensus has been reached as to the best practices for using TDM to optimize efficacy and minimize toxicity for most of these agents. Fluoroquinolones (e.g. ciprofloxacin) and p-lactams (e.g. penicillins), display little correlation between serum concentration and toxicity. The efficacy of many of these common antibiotics follows a time-dependent rather than a concentration-dependent pattern (i.e. serum concentrations must simply remain above the MIC for a certain percentage of time to obtain killing); thus measurement of drug peak or trough concentrations is not routinely necessary. TDM is recommended for management of patients with renal dysfunction, severe hepatic disease, or suspicion of atypical pharmacokinetics (e.g. poor absorption, altered distribution). Several specific antibiotic classes were reviewed extensively in the previous version of this chapter, to which readers are referred for further information.

Antifungal Agents

The incidence of fungal infection is increasing as is the prevalence of susceptible immune-compromised individuals (e.g. transplant recipients, HIV-positive patients). The most common pathogens are species of Candida yeasts or Aspergillus molds. Recent advances have expanded the number of fungicidal drugs available to combat such infections; however, the relative novelty of these agents is accompanied by a scarcity of data regarding optimal use of TDM for patient management.

5-Flucytosine

One of the first antifungals developed, the pyrimidine analog 5-flucytosine (ancobon), is a broad-spectrum agent that is co-administered with another fungicidal drug (typically amphotericin B) to prevent emergence of resistant pathogen populations. Toxicity of 5-flucytosine is well correlated with serum concentrations greater than 100 mg/L and presents as myelo-suppression (e.g. thrombocytopenia) or hepatic dysfunction evidenced by elevated transaminases.

Evidence for the utility of TDM for 5-flucytosine is more convincing than evidence for most other antifungal agents. Its bioavailability is excellent, but its renal elimination is variable and may be affected by the nephrotoxicity of amphotericin B. TDM is therefore recommended at the onset of therapy (to ensure that concentrations are within the target range) and in patients with renal dysfunction or evidence of toxicity. Because of its short half-life, the drug is administered in multiple doses daily; it is recommended to draw TDM samples at peak serum concentrations, roughly 2 hours after a dose. Target concentrations for efficacy appear to vary with the pathogen and the extent of infection but are approximately 30–80 mg/L for most patients.

Triazoles

The Triazole group of antifungal drugs includes fluconazole (diflucan), itraconazole (sporanox), voriconazole (Vfend), and posaconazole (noxafil). These broad-spectrum compound skill by inhibiting synthesis of the major fungal sterol, ergosterol. All Triazoles are available for oral or intravenous administration, except posaconazole, which currently is approved only in the oral formulation. Bioavailability canvary greatly, thus specific recommendations have been put forth for taking these agents while fasting (voriconazole), with acidic food, such as a cola (itraconazole), or with a high fat meal (posaconazole). Efficacy of triazoles correlates best with the ratio of drug AVC to pathogen MIC and appears optimal for eliminating invasive fungal infections when AVC/MIC is greater than 25. Target concentrations for prophylactic therapy are likely lower than for invasive infections, but have not been as well characterized.

All triazole agents are known to inhibit one or more of the CYP enzymes (specifically, CYP3A4, CYP2C9, or CYP2C19); thus their administration can greatly affect serum concentrations of other drugs (e.g. immuno-suppressants). As substrates of these same enzymes, triazole antifungals are subject to induction or inhibition of metabolism; thus co-medication with interacting compounds is a common rationale for performing TDM on triazoles. Currently, relatively few institutions are able to perform such TDM analyses; bioassay has historically been the most common method used, but newer assays are HPLC or LC-MS/MS based.

Of the individual compounds, fluconazole is the only triazole for which routine TDM does not appear necessary. Fluconazole concentrations are reasonably predictable based on dose, thus TDM is recommended only for special populations (e.g. children), or when concerns of poor absorption or noncompliance arise. In contrast, Itraconazole shows widely variable absorption and nonlinear kinetics, making TDM necessary for optimal therapy. The major metabolite, hydroxyitracona-zole, shows comparable antifungal effect to the parent compound, and must therefore be included in non-bioassay methods. Recommended steady-state trough concentrations for it raconazole are greater than 0.5 mg/L (HPLC) or greater than 5 mg/L (bioassay); no upper limit has been defined given the poor correlation of serum concentration with toxicity.

The newer triazoles, voriconazole and posaconazole, show broader spectra of activity and are effective against fluconazole and itraconazole resistant fungi. As with itraconazole, absorption of these two triazoles is extremely variable and can be greatly affected by food intake. Voriconazole shows nonlinear kinetics; posaconazole generally follows linear kinetics but can convert to nonlinear behavior (saturation) at high doses. Both agents show progressively greater risk of toxicity as serum concentrations increase, but there does not appear to be a single cutoff that clearly delineates toxic concentrations from nontoxic. Recommended steady-state trough concentrations for voriconazole are 1–6 mg/L; targets for posaconazole are as yet poorly defined, although concentrations greater than 1.5 mg/L appear to be effective against invasive fungal infections.

Other Antifungal Agents

Its bioavailability is excellent, but its renal elimination is variable and may be affected by the nephrotoxicity of amphotericin B. TDM is therefore recommended at the onset of therapy (to ensure that concentrations are within the target range) and in patients with renal dysfunction or evidence of toxicity. Because of its short half-life, the drug is administered in multiple doses daily; it is recommended to draw TDM samples at peak serum concentrations, roughly 2 hours after a dose. Target concentrations for efficacy appear to vary with the pathogen and the extent of infection but are approximately 30–80 mg/L for most patients.

Anti-retrovirals

The prevalence of infection with HIV has led to the development of several classes of drugs targeting this disease, collectively termed anti-retroviral agents. The major categories include nucleoside/nucleotide reverse transcriptase inhibitors (NRTIs), non-nucleoside reverse transcriptase inhibitors (NNRTIs), protease inhibitors (PIs), and entry/fusion inhibitors.

Current guidelines for treatment of anti-retroviral-naïve patients recommend the use of drug combinations termed highly active anti-retroviral therapy (HAART). This generally involves the use of two NRTIs, plus one or more agents from the other categories. Management of previously treated individuals can be more complex, as therapeutic options tend to be limited by viral strains with resistance to specific agents, or patients who are intolerant of certain drugs. Clinical response is assessed by monitoring viral load (i.e. the number of copies of HIV RNA) and the count of CD4$^+$ T-lymphocytes. Several factors indicate that TDM of anti-retrovirals can aid long-term patient management. First, these agents exhibit wide inter-individual variability in serum drug concentrations for a given dose, suggesting that there is risk of under-treatment or toxicity if serum concentrations are not assessed. Second, both the success of therapy and the prevention of viral drug resistance depend heavily on patient compliance.

Third, several anti-retroviral agents are capable of inhibiting or inducing various CYP isoforms. Patients generally are on multiple medications for HIV, opportunistic infections, and comorbidities; thus there is ample opportunity for drug interaction.

Successful use of TDM requires analytical methods capable of quantitating drugs of interest without interference from other compounds. This is extremely important for anti-retrovirals, given the large number of medications commonly administered to HIV-positive patients. Where available, LC-MS/MS methods are generally preferred for their ability to specifically monitor multiple agents with minimal interference. However, the complexity and expense of LC-MS/MS can prevent its use in many laboratories, notably in the developing world, where HIV infection rates are highest. For this and other reasons, assays for anti-retroviral TDM are currently performed at only a few sites, although the need for better availability is well recognized. Efforts to expand access to testing are under way, such as measuring drug concentrations from dried blood spots to facilitate sample transport and minimize infection risk.

PROTEASE INHIBITORS

Protease inhibitors inhibit viral propagation by interfering with the processing of HIV polypeptide precursors, thus disrupting a step that is mandatory for formation of mature viral particles and continuation of the infection cycle. Oral bioavailability tends to vary greatly depending on formulation and food intake. Most PIs are highly protein bound, and *in vivo* efficacy (which involves entry into cells) may require higher serum concentrations than those predicted by *in vitro* measures of viral susceptibility. PIs in current use include indinavir, saquinavir, atazanavir, lopinavir, nelfinavir, and ritonavir; nelfinavir has an active metabolite, M8, which should be included in TDM considerations.

Most of these agents are CYP substrates, and several are capable of modulating the activity of specific CYPs. Enzyme inducers (e.g. lopinavir, nelfinavir), and inhibitors (e.g. atazanavir, ritonavir) may affect their own metabolism, as well as that of co-medications. This has been exploited therapeutically in so-called boosted regimens, wherein a PI is administered alongside low-dose ritonavir—a potent CYP3A4 inhibitor to prolong exposure to the first agent. This strategy enhances the efficacy of the boosted PI, allowing use of less drug (likely reducing expense) while potentially minimizing toxicity, because the area under the curve (AUC) of the PI is increased without a dramatic rise in peak concentrations.

Particularly for treatment-experienced patients, current anti-retroviral TDM assesses both the amount of drug present and the susceptibility of the HIV isolate to that agent. This strategy, termed the inhibitory quotient (IQ), has been expressed as the phenotypic IQ [Cmin/IC50 (half maximal inhibitory concentration)], the virtual IQ (vIQ; Cmin/virtual IC50), the genotypic IQ (gIQ; Cmin/number of mutations), and normalized IQ based on population susceptibility.

Although, additional studies are required to delineate the preferred measure of IQ, it appears that the use of IQ to optimize anti-retroviral therapy is more success-

ful than examination of pharmacologic or virologic parameters alone. Effective IQ concentrations are drug specific and likely regimen specific (e.g. boosted vs. non-boosted); thus target IQs for individual agents must be carefully assessed.

Non-nucleoside reverse transcriptase inhibitors specifically target the reverse transcriptase enzyme that transcribes viral RNA into DNA, thus preventing viral incorporation into the host genome. Unlike the NRTIs, these agents are not nucleoside or nucleotide analogs, and they do not bind reverse transcriptase at its active site. Compared with PIs, NNRTIs appear to display less marked inter-individual variability in serum concentrations, but evidence suggests that their use can be improved by robust TDM. Common NNRTIs include efavirenz and nevirapine.

Efavirenz and nevirapine induce metabolic activity via CYP3A4 and CYP2B6, the same enzymes responsible for NNRTI metabolism. Management of drug interactions, therefore is one of the more obvious reasons to request TDM for these agents. Much like the PIs, target concentrations for TDM of NNRTIs are still being defined; use of IQ strategies appears helpful in achieving effective clinical responses, particularly in treatment-experienced patients. Some evidence suggests that high serum NNRTI concentrations correlate with onset of toxicity, specifically, central nervous system effects in the case of efavirenz, or liver enzyme elevations and rash for nevirapine. Although, the association of serum concentration with toxicity has been challenged, TDM guided dose reduction trials have successfully decreased adverse effects, supporting the utility of TDM in optimizing NNRTI therapy. NRTIs include some of the first anti-HIV therapies devised, such as zidovudine, didanosine, and stavudine, as well as several newer agents (e.g. abacavir, tenofovir).

Analysis of Antibiotics

Gentamicin, tobramycin, and vancomycin are most commonly analyzed by a nonisotopic immunoassay, such as fluorescence polarization immunoassay (FPIA). This method is highly sensitive and specific for these drugs, is highly automated, and requires only a moderate complexity of skill for performing the analysis.

A general rule of thumb for timing of TDM blood samples is that specimens for peak drug levels are drawn 1 hour after an oral dose is given and the trough drug level specimens are drawn at the t1/2 or just prior to giving the next dosage. This rule is not true for drugs, such as phenobarbital, phenytoin, digoxin, lithium, and the aminoglycoside antibiotics or for pediatric or some elderly patients, whose fluid levels and metabolic and renal function are different than adults. Most dosing and timing information is derived from study of young healthy adults, but adaptations have been made for pediatric and geriatric patients, who tend to have a decreased drug clearance.

Specimen collection for analysis of antibiotics allows for serum and other types of body fluids. The specimen of choice for gentamicin and tobramycin is serum, but EDTA plasma can be used. Heparin has been shown to deactivate gentamicin by forming an inactive complex that interferes with some immunoassay procedures.

Most vancomycin methods call for serum but allow heparinized and EDTA plasma. Often only vancomycin trough levels are monitored for therapeutic range due to the drug's long distribution phase.

The typical method of choice for analysis of chloramphenicol is by high-performance liquid chromatography (HPLC) in order to differentiate parent drug from active metabolite. Immunoassay methods are now also available for chloramphenicol as for other antibiotics. You should always refer to manufacturer's information regarding specific sources of pre-analytical and analytical interferences.

The specimen of choice for chloramphenicol testing is serum, but heparinized and EDTA plasma or CSF can be analyzed. Typically the trough level is used to evaluate therapeutic effects and the peak level, drawn 1–2 hours post-dose, is used to monitor toxic levels of chloramphenicol. Often a clotted blood sample is to be collected, but the container should not have gel separation barriers, which leach out some drugs. Likewise, some drugs, such as lidocaine, propranolol, and tricyclic antidepressants are disturbed by the plasticizer found in some stoppers (TBEP), so special collection tubes may be required.

Antibiotics are typically reported in whole numbers as micrograms per milliliter, with different expected ranges for samples drawn at peak and trough times. It is important to report these results in the standardized format in order to avoid confusion on the part of healthcare providers when interpreting therapeutic drug levels.

Cardioactive Drugs

Many agents used to treat various cardiovascular conditions are predominantly assessed for efficacy by biomarkers (e.g. monitoring cholesterol for statin therapy) or by clinical measures (e.g. blood pressure for anti-hypertensives). For many of these drugs, the therapeutic window is sufficiently wide to obviate the requirement for TDM, or poor correlation is noted between serum concentration and clinical effect or toxicity. Although, laboratory measurements for such agents are still useful in ascertaining compliance for such agents, this section will focus on cardioactive medications for which TDM has been shown to be clinically useful in optimizing therapy or preventing toxicity. Pharmacokinetic parameters of select cardioactive drugs are listed in Table 16.5.

The major cardioactive drugs requiring TDM are the antiarrhythmic agents and the glycoside digoxin. These compounds have benefited from well-established monitoring guidelines for over a decade; the guidelines are still valid, and the essential importance of TDM for cardioactive therapeutics has not diminished. However, prescription trends for cardioactive agents have shifted in recent years, resulting in fewer prescriptions for older, relatively difficult-to-manage drugs. Key points pertaining to current TDM recommendations are summarized here.

Table 16.5 Pharmacokinetic parameters of cardioactive drugs

Drug	Therapeutic range, mg/L*	Minimum toxic concentration, mg/L	Mean half-life, hours	Mean volume of distribution, L/kg	Protein binding, %	Enzymes involved in metabolism
Amiodarone	0.5–2	>2.5	45 days	60	99	CYP3A4, 2C8
Digitoxin	0.01–0.03	>0.045	150	0.5	90	CYP3A4
Digoxin (in heart failure)	0.5–2 flg/L0 5–0.8 flg/L	>3	40	5	25	CYP3A4
Disopyramide	2–5	>7	8	0.6	65	CYP2D6, 3A4
Flecainide	0.2–1	>1	14	5	45	CYP2D6
Lidocaine	1.5–5	6	1.8	1.1	70	CYP2D6, 3A4, Pg
Mexiletine	0.5–2	>2	10	5	60	CYP2D6, IA2
Procainamide	4–8	>10	6	1.9	20	NAT
N-acetylprocainamide	10–20	>40	8	NA	NA	NA
Quinidine	2–5	>6	6	3	85	CYP3A4
Sotalol	1–3	NA	12	2	NA	NA

NA, data not available. *Except where noted.

Antiarrhythmic Agents

Arrhythmias, disturbances of the normal cardiac sinus rhythm, can be associated with substantial morbidity and mortality; atrial fibrillation is the most common form of serious arrhythmia. A variety of agents are available to treat atrial fibrillation and other medically significant arrhythmias.

Many of these drugs act via regulation of cation channels (Na^+, K^+, or Ca^{2+}) and are associated with the potential for serious side effects and drug-drug interactions. Monitoring of clinical parameters (e.g. thyroid function tests for amiodarone therapy) is essential but can be complemented by TDM measurements. Antiarrhythmic agents for which TDM is commonly performed tend to show onset of toxicity at concentrations only slightly above or even coincident with the upper range of the therapeutic window.

The antiarrhythmic agents are classified according to function. Class I compounds primarily affect sodium channel function, although several members of the class have other activities as well. Moderate Na^+ channel blockers (i.e. class IA agents) include quinidine, procainamide, and disopyramide; procainamide should be monitored in conjunction with its active metabolite, N-acetylprocainamide. Many of these agents can be measured by immunoassays compatible with high-throughput autoanalyzers, making TDM convenient for most providers. However, the use of class IA agents has fallen off in recent years, most notably in the case of quinidine. This trend may reflect cardiac toxicity associated with these agents, including risk of a potentially lethal arrhythmia, torsades de pointes.

Class IE agents (weak Na^+ channel blockers) include lidocaine, tocainide, and mexiletine; these agents are used in acute management of cardiac conditions (e.g. life-threatening ventricular arrhythmia, digitalis toxicity), but are less likely to be used in settings requiring prolonged TDM. Serum concentrations are typically measured to ensure adequate therapy and to minimize toxicity. Of note, lidocaine binds primarily to AAG, which is often elevated in acute situations, such as myocardial infarction, possibly affecting free concentrations of the drug. Use of strong Na^+ channel blockers (class IC agents) has increased slowly over time, possibly in part because of their comparatively lower association with torsades de pointes [a form of polymorphic ventricular tachycardia associated with a long QT interval on electrocardiogram (ECG)] or other serious arrhythmias. Class IC agents include flecainide and propafenone. TDM for these agents is primarily recommended to prevent concentration-dependent toxicity (flecainide) and to ensure adequate concentrations after first-pass metabolism (propafenone). Class III antiarrhythmics, which act primarily via K^+ channel blockade, include amiodarone, dofetilide, and sotalol.

Amiodarone (cordarone, pacerone) has rapidly gained popularity for the management of atrial fibrillation; it is less prone to inducing arrhythmia than many of the class I agents but is nonetheless associated with adverse events, such as pulmonary fibrosis, hepatic failure (both uncommon, but serious), and disruption of thyroid function (relatively common, but generally manageable). Most of these complications are related to the extent of exposure to amiodarone and may reverse after reduction or elimination of the drug. TDM for amiodarone should include measurement of its active metabolite, desethylamiodarone, although recommended therapeutic ranges tend to address only the parent drug.

Acceptance of TDM for cardioactive agents is not universal. Although, the benefits of a robust program have been shown. Common situations that call strongly for the use of TDM include management of patients with comorbidities, such as renal failure (not uncommon in the elderly populations most prone to arrhythmia) and those experiencing physiologic change, for example, rapid weight fluctuations. In addition, many antiarrhythmic agents affect both metabolic (e.g. CYP enzymes) and transporter (e.g. P-glycoprotein) activities; thus the potential for serious drug-drug interactions is very real.

Digoxin

Obtained from digitalis plants, such as foxglove, digoxin (lanoxin) is a cardiac glycoside used in treatment of arrhythmias and heart failure. Cardiac glycosides (i.e. cardioactive agents containing one or more sugar moieties) are a group of related compounds found in a variety of plants, many of which are poisonous (e.g. oleandrin, the toxic component of oleander). Thus, it is not surprising that digoxin use is accompanied by the risk of serious toxicity, necessitating the use of TDM to avert such concerns.

Digoxin is thought to act through several mechanisms, including inhibition of the Na^+–K^+–ATPase that regulates cation flux in myocardial cells. Its direct and indirect activities coordinate to slow heart rate, increase the strength and velocity of cardiac contraction, and regulate nervous (sympathetic) and endocrine (renin-angiotensin) systems, affecting cardiovascular function. Digoxin use has declined in recent years, but the drug is still prescribed, particularly in congestive heart failure, where it is successful in relieving symptoms although without substantial improvement in mortality, and for treatment of atrial rhythm disturbances. Clinical response to digoxin is thought to correlate better with tissue concentrations than with serum concentrations.

The relationship between tissue and serum stores can be highly variable, thus serum measurements are an unreliable predictor of efficacy. The practice of titrating dose to target serum concentrations is now discouraged, following large studies showing that low digoxin concentrations (<0.9 mg/L) can produce adequate clinical responses. However, TDM remains essential in assessing risk of digoxin toxicity, particularly in patients with suspicious symptoms. Certain populations (e.g. women, the elderly) are at increased risk for elevated digoxin concentrations and thus toxicity, which begins with nonspecific effects (nausea, vomiting, and anorexia), but can progress to severe, potentially lethal cardiac manifestations (tachycardia, ventricular fibrillation) A greenish-yellow visual distortion has been described; although relatively uncommon, this is highly suspicious for digoxin toxicity. Patients with serum electrolyte imbalance (high calcium, low magnesium, or low potassium) or renal dysfunction are predisposed to developing toxicity, even at digoxin concentrations within the therapeutic window.

If samples are collected at the appropriate time, high serum digoxin correlates with toxicity. Digoxin distributes extensively into tissue, a process that requires several hours after a dose is administered. For this reason, TDM samples must be drawn at least 8 hours after the last dose (i.e. the time of peak tissue concentration); serum drawn earlier will provide elevated results that are not representative of the true serum concentration after distribution. Similarly, because of its long half-life, digoxin requires 8–10 days after a dose adjustment to reach steady state. Reviews of current TDM practices have shown that digoxin sampling is often performed inappropriately, leading to potential confusion and mismanagement of patients. Digoxin-binding agents (e.g. digibind, digifab) are available for treatment of toxicity. These are modified antibodies specific to digoxin that sequester the drug to prevent its physiologic effects. It should be noted that these agents only mildly enhance elimination of digoxin; thus the anti-dote bound drug remains in serum for some time after treatment.

For this reason, assays measuring total digoxin concentrations will still reflect the sum of digoxin bound to antidote plus serum protein-bound digoxin. The active fraction (i.e., that which is not bound to the antidote antibody fragments) can be determined by measuring free digoxin concentrations.

As a substrate for CYP3A4 and P-glycoprotein, digoxin is subject to a variety of drug-drug interactions, particularly in the setting of heart disease, where many patients require multiple medications. It is interesting to note that herbal products not only can affect digoxin therapy, but can also interfere with common analytical methods used to detect digoxin. Certain traditional herbal therapies containing a closely related cardiac glycoside can cause false elevation of immunoassay results for digoxin; similarly, patients experiencing oleander poisoning can show positive digoxin results due to antibody cross-reactivity. There is a positive clinical utility for antibody cross-reactivity, however, as it has been shown that digoxin-binding antidotes can successfully treat poisoning by oleander or related plants.

Digitoxin, a cardiac glycoside that is closely related to digoxin, is similarly effective in therapy of congestive heart failure. The mechanism of action and clinical efficacy of digitoxin are similar to those of digoxin; however, its pharmacokinetic parameters may be preferable for certain patients. Specifically, digitoxin undergoes hepatic metabolism, and its elimination is less heavily dependent on renal function than digoxin, which is excreted largely unchanged in urine. Thus, patients with renal disease do not accumulate digitoxin; however, hepatic metabolism presents the potential for additional drug-drug interactions.

Toxicity of Cardioactive Drugs

Toxic effects of cardioactive drugs, such as digoxin include changes in heart rate and contractions (including PVCs), nausea, visual distortion, central nervous system depression, seizures, decreased blood pressure, and/or decreased cardiac output of blood. Toxic effects of excessive procainamide are similar and includes lowing of heart muscle contractions and rate and changes in normal rhythm. Thus, it is noted that some of the symptoms of toxicity are the same as undertreatment of the underlying illness. In addition, if drug elimination is slowed due to impaired circulation, congestive heart failure, or impaired hepatic or renal function, the usual dosing interval of the drug may be too frequent and drug toxicity can result from higher than expected drug levels. Providing serum drug concentrations, as well as hepatic and renal function test results, may be necessary to determine the cause of the symptoms.

Methods of Analysis for Therapeutic Drugs

There is no one method that can be used to measure all drugs and toxic compounds. However, since medications are usually only present in small amounts in the patient's body, as compared to glucose or urea, the method must be sensitive to these minute levels of drug. As mentioned earlier with antibiotic assays, one common type of immunoassay is fluorescent polarization immunoassay. This method can also be used for quantification of drugs of abuse, hormones, and some toxins.

When drug concentration is measured, the value reflects both the protein bound and non-protein-bound or free drug. The free drug concentration will reflect the pharmacological response but, because the total and free drug concentrations are often similar, total drug concentration will be adequate for TDM. However, there are circumstances when the measurement of free drug levels would be of clinical value, such as when the free drug level is considerably less than total drug concentration or when two drugs compete for binding sites on albumin. In the latter circumstance, the drug with the lower affinity for albumin will reach higher free drug concentrations in the plasma, and the free drug level should be monitored for possible toxic effects. The amount of free drug in a patient sample is determined by analyzing a protein-free filtrate produced by a selective filtering membrane. The filtering membrane will allow only the non-protein-bound substances to pass through to be analyzed.

ENZYME-MULTIPLIED IMMUNOASSAY

In enzyme-multiplied immunoassay technique (EMIT), enzyme-labeled digoxin competes with digoxin in the patient sample for a limited amount of antibody specific to digoxin. Generally, all the patient digoxin binds with antibody and there are plenty of antibodies leftover to react with the enzyme-labeled digoxin. When antibody binds to the enzyme-labeled digoxin, the enzyme is inhibited and won't react with its substrate, preventing formation of product. There is generally leftover free enzyme-labeled digoxin. This will react with the substrate to form a product that is measured spectrophotometrically. An increase in absorbance due to the product in the reaction is directly proportional to amount of patient drug.

Immunosuppressants

Immunosuppressants, drugs capable of suppressing immune responses, are used to treat autoimmune disease,

allergies, multiple myeloma, and chronic nephritis, and in organ transplantation. Therapeutic ranges and toxic thresholds are proposed and are widely utilized to optimize dosing of these drugs. TDM is important for optimizing immunosuppressant therapy because serious consequences of under dosing (e.g. graft rejection) and overdosing (e.g. risk of opportunistic infections) are known. TDM can also prevent drug-related toxicity (e.g. kidney damage) and can be used to evaluate compliance. The common immunosuppressants currently monitored clinically to support initiation and maintenance of immunosuppression in solid organ and bone marrow transplant patients, including two calcineurin inhibitors (cyclosporine, tacrolimus), an inosine-5'-monophosphate dehydrogenase (IMPDH) inhibitor (mycophenolate mofetil), and two mammalian target of rapamycin (mTOR) inhibitors (sirolimus and everolimus). Pharmacokinetic parameters for immunosuppressants are summarized in Table 16.6.

Cyclosporine

Cyclosporine, also known as cyclosporin A, cicloral, gengraf, neoral, restasis, and sandimmune, is a fat-soluble cyclic peptide composed of 11 amino acids, some of novel structure, isolated from the fungus *Trichoderma polysporum*. It is available in many formulations and brand names (e.g. sandimmune, neoral, and gengraf). The compound has been shown effective in suppressing acute rejection in recipients of allograft organ transplants, and is approved for use in renal, cardiac, hepatic, pancreatic, and bone marrow transplants. Although, not discussed further here, cyclosporine is also used to treat keratoconjunctivitis sicca, and to manage immune-mediated conditions such as psoriasis and rheumatoid arthritis.

Cyclosporine is considered a calcineurin inhibitor, but in reality, it provides immunosuppression by blocking

Table 16.6	Pharmacokinetic parameters of immunosuppressant drugs				
Drug	Minimum effective concentration, MEC, µg/L	Minimum toxic concentration, MTC*, µg/L	Average half-life, hours	Average volume of distribution, L/kg	Average protein binding, %
Cyclosporin A	50	350*	8.4	3–5	90
Everolimlls	3	15	24	NA	74
Mycophenolic acid	1.3 mg/L	12 mg/L	18	4	97
Sirolimus	4	20*	62	12	90
Tacrolimlls	3	20*	21	0.85	85

*Trough (pre-dose) concentrations. The minimum effective and toxic concentrations are intended to provide general guidelines, but should not be applied to clinical practice without consideration of the analytical technique used, the clinical indication, the clinical status of the patient, time post-transplant (for tissue or organ transplant recipients), time of specimen collection relative to drug administration, and co-medications. In general. Therapeutic ranges are higher in the immediate post-transplant period (0–3 months) and lower during maintenance therapy. They may also be lower for combination therapies and specialized protocols. UCT, uridine diphosphate glucuronosyl transferase.

the activation of T-lymphocytes via a multifaceted mechanism. Cyclosporine crosses the lymphocyte membrane freely, where it forms a pharmacologically active complex with the intracellular immunophilin receptor cyclophilin. This complex, but not cyclosporine by itself, inhibits the Ca^{2+}/calmodulin-activated form of serine/threonine phosphatase calcineurin, thereby inhibiting the activation of nuclear factor of activated T (NFAT) in T-cells. Inhibition of NFAT activation mediated by cyclosporine leads to the down regulation of transcription of genes for cytokines such as interleukin (IL)-2, IL-3, IL-4, and IL-12; inflammatory mediators, such as tissue necrosis factor-alpha (TNF-α); and growth factors, such as granulocyte and/or macrophage colony-stimulating factor.

Inhibition of calcineurin by the cyclosporine-cyclophilin complex produces other important intracellular effects that contribute to the overall immunosuppressive effect. The intracellular mechanism(s) by which cyclosporine produces side effects, such as acute nephrotoxic effects including reduced renal blood flow, afferent arteriolar vasoconstriction, decreased glomerular filtration rate, and increased renal vascular resistance-remains unknown but appears to be related to altered release of vasoactive factors and effects on transcriptional regulation.

Cyclosporine formulations are not bioequivalent and cannot be used interchangeably. Formulations are described as 'modified' (Gengraf, Neoral) or 'non-modified' (sandimmune), wherein the modified forms (microemulsion formulations) are better absorbed. However, all formulations are considered to have erratic and incomplete absorption after oral administration, ranging from 5–60%, and averaging 30%. Peak concentrations are reached in 2–6 hours after oral administration with the non-modified formulations, and in 1–2 hours with the modified forms. With the non-modified form, a second peak is sometimes observed at 5–6 hours after administration. Cyclosporine is highly protein bound (approximately 90%), primarily to lipoprotein concentrates in erythrocytes, and has a relatively high volume of distribution (Vd = 3 to 5 L/kg). Cyclosporine undergoes extensive metabolism mediated by CYP3A4. Many of the 31 known metabolites of cyclosporine are inactive. One of the major metabolites, hydroxylated at the number 1 amino acid, retains approximately 10% of the immunosuppressive activity of the parent compound. The combination of variable expression of CYP3A4 and the associated multidrug efflux pump known as P-glycoprotein in the small intestine is thought to form a natural barrier to the absorption of cyclosporine after oral administration, and is thought to explain much of the extensive interpatient range of bioavailability. Because many other drugs are substrates for these two systems, the gastrointestinal tract is an important site for drug-drug interactions. Elimination of cyclosporine is biphasic and is primarily biliary. Terminal half-life is variable with formulation and patient, ranging from 5–18 hours for the modified forms and from 10–27 hours for the non-modified forms.

Therapeutic drug monitoring is best performed with whole blood. The degree of concentration in erythrocytes is temperature dependent *in vitro*; for this reason, measurement of plasma concentration is not recommended. Whole blood concentration of the parent drug (cyclosporine) correlates with the degree of immunosuppression and toxicity, but a poor relationship is seen between dose and blood concentration. Immunoassay methods were historically nonspecific because polyclonal antibodies were approximately 30% cross-reactive with several metabolites, leading to falsely elevated concentrations in some patients.

Conventional therapeutic trough blood concentrations of cyclosporine for renal transplants are 150–300 µg/L immediately post-transplant, and 100–200 µg/L thereafter. Efforts to minimize toxicity have led to evaluation of lower cyclosporine target ranges, such as 50–100 µg/L. Rates of acute rejection have not been different with low-dose versus conventional dosing; hence, prescribing patterns are being redefined to minimize cyclosporine exposure. Higher target concentrations are commonly used for cardiac, hepatic, and pancreatic transplants.

Although, trough concentration monitoring of cyclosporine was shown to be less effective than interval AVC of the drug in providing a precise estimate of drug exposure, the impracticality of measuring a full AVC using a series of samples collected over the 12-hours dose interval prevented this more accurate and precise determination of cyclosporine exposure from ever becoming a widely used monitoring test. Another approach is based on the association of most of the variability in cyclosporine pharmacokinetics during the first few hours following oral administration. This approach measures either the area under the blood cyclosporine concentration-time curve in the first 4 hours post-dose or the blood cyclosporine concentration at 2 hours post-dose, known as C2 monitoring. It has been reported that patients with C2 concentrations higher than 1300 µg/L during the first week post-kidney transplant were free of acute rejection, although specific target ranges for C2 monitoring are not well established. However, C2 monitoring is logistically challenging and has not been proven to improve outcomes over traditional pre-dose monitoring. Many drugs alter the disposition of cyclosporine. Drugs that inhibit CYP3A enzyme activity and block P-glycoprotein have been found to decrease cyclosporine metabolism and reduce the barrier to absorption from the gastrointestinal tract, thereby causing increased blood concentration.

Tacrolimus

Tacrolimus (proprietary names Prograf, Advagraf, and Protopic, and formerly known as FK506); it is a potent immunosuppressant that consists of a 23-member carbon ring and a hemi ketal-masked α, β-diketoamide function.

Structurally, tacrolimus is similar to the other macrolides sirolimus and everolimus. Tacrolimus is approved for prophylaxis of organ rejection in patients receiving allogeneic liver transplants and for use as an immunosuppressant in kidney transplantation. This potent immunosuppressant has been used effectively in other solid organ transplant patients, for prevention of graft-versus-host disease in allogeneic stem cell transplant recipients, and in pancreatic islet transplantation, as well as for atopic dermatitis.

As with cyclosporine, tacrolimus exerts its immunosuppressive effects following the formation of a complex with immunophilins. The complex of tacrolimus and FKBP12 in lymphocytes suppresses the synthesis of cytokines and inflammatory mediators by the same mechanisms as with cyclosporine (see cyclosporine section for details and references). Tacrolimus is administered in much lower doses than cyclosporine because of its substantially higher potency.

Absorption from the small intestine is generally low, averaging 25%, but is highly variable from patient to patient and with time post-transplant. Low tacrolimus bioavailability, as with cyclosporine, is probably due to the presence of CYP3A4 and P-glycoprotein in the small intestinal enterocytes. Peak concentrations are observed 0.5–4 hours after administration. The distribution in blood is characterized by extensive uptake by the cells. The whole blood-to-plasma ratio varies from 15–35, but the Vd is 1–2 kg/L if based on blood. Approximately, 99% of tacrolimus in plasma is bound to proteins, primarily α 1-acid glycoprotein, lipoproteins, albumin, and globulins. The major route of elimination is fecal excretion of metabolites. The elimination half-life of tacrolimus is variable, averaging 8–12 hours, but it can range from 4–41 hours. As with cyclosporine, CYP3A4 is primarily responsible for tacrolimus metabolism; nine metabolites have been identified, including one active metabolite, 31-O-desmethyl tacrolimus. This metabolite is generally present at very low concentrations and therefore is negligible in most patients. An exception, however, is seen in liver transplant patients with hyperbilirubinemia, in whom significant high bias in the immunoassay results may occur because of metabolite accumulation that results from impaired bile clearance.

Therapeutic drug monitoring for tacrolimus is similar to that for cyclosporine. The relationship between tacrolimus dose, trough blood concentration, and clinical outcomes-including acute rejection, nephrotoxicity, and toxicity requiring dose reduction, was investigated in a prospective multicenter study in liver transplant patients. A significant inverse correlation between tacrolimus trough blood concentration and risk of acute rejection during the first week following liver transplantation was shown using logistic regression analysis. Nephrotoxicity and other side effects were significantly correlated with increasing tacrolimus trough blood concentrations during this period. Receiver operator characteristic curve analyses showed that tacrolimus trough blood concentrations could differentiate between toxicity and nonevents. However, these relationships are somewhat controversial. Despite the fact that tacrolimus exposure is best predicted by the AUC, most TDM occurs with single pre-dose blood samples and, as with cyclosporine, whole blood is the preferred specimen. The originally proposed therapeutic range for tacrolimus was 5–20 µg/L, although efficacy has been demonstrated at lower concentrations, particularly for protocols designed to minimize renal toxicity by lowering concentrations of calcineurin inhibitors.

Inosine-5'-monophosphate Dehydrogenase Inhibitor

Mycophenolate mofetil (MMF) (proprietary names CellCept and Myfortic) is the 2-morpholinoethyl ester prodrug form of the active immunosuppressant mycophenolic acid (MPA).

The latter is a fermentation product of several *Penicillium* species that has antifungal, antibacterial, antitumor, and immunosuppressive activity in animal models. Following demonstration of its immunosuppressive efficacy in human renal transplant patients and in combination with cyclosporine and corticosteroids, formal clinical trials were conducted.

Mycophenolate mofetil is also used with cardiac and liver transplantation, particularly for patients who do not tolerate cyclosporine or tacrolimus well, to treat Crohn's disease, and to manage psoriasis. MPA is a reversible and uncompetitive inhibitor of IMPDH. A very important characteristic of proliferating lymphocytes is the greatly increased rate of de novo purine biosynthesis. The sustained and markedly increased rate of guanine nucleotide production catalyzed by IMPDH is the rate limiting step in de novo purine biosynthesis that cannot be provided by the salvage pathway in proliferating lymphocytes.

Thus, the proliferative response of activated T-cells is dependent on a continuous and increased supply of intracellular guanine nucleotide pool. T-cell proliferation is arrested by the suppression of guanine nucleotide production when IMPDH is inhibited by MPA. The mechanism of action whereby MPA produces its immunosuppressive effects in proliferating T-lymphocytes, is thus clearly distinct from that of the calcineurin and mTOR inhibitors.

Mycophenolate mofetil has near complete bioavailability after oral administration and is rapidly hydrolyzed by widely distributed esterases in blood and tissues to produce MPA. MPA usually reaches maximal concentrations within an hour of oral administration of MMF. Distribution of the drug is rapid and is essentially complete in most patients within 2–3 hours of oral administration. In whole blood, more than 99.9% of the drug is in the plasma compartment and is highly protein bound. The volume of distribution for MPA is 4 L/kg, and the half-life is, on average, 18 hours. Clearance of MPA is affected by (1) glucuronidation, (2) enterohepatic circulation (EHC), and (3) the quantity of its free fraction.

Enterohepatic circulation is considered to be a significant contributor to the dose interval kinetics of MPA, especially the post-distribution phase of the concentration-time curve. The contribution of EHC to the MPA AUC is about 37%, ranging from 10–61%, based on the effects of concomitant administration of cholestyramine. The appearance of a secondary MPA concentration peak anywhere from 4–12 hours following the morning dose of MMF is believed to result from EHC. The rate-limiting step in the clearance of MPA is its conversion to the phenolic glucuronide metabolite mycophenolic acid glucuronide (MPAG) via the catalytic action of UGT in the liver, gastrointestinal tract, and possibly other tissues such as kidney. MPAG is the primary metabolite of MPA and is pharmacologically inactive. The acyl glucuronide and 7-O-glucoside are metabolites that are produced in much smaller quantities than MPA or MPAG. The glucoside metabolite has no pharmacologic activity, but the acyl glucuronide is under evaluation for its potential toxic effects. MPAG is cleared by the kidney and accumulates to as much as several hundred-fold higher plasma concentration as the steady state trough concentration of MPA in uremic patients.

The specimen of choice for TDM of MPA is plasma or serum. A well-accepted therapeutic range for pre-dose MPA is 1.0–3.5 mg/L when combined with cyclosporine, and 1.9–4.0 mg/L when combined with tacrolimus. The therapeutic range based on AUC measurements is 30–60 mg/h.L.

Timing of specimen collection relative to drug administration is important in ensuring that MMF is fully hydrolyzed in vivo. It has been shown that MMF can become hydrolyzed *in vitro*, which may lead to determinations that overestimate the proportion of active MPA in vivo. Because MPA is avidly and extensively bound to albumin in plasma, investigators have studied the utility of monitoring the free fraction for patients with poor kidney function, hypoalbuminemia, and hyperbilirubinemia. In stable transplant patients, the MPA free fraction ranges from 1–3%. Increased free fraction will cause enhanced clearance of MPA, resulting in lower total MPA concentrations that return to baseline values when the condition that caused the change in free fraction becomes normal. In chronic renal failure, the total MPA concentration is often within the guidelines for effective immunosuppression, but the free concentrations can be substantially elevated, placing the patient at increased risk for overimmunosuppression. It is hypothesized that chronic uremia causes a reduction in intrinsic clearance that results in zero-order kinetics for MPA elimination. Severely decreased creatinine clearance <25 mL/min) is associated with reduced exposure to MPA, and moderate loss of renal function appears to increase MPA-AUC.

The primary sites and effects of drug-drug interactions involving other medications and MPA are likely to include decreased absorption in the gastrointestinal tract, inhibition of EHC, and inhibition of transport of the primary phenolic glucuronide metabolite. Meal consumption just before oral intake of MMF delays absorption, causing a reduction in maximal concentration of about 25%. Administration of antacids containing magnesium and aluminum hydroxides has been reported to reduce peak concentration of MPA by 33% and AUC by 17%. The two interactions with the greatest reported effects are cholestyramine and ferrous sulfate.

Cholestyramine produces a 40% reduction in the MPA-AUC when co-administered with MMF. The common iron supplement ferrous sulfate lowers the MPA-AUC by about 90%. Metronidazole, norfloxacin, and rifampin are among the other drugs that reduce exposure to MPA. Long-term effects of these drug interactions are under investigation. It has been suggested that corticosteroids cause enhanced clearance of MPA via induction of UGT activity. This is based on the observed 33% increase in the dose-corrected MPA trough concentration in a cohort of stable renal transplant patients at 12 months, following corticosteroid withdrawal, compared with the value at 6 months during maintenance therapy with corticosteroids. Inhibition of multidrug resistance protein 2 (MRP2) activity through co-administration of cyclosporine reduces the secondary peak and the overall AUC of MPA.

Inhibition of transport of MPAG from liver into bile is the presumed mechanism for the significant lowering of MPA concentration and raising of MPAG concentration by concomitant cyclosporine. This drug-drug interaction results in MPA-AUC values, adjusted for MMF dose, that are approximately 45% higher in patients on concomitant tacrolimus versus those on concomitant cyclosporine.

Immunoassays are now available to support TDM, although most TDM currently occurs through the use of chromatographic assays. A new functional method that uses IMPDH, the natural target receptor of MPA, is also available.

Sirolimus

Sirolimus (proprietary name Rapamune, formerly known as Rapamycin) is a macrocyclic antibiotic with immunosuppressive activity. Structurally, sirolimus is a lipophilic macrocyclic lactone composed of a 31-member macrolide ring.

Sirolimus inhibits T-lymphocyte activation and proliferation by inhibiting the mTOR through a mechanism of action unique from calcineurin or IMPDH inhibitors. The complex of sirolimus and the intracellular immunophilin FK-BPI2 modulates the immune response by combining with the specific cell-cycle regulatory protein mTOR and inhibiting its activation, and inhibiting progression from the G1 to the S phase of the cell cycle.

Formulations of sirolimus are not bioequivalent, although tablet and solution formulations were shown to be clinically equivalent. Sirolimus is rapidly absorbed from the gastrointestinal tract, with average time to reach maximal concentration in whole blood of about 2 hours, the average bioavailability of sirolimus is 15%. As with calcineurin inhibitors, the low bioavailability is attributable to extensive intestinal and hepatic metabolism by CYP3A4 and to counter transport by the multi-drug efflux pump P-glycoprotein in the gastrointestinal tract. This absorption barrier varies considerably from patient to patient and within patients and is the site of clinically important drug-drug and drug-food interactions. Sirolimus distributes primarily into red blood cells (95%), with only 3% and 2% distributing into plasma and other blood cellular components, respectively. Extensive and avid binding of sirolimus to the ubiquitously distributed intracellular FK-binding proteins accounts for the high blood-to-plasma sirolimus concentration ratio. Approximately, 92% of the sirolimus within the plasma fraction is bound to circulating protein, primarily albumin. Metabolism of sirolimus by the human body is driven by oxidative metabolism by CYP3A4 in the gastrointestinal tract and liver. At least seven metabolites are characterized as 41-O- and 7-O-demethyl, hydroxy, hydroxy-demethylated, and di-demethylated sirolimus, which are thought to be pharmacologically inactive. Elimination occurs primarily through the biliary tract, with average half-life of 62 hours in adults and substantially shorter (approximately 11 hours) in children.

The specimen of choice for sirolimus TDM is whole blood. The relationship between pre-dose sirolimus concentrations has been investigated in renal transplant patients who received concomitant full-dose cyclosporine and corticosteroid therapy. According to this study, the minimum effective sirolimus concentration, below which a significant increase in risk for acute rejection is seen, is 4–5 µg/L. The threshold concentration of 13–15 µg/L has been identified, above which the risks for concentration-related side effects of thrombocytopenia <100,000 platelets/mm^3), leukopenia <4000 leukocytes/mm), and hypertriglyceridemia (>300 mg/dL serum triglycerides) are increased. In general, a well-accepted range is 4–12 µg/L when sirolimus is used in conjunction with cyclosporine and corticosteroids. Alternative ranges proposed include 5–10 µg/L when sirolimus is combined with MMF and corticosteroids, and 12–20 µg/L when used with just corticosteroids. Drug-drug interactions revolving around CYP3A4 and P-glycoprotein, as described earlier, apply for sirolimus as well and have been reviewed extensively.

Chromatographic methods with ultraviolet (UV) and mass spectrometric detection have been validated and are used in laboratories worldwide.

EVEROLIMUS

Everolimus (proprietary names Afinitor and Certican) also known as SDZ RAD and RADOO1, is a structural analog of sirolimus with potent immunosuppressive activity when used in conjunction with cyclosporine. The primary difference between everolimus and sirolimus is the half-life, which is approximately half that of sirolimus, theoretically leading to more rapid attainment of steady-state concentrations. Everolimus is a semisynthetic lipophilic macrocyclic lactone macrolide. Similar to sirolimus, everolimus forms a complex with intracellular immunophilin FK-BP12 that modulates the immune response by combining with the specific cell-cycle regulatory protein mTOR and inhibiting its activation. This inhibition results in suppression of cytokine-driven T-lymphocyte proliferation, inhibiting progression from the G1 to the S phase of the cell cycle. Everolimus is metabolized through oxidation by CYP3A4 in the gastrointestinal tract and liver. At least 20 metabolites have been identified.

Cyclosporine inhibits the metabolism of everolimus, requiring everolimus dose reduction when co-administered. Everolimus does not affect cyclosporine metabolism. A review of drug-drug interactions observed with everolimus has been published. The primary side effect of concern with everolimus therapy is hyperlipidemia and thrombocytopenia of concentrations >8 µg/L.

Everolimus is administered orally as an oral micro-suspension. Everolimus is rapidly absorbed from the gastrointestinal tract, with the average time to reach maximal concentration in whole blood of about 3 hours. Low bioavailability is predicted by extensive intestinal and hepatic metabolism by CYP3A4 and counter transport by the multidrug efflux pump P-glycoprotein in the gastrointestinal tract. This absorption barrier varies considerably from patient to patient and within patients and is the site of clinically important drug-drug and drug-food interactions. Peak concentrations are observed in adults approximately 30 minutes after dosing. The apparent elimination half-life of everolimus is 32 hours. Proportionality between dose and blood concentration increases with increasing dose, and higher dosing appears to increase bioavailability. Steady-state trough blood concentration on a 3 mg/day dose in an adult is likely to be in the range of 5–20 µg/L. The proposed therapeutic dose for kidney transplant patients co-medicated with cyclosporine is 1.5 mg/day, and the target therapeutic range is 3–8 µg/L.

The specimen of choice for supporting TDM of evero-limus is currently pre-dose whole blood. Everolimus can be determined by immunoassay or by multiple HPLC methods with UV or mass spectrometric detection.

Psychiatric Therapies

Psychoactive drugs, including lithium, have a long history of use in treating psychiatric disorders. Psychoactive drugs are those that affect the mind or behavior. It has been long recognized that some psychoactive drugs require frequent therapeutic monitoring. A classic therapeutic drug in this category is lithium, which has serious toxic side-effects that begin when levels just exceed the upper limit of the the rapeuticrange. The traditional method of analysis for lithium, since it is a univalent metal, is by ion-selective electrode (ISE). Newer spectrophotometric methods provide a useful alternative to ISE and employ a more fully automated analyzer.

Other common psychoactive drugs that require some therapeutic monitoring include tricyclic antidepressants, amitriptyline, desipramine, imipramine, and nortriptyline. Alternative psychoactive drugs are available on the market, but there is a lack of defined concentration-effect relationship for newer psychoactive drugs.

Anti-asthmatic Drugs

Anti-asthmatic drugs, such as theophylline and the-obromine, are used for treatment of neonatal breathing disorders or of respiratory conditions that affect adults or children, such as asthma. Theophylline's action is in bronchodilation and smooth muscle relaxation.

Bronchodilation is the term for respiratory airway opening. Anti-asthmatic drugs are usually given intra-venously for initial therapy, followed by a regimen of oral dosages. Toxicity causes nausea, vomiting, diarrhea, headache, cardiac rhythm problems, and seizures. Theophylline is commonly measured with immuno-assay, while theobromine is generally measured by high-pressure liquid chromatography.

Anti-neoplastic Drugs

Methotrexate is an anti-neoplastic agent that historically has been measured with TDM. It is a nonspecific cellular growth regulator that is useful in the treatment of various neoplasms as well as some severe chronic skin disorders. Methotrexate inhibits DNA synthesis in rapidly dividing tumor cells with some effect on certain healthy cells. Leucovorin is administered to counteract some of the side effects from methotrexate toxicity. This drug is generally given in a single high dose intravenously. Toxic effects include bone marrow suppression, GI inflammation, and hepatic cirrhosis. Methotrexate is commonly measured by immunoassay.

Analgesics

Analgesics are substances that relieve pain without causing loss of consciousness. When used in excess, analgesics such as acetaminophen and salicylate can result in a toxic response.

Acetaminophen

Acetaminophen has analgesic and antipyretic actions. In common with the group of drugs referred to as non-steroidal anti-inflammatory drugs (NSAIDs; e.g. aspirin, ibuprofen, indomethacin), the pharmacologic actions of acetaminophen are related to its competitive inhibition of cyclooxygenase enzymes. This results in decreased production of prostaglandins, which are important mediators of inflammation, pain (low to moderate), and fever. Contrary to other NSAIDs, acetaminophen has very weak anti-inflammatory activity, a consequence of its weak inhibition of peripheral tissue cyclooxygenase compared with that in the brain. In normal doses, acetaminophen is safe and effective, but it may cause severe hepatic toxicity or death when consumed in overdose quantities.

Less frequently, nephrotoxicity may also occur. The initial clinical findings in acetaminophen toxicity are relatively mild and nonspecific (nausea, vomiting, and abdominal discomfort) and thus are not predictive of impending hepatic necrosis, which typically begins 24–36 hours after toxic ingestion and becomes most severe by 72–96 hours. Although, uncommon with severe overdose, coma and metabolic acidosis may occur before development of hepatic necrosis. Antidotal therapy with N-acetylcysteine (NAC; mucomyst) is most effective when administered before hepatic injury occurs, as signified by elevations of aspartate aminotransferase (AST) and alanine transaminase (ALT). Thus, the measurement of serum acetaminophen concentration becomes paramount for proper assessment of the severity of overdose and for appropriate decision making for antidotal therapy. The Rumack-Matthew nomogram relates serum acetaminophen concentration and time following acute ingestion to the probability of hepatic necrosis (Fig. 16.3).

Several qualifications pertain to the use of this nomogram. First, blood samples should not be obtained earlier than 4 hours after ingestion to ensure that absorption is complete. Second, the nomogram applies only to acute and not to chronic ingestion. Toxicity from chronic ingestion of acetaminophen or other drugs is cumulative and typically occurs at lower blood concentrations than in acute overdose. Third, the nomogram is not useful if the time of ingestion is unknown or is considered unreliable. In this case, when the exact time of ingestion is unknown, clinicians should err on the side of treating with NAC until the acetaminophen concentration is non-detectable and no transaminase elevation is seen. Fourth, if acetaminophen is ingested with another substance that may delay absorption (i.e. an anticholinergic), the patient should be clinically monitored for clinical effects. If, for example, noanticholinergic signs or symptoms develop after the

4-hours, acetaminophen concentration is measured, one may assume that absorption will not be delayed and the concentration can be plotted normally. If however, the patient develops anticholinergic signs and symptoms, and the acetaminophen concentration is detectable, that patient should be treated with NAC as absorption is most likely delayed, and the concentration should not be plotted. Fifth, alcoholic patients, fasting or malnourished patients, and patients on long-term therapy with microsomal enzyme-inducing drugs (anticonvulsants) may have increased susceptibility to acetaminophen hepato-toxicity, presumably as a result of induction of cytochrome P450 and, in the case of alcoholics or fasting patients, depletion of glutathione. In these cases, it has been proposed that the decision line in the nomogram should be lowered by 50–70%. Others do not advocate any change in the therapeutic decision line for such patients with acute ingestion. These risk factors may be more important in chronic acetaminophen poisoning. Although, therapeutic guidelines for chronic, acetaminophen poisoning have not been established, it is recommended to administer NAC, if the AST is elevated or acetaminophen is given at >10 µg/mL.

Acetaminophen is normally metabolized in the liver to glucuronide (50–60%) and sulfate (approximately 30%) conjugates. A smaller amount (approximately 10%) is metabolized by a cytochrome P450 mixed-function oxidase pathway that is thought to involve formation of a highly reactive intermediate (Fig. 16.4), N-acetyl

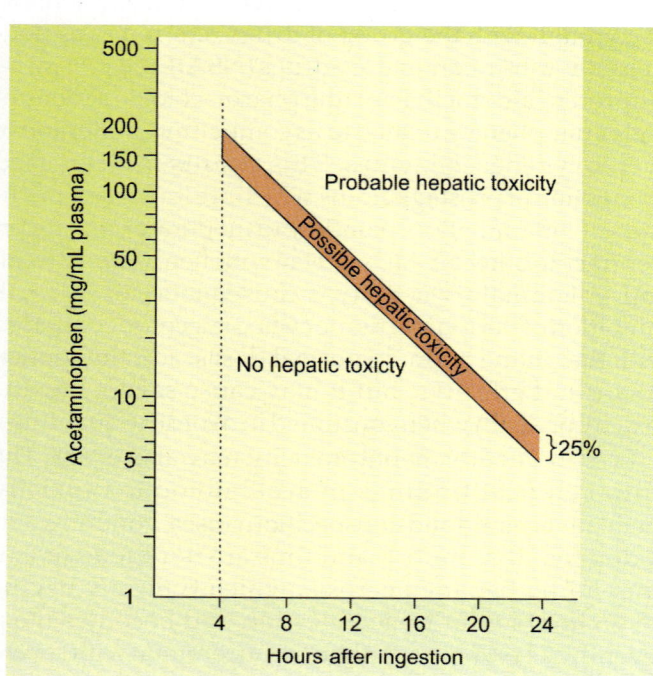

Fig. 16.3: Rumack-Matthew nomogram

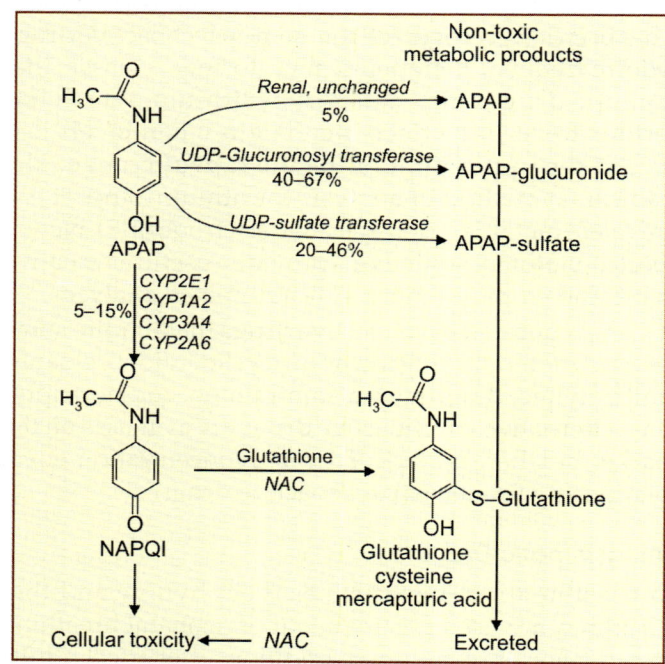

Fig. 16.4: Pathways of acetaminophen metabolism. APAP (N-acetyl–p-aminophenol/acetaminophen), NAPQI (N-acetyl-p-benzo-quinone imine), and NAC (N-acetyl-L-cysteine)

benzoquinoneimine (NAPQI). This intermediate normally undergoes electrophilic conjugation with glutathione and then subsequent transformation to cysteine and mercapturic acid conjugates of acetaminophen. With acetaminophen overdose, the sulfation pathway becomes saturated; consequently, a greater portion is metabolized by the P450 mixed-function oxidase pathway. When the tissue stores of glutathione become depleted, arylation of cellular molecules by the benzoquinoneimine intermediate leads to hepatic necrosis.

Specific therapy for acetaminophen overdose is the administration of NAC, which probably acts as a glutathione substitute. NAC may also provide substrate to replenish hepatic glutathione or to enhance sulfate conjugation, or both.

The time of administration of NAC is critical. Maximum efficacy is observed when NAC is administered within 8 hours, but efficacy then declines sharply between 18 hours and 24 hours after ingestion. The antidote provides definite beneficial effects even after liver injury has occurred, presumably through its ability to improve tissue oxygen delivery and use. NAC can be given by both oral and intravenous routes.

Oral dosing consists of a 140 mg/kg loading dose followed by 70 mg/kg every 4 hours for 17 doses. Intravenous dosing consists of a 150 mg/kg loading dose followed by 50 mg/kg over 4 hours, then 100 mg/kg infused over 16 hours. If serum acetaminophen analytical services are not available locally within 8 hours of suspected ingestion, treatment with NAC should begin.

An area of some controversy is whether acetaminophen screening should be performed on all intentional overdose patients. One of the most worrisome aspects of acetaminophen poisoning is that initial clinical symptoms (e.g., nausea, vomiting, abdominal pain) may be vague or even absent in the first 24 hours. This possible delay in diagnosis is particularly problematic because the antidote, NAC, has been shown to be most effective when initiated within the first 8 hours.

Many spectrophotometric methods are available for the determination of acetaminophen. In general, these methods are relatively easy to perform but are subject to various interferences, such as bilirubin or bilirubin by-products absorbing at similar wavelengths. Some methods measure the nontoxic metabolites and the potentially toxic parent acetaminophen, and thus may produce especially misleading results. Therefore, only methods specific for parent acetaminophen should be used. Immunoassays are widely used for this purpose, as they are rapid, easily performed, and accurate. A different spectrophotometric approach uses arylacylamide amidohydrolase to hydrolyze acetaminophen (but not conjugates) to p-aminophenol and acetate. Subsequent formation of the absorbing species depends on the reaction of generated p-aminophenol with 8-hydroxy quinoline or O-cresol. Arylacylamide amidohydrolase methods are susceptible to interference by NAC, bilirubin, and immunoglobulin (Ig)-M monoclonal immunoglobulins. Most chromatographic methods are very accurate and are considered reference procedures. A qualitative, one-step lateral flow immunoassay (cutoff of 25 μg/mL) may be suitable for point-of-care application, yet it has a low positive predictive value.

Salicylate

Acetylsalicylic acid (aspirin) has analgesic, antipyretic, and anti-inflammatory properties. These therapeutic benefits derive from its ability to inhibit biosynthesis of prostaglandins by acetylation of active site serine and subsequent irreversible inhibition of cyclo-oxygenase enzymes (COX-1; COX-2 isoenzymes). Salicylate, the metabolite of aspirin, also reduces prostaglandin synthesis by uncertain mechanisms. Because of these therapeutic benefits and the general lack of serious side effects at normal doses, aspirin is widely available and frequently consumed. Therapeutic serum salicylate concentrations are generally lower than 60 mg/L for analgesic-antipyretic effects, and 150–300 mg/L for anti-inflammatory actions.

Aspirin also interferes with platelet aggregation and thus prolongs bleeding time. The platelet inhibitory effect is a consequence of the ability of aspirin to acetylate and irreversibly inhibit platelet cyclo-oxygenase, thereby reducing the formation of thromboxane A2, a potent mediator of platelet aggregation. Platelets have little or no capacity for proteinsynthesis; therefore, the duration of this enzyme inhibition isthe normal life span of the platelets (8 to 11 days). Because of this platelet inhibitory activity, low-dose aspirin has been recommended as prophylactic therapy for some individuals at risk for thromboembolic disease. An epidemiologic association has been noted between aspirin ingestion and Reye syndrome in children and adolescents with viral infection (e.g. varicella, influenza). Therefore, aspirin use iscontraindicated in these patients.

Absorption of normal doses of regular aspirin from the GI tract is generally rapid, with peak serum concentration achieved within 2 hours. This peak value may be delayedfor 12 hours or longer for enteric-coated or slow-release formulations. Moreover, toxic doses of aspirin may form concretions or bezoars and produce pylorospasm, thereby delaying absorption. Serum salicylate in such instances may not reach maximum concentration for 6 hours or longer, an important consideration when assessment of the severity of toxicity is based on such measurements. Once absorbed, aspirin has a very short half-life (t1/2 = 15 minutes) because of its rapid hydrolysis to salicylate.

Salicylate is eliminated mainly by conjugation with glycine to form salicyluric acid, and to a lesser extent with glucuronic acid to form phenol and acyl glucuronides. A very small amount is hydroxylated to gentisic acid. These metabolic pathways may become saturated even at high therapeutic doses. Consequently, serum salicylate concentration may increase disproportionately with dosage. At high therapeutic or toxic doses, the salicylate elimination half-life is prolonged (15–30 hours vs 2–3 hours at low dose) and a much larger portion of the dose is excreted in urine as salicylate. Salicylates directly stimulate the central respiratory center and thereby cause hyperventilation and respiratory alkalosis. Moreover, salicylates cause uncoupling of oxidative phosphorylation. As a result, heat production (hyperthermia), oxygen consumption, and metabolic rate may be increased. In addition, salicylates enhance anaerobic glycolysis but inhibit the Krebs cycle and transaminase enzymes, all of which lead to accumulation of organic acids and thus to metabolic acidosis.

The primary acid-base disturbance observed with salicylate overdosage depends on age and severity of intoxication. Respiratory alkalosis predominates in children over age 4 and in adults, except in very severe cases that may progress through a mixed respiratory alkalosis-metabolic acidosis to metabolic acidosis. Among 97 adult patients who had plasma salicylate concentrations greater than 700 mg/L, 19% were found to have respiratory alkalosis, 61% had combined respiratory alkalosis and metabolic acidosis, and 15% had metabolic acidosis. Mortality was associated with acidemia. In children younger than age 4, the initial period of respiratory alkalosis is very brief and therefore may not be observed; in such cases, metabolic acidosis predominates. CNS depression is more pronounced when acidemia is severe, which is a consequence of increased brain uptake of non-ionized salicylic acid. Respiratory acidosis, a result of severe CNS depression or pulmonary edema, may sometimes occur and is indicative of a poor prognosis.

Salicylates remain readily available in numerous over-the-counter products. In any patient with a history of salicylate ingestion or possessing characteristic signs or symptoms of salicylate poisoning, a serum salicylate concentration should be obtained. Early identification of salicylate toxicity can belief saving. Following acute salicylate overdose, patients initially may be asymptomatic, especially if that product is enteric coated.

Salicylate toxic patients may develop nausea, vomiting, abdominal pain, tinnitus, tachypnea, oliguria, and altered mental status ranging from lethargy to coma. Chronic intoxication can present in a similar fashion as acute exposures, yet such exposures typically are more insidious and therefore are often misdiagnosed.

Interpretation of salicylate concentrations as a guide for clinical management decisions can be difficult. Perhaps the most well-known attempt at utilizing salicylate concentrations to predict the severity of salicylate toxicity was the nomogram developed by Done. After examining both the clinical symptoms and the salicylate concentrations in patients who had a single acute overdose, Done created a nomogram that predicted severity of poisoning based on the salicylate concentration drawn at a given time from ingestion.

Treatment for salicylate intoxication is directed toward (1) decreasing further absorption, (2) increasing elimination, and (3) correcting acid-base and electrolyte disturbances. Activated charcoal binds aspirin and prevents its absorption.

Elimination of salicylate may be enhanced by alkaline diuresis and in severe cases by hemodialysis. Sodium bicarbonate may be given to alleviate metabolic acidosis. Indications for hemodialysis include serum salicylate >1000 mg/L, severe CNS depression, intractable metabolic acidosis, hepatic failure with coagulopathy, and renal failure.

A urine drug screen may be helpful in detecting the presence of drugs included as part of combination medications with aspirin (e.g. antihistamines, sympathomimetic amines, and propoxyphene) or that otherwise are coingested. Classic methods for the measurement of salicylate in serum are based on the method of Trinder. These procedures rely on the reaction between salicylate and Fe^{3+} to form a colored complex that is measured at 540 nm.

Other methods for salicylate quantitation include fluorescent polarization immunoassay and a salicylate hydroxylase-mediated photometric procedure. These procedures are subject to some of the same interferences as the Trinder method, but the salicylate hydroxylase method is considered more specific and has been adapted to automated analyzers.

The reference method for salicylates is HPLC, which imparts a high level of specificity due to unique retention times in the column based on solubility in the mobile and stationary phases. High-pressure liquid chromatography can be moderate in cost, but more complex technology and training is required when compared to other automated systems. Turnaround time with HPLC can be longer than with other automated systems.

ETHANOL AND ALCOHOL TESTING

Some key facts about ethanol and other toxic alcohols will be helpful to consider as you think about this case scenario. First, ethanol is the most common toxicological agent involved in medicolegal cases, because it is legally obtained by adults and a common aspect of many social environments. It is a commonly measured analyte in the laboratory. Second, excessive exposure to ethanol can be lethal. It is often involved in automobile accidents and other legal situations, such as domestic violence.

Finally, ethanol, even in small amounts, can interfere or cause enhanced reactions with other medications, such as hypnotics or analgesics, so that patients who are going to receive treatment, such as surgery may need to have their alcohol level measured prior to administration of other medications.

Physiological Effects of Alcohol toxicity

Ethanol and other alcohols are small molecules that are soluble in water. Because they are easily distributed from the blood circulation to cerebrospinal fluid, disturbances to the CNS are common. Small amounts of alcohol depress the CNS and provide sensations of relaxation. Judgment, emotional release, reasoning, and recognition are all aspects controlled by cerebral functions, and these are affected by ethanol intake. Impaired cerebellar reflexes, including problems with balance and coordination as well as slower motor response times, occur when blood ethanol levels are 80 mg/dL or greater. The classic inability to walk in a straight line or balance on one foot has been used as a simple method to assess this type of impairment.

Toxicity of Ethanol

Toxicity and CNS disturbance increase proportionately with levels of alcohol. For example, blood ethanol concentrations of 10–100 mg/dL can cause diminished inhibitions, loss of self-control, and weakening of will power. Blood ethanol concentrations of 100–300 mg/dL are associated with problems walking, slurred speech, and dulled and distorted perceptions. Nausea and vomiting are usually triggered when alcohol toxicity begins. Severe CNS depression occurs with toxic levels of blood ethanol greater than or equal to 300 mg/dL.

METABOLISM AND EXCRETION OF ETHANOL

Small amounts of ethanol are metabolized in the gastric lining before absorption. Of the remaining ethanol, 90% is metabolized in the liver to acetaldehyde by hepatic alcohol dehydrogenase (ADH). The resulting acetaldehyde is converted to acetic acid by aldehyde dehydrogenase. In small or moderate amounts, the metabolites are nontoxic and readily excreted. Food contents in the stomach can slow absorption of alcohol, allow for more gastric metabolism of ethanol, and help to maintain lower blood alcohol concentrations. However, aspirin and gastric hyperacidity medication, such as cimetidine can inhibit gastric ADH activity and thereby slow metabolism. ADH is not 100% specific for ethanol and can also metabolize other alcohols, including methyl alcohol.

Ten percent of the ethanol in circulation is not metabolized, but is excreted unchanged in breath and urine. Thus, ethanol can be tested in urine or in breath samples along with blood samples. Ethanol induces diuresis, helping in renal excretion of ethanol and its metabolites.

Specimen Handling for Forensic Blood Alcohol Testing

Test results that will be used as legal evidence must be collected following strict guidelines, including the transport, storage, and handling conditions and the personnel involved in each of these steps. Frequently the specimen is kept in a locked box until testing occurs. The specimen must have documentation called a **chain of custody**. This is additional documentation of the condition of a specimen, all procedures performed, and personnel who have encountered a test specimen. It is used to document the integrity of the legal evidence as obtained from the test result.

This is also sometimes referred to as a chain of evidence. In addition, a **definitive test** method should be used rather than a **presumptive test** method of analysis. Presumptive tests are procedures with minimal complexity of instrumentation or personnel requirements so that the results can be quickly determined. Often presumptive tests have high sensitivity but lower specificity, and results must be verified by another methodology. A definitive test is a highly sensitive and specific test in which results can be used as legal evidence. Definitive test methodology is often the reference method, which requires more sophisticated instrumentation and personnel training.

For forensic blood alcohol testing in some states, a physician is required to draw a forensic specimen in the presence of the law enforcement officer, who will identify the patient and the specimen. In other situations, the officer of the law draws the specimen. The chain-of-custody documentation must be maintained. Prior to collection of the specimen for blood alcohol, cleaning of the skin puncture site should be performed with a nonalcoholic solution. The typical wipe contains isopropanol and should not be used. The sample must be collected in a closed system and may be arterial, venous, or capillary whole blood. The recommended sample tube is the 7 mL tube containing sodium fluoride and potassium oxalate as an anticoagulant. Some methods allow for use of serum. The container must be kept sealed until analysis. Lipemia, icterus, and hemolysis generally pose very little interference and are not considered problems in the collection phase. Some methods allow for use of freshly collected urine, maintained in a sealed container. As always, complete and accurate identification of the sample is important.

While enzymatic spectrophotometry is generally the method of analysis for medical testing of ethanol, a legal alcohol level is measured by gas-liquid chromatography (GLC), the reference method. Chromatography provides separation of ethanol from other alcohols within a low-temperature column using a carrier gas.

Little or No sample preparation is required, and the sample includes the air above the meniscus of serum or plasma. This is referred to as headspace analysis. The resulting output is determined as a unique retention time when compared to standard alcohol solutions. This method is specific for all alcohols, including methanol.

Chromatography is a technique for separation and quantification of alcohol molecules in body fluids. Chromatography involves the interaction of the sample mixture with a mobile phase, often a liquid or a gas, and a stationary phase, such as resin beads in a column. Detection of separated components can be achieved by using different solvents that selectively elute certain compounds, to be quantified spectrophotometrically or by flame ionization. Examples of other analytes that are separated and analyzed by chromatography include therapeutic drugs, such as chloramphenicol and drugs of abuse.

The more common method for measuring blood alcohol is a spectrophotometric method utilizing an enzyme that catalyzes the conversion of ethanol to measured product. This method is considered adequate for providing information for medical decisions, although it is not considered specific enough for forensic cases.

Drug-of-abuse Testing

Drug-of-abuse testing is ordered by physicians based on behaviors or signs exhibited by the patient. Since the patient may be uncooperative, a sample for drug testing should be relatively easy to obtain, such as urine or saliva, particularly, if it is to be used for legal purposes. Blood or other body fluids may be analyzed also. Drugs of abuse are frequently involved in situations of trauma, including those involving legal situations. Motor-vehicular crimes are often associated with alcohol and drug-of-abuse

intoxication. Thus, forensic testing for drugs of abuse is critical in providing legal evidence. Proper identification of the patient and sample, maintaining a chain of custody for the evidence, and following standardized procedures for maintaining the integrity of the sample during processing, testing, and reporting are critical in drug-of-abuse testing just as in legal alcohol testing.

There are thousands of potentially toxic drugs or toxins, and it is impossible to test for all of them. Consulting with the emergency department and the ordering physicians can determine what are the most important or likely drugs of abuse and toxins suspected for patients in the region. A negative result for a drug screen means that it is negative or below detectable levels only for the drugs that were tested. A good drug screen report should also list which drugs are tested for, so that a negative result is not misleading.

Drugs of abuse are typically medications obtained without a prescription, or taken by a person other than the one for whom they were prescribed, or are illicit drugs. The most common drugs of abuse vary from region to region and change with current times. Currently throughout the country, marijuana and methamphetamine are common drugs of abuse, as are prescription drugs such as oxycodone (Oxycontin) or diazepam (valium).

Drugs of abuse are grouped by chemical similarity, methodology of analysis, and physiological effects. The following list groups common drugs of abuse within categories:

1. **Central nervous system stimulants:** These drugs stimulate the CNS, raise heart and respiration rates, depress appetite, and give a feeling of euphoria. Drugs or drug classes commonly analyzed in this group include cocaine and its metabolite, benzoylecgonine, and amphetamines, and methamphetamines. Methamphetamine use has been steadily rising and is common in rural and metropolitan areas. Drugs in this category taken in overdoses or over long periods of time cause serious nervous system and cardiac side effects.

2. **Central nervous system depressants:** These drugs relax nerves, lower heart rate and respiratory rate, reduce pain, and give a feeling of euphoria. These include narcotics, hypnotics, sedatives, and tranquilizers. Drugs or Drug classes in this group include barbiturates; methaqualone; benzodiazepines, including valium; and oxycodone and other opiates, including morphine heroin (which metabolizes to morphine), codeine (methyl morphine), and methadone. Drugs in this category taken in overdoses cause respiratory depression and acidosis.

3. **Hallucinogens or Psychoactives:** Psychoactive drugs include cannabinoids and phencyclidine (PCP). Cannabinoids are drug forms derived from the cannabis plant, such as marijuana and its active forms, $\Delta 9$-tetrahydrocannabinoid (THC) and 11-nor-$\Delta 9$-THC carboxylic acid. Long-term abuse of psychoactive drugs can cause memory loss.

4. **Antidepressants:** Antidepressants include lithium, tricyclic antidepressants, and others.

When considering how sensitive and specific drug testing should be, one needs to consider the intended use of the test results. Two main uses are for medical or for legal purposes. Often a quick and relatively simple method can be highly sensitive but less specific, with cross reaction with similar groups of drugs, but also have more analytical interferences. Drug-of-abuse screening tests require a high sensitivity, which often compromises analytical specificity, in order to provide quick turn-around time, low cost and low technological needs. Screening tests are considered presumptive and may be strictly qualitative (with positive or negative results).

Confirmatory tests are needed for definitive results, especially for forensic or legal situations. Chain-of-custody considerations also must be made for results of legal concern.

The technologist needs to consider what instrumentation should be used for drug testing based on anticipated test volume, staffing, cost per test, and many other considerations. Some immunoassay methods have been incorporated into analyzers already in use. Other methods are simple spot tests that don't require sophisticated instruments but may require a confirmatory test before any results are reported. Thus, all positive tests may need to be retested by an alternate method, which would slow down turnaround time and increase costs. The definitive or reference methods often utilize gas chromatography, which is time consuming and highly technical and is not likely to be a realistic consideration for many laboratories.

The standard for drug testing in clinical toxicology is an immunoassay screen conducted with a urine sample, followed by confirmation by gas chromatography with mass spectrometric detection. Qualitative results in the immunoassay method are determined based on federal guidelines for cutoff values. If a drug is present, but determined to be below the recommended cutoff value based on a standard calibration curve, the positive result may be due to cross reactivity from similar drugs or chemicals. This would be considered a false positive for the drug and therefore not to be reported. Other screening tests for drugs of abuse include spot tests by UV spectrophotometry or enzyme-linked immunosorbent assay or by thin-layer chromatography (TLC). Drugs of abuse can also be presumptively quantified using immunoassays or HPLC or quantified by a definitive assay using as chromatography. Column chromatography with mass spectrometry detection provides a high level of specificity and can be used for less common drugs that are not detected with routine immunoassays.

Point-of-care Drug Testing Devices

On-site urinalysis drug-testing devices have been used in emergency departments and clinics and for forensic purposes. The false-negative rate for some of these point-of-care devices has been found to be less than 1% and the false-positive rate less than 1.75% for all drug classes, making them useful for impaired driving (DUI) investigations by law enforcement officers. They tend to have a high cost per test but do not require purchase of new automated analyzers.

A commonly used point-of-care spot test is a competitive homogeneous immunoassay. In this method, the patient drug competes with a reagent drug complexed with colloidal gold for a limited amount of antibody. A second antibody, an antidrug antibody, is bound to nylon membrane in a discrete zone and reacts with any residual drug—colloidal gold. Buffer is added, and a violet color indicates patient drug level that exceeded the threshold. Eight different drugs can be tested for in this system. These methods do have some interference, with a likelihood of false positives due to cross reaction with similar chemicals. Spot tests use high-affinity monoclonal antibodies that are specific to drug classes, but cross reaction with related chemicals and over-the-counter medications are possible.

AUTOMATED IMMUNOASSAY METHODS

Automated immunoassay techniques are often the method employed for drug screens, just as they are for therapeutic drugs. Considerable improvements in specificity and sensitivity have been made with newer generations of the immunoassays. The precision of several commercial immunoassay systems for drug-of-abuse screening is adequate to detect drugs below standardized lower limits of detection, but care should be used to interpret the results based on manufacturer's recommendations and federal guidelines for cutoff values. Knowledge of the positive predictive values of screening immunoassays at lower cutoff concentrations could enable efficient use of confirmatory testing resources and improved detection of illicit drug use.

In a commonly employed enzyme immunoassay, enzyme-labeled drug competes with patient drug for a limited amount of specific antibody. Excess free enzyme-labeled drug reacts with substrate to form product. Color reaction is directly proportional to amount of patient drug. Thresholds are set so that qualitative results can be determined. Although, monoclonal antibody is used with specificity to drug classes, cross reaction with similar drugs is possible. For example, in a test for anamphetamine, methamphetamine will enter into the reaction, as will other amphetamines, thus making this enzyme immunoassay a presumptive test.

CHROMATOGRAPHY METHODS

Thin-layer chromatography is also used as a presumptive screen for drugs of abuse. It can be used to screen for a variety of drugs in one process. In TLC, drugs migrate in a mobile phase on a silica gel support medium to a specific position depending on solubility in the two phases. Additional development of color or UV fluorescence provides further identification. Semi quantification of the drug may be achieved with densitometry. Although, TLC separation is highly specific for drug classes, cross reaction with related chemicals is possible. For example, poppy seeds from food will often appear as a positive test for morphine. Therefore, TLC is a presumptive test that requires confirmation. It can often differentiate between types of amphetamine drugs and so may be used in conjunction with immunoassay methods to narrow the type of amphetamine drug class detected.

Results admissible for legal purposes must maintain scrupulous patient identification and follow specimen collection and handling protocols. Evidence chain of custody must be maintained. Definitive test methods, often the reference method, are required to assure the highest analytical specificity and sensitivity of results to be provided as legal evidence. Gas or liquid chromatography often is the definitive method for plasma ethanol and urinary drugs of abuse. Gas chromatography with mass spectrometry has even been adapted to detect and quantitate up to 18 common drugs of abuse or their metabolites in hair samples.

Assessing patients with acute impairment often involves detecting large doses of drugs of abuse. However, sometimes the situation calls for monitoring of lingering doses or chronic use of drugs. In general, the detection time is longest in hair, followed by urine, sweat, oral fluid, and blood. In saliva, blood, or plasma, most drugs of abuse can be present for 1–2 days. In urine, the detection time of a single dose is 1.5–4 days. In chronic users, most drugs of abuse can be detected in urine for approximately 1 week after last use, but up to 4 weeks for some drugs. Hair may be the sample of choice for monitoring chronic drug use since drugs can be detected over a longer time frame in hair samples. Although, the

standard for drug testing in toxicology is conducted with urine samples, in recent years, more sensitive analytic techniques have enabled the analysis of drugs in saliva. Saliva is becoming increasingly useful for the detection of drugs, since it is a noninvasive specimen to collect and, because collection is directly observed, it is difficult to adulterate. A point-of-collection oral fluid drug analysis kit has been developed for use in many drug-testing situations, including common drugs of abuse, such as opiates, cannabinoids, and amphetamines.

To determine the best specimen to collect and appropriateness of specific drug requests, specific information should be available from the ordering physician. For example, the time and date of suspected drug exposure help to determine the best specimen to collect. The suspected toxin or group of toxins for screening needs to be determined since drug-of-abuse panels are still limited to certain groups or categories. Sometimes, other pertinent physical information is helpful as well.

Regardless of the type of testing employed by the laboratory for drug-of-abuse testing, a method validation and method comparison study must be completed prior to implementation. This should comply with guidelines established by the national clinical laboratory standards institute and meet clinical laboratory improvement amendments (CLIA) regulations.

In addition, a detailed operating procedure must be written and implemented along with training of personnel who will be involved in the specimen collection, transport, and preparation as well as analysis and reporting. This procedure should include maintenance and operation of equipment, when applicable, as well as quality control sample testing, documentation, and rules for corrective action, as well as other aspects of quality assessment.

HEAVY METAL TOXICITY

Heavy metal exposure, such as from mercury and lead, can be acute or chronic. Heavy metals can cause serious toxicological consequences that may be initially confused with drug-of-abuse or alcohol exposure due to behavioral and neurological manifestations. For example, high doses of lead can cause systolic hypertension and encephalopathy, while high or chronic exposure to mercury can cause psychotic behavior. Encephalopathy is a general term for disease of the brain, while neuropathy means disease of the nerves or neurons that may impair voluntary nerve function or functions of the brain. Psychosis or confusion, complete disorientation, and loss of reasoning power, can be a result of heavy metal neurotoxicity. In addition, chronic low-dose exposure to heavy metals is a concern for proper neurological and other organ development in the young. Therefore, physical examination and history can be helpful in determining if heavy metal toxicity is suspected. Specific laboratory tests are required to confirm heavy metal toxicity. A detailed account of lead poisoning can be referred to in hematology books, it is often seen as basophilic stippling, since in typical doses lead exhibits hematologic changes. Table 16.7 lists common toxic metals, their clinical manifestations and a brief description of testing methods.

MERCURY EXPOSURE

Exposure to mercury can lead to neurological impairment, renal tubular acidosis, and gastrointestinal symptoms. Mercury binds to structural and metabolic proteins to produce tissue impairment, such as renal tubular or myelin damage. Clinically, patients present with symptoms of headache, tremor, abdominal cramps, diarrhea, neuropathy, proteinuria, and liver impairment.

Mercury may be found in the environment from mining and other industrial processes. The metal may also be found in seafood, thermometers, barometers,

and dental amalgam. Mercury may be found in non-symptomatic, healthy individuals as a result of diet and environmental exposure. Mercury exposure screening may not be appropriate for asymptomatic individuals or individuals without a history of recent exposure. Screening of individuals who have had occupational exposure may be appropriate.

Whole blood is the specimen of choice for recent exposure. A 12- or 24-hour timed urine collection in a mercury-free container is the specimen of choice for long-term exposure. The timed urine may be helpful in determining recent or long-term exposure and the need for therapy. Although, there is no antidote to mercury, early chelation therapy may be used to lessen the effects of exposure. Dimercaprol has been used effectively as a chelat or of inorganic and aryl organic mercury.

Laboratory analysis for mercury uses atomic absorption spectrophotometry (AAS) methodology. Tests for mercury are not generally available from the routine clinical laboratory. They are provided by reference laboratories. The toxic effects and laboratory testing methodologies for other potentially toxic heavy metals are listed in Table 16.7.

Table 16.7	Toxic heavy metals	
Metal	**Pathology**	**Test methodology**
Aluminum	Pulmonary and nervous system impairment. High doses of this mineral usually required to cause adverse effects. Hemosiderosis and hepatic cirrhosis.	Electrothermal atomic absorption spectroscopy (AAS)
Arsenic	Interferes with protein sulfhydryl group in protein co-enzymes, reduces oxidative phosphorylation and ATP production	AAS Qualitative tests: Gutzeit and Reinsch tests
Cadmium	Binds sulfhydryl groups to inhibit enzymes. Pulmonary and nervous system impairment. Affects kidney function, resulting in proteinuria.	Electrothermal AAS
Lead	Binds sulfhydryl groups of proteins Symptom triad of colic, anemia, and encephalopathy	Anodic stripping voltammetry Electrothermal AAS Free erythrocyte protoporphyrin Erythrocyte zinc protoporphyrin Delta-aminolevulinic acid Delta-aminolevulinic acid synthetase Delta-aminolevulinic acid dehydratase
Mercury	Reacts with protein sulfhydryl groups Neurological, gastrointestinal, and renal impairment	AAS
Nickel	Pulmonary and nervous system impairment Dermatitis	Electrothermal AAS
Thallium	Has a great affinity for K and, thus, interrupts oxidative phosphorylation. Binds sulfhydryl groups to inhibit enzymes	Electrothermal AAS
Iron	High doses of this mineral usually required to cause adverse effects. Hemosiderosis and hepatic cirrhosis	Colorimetric, AAS

BIBLIOGRAPHY

1. Andersson BS, de Lima M, Thall PF, Wang X, Couriel D, Korbling M, et al. Once daily Lv. busulfan and fludarabine (Lv. Bu-Flu) compares favorably with Lv. busulfan and cyclophosphamide (Lv. BuCy2) as pretransplant conditioning therapy in AML/MDS. BioI Blood Marrow Transplant 2008; 14: 672–84.

2. Andes D, Pascual A, Marchetti O. Antifungal therapeutic drug monitoring: established and emerging indications. Antimicrob Agents Chemother 2009; 53: 24–34.

3. Atkinson JH, Patel SM, Meyer JM, Slater MA, Zisook S, Capparelli E. Is there a therapeutic window with some antidepressants for analgesic response? Curr Pain Headache Rep 2009;13: 93–9.

4. Back D, Gibbons S, Khoo S. An update on therapeutic drug monitoring for antiretroviral drugs. TIler Drug Monit 2006; 28: 468–73.

5. Bartelink IH, Bredius RG, Ververs TT, et al. Once-daily intravenous busulfan with therapeutic drug monitoring compared to conventional oral busulfan improves survival and engraftment in children undergoing allogeneic stem cell transplantation. BioI Blood Marrow Transplant 2008; 14: 88–98.

6. Barten MJ, Tarnok A, Garbade J, Bittner HB, Dhein S, Mohr F\v, et al. Pharmacodynamics of T-cell function for monitoring immunosuppression. Cell Prolif 2007; 40: 50–63.

7. Baumann P, Hiemke C, Ulrich S, Eckermann G, Gaertner I, Gerlach M, et al. The AGNP-TDM expert group consensus guidelines: therapeutic drug monitoring in psychiatry. Pharmacopsychiatry 2004; 37: 243–65.

8. Begg EJ, Barclay ML, Kirkpatrick CM. "The therapeutic monitoring of antimicrobial agents. Br J ClinPharmacol 2001; 52 (Suppl 1): 35S-43S.

9. Belitsky P, Dunn S, Johnston A, Levy G. Impact of absorption profiling on efficacy and safety of cyclosporin therapy in transplant recipients. ClinPharmacokinet 2000; 39: 117–25.

10. Belz GG, Breithaupt-Grogler K, Osowski U. Treatment of congestive heart failure-current status of use of digitoxin. Eur J Clin Invest 2001;31 (SuppI2):10-7.

11. Belz S, Frickel C, Wolfrom C, Nau H, Henze G. High-performance liquid chromatographic determination of methotrexate, 7-hydroxymethotrexate, 5-methyltetra-hydrofolic acid and folinic acid in serum and cerebrospinal fluid. J Chromatogr B Biomed Appl 1994; 661: 109–18.

12. Benedetti MS. Enzyme induction and inhibition by new Anti-epileptic drugs: a review of human studies. Fundam Clin Pharmacol 2000; 14: 301–19.

13. Bengtsson F. Therapeutic drug monitoring of psychotropic drugs: TDM "nouveau:' Ther Drug Monit 2004; 26: 145–51.

14. Bhorade SM, Janata K, Vigneswaran WT, Alex CG, Garrity ER. CylexImmuKnow assay levels are lower in lung transplant recipients with infection. J Heart Lung Transplant 2008; 27: 990–4.

15. Bialer M, Johannessen SI, Kupferberg HJ, Levy RH, Perucca E, Tomson T. Progress report on new Anti-epileptic drugs: a summary of the Eighth Eilat Conference (EILAT VIII). Epilepsy Res 2007; 73: 1–52.

16. Blum RA, Comstock TJ, Sica DA, Schultz RW, Keller E, Reetze P, et al. Pharmacokinetics of gabapentin in subjects with various degrees of renal function. ClinPharmacolTher 1994; 56: 154–9.

17. Boffito M, Acosta E, Burger D, Fletcher CV, Flexner C, Garaffo R, et al. Current status and future prospects of therapeutic drug monitoring and applied clinical pharmacology in antiretroviral therapy. Antivir Ther 2005; 10: 375–92.

18. Boffito M, Acosta E, Burger D, Fletcher CV, Flexner C, Garaffo R, et al. Therapeutic drug monitoring and drug-drug interactions involving antiretroviral drugs. AntivirTher 2005; 10: 469–77.

19. Booth BP, Rahman A, Dagher R, Griebel D, Lennon S, Fuller D, et al. Population pharmacokinetic-based dosing of intravenous busulfan in pediatric patients. J ClinPharmacoI 2007; 47: 101–11.

20. Brandhorst G, Marquet P, Shaw LM, Liebisch G, Schmitz G, Coffing MJ, et al. Multicenter evaluation of a new inosine monophosphate dehydrogenase inhibition assay for quantification of total mycophenolic acid in plasma. Ther Drug Monit 2008; 30: 428–33.

21. Brauch H, Murdter TE, Eichelbaum M, Schwab M. Pharma-cogenomics of tamoxifen therapy. Clin Chem 2009; 55: I 770–82.

22. Brooks AJ, Begg EJ, Zhang M, et al. Red blood cell methotrexate polyglutamate concentrations in inflammatory bowel disease. Ther Drug Monit 2007; 29: 619–25.

23. Bruggemann RJ, Donnelly JP, Aarnoutse RE, et al. Therapeutic drug monitoring of voriconazole. Ther Drug Monit 2008; 30: 403–11.

24. Brunetti L, Santell JP, Hicks RW. The impact of abbreviations on patient safety. JtComm J Qual Patient Saf 2007; 33: 576–83.

25. Brunton LL, Lazo JS, Parker KL, eds. Goodman and Gilman's the pharmacological basis of therapeutics, II th edition. New York: McGraw-Hill Professional, 2005.

26. Buchthal F, Svensmark 0, Schiller PJ. Clinical and electroen-cephalographic correlations with serum levels of diphenyl-hydantoin. Arch Neurol 1960;2:624-30.

27. Budde K, Glander P, Bauer S, Braun K, Waiser J, Fritsche L, et al. Pharmacodynamic monitoring of mycophenolate mofetil. Clin Chern Lab Med 2000; 38: 1213–6.

28. Bullingham RE, Nicholls AJ, Kamm BR. Clinical pharmaco-kinetics of mycophenolate mofetil. Clin Pharmacokinet 1998; 34: 429–55.

29. Burton ME, Shaw LM, Schentag JJ, Evans WE, eds. Applied pharmacokinetics and pharmacodynamics: principles of therapeutic drug monitoring, 4th edition. Philadelphia, Pa: Lippincott, Williams, & Wilkins, 2006.

30. Busauschina A, Schnuelle P, van der Woude FJ. Cyclosporine nephrotoxicity. Transplant Proc 2004; 36: 229S-33S.

31. Camm AJ. Safety considerations in the pharmacological management of atrial fibrillation. Int J Cardiol 2008; 127: 299–306.

32. Campbell TJ, Williams KM. Therapeutic drug monitoring: antiarrhythmic drugs. Br J Clin Pharmacol 2001;52(Suppl 1): 2IS-34S.

33. Cloyd JC, Miller KW, Leppik IE. Primidone kinetics: effects of concurrent drugs and duration of therapy. ClinPharmacol Ther 1981; 29: 402–7.

34. Cohen JM, Whittaker E, Walters S, Lyall H, Tudor-Williams G, Kampmann B. Presentation, diagnosis and management of tuberculosis in HIV-infected children in the UK. HIV Med 2008; 9: 277–84.

35. Cole E, Midtvedt K, Johnston A, Pattison J, O'Grady C. Recommendations for the implementation of Neoral C (2) monitoring in clinical practice. Transplantation 2002; 73: S19-22.

36. Coulthard KP, Peckham DG, Conway SP, Smith CA, Bell J, Turnidge J. Therapeutic drug monitoring of once daily tobramycin in cystic fibrosis-caution with trough concentrations. J Cyst Fibros 2007; 6: 125–30.

37. Darley ES, MacGowan AP. The use and therapeutic drug monitoring of teicoplanin in the UK. ClinMicrobiolInfect 2004; 10: 62–9.

38. Dasgupta A. Herbal supplements and therapeutic drug monitoring: focus on digoxin immunoassays and inter-actions with St. John's wort. Ther Drug Monit 2008; 30: 212–7.

39. Dasgupta A. Usefulness of monitoring free (unbound) concentrations of therapeutic drugs in patient management. Clin Chim Acta 2007; 377: 1–13.

40. deJonge H, Naesens M, Kuypers DR. New insights into the pharmacokinetics and pharmacodynamics of the calcineurin inhibitors and mycophenolic acid: possible consequences for therapeutic drug monitoring in solid organ transplantation. Ther Drug Monit 2009; 31: 416–35.

41. de Lima M, Couriel D, Thall PF, et al. Once-daily intravenous busulfan and fludarabine: clinical and pharmacokinetic results of a myeloablative, reduced-toxicity conditioning regimen for allogeneic stem cell transplantation in AML and MDS. Blood 2004; 104: 857–64.

42. Dervieux T, Meyer G, Barham R, Matsutani M, Barry M, BoulieuR, et al. Liquid chromatography-tandem mass spectrometry analysis oferythrocytethiopurine nucleotides and effect of thiopurinemethyltransferase gene variants on these metabolites in patientsreceiving azathioprine/6-mercaptopurine therapy. ClinChern 2005; 51: 2074–84.

43. Devinsky 0, Vazquez B, Luciano D. New Anti-epileptic drugs for children: felbamate, gabapentin, lamotrigine, and vigabatrin. J Child Neurol 1994; 9 (Suppl 1):S33-45.

44. Dreifuss FE, Penry JK, Rose Sw, Kupferberg HI. Dyken P, Sato S. Serum clonazepam concentrations in children with absence seizures. Neurology 1975; 25: 255–8.

45. Duffus J. Glossary for chemists of terms used in toxicology. Pure Appl Chem 1993; 65: 2003–122.

46. Ecker GF, Stockner T, Chiba P. Computational models for prediction of interactions with ABC-transporters. Drug Discov Today 2008;13: 311-7.

47. Einollahi B, Taheri S, Lessan-Pezeshki M, Pourfarziani V, Hosseini MS, Nemati E, et al. Approach to a target value for 2-hours post dose cyclosporine (C2) during the first week post renal transplantation. Ann Transplant 2009; 14: 18–22.

48. Eisen HI, Tuzcu EM, Dorent R, Kobashigawa I, Mancini D, ValantinevonKaeppler HA, et al. Everolimus for the prevention of allograft rejection and vasculopathy in cardiac-transplant recipients. N Engl J Med 2003; 349: 847–58.

49. Ekberg H, Tedesco-Silva H, Demirbas A, Vitko S, Nashan B, Gurkan A, et al. Reduced exposure to calcineurin inhibitors in renal transplantation. N Engl J Med 2007; 357: 2562–75.

50. Ellwood M, Lichtenfeld L, Parker RM, Tuncer D, Solis P, Fusco- Walker SI. et al. Enhancing prescription medicine adherence: a national action plan. Bethesda, Md: National Council on Patient Information and Education, 2007.

51. Fang MC, Stafford RS, Ruskin IN, Singer DE. National trends in antiarrhythmic and anti thrombotic medication use in atrial fibrillation. Arch Intern Med 2004;164: 55–60.

52. Ferrari S, Sass 0Ii V, Orlandi M, Strazzari S, Puggioli C, Battistini A, et al. Serum methotrexate (MTX) concentrations and prognosis in patients with osteosarcoma of the extremities treated with a multi drug neoadjuvant regimen. I Chemother 1993;5: 135–41.

53. Filler G, Lepage N, Delisle B, Mai I. Effect of cyclosporine on mycophenolic acid area under the concentration-time curve in pediatric kidney transplant recipients. TIler Drug Monil 2001; 23: 514–9.

54. Fukuoka N, Tsukamoto T, Uno J, Kimura M, Morita S. Influence of coadministeredanti epileptic drugs on serum zonisamide concentrations in epileptic patients: quantitative analysis based on suitable transforming factor. Bioi Pharm Bull 2003;26: 1734–8.

55. Geddes M, Kangarloo SB, Naveed F, Quinlan D, Chaudhry MA, Stewart D, et al. High busulfan exposure is associated with worse outcomes in a daily Lv. busulfan and fludarabine allogeneic transplant regimen. Bioi Blood Marrow Transplant 2008;14: 220–8.

56. Gelow 1M, Fang Ie. Update in the approach to and management of heart failure. South Med J 2006;99:1346-55; quiz 56-7, 84.

57. Gervasini G, Carrillo lA, Benitez J. Potential role of cerebral cytochrome P450 in clinical pharmacokinetics: modulation by endogenous compounds. ClinPharmacokinet 2004; 43: 693–706.

58. Ghanbari F, Rowland-Yeo K, Bloomer IC, Clarke SE, Lennard MS, Tucker GT, et al. A critical evaluation of the experimental design of studies of mechanism based enzyme inhibition, with implications for in vitro-in vivo extrapolation. Curr Drug Metab 2006; 7: 315–34.

59. Gillman PK. A review of serotonin toxicity data: implications for the mechanisms of antidepressant drug action. Bioi Psychiatry 2006;59: 1046–51.

60. Gillman PK. Tricyclic antidepressant pharmacology and therapeutic drug interactions updated. Br J Pharmacol 2007;151: 737–48.

61. Goetz MP, Kamal A, Ames MM. Tamoxifen pharma-cogenomics: the role of CYP2D6 as a predictor of drug response. Clin Pharmacol Ther 2008; 83: 160–6.

62. Gonzalez-Esquivel DF, Ortega-Gavilan M, Alcantara-Lopez G, lung-Cook H. Plasma level monitoring of oxcarbazepine in epileptic patients. Arch Med Res 2000; 31: 202–5.

63. Goodwin ML, Drew RH. Antifungal serum concentration monitoring: an update. I Antimicrob Chemother 2008; 61: 17–25.

64. Grime KH, Bird J, Ferguson D, Riley RI. Mechanism-based inhibition of cytochrome P450 enzymes: an evaluation of early decision making in vitro approaches and drug-drug interaction prediction methods. Eur I Ph arm Sci 2009; 36: 175–91.

65. Grinyo 1M, Cruzado 1M, Millan 0, Cal des A, Sabate I, Gil-Vernet S, et al. Low-dose cyclosporine with mycophenolate mofetil induces similar calcineurin activity and cytokine inhibition as doesstandarddose cyclosporine in stable renal allografts. Transplantation 2004; 78: 1400–3.

66. Grochow LB, lones RI, Brundrett RB, Braine HG, Chen TL, Saral R, et al. Pharmacokinetics of busulfan: correlation with veno-occlusive disease in patients undergoing bone marrow transplantation. Cancer Chemother Pharmacol 1989; 25: 55–61.

67. Johnson MD, Zuo H, Lee KH, et al. Pharmacological characterization of 4-hydroxy-N-desmethyl tamoxifen, a novel active metabolite of tamoxifen. Breast Cancer Res Treat 2004; 85: 151–9.

68. Johnston A, Holt OW Therapeutic drug monitoring of immunosuppressant drugs. Br J ClinPharmacol 1999; 47: 339–50.

69. Juang P. Update on new antifungal therapy. AACN AdvCrit Care 2007; 18: 253–60; quiz 61–2.

70. Juenke J, McMillin GA. Analytical support of classical anticonvulsant drug monitoring beyond immunoassay: application of chromatographic methods. In: Dasgupta A, ed. Advances in chromatographic techniques for therapeutic drug monitoring. Boca Raton, Fla: CRC Press, 2009; 87–103.

71. Justesen US. Protease inhibitor plasma concentrations in HIV antiretroviral therapy. Dan Med Bull 2008; 55: 165–85.

72. Kahan BD, Napoli KL, Kelly PA, Podbielski J, Hussein I, Urbauer DL, et al. Therapeutic drug monitoring of sirolimus: correlations with efficacy and toxicity. Clin Transplant 2000; 14: 97–109.

73. Kapoor N, Kirkpatrick 0, Blaese RM, Oleske J, Hilgartner MH, Chaganti RS, et al. Reconstitution of normal megakaryocytopoiesis and immunologic functions in Wiskott-Aldrich syndrome by marrow transplantation following myeloablation and immunosuppression with busulfan and cyclophosphamide. Blood 1981; 57: 692–6.

74. Minami K, Uezono Y, Ueta Y. Pharmacological aspects of the effects of tramadol on G-protein coupled receptors. J Pharmacol Sci 2007; 103: 253–60.

75. Mitchell PB. Therapeutic drug monitoring of non-tricyclic antidepressant drugs. Clin Chem Lab Med 2004; 42: 1212–8.

76. Mitchell PB. Therapeutic drug monitoring of psychotropic medications. Br J Clin Pharmaco I2001; 52(Suppl 1): 45S–54S.

77. Moore J, Middleton L, Cockwell P, Adu D, Ball S, Little MA, et al. Calcineurin inhibitor sparing with mycophenolate in kidney transplantation: a systematic review and meta-analysis. Transplantation 2009; 87: 591–605.

78. Morii M, Ueno K, Ogawa A, Kato R, Yoshimura H, Wada K, et al. Impairment of mycophenolate mofetil absorption by iron ion. Ciin Pharmacol Ther 2000; 68: 613–6.

79. Moyer TP, Temesgen Z, Enger R, Estes L, Charlson j, Oliver L, et al. Drug monitoring of antiretroviral therapy for H1V-1 infection: method validation and results of a pilot study. Clin Chem 1999; 45: 1465–76.

80. Musenga A, Saracino MA, Sani G, Raggi MA. Antipsychotic and Anti-epileptic drugs in bipolar disorder: the importance of therapeutic drug monitoring. Curr Med Chem 2009; 16: 1463–81.

81. Nafziger AN, BertinojS Jr. Utility and application of urine drug testing in chronic pain management with opioids. Clin j Pain 2009; 25: 73–9.

82. Nashan B. Review of the proliferation inhibitor everolimus. Expert Opinlnvestig Drugs 2002; 11: 1845–57.

83. Neef C, Touw DJ, Harteveld AR, Eerland n, Uges DR. Pitfalls in TDM of antibiotic drugs: analytical and modelling issues. Ther Drug Monit 2006; 28: 686–9.

84. Newman RA, Yang P, Pawl us AD, Block KI. Cardiac glycosides as novel cancer therapeutic agents. Mol1nterv 2008; 8: 36–49.

85. Nowak 1, Shaw LM. Mycophenolic acid binding to human serum albumin: characterization and relation to pharma-codynamics. Clin Chem 1995; 41: 1011–7.

86. Oellerich M, Armstrong VW. The role of therapeutic drug monitoring in individualizing immunosuppressive drug therapy: recent developments. Ther Drug Monit 2006; 28: 720–5.

87. O'Kane Dj, Weinshilboum RM, Moyer TP. Pharma-cogenomics and reducing the frequency of adverse drug events. Pharmacogenomics 2003; 4: 1–4.

88. Pacher P, Kecskemeti V. Cardiovascular side effects of new antidepressants and antipsychotics: new drugs, old concerns? Curr Pharm Des 2004; 10: 2463–75.

89. Patsalos PN, Berry Dj, Bourgeois BF, Cloydj C, Glauser TA, Johannessen SI, et al. Anti-epileptic drugs-best practice guidelines for therapeutic drug monitoring: a position paper by the subcommission on therapeutic drug monitoring, ILAE Commission on Therapeutic Strategies. Epilepsia 2008; 49: 1239–76.

90. Pavek P, Dvorak Z. Xenobiotic-induced transcriptional regulation of xenobiotic metabolizing enzymes of the cytochrome P450 superfamily in human extrahepatic tissues. Curr Drug Metab 2008; 9: 129–43.

91. Peloquin CA. Therapeutic drug monitoring in the treatment of tuberculosis. Drugs 2002; 62: 2169–83.

92. Perucca E. Pharmacokinetic profile of topiramate in comparison with other new Anti-epileptic drugs. Epilepsia 1996; 37(SuppI2): S8–13.

93. Pette M, Pette DF, Muraro PA, Martin R, McFarland HE In vitro modulation of human, auto reactive MBP-specific CD4 + T-cell clones by cyclosporin A. j Neuroimmunol 1997; 76: 9 1–9.

94. Pike MG, Franklin CL, Mays DC, Lipsky n, Lowry PW, SandbornWj. Improved methods for determining the concentration of 6-thioguanine nucleotides and 6-methylmercaptopurine nucleotides in blood. jChromatogr B Biomed Sci AppI 2001; 757: 1–9.

95. Pippenger CE, Penry jK, White BG, Daly DD, Buddington R. Interlaboratory variability in determination of plasma Anti-epileptic drug concentrations. Arch Neurol 1976; 33: 351–5.

96. Pollard S, Nashan B, johnston A, Hoyer P, Belitsky P, Keown P, et al. A pharmacokinetic and clinical review of the potential clinical impact of using different formulations of cyclosporin A, Berlin, Germany, November 19, 2001. Clin Ther 2003; 25: 1654-69.

97. Pomfret EA, Feng S, Hale DA, Magee jC, Mulligan M, KnechtleSj. The Art and science of immunosuppression: the fifth annual American Society of Transplant Surgeons' state-of-the-art winter symposium. Am j Transplant 2006; 6: 275–80.

98. Raggi MA, Mandrioli R, Sabbioni C, Pucci V. Atypical antipsychotics: pharmacokinetics, therapeutic drug monitoring and pharmacological interactions. Curr Med Chem 2004: 11: 279–96.

99. Rajapakse S. Management of yellow oleander poisoning. Clin Toxicol (Phila) 2009; 47: 206–12.

100. Ramsay RE, Wilder Bj, Uthman BM, Garnett WR, PellockjM. Barkley GL, et al. Intramuscular fosphenytoin (Cerebyx) in patients requiring a loading dose of phenytoin. Epilepsy Res 1997; 28: 181–7.

101. Ramsay RE. Clinical efficacy and safety of gabapentin Neurology 1994; 44: S23-30; discussion SI-2.

102. Rao A, Luo C, Hogan PG. Transcription factors of the NFAT family: regulation and function. Annu Rev 1mmunol 1997, 15: 707–47.

103. Rasmussen BB, Brosen K. Is therapeutic drug monitoring a case for optimizing clinical outcome and avoiding interactions of the selective serotonin reuptake inhibitors? Ther Drug Monit 2000; 22: 143–54.

104. Rea RS, Capitano B, Bies R, Bigos KL, Smith R, Lee H. Suboptimal aminoglycoside dosing in critically ill patients. Ther Drug Monit 2008; 30: 674–81.

105. Reiling MV, Fairclough D, Ayers D, Crom WR, Rodman jH, Pui CH, et al. Patient characteristics associated with high-risk methotrexate concentrations and toxicity. jClinOncol 1994; 12: 1667–72.

106. Rendon A, Nunez M, jimenez-Nacher I, Gonzalez de Requena D, Gonzalez- Lahoz J, Soriano V. Clinical benefit of interventions driven by therapeutic drug monitoring. HIV Med 2005; 6: 360–5.

107. Ritter jK, Kessler FK, Thompson MT, Grove AD, Auyeung Dj, Fisher RA. Expression and inducibility of the human bilirubin UDP glucuronosyltransferase UGTIA1 in liver and cultured primary hepatocytes: evidence for both genetic and environmental influences. Hepatology 1999; 30: 476–84.

108. Roberts jA, Lipman j. Antibacterial dosing in intensive care: pharmacokinetics, degree of disease and pharmacodynamics of sepsis. Clin Pharmacokinet 2006; 45: 755–73.

109. Rossanoj W, Denfield SW, Kim n, Price jF, Jefferies jL, Decker jA, et al. Assessment of the Cylex ImmuKnow cell function assay in pediatric heart transplant patients. j Heart Lung Transplant 2009; 28: 26-31.

110. Rothenburger M, Zuckermann A, Bara C, Hummel M, Struber M, Hirt S, et al. Recommendations for the use of everolimus (Certican) in heart transplantation: results from the second German-Austrian Certican Consensus Conference. j Heart Lung Transplant 2007; 26: 305–11.

111. Rowland M, Tozer T. Clinical pharmacokinetics: concepts and application. Philadelphia: Lea & Febiger, 1995.

112. Rybak M, Lomaestro B, Rotschafer)C, Moellering R jr, Craig W, Billeter M, et al. Therapeutic monitoring of vancomycin in adult patients: a consensus review of the American Society of Health- System Pharmacists, the Infectious Diseases Society of America, and the Society of Infectious Diseases Pharmacists. Am j Health Syst Pharm 2009; 66: 82–98.

113. Ryu SG, Lee jH, Choi Sj, Lee jH, Lee YS, Seol M, et al. Randomized comparison of four-times-daily versus once-daily intravenous busulfan in conditioning therapy for hematopoietic cell transplantation. Bioi Blood Marrow Transplant 2007; 13: 1095–105.

114. Saad AH, DePestel DD, Carver PI. Factors influencing the magnitude and clinical significance of drug interactions between azole antifungals and select immunosuppressants. Pharmacotherapy 2006; 26: 1730–44.

115. Sanchez-Fructuoso AI. Everolimus: an update on the mechanism of action, pharmacokinetics and recent clinical trials. Expert Opin Drug MetabToxicol 2008; 4: 807-19.

116. Santos GW, TutschkaPj, Brookmeyer R, Saral R, Beschorner WE, Bias WB, et al. Marrow transplantation for acute nonlymphocytic leukemia after treatment with busulfan and cyclophosphamide. N Engl j Med 1983; 309: 1347–53.

117. SoldinSj, Steele BW, Witte DL, Wang E, Elin RI. Lack of specificity of cyclosporine immunoassays: results of a College of American Pathologists study. Arch Pathol Lab Med 2003; 127: 19–22.

118. SoldinSj, Wang E, Verjee Z, Elin RI. Phenytoin overview-metabolite interference in some immunoassays could be clinically important: results of a College of American Pathologists study. Arch Pat hoI Lab Med 2003; 127: 1623–5.

119. Spina E, Perugi G. Anti-epileptic drugs: indications other than epilepsy. Epileptic Disord 2004; 6: 57–75.

120. Spina E, Santoro V, D'Arrigo C. Clinically relevant pharmacokinetic drug interactions with second-generation antidepressants: an update. Clin TIler 2008; 30: 1206–27.

121. Stenton SB, Partovi N, Ensom MH. Sirolimus: the evidence for clinicalpharmacokinetic monitoring. ClinPharmacokinet 2005; 44: 769–86.

122. Stevens DL. Association between selective serotonin-reuptake inhibitors, second-generation antipsychotics, and neuroleptic malignant syndrome. Ann Pharmacother 2008; 42: 1290–7.

123. Straatman Lp, Coles IG. Pediatric utilization of rapamycin for severecardiac allograft rejection. Transplantation 2000; 70: 541–3.

124. Streit F, Armstrong VW, Oellerich M. Rapid liquid chromatography tandem mass spectrometry routine method for simultaneous determination of sirolimus, everolimus, tacrolimus, and cyclosporin A in whole blood. Clin Chem 2002; 48: 955–8.

125. Striano S, Striano 1', Capone D, Pisani F. Limited place for plasma monitoring of new Anti-epileptic drugs in clinical practice. Med Sci Monit 2008;14: RAI73-8.

126. Takada M, Goto 1', Kotake 1', Saito M, Kawato N, Nakai M, et al. Appropriate dosing of antiarrhythmic drugs in Japan requires therapeutic drug monitoring. J Clin Pharm Ther 2005; 30: 5–12.

127. Taylor PI. Therapeutic drug monitoring of immuno-suppressant drugs by high-performance liquid chromato

graphy-mass spectrometry. Ther Drug Monit 2004; 26: 215–9.

128. Trescot AM, Helm S, Hansen H, Benyamin R, Glaser SE, Adlaka R, et al. Opioids in the management of chronic non-cancer pain: an update of American Society of the Interventional Pain Physicians' (ASIpp) guidelines. Pain Physician 2008; II: 55–62.

129. Trivedi MH, Lin EH, Katon WI. Consensus recommendations for improving adherence, self-management, and outcomes in patients with depression. CNS Spectr 2007;12:1-27.

130. Valdes R Ir, Iortani SA, Gheorghiade M. Standards of laboratory practice: cardiac drug monitoring. National Academy of Clinical Biochemistry. Clin Chern 1998; 44: 1096–109.

131. vanGelder 1', Le Meur Y, Shaw LM, Oellerich M, DeNofrio D, Holt C. et al. Therapeutic drug monitoring of mycophenolate mofetil in transplantation. Ther Drug Manit 2006;28: 145-54.

132. vanLuin M, Kuks pF, Burger DM. Use of therapeutic drug monitoring in HIV disease. CurrOpin HIV AIDS 2008; 3: 266–71.

133. van Rossum HH, de Fijter IW, van Pelt I. Pharmacodynamic monitoring of calcineurin inhibition therapy: principles, performance, and perspectives. TIler Drug Monit 2010; 32: 3–10.

134. Venkataramanan R, Shaw LM, Sarkozi L, Mullins R, Pirsch I, MacFarlane G, et al. Clinical utility of monitoring tacrolimus blood concentrations in liver transplant patients. I ClinPharmacol 2001;41: 542-51.

135. Venkataramanan R, Swaminathan A, Prasad 1', Iain A, Zuckerman S, Warty V, et al. Clinical pharmacokinetics of tacrolimus. ClinPharmacokinet 1995;29:404-30.

136. Visser K, Katchamart W, Loza E, et al. Multinational evidence-based recommendations for the use of methotrexate in rheumatic disorders with a focus on rheumatoid arthritis: integrating systematic literature research and expert opinion of a broad international panel of rheumatologists in the 3E Initiative. Ann Rheum Dis 2009;68: 1086–93.

137. Wallemacq 1', Armstrong VW, Brunet M, Haufroid V, Holt DW, IohnstonA, et al. Opportunities to optimize tacrolimus therapy in solid organ transplantation: report of the European Consensus Conference. Ther Drug Monit 2009; 31: 139–52.

138. Wang PW, Ketter TA. Pharmacokinetics of mood stabilizers and new anticonvulsants. Psychopharmacol Bull 2002; 36: 44–66.

139. Waring WS. Management of lithium toxicity. Toxicol Rev 2006; 25: 221–30.

140. Warner A, Privitera M, Bates D. Standards of laboratory practice: Anti-epileptic drug monitoring. National Academy of Clinical Biochemistry. Clin Chern 1998; 44: 1085–95.

141. Weinshilboum R. Inheritance and drug response. N Engl, Med 2003; 348: 529–37.

142. Weinshilboum RM, Sladek SL. Mercaptopurine pharmacogenetics: monogenic inheritance of erythrocyte thiopurine methyl transferase activity. Am I Hum Genet 1980; 32: 651–62.

143. Wille SM, Cooreman SG, Neels HM, Lambert WE. Relevant issues in the monitoring and the toxicology of antidepressants. Crit Rev Clin Lab Sci 2008; 45: 25–89.

144. Williams j, Bialer M, Iohannessen SI, Kramer G, Levy R, Mattson RH, et al. Interlaboratory variability in the quantification of new generation Anti-epileptic drugs based on external quality assessment data. Epilepsia 2003; 44: 40–5.

145. Wilson IF, Tsanaclis LM, Williams j, et al. Evaluation of assay techniques for the measurement of anti epileptic drugs in serum: a study based on external quality assurance measurements. Iher Drug Monit 1989; 11: 185–95.

146. Woodbury DM, Penfy IK, Schmidt Rp, eds. Anti-epileptic drugs. Amsterdam: North-Holland Publishing, 1972.

147. Yang Z, Peng Y, Want S. Immunosuppressants: pharmacokinetics, methods of monitoring and role of high performance liquid chromatography/mass spectrometry. ClinAppllmmunol Rev 2005; 5: 405–30.

148. Yasui-Furukori N, Furukori H, Saito M, Inoue Y, Kaneko S, Tateishi T. Poor reliability of therapeutic drug monitoring data for haloperidol and bromperidol using enzyme immunoassay. Ther Drug Monit 2003; 25: 709–14.

149. Yatscoff RW, Rosano TG, Bowers LD. The clinical significance of cyclosporine metabolites. Clin Biochem 1991; 24: 23–35.

150. Yip JS, Woodward M, Abreu MT, Sparrow MP. How are azathioprine and 6-mercaptopurine dosed by gastroenterologists? Results of a survey of clinical practice. Inflamm Bowel Dis 2008; 14: 514–8.

151. Zahir H, Nand RA, Brown KF, Tattam BN, McLachlan AJ. Validationof methods to study the distribution and protein binding of tacrolimus in human blood. J PharmacolToxicol Methods 2001; 46: 27–35.

152. Zhang G Jr, Bartlett MG. Bioanalytical methods for the determination of antipsychotic drugs. Biomed Chromatogr 2008; 22: 671–87.

153. Zimmerman JJ. Exposure-response relationships and drug interactions of sirolimus. AAPS J 2004; 6: e28.

17

Tumor Markers

INTRODUCTION

Tumor markers, by broad definition, are biochemical analytes that are useful for cancer detection, tumor growth prediction, or progression of the illness. They are most commonly used in diagnosis of lymphoma, leukemia, and colorectal, pulmonary, gastric, pancreatic, breast, liver, or prostatic carcinomas. Tumors are rapidly dividing cells, often unresponsive to normal physiological stimuli, and may appear in the wrong place. The center of a tumor is typically dead or dying cells that exude substances that can be analyzed and are therefore a marker for presence of tumor. Other types of tumor markers arise from cellular products, receptors, or genetic markers. Different terms are used to discuss unusual cell growth, including neoplasia, anaplasia, carcinoma, adenoma, and metastases.

Tumor markers can help the physician in monitoring for recurrences of malignancy and spreading tumors or metastases in the patient. Most tumor markers are not good analytes for screening tests, as in general they are not specific to malignancies. They can also be found in abnormal concentrations in conditions other than malignancies. However, once a diagnosis of a particular malignancy is made, these antigens can be very helpful in determining whether or not treatment is effectively reducing the tumor mass. Once the presence of a tumor is detected, the oncologist will order a baseline tumor marker measurement. Which marker is assayed will depend on the tumor's primary location. Then, during treatment, serial assays will be done to determine whether or not the treatment is working. Effective treatment will drop the level of the tumor marker precipitously and the level will remain within the reference range. Rising levels after treatment are often associated with recurrence or metastases.

Neoplasia is a general term for accelerated growth of tissue, which could be benign or malignant. Malignant growth is completely unrestricted and tends toward **metastasis**, or spreading past normal tissue boundaries into distant organs or sites. **Anaplasia** is a general term for loss of cell differentiation and change in cell and tissue structure from typical or normal. Other terms that relate to the origin or type of tumor include carcinoma and adenoma. A carcinoma is a malignant growth arising from skin or organ tissue epithelium, while an adenoma is a benign growth arising from glandular epithelium.

There are several categories of **tumor markers** based on their chemical makeup or general nature in the human body. Some of the oldest biochemical tests used as tumor markers are proteins, enzymes, and hormones. Newer laboratory techniques have yielded additional types of tumor marker testing such as carbohydrate markers, blood group antigens, receptors, and genetic markers.

ENZYMES

Enzymes were one of the first groups of tumor markers identified. Their elevated activities were used to indicate the presence of cancer. Measurement of enzymes was relatively easy using spectrophotometric determination of enzymatic activities. With the introduction of radioimmunoassay (RIA) in the late 1950s, the mass of an enzyme could be measured as a protein antigen instead of its catalytic activity. With few exceptions, an increase in the activity or mass of an enzyme or isoenzyme is not specific or sensitive enough to be used to identify the type of cancer or the specific organ involvement. An exception is prostate-specific antigen (PSA). PSA has mild protease activity and amino acid sequence homology with serine proteases of the kallikrein family. It is expressed by normal, benign, hyperplastic, and cancerous prostate glands and minimally by other tissue. Until the application of PSA as a marker for prostate cancer, tumor enzymes had lost most of their popularity for use as cancer markers. Enzymes were used historically as tumor markers before the discovery of oncofetal antigens and the advent of monoclonal antibodies. Abnormalities of enzymes as a marker for cancer include expression of the fetal form of the enzyme (isozyme) and ectopic production of enzymes.

Enzymes are present in much higher concentrations inside the cell. Enzymes are released into the systemic circulation as the result of tumor necrosis or following a change in membrane permeability of cancer cells. Increased enzymes are also observed in the blockage of pancreatic or biliary ducts and in renal insufficiency. The intracellular location of the enzyme may determine the rate of release. By the time enzymes are released into the systemic circulation, tumor metastasis may have occurred. Most enzymes, are not unique for a specific organ. Therefore, enzymes are most suitable as non-specific tumor markers. Elevated enzymes may signal the presence of malignancy.

Isoenzymes and multiple forms of enzymes may provide additional organ specificity. Table 17.1 summarizes various enzymes, their associated types of malignancy, and the assays used to measure their activity (Act) or their mass concentration (immunoassay). Enzymes are traditionally measured by their activities. With the introduction of antibody techniques, some enzymes, such as PSA, are measured as protein antigens rather than by their enzyme activity.

ALKALINE PHOSPHATASE

Alkaline phosphatase may arise from liver, bone, or placenta. The alkaline phosphatase in the sera of normal adults comes primarily from the liver or biliary tract. Elevated alkaline phosphatase is seen in primary or secondary liver cancer. Quantification may be helpful in evaluating metastatic cancer with bone or liver involvement. Greatest elevations are seen in patients with osteoblastic lesions, such as in those with prostatic cancer with bone metastases. Minimal elevations are seen in patients with osteolytic lesions, such as those with breast cancer with bone metastases.

In liver metastases, serum alkaline phosphatase shows a better correlation with the extent of liver involvement than the results of other liver tests. To determine the origin of elevated alkaline phosphatase, tests of other liver enzymes may be performed. Elevations in 5'-nucleotidase or γ-glutamyltransferase suggest that the elevated alkaline phosphatase is of liver, not

Table 17.1	Enzymes as tumor markers	
Enzyme	Assay	Type of cancer
Alcohol dehydrogenase	Act	Liver
Aldolase	Act	Liver
Alkaline phosphatase	Act	Bone, liver, leukemia, sarcoma
Alkaline phosphatase-placental	Act	Ovarian, lung, trophoblastic, gastrointestinal, seminoma, Hodgkin's
Amylase	Act	Pancreatic, various
Aryl sulfatase B	Act	Colon, breast
Creatine kinase-BB	IMA	Prostate, lung (small cell), breast, colon, ovarian
Esterase	Act	Breast
Galactosyltransferase	Act	Colon, bladder, gastrointestinal, various
γ-glutamyltransferase	Act	Liver
Hexokinase	Act	Liver
Lactate dehydrogenase	Act	Liver, lymphoma, leukemia, various
Leucine aminopeptidase	Act	Pancreatic, liver
Neuron-specific enolase	IMA	Lung (small cell), neuroblastoma, carcinoid, melanoma, pheochromocytoma, pancreatic
5'-Nucleotidase	Act/IMA	Liver
Prostatic acid phosphatase	Act/IMA	Prostate
PSA	IMA	Prostate
Pyruvate kinase	Act	Liver, various
Ribonuclease	Act	Various (ovarian, lung, large bowel)
Sialyltransferase	Act	Breast, colon, lung
Terminal deoxytransferase	Act	Leukemia
Thymidine kinase	Act/IMA	Various, leukemia, lymphoma, lung (small cell)

bone origin. Determination of alkaline phosphatase isoenzymes may provide additional specificity. The liver isoenzyme is thermally more stable than the bone isoenzyme.

Other malignancies, such as leukemia, sarcoma, and lymphoma complicated with hepatic infiltration, may also elevate alkaline phosphatase. Placental alkaline phosphatase (PALP) is synthesized by the trophoblast and is elevated in the sera of pregnant women. It is elevated in a variety of malignancies, including ovarian, lung, trophoblastic, and gastrointestinal cancers, seminoma, and Hodgkin's disease.

NEURON-SPECIFIC ENOLASE

Neuron-specific enolase (NSE) is the γ-subunit of the glycolytic enzyme phosphopyruvate hydrolase, which exists as a homodimer (γγ) and a heterodimer (αγ). The enzyme is found in neuronal tissue and cells of the diffuse neuroendocrine system. NSE therefore is associated with tumors of neuroendocrine origin. NSE is released into the blood as a result of cell lysis as opposed to secretion. NSE is also released into CSF with neuronal injury. NSE is found in tumors associated with neuroendocrine origin, including small cell lung cancer (SCLC), neuroblastoma, pheochromocytoma, carcinoid, medullary carcinoma of the thyroid, melanoma, and pancreatic endocrine tumor.

Serum NSE concentrations have been measured by immunoassay. Using a cutoff of 12.5 µg/mL, NSE has a clinical sensitivity of 80% in patients with SCLC with a clinical specificity of 80–90%. The NSE concentration appears to correlate with stage and provides a useful prognosis for disease progression. The value of NSE in detecting disease relapse has not been proved. Although the findings are mixed, NSE appears to be useful in monitoring chemotherapy and correlates with disease state. Immunostaining of NSE may provide the diffe-rential diagnosis between SCLC and other histologic carcinoma types.

Among children with advanced neuroblastoma, more than 90% have been reported to have elevated serum concentrations of NSE. High concentrations of NSE are associated with poor prognosis, and concentrations seem to correlate with the stage of the disease. Monitoring therapy using serum NSE is controversial, particularly with respect to the issue of specificity. However, elevated concentrations of NSE in children with stage IV neuro-blastoma were associated with a poorer outcome.

Prostatic Acid Phosphatase

The acid phosphatases include all phosphatases that hydrolyze phosphate esters with an optimum pH of less than 7.0. They are present in the lysozymes of secretory epithelial cells. Although, acid phosphatase is produced primarily by the (1) prostate gland, it is also found in (2) erythrocytes, (3) platelets, (4) leukocytes, (5) bone marrow, (6) bone, (7) liver, (8) spleen, (9) kidney, and (10) intestine. Prostatic acid phosphatase (PAP), with an optimum pH of 5–6, is very labile at a pH of greater than 7.0 and a temperature greater than 37°C. It can be distinguished from other acid phosphatases by using tartrate, which strongly inhibits the prostatic form. Another approach is to select substrates that are more specific for PAP, including thymolphthalein monophosphate (Roy method—most specific) and β-naphthol phosphate. Acid phosphatase was first used as a tumor marker. PAP was measured first by its enzymatic activity, then with the use of counter immune-electrophoresis, and subsequently by RIA. Elevated serum PAP may be seen in malignant conditions, such as osteogenic sarcoma, multiple myeloma, and bone metastases of other cancers. It also may be elevated in some benign conditions, such as BPH, osteoporosis, and hyperparathyroidism. For clinical use, PAP has been replaced by PSA. PAP is not as sensitive as PSA for detection of early cancer. It is less likely to be elevated in BPH than is PSA. However, as an individual marker, PAP may be useful for disease management in the rare patient whose tumor does not secrete PSA, and it may have utility when combined with other markers for improving prostate cancer detection or predicting recurrence after radical prostatectomy. Currently, the method of choice for PAP is measurement of its enzymatic activity.

KALLIKREINS

Kallikreins constitute a subgroup of the serine protease enzyme family, three members of which have been assigned a specific biological role.

The human kallikrein (hK) gene locus spans a region of approximately 300 kb of chromosome 19q13.4, which contains 15 tandemly localized kallikrein genes (KLK1 to KLK15) with no intervention from other genes. This is the largest cluster of serine proteases within the human genome.

Members of the kallikrein family are identified by various similar features. All have a nearly identical genetic structure (5′ untranslated region, intron-exon size and organization), and the catalytic triad of serine proteases is conserved by all members, with the histidine always occurring near the end of the second exon, the aspartate in the middle of the third exon, and the serine residue at the beginning of the fifth exon.

All kallikreins are produced as pre-propeptides with a 17–20 amino acid signal sequence and a 4–9 amino acid activation peptide. They contain 10–12 conserved cysteines that form 5–6 disulfide bonds. Finally, most if not all genes are under steroid hormone control. Kallikreins are expressed in a wide variety of tissues, including (1) prostate, (2) breast, (3) ovary, and (4) testis. 306F or example, KLK3 (PSA) is highly expressed in prostate and is discussed in detail later in the chapter. KLK3 also has minor expression in breast, thyroid, salivary glands, lung, and trachea, and KLKll and KLK12 are highly expressed in more than 10 tissues, with minor expression in at least four others.

Only 3 of the 15 kallikreins have been assigned a specific biological role. The major biological role of human kallikrein 1 (hK1) is the release of lysyl-bradykinin (kallidin) from low molecular weight kininogen; however, it has been implicated in the processing of peptide hormones, including proinsulin, low-density lipoprotein (LDL), prorenin, the precursor of atrial natriuretic peptide, and vasoactive intestinal peptide. The role of hK2 has only recently been investigated with seminal plasma hK2 found to cleave seminogel in I and II, but at different sites than hK3 (PSA). Furthermore, a role for hK2 in the regulation of growth factors through the proteolysis of insulin-like growth factor binding protein 3 (IGFBP-3) has been suggested. hK3, also known as PSA, is found not only in prostate tissue (discussed later), but in relatively high concentrations in nipple aspirate fluid, breast cyst fluid, breast milk, amniotic fluid, and tumor extracts. Its presence in these fluids and tissues suggests a biological function in the breast and a possible role in fetal development; however, no specific function in these tissues has been identified to date.

The role of kallikreins as tumor markers is rather varied. Several kallikreins have been associated with hormonal malignancies, such as (1) prostate, (2) breast, (3) testicular, and (4) ovarian cancers. hK6 has been investigated as a serum marker for the diagnosis, prognosis, and monitoring of ovarian cancer, and as a cytosolic marker for prognosis in breast cancer. Serum hK5, hK6, hKl0, and hKll have also been investigated for the diagnosis and monitoring of ovarian cancer, and a high concentration of cytosolic hKI0 in ovarian tumor and breast cells is a poor prognostic marker. Kallikrein gene expression is associated with both positive and negative prognoses in various cancers, including prostate, ovarian, and breast cancers.

Reverse-transcriptase polymerase chain reaction (RT-PCR), northern and western blotting, and immunoassays have been used for detection of kallikrein mRNA and protein in tissue extracts of (1) ovarian, (2) breast, (3) testicular, and (4) prostate tumors. Immunohisto-chemical techniques have been used for the detection of KLK7 in ovarian tumors and KLK10 in ovarian and testicular tumors. Serum concentrations of KLK3 (PSA) and KLKII are evaluated by immunoassay.

PROSTATE-SPECIFIC ANTIGEN

Prostate-specific antigen is found in normal, benign, hypertrophic, and malignant prostatic tissues. Originally, it was thought that PSA was solely expressed in prostate tissue. However, it was later found that PSA also is expressed in numerous other tissues, most notably hormonally regulated tissue, such as breast tissue. Low concentrations of PSA are detectable in sera from women as well as in nipple aspirate fluid.

PSA is a single-chain glycoprotein that is 7% carbohydrate. It has 237 amino acid residues and four carbohydrate sidechains with linkages at amino acid 45 (asparagine), 69 (serine), 70 (threonine), and 71 (serine). The N-terminal amino acid is isoleucine, and the C-terminal residue is proline. Its MW is 28,430 Da, and it has isoelectric points from 6.8–7.2 because of its various iso forms.

PSA is secreted into the lumina of the prostatic duct. In seminal fluid, PSA cleaves seminal vesicle-specific proteins into several low molecular weight proteins as part of the process of liquefaction of the seminal coagulum. Therefore, PSA possesses chymotrypsin-like and trypsin-like activity.

The metabolic clearance rate of PSA follows a two compartment model, with initial half-lives of 1.2 and 0.75 hours for free PSA and total PSA and subsequent half-lives of 22 and 33 hours. Because of this relatively long half-life, at least 2–3 weeks may be necessary for the serum PSA to return to base line concentrations after certain procedures, including transrectal biopsy, transurethral resection of the prostate, and radical prostatectomy. Benign prostatic conditions, such as benign prostatic hyperplasia (BPH) and prostatitis, can also elevate PSA concentrations.

PSA is an extremely useful tumor marker and is used to detect and monitor treatment of prostate cancer. PSA testing by itself is limited in the screening or detection of early prostate cancer because PSA is specific for prostatic tissue but not for prostatic cancer. BPH is a common disease in men 50 years of age and older.

The metabolic clearance rate of PSA follows a two compartment model, with initial half-lives of 1.2 and 0.75 hours for free PSA and total PSA and subsequent half-lives of 22 and 33 hours. Because of this relatively long half-life, at least 2–3 weeks may be necessary for the serum PSA to return to base line concentrations after certain procedures, including transrectal biopsy, transurethral resection of the prostate, and radical prostatectomy.

Benign prostatic conditions, such as BPH and prostatitis, can also elevate PSA concentrations. Although, the DRE typically causes no clinically important effects on serum PSA concentrations in most patients, in some it may lead to a twofold elevation. 5 α-reductase inhibitors, such as finasteride, for treatment of BPH cause a decrease in PSA concentrations of approximately 50%; thus results should be adjusted. Significant physiologic variation in serum PSA concentrations (up to 30%) has also been noted.

PSA is an extremely useful tumor marker and is used to detect and monitor treatment of prostate cancer.

PSA has been found to correlate with clinical stages of prostate cancer. For example, higher PSA concentrations and higher percentages of patients with elevated PSA concentrations are associated with advanced stages. PSA has also been found to correlate with pathologic stages of tumor extension and metastases, cancer volume, and cancer grade. Approximately, 80% of men with PSA concentrations <4 µg/L at diagnosis have organ-confined disease; this decreases to 70% and 50% for PSA concentrations of 4–10 µg/L and >10 µg/L, respectively. Because significant overlap occurs in PSA concentrations among stages, PSA cannot be used to determine the pathologic stage in a given individual. Therefore, PSA by itself should not be used to decide whether a patient has prostate cancer confined to the organ and therefore is a likely candidate for radical prostatectomy or other treatment, or active surveillance. The concentration of PSA can serve as a guide and is more useful in evaluating the presence of metastases. Patients with PSA concentrations less than 20 µg/L rarely have bone metastases.

The greatest clinical use for PSA is in the monitoring of definitive treatment of prostate cancer. This treatment includes radical prostatectomy, radiation therapy, and antiandrogen therapy. PSA is produced almost exclusively by prostatic tissue; thus after radical prostatectomy, the PSA concentration should fall below the detection limit of the assay. This may require 2–3 weeks owing to the half-life of PSA. If the half-life is longer than usual, it must be assumed that residual tumor is present, although detectable PSA may also reflect benign prostatic tissue. Biochemical recurrence has been defined as two postprostatectomy PSA concentrations 0.2 µg/L. A cut point of 0.4 µg/L is also used. Increasing PSA after radical prostatectomy is a strong indication of disease recurrence.

The time between PSA concentration elevation and clinical evidence of recurrence (metastases) averages 8 years. PSA doubling time is also useful in assessing risk of progression to metastasis with a low likelihood if the doubling time is greater than 10–15 months.

Unlike surgery, treatment with external beam radiation does not affect all tissues; therefore, PSA concentrations fall but do not become undetectable.

Hormone therapy includes (1) bilateral orchiectomy, (2) treatment with luteinizing hormone-releasing hormone agonists, and (3) antiandrogen therapy. PSA testing is useful for predicting prognosis and monitoring treatment response to this type of therapy in patients with metastatic prostate cancer. The concentration of PSA is inversely proportional to the survival time and increases with cancer progression, decreases in remission, and remains unchanged in stable disease. Androgen deprivation therapy may have a direct effect on PSA concentration that is independent of the antitumor effect. Production of PSA may be under the influence of androgenic hormones, such as dihydrotestosterone. Thus, PSA concentrations in patients who receive antiandrogen therapy may have a different meaning than they do in patients receiving other types of therapies.

Sandwich immunoassays are used to measure PSA and are commercially available. Most of them use non-isotopic labels, such as enzyme, fluorescence, or chemiluminescence. Most of these assays are automated on an immunoassay system. Different assays and even the same assay with different lots of reagent may produce different results. Such differences are due to changes in (1) assay calibration, (2) production lot variation, (3) assay reaction time, (4) reagent matrices, (5) assay limit of detection, and (6) imprecision.

Antibodies react with different PSA epitopes; therefore, some antibodies react dissimilarly with various molecular forms of PSA. Currently, most PSA assays are standardized to the Hybritech PSA method or to standards introduced by the World Health Organization (WHO) in 1999. The two international preparations consist of 100% free PSA and 90% prostate-specific antigen-antichymotrypsin (PSA-ACT) complex and 10% free PSA. Because of differences in the molar absorptivities used, PSA results from Hybritech standardized assays are approximately 20% higher than results from WHO standardized assays.

One of the most valuable applications of PSA is the detection of residual or recurrent disease following radical prostatectomy. Traditionally, 0.1 µg/L has been used as the lower limit of detection, which was based on assay analytical characteristics as well as clinical need. Ultrasensitive PSA assays can be defined as those with a functional sensitivity (20% CV) of 0.01 µg/L or lower. One PSA assay has been labeled as a third-generation assay, and many automated assays now achieve limits of detection close to 0.001 µg/L. Although, cancer recurrence may be detected earlier, the effect on clinical management is unclear, and no assay has a specific FDA claim for earlier detection of recurrence.

Free PSA is not typically used as a single measurement but is expressed as a ratio or percentage of total PSA.

Because of assay differences among manufacturers, total and free PSA should be measured in the same specimen using assays from the same diagnostics company. Percentage of free prostatic-specific antigen (fPSA) is approved by the United States Food and Drug Administration (FDA) as an aid in distinguishing prostate cancer from benign prostatic conditions in men aged 50 and older with a total PSA between 4 µg/L and 10 µg/L with a nonsuspicious digital rectal examination (DRE). The complexed PSA (cPSA) assay measures PSA-ACT and other minor PSA complexes by rendering free PSA nonreactive with a free PSA-specific antibody. The two FDA intended uses are the same as for total PSA: (1) as an aid in the detection of prostate cancer in men aged 50 years or older in conjunction with DRE, and (2) for serial measurements to aid in the management of prostate cancer patients. A cPSA concentration of 3.2 µg/L is equivalent to a PSA cutoff of 4.0 µg/L, and a PSA threshold of 2.5 µg/L corresponds to a cPSA concentration of 2.2 µg/L.

Human Glandular Kallikrein 2

Human kallikrein 2 (hK2) and PSA (human kallikrein 3) are serine proteases that share 80% identity in protein sequence and are almost exclusively found in prostatic epithelium.

Similar to PSA, hK2 concentrations are 100,000-fold higher in seminal fluid than in serum hK2 has the ability to form complexes with endogenous anti-proteases. One important inhibitor is the protein C inhibitor (PCI), which is the major ligand complexed to hK2 in seminal fluid, but in vitro, hK2 also forms complexes with α2 antiplasmin, α2 macroglobulin, ACT, anti-thrombin III, Cl-inactivator, and plasminogen activator inhibitor-l. Gel filtration studies have suggested that hK2 occurs mainly in a free, non-complexed form in serum, whereas only a minor proportion (5–20%) may be complexed with protease inhibitors. In vitro, recombinant hK2 activates pro PSA into mature, catalytic active form.

Immunohistochemical studies have demonstrated that tissue expression of hK2 shows intense staining in high-grade cancers and lymph node metastases, whereas it shows weaker alone or hK2* total PSA/free PSA has been shown to be a significantly better predictor of organ-confined disease than tPSA. In addition to the improvement in staging accuracy, hK2 discriminated aggressive, poorly differentiated prostate cancer from less aggressive, well-differentiated prostate cancer. Although serum hK2 is independently indicative of prostate cancer of unfavorable prognosis, a model combining total and free PSA and total hK2 had superior discrimination. Currently, two major hK2 immunoassays are available.

THE UROKINASE-PLASMINOGEN ACTIVATOR SYSTEM

The urokinase-plasminogen activator system consists of three main components: urokinase-plasminogen activator (uPA, a 53 kDa serine protease), the uPA membrane-bound receptor (uPAR), and the uPA inhibitors, plasminogen activator inhibitor (PAI)-1 and PAI-2.

The urokinase-plasminogen activator is produced as a single inactive polypeptide, which is activated by cleavage between lysine 158 and isoleucine. The cleavage is catalyzed by a number of proteases, including cathepsins B and L and hK2. The active form of uPA consists of an A chain, which interacts with its cell surface receptor, uPAR, and a catalytically active B chain. The most thoroughly characterized activity of uPA is the conversion of plasminogen to active plasmin, which degrades extracellular matrix (ECM) components and activates matrix metalloproteinases (MMPs), which further degrade the ECM and activate and release specific growth factors [fibroblast growth factor (FGF)2 and transforming growth factor (TGF)-P]. The activity of uPA is controlled in vivo by two inhibitor molecules: PAI-1 and PAI-2. PAI-1 and PAI-2 not only act to inhibit uPA but also have a number of other functions, including angiogenesis, cell adhesion and migration, and inhibition of apoptosis.

Urokinase-plasminogen activator has been used as a prognostic marker in breast cancer and a number of other cancers. The prognostic impact of uPA appears to be independent of other traditionally used markers, such as (1) axillary nodestatus, (2) tumor size, (3) tumor grade, and (4) estrogen receptor (ER) status. uPA is a more potent predictor of overall survival than tumor size, tumorgrade, or ER status, and is equally powerful as nodal status. Patients who benefit most from uPA measurement are those who are newly diagnosed with histologically negative local nodes. The long-term survival of this group is 70–80% with local therapy alone, and no further benefit is gained from adjuvant chemotherapy. uPA may be able to detect the small number of patients most at risk for recurrent disease and spare other cured patients from unnecessary chemotherapy.

American society of clinical oncology (ASCO) has recommended uPA/PAI, measured by enzyme-linked immunosorbent assay (ELISA) on 300 mg of breast cancer tissue, to determine prognosis in newly diagnosed node-negative patients; concentrations of both markers may aid in determining the benefit of chemotherapeutic treatment.

HORMONES

Hormones have been recognized as tumor markers for more than 50 years. The introduction of specific RIA methods for a particular hormone that has very little cross-reactivity with similar hormones made it possible to monitor the treatment of cancer patients. With the introduction and use of monoclonal antibodies, measurement of hormones is now accurate and precise. The production of hormones in cancer involves two separate routes. First, the endocrine tissue that normally produces it can produce excess amounts of a hormone. Second, a hormone may be produced at a distant site by a non-endocrine tissue that normally does not produce the hormone. The latter condition is called ectopic syndrome. For example, the production of adreno-corticotropic hormone (ACTH) is normotropic by the pituitary and is ectopic by the small cell of the lung. Consequently, elevation of a given hormone is not diagnostic of a specific tumor, because a hormone may be produced by a variety of cancers.

Multiple endocrine neoplasia (MEN) syndromes (MEN-1, MEN-2A, and MEN-2B) are familial disorders inherited in an autosomal dominant fashion that are manifested by both benign and malignant tumors. Various poly peptidehormones, such as (1) ACTH, (2) calcitonin, (3) gastrin, (4) glucagon, (5) insulin, (6) secretin, and (7) vasoactive intestinal polypeptide, may be produced by the pancreatic islet cell and pituitary tumors found in MEN-1 and by medullary thyroid cancer found in MEN-2A and -2B and in familial medullary thyroid cancer (FMTC), a variant of MEN- 2A. Examples of hormones that are used as tumor markers are listed in Table 17.2.

Adrenocorticotropic Hormone

Elevated plasma concentrations of ACTH could be the result of pituitary or ectopic production. A high concentration of ACTH (>200 ng/L) is suggestive of ectopic

origin. Failure of dexamethasone to suppress cortisol is also indicative of ectopic production. About half of the ectopic production of ACTH is a result of small cell carcinoma of the lung. Other conditions that elevate ACTH concentrations have been reported, including pancreatic, breast, gastric, and colon cancer, and benign conditions, such as chronic obstructive pulmonary disease, mental depression, obesity, hypertension, diabetes mellitus, and stress. The value of ACTH in the monitoring of therapy is still unknown.

Traditional RIA measures precursors pro-ACTH and pro-opiomelanocortin (POMC), as well as the intact molecule and ACTH fragments that may be beneficial for ectopic ACTH-producing tumors, whereas reactivity of the immunometric assay depends on the antibodies used and may measure ACTH as well as its precursors.

Calcitonin

Calcitonin is a polypeptide with 32 amino acids; it has an MW of about 3400 Da and is produced by C cells of the thyroid. Normally, calcitonin is secreted in response to increased serum calcium. It inhibits the release of calcium from bone and thus lowers the serum calcium concentration. The serum half-life is about 12 minutes. The concentration in healthy individuals is less than 0.1 µg/L. An elevated concentration is usually associated with medullary carcinoma of the thyroid. Approximately 75% of medullary thyroid carcinoma (MTC) cases are sporadic, and 25% are familial. Most familial MEN-2A, MEN-2B, and FMTC cases are the result of mutations of the RET proto-oncogene, a receptor tyrosine kinase, and almost all develop MTC.

Calcitonin is most useful for diagnosing sporadic MTC or for identifying the index case in familial MTC; genetic testing has supplanted calcitonin for screening family members of the index case. Calcitonin is used for monitoring MTC. Provocative testing with intravenous administration of calcium and/or pentagastrin produces increased calcitonin concentrations and is used to increase the sensitivity and specificity of MTC detection. Microscopic or occult malignancy has been detected in patients having a negative radioisotopic scan and normal thyroid glands on physical examination.

Calcitonin concentrations appear to correlate with indicators of the extent of disease, such as tumor volume and tumor involvement in local and distant metastases. Calcitonin is useful for monitoring treatment and detecting the recurrence of disease. Calcitonin concentrations are also elevated in some patients with carcinoid tumors and cancers of the lung, breast, kidney, and liver. The usefulness of calcitonin as a tumor marker in these malignancies has not been proven. Calcitonin elevation

Table 17.2	Hormones as tumor markers
Hormone	Type of cancer
ACTH	Cushing's syndrome, lung (small cell)
Antidiuretic hormone	Lung (small cell), adrenal cortex, pancreatic, duodenal
Bombesin	Lung (small cell)
Calcitonin	Medullary thyroid
Gastrin	Glucagonoma
Growth hormone	Pituitary adenoma, renal, lung
hCG	Embryonal, choriocarcinoma, testicular (non-seminoma)
Human placental lactogen	Trophoblastic, gonads, lung, breast
Neurophysins	Lung (small cell)
Parathyroid hormone	Liver, renal, breast, lung
Prolactin	Pituitary adenoma, renal, lung
Vasoactive intestinal peptide	Pancreas, bronchogenic, pheochromocytoma, neuroblastoma

has been reported in other nonmalignant conditions, such as (1) pulmonary disease, (2) pancreatitis, (3) hyperparathyroidism, (4) pernicious anemia, (5) Paget's disease of bone, and (6) pregnancy.

Human Chorionic Gonadotropin

Elevated human chorionic gonadotropin (hCG) concentrations are seen in pregnancy, trophoblastic disease, and germ cell tumor. It is a useful tumor marker for tumors of the placenta (trophoblastic tumors) and for some tumors of the testes. It is also useful for diagnosing and monitoring pregnancy.

Human chorionic gonadotropin is a glycoprotein secreted by the syncytiotrophoblastic cells of the normal placenta. hCG consists of two dissimilar α and β subunits. The β-subunit is common to several other hormones: luteinizing hormone (LH), follicle-stimulating hormone (FSH), and thyroid-stimulating hormone (TSH). The β-subunit is unique to hCG, and the 28–30 amino acids making up the carboxyl terminal are antigenically distinct. hCG has an MW of 45,000 Da. Additional serum forms, including hyper glycosylated (hCGh) and nicked hCG (hCGn) and the urine form hCG β core fragment (hCG–β cf) have relevant clinical usefulness. The upper reference limit in men and non-pregnant women is 5.0 IU/L. hCG assays with a detection limit <2 lU/L, crossreactivity with LH <2%, and equimolar recognition of hCG and hCG-β (or a separate assay for hCG-β) are desired for tumor marker use. Production of the two hCG-subunits is under separate genetic control. In early pregnancy, the free β-subunit is produced together with intact (a whole molecule of) hCG. In late pregnancy, the free a subunit predominates. Trophoblastic tumors of placental and germ cell origin primarily produce intact hCG, while differential production of the subunits, primarily the free β subunit, has been observed in non-trophoblastic cancer patients.

Patients with trophoblastic tumors typically have elevated concentrations of hCG (>1 million IU/L). It is also elevated in 70% of those with non-seminomatous testicular germ cell tumors, and less frequently in those with seminoma. Elevated serum concentrations of hCG are also found in 45–60% of (1) biliary and (2) pancreatic cancers and in 10–30% of many other cancers, including (3) bladder, (4) renal, (5) prostate, (6) liver, (7) colorectal, (8) non-small cell lung, (9) breast, and (10) head and (11) neck cancers, and (12) hematologic malignancies. Most neuroendocrine tumors produce hCG β, while carcinoid tumors produce hCG. Elevations have also been reported in benign conditions, such as cirrhosis, duodenal ulcer, and inflammatory bowel disease. hCG is useful in identifying patients with trophoblastic tumors and,

together with AFP, in detecting non-seminomatous testicular tumors. Concentrations of hCG correlate with tumor volume and disease prognosis. The hyper glycosylated form of hCG may aid in the early detection of new or recurrent active trophoblastic malignancy and may discriminate quiescent gestational trophoblastic disease from active gestational trophoblastic neoplasia/choriocarcinoma. Because hCG does not cross the blood-brain barrier, the normal cerebrospinal fluid-to-serum ratio is 1:60. Higher concentrations in cerebrospinal fluid may indicate metastases to the brain. Furthermore, the response to therapy for patients with central nervous system metastasis may be observed by monitoring the CSF hCG concentration.

hCG is most useful for monitoring treatment and progression of trophoblastic disease. Concentrations of hCG correlate with tumor volume. A patient with an initial hCG concentration greater than 400,000 lU/L is considered at high risk for treatment failure. After surgical removal of the tumor, hCG concentration is expected to decline. The normal half-life of serum hCG is about 12–20 hours. Slowly decreasing or persistent concentrations of hCG may indicate the presence of residual disease. During chemotherapy, weekly hCG measurement is recommended. After remission is achieved, yearly hCG measurement is recommended to detect relapse.

Most hCG assays use an immunometric ('sandwich') format. The hCG assay measures the intact (whole) molecule when an antibody for the α-subunit and an antibody for the β-subunit are used in the immunometric format. This type of assay does not measure free ex or β-subunits, because free subunits cannot form a sandwich with both antibodies. The total β-hCG assay measures both intact hCG and free β-subunits.

As a tumor marker, a total β-hCG assay is preferred, because many cancer patients produce notable amounts of free β-subunit. World Health Organization international reference reagents (IRRs) for hCG iso forms, including (1) intact hCG, (2) nicked hCG, (3) hCG-β, (4) nicked hCG-β, (5) hCG-β cf, and (6) hCG-α, have been developed, and studies with these preparations have indicated that varying specificity of these variants in commercial hCG assays contributes to methodologic differences. None of the commercially available hCG assays have been approved by the FDA for use as a tumor marker assay. Heterophile antibodies and anti-animal antibodies, such as human anti-mouse antibodies (HAMAs) can cause false-positive or -negative results in immunoassays, including those for hCG. Urine hCG testing, among other approaches, can help distinguish true positives from assay interference.

ONCOFETAL ANTIGENS

Oncofetal antigens are proteins produced during fetal life. These proteins are present in high concentration in the sera of fetuses and decrease to low concentration or disappear after birth. In cancer patients, these proteins often reappear, revealing that certain genes are reactivated as the result of the malignant transformation of cells. Oncofetal antigens that have been used as tumor markers are listed in Table 17.3.

α-Fetoprotein

α-fetoprotein (AFP) is a marker for hepatocellular and germ cell (non-seminoma) carcinoma. AFP is a glycoprotein with a molecular mass of 70 kDa. It consists of a single polypeptide chain and is 4% carbohydrate. AFP is synthesized in large quantities during embryonic development by the fetal yolk sac and liver. It is one of the major proteins in the fetal circulation, but its maximum concentration is about 10% that of albumin. AFP is closely related both genetically and structurally to albumin, having extensive homologies in amino acid sequence. The genes coding for both proteins have been localized to chromosome 4q. As albumin synthesis increases during later fetal development, AFP concentrations in fetal serum begin to decline. They finally reach the trace concentrations found in normal adults 18 months after birth.

For tumor-derived AFP, the composition of carbohydrate on AFP depends on the activity of saccharide transferase within tumor cells. Differences in carbohydrate side chains on AFP may be determined by the binding of AFP to lectins, such as concanavalin A (Con A) and lens culinaris agglutinin (LCA). Molecular variants of AFP can be separated into the liver type and the yolk sac type; they differ from each other in terms of their carbohydrate moiety. The yolk sac type of AFP contains an additional sugar, N-acetylglycosamine; this blocks the Con A binding site on the AFP. Therefore, the yolk sac type of AFP shows a high percentage (50–70%) of Con A nonreactive (CNR) fraction, whereas the liver type, which lacks this additional sugar, shows a low CNR fraction (10–20%). LCA binds to the fucosylated form of the first core N-acetyl glucose, which is present in both liver and yolk sac types of tumor-derived AFP, but not in AFP generated by benign liver disease.

The serum AFP concentration is less than 10 µg/L in healthy adults. During pregnancy, maternal AFP concentrations increase from 12 weeks gestation to a peak of about 500 µg/L during the third trimester. Fetal serum AFP reaches a peak of 2 g/L at 14 weeks and then declines to about 70 mg/L at term. In addition to pregnancy, elevated concentrations of serum AFP are associated with benign liver conditions, such as hepatitis and cirrhosis. Most patients with these benign diseases (95%) have AFP concentrations less than 200 µg/L. Except in the pregnant patient, AFP concentrations greater than 1000 µg/L are indicative of cancer. At these concentrations of AFP, about half of hepatocellular carcinomas may be detected. However, because the serum concentration of AFP correlates with the size of the tumor, detection of hepatocellular carcinoma is more useful at the earlier stages, when the tumor is small enough to be respectable <5 cm than when the tumor is large. To detect small tumors, the cutoff for AFP is typically set at a low concentration; a cutoff point of 10 to 20 µg/L has been recommended. However, at this concentration, hepatitis and cirrhosis must be considered as possible causes of elevation.

AFP is also useful for determining prognosis and for monitoring therapy for hepatocellular carcinoma. The concentration of AFP is a prognostic indicator of survival. Elevated AFP concentrations (>10 µg/L) and serum bilirubin concentrations greater than 2 mg/dL are associated with shorter survival time.

Total AFP can be separated into three glycoforms: AFP-L1, AFP-L2, and AFP-L3, based on reactivity to LCA. The L1 fraction of total AFP is present in patients with chronic hepatitis and liver cirrhosis, and it constitutes the majority of total AFP in non-malignant liver disease. AFP-L1 has low reactivity with LCA.

α-fetoprotein-L2 is mostly derived from yolk sac tumors and has an intermediate affinity to LCA. AFP-L3 is produced by cancer cells and has an additional (α-1-6-fucose residue attached at the reducing terminus of N-acetylglycosamine. AFP-L3% is calculated as the proportion of measured AFP-L3 to total AFP.

The AFP-L3% test is indicated for use in risk assessment for the development of hepatocellular carcinoma in patients who have chronic liver disease. A cutoff of 10%

Table 17.3	Oncofetal antigens as tumor markers
Name	**Type of cancer**
AFP	Hepatocellular, germ cell (non-seminoma)
Oncofetal	Colon antigen
Carcinofetal ferritin	Liver
CEA	Colorectal gastrointestinal, CHO pancreatic, lung, breast
Pancreatic	Pancreatic oncofetal
Squamous cell antigen	Cervical, lung, skin, head and neck (squamous)
Tennessee antigen	Colon, gastrointestinal, bladder
Tissue polypeptide	Various (breast, colorectal, ovarian, antigen bladder)

is used, and those patients with chronic liver disease and an elevated AFP-L3% have a sevenfold increased risk of developing hepatocellular carcinoma within 21 months. The test is useful for early detection, particularly in the AFP range of 20–200 µg/L, as has been shown in patients with hepatitis C-related cirrhosis, where hepatocellular incidence was higher in patients with elevated AFP-L3% compared with those with elevated AFP concentrations. AFP-L3% correlates with tumor staging and aggressiveness. Although, AFP-L3% is useful in detection and prognosis, it can be used only when AFP concentrations are elevated.

The AFP concentration is a good indicator for monitoring therapy and the change in clinical status. Elevated AFP concentrations after surgery may indicate incomplete removal of the tumor or the presence of metastasis. Falling or rising AFP concentrations after therapy may determine the success or failure of the treatment regimen. A notable increase in AFP concentrations in patients considered free of metastatic tumor may indicate the development of metastasis.

The combination of AFP and hCG is useful in classifying and staging germ cell tumors. Germ cell tumors may be predominantly one type of cell or may be a mixture of seminoma, yolk sac, choriocarcinomatous elements (embryonal carcinoma), and teratoma. Serum concentrations of AFP are elevated in yolk sac tumors, whereas hCG is elevated in choriocarcinoma. Both are elevated in embryonal carcinoma. In seminomas, AFP is not elevated, whereas hCG is elevated in 10–30% of patients who have syncytiotrophoblastic cells in the tumor. Neither marker is elevated in teratoma. One or Both of the markers are elevated in about 90% of patients with non-seminomatous testicular tumor. Elevations were noted in less than 20% of patients with stage–I disease, 50–80% with stage–II disease, and 90–100% with stage–III disease. These markers correlate with tumor volume and the prognosis of disease.

The combined use of these markers is useful in monitoring patients with germ cell tumors: elevation of either marker indicates recurrence of disease or development of metastasis.

The success of chemotherapy can be assessed by calculating the decrease in concentration of both markers using the half-lives of AFP (5 days) and hCG (12–20 hours).

Serum AFP is determined by immunometric assay on many automated immunoassay systems. AFP is reported using units of ng/mL (µg/L) primarily and kIU/L. One international unit (IV) of AFP is equivalent to 1.21 ng. A detection limit of 1 ng/mL is recommended for clinical use. AFP-L3% is measured using a liquid-phase binding method that incorporates LCA binding and anion-conjugated antibodies separated by anion-exchange chromatography and detected fluorometrically. AFP-L3% is calculated from the concentration of AFP-L3 fraction and the sum of the two fractions that constitute total AFP.

CARCINOEMBRYONIC ANTIGEN

Carcinoembryonic antigen (CEA) is a marker for colorectal, gastrointestinal, lung, and breast carcinoma. CEA is a glycoprotein with a molecular mass of 150–300 kDa; it contains 45–55% carbohydrate. It is a single polypeptide chain consisting of 641 amino acids, with lysine in the N-terminal position. The heterogeneity of CEA can be demonstrated by using isoelectric focusing to separate the variants.

CEA consists of a large family of related cell surface glycoproteins. CEA proteins are encoded by about 10 genes located on chromosome. Up to 36 different glycoproteins have been identified in the CEA family. The major proteins are CEA and nonspecific cross-reacting antigen (NCA). The domain structures of CEA, NCA 50, and the heavy chain of immunoglobulin (Ig)G are very similar. Thus, CEA is part of the immunoglobulin gene 'superfamily'.

The CEA concentration is elevated in a variety of cancers, such as colorectal (70%), lung (45%), gastric (50%), breast (40%), pancreatic (55%), ovarian (25%), and uterine (40%) carcinomas. Because of the elevations associated with benign disease (i.e. false-positive results) and the number of tumors that do not produce CEA (i.e. false-negative results), CEA testing should not be used for screening. CEA testing may be useful as an adjunct to clinical staging. Persistently elevated concentrations that are 5–10 times the upper reference limit strongly suggest the presence of colon cancer but may be associated with other cancers. In colon cancer, CEA concentrations correlate with the stage of disease. CEA concentrations are elevated in 28% of patients with stage A colorectal cancer and in 45% of those with stage B.

The pretreatment CEA concentration is prognostic of the development of metastasis. A high concentration of CEA is associated with a greater likelihood of developing metastasis. Evidence suggests that CEA is a cellular adhesion molecule that may potentiate invasion and metastasis.

After successful initial therapy, CEA concentrations decline. During remission, CEA concentrations are stable. Rising CEA concentrations may indicate recurrence of disease. The lead time from CEA elevation to clinical recurrence is about 5 months. A repeat laparotomy can be performed to confirm the relapse, which is detected in 90% of cases. In the monitoring of metastatic colon cancer, CEA is useful in following patients throughout therapy and the clinical course of the disease.

CEA is also useful in monitoring breast, lung, gastric, and pancreatic carcinomas. In breast cancer, elevated CEA is associated with metastatic disease. Early or localized breast cancer does not show CEA elevation and is less sensitive than cancer antigen (CA) 15-3 and CA 27.29. CEA is most useful in monitoring metastatic breast cancer during therapy and in detecting the development of bone or lung metastasis. An increasing serum CEA concentration may reflect treatment failure when measurable disease is not present in lung cancer, CEA determination is helpful in diagnosing non-small cell lung carcinoma (>65% of patients have elevated CEA) and in monitoring lung cancer.

As with AFP, most assays use the immunometric format for determination of serum CEA. Polyclonal and monoclonal antibodies and combinations of the two types have been used in CEA immunoassays. In the healthy population, the upper limit of CEA is about 3 µg/L for nonsmokers and 5 µg/L for smokers. Because the concentration of CEA measured is method dependent, values should always be compared using the same method. When methods are changed, all patients who are being monitored should be tested in parallel using both old and new methods. CEA concentration is elevated in some patients with benign conditions, such as cirrhosis (45%), pulmonary emphysema (30%), rectal polyps (5%), benign breast disease (15%), and ulcerative colitis (15%).

CARBOHYDRATE MARKERS

Carbohydrate-related tumor markers may be (1) antigens on the tumor cell surface, or (2) secreted by the tumor cells. Monoclonal antibodies against these antigens have been developed. These markers have been found to be clinically useful as tumor markers and tend to be more specific than naturally secreted markers, such as enzymes and hormones. Biochemically, they are high molecular weight mucins (Table 17.4) or blood group antigens (Table 17.5).

Table 17.4	Mucin tumor markers
Name	Type of cancer
CA 125	Ovarian, endometrial
Episialin	
• CA 15-3	Breast, ovarian
• CA 549	Breast, ovarian
• CA 27.29	Breast
MCA	Breast, ovarian
DU-PAN-2	Pancreatic, ovarian, gastrointestinal, lung

Table 17.5	Blood group antigen-related cancer markers
Name	Type of cancer
CA 19-9	Pancreatic, gastrointestinal, hepatic
CA 19-5	Pancreatic, gastrointestinal, pancreatic, ovarian
CA 50	gastrointestinal, colon
CA 72-4	Ovarian, breast, gastrointestinal, colon
CA 242	Gastrointestinal, pancreatic

CA 15-3, CA 549, and CA 27.29 assays detect a high molecular weight glycoprotein mucin expressed by the mammary epithelium known as episialin, and thus are used as markers for breast carcinoma. Circulating episialin antigen is a heterogeneous molecule. CA 15-3, CA 549, and CA 27.29 assays detect similar yet different epitopes on the episialin.

CA 15-3

CA 15-3 is a marker for breast carcinoma. It is detected by a murine monoclonal antibody (MAb) DF3 produced against a membrane-enriched extract of a human breast cancer metastatic to liver. Another monoclonal antibody, 115D8, was developed against the human milk fat globule membrane. Circulating DF3-reactive antigen is a heterogeneous molecule with a molecular mass of 300 to 450 kDa. The gene for this molecule is located on chromosome 1q. cDNA cloning indicates that the DF3 peptide coreconsists of a highly conserved 60-bp tandem repeat sequence. The polymorphism of the antigen is the result of different numbers of repeats in the peptide core. The DF3 antibody recognizes the epitope within this 20 amino acid repeating sequence of the peptide core.

CA 15-3 should not be used to diagnose primary breast cancer because the incidence of elevation (23%) is fairly low. CA 15-3 is most useful in monitoring therapy and disease progression in metastatic breast cancer patients. In healthy subjects, the upper limit of CA 15-3 concentrations is 25 kU/L.

Two antibodies are used in CA 15-3 immunoassays. The MAb 115D8 is attached to a solid support, whereas MAb DF3 is labeled. Assays using alternative antibodies against the same common antigen are also available for clinical use.

CA 549

CA 549 is a marker for breast carcinoma. It is an acidic glycoprotein with an isoelectric point of pH 5.2. By sodium dodecyl sulfate/polyacrylamide gel electrophoresis under reducing conditions, CA 549 can be separated into two species with molecular masses of 400 and 512 kDa. In a population of healthy women, 95% of the population has CA 549 concentrations below 11 kU/L. Pregnancy and benign breast disease show minimum elevation.

Similar to CA 15-3, CA 549 is not useful in detecting early breast carcinoma, because the proportion of patients with elevated CA 549 concentrations is low. Using ROC analysis,

CA 549 is better than CEA in identifying active breast cancer. CA 549 is useful in detecting recurrence of breast cancer in patients after initial therapy followed by adjuvant therapy.

Increasing CA 549 concentration after an initial decrease or stabilization indicates the development of metastases. In the monitoring of advanced breast cancer patients, CA 549 correlates with disease progression and regression and helps detect metastases.

CA 27.29

CA 27.29 is a marker for breast carcinoma. It is recognized by a monoclonal antibody, B27.29, which is produced against an antigen in ascites of patients with metastatic breast carcinoma. The minimum epitope to which B27.29 reacts is the 8 amino acid sequence (SAPDTRPA) within the 20 amino acid tandem repeating sequence of the mucin core. The reactive sequence of the B27.29 overlaps with the sequence of DF3 used in the CA 15-3 assay. In inhibition studies using labeled MAb, B27.29 effectively competes with DF3 for binding to both CA 27.29 and CA 15-3 antigens.

CA 27.29 has been approved by the FDA for clinical use in the detection of recurrent breast cancer in patients with stage–II or stage–III disease and for monitoring response to therapy in patients with stage IV (metastatic) disease. CA 27.29 performance appeared to be better than that of CA 15-3 in detecting patients with recurrent breast cancer.

The CA 27.29 immunoassay has both competitive and sandwich formats that incorporate the B27.29 monoclonal antibody. Assays utilizing alternative antibodies against the same common antigen are also available for clinical use.

Mucin-like Carcinoma-associated Antigen

Mucin-like carcinoma-associated antigen (MCA) is a marker for breast carcinoma, it was identified on the surface of a breast carcinoma cell line by the monoclonal antibody b-12. MCA is a glycoprotein with a molecular mass of 350 kDa. Epitopes on this moleculeare also recognized by DF3 and 115D8 antibodies of the CA15-3 assay.

Mucin-like carcinoma-associated antigen concentrations increase throughout pregnancy. In contrast, CA 15-3 increases only slightly during pregnancy. MCA concentration is elevated in 60% of metastatic breast cancer patients. However, elevated concentrations are also found in (1) ovarian, (2) cervical, (3) endometrial, and (4) prostate carcinoma.

Minimum elevation is observed in benign breast disease. MCA concentrations correlate with CA 15-3 concentrations but not with CEA concentrations. In monitoring metastatic breast cancer patients, changes in MCA concentrations parallel changes in CA 15-3 concentrations.

CA 125

CA 125 is a marker for monitoring ovarian cancer. It is a high molecular mass (greater than 200 kDa) glycoprotein recognized by the monoclonal antibody OC 125. It contains 24% carbohydrate and is expressed by epithelial ovarian tumors and other pathologic and normal tissues of mllerian duct origin.

The primary FDA-indicated use for CA 125 is to monitor response to therapy in patients with epithelial ovarian cancer. The second FDA-indicated use is to detect residual or recurrent disease in patients who have undergone first-line therapy and would be considered for second-look procedures. However, second-look laparotomy is now considered controversial except for use in clinical trials, or when surgical findings would alter disease management. In a healthy population, the upper limit of CA 125 is 35 kU/L. CA 125 is elevated in non-ovarian carcinoma, including endometrial, pancreatic, lung, breast, and colorectal and other gastrointestinal tumors. CA 125 is useful for determining the prognosis of endometrial carcinoma. It is also elevated in women in the follicular phase of the menstrual cycle and with benign conditions, such as cirrhosis, hepatitis, endometriosis, pericarditis, and early pregnancy. It cannot be used to differentiate ovarian cancer from other malignancies. CA 125 is not useful in screening for ovarian cancer in asymptomatic populations, but screening is recommended in at-risk women with a family history of hereditary ovarian cancer, in conjunction with pelvic examination and ultrasound testing. Strategies to improve the clinical usefulness of CA 125 for screening/early detection of ovarian cancer to achieve needed high sensitivity and very high specificity include combining with transvaginal sonography, assessing changes in concentrations measured over time, and using multi-marker panels.

In ovarian carcinoma, CA 125 is elevated in 50% of patients with stage–I disease, 90% with stage–II, and more than 90% with stages–III and IV. The concentration of CA 125 correlates with tumor size and staging. CA 125 is also useful in differentiating benign from malignant disease in patients with palpable ovarian masses. This differentiation is important because surgical intervention for malignant ovarian masses is far more extensive than that for benign masses. Preoperative CA 125 concentration less than 65 kU/L is associated with a significantly greater 5-year survival rate (42%) when compared with a concentration greater than 65 kU/L (5%). Postoperative CA 125 concentrations and rate of decline are also predictors of survival. The half-life of CA 125 is normally 4.8 days.

CA 125 is useful for detecting residual disease in cancer patients following initial therapy. The sensitivity of CA 125 for detecting tumors before repeat laparotomy is 50%, and the specificity is 96%. After chemotherapy, CA 125 concentrations provides an indication of disease prognosis. A decrease in the CA 125 concentration by a factor of 10 after the first cycle of chemotherapy is indicative of response. Persistent elevation of CA 125 concentrations after three cycles of chemotherapy indicates a poor prognosis. In the detection of recurrent metastasis, use of CA 125 concentration as an indicator is about 75% accurate. The lead time from CA 125 elevation to clinically detectable recurrence is about 3–4 months. CA 125 correlates with disease progression or regression in 80–90% of cases.

An immunoradiometric assay for CA 125 which incorporated the OC 125 antibody for both capture and detection, allowing recognition of multiple CA 125 determinants were first developed. A second-generation assay (CA 125II) typically uses the monoclonal antibody, M11, as the capture antibody and OC 125 as the conjugate antibody. Other FDA-cleared assays for CA 125, which employ antibodies other than the OC 125 and M11 antibodies, are available on automated immunoassay platforms. Results from different assays are not interchangeable, and individual patients should be monitored with a single assay.

Human Epididymis Protein 4

Human epididymis protein 4 (HE4) is a marker for ovarian cancer. The gene for HE4, *Homo sapiens* epididymis specific, WFDC2, was initially discovered using microarrays to be over expressed in epididymal tissue and later in ovarian cancer tissue. Tumor expression is histologic dependent with most serious and endometrioid tumors expressing HE4 and only 50% of clear cell and 0% of mucinous tumors. The protein is characterized as part of the four-disulfide core protein family and contains whey acid protein domains (WAPs). These proteins typically are secreted and are protease inhibitors, although this function has not been ascribed to HE4, and its physiologic role is unknown. Subsequent studies have shown that HE4 is not specific for ovarian tumors. Generation of the monoclonal antibodies 2H5 and 3D8 to epitopes on HE4 has allowed development of a sandwich ELISA and measurement in serum.

At an HE4 concentration of 150 pM, 95% of healthy women were below this cutoff, while 79% of women with ovarian cancer were above this cutoff. Elevations in other subjects include breast (13%), endometrial (26%), gastrointestinal (16%), and lung cancers (42%), as well as benign gynecologic disease (7%) and other benign disease (24%). The assay is FDA cleared for monitoring recurrence or progressive disease in patients with epithelial ovarian cancer. In serial samples from 80 ovarian cancer patients in which a 25% increase in HE4 concentration was used to define a positive change, 60% of patients with disease progression had an increase greater than 25%, and 75% had a change of 25% or less or did not have disease progression. Results comparing HE4 and CA 125 to distinguish women with ovarian cancer from normal women or those with benign processes appear to depend on the population studied, although combining the two markers may allow more accurate prediction of cancer than use of the individual markers. An algorithm incorporating HE4 and CA 125 has been reported to successfully classify women with a pelvic mass as at high or low risk for epithelial ovarian cancer.

HE4 is measured by an enzyme immunoassay, with 2H5 as the capture antibody and 3D8 as the detector antibody. This assay is not recommended for patients with mucinous or germ cell ovarian cancer.

Duke pancreatic monoclonal antigen type 2

Duke pancreatic monoclonal antigen type 2 (DU-PAN-2) is a marker for pancreatic cancer. The epitope recognized by the antibody DU-PAN-2 is a mucin. Its molecular mass is between 100 and 500 kDa, and it is 80% carbohydrate. The core protein (eDNA) has been cloned and sequenced, and the predicted amino acid sequence reveals a protein of 126 kDa containing 1295 amino acid residues with 42 tandem repeats. DU-PAN-2 antigen is found mainly in the (1) glandular epithelia of the pancreatic and biliary systems and in the (2) breast and (3) bronchial ducts. Less expression is found in cells of the (4) salivary glands, (5) stomach, (6) colon, and (7) intestine.

Serum DU-PAN-2 concentrations are elevated in patients with pancreatic (54–61%), biliary tract (44–47%), and hepatocellular (44%) carcinomas. Comparative studies between DU-PAN-2 and CA 19-9 concentrations in pancreatic cancer show similar elevations in 70–80% of patients. DU-PAN-2 and CA 19-9 concentrations correlate well, except in patients who are Lea-b and therefore do not express.

CA 19-9

CA 19-9 is a marker for gastrointestinal cancers and is used primarily to test for pancreatic carcinoma. It has been approved by the FDA for quantitative measurement in serum and as an aid in monitoring pancreatic cancer patients.

This carbohydrate antigen is a glycolipid, specifically, sialylated lacto-N-fucopenteose II ganglioside, that is a sialylated derivative of the Le^a blood group antigen and is denoted as Le^{xa}. Expression of the antigen requires the Lewis gene product, 1,4-fucosyl transferase. CA 19-9 is synthesized by normal human pancreatic and biliary ductular cells and by gastric, colon, endometrial, and salivary epithelia. In serum, it exists as a mucin—a high molecular mass (200–1000 kDa) glycoprotein complex. Patients who are genotypically Le^{a-b} (about 5%) do not express CA 19-9. The monoclonal antibody against CA 19-9 was developed from a human colon carcinoma cell line, SW-1116.

The CA 19-9 upper reference limit is 37 kU/L, as determined from the 99th percentile of normal subjects. This cutoff discriminates between pancreatic cancer and benign pancreatic disease with clinical sensitivities of 69 to 93% and clinical specificities of 76–99%. Elevated CA 19-9 concentrations (>37 kU/L) are found in patients with pancreatic (80%), hepatobiliary (67%), gastric (40–50%), hepatocellular (30–50%), colorectal (30%), and breast (15%) cancers. Some patients (10–20%) with pancreatitis and other benign gastrointestinal diseases have elevated concentrations up to 120 kU/L. CA 19-9 is useful in monitoring pancreatic and colorectal and gastric cancers.

CA 19-9 concentrations correlate with pancreatic cancer staging. With a cutoff of 37 kU/L, 67% of patients with resectable and 87% of those with unresectable pancreatic cancers have elevated concentrations.

When the cutoff is raised to 1000 kU/L, 35% of patients with unresectable tumors and only 5% of those with resectable tumors have elevated CA 19-9 concentrations. CA 19-9 is also useful for establishing prognosis for pancreatic cancer at initial diagnosis, as concentrations have independent predictive value for determination of respectability and of overall survival. Elevated or increasing concentrations can indicate recurrence 1–7 months before it is detected by radiographs or clinical findings. Unfortunately, early detection of relapse may not be useful because effective therapy for pancreatic cancer is not available.

Several companies have produced CA 19-9 immunoassays. Considerable differences among assays are noted, and assay results are not interchangeable for individual patients. Typically, the CA 19-9 antibody is used as both the capture and the signal antibody.

CA 50

CA 50 is a marker for pancreatic and colorectal carcinoma. It is a monoclonal antibody developed against the human colon adenocarcinoma cell line COLO 205. The CA 50

antibody recognizes an epitope on two carbohydrate moieties: sialosylfucosyllactotetraose (sialylated Le^a) and sialosyllactotetraose (sialylated Le^a lacking fucose). This antigen exists as a glycoprotein in serum and also as gangliosides in tissue. Sialylated Le^a is the predominant form of CA 50 in epithelial carcinoma and is recognized by CA 19-9.

Elevated CA 50 concentrations have been reported in benign diseases of the pancreas (12–46%), biliary tract (35–38%), and liver (22–59%). In pancreatic cancer, 80–97% of patients have elevated concentrations. In colon cancer, elevated concentrations were reported in various stages. In digestive tract carcinoma, elevated concentrations were seen in esophageal (41–71%), gastric (41–78%), biliary (58–70%), and hepatocellular (14–78%) cancers. Other malignancies were reported to have lower percentages of elevation, including breast, lung, renal, prostate, bladder, and ovarian cancers. Similar performances and good correlations were reported between CA 50 and CA 19-9 concentrations.

The original inhibition test has been replaced by an immunoradiometric assay and a time-resolved fluorescent immunoassay. The upper reference interval for healthy subjects varies from 14–20 kU/L, depending on the method.

CA 72-4

CA 72-4 is a marker for carcinomas of the gastrointestinal tract and of the ovary. The 72-4 assay utilizes the monoclonal antibody B72.3 developed from the membrane-enriched fraction of breast carcinoma in a patient with liver metastasis. The B72.3 reactive antigen was purified and called TAG-72 (tumor-associated glycoprotein). Further purification of TAG-72 from LS-174T human colon carcinoma xenograft produced a new generation of monoclonal antibodies with higher affinity. These antibodies, denoted 'cc' for 'colon carcinoma'.

A cutoff of 6 kU/L is used in the CA 72-4 assay. A poor clinical correlation between CEA and CA 72-4 concentrations was found in gastric cancer. CEA and CA 72-4 concentrations may be complementary. The plasma clearance of TAG-72 was studied by measuring serial TAG-72 concentrations in patients with primary carcinoma of the breast and with gastric, colorectal, and ovarian cancers. After removal of the tumor, the average time required for the concentration to decrease to 4 kU/L was 23.3 days. This suggests that TAG-72 may be useful in detecting residual tumor in these cancer patients.

CA 72-4 is measured using an immunoradiometric assay (IRMA), it uses two monoclonal antibodies B72.3 is the conjugate, whereas cc49 is the capture antibody. An automated eletrochemiluminescence method is also available.

CA 242

CA 242 is a marker for pancreatic and colorectal cancer. It is a monoclonal antibody developed from a human colorectal carcinoma cell line, COLO 205. The antigenic determinant is a sialylated carbohydrate. CA 242 recognizes the epitopes of CA 50 and CA 19-9. CA 242 is found in the apical border of ductal cells of the human pancreas and in epithelial and goblet cells of the colonic mucosa.

At a concentration of 20 U/L, elevated CA 242 concentrations were found in 5–33% of patients with benign colon, gastric, patients with malignant pancreatic cancer; in 55–85% of patients with colorectal cancer; and in 44% of patients with gastric cancer. The correlation coefficients (R2) of CA 242, CA 50, and CA 19-9 concentrations in patients with colorectal, liver, pancreatic, and biliary tract disease ranged from 0.81–0.95. CA 242 and CEA appeared to have higher percentages of elevation in colorectal cancer than did CA 50 and CA 19-9. CA 242 seems to be less efficient than CA 19-9 or CA 50 in the detection of pancreatic cancer; however, this may depend on the cutoff.

An immunometric assay which is uses the C241 antibody against sialylated Lewis as the capture antibody and the CA 242 antibody as the conjugate. The upper reference limit is 29 U/mL.

PROTEINS

Several proteins having tumor marker potential are listed in Table 17.6. Included in this group of tumor markers are proteins that are not enzymes or hormones, and are not high in carbohydrate content. Additional research is required to assess the clinical usefulness of most of these markers.

Immunoglobulin

Monoclonal immunoglobulin has been used as a marker for multiple myeloma, monoclonal paraproteins appear as sharp bands in the globulin region of serum electrophoretic patterns. More than 95% of patients with multiple myeloma have such an electrophoretic pattern. Appearance of nonmalignant monoclonal immunoglobulins increases with age, reaching 5% in patients older than 75 years. These nonmalignant monoclonal bands are usually lower in concentration than malignant bands and are not associated with Bence Jones protein. Bence Jones protein is a free monoclonal immunoglobulin light chain in the urine. The concentration of monoclonal immunoglobulin at initial diagnosis is a prognostic indicator of disease progression. During treatment, the serum concentration of urinary Bence Jones protein may reflect the success of therapy. Lower concentrations are associated with more favorable outcomes.

BLADDER CANCER MARKERS

The most common type of cell seen is transitional cell carcinoma (TCC), and the most frequent symptom is hematuria. Bladder cancer is staged pathologically and is treated on the basis of the extent of tumor invasion. Carcinoma in situ (stage–Tis) and superficial bladder cancers (stages–Ta and T1) occur on the epithelial lining and do not invade the muscle layer. Stage Ta tumors are confined to the mucosa, and stage–T1 tumors superficially invade the lamina propria. Stage–T2 tumors extend into the muscle layer, and T3 tumors invade beyond the muscle layer. Stage–T4 tumors have metastasized to local nodes or distant organs.

Urinary Bladder Tumor Markers

Bladder cancer is detected through cystoscopy or cytology of shed cells, or by non-cellular markers, such

Table 17.6 Proteins as tumor markers	
Name	**Type of cancer**
β 2-microglobulin	Multiple myeloma, B-cell lymphoma, chronic lymphocytic leukemia, Waldenstrom's smacroglobulinemia
C-peptide	Insulinoma
Ferritin	Liver, lung, breast, leukemia
HER-2/neu	Breast
Immunoglobulin	Multiple myeloma, lymphomas
Melanoma-associated antigen	Melanoma
Pancreas-associated antigen	Pancreatic, stomach
Pregnancy-specific protein 1	Trophoblastic, germ cell
Pro-gastrin releasing peptide	Small cell lung
Prothrombin precursor	Hepatocellular
Soluble mesothelin-related peptides	Mesothelioma, ovarian
Tumor-associated trypsin inhibitor	Lung, gastrointestinal, ovarian

as NMP22, complement factor-H (CFH), and fibronectin. Tumor antigens present in urine are the easiest to analyze; however, they cannot be used as the sole mechanism for tumor detection.

They should be used in a complementary manner with cystoscopy and cytology. Two bladder cancer-related tests that are fluorescence based have been cleared by the FDA. (1) Immunocyt uses three fluorescently labeled monoclonal antibodies and microscopy to identify bladder cancer markers on cells found in urine. This test appears most useful with cytology in identifying low-grade tumors. (2) Uro Vysion as a fluorescence in situ hybridization (FISH) technique, uses fluorescently labeled probes to detect aneuploidy of chromosomes 3, 7, and 17, and deletion of the 9p21 locus that contains the tumor suppressor p16, which is the most common alteration seen in urothelial carcinoma.

Bladder Tumor-associated Analytes

A qualitative, lateral flow immunoassay for bladder tumor-associated (BTA) analytes in urine, termed the BTA stat test, has been developed. The antigen detected in the BTA stat assay is human complement factor H-related protein (hCFHrp), which is a variant of human complement factor H (hCFH). hCFH functions in the alternative complement pathway by interacting with complement factor C3b to prevent cell lysis. Bladder tumor associated antigen may allow tumor cells to evade the host immune system.

Soluble Mesothelin-related Peptides

Mesothelioma is a rare cancer of the mesothelial surfaces of the pleural and peritoneal cavities or the pericardium that is linked to asbestos exposure. Mesothelin is a cell surface glycoprotein expressed on mesothelial cells, and mesothelin fragments, which are soluble mesothelin-related peptides (SMRPs), can be found in the circulation of patients with mesothelial tumor. An ELISA assay has been developed that measures serum soluble molecules related to the mesothelin/megakaryocyte potentiating factor (MPF) family of proteins recognized by the monoclonal antibody OV569. The assay also incorporates the 4H3 monoclonal antibody. It is intended as an aid in monitoring patients who have been diagnosed with epithelioid mesothelioma. A cutoff of 2.5 nmol/L was derived from the 99th percentile of healthy subjects. In addition to patients with mesothelioma (52%), approximately 10–15% of patients with other cancers, including ovarian, lung, colon, and pancreas cancers, may have elevations in SMRp29 compared with 5% of individuals exposed to asbestos. SMRP increases with increasing stage of malignant pleural mesothelioma. SMRPs have also been reported to be higher in malignant pleural mesothelioma pleural effusions compared with benign or other nonmalignant pleural mesothelioma pleural effusions.

Thyroglobulin and Antibodies

Thyroglobulin (Tg) is produced by the thyroid gland as the precursor to thyroid hormone. The main use of Tg measurement is as a tumor marker for patients with a diagnosis of differentiated thyroid cancer. Approximately two-thirds of these patients have an elevated preoperative Tg concentration. An elevated preoperative concentration of Tg confirms the tumor's ability to secrete Tg and validates the use of postoperative measurement of Tg to monitor for tumor recurrence. Postoperatively, the most sensitive time to detect residual tumor or metastasis is after TSH stimulation. In well-differentiated tumors, a tenfold increase in Tg concentrations is seen after TSH stimulation. Poorly differentiated tumors that do not concentrate iodide may display a blunted response to TSH stimulation. Tg monitoring generally is not useful in patients who do not have elevated preoperative Tg. Anti-thyroglobulin antibodies have been proposed to monitor residual disease and/or recurrence. Serial anti-Tg measurements may be an independent prognostic indicator of therapy, because an increase in anti-Tg antibodies may suggest recurrence of the tumor.

Immunometric assays (IMAs) and RIAs are the two main methods used for the measurement of Tg. IMA assays have the advantage of having a shorter incubation time and are automatable; however, they suffer from greater interferences. The main interferons in both assays are anti-thyroglobulin antibodies, which typically cause an underestimation of Tg concentrations in the IMA. Anti-thyroglobulin antibodies can be measured directly in all patients; if both IMA and RIA are used to measure Tg, a discordant result suggests the presence of anti-thyroglobulin antibodies.

RECEPTORS AND OTHER MARKERS
Estrogen and Progesterone Receptors

Estrogen and progesterone receptors are used in breast cancer as indicators for hormonal therapy. Patients with positive estrogen and progesterone receptors tend to respond to hormonal treatment. Those with negative receptors will be treated using other therapies, such as chemotherapy. Hormone receptors also serve as prognostic factors in breast cancer. Patients positive for hormone receptors tend to survive longer.

Estrogen receptors (ERs) and progesterone receptors (PRs) are members of the nuclear steroid hormone receptor family, and are involved in hormone-directed transcriptional activation. The general structure of nuclear steroid hormone receptors, including ERs and PRs, consists of a large N-terminal domain containing transcriptional activation domains, a DNA-binding domain, a hinge region, and the hormone binding domain at the C-terminus. Both ERs and PRs are present in a large protein complex, and upon hormone binding, some members of the complex dissociate, and the receptors bind to their respective response elements and activate transcription.

Estrogen and progesterone each have at least two separate receptors. Estrogen has ERα and ERβ, which are transcribed from separate genes. ERα and ERβ show 96% and 58% homology in their DNA- and hormone-binding domains, respectively, with a more divergent sequence in the N-terminal region. Two forms of PR-PR-A and PR-B also exist, and both are transcribed from the same gene. PR-A lacks the first 165 amino acids of PR-B. ERs and PRs are found in target tissue cells, such as the uterus, pituitary gland, hypothalamus, and breast, and appear to be involved in tumor development and progression. Furthermore, ER status and PR status correlate with both prognosis and treatment response; therefore, ER and PR measurement is clinically useful.

Measurement of ER content in breast tumor tissue is useful primarily in determining the probability of hormonal therapy and also as a prognostic indicator. ERs and PRs are routinely measured in all newly diagnosed breast cancers.

The routinely used ELISA method for quantitation of ER predominantly detects ERα. The fact that ERβ seems to attenuate ERα signaling, coupled with the fact that there is an inverse relationship between ERβ and PR and ERα proteins, suggests a possible mechanism for ER-positive tumors that do not respond to hormonal treatment.

The PR assay is a useful adjunct to the assay of ERs. Because PR synthesis appears to be dependent on estrogen action, measurement of PR activity provides confirmation that all steps of estrogen action are intact. Indeed, metastatic breast cancer patients with both ER- and PR-positive tumors have a response rate of 75% to endocrine therapy, where as those with ER-positive and PR-negative tumors have a 40% response rate. In addition, only 25% of ER-negative/PR-positive patients respond to endocrine therapy, whereas less than 5% of ER-negative/PR-negative patients respond. The percentage of positive specimens is greater in postmenopausal women than in those who are premenopausal.

Immunohistochemistry assay is used to measure steroid hormone receptors in breast tumor tissue specimens. The classical quantitative biochemical method, the multiplepointdextran-coated (DCC) titration assay, and enzyme immunoassays are obsolete. Immunohistochemical assays are simple and less expensive and can use small amounts of tissue from frozen tissue sections, paraffin-embedded tissue, fine-needle aspirates, and malignant effusions. However, assay interpretations can be subjective, and use of different antibodies can yield different results.

The primary monoclonal antibody is incubated with a thin section of tissue mounted on a microscope slide. Localization and visualization of receptor material are subsequently accomplished by an indirect immuno-peroxidase technique. Semiquantitative scoring is based on the percentage of cells with nuclear staining and may include the intensity of staining.

Specimens with staining in at least 20% of malignant cells are usually considered to have a favorable response, with 10–19% borderline, and <10% unfavorable. Immunohistochemistry is not influenced by the presence of estrogens, anti-estrogens, or steroid-binding proteins and can evaluate receptor content specific to malignant cells and not in other nonmalignant breast tissue.

Androgen Receptors

Androgens, namely, testosterone and dihydrotestosterone (DHT), are involved in growth and maintenance of the prostate gland. Testosterone and DHT exert their effects through the androgen receptor (AR), a classical nuclear steroid hormone receptor. The AR activates the transcription of genes containing androgen response elements, and thereby modulates prostate growth and development. The role of the AR in development and progression of prostate cancer is suggested by the fact that antiandrogen therapy is highly but transiently effective, and antiandrogen therapy can stimulate prostate cancer cells, as seen in antiandrogen withdrawal syndrome.

Two polymorphic repeats have been identified: a CAG repeat and a GGN repeat that correlate with prostate cancer development. Shorter CAG repeats are associated with greater cancer risk and increased prostate cancer aggressiveness. Also, mutations have been found that cause inappropriate activation of the AR by estrogens, progestins, glucocorticoids, and antiandrogens that promote prostate cancer cell growth, suggesting that these mutations play a role in cancer progression and development of resistant tumors.

BIBLIOGRAPHY

1. Aaronson SA. Grmvth factors and cancer. Science 1991;254: 1146–53.
2. Abelev GI. Perova SD, Khramkova NI, et al. Production of embryonal alpha-globulins by transplantable mouse hepatomas. Transplantation 1963; 1: 174–8.

3. Adam B-L. Qu Y. Davies JW. et al. Serum protein finger-printing coupled with a pattern-matching algorithm distinguishes prostate cancer from benign prostate hyperplasia and healthy men. Cancer Res 2002; 62: 3609–14.

4. Agendia Inc. MammaPrint. Available at: http://usa. agendia. com/ (accessed May 2, 2011).

5. Albain A. Barlo W. Shak S. et al. Prognostic and predictive value of the 21-gene recurrence score assay in postmeno-pausal, node-positive. estrogen receptor-positive breast cancer. Lancet Oncol 2010; 11: 55–65.

6. Alberti L, Carniti C. Miranda C. et al. RET and NTRKI proto-oncogenes in human diseases. J Cell PhysioI2003;195:168-86.

7. Allegra CJ, Jessup JM. Somerfield MR. et al. American Society of Clinical Oncology provisional clinical opinion: testing for KRAS gene mutations in patients with metastatic colorectal carcinoma to predict response to anti-epidermal growth factor receptor monoclonal antibody therapy. J Clin Oncol 2009; 27: 2091–6.

8. American Society for Therapeutic Radiology and Oncology Consensus Panel. Consensus statement: guidelines for PSA following radiation therapy. Int J RadiatOncolBioI Phys 1997; 37: 1035–41.

9. Andreasen PA. Kjoller L. Christensen L. et al. The urokinase-type plasminogen activator system in cancer metastasis: a review. Int J Cancer 1997; 72: 1–22.

10. Andriole GL. Grubb RL III, Buys SS, et al. Mortality results from a randomized prostate-cancer screening trial. N Engl J Med 2009; 360: 1310–9.

11. Angelopoulou K. Diamandis EP. Sutherland DJ. et al. Prevalence of serum antibodies against the p53 tumor suppressor gene protein in various cancers. Int J Cancer 1994; 58: 480–7.

12. Ariyaratana S, Loeb DM. The role of the Wilms tumour gene (WTl) in normal and malignant haematopoiesis. Expert Rev Mol Med 2007; 9: 1–17.

13. Austin LA. Heath H. Calcitonin: physiology and patho-physiology. N Engl J Med 1981; 304: 269–78.

14. Babaian RJ, Fritsche H. Ayala A. et al. Performance of a neural network in detecting prostate cancer in the prostate-specific antigen reflex range of 2.5 to 4.0 ng/mL. Urology 2000; 56: I 000-6.

15. Babaian RJ, Fritsche HA. Zhang Z. et al. Evaluation of ProstAsure index in the detection of prostate cancer: a preliminary report. Urology 1998; 51: 132–6.

16. Babaian RJ, Johnston DA, Naccarato W. et al. The incidence of prostate cancer in a screening population with a serum prostate specific antigen between 2.5 and 4.0 ng/ml: relation to biopsy strategy. J UroI 2001; 165: 757–60.

17. Barak V. Goike H. Panaretakis KW. Einarsson R. Clinical utility of cytokeratins as tumor markers. ClinBiochem 2004; 37: 529–40.

18. Bar-Sagi D. A Ras by any other name. Mol Cell Bioi 2001; 21: 1441–3.

19. Bartlett NL. Freiha FS. Torti FM. Serum markers in germ cell neoplasms. Hematol On col Clin North Am 1991; 5: 1245–60.

20. Bast RC Jr. Brewer M. Zou C. et al. Prevention and early detection of ovarian cancer: mission impossible? Recent Results Cancer Res 2007; 174: 91–100.

21. Bates SE, Longo DL. Use of serum tumor markers in cancer diagnosis and management. Semin Oncol 1987; 14: 102–38.

22. Bates SE. Clinical applications of serum tumor markers. Ann Intern Med 1991; 115: 623–38.

23. Belanger A. van Halbeek H. Graves HDB. et al. Molecular mass and carbohydrate structure of prostate specific antigen: studies for establishment of an international PSA standard. Prostate 1995; 27: 187–97.

24. Bence-Jones H. Papers on chemical pathology. Lecture III. Lancet I 847; ii: 269–72.

25. Benson MC. Whang IS. Pantuck A. et al. Prostate specific antigen density: a means of distinguishing benign prostatic hypertrophy and prostate cancer. J UroI 1992; 147: 815–16.

26. Bergers G. Benjamin LE. Tumorigenesis and the angiogenic switch. Nat Rev Cancer 2002; 3: 401–10.

27. Berkowitz RS. Goldstein DP. Gestational trophoblastic disease. In: Mossa AR. Schimpff SC. Robson MC. eds. Comprehensive textbook of oncology. Baltimore: Williams & Wilkins. 1991: 1046–51.

28. Bernini GP, Moretti A, Ferdeghini M. et al. A new human chromogranin "1\' immunoradiometric assay for the diagnosis of neuroendocrine tumours. Br J Cancer 2001; 84: 636–42.

29. Beyer HL. Geschwindt RD. Glover CL. et al. MESOMARK: a potential test for malignant pleural mesothelioma. ClinChem 2007; 53: 666–72.

30. Birken S. Berger P. Bidart JM. et al. Preparation and characterization of new WHO reference reagents for human chorionic gonadotropin and metabolites. ClinChem 2003; 49: 144–54.

31. Bjorklund B. Bjorklund V. Antigenicity of pooled human malignant and normal tissues by cyto-immunologic techniques: presence of an insoluble heat labile tumor antigen. Arch Allergy 1957; 10: 153–84.

32. Black MH. Diamandis EP. The diagnostic and prognostic utility of prostate-specific antigen for diseases of the breast. Breast Cancer Res

33. Bloom G. Yang IV. Boulware D. et al. Multi-platform. multi-site. microarray-based human tumor classification. Am J Pat hoi 2004;164: 9–16.

34. Bombardieri E, Gion M. Mucin-like cancer associated antigen (MCA) as available circulating tumor marker for breast cancer. [n: Sell S. ed. Serological cancer markers. Totowa NJ: Humana Press, 1992: 341–54.

35. Bonfrer JMG. Working group on tumor marker criteria (WGTMC). Tumour BioI 1990; II : 287–88.

36. Bouchalova K. Cizkova M. Cwiertka K. Trojanec R. Hajduch M. Triple negative breast cancer-current status and prospective targeted treatment based on HERI (EGFR). TOP2A and C-MYC gene assessment. Biomed Pap Med Fac Univ Palacky Olomouc Czech Repub 2009; 153: 13–7.

37. Bray KR. Koda JE. Gaur PK. Serum concentrations and biochemical characteristics of cancer associated antigen (CA) 549, a circulating breast cancer marker. Cancer Res 1987; 47: 5853–60.

38. Brown WHo A case of pluriglandular syndrome. Lancet 1928; ii: I 022–4.

39. Buccheri G. Ferrigno D. Lung tumor markers of cytokeratin origin: an overview. Lung Cancer 2001; 34: S65–9.

40. Bunting PS. [s there still a role for prostatic acid phosphatase? CSCC Position Statement, Canadian Society of Clinical Chemists. ClinBiochem 1999; 32: 591–4.

41. Bussemakers MJ, van Bokhoven A. Verhaegh GW. et al. DD3: a new prostate-specific gene. highly overexpressed in prostate cancer. Cancer Res 1999; 59: 5975–9.

42. Buyse M. Loi S. Van't Veer L. et al. Validation and clinical utility of a 70-gene prognostic signature for women with node-negative breast cancer. J Natl Cancer Inst 2006;98: 1183–92.

43. Callagy GM. Webber MJ, Pharoah PD, Caldas C. Meta-analysis confirms BCL2 is an independent prognostic marker in breast cancer. BMC Cancer 2008; 8:153.

44. Cancer Facts and Figures 2010. Atlanta, Ga: American Cancer Society, 2010: 1–62.

45. Cao Y. Tumor angiogenesis and molecular targets for therapy. Front Biosci 2009; 14: 3962–73.

46. Carmeliet P. Angiogenesis in health and disease. Nat Med 2003; 9: 653–60.

47. Carter HB, Pearson ID, Metter EI. et al. Longitudinal evaluation of prostate specific antigen levels in men with and without prostate disease. lAMA 1992; 267: 2215–20.

48. Catalona WI. Partin AW, Slawin KM, et al. Use of the percentage of free prostate-specific antigen to enhance differentiation of prostate cancer from benign prostatic disease: a prospective multicenter clinical trial. lAMA 1998: 297: 1542–7.

49. Catalona WI. Smith DS, Ratliff TL, et al. Measurement of prostate specific antigen in serum as a screening test for prostate cancer. N Engl I Med 1991; 324: 1156–61.

50. Cavaliere A, Bucciarelli E, Sidoni A, et al. Estrogen and progesterone receptors in breast cancer: comparison between enzyme immunoassay and computer-assisted image analysis of immunocytochemical assay. Cytometry 1996; 26: 204–8.

51. Chan AK, Chiu RW, Lo YM; Clinical Sciences Reviews Committee of the Association of Clinical Biochemists. Cell-free nucleic acids in plasma, serum and urine: a new tool in molecular diagnosis. Ann Clin Biochem 2003; 40: 122–30.

52. Chan DW, Beveridge RA, Bhargava A, et al. Breast cancer marker CA549: a multicenter study. Am I Clin Pathol 1994; 101: 465–70.

53. Chan DW, Beveridge RA, Bruzek DI, et aL Monitoring breast cancer with CA 549. Clin Chern 1988; 34: 2000–4.

54. Chan DW, Beveridge RA, Muss H, et al. Use of TRUQUANT BR RIA for early detection of breast cancer recurrence in patients with stage II and stage III disease. I Clin Oncol 1997; 15: 2322–8.

55. Chan DW, Bruzek DI. Oesterling IE, et al. Prostatic-specific antigen as a marker for prostatic cancer: a monoclonal and a polyclonal immunoassay compared. Clin Chern 1987; 33: 1916–20.

56. Chan DW, Kelsten M, Rock R, Bruzek D. Evaluation of a monoclonal immunoenzymometric assay for alpha-fetoprotein. Clin Chern 1986; 32: 1318-22.

57. Chan DW, Maioyc. Affinity chromatographic separation of alpha-fetoprotein variants: development of a minicolumn procedure and application to cancer patients. ClinChern 1986:32:2143-6.

58. Chan DW, Sokoll LI. WHO first international standards for prostatespecific antigen: the beginning of the end for assay discrepancies? [Editorial] ClinChern 2000;46:1291-2.

59. Chin KF, Greenman I, Reusch P, et al. Vascular endothelial growth factor and soluble Tie-2 receptor in colorectal cancer: associations with disease recurrence. Eur I SurgOncol 2003: 29: 497–505.

60. Chu TM. Prostate specific antigen. In: Sell S, ed. Serological cancer markers. Totowa NI: Humana Press, 1992: 99–115.

61. Clark GI, Der CT. Ras proto-oncogene activation in human malignancy. In: Garret G, Sell S, eds. Cellular cancer markers. Totowa NI: Humana Press, 1995: 17–52.

62. Cole LA, Butler SA, Khanlian SA, et al. Gestational trophoblastic diseases. 2. HyperglycosylateddhCG as a reliable marker of active neoplasia. Gynecol Oncol 2003; 102: 151–9.

63. Correale M, Abbate I, Gargano G, et al. Analytical and clinical evaluation of a new tumor marker in breast cancer: CA 27.29. Int I BioI Markers 1992; 7: 43–6.

64. Cristofanilli M, Budd GT, Ellis MI. et aL Circulating tumor cells, disease progression, and survival in metastatic breast cancer. N Engl I Med 2004: 351: 781–91.

65. Darson MF, Pacelli A, Roche P, et al. Human glandular kallikrein 2 expression in prostate adenocarcinoma and lymph node metastases. Urology 1999; 53: 939–44.

66. De Bie SH, Ferreira TC, Pauwels EKI. Cleton Fl. Immuno-scintigraphy for cancer detection: "a thousand ills require a thousand cures." I Cancer Res ClinOnco\ 1992;118:1-15.

67. de Kok IB, Verhaegh GW, Roelofs RW, et al. DD3(PCA3), a very sensitive and specific marker to detect prostate tumors. Cancer Res 2002; 62: 2695–8.

68. de Medeiros SF, Norman RI. Human choriogonadotrophin protein core and sugar branches heterogeneity: basic and clinical insights. Hum Reprod Update 2009; 15: 69–95.

69. Deras IL, Aubin SMI, Blase A, et al. PCA3-a molecular urine assay for predicting biopsy outcome. I UroI 2008; 179: 1587–92.

70. Diamandis EP, Fritsche HA, Lilja H, Chan DW, Schwartz MK, eds. Tumor markers: physiology, pathobiology, technology and clinical applications. Washington, DC: AACC Press, 2002.

71. Diamandis EP, Scorilas A, Fracchioli S, et al. Human kallikrein 6 (hK6): a new potential serum biomarker for diagnosis and prognosis of ovarian carcinoma. I Clin Oncol 2003; 21: 1035–43.

72. Diamandis EP, Yousef GM. Human tissue kallikreins: a family of new cancer biomarkers. Clin Chern 2002; 48: 1198–205.

73. Diamandis EP. Prostate-specific antigen: its usefulness in clinical medicine. Trends Endocrinol Metab 1998: 8: 310–6.

74. Drapkin R, von Horsten HH, Lin Y, et al. Human epididymis protein 4 (HE4) is a secreted glycoprotein that is over expressed by serous and endometrioid ovarian carcinomas. Cancer Res 2005; 65: 2162–9.

75. Duffy MI, Maguire TM, McDermott EW, et al. Urokinase plasminogen activator: a prognostic marker in multiple types of cancer. I Surg Oncol 1999; 1: 130–5.

76. Duman-Scheel M. Netrin and DCC: axon guidance regulators at the intersection of nervous system development and cancer. Curr Drug Targets 2009: 10:602-10.

77. Einhorn N, Bast RC Ir, Knapp RC, et al. Preoperative evaluation of serum CA 125 levels in patients with primary epithelial ovarian cancer. Obstet Gynecol 1986; 67: 414–6.

78. Eissa S, Swellam M, Sadek M, et al. Comparative evaluation of the nuclear matrix protein, fibronectin, urinary bladder cancer antigen and voided urine cytology in the detection of bladder tumors. I Urol 2002; 168: 465–9.

79. Haglund C, Kuusela P, Roberts P, Jalanko H. CA 50. In: Sell S, ed. Serological cancer markers. Totowa, NJ: Humana Press, 1992: 375–86.

80. Hakomori S-I. Tumor associated carbohydrate markers. In: Sell S, ed. Serological cancer markers. Totowa NJ: Humana Press, 1992: 207–32.

81. Hall PA, McCluggage WG. Assessing p53 in clinical contexts: unlearned lessons and new perspectives. J Pathol 2006; 208: 1–6.

82. Han M, Piantadosi S, Zahurak ML, et al. Serum acid phosphatase level and biochemical recurrence following radical prostatectomy for men with clinically localized prostate cancer. Urology 2001; 57: 707–11.

83. Hanahan D, Weinberg RA. The hallmarks of cancer. Cell 2000; 100: 57–70.

84. Harbeck N, Schmitt M, Kates RE, et al. Clinical utility of urokinase type plasminogen activator and plasminogen activator inhibitor-l determination in primary breast cancer tissue for individualized therapy concepts. Clin Breast Cancer 2002; 3: 196–200.

85. Harper PS. Research samples from families with genetic diseases: a proposed code of conduct. Br Med J 1993; 306: 1391–3.

86. Hostetter RB, Augustus LB, Mankarious R, et al. Carcino-embryonic antigen as a selective enhancer of colorectal cancer metastasis. J Natl Cancer Inst 1990; 82: 380–5.

87. Hotakainen K, Tanner P, Alfthan H, Haglund C, Stenman UH. Comparison of three immunoassays for CA 19-9. Clin Chim Acta 2009; 400: 123–7.

88. International HapMap Consortium. The International HapMap Project. Nature 2003; 426: 789–96.

89. Jacobs I, Bast RC. The CA 125 tumor-associated antigen: a review of the literature. Hum Reprod 1989; 4: 1–12.

90. Janicke F, Prechtl A, Thomssen C. Randomized adjuvant chemotherapy trial in high-risk, lymph node-negative breast cancer patients identified by urokinase-type plasminogen activator and plasminogen activator inhibitor type 1. J Natl Cancer Inst 2001; 93: 913–20.

91. Johnson PJ, Lo YM. Plasma nucleic acids in the diagnosis and management of malignant disease. Clin Chern 2002; 48: 1186–93.

92. Kastan MB, Canman CE, Leonard C/. P53, cell cycle control and apoptosis: implications for cancer. Cancer Metastasis Rev 1995; 14: 3–15.

93. Kastan MB, Sidransky D, Vogelstein B, Craig RW. Participation of p53 protein in the cellular response to DNA damage. Cancer Res 1991; 51: 6304–11.

94. Kato H. Squamous cell carcinoma antigen. In: Sell S, ed. Serological cancer markers. Totowa NJ: Humana Press, 1992: 437–51.

95. Kelsten ML, Chan DW, Bruzek DJ, Rock RC. Monitoring hepatocellular carcinoma by using a monoclonal immuno-enzymometric assay for alpha-fetoprotein. Clin Chern 1988; 34: 76–81.

96. Lakhani VT, You YN, Wells SA. The multiple endocrine neoplasia syndromes. Annu Rev Med 2007; 58: 253–65.

97. Lamerz R. CAI9-9: GICA (gastrointestinal cancer antigen). In: Sell S, ed. Serological cancer markers. Totowa, NJ: Humana Press, 1992: 309–39.

98. Lander ES, Linton LM, Birren B, et al. Initial sequencing and analysis of the human genome. Nature 2001; 409: 860–921.

99. Lee W-H, Shew JY, Hong RD, et al. The retinoblastoma susceptibility gene encodes a nuclear phosphoprotein associated with DNA binding activity. Nature 1987; 329: 642–4.

100. Lemal A, Siegel R, Xu J, Ward E. Cancer statistics, 2010. CA Cancer J Clin 2010; 60: 277–300.

101. Leppert M, Dobbs M, Scrambler P, et al. The gene for familial polyposis coli maps to the long arm of chromosome 5. Science 1987; 238: 1411–3.

102. Lev Z, Kislitsin D, Rennert G, Lerner A. Utilization of K-ras mutations identified in stool DNA for the early detection of colorectal cancer. J Cell Biochem Suppl 2000; 34: 35–9.

103. Levine A], Momand J, Finlay CA. The p53 tumour suppressor gene. Nature 1999; 351: 453–6.

104. Li D, Mallory T, Satomura S. AFP- L3: a new generation of tumor marker for hepatocellular carcinoma. ClinChimActa 2001; 313: 15–9.

105. Li J, Dowdy S, Tipton T, et al. HE4 as a biomarker for ovarian and endometrial cancer management. Expert Rev Mol Diagn 2009; 9: 555–66.

106. Li J, Yen C, Liaw D, et al. PTEN, a putative protein tyrosine phosphatase gene mutated in human brain, breast, and prostate cancer. Science 1997; 275: 1943–7.

107. Li JL, Zhang Z, Rosenzweig J, et al. Proteomics and bioinformatics approaches for identification of serum biomarkers to detect breast cancer. Clin Chern 2002; 48: 1296–304.

108. Lilja H, Christens on A, Dahlen U, et al. Prostate specific antigen in human serum occurs predominantly in complex with alpha-1- antichymotrypsin. Clin Chern 1991; 37: 1618–25.

109. Lin F, van Rhee F, Goldman JM, et al. Kinetics of increasing BCR-ABL transcript numbers in chronic myeloid leukemia patients who relapse after bone marrow transplantation. Blood 1996; 7: 4473–8.

110. Oesterling JE, Jacobsen SJ, Chute GG, et al. Serum prostate specific antigen in a community based population of healthy men: establishment of age-specific reference ranges. JAMA 1993; 270: 860–4.

111. Overall CM, Lopez-Otin e. Strategies for MMP inhibition in cancer: innovations for the post-trial era. Nat Rev Cancer 2002; 2: 657–72.

112. Owen WE, Roberts RF, Roberts WL. Performance characteristics of the LiBASys des-gamma-carboxy prothrombin assay. Clin Chim Acta 2008; 339: 183–5.

113. Ozturk M. p53 mutation in hepatocellular carcinoma after aflatoxin exposure. Lancet 1991; 338: 1356–9.

114. Paech K, Webb P, Kuiper GG, et al. Differential ligand activation of estrogen receptors ER alpha and ER beta at AP 1 sites. Science 1997; 277: 1508-1 O.

115. Paik S, Shak S, Tang G, et al. A multigene assay to predict recurrence of tamoxifen-treated, node-negative breast cancer. N Engl J Med 2004; 351: 2817–26.

116. Paik S, Tang G, Shak S, et al. Gene expression and benefit of chemotherapy in women with node-negative, estrogen receptorpositive breast cancer. J Clin Oncol 2006; 24: 3726–34.

117. Paik S. Development and clinical utility of a 21-gene recurrence score prognostic assay in patients with early breast cancer treated with tamoxifen. Oncologist 2007; 12: 631–5.

118. Palmer-Toy D, Kuzdzal S, Chan DW. Proteomic approaches to tumor marker discovery. In: Diamandis EP, Fritsche HA, Lilja H, Chan DW, Schwartz MK, eds. Tumor markers: physiology, pathobiology, technology and clinical applications. Washington, DC: AACC Press, 2002:391-400.

119. Quintas-Cardama A, Cortes J. Molecular biology ofbcr-abl1-positive chronic myeloid leukemia. Blood 2009; 113: 1619–30.

120. Quyn AI, Steele RJ, Carey FA, Nathke IS. Prognostic and therapeutic implications of Apc mutations in colorectal cancer. Surgeon 2008; 6: 350–6.

121. Radich JP, Gehly G, Gooley T, et al. Polymerase chain reaction detection of the BCR-ABL fusion transcript after allogeneic marrow transplantation for chronic myeloid leukemia: results and implications in 346 patients. Blood 1995; 5: 2632–8.

122. Rai AJ, Zhang Z, Rosenzweig J, et al. Proteomic approaches to tumor marker discovery: identification of biomarkers for ovarian cancer. Arch Pat hoi Lab Med 2002; 26: 1518–26.

123. Recker F, Kwiatkowski MK, Piironen T, et al. Human glandular kallikrein as a tool to improve discrimination of poorly differentiated and non-organ-confined prostate cancer compared with prostate specific antigen. Urology 2000; 55: 481–5.

124. Reddish MA, Helbrecht N, Almeida AF, et al. Epitope mapping of Mab within the peptide core of the malignant breast carcinoma associated mucin antigen coded for by the human MUC 1 gene. J Tumor Marker Oncol 1992; 7: 19–27.

125. Riethdorf S, Fritsche H, Muller V, et al. Detection of circulating tumor cells in peripheral blood of patients with metastatic breast cancer: a validation study of the cell search system. Clin Cancer Res 2007; 13: 920–8.

126. Riou GF, Bourhis J, Le MG. The c-myc proto-oncogene in invasive carcinomas of the uterine cervix: clinical relevance of overexpression in early stages of the cancer. Anticancer Res 1990; 10: 1225–31.

127. Roach M 3rd, Hanks G, Thames H Jr, et al. Defining biochemical failure following radiotherapy with or without hormonal therapy in men with clinically localized prostate cancer: recommendations of the RTOG-ASTRO Phoenix Consensus Conference. Int J RadiatOncolBioi Phys 2006; 65: 965–74.

128. Rochefort H, Garcia M, Glondu M, et al. Cathepsin D in breast cancer: mechanisms and clinical applications, a 1999 overview. Clin Chim Acta 2000; 291: 157–70.

129. Sterling RK, Jeffers L, Gordon F, et al. Clinical utility of AFP-L3% measurement in North American patients with HCV-related cirrhosis. Am J GastroenteroI 2007; 102: 2196–205.

130. Steuber T, Vickers AJ, Serio AM, et al. Comparison of free and total forms of serum human kallikrein 2 and prostate-specific antigen for prediction of locally advanced and recurrent prostate cancer. Clin Chem 2007; 53: 233–40.

131. Stigbrand T, Wahren B. Alkaline phosphatase as tumor markers. In: Sell S, ed. Serological cancer markers. Totowa NJ: Humana Press, 1992: 135–49.

132. Sturgeon CM, Berger P, Bidart JM, et al. Differences in recognition of the 1st WHO international reference reagents for hCG-related isoforms by diagnostic immunoassays for human chorionic gonadotropin. Clin Chem 2009; 55: 1484–91.

133. Sturgeon CM, Duffy MJ, Stenmab UH, et al; National Academy of Clinical Biochemistry. National Academy of Clinical Biochemistry laboratory medicine practice guidelines for use of tumor markers in testicular, prostate, colorectal, breast, and ovarian cancers. Clin Chem 2008; 54: ell-79.

134. Sulis ML, Parsons R. PTEN: from pathology to biology. Trends Cell BioI 2003; 13: 478–83.

135. Treat 2000; 59: 1-14.

136. Swarup V, Rajeswari MR. Circulating (cell-free) nucleic acids-apromising, non-invasive tool for early detection of several humandiseases. FEBS Lett 2007; 581: 795–9.

137. Taketa K. Alpha-fetoprotein in the 1990s. In: Sell S, ed. Serologicalcancer markers. Totowa, NJ: Humana Press, 1992: 31–46.

138. Takeuchi H, Bilchik A, Saha S, et al. c-MET expression level inprimary colon cancer: a predictor of tumor invasion and lymph nodemetastases. Clin Cancer Res 2003; 9:14808.

139. Tatarinov Y. New data on the embryo-specific antigenic componentsof human blood serum. Vopr Med Khim 1964; 10: 584–8.

140. Thompson 1M, Goodman PJ, Tangen CM, et al. The influence offinasteride on the development of prostate cancer. N Engl J Med 2003; 349: 215–24.

141. Thompson 1M, Pauler OK, Goodman PJ, et al. Prevalence of prostatecancer among men with a prostate-specific antigen level ~4.0 ng per milliliter. N Engl J Med 2004; 350: 2239–46.

142. TolgayOcall, Dolled-Filhart M, D'Aquila TG, et al. Tissuemicroarray-based studies of patients with lymph node negative breastcarcinoma show that met expression is associated with worse outcomebut is not correlated with epidermal growth factor family receptors.Cancer 2003; 97: 1841–8.

143. Wolf AM, Wender RC, Etzioni RB, et al. American Cancer Societyguideline for the early detection of prostate cancer: update 2010. CA Cancer J Clin 2010; 60: 70–98.

144. Wooster R, Neuhausen SL, Mangion J, et al. Localization of a breastcancer susceptibility gene, BRCA 2, to chromosome 13qI2-13. Science 1994; 265: 2088–90.

145. Yin BW, Lloyd KO. Molecular cloning of the CA 125 ovarian cancerantigen: identification as a new mucin, MUCI6. J BioI Chem 2001; 276: 27371–5.

146. Yousef GM, Diamandis EP. The new human tissue kallikrein genefamily: structure, function, and association to disease. Endocr Rev 2001; 2: 184–204.

147. Yousef GM, Polymeris ME, Grass L, et al. Human kallikrein 5: apotential novel serum biomarker for breast and ovarian cancer. Cancer Res 2003; 63: 3958–65.

148. Yousef GM, Polymeris ME, Yacoub GM, et al. Parallel overexpression of seven kallikrein genes in ovarian cancer. Cancer Res 2003; 63: 2223–7.

149. Zeltzer PM, Marangos PJ, Evans AE, Schneider SL. Serum neuronspecificenolase in children with neuroblastoma. Cancer 1986; 57: 1230–4.

150. Zemzoum I, Kates RE, Ross JS, et al. Invasion factors uPA/PAI-I andHER2 status provide independent and complementary information onpatient outcome in node-negative breast cancer. J Clin Oncol 2003; 21: 1022–8.

151. Zhang Z. Combining multiple biomarkers in clinical diagnostics: areview of methods and issues. In: Diamandis EP, Fritsche HA, Lilja H,Chan OW, Schwartz MK, eds. Tumor markers: physiology,pathobiology, technology and clinical applications. Washington, DC:AACC Press, 2002: 133–9.

18

Vitamins

INTRODUCTION

Vitamins have a wide range of functions in biologic tissue, serving as cofactors in many enzymatic reactions, so that these enzymes have low catalytic activity in cellular reactions if vitamins are not present. These compounds and their biologically inactive precursors must be partially obtained from food sources and, in some instances, from bacterial synthesis. When cellular vitamin and activity levels from diet or intestinal absorption are inadequate, it is termed vitamin deficiency. The term vitamin has an historical basis in deficiency states that were relieved by specific food intake. The most notable examples are scurvy (vitamin C, sailors and lime consumption, limeys); rickets (vitamin D in the early industrial age); beriberi (alcoholics and thiamine); pellagra (niacin) and night blindness (vitamin A); megaloblastic anemia (folic acid or vitamin B12); spina bifid a (folic acid); and pernicious anemia with neuropathy (vitamin B12).

Abnormal increases of metabolism requiring high supplies of one of these cofactors may be termed vitamin insufficiency or vitamin dependency, depending on the level of supply demanded for physiologic function.

Variabilities in clinical expression of vitamin abnormalities result from differences in any of the following: in specific cause, degree, and duration of vitamin inadequacy, the simultaneous presence of nutritional insufficiencies, and/or the increased metabolic demands imposed by conditions, such as pregnancy, infection, and cancer. The clinical symptoms of vitamin deficiencies are usually nonspecific in early stages and in mild, chronic deficiency states. A combination of dietary history, physical examination, and laboratory measurements is often required to diagnose vitamin deficiency. Vitamin metabolism is complex and vitamin supplementation of foods is common. It is not unusual to find vitamin toxicities from inappropriate use of vitamin supplementation. For simplicity, vitamins of diverse chemical structure are classified as either water soluble or fat soluble. Fat-soluble vitamins include A, D, E, and K. Those vitamins soluble in water include the B complex of vitamins; thiamine, riboflavin, niacin, vitamins B6 and B12, biotin, folate, and vitamin C. Water-soluble vitamins are readily excreted in the urine and are less likely than fat-soluble vitamins to accumulate to toxic levels in the body. Vitamins, classified as fat or water soluble, and the symptoms usually seen in deficiency states are shown in Table 18.1.

For dietary requirements, sources, functions, effects of deficiencies and toxicities, blood levels, and usual therapeutic dosages for vitamins daily intakes (Table 18.2).

Dietary requirements for vitamins (and other nutrients) are expressed as daily recommended intake (DRI). There are 3 types of DRI:

- Recommended daily allowances (RDAs) are set to meet the needs of 97–98% of healthy people.
- Adequate intake (AI): When data to calculate an RDA are insufficient, AIs are based on observed or experimentally determined estimates of nutrient intake by healthy people.
- Tolerable upper intake levels (ULs) are the largest amount of a nutrient that most adults can ingest daily without risk of adverse health effects.

Chemical determination of human vitamin states has been approached in the following ways—(1) measurement of active cofactors or precursors in biologic fluids or blood cells, (2) measurement of urinary metabolites of the vitamin, (3) measurement of a biochemical function

Table 18.1	Vitamin and deficiency states
Vitamin name	**Clinical deficiency**
Fat-soluble vitamins	
Vitamin A1	Night blindness, growth retardation, abnormal taste response, dermatitis, recurrent infections
Vitamin E	Mild hemolytic anemia (newborn), red blood cell fragility, ataxia
Vitamin D	Rickets (young), osteomalacia (adult
Vitamin K	Hemorrhage (ranging from easy bruising to massive bruising), especially post-traumatic bleeding
Water-soluble vitamins	
Vitamin B1	Infants: Dyspnea, cyanosis, diarrhea, vomiting Adults: Beriberi (fatigue, peripheral neuritis), Wernicke-Korsakoff syndrome (apathy, ataxia, visual problems)
Vitamin B2	Angular stomatitis (mouth lesions), dermatitis, photophobia, neurologic changes
Niacin/Niacinamide	Pellagra (dermatitis, mucous membrane inflammation, weight loss, disorientation)
Folic acid	Megaloblastic anemia
Vitamin B12	Megaloblastic anemia, neurologic abnormalities
Vitamin C	First, vague aches and pains; if long term, scurvy (hemorrhages into skin, alimentary and urinary tract, anemia, wound healing delayed)

Table 18.2	Recommended daily intakes for vitamins and sources, functions, and effects of vitamins		
Nutrient	**Principal sources**	**Functions**	**Effects of deficiency and toxicity**
Folate (folic acid)	Raw green leafy vegetables, fruits, organ meats (e.g. liver), enriched cereals and breads	Maturation of RBCs Synthesis of purines, pyrimidines, and methionine Development of fetal nervous system	Deficiency: Megaloblastic anemia, neural tube birth defects, and confusion
Niacin (nicotinic acid, nicotinamide)	Liver, red meat, fish, poultry, legumes, whole-grain or enriched cereals and breads	Oxidation-reduction reactions Carbohydrate and cell metabolism	Deficiency: Pellagra (dermatitis, glossitis, GI and CNS dysfunction); toxicity—flushing
Riboflavin (vitamin B2)	Milk, cheese, liver, meat, eggs, enriched cereal products	Many aspects of carbohydrate and protein metabolism Integrity of mucous membranes	Deficiency: Cheilosis, angular stomatitis, corneal vascularization
Thiamin (vitamin B1)	Whole grains, meat (especially pork and liver), enriched cereal products, nuts, legumes, potatoes	Carbohydrate, fat, amino acid, glucose, and alcohol metabolism Central and peripheral nerve cell function, myocardial function	Deficiency: Beriberi (peripheral neuropathy, heart failure), Wernicke-Korsakoff syndrome
Vitamin A (retinol)	As preformed vitamin: Fish liver oils, liver, egg yolks, butter, vitamin A—fortified dairy products As provitamin carotenoids: dark green and yellow vegetables, carrots, yellow and orange fruits	Formation of rhodopsin (a photoreceptor pigment in the retina) Integrity of epithelia Lysosome stability Glycoprotein synthesis	Deficiency: Night blindness, perifollicular hyperkeratosis, xerophthalmia, keratomalacia, increased morbidity and mortality in young children Toxicity: Headache, peeling of skin, hepatosplenomegaly, bone thickening, intracranial hypertension, papilledema, hypercalcemia
Vitamin B6 group (pyridoxine, pyridoxal, pyridoxamine)	Organ meats (e.g. liver), whole-grain cereals, fish, legumes	Many aspects of nitrogen metabolism (e.g. transaminations, porphyrin and heme synthesis, tryptophan conversion to niacin) Nucleic acid biosynthesis Fatty acid, lipid, and amino acid metabolism	Deficiency: Seizures, anemia, neuropathies, seborrheic dermatitis Toxicity: peripheral neuropathy

Contd.

Table 18.2	Recommended daily intakes for vitamins and sources, functions, and effects of vitamins (Contd.)		
Nutrient	Principal sources	Functions	Effects of deficiency and toxicity
Vitamin B12 (cobalamins)	Meats [especially beef, pork, and organ meats (e.g. liver)], poultry, eggs, fortified cereals, milk and milk products, clams, oysters, mackerel, salmon	Maturation of RBCs, neural function, DNA synthesis, myelin synthesis and repair	Deficiency: Megaloblastic anemia, neurologic deficits (confusion, paresthesias, ataxia)
Vitamin C (ascorbic acid)	Citrus fruits, tomatoes, potatoes, broccoli, strawberries, sweet peppers	Collagen formation Bone and blood vessel health Carnitine, hormone, and amino acid formation, wound healing	Deficiency: Scurvy (hemorrhages, loose teeth, gingivitis, bone defects)
Vitamin D (cholecal-ciferol, ergocalciferol)	Direct ultraviolet B irradiation of the skin (main source), fortified dairy products (main dietary source), fish liver oils, fatty fish, liver	Calcium and phosphate absorption Mineralization and repair of bone Tubular reabsorption of calcium Insulin and thyroid function, improvement of immune function, reduced risk of autoimmune disease	Deficiency: Rickets (sometimes with tetany), osteomalacia Toxicity: hypercalcemia, anorexia, renal failure, metastatic calcifications
Vitamin E group (alpha-tocopherol, other tocopherols)	Vegetable oils, nuts	Intracellular antioxidant Scavenger of free radicals in biologic membranes	Deficiency: Red blood cell hemolysis, neurologic deficits Toxicity: Tendency to bleed
Vitamin K group (phylloquinone, menaquinones)	Green leafy vegetables (especially collards, spinach, and salad greens), soy beans, vegetable oils Bacteria in the GI tract after neonatal period	Formation of prothrombin, other coagulation factors, and bone proteins	Deficiency: Bleeding due to deficiency of prothrombin and other factors, osteopenia

requiring the vitamin (e.g. enzymatic activity), with and without *in vitro* addition of the cofactor form, (4) measurement of urinary excretion of vitamin or metabolites after a test load of the vitamin, (5) measurement of urinary metabolites of a substance, the metabolism of which requires the vitamin after administration of a test load of the substance. Reduced serum concentrations of a vitamin do not always indicate a deficiency that interrupts cellular function. Conversely, values within the reference interval do not always reflect adequate function. Interpretation of laboratory values must be done with knowledge of the biochemistry and physiology of vitamins.

FAT-SOLUBLE VITAMINS

Vitamin A

Vitamin A is the nutritional term for the group of compounds with a 20-carbon structure containing a methyl-substituted cyclohexenyl ring (β-ionone ring) and an isoprenoid side-chain (Fig. 18.1), with a hydroxyl

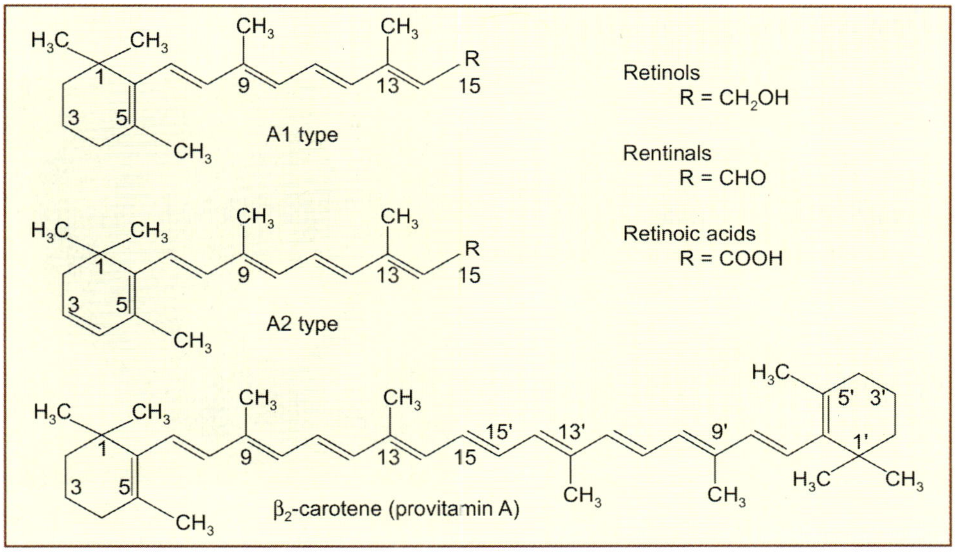

Fig. 18.1: Vitaminic forms of A1, A2, and β-carotene

group (retinol), an aldehyde group (retinal), a carboxylic acid group (retinoic acid), or an ester group (retinyl ester) at the terminal C15.

Retinol and retinoic acid are derived directly from dietary sources, primarily as retinyl esters, or from metabolism of dietary carotenoids (pro-vitamin A), primarily beta carotene. Major dietary sources of these compounds include animal products and pigmented fruits and vegetables (carotenoids). Vitamin A is stored in the liver and transported in the circulation complexed to retinal-dinding protein (RBP) and transthyretin. Vitamin A and related retinoic acids area group of compounds essential for vision, cellular differentiation, growth, reproduction, and immune system function. A clearly defined physiologic role for retinol is in vision. Retinol is oxidized in the rods of the eye to retinal, which, when complexed with opsin, forms rhodopsin, allowing dim-light vision. This vitamin and vitamin D act through specific nuclear receptors in the regulation of cell proliferation.

VITAMIN A DEFICIENCY

Vitamin A deficiency can result from inadequate intake, fat malabsorption, or liver disorders. Deficiency impairs immunity and hematopoiesis and causes rashes and typical ocular effects (e.g. xerophthalmia, night blindness). Diagnosis is based on typical ocular findings and low vitamin A levels. Treatment consists of vitamin A given orally or, if symptoms are severe or malabsorption is the cause, parenterally.

Etiology

Primary vitamin A deficiency is usually caused by prolonged dietary deprivation. It is endemic in areas, such as southern and eastern Asia, where rice, devoid of beta-carotene, is the staple food. Xerophthalmia due to primary deficiency is a common cause of blindness among young children in developing countries.

Secondary vitamin A deficiency may be due to decreased bioavailability of provitamin A carotenoids or interference with absorption, storage, or transport of vitamin A. Interference with absorption or storage is likely in celiac disease, cystic fibrosis, pancreatic insufficiency, duodenal bypass, chronic diarrhea, bile duct obstruction, giardiasis, and cirrhosis. Vitamin A deficiency is common in prolonged protein-energy undernutrition not only because the diet is deficient, but also because vitamin A storage and transport is defective.

Signs and Symptoms

Impaired dark adaptation of the eyes, which can lead to night blindness, is an early symptom of vitamin A deficiency. Xerophthalmia (which is nearly pathog-

nomonic) results from keratinization of the eyes. It involves drying (xerosis) and thickening of the conjunctivae and corneas. Superficial foamy patches composed of epithelial debris and secretions on the exposed bulbar conjunctiva (Bitot spots) develop (Fig. 18.2). In advanced deficiency, the cornea becomes hazy and can develop erosions, which can lead to its destruction (keratomalacia). Keratinization of the skin and of the mucous membranes in the respiratory, GI, and urinary tracts can occur. Drying, scaling, and follicular thickening of the skin and respiratory infections can result, immunity is generally impaired. The younger the patient, the more severe are the effects of vitamin A deficiency. Growth retardation and infections are common among children. Mortality rate can exceed 50% in children with severe vitamin A deficiency.

Diagnosis

Ocular findings suggest vitamin A deficiency. Dark adaptation can be impaired in other disorders (e.g. zinc deficiency, retinitis pigmentos a, severe refractive errors, cataracts, diabetic retinopathy). If dark adaptation is impaired, rod scotometry and electroretinography are done to determine whether vitamin A deficiency is the cause.

Serum levels of retinol are measured. Normal range is 1–3 µmol/L. However, levels decrease only after the deficiency is advanced because the liver contains large stores of vitamin A. Also, decreased levels may result from acute infection, which causes retinol-binding protein and transthyretin (also called pre-albumin) levels to decrease transiently.

Treatment

Dietary deficiency of vitamin A is traditionally treated with vitamin A palmitate in oil 60,000 IU po once a day

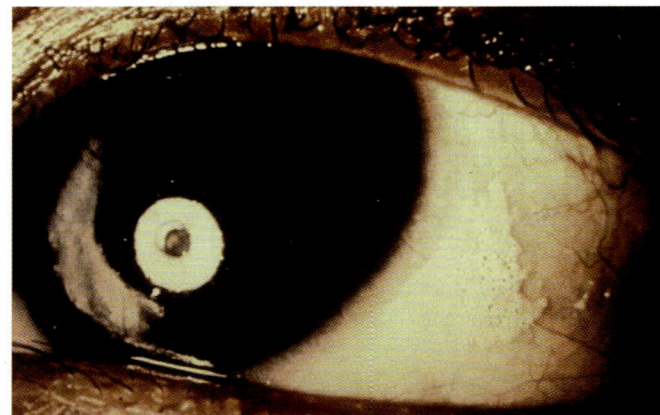

Fig. 18.2: Chronic dryness of the conjunctival membrane with keratinized patches known as Bitot spots

for 2 days, followed by 4500 IU po once a day. If vomiting or malabsorption is present or xerophthalmia is probable, a dose of 50,000 IU for infants <6 months, 100,000 IU for infants 6–12 months, or 200,000 IU for children >12 months and adults should be given for 2 days, with a third dose at least 2 weeks later. The same doses are recommended for infants and children with complicated measles.

Vitamin A deficiency is a risk factor for severe measles; treatment with vitamin A can shorten the duration of the disorder and may reduce the severity of symptoms and risk of death. The WHO recommends that all children with measles in developing countries should receive 2 doses of vitamin A, (100,000 IU for children <12 months and 200,000 IU for those >12 months) given 24 h apart. Infants born of HIV-positive mothers should receive 50,000 IU (15,000 RAE) within 48 hours of birth. Prolonged daily administration of large doses, especially to infants, must be avoided because toxicity may result. For pregnant or breast-feeding women, prophylactic or therapeutic doses should not exceed 10,000 IU (3000 RAE)/day to avoid possible damage to the fetus or infant.

Vitamin A Toxicity

Vitamin A toxicity can be acute (usually due to accidental ingestion by children) or chronic. Both types usually cause headache and increased intracranial pressure. Acute toxicity causes nausea and vomiting. Chronic toxicity causes changes in skin, hair, and nails; abnormal liver test results; and, in a fetus, birth defects. Diagnosis is usually clinical. Unless birth defects are present, adjusting the dose almost always leads to complete recovery.

Acute vitamin A toxicity in children may result from taking large doses [>300,000 IU (>100,000 RAE)], usually accidentally. In adults, acute toxicity has occurred when arctic explorers ingested polar bear or seal livers, which contain several million units of vitamin A.

Chronic vitamin A toxicity in older children and adults usually develops after doses of >100,000 IU (>30,000 RAE)/day have been taken for months. Megavitamin therapy is a possible cause, as are massive daily doses [150,000–350,000 IU (50,000–120,000 RAE)] of vitamin A or its metabolites, which are sometimes given for nodular acne or other skin disorders. Adults who consume >4500 IU (>1500 RAE)/day of vitamin A may develop osteoporosis. Infants who are given excessive doses [18,000–60,000 IU (6,000–20,000 RAE)/day] of water-miscible vitamin A may develop toxicity within a few weeks. Birth defects occur in children of women receiving isotretinoin (which is related to vitamin A) for acne treatment during pregnancy.

Although, carotene is converted to vitamin A in the body, excessive ingestion of carotene causes carotenemia, not vitamin A toxicity. Carotenemia is usually asymptomatic but may lead to carotenosis, in which the skin becomes yellow. When taken as a supplement, beta-carotene has been associated with increased cancer risk; risk does not seem to increase when carotenoids are consumed in fruits and vegetables.

Signs and Symptoms

Although, symptoms of vitamin A toxicity may vary, headache and rash usually develop during acute or chronic toxicity. Acute toxicity causes increased intracranial pressure. Drowsiness, irritability, abdominal pain, nausea, and vomiting are common. Sometimes, the skin subsequently peels.

Early symptoms of chronic toxicity are sparsely distributed, coarse hair; alopecia of the eyebrows; dry, rough skin; dry eyes; and cracked lips. Later, severe headache, pseudotumor cerebri, and generalized weakness develop. Cortical hyperostosis of bone and arthralgia may occur, especially in children. Fractures may occur easily, especially in the elderly. In children, toxicity can cause pruritus, anorexia, and failure to thrive. Hepatomegaly and splenomegaly may occur. In carotenosis, the skin (but not the sclera) becomes deep yellow, especially on the palms and soles.

Diagnosis

Diagnosis of vitamin A toxicity is clinical. Blood vitamin levels correlate poorly with toxicity. However, if clinical diagnosis is equivocal, laboratory testing may help. In vitamin A toxicity, fasting serum retinol levels may increase from normal (1–3 μmol/L) to (>3.49 μmol/L), sometimes to (>69.8 μmol/L). Hypercalcemia is common.

Differentiating vitamin A toxicity from other disorders may be difficult. Carotenosis may also occur in severe hypothyroidism and anorexia nervosa, possibly because carotene is converted to vitamin A more slowly.

Treatment

Vitamin A is stopped.

VITAMIN E

Vitamin E is the nutritional term for the group of naturally occurring tocopherols and to cotrienols that have biological activity similar to RRR—a tocopherol (formerly D-α-tocopherol). Both groups have a common 6-chromanol nucleus substituted with methyl groups at positions 2 and 8 and with a phytyl tail of isoprenoid units at position 2. The isoprenoid chain is saturated in the tocopherols, but is unsaturated at positions 3', 7', and 11' for to cotrienols (Fig. 18.3).

Vitamin E is a powerful antioxidant and the primary defense against potentially harmful oxidations that cause disease and aging, protecting unsaturated lipids from peroxidation (cleavage of fatty acids at unsaturated sites by oxygen addition across the double bond and formation of free radicals). The role of vitamin E in protecting the erythrocyte membrane from oxidant stress is presently its major documented role in human physiology. It has been shown to strengthen cell membranes and augment such functions as drug metabolism, heme biosynthesis, and neuromuscular function. About 40% of ingested to copherolis absorbed, affected mainly by the amount and degree of unsaturated dietary fat, largely determining the physiologic requirement. Absorbed vitamin E is associated with circulating chylomicrons, very-low-density lipoprotein, and chylomicron remnants. Dietary sources of tocopherols include vegetable oil, fresh leafy vegetables, egg yolk, legumes, peanuts, and margarine. Diets suspect for vitamin E deficiency are those low in vegetable oils, fresh green vegetables, or unsaturated fats.

Vitamin E Deficiency

Dietary vitamin E deficiency is common in developing countries; deficiency among adults in developed countries is uncommon and usually due to fat malabsorption. The main symptoms are hemolytic anemia and neurologic deficits. Diagnosis is based on measuring the ratio of plasma alpha-tocopherol to total plasma lipids; a low ratio suggests vitamin E deficiency. Treatment consists of oral vitamin E, given in high doses if there are neurologic deficits or if deficiency results from malabsorption. Vitamin E deficiency causes fragility of RBCs and degeneration of neurons, particularly peripheral axons and posterior column neurons.

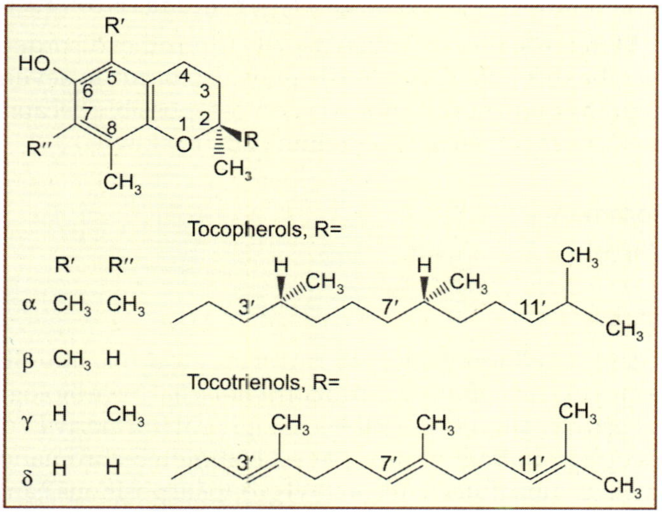

Etiology

Inadequate intake of vitamin E is the most common cause of vitamin E deficiency in developing countries and in developed countries, the most common causes are the disorders that cause fat malabsorption, including abetalipoproteinemia (Bassen–Kornzweig syndrome, due to genetic absence of apolipoprotein B), chronic cholestatic hepatobiliary disease, pancreatitis, short bowel syndrome, and cystic fibrosis. A rare genetic form of vitamin E deficiency without fat malabsorption results from defective liver metabolism.

Signs and Symptoms

The main symptoms of vitamin E deficiency are mild hemolytic anemia and nonspecific neurologic deficits. Abetalipoproteinemia results in progressive neuropathy and retinopathy in the first 2 decades of life.

Vitamin E deficiency may contribute to retinopathy of prematurity (also called retrolental fibroplasia) in premature infants and to some cases of intraventricular and subependymal hemorrhage in neonates. Affected premature neonates have muscle weakness.

In children, chronic cholestatic hepatobiliary disease or cystic fibrosis causes neurologic deficits, including spinocerebellar ataxia with loss of deep tendon reflexes, truncal and limb ataxia, loss of vibration and position senses, ophthalmoplegia, muscle weakness, ptosis, and dysarthria. In adults with malabsorption, vitamin E deficiency very rarely causes spinocerebellar ataxia because adults have large vitamin E stores in adipose tissue.

Diagnosis

Without a history of inadequate intake or a predisposing condition, vitamin E deficiency is unlikely. Confirmation usually requires measuring the vitamin level. Measuring RBC hemolysis in response to peroxide can suggest the diagnosis but is nonspecific. Hemolysis increases as vitamin E deficiency impairs RBC stability.

Measuring the serum alpha-tocopherol level is the most direct method of diagnosis. In adults, vitamin E deficiency is suggested if the alpha-tocopherol level is <11.6 µmol/L. Because abnormal lipid levels can affect vitamin E status, a low ratio of serum alpha-tocopherol to lipids (<0.8 mg/g total lipid) is the most accurate indicator in adults with hyperlipidemia.

In children and adults with abetalipoproteinemia, serum alpha-tocopherol levels are usually undetectable.

Fig. 18.3: Vitaminic forms of vitamin E

Treatment

If malabsorption causes clinically evident deficiency, alpha-tocopherol 15–25 mg/kg by mouth once a day should be given. Or mixed tocopherols (200–400 IU) can be given. However, larger doses of alpha-tocopherol given by injection are required to treat neuropathy during its early stages or to overcome the defect of absorption and transport in abetalipoproteinemia.

Vitamin E Toxicity

Many adults take relatively large amounts of vitamin E (alpha-tocopherol 400–800 mg/day) for months to years without any apparent harm. Occasionally, muscle weakness, fatigue, nausea, and diarrhea occur. The most significant risk is bleeding. However, bleeding is uncommon unless the dose is >1000 mg/day or the patient takes oral coumarin or warfarin. Thus, the upper limit for adults aged ≥19 years is 1000 mg for any form of alpha-tocopherol.

VITAMIN D

Vitamin D and its metabolites may be categorized as cholecalciferols or ergocalciferols (Fig. 18.4). Cholecalciferol (vitamin D3) is the parent compound of the naturally occurring family and is produced in the skin from 7-dehydrocholesterol on exposure to the ultraviolet B portion of sunlight. Latitude, season, aging, sunscreen use, and skin pigmentation influence production of vitamin D3 by the skin. Vitamin D2 (ergocalciferol), the parent compound of the other family, is manufactured by irradiation of ergosterol produced by yeasts. Vitamin D occurs in foods as cholecalciferol or ergocalciferol. The most active metabolite of vitamin D is 1,25(OH)2D3. It stimulates intestinal absorption of calcium and phosphate for bone growth and metabolism and, together with parathyroid hormone, stimulates bone to increase the mobilization of calcium and phosphate. 1,25(OH)2D3 has an important proapoptotic effect, acting through a vitamin D hormonal system, that depends on binding of the active ligand to a vitamin D receptor. This led to important drug discovery developments in which calcium and phosphate release is minimized and proliferative and anti-inflammatory effects of D-analogues are modulated. In northern climates, it is difficult to receive enough ultraviolet exposure to fully meet minimum requirements (2 h/d). Major dietary sources of vitamin D include irradiated foods and commercially prepared milk. Small amounts are found in butter, egg yolks, liver, sardines, herring, tuna, and

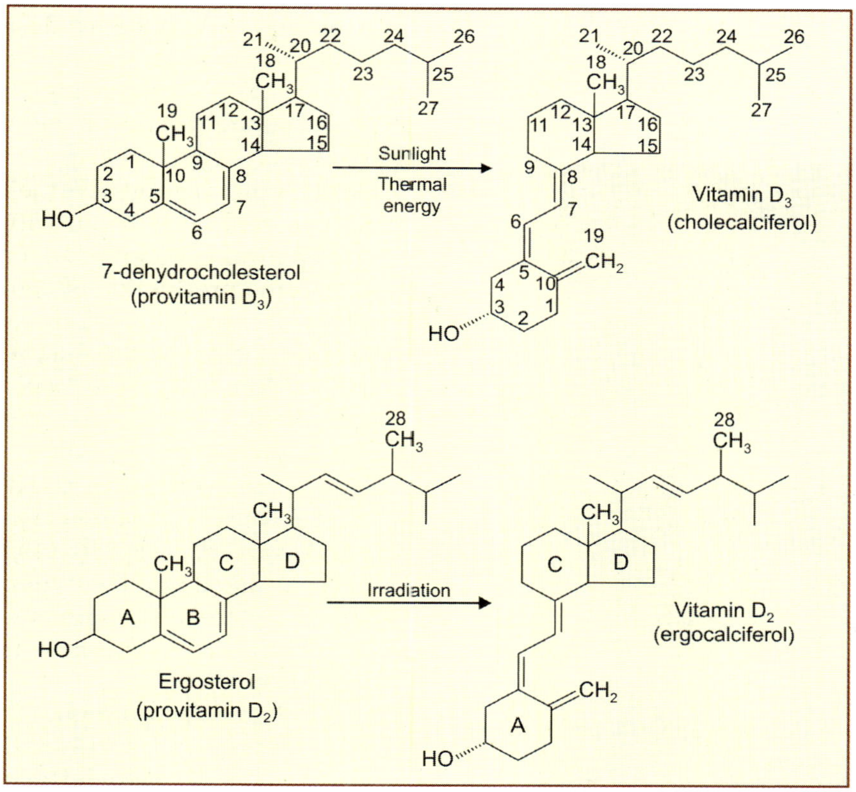

Fig. 18.4: Structures of vitamin D3 (cholecalciferol) and vitamin D (ergocalciferol) and their precursors. 7- cholecalciferol is produced in the skin from 7-dehydrocholesterol on exposure to sunlight. Ergocalciferol is produced commercially by irradiation of ergosterol

salmon. The RDA of vitamin D for adults is 15–20 mg/d, depending on age. Absorbed in the small intestine, vitamin D requires bile salts for absorption. It is stored in the liver and excreted in the bile. Severe deficiency in children causes a failure to calcify cartilage at the growth plate in metaphysical bone formation, leading to the development of rickets. In adults, the deficiency leads to undermineralization of bone matrix in remodeling, resulting in osteomalacia.

Vitamin D Deficiency and Dependency

Inadequate exposure to sunlight predisposes to vitamin D deficiency. Deficiency impairs bone mineralization, causing rickets in children (Fig. 18.5) and osteomalacia in adults and possibly contributing to osteoporosis. Diagnosis involves measurement of serum 25(OH)D (D2+D3). Treatment usually consists of oral vitamin D; calcium and phosphate are supplemented as needed. Prevention is often possible. Rarely, hereditary disorders cause impaired metabolism of vitamin D (dependency).

Vitamin D deficiency is common worldwide. It is a common cause of rickets and osteomalacia, but these disorders may also result from other conditions, such as chronic kidney disease, various renal tubular disorders, familial hypophosphatemic (vitamin D resistant) rickets, chronic metabolic acidosis, hyperparathyroidism, hypoparathyroidism, inadequate dietary calcium, and disorders or drugs that impair the mineralization of bone matrix.

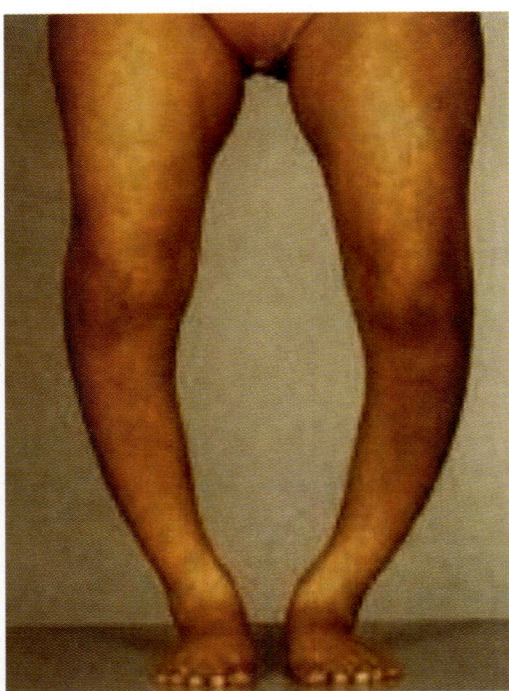

Fig. 18.5: Rickets in children

Vitamin D deficiency causes hypocalcemia, which stimulates production of parathyroid hormone (PTH), causing hyperparathyroidism. Hyperparathyroidism increases absorption, bone mobilization, and renal conservation of calcium but increases excretion of phosphate. As a result, the serum level of calcium may be normal, but because of hypophosphatemia, bone mineralization is impaired.

Etiology

Vitamin D deficiency may result from the inadequate exposure to sunlight, inadequate intake of vitamin D, reduced absorption of vitamin D, and abnormal metabolism of vitamin D and resistance to the effects of vitamin D.

Inadequate direct sunlight exposure or sunscreen use and inadequate intake usually occur simultaneously to result in clinical deficiency. Susceptible people include (1) the elderly (who are often undernourished and are not exposed to enough sunlight), (2) certain communities (e.g. women and children who are confined to the home or who wear clothing that covers the entire body and face).

Inadequate vitamin D stores are common among the elderly, particularly those who are house bound, institutionalized, or hospitalized or who have had a hip fracture. Recommended direct sunlight exposure is 5–15 minutes (suberythemal dose) to the arms and legs or to the face, arms, and hands, at least 3 times a week. However, many dermatologists do not recommend increased sunlight exposure because risk of skin cancer is increased.

Malabsorption can deprive the body of dietary vitamin D; only a small amount of 25(OH)D is recirculated enterohepatically. Vitamin D deficiency may result from defects in the production of 25(OH)D or 1,25(OH)2D. People with chronic kidney disease commonly develop rickets or osteomalacia because renal production of 1,25(OH)2D is decreased and phosphate levels are elevated. Hepatic dysfunction can also interfere with production of active vitamin D metabolites.

Type I hereditary vitamin D dependent rickets is an autosomal recessive disorder characterized by absent or defective conversion of 25(OH)D to 1,25(OH)2D in the kidneys. X-linked familial hypophosphatemia reduces vitamin D synthesis in the kidneys. Many anticonvulsants and use of glucocorticoids increase the need for vitamin D supplementation.

Type II hereditary vitamin D dependent rickets has several forms and is due to mutations in the 1,25(OH)2D receptor. This receptor affects the metabolism of gut, kidney, bone, and other cells. In this disorder, 1,25(OH)2D is abundant but ineffective because the receptor is not functional.

Signs and Symptoms

Vitamin D deficiency can cause muscle aches, muscle weakness, and bone pain at any age. Vitamin D deficiency in a pregnant woman causes deficiency in the fetus. Occasionally, deficiency severe enough to cause maternal osteomalacia results in rickets with metaphyseal lesions in neonates. In young infants, rickets causes softening of the entire skull (craniotabes). When palpated, the occiput and posterior parietal bones feel like a ping pong ball. In older infants with rickets, sitting and crawling are delayed, as is fontanelle closure; there is bossing of the skull and costochondral thickening. Costochondral thickening can look like bead-like prominences along the lateral chest wall (rachitic rosary). In children 1–4 years, epiphyseal cartilage at the lower ends of the radius, ulna, tibia, and fibula enlarge; kyphoscoliosis develops, and walking is delayed. In older children and adolescents, walking is painful; in extreme cases, deformities such as bowlegs and knock-knees develop. The pelvic bones may flatten, narrowing the birth canal in adolescent girls.

Tetany is caused by hypocalcemia and may accompany infantile or adult vitamin D deficiency. Tetany may cause paresthesias of the lips, tongue, and fingers; carpopedal and facial spasm; and, if very severe, seizures. Maternal deficiency can cause tetany in neonates. Osteomalacia predisposes to fractures. In the elderly, hip fractures may result from only minimal trauma.

Diagnosis

X-rays of the radius and ulna plus serum levels of calcium, phosphate, alkaline phosphatase, PTH, and 25(OH)D are needed to differentiate vitamin D deficiency from other causes of bone demineralization.

Assessment of vitamin D status and serologic tests for syphilis can be considered for infants with craniotabes based on the history and physical examination, but most cases of craniotabes resolve spontaneously. Rickets can be distinguished from chondrodystrophy because the latter is characterized by a large head, short extremities, thick bones, and normal serum calcium, phosphate, and alkaline phosphatase levels. Tetany due to infantile rickets may be clinically indistinguishable from seizures due to other causes. Blood tests and clinical history may help distinguish them.

X-rays

Bone changes, seen on X-rays, precede clinical signs. In rickets, changes are most evident at the lower ends of the radius and ulna. The diaphyseal ends lose their sharp, clear outline; they are cup-shaped and show a spotty or fringy rarefaction. Later, because the ends of the radius and ulna have become non-calcified and radiolucent, the distance between them and the metacarpal bones appears increased. The bone matrix elsewhere also becomes more radiolucent. Characteristic deformities result from the bones bending at the cartilage-shaft junction because the shaft is weak. As healing begins, a thin white line of calcification appears at the epiphysis, becoming denser and thicker as calcification proceeds. Later, the bone matrix becomes calcified and opacified at the subperiosteal level.

In adults, bone demineralization, particularly in the spine, pelvis, and lower extremities, can be seen on X-rays; the fibrous lamellae can also be seen, and incomplete ribbonlike areas of demineralization (pseudo fractures, looser lines, and Milkman syndrome) appear in the cortex.

Laboratory Tests

Because levels of serum 25(OH)D reflect body stores of vitamin D and correlate with Signs and symptoms of vitamin D deficiency better than levels of other vitamin D metabolites, the best way to diagnose vitamin D deficiency is generally considered to be 25(OH)D (D2+D3) levels.

Target 25(OH)D levels about 50–60 nmol/L for maximal bone health; whether higher levels have other benefits remains uncertain, and higher absorption of calcium may increase risk of coronary artery disease. If the diagnosis is unclear, serum levels of 1,25(OH)2D and urinary calcium concentration can be measured. In severe deficiency, serum 1,25(OH)2D is abnormally low, usually undetectable. Urinary calcium is low in all forms of the deficiency except those associated with acidosis. In vitamin D deficiency, serum calcium may be low or, because of secondary hyperparathyroidism, may be normal. Serum phosphate usually decreases, and serum alkaline phosphatase usually increases. Serum PTH may be normal or elevated. Type I hereditary vitamin D dependent rickets results in normal serum 25(OH)D, low serum 1,25(OH)2D and calcium, and normal or low serum phosphate.

Treatment

Calcium deficiency (which is common) and phosphate deficiency should be corrected. As long as calcium and phosphate intake is adequate, adults with osteomalacia and children with uncomplicated rickets can be cured by giving vitamin D3 40 μg 1600 IU by mouth once a day. Serum 25(OH)D and 1,25(OH)2D begin to increase within 1 or 2 days. Serum calcium and phosphate increase and serum alkaline phosphatase decreases within about

10 days. During the third week, enough calcium and phosphate are deposited in bones to be visible on X-rays. After about 1 months, the dose can usually be reduced gradually to the usual maintenance level of 15 µg (600 IU) once a day.

If tetany is present, vitamin D should be supplemented with IV calcium salts for up to 1 week. Some elderly patients need vitamin D3 25 to > 50 µg (1000 to ≥2000 IU) daily to maintain a 25(OH)D level >20 ng/mL (> 50 nmol/L); this dose is higher than the recommended daily allowance for people <70 years (600 IU) or >70 years (800 IU). The current upper limit for vitamin D is 4000 IU/day. Higher doses of vitamin D2 (e.g. 25,000–50,000 IU every week or every month) are sometimes prescribed; because vitamin D3 is more potent than vitamin D2, it is now preferred.

Because rickets and osteomalacia due to defective production of vitamin D metabolites are vitamin D-resistant, they do not respond to the doses usually effective for rickets due to inadequate intake. Endocrinologic evaluation is required because treatment depends on the specific defect. When 25(OH)D production is defective, vitamin D3 50 µg (2000 IU) once a day increases serum levels and results in clinical improvement. Patients with kidney disorders often need 1,25(OH)2D (calcitriol) supplementation.

Type I hereditary vitamin D-dependent rickets responds to 1,25(OH)2D 1–2 µg by mouth once a day. Some patients with type II hereditary vitamin D-dependent rickets respond to very high doses (e.g. 10–24 µg/day) of 1,25(OH)2D; others require long-term infusions of calcium.

Vitamin D Toxicity

Usually, vitamin D toxicity results from taking excessive amounts. In vitamin D toxicity, resorption of bone and intestinal absorption of calcium is increased, resulting in hypercalcemia. Marked hypercalcemia commonly causes symptoms. Diagnosis is typically based on elevated blood levels of 25(OH)D. Treatment consists of stopping vitamin D, restricting dietary calcium, restoring intravascular volume deficits, and, if toxicity is severe, giving corticosteroids or bisphosphonates. Because synthesis of 1,25(OH)2D (the most active metabolite of vitamin D) is tightly regulated, vitamin D toxicity usually occurs only if excessive doses (prescription or megavitamin) are taken. Vitamin D 1000 µg (40,000 IU)/day causes toxicity within 1–4 months in infants. In adults, taking 1250 µg (50,000 IU)/day for several months can cause toxicity. Vitamin D toxicity can occur iatrogenically when hypoparathyroidism is treated too aggressively.

Signs and Symptoms

The main symptoms of vitamin D toxicity result from hypercalcemia. Anorexia, nausea, and vomiting can develop, often followed by polyuria, polydipsia, weakness, nervousness, pruritus, and eventually renal failure. Proteinuria, urinary casts, azotemia, and metastatic calcifications (particularly in the kidneys) can develop.

Diagnosis

A history of excessive vitamin D intake may be the only clue differentiating vitamin D toxicity from other causes of hypercalcemia. Elevated serum calcium levels of 3–4 mmol/L are a constant finding when toxic symptoms occur. Serum 25(OH)D levels are usually elevated to >375 nmol/L. Levels of 1,25(OH)2D, which need not be measured to confirm the diagnosis, may be normal. Serum calcium should be measured often (weekly at first, then monthly) in all patients receiving large doses of vitamin D, particularly the potent 1,25(OH)2D.

Treatment

After stopping vitamin D intake, hydration (with IV normal saline) and corticosteroids or bisphosphonates (which inhibit bone resorption) are used to reduce blood calcium levels.

VITAMIN K

Compounds in the vitamin K series are 2-methyl-1, 4-napthoquinones, which are substituted with side chains at carbon 3. Phylloquinon (K, type) synthesized in plants and menaquinones (K2 type) of bacterial origin are the two principal natural classes of vitamin K (Fig. 18.6).

Vitamin K (from the German word 'Koagulation') is the group of substances essential for the formation of prothrombin and at least five other coagulation proteins, including factors VII, IX, and X and proteins C and S. The quinone-containing compounds are a generic

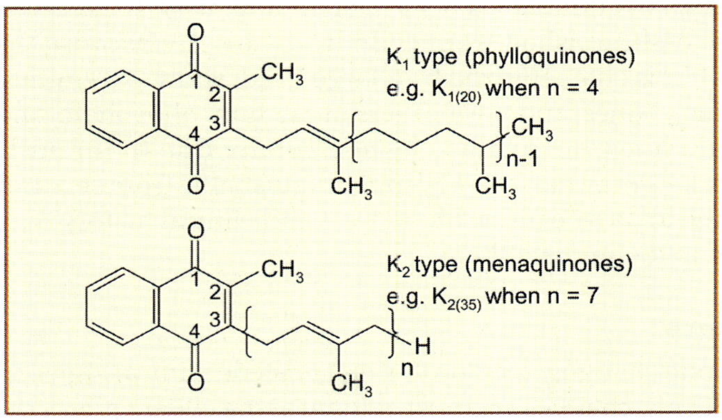

Fig. 18.6: Vitaminic forms of vitamin K

description for menadione and derivatives exhibiting this activity. Vitamin K helps convert precursor forms of these coagulation proteins to functional forms; this transformation occurs in the liver. Dietary vitamin K is absorbed primarily in the terminal ileum and, possibly, the colon. Vitamin K is synthesized by intestinal bacteria; this synthesis provides 50% of the vitamin K requirement.

Major dietary sources are cabbage, cauliflower, spinach and other leafy vegetables, liver, soybeans, and vegetable oils. Uncomplicated dietary vitamin K deficiency is considered rare in healthy children and adults.

Vitamin K Deficiency

Vitamin K deficiency results from extremely inadequate intake, fat malabsorption, or use of coumarin anticoagulants. Deficiency is particularly common among breast fed infants. It impairs clotting. Diagnosis is suspected based on routine coagulation study findings and confirmed by response to vitamin K. Treatment consists of vitamin K given orally or, when fat malabsorption is the cause or when risk of bleeding is high, parenterally. Vitamin K deficiency decreases levels of prothrombin and other vitamin K-dependent coagulation factors, causing defective coagulation and, potentially, bleeding. Worldwide, vitamin K deficiency causes infant morbidity and mortality.

Vitamin K deficiency causes hemorrhagic disease of the newborn, which usually occurs 1–7 days post-partum. In affected neonates, birth trauma can cause intracranial hemorrhage. A late form of this disease can occur in infants about 2–12 weeks old, typically in infants who are breast fed and are not given vitamin K supplements. If the mother has taken phenytoin anticonvulsants, coumarin anticoagulants, or cephalosporin antibiotics, the risk of hemorrhagic disease is increased.

In **healthy adults,** dietary vitamin K deficiency is uncommon because vitamin K is widely distributed in green vegetables and the bacteria of the normal gut synthesize menaquinones.

Etiology

Neonates are prone to vitamin K deficiency because of (1) the placenta transmits lipids and vitamin K relatively poorly, (2) the neonatal liver is immature with respect to prothrombin synthesis, (3) breast milk is low in vitamin k, containing about 2.5 μg/L (cow's milk contains 5000 μg/L), and (4) the neonatal gut is sterile during the first few days of life. In **adults,** vitamin K deficiency can result from (1) fat malabsorption (e.g. due to biliary obstruction, malabsorption disorders, cystic fibrosis, or resection of the small intestine), and (2) use of coumarin anticoagulants.

Coumarin anticoagulants interfere with the synthesis of vitamin K-dependent coagulation proteins (factors II, VII, IX, and X) in the liver. Certain antibiotics (particularly some cephalosporins and other broad-spectrum antibiotics), salicylates, megadoses of vitamin E, and hepatic insufficiency increase risk of bleeding in patients with vitamin K deficiency. Inadequate intake of vitamin K is unlikely to cause symptoms.

Signs and Symptoms

Bleeding is the usual manifestation. Easy bruisability and mucosal bleeding (especially epistaxis, GI hemorrhage, menorrhagia, and hematuria) can occur. Blood may ooze from puncture sites or incisions. Hemorrhagic disease of the newborn and late hemorrhagic disease in infants may cause cutaneous, GI, intrathoracic, or, in the worst cases, intracranial bleeding. If obstructive jaundice develops, bleeding if it occurs usually begins after the 4th or 5th day. It may begin as a slow ooze from a surgical incision, the gums, the nose, or GI mucosa, or it may begin as massive bleeding into the GI tract.

Diagnosis

Vitamin K deficiency or antagonism (due to coumarin anticoagulants) is suspected when abnormal bleeding occurs in a patient at risk. Blood coagulation studies can preliminarily confirm the diagnosis. Prothrombine time (PT) is prolonged and international normalized ratio (INR) is elevated, but partial thromboplastin time (PTT), thrombin time, platelet count, bleeding time, and levels of fibrinogen, fibrin-split products, and d-dimer are normal. If phytonadione [United States Pharmacopeia (USP) generic name for vitamin K1] 1 mg interavenous (IV) significantly decreases PT within 2–6 hours, a liver disorder is not the likely cause, and the diagnosis of vitamin K deficiency is confirmed.

Some centers can detect vitamin K deficiency more directly by measuring the serum vitamin level. The serum level of vitamin K1 ranges from 0.2–1.0 ng/mL in healthy people consuming adequate quantities of vitamin K1 (50–150 μg/day). Knowing vitamin K intake can help interpret serum levels; recent intake affects levels in serum but not in tissues.

Treatment

Whenever possible, phytonadione should be given by mouth or SC. The usual adult dose is 1–20 mg. INR usually decreases within 6–12 hours. The dose may be repeated in 6–8 hours if INR has not decreased satisfactorily. Phytonadione 1–10 mg by mouth is indicated for non-emergency correction of a prolonged INR in patients taking anticoagulants. Correction usually occurs within

6–8 hours. When only partial correction of INR is desirable (e.g. when INR should remain slightly elevated because of a prosthetic heart valve), lower doses (e.g. 1–2.5 mg) of phytonadione can be given. In infants, bleeding due to vitamin K deficiency can be corrected by giving phytonadione 1 mg SC or intramuscular (IM) once. The dose is repeated if INR remains elevated. Higher doses may be necessary if the mother has been taking oral anticoagulants.

Vitamin K Toxicity

Vitamin K1 (phylloquinone) is not toxic when consumed orally, even in large amounts. However, menadione (a synthetic, water-soluble vitamin K precursor) can cause toxicity and should not be used to treat vitamin K deficiency.

WATER SOLUBLE VITAMINS

Thiamine

Thiamine (vitamin B1) or thiamin acts as a coenzyme in decarboxylation reactions in major carbohydrate pathways and in branched-chain amino acid metabolism. The structure of thiamine (vitamin B1) [3-(4-amino-2-methylpyrimidyl-5-methyl)-4-methyl-5-(β-hydroxyethyl) thiazole] is that of a pyrimidine ring, bearing an amino group, linked by a methylene bridge to a thiazole ring (Fig. 18.7). Thiamine rapidly absorbed from food in the small intestine and excreted in the urine. The clinical condition associated with chronic thiamine deficiency is beriberi. Although, usually occurring in underdeveloped countries of the world, beriberi may be found in the United States among persons with chronic alcoholism. Decreased intake, impaired absorption, and increased requirements all appear to play a role in the development of thiamine deficiency in persons with alcoholism. The RDA of thiamine is 1.2 mg/d for adult males and 1.1 mg/d for adult females. Thiamine functional activity is best measured by erythrocyte transketolase activity, before and after the addition of thiamine pyrophosphate (TPP). Thiamine deficiency is present if the increase in activity after the addition of TPP is greater than 25%.

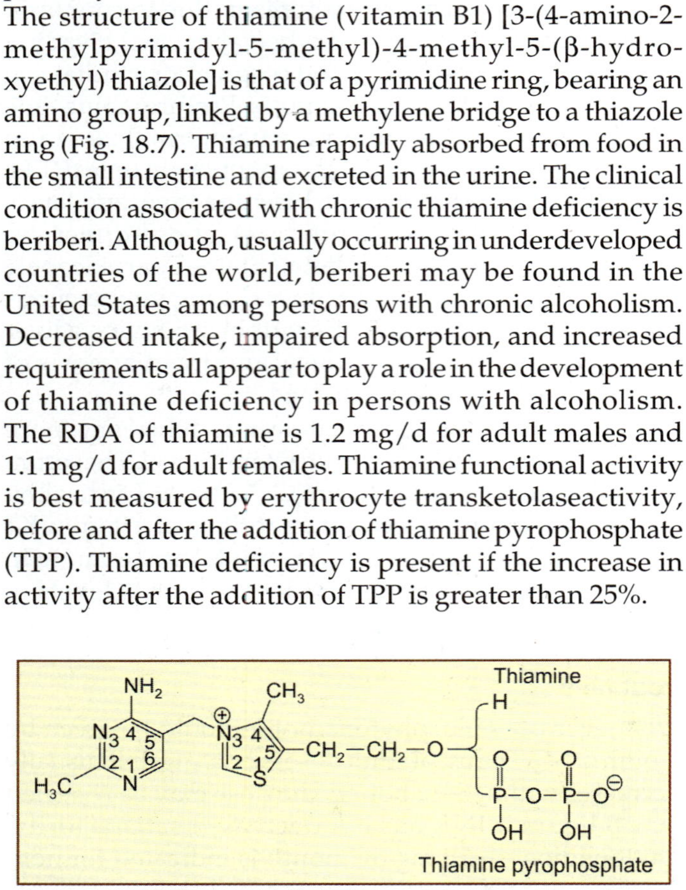

Fig. 18.7: Thiamine and the pyrophosphate coenzyme

Thiamin Deficiency

Thiamin deficiency beriberi is most common among people subsisting on white rice or highly refined carbohydrates in developing countries and among alcoholics. Symptoms include diffuse polyneuropathy, high-output heart failure, and Wernicke-Korsakoff syndrome. Thiamin is given to help diagnose and treat the deficiency.

Etiology

- **Primary thiamin deficiency** is caused by inadequate intake of thiamin. It is commonly due to a diet of highly refined carbohydrates (e.g. polished rice, white flour, and white sugar) in developing countries. It also develops when intake of other nutrients is inadequate, as may occur in young adults with severe anorexia; it often occurs with other B vitamin deficiencies.
- **Secondary thiamin deficiency** is caused by (1) increased demand (e.g. due to hyperthyroidism, pregnancy, lactation, strenuous exercise, or fever), (2) impaired absorption (e.g. due to prolonged diarrhea), and (3) impaired metabolism (e.g. due to hepatic insufficiency). In alcoholics, many mechanisms contribute to thiamin deficiency; they include decreased intake, impaired absorption and use, increased demand, and possibly an apo-enzyme defect.

Pathophysiology

Thiamin deficiency causes degeneration of peripheral nerves, thalamus, mammillary bodies, and cerebellum. Cerebral blood flow is markedly reduced, and vascular resistance is increased. The heart may become dilated; muscle fibers become swollen, fragmented, and vacuolized, with interstitial spaces dilated by fluid. Vasodilation occurs and can result in edema in the feet and legs. Arteriovenous shunting of blood increases. Eventually, high-output heart failure may occur.

Signs and Symptoms

Early symptoms are nonspecific: fatigue, irritability, poor memory, sleep disturbances, precordial pain, anorexia, and abdominal discomfort. **Dry beriberi** refers to peripheral neurologic deficits due to thiamin deficiency. These deficits are bilateral and roughly symmetric, occurring in a stocking-glove distribution. They affect predominantly the lower extremities, beginning with paresthesias in the toes, burning in the feet (particularly severe at night), muscle cramps in the calves, pains in the legs, and plantar dysesthesias. Calf muscle tenderness, difficulty rising from a squatting position, and decreased vibratory sensation in the toes are early signs. Muscle wasting occurs. Continued deficiency worsens polyneuropathy, which can eventually affect the arms.

Wernicke–Korsakoff syndrome, which combines Wernicke encephalopathy and Korsakoff psychosis, occurs in some alcoholics who do not consume foods fortified with thiamin. Wernicke encephalopathy consists of psychomotor slowing or apathy, nystagmus, ataxia, ophthalmoplegia, impaired consciousness, and, if untreated, coma and death. It probably results from severe acute deficiency superimposed on chronic deficiency. Korsakoff psychosis consists of mental confusion, dysphonia, and confabulation with impaired memory of recent events. It probably results from chronic deficiency and may develop after repeated episodes of Wernicke encephalopathy.

Cardiovascular (wet) beriberi is myocardial disease due to thiamin deficiency. The first effects are vasodilation, tachycardia, a wide pulse pressure, sweating, warm skin, and lactic acidosis. Later, heart failure develops, causing orthopnea and pulmonary and peripheral edema. Vasodilation can continue, sometimes resulting in shock.

Infantile beriberi occurs in infants (usually by age 3–4 weeks) who are breast fed by thiamin-deficient mothers. Heart failure (which may occur suddenly), aphonia, and absent deep tendon reflexes are characteristic. Because thiamin is necessary for glucose metabolism, glucose infusions may precipitate or worsen symptoms of deficiency in thiamin-deficient people.

Diagnosis

Diagnosis of thiamin deficiency is usually based on a favorable response to treatment with thiamin in a patient with symptoms or signs of deficiency. Similar bilateral lower extremity polyneuropathies due to other disorders (e.g. diabetes, alcoholism, vitamin B12 deficiency, heavy metal poisoning) do not respond to thiamin. Single-nerve neuritides (mononeuropathies; e.g. sciatica) and multiple mononeuropathies (mononeuritis multiplex) are unlikely to result from thiamin deficiency. Electrolytes, including magnesium, should be measured to exclude other causes. For confirmation in equivocal cases, erythrocyte transketolase activity and 24-hours urinary thiamin excretion may be measured. Diagnosis of cardiovascular beriberi can be difficult if other disorders that cause heart failure are present. A therapeutic trial of thiamin can help.

Treatment

Ensuring that dietary supplies of thiamin are adequate is important regardless of symptoms. Because IV glucose can worsen thiamin deficiency, alcoholics and others at risk of thiamin deficiency should receive IV thiamin 100 mg before receiving IV glucose solutions.

The thiamin dose is 10–20 mg by mouth once a day for 2 weeks for mild polyneuropathy, for moderate or advanced neuropathy 20–30 mg/day, continued for several weeks after symptoms disappear, for edema and congestion due to cardiovascular beriberi: 100 mg IV once a day for several days.

For **Wernicke–Korsakoff syndrome,** thiamin 50–100 mg IM or IV bid must usually be given for several days, followed by 10–20 mg once a day until a therapeutic response is obtained. Anaphylactic reactions to IV thiamin are rare. Symptoms of ophthalmoplegia may resolve in a day; improvement in patients with Korsakoff psychosis may take 1–3 months. Recovery from neurologic deficits is often incomplete in Wernicke-Korsakoff syndrome and in other forms of thiamin deficiency. Because thiamin deficiency often occurs with other B vitamin deficiencies, multiple water-soluble vitamins are usually given for several weeks. Patients should continue to consume a nutritious diet, supplying 1–2 times the daily recommended intake of vitamins; all alcohol intake should stop.

RIBOFLAVIN

Riboflavin (vitamin B2) functions primarily as a component of two coenzymes, flavin mononucleotide (FMN) and flavin adenine dinucleotide (FAD). These two coenzymes catalyze various oxidation–reduction reactions. The parent compound [riboflavin, 7, 8-dimethyl-10-(I'-Dribityl) isoalloxazine] is a yellow fluorescent compound whose major physiologic role is to act as a precursor for FMN (riboflavin-5'-phosphate) and FAD. FMN is formed from riboflavin by flavokinase-catalyzed phosphorylation, and FAD is formed from FMN and ATP by the action of FAD synthetase, also called pyrophosphorylase (Fig. 18.8).

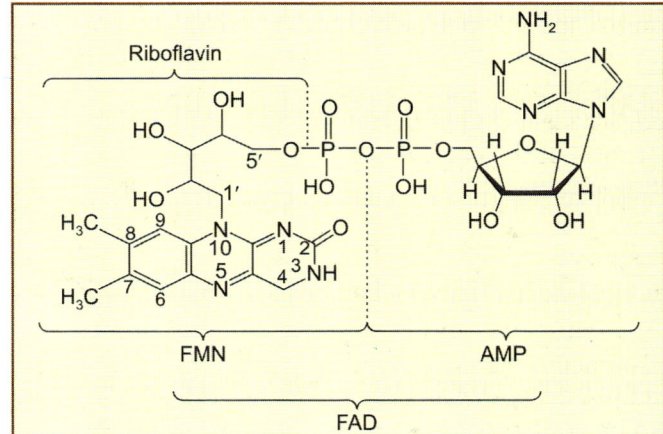

Fig. 18.8: Riboflavin and flavin mononucleotide (FMN) as components of flavin adenine dinucleotide (FAD)

Dietary riboflavin is absorbed in the small intestine. The body stores of a well-nourished person are adequate to prevent riboflavin deficiency for 5 months. Excess riboflavin is excreted in the urine and has no known toxicity. Foods high in riboflavin include milk, liver, eggs, meat, and leafy vegetables. Riboflavin deficiency occurs with other nutritional deficiencies, alcoholism, and chronic diarrhea and malabsorption. Certain drugs antagonize the action or metabolism of riboflavin, including phenothiazine, oral contraceptives, and tricyclic antidepressants. The RDA of riboflavin is 1.3 mg/d for adult males and 1.1 mg/d for adult females. Reduced glutathione reductase activity greater than 40% is an indication of deficiency.

RIBOFLAVIN DEFICIENCY

Riboflavin deficiency usually occurs with other B vitamin deficiencies.

Etiology

Primary riboflavin deficiency results from inadequate intake of fortified cereals, milk and other animal products. secondary riboflavin deficiency is most commonly caused as a result of chronic diarrhea, malabsorption syndromes, liver disorders, hemodialysis, peritoneal dialysis, long-term use of barbiturates and chronic alcoholism.

Signs and Symptoms

The most common signs of riboflavin deficiency are pallor and maceration of the mucosa at the angles of the mouth (angular stomatitis) and vermilion surfaces of the lips (cheilosis), eventually replaced by superficial linear fissures. The fissures can become infected with *Candida albicans,* causing grayish white lesions (perlèche). The tongue may appear magenta. Seborrheic dermatitis develops, usually affecting the nasolabial folds, ears, eyelids, and scrotum or labia majora. These areas become red, scaly, and greasy. Rarely, neovascularization and keratitis of the cornea occur, causing lacrimation and photophobia.

Diagnosis

The lesions characteristic of riboflavin deficiency are nonspecific. Riboflavin deficiency should be suspected if characteristic signs develop in a patient with other B vitamin deficiencies. Diagnosis of riboflavin deficiency can be confirmed by a therapeutic trial or laboratory testing, usually by measuring urinary excretion of riboflavin.

Treatment

Riboflavin 5–10 mg by mouth once a day is given until recovery. Other water-soluble vitamins should also be given.

VITAMIN B6

Pyridoxine (pyridoxol), pyridoxamine, and pyridoxal are the three natural forms of vitamin B6. They are converted to pyridoxal phosphate, which is required for synthesis, catabolism, and interconversion of amino acids. The vitamin B6 group comprises three natural forms: pyridoxine (pyridoxol) (PN), pyridoxamine (PM), and pyridoxal (PL), which are 4-substituted 2-methyl-3-hydroxyl-5- hydroxymethyl pyridines (Fig. 18.9).

The major dietary sources of vitamin B6 are meat, poultry, fish, potatoes, and vegetables; dairy products and grains contribute lesser amounts. Readily absorbed from the intestinal tract, vitamin B6 is excreted in the urine in the form of metabolites. Vitamin B6 deficiency rarely occurs alone; it is more commonly seen in patients deficient in several B vitamins. Those particularly at risk for deficiency are patients with uremia, liver disease, absorption syndromes, malignancies, or chronic alcoholism. High intake of proteins increases the requirements for vitamin B6. Deficiency is associated with hyper homocysteinemia. Vitamin B6 has low toxicity because of its water-soluble nature; however, extremely high doses may cause peripheral neuropathy. The RDA of vitamin B6 is 1.3–1.7 mg/d for adult males and 1.3– 1.5 mg/d for adult females, depending on age.

Vitamin B6 Deficiency and Dependency

Because vitamin B6 is present in most foods, dietary deficiency is rare. Secondary deficiency may result from various conditions. Symptoms can include peripheral neuropathy, a pellagra-like syndrome, anemia, and seizures, which, particularly in infants, may not resolve when treated with anticonvulsants. Impaired metabolism (dependency) is rare; it causes various symptoms, including seizures, intellectual disability, and anemia.

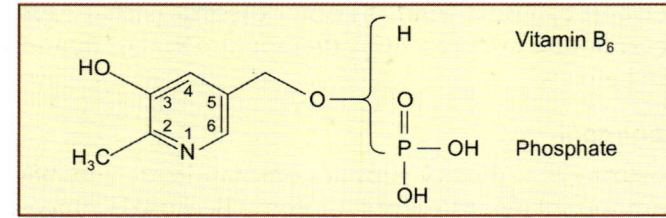

Fig. 18.9: Free and phosphorylated forms of vitamin B6• R = CH_2OH for pyridoxine, CH_2NH_2 for pyridoxamine, and CHO for pyridoxal

Diagnosis is usually clinical; no laboratory test readily assesses vitamin B6 status. Treatment consists of giving oral vitamin B6 and, when possible, treating the cause.

Etiology

Dietary vitamin B6 deficiency, though rare, can develop because extensive processing can deplete foods of vitamin B6. Secondary **vitamin B6 deficiency** most often results from (1) protein-energy undernutrition, (2) malabsorption, (3) alcoholism, (4) use of pyridoxine-inactivating drugs (e.g. anticonvulsants, isoniazid, cycloserine, hydralazine, corticosteroids, penicillamine) and (5) excessive loss during hemodialysis. Rarely, secondary deficiency results from increased metabolic demand (e.g. in hyperthyroidism).

Signs and Symptoms

Vitamin B6 deficiency causes peripheral neuropathy and a pellagra-like syndrome, with seborrheic dermatitis, glossitis, and cheilosis, and, in adults, can cause depression, confusion, EEG abnormalities, and seizures. Rarely, deficiency or dependency causes seizures in infants. Seizures, particularly in infants, may be refractory to treatment with anticonvulsants. Normocytic, microcytic, or sideroblastic anemia can also develop.

Diagnosis

Diagnosis of vitamin B6 deficiency is usually clinical. There is no single accepted laboratory test of vitamin B6 status; measurement of serum pyridoxal phosphate is most common.

Treatment

For secondary vitamin B6 deficiency, causes (e.g. use of pyridoxine-inactivating drugs, malabsorption) should be corrected if possible. Usually, pyridoxine 50–100 mg by mouth once a day corrects the deficiency in adults. Most people taking isoniazid should also be given pyridoxine 30–50 mg by mouth once a day. For deficiency due to increased metabolic demand, amounts larger than the daily recommended intake may be required. For most cases of inborn errors of metabolism, high doses of pyridoxine may be effective.

Vitamin B6 Toxicity

The ingestion of megadoses (>500 mg/day) of pyridoxine (e.g. taken to treat carpal tunnel syndrome or premenstrual syndrome although efficacy is unproved) may cause peripheral neuropathy with deficits in a stocking-glove distribution, including progressive sensory ataxia and severe impairment of position and vibration senses. Senses of touch, temperature, and pain are less affected. Motor and central nervous systems are usually intact.

Treatment of vitamin B6 toxicity is to stop taking vitamin B6. Recovery is slow and, for some patients, incomplete.

NIACIN

The term niacin refers to nicotinic acid (pyridine-3-carboxylic acid), its amide nicotinamide, and derivatives that show the same biological activity as nicotinamide. A distinction between the two primary vitamin forms has to be considered, however, when some aspects of their metabolism and especially their different pharmacologic actions at high doses are considered. Structures of both vitamers and the two coenzyme forms containing the nicotinamide moiety are given (Fig. 18.10). The requirement for niacin in humans is met, to some extent, by the conversion of dietary tryptophan to niacin. Niacin is absorbed in the small intestine, and excess is excreted in the form of metabolites in the urine.

Niacin Deficiency

Dietary niacin deficiency pellagra (Fig. 18.11) is uncommon in developed countries. Clinical manifestations include the three Ds—(1) localized pigmented rash (dermatitis); (2) gastroenteritis (diarrhea); and (3) widespread neurologic deficits, including cognitive decline (dementia). Diagnosis is usually clinical, and dietary supplementation (oral or, if needed, IM) is usually successful.

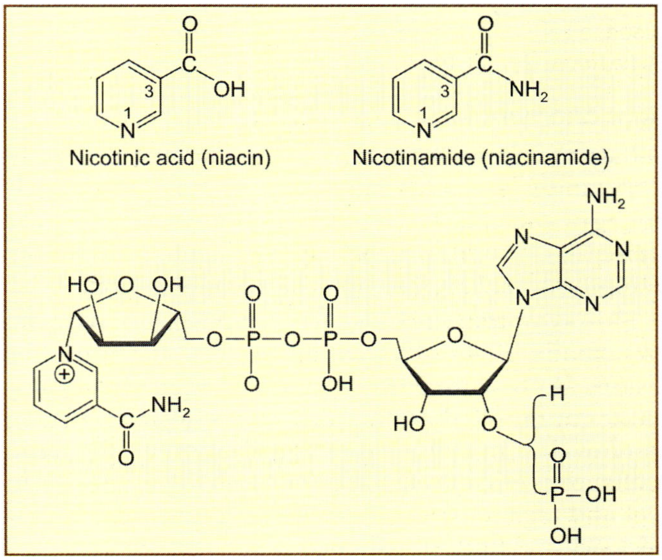

Fig. 18.10: Niacin, niacinamide, and coenzyme

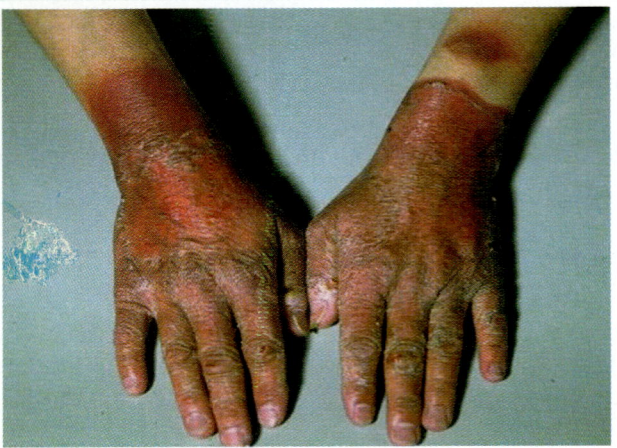

Fig.18.11: Erythematous to brown plaques on the sun-exposed dorsal surface of both hands resulting from niacin deficiency

Etiology

Primary niacin deficiency results from extremely inadequate intake of both niacin and tryptophan, which usually occurs in areas where maize (Indian corn) constitutes a substantial part of the diet. Bound niacin, found in maize, is not assimilated in the GI tract unless it has been previously treated with alkali, as when tortillas are prepared. Corn protein is also deficient in tryptophan. The high incidence of pellagra in India among people who eat millet with a high leucine content has led to the hypothesis that amino acid imbalance may contribute to deficiency. Deficiencies of protein and many B vitamins commonly accompany primary niacin deficiency.

Secondary niacin deficiency may be due to diarrhea, cirrhosis, or alcoholism. Pellagra also may occur in carcinoid syndrome (tryptophan is diverted to form 5-hydroxytryptophan and serotonin) and in Hartnup disease (absorption of tryptophan by the intestine and kidneys is defective).

Signs and Symptoms

Pellagra is characterized by skin, mucous membrane, CNS, and gastrointestinal (GI) symptoms. Advanced pellagra can cause a symmetric photosensitive rash, stomatitis, glossitis, diarrhea, and mental aberrations. Symptoms may appear alone or in combination.

Skin symptoms include several types of lesions, which are usually bilaterally symmetric. The distribution of lesions at pressure points or sun-exposed skin is more pathognomonic than the form of the lesions. Lesions can develop in a glove like distribution on the hands (pellagrous glove) or in a boot-shaped distribution on the feet and legs (pellagrous boot). Sunlight causes Casal necklace and butterfly-shaped lesions on the face.

Mucous membrane symptoms affect primarily the mouth but, may also affect the vagina and urethra.

Glossitis and stomatitis characterize acute deficiency. As the deficiency progresses, the tongue and oral mucous membranes become reddened, followed by pain in the mouth, increased salivation, and edema of the tongue. Ulcerations may appear, especially under the tongue, on the mucosa of the lower lip, and opposite the molar teeth.

GI symptoms early in the deficiency include burning in the pharynx and esophagus and abdominal discomfort and distention. Constipation is common. Later, nausea, vomiting, and diarrhea may occur. Diarrhea is often bloody because of bowel hyperemia and ulceration.

CNS symptoms include psychosis, encephalopathy (characterized by impaired consciousness), and cognitive decline (dementia). Psychosis is characterized by memory impairment, disorientation, confusion, and confabulation; the predominant symptom may be excitement, depression, mania, delirium, or paranoia.

Diagnosis

Diagnosis of niacin deficiency is clinical and may be straightforward when skin and mouth lesions, diarrhea, delirium, and dementia occur simultaneously. More often, the presentation is not so specific. Differentiating the CNS changes from those in thiamin deficiency is difficult. A history of a diet lacking niacin and tryptophan may help establish the diagnosis. A favorable response to treatment with niacin can usually confirm it.

If available, laboratory testing can help confirm the diagnosis, particularly when the diagnosis is otherwise unclear. Urinary excretion of N1-methylnicotinamide (NMN) is decreased; <5.8 µmol/day suggests a niacin deficiency.

Treatment

Because multiple deficiencies are common, a balanced diet, including other B vitamins (particularly riboflavin and pyridoxine), is needed.

Nicotinamide is usually used to treat niacin deficiency, because nicotinamide, unlike nicotinic acid (the most common form of niacin), does not cause flushing, itching, burning, or tingling sensations. Nicotinamide is given in doses in doses of 250–500 mg by mouth daily.

Niacin Toxicity

Niacin (nicotinic acid) in large amounts is sometimes used to lower low-density lipoprotein (LDL) cholesterol and triglyceride levels and to increase high-density lipoprotein (HDL) cholesterol levels. Symptoms may include flushing and, rarely, hepatotoxicity.

Immediate and sustained-release preparations of niacin (but not nicotinamide) may affect lipid levels. However, whether niacin reduces risk of coronary artery disease and stroke is unclear.

At intermediate doses (1000 mg/day), niacin has the following effects: higher doses of niacin (3000 mg/day) reduce LDL cholesterol 15–20%, but may cause jaundice, abdominal discomfort, blurred vision, worsening of hyperglycemia, and precipitation of preexisting gout. People with a liver disorder probably should not take high-dose niacin.

Flushing, which is prostaglandin-mediated, is more common with immediate-release preparations. It may be more intense after alcohol ingestion, aerobic activity, sun exposure, and consumption of spicy foods. Flushing is minimized if niacin is taken after meals or if aspirin (325 mg, which may work better than lower doses) is taken 30–45 minutes before niacin. The chance of severe flushing can be reduced by starting immediate-release niacin at a low dose (e.g. 50 mg 3 times a day) and increasing it very slowly.

Hepatotoxicity may be more common with some sustained-release preparations. Some authorities recommend checking levels of uric acid, blood glucose, and plasma aminotransferases every 6–8 weeks until the dose of niacin has been stabilized.

FOLIC ACID

Folic acid serves as a carrier of one-carbon groups in many metabolic reactions. It is required for the biosynthesis of compounds, such as choline, serine, glycine, purines, and deoxythymidine monophosphate (dTMP). Folate and folic acid are generic terms for a family of compounds that function as coenzymes in the processing of one carbon units and that are derived from pteroic acid (Pte), to which one or more molecules of glutamic acid are attached. Pteroic acid is composed of a pteridine ring joined to a p-aminobenzoic acid residue (Fig. 18.12).

Folates are involved in RBC maturation and synthesis of purines and pyrimidines. They are required for development of the fetal nervous system. Absorption occurs in the duodenum and upper jejunum. Enterohepatic circulation of folate occurs.

Folate supplements do not protect against coronary artery disease or stroke (even though they lower homocysteine levels); current evidence does not support claims that folate supplementation increases or reduces the risk of various cancers. The upper limit for folate intake is 1000 µg; higher daily doses (up to 4 mg) are recommended for women who have had a baby with a neural tube defect. Folate is essentially nontoxic. Women taking both oral contraceptives and anticonvulsants may need to take folate supplements to maintain birth control effectiveness.

Folate levels may be measured in serum using a microbiologic assay with *Lactobacillus casei* or a competitive protein-binding assay for levels in serum and erythrocytes. When folate deficiency develops, serum levels fall first, followed by a decrease in erythrocyte folate levels and ultimately hematologic manifestation. Measuring both serum and erythrocyte levels is helpful because serum levels indicate circulating folate and erythrocyte levels better approximate stores.

Serum contains endogenous binding proteins that can bind folate and result in falsely low serum folate concentration measurements. Although, measurement of red blood cell folate concentration has advantages over the serum assay for the diagnosis of megaloblastic anemia, analytic problems may result from the various forms of folate in erythrocytes. Folate in the serum is almost exclusively present in the monoglutamate form;

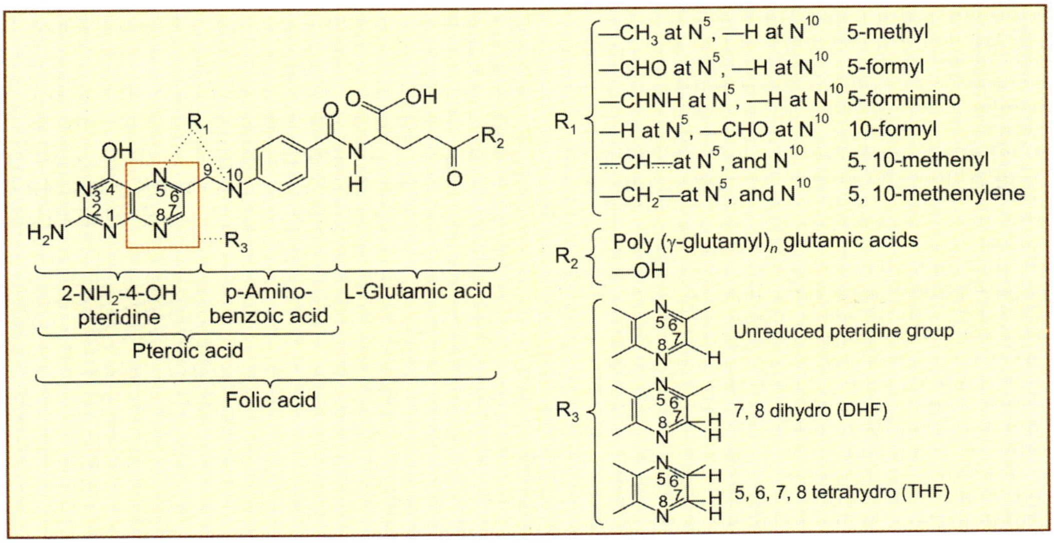

Fig. 18.12: Structure and relationships of folic acid and its derivatives

however, in red blood cells, it is in the poly glutamate form and as high-molecular-weight complexes.

Folate Deficiency

Folate deficiency is common. It may result from inadequate intake, malabsorption, or use of various drugs. Deficiency causes megaloblastic anemia (indistinguishable from that due to vitamin B12 deficiency). Maternal deficiency increases the risk of neural tube birth defects. Diagnosis requires laboratory testing to confirm. Measurement of neutrophil hyper segmentation is sensitive and readily available. Treatment with oral folate is usually successful.

Etiology

The most common causes of folate deficiency are; inadequate intake (usually in patients with under nutrition or alcoholism), increased demand (e.g. due to pregnancy or lactation), and impaired absorption (e.g. in celiac disease or due to certain drugs). Deficiency can also result from inadequate bioavailability and increased excretion (Table 18.3).

Prolonged cooking destroys folate, predisposing to inadequate intake. Intake is sometimes barely adequate (e.g. in alcoholics). Liver stores provide only a several-month supply.

Alcohol interferes with folate absorption, metabolism, renal excretion, and enterohepatic reabsorption and reduces healthy food intake. 5-fluorouracil, metformin, methotrexate, phenobarbital, phenytoin, sulfasalazine, triamterene, and trimethoprim impair folate metabolism.

Signs and Symptoms

Folate deficiency may cause glossitis, diarrhea, depression, and confusion. Anemia may develop insidiously and, because of compensatory mechanisms, be more severe than symptoms suggest.

Folate deficiency during pregnancy increases the risk of fetal neural tube defects and perhaps other brain defects.

Diagnosis

Complete blood count (CBC) may indicate megaloblastic anemia indistinguishable from that of vitamin B12 deficiency. If serum folate is <7 nmol/L, deficiency is likely. Serum folate reflects folate status unless intake has recently increased or decreased. If intake has changed, erythrocyte (RBC) folate level better reflects tissue stores. A level of <305 nmol/L indicates inadequate status.

Also, an increase in the homocysteine level suggests tissue folate deficiency (but the level is also affected by vitamin B12 and vitamin B6 levels, renal insufficiency, and genetic factors). A normal methylmalonic acid (MMA) level may differentiate folate deficiency from vitamin B12 deficiency because MMA levels rise in vitamin B12 deficiency but not in folate deficiency.

Treatment

Folate 400–1000 μg by mouth once a day replenishes tissues and is usually successful even if deficiency has resulted from malabsorption. The normal requirement is 400 μg a day. (Caution: In patients with megaloblastic anemia, vitamin B12 deficiency must be ruled out before treating with folate. If vitamin B12 deficiency is present, folate supplementation can alleviate the anemia but does not reverse, and may even worsen, neurologic deficits.)

For pregnant women, the recommended daily allowance is 600 μg/day. For women who have had a fetus or infant with a neural tube defect, the recommended dose is 4000 μg/day, started 1 month before conception (if possible) and continued until 3 months after conception.

VITAMIN B12

Vitamin B12 (cobalamin) refers to a large group of cobalt containing compounds. Intestinal absorption of vitamin B12 takes place in the ileum and is mediated by a unique binding protein called intrinsic factor, which is secreted by the stomach. Vitamin B12 participates as a coenzyme in enzymatic reactions necessary for hematopoiesis and fatty acid metabolism. Vitamin B12 composed of tetrapyrrole rings surrounding central cobalt atoms and nucleotide side chains attached to the cobalt. The cobalamin tetrapyrrole ring, exclusive of cobalt and other

Table 18.3	Causes of folate deficiency
Cause	Source
Inadequate intake	Diet lacking raw green vegetables or enriched grains, chronic alcoholism, TPN
Impaired absorption	Celiac disease, sprue, other malabsorption syndromes, anticonvulsants, congenital or acquired folate malabsorption
Inadequate utilization	Folate antagonists (metformin, methotrexate, triamterene, trime thoprim), anticonvulsants, congenital or acquired enzyme deficiency, alcoholism
Increased demand	Pregnancy, lactation, infancy, increased metabolism
Increased excretion	Renal dialysis (peritoneal or hemodialysis)

side chains, is called a corrin. All compounds containing this corrin nucleus are corrinoids. The cobalt-corrin complex is termed cobamide. In cobalamins, 5,6-dimethylbenzimidazole riboside is bound to the cobalt atom by one of its imidazole nitrogens, and its 2'-ribose carbon is linked with an ester of aminoisopropanol and propionic acid to the corrin ring (Fig. 18.13).

Excess vitamin B12 is excreted in the urine. Vitamin B12 bears a corrin ring (containing pyrroles similar to porphyrin) linked to a central cobalt atom. Different corrinoid compounds, or cobalamins, are distinguished by the substituent linked to the cobalt. The active cofactor forms of vitamin B12 are methylcobalamin and deoxyadenosylcobalamin. The primary dietary sources for vitamin B12 are from animal products (e.g. meat, eggs, and milk). Therefore, total vegetarian diets are likely to be deficient or low in vitamin B12. Animals derive vitamin B12 from intestinal microbial synthesis. The average daily diet contains 3–30 μg of vitamin B12, of which 1–5 μg is absorbed.

The frequency of dietary deficiency increases with age, occurring in more than 0.5% of people older than 60, 70, although, the symptoms resulting from dietary deficiency are rare. Most vitamin B12 absorption occurs through a complex with intrinsic factor, a protein secreted by gastric parietal cells. This intrinsic factor–B12 complex binds with specific ileal receptors. 'Blocking' intrinsic factor antibodies prevents binding of vitamin B12 to intrinsic factor, and 'binding' antibodies can combine with either free intrinsic factor or the intrinsic factor B12 complex,

preventing attachment of the complex to ileal receptors and intestinal uptake of the vitamin. Parietal cell antibodies have also been identified as a cause of pernicious anemia. After release from the intrinsic factor complex within the mucosal cell, vitamin B12 circulates in plasma bound to specific transport proteins and is deposited in liver, bone marrow, and other tissues. There is a significant enterohepatic circulation of vitamin B12. Plasma contains both types of transport proteins, transcobalamins, and the three forms of vitamin B12 (hydroxocobalamin, methylcobalamin, and deoxyadenosylcobalamin).

In the Schilling test, the patient receives a small, oral dose of radiolabeled vitamin B12. Parenteral B12 is given simultaneously to saturate binding sites. Serum and urine are collected at intervals, and labeled B12 is measured in the specimens. Patients who cannot absorb vitamin B12 (usually a deficiency of intrinsic factor, as in perniciousanemia) cannot absorb the labeled B12 and, therefore, have low levels in the blood and urine.

The term pernicious anemia is now most commonly applied to vitamin B12 deficiency resulting from lack of intrinsic factor. Antibodies to intrinsic factor and parietal cells are common in patients with pernicious anemia, their healthy relatives, and patients with other auto-immune disorders. Deficiency of B12 can occasionally occur in strict vegetarians because of dietary deficiency.

A loss of vitamin B12 also occurs in individuals infected with fish tapeworm or because of malabsorption diseases, such as sprue or celiac disease. Low vitamin B12 levels occur with folate deficiency, and a vitamin B12 deficiency can be masked by large doses of folate. Toxicity of vitamin B12 has not been reported.

The RDA of vitamin B12 for adults is 2.4 μg/d. Assay methods for B12 are either microbiologic assay using *Lactobacillus leichmannii* competitive protein-binding radioimmunoassay (RIA) or an enzyme immunoassay.

Deficiency of vitamin B12 causes two major disorders; megaloblastic anemia (pernicious anemia) and a neurologic disorder called combined systems disorder. The neurologic manifestations are variable and may be subtle. For this reason, vitamin B12 deficiency should be considered a cause of any unexplained macrocytic anemia or neurologic disorder, especially in an elderly person. Serum vitamin B12 may be used in the initial assessment. Methylmalonic acid levels may be more definitive because the lower reference limit of B12 is unclear. Patients with pernicious anemia usually have atrophic gastritis and have an increased incidence of gastric carcinoma. The reference range for vitamin B12 is 81.2–590.4 pmol/L. The most common methods for determination of vitamin B12 are the competitive

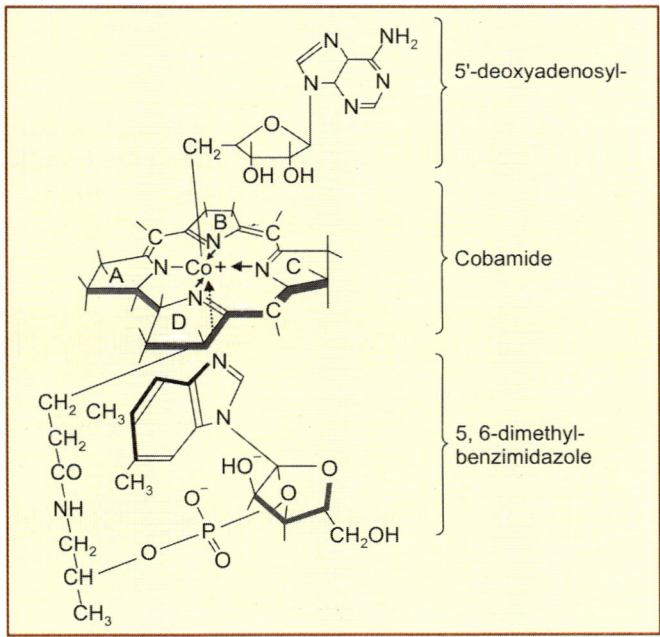

Fig. 18.13: The structure of 5'-deoxyadenosyl cobalamin

protein-binding RIAs, which are based on the principle that vitamin B12 released from endogenous binding proteins can be measured by its competition with co-labeled B12 for a limited amount of specific binding protein.

The binding proteins typically used are animal intrinsic factors. Special measures must be taken to eliminate interference caused by other, nonspecific protein binders of vitamin B12. Several non-radioisotopic assays for vitamin B12 have been developed for routine laboratory use.

Vitamin B12 Deficiency

Dietary vitamin B12 deficiency usually results from inadequate absorption, but deficiency can develop in vegans who do not take vitamin supplements. Deficiency causes megaloblastic anemia, damage to the white matter of the spinal cord and brain, and peripheral neuropathy. Diagnosis is usually made by measuring serum vitamin B12 levels. The Schilling test helps determine etiology. Treatment consists of oral or parenteral vitamin B12. Folate (folic acid) should not be used instead of vitamin B12 because folate may alleviate the anemia but allow neurologic deficits to progress.

Etiology

Vitamin B12 deficiency can result from; **inadequate vitamin B12 intake** is possible in vegans, but is otherwise unlikely. Breastfed babies of vegan mothers may develop vitamin B12 deficiency by age 4–6 months because in these babies, liver stores (which are normally extensive in other babies) are limited and their rapid growth rate results in high demand.

Inadequate vitamin B12 absorption is the most common cause of deficiency (Table 18.4). In the elderly, inadequate absorption most commonly results from decreased acid secretion. In such cases, crystalline vitamin B12 (such as that available in vitamin supplements) can be absorbed, but food-bound vitamin B12 is not liberated and absorbed normally.

Inadequate absorption may occur in blind loop syndrome (with overgrowth of bacteria) or fish tapeworm infestation; in these cases, bacteria, or parasites use ingested vitamin B12, so that less is available for absorption. Vitamin B12 absorption may be inadequate if ileal absorptive sites are destroyed by inflammatory bowel disease or are surgically removed.

Less common causes of inadequate vitamin B12 absorption include chronic pancreatitis, gastric or bariatric surgery, malabsorption syndromes, acquired immunodeficiency syndrome (AIDS), use of certain drugs (e.g. antacids, metformin), repeated exposure to nitrous oxide, and a genetic disorder causing malabsorption in the ileum (Imerslund–Graesbeck syndrome). Less commonly, **decreased utilization of vitamin B12** or **use of certain drugs** causes vitamin B12 deficiency (Table 18.4).

Pernicious anemia is often used synonymously with vitamin B12 deficiency. However, pernicious anemia specifically refers to anemia resulting from vitamin B12 deficiency caused by an autoimmune metaplastic atrophic gastritis with loss of intrinsic factor. Patients with classic pernicious anemia, most commonly younger adults, are at increased risk of stomach and other GI cancers.

Signs and Symptoms

Anemia usually develops insidiously. It is often more severe than its symptoms indicate because its slow evolution allows physiologic adaptation. Occasionally, splenomegaly and hepatomegaly occur. Various GI symptoms, including weight loss and poorly localized abdominal pain, may occur. Glossitis, usually described as burning of the tongue, is uncommon. Neurologic symptoms develop independently from and often without hematologic abnormalities.

Subacute combined degeneration refers to degenerative changes in the nervous system due to vitamin B12 deficiency; they affect mostly brain and spinal cord white matter. Demyelinating or axonal peripheral neuropathies can occur.

Table 18.4	Causes of vitamin B12 deficiency
Cause	**Source**
Inadequate diet	Vegan diet, breast-feeding of infants by vegan mothers, fad diets
Impaired absorption	Lack of intrinsic factor (due to autoimmune metaplastic atrophic gastritis, destruction of gastric mucosa, gastric surgery, or gastric bypass surgery)
	Intrinsic factor inhibition
	Decreased acid secretion, small-bowel disorders (e.g. inflammatory bowel disease, celiac disease, cancer, biliary or pancreatic disorders)
	Competition for vitamin B12 (in fish tapeworm infestation or blind loop syndrome), AIDS
Inadequate utilization	Enzyme deficiencies, liver disorders, transport protein abnormality
Drugs	Antacids, metformin, nitrous oxide (repeated exposure)

In early stages, decreased position and vibratory sensation in the extremities is accompanied by mild to moderate weakness and hyporeflexia. In later stages, spasticity, extensor plantar responses, greater loss of position and vibratory sensation in the lower extremities, and ataxia emerge. These deficits may develop in a stocking-glove distribution. Tactile, pain, and temperature sensations are usually spared but may be difficult to assess in the elderly.

Some patients are also irritable and mildly depressed. Paranoia (megaloblastic madness), delirium, confusion, and, at times, postural hypotension may occur in advanced cases. The confusion may be difficult to differentiate from age-related dementias, such as Alzheimer disease.

Diagnosis

It is important to remember that severe neurologic disease may occur without anemia or macrocytosis. Diagnosis of vitamin B12 deficiency is based on CBC and vitamin B12 and folate levels. CBC usually detects megaloblastic anemia. Tissue deficiency and macrocytic indexes may precede the development of anemia. A vitamin B12 level <145 pmol/L indicates vitamin B12 deficiency. The folate level is measured because vitamin B12 deficiency must be differentiated from folate deficiency as a cause of megaloblastic anemia; folate supplementation can mask vitamin B12 deficiency and may alleviate megaloblastic anemia but allow the neurologic deficits to progress or even accelerate.

When clinical judgment suggests vitamin B12 deficiency but the vitamin B12 level is low-normal 145–260 pmol/L or hematologic indexes are normal, other tests can be done. They include measuring the following:

- *Serum methylmalonic acid levels:* An elevated MMA level supports vitamin B12 deficiency, but may be due to renal failure. MMA levels can also be used to monitor the response to treatment. MMA levels remain normal in folate deficiency.
- *Homocysteine levels:* Levels may be elevated with either vitamin B12 or folate deficiency.
- Less commonly, *holotranscobalamin II (transcobalamin II–B12 complex) content:* When holotranscobalamin II is <30 pmol/L, vitamin B12 is deficient.

After vitamin B12 deficiency is diagnosed, additional tests (e.g. Schilling test) may be indicated for younger adults but usually not for the elderly. Unless dietary vitamin B12 is obviously inadequate, serum gastrin levels or autoantibodies to intrinsic factor may be measured; sensitivity and specificity of these tests may be poor.

Schilling Test

The schilling test is useful only if diagnosing intrinsic factor deficiency is important, as in classic pernicious anemia. This test is not necessary for most elderly patients. The Schilling test measures absorption of free radiolabeled vitamin B12. Radiolabeled vitamin B12 is given orally, followed in 1–6 hours by 1000 µg (1 mg) of parenteral vitamin B12, which reduces uptake of radiolabeled vitamin B12 by the liver. Absorbed radiolabeled vitamin B12 is excreted in urine, which is collected for 24 hours. The amount excreted is measured, and the percentage of total radiolabeled vitamin B12 is determined. If absorption is normal, ≥9% of the dose given appears in the urine. Reduced urinary excretion (<5% if kidney function is normal) indicates inadequate vitamin B12 absorption. Improved absorption with the subsequent addition of intrinsic factor to radiolabeled vitamin B12 confirms the diagnosis of pernicious anemia.

The test is often difficult to do or interpret because of incomplete urine collection or renal insufficiency. In addition, because the Schilling test does not measure absorption of protein-bound vitamin B12, the test does not detect defective liberation of vitamin B12 from foods, which is common among the elderly. The Schilling test repletes vitamin B12 and can mask deficiency, so it should be done only after all other diagnostic tests and therapeutic trials. If malabsorption is identified, the Schilling test can be repeated after a 2-weeks trial of an oral antibiotic. If antibiotic therapy corrects malabsorption, the likely cause is intestinal overgrowth of bacteria (e.g. blind-loop syndrome).

Treatment

Vitamin B12 1000–2000 µg by mouth can be given once a day to patients who do not have severe deficiency or neurologic symptoms or signs. A nasal gel preparation of vitamin B12 is available at a higher price. Large oral doses can be absorbed by mass action, even when intrinsic factor is absent. If the MMA level (sometimes used to monitor treatment) does not decrease, patients may not be taking vitamin B12.

For more severe deficiency, vitamin B12 1 mg IM is usually given 1–4 times/week for several weeks until hematologic abnormalities are corrected; then it is given once a month.

Although, hematologic abnormalities are usually corrected within 6 weeks (reticulocyte count should improve within 1 week), resolution of neurologic symptoms may take much longer. Neurologic symptoms that persist for months or years become irreversible. In most elderly people with vitamin B12 deficiency and dementia, cognition does not improve after treatment. Vitamin B12 treatment must be continued for life unless the pathophysiologic mechanism for the deficiency is corrected. Infants of vegan mothers should receive supplemental vitamin B12 from birth.

BIOTIN

Biotin (also known as vitamin H) is the prosthetic group for a number of carboxylation reactions (e.g. pyruvate, acetyl- CoA, propionyl Co-A, decarboxylases). Biotin is cis-tetrahydro-2-oxothieno [3,4-d] -imidazoline-4- valeric acid (Fig. 18.14). The vitamin in most organisms occurs mainly bound to protein. The ε-amino group of the lysyl side-chain of protein is linked via an amide function involving the carboxyl group of the valeryl side-chain of biotin. In addition, some biotin is linked non-covalently as a complex with avidin, a protein in egg white.

Dietary biotin is absorbed in the small intestine, but it is also synthesized in the gut by bacteria. Numerous foods contain biotin, although no food is especially rich (up to 20 µg/100 g). The dietary intake of biotin, while low in the neonatal period, increases as newborns switch from colostrum to mature breast milk. Biotin deficiency can be produced by ingestion of large amounts of avidin, found in raw egg whites that bind to biotin.

Biotin deficiency has been noted in patients receiving long-term parenteral nutrition (PN) and in infants with genetic defects of carboxylase and biotinidase enzymes. The AI for biotin is 30 µg/d.

Assays had been performed using microbiology functional assay and the *Lactobacillus* organism. Newer methods of isotopic dilution, chemiluminescent, and photometric assays are now available but rarely use din hospital laboratories. Specimens are usually sent to reference laboratory for analysis.

Reference ranges of 82–2.05 nmol/L have been established in whole blood and serum. Assays had been performed using microbiology functional assay and the *Lactobacillus* organism. Newer methods of isotopic dilution, chemiluminescent, and photometric assays are now available but rarely used in hospital laboratories. Specimens are usually sent to a reference laboratory for analysis.

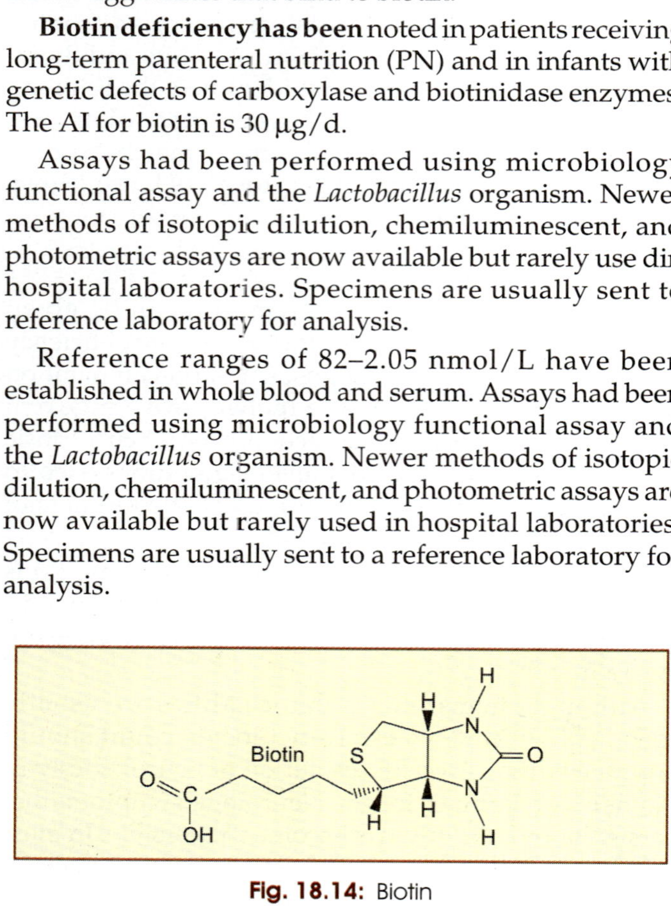

Fig. 18.14: Biotin

PANTOTHENIC ACID

Pantothenic acid is a component of coenzyme A (CoA) that is required for the metabolism of fat, protein, and carbohydrate via the citric acid cycle. Pantothenic acid is of ubiquitous occurrence in nature, where it is synthesized by most microorganisms and plants from pantoic acid (D-2,4-dihydroxy-3,3-dimethylbutyric acid) derived from L-valine, and from β-alanine derived from L-aspartate. Addition of cysteamine at the C-terminal end and phosphorylation at C4 of pantoic acid form 4'-phosphopantetheine, which serves as a covalently attached prosthetic group of acyl carrier proteins; when attached to ribose 3'-phosphate and adenine, CoA is formed (Fig. 18.15).

A growth factor occurring in all types of animal and plant tissue was first designated as vitamin B3 and later named pantothenic acid (from Greek for 'everywhere'). Dietary sources include liver and other organ meats, milk, eggs, peanuts, legumes, mushrooms, salmon, and whole grains. Approximately 50% of pantothenate in food is available for absorption. Pantothenate is metabolically converted to 42-phosphopantetheine, which becomes covalently bound to either serum acyl carrier protein or coenzyme A. Coenzyme A is a highly important acyl-group transfer coenzyme involved in many reaction types. The AI for pantothenic acid in adults is 5 mg/d. Whole blood pantothenate of less than 100 µg/dL and urinary excretion of less than 1 mg/d are regarded as indicative of deficiency. Reference range for urine is 5–68 µmol/d. Assays using a load test look for excretion of the acetylated p-aminobenzoic acid that is formed.

ASCORBIC ACID

Ascorbic acid (vitamin C) serves as a reducing agent in several important hydroxylation reactions in the body (Fig. 18.16), the term vitamin C refers to all molecules that exhibit antiscorbutic properties in humans and includes both ascorbic acid and its oxidized form, dehydroascorbic acid (DHA). The most commonly discussed vitamin, is a strong reducing compound that has to be acquired via dietary ingestion. Major dietary sources include fruits (especially citrus) and vegetables (e.g. tomatoes, green peppers, cabbage, leafy greens, and potatoes). Ascorbic acid is important in formation and stabilization of collagen by hydroxylation of proline and lysine for cross-linking and conversion of tyrosine to catecholamines (by dopamine β-hydrolase). It increases the absorption of certain minerals, such as iron, and is absorbed in the upper small intestine and distributed throughout the water-soluble compartments of the body. The deficiency state, known as scurvy, is characterized by hemorrhagic disorders, including swollen, bleeding gums and impaired wound healing and anemia.

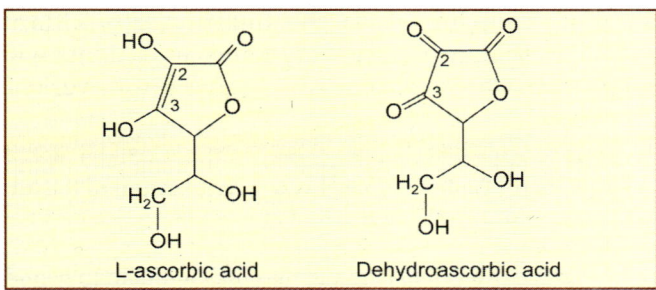

Fig. 18.15: Pantothenate and 4'-phosphopantetheine as components of CoA

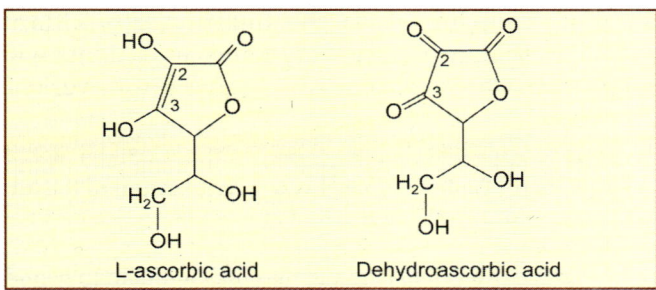

Fig. 18.16: L-ascorbic and dehydroascorbic acids

increased sensitivity and specificity. The reference range for ascorbic acid is 23–34 µmol/L. The RDA for vitamin C is 90 mg/d for adult males and 75 mg/d for adult females.

Vitamin C Deficiency

In developed countries, vitamin C deficiency can occur as part of general undernutrition, but severe deficiency (causing scurvy) is uncommon. Symptoms include fatigue, depression, and connective tissue defects (e.g. gingivitis, petechiae, rash, internal bleeding, impaired wound healing). In infants and children, bone growth may be impaired. Diagnosis is usually clinical. Treatment consists of oral vitamin C. Severe vitamin C deficiency results in scurvy, a disorder characterized by hemorrhagic manifestations and abnormal osteoid and dentin formation.

Etiology

The need for dietary vitamin C is increased by febrile illnesses, inflammatory disorders (particularly diarrheal disorders), achlorhydria, smoking, hyperthyroidism, iron deficiency, cold or heat stress, surgery, burns, and protein deficiency. Heat (e.g. sterilization of formulas, cooking) can destroy some of the vitamin C in food.

Pathophysiology

When vitamin C is deficient, formation of intercellular cement substances in connective tissues, bones, and dentin is defective, resulting in weakened capillaries with subsequent hemorrhage and defects in bone and related structures. Bone tissue formation becomes impaired, which, in children, causes bone lesions and poor bone

Although, urine is the primary route of excretion, measurement of urinary ascorbate is not recommended for status assessment. Drugs known to increase urinary excretion of ascorbate include aspirin, aminopyrine, barbiturates, hydantoin, and paraldehyde. Ascorbic acid requirements are more increased with acute stress injury and chronic inflammatory states, but are also increased with pregnancy and oral contraceptive use. Excessive intake may interfere with vitamin B12 metabolism and drug actions (e.g. aminosalicylic acid, tricyclic antidepressants, and anticoagulants).

The most widely used assay for ascorbic acid is the 2,4-dinitrophenylhydrazine method. In this procedure, ascorbic acid is first oxidized to dehydroascorbic acid and 2, 3-diketogulonic acid with the formation of a colored product that absorbs at 520 nm. This method measures the total vitamin C content of the sample because ascorbic acid, dehydroascorbic acid, and diketogulonic acid are also measured, and it is subject to interference from amino acids and thiosulfates. High-performance liquid chromatography (HPLC) has been developed to give

growth. Fibrous tissue forms between the diaphysis and the epiphysis, and costochondral junctions enlarge. Densely calcified fragments of cartilage are embedded in the fibrous tissue. Subperiosteal hemorrhages, sometimes due to small fractures, may occur in children or adults.

Signs and Symptoms

In adults, symptoms of vitamin C deficiency develop after weeks to months of vitamin C depletion. Lassitude, weakness, irritability, weight loss, and vague myalgias and arthralgias may develop early.

Symptoms of scurvy (related to defects in connective tissues) develop after a few months of deficiency. Follicular hyperkeratosis, coiled hair, and perifollicular hemorrhages may develop. Gums may become swollen, purple, spongy, and friable; they bleed easily in severe deficiency. Eventually, teeth become loose and avulsed. Secondary infections may develop. Wounds heal poorly and tear easily, and spontaneous hemorrhages may occur, especially as ecchymoses in the skin of the lower limbs or as bulbar conjunctival hemorrhage. Other signs and symptoms include femoral neuropathy due to hemorrhage into femoral sheaths (which may mimic deep venous thrombosis), lower extremity edema, and painful bleeding or effusions within joints. In infants, symptoms include irritability, pain during movement, anorexia, and slowed growth. In infants and children, bone growth is impaired, and bleeding and anemia may occur.

Diagnosis

Skeletal X-rays can help diagnose childhood (but not adult) scurvy. Changes are most evident at the ends of long bones, particularly at the knee. Early changes resemble atrophy. Loss of trabeculae results in a ground-glass appearance. The cortex thins. A line of calcified, irregular cartilage (white line of Fraenkel) may be visible at the metaphysis. A zone of rarefaction or a linear fracture proximal and parallel to the white line may be visible as only a triangular defect at the bone's lateral margin but is specific. The epiphysis may be compressed. Healing subperiosteal hemorrhages may elevate and calcify the periosteum.

Laboratory diagnosis, which requires measuring blood ascorbic acid. Levels of $<34\,\mu mol/L$ are considered marginal; levels of $<11\,\mu mol/L$ indicate vitamin C deficiency. Measurement of ascorbic acid levels in the WBC-platelet layer of centrifuged blood is not widely available or standardized.

In adults, scurvy must be differentiated from arthritis, hemorrhagic disorders, gingivitis, and protein-energy undernutrition. Hyperkeratotic hair follicles with surrounding hyperemia or hemorrhage are almost pathognomonic. Bleeding gums, conjunctival hemorrhages, most petechiae, and ecchymoses are nonspecific.

Treatment

For scurvy in adults, ascorbic acid 100–500 mg by mouth 3 times a day is given for 1–2 weeks, until signs disappear, and followed by a nutritious diet supplying 1–2 times the daily recommended intake.

In scurvy, therapeutic doses of ascorbic acid restore the functions of vitamin C in a few days. The signs and symptoms usually disappear over 1–2 weeks. Chronic gingivitis with extensive subcutaneous hemorrhage persists longer.

Vitamin C Toxicity

Up to 10 g/day of vitamin C are sometimes taken for unproven health benefits, such as preventing or shortening the duration of viral infections or slowing or reversing the progression of cancer or atherosclerosis. Such doses may acidify the urine, causes nausea and diarrhea, interfere with the healthy antioxidant-prooxidant balance in the body, and, in patients with thalassemia or hemochromatosis, promote iron overload.

BIBLIOGRAPHY

1. Adams JF, Tanke! HI, MacEwan F. Estimation of the total body vitamin BI2 in the live subject. Clin Sci 1970; 39: 107–13.
2. Allen RH. Megaloblastic anemias. In: Goldman L, Bennett JC, eds. Cecil textbook of medicine. Philadelphia: WB Saunders, 2000: 859–67.
3. Anderson RA. Chromium in the prevention and control of diabetes. Diabetes Metab 2000; 26: 22–7.
4. Bailey LB. New standard for dietary folate intake in pregnant women. Am I Clin Nutr 2000; 71:1304S-7S.
5. Baines M. Davies G. The evaluation of erythrocyte thiamindiphosphate as an indicator of thiamin status in man and its comparison with erythrocyte transketolase activity measurements. Ann Clin Biochem 1988; 25(Pt 6): 698–705.
6. Baker EM. Hodges RE. Hood J, Sauberlich HE. March SC. CanhamIE. Metabolism of 14C- and 3H-labeled L-ascorbic acid in human scurvy. Am I Clin Nutr 1971; 24: 444–54.
7. Ball GFM. Pantothenic acid: water-soluble vitamin assays in human nutrition. New York: Chapman and Hall. 1994.
8. Banerjee R. Vlasie M. Controlling the reactivity of radicalinter mediates by coenzyme B (l2)-dependent methylmalonyl-Co Amutase. Biochem Soc Trans 2002; 30: 621–4.
9. Banno K. Measurement of pantothenic acid and hopantenic acid by gas chromatography-mass spectroscopy. Methods Enzymol 1997; 279: 213–9.
10. Barber RC, Lammer EJ, Shaw GM. Greer KA. Finnell RH. The role of folate transport and metabolism in neural tube defect risk. Mol Genet Metab 1999; 66:1 9.
11. Barclay MN. MacPherson A. Dixon I. Selenium content of a range of UK foods. I Food Compos Anal 1995; 8: 307–8.

12. Bates CI. Vitamin analysis. Ann Clin Biochem 1997;34 (Pt 6): 599–626.

13. Batista BL. Rodrigues IL. Nunes IA. Souza VC. Barbosa Fir. Exploiting dynamic reaction cell inductively coupled plasma mass spectrometry (DRC-ICP-MS) for sequential determination of trace elements in blood using a dilute-and-shoot procedure. Anal ChimActa 2009; 639: 13–8.

14. BauernfeindIe. The tocopherol content of food and influencing factors. CRC Crit Rev Food SciNutr 1977; 8: 337–82.

15. Beattie IH. Peace HS. The influence of a low-boron diet and boron supplementation on bone. major mineral and sex steroid metabolism in postmenopausal women. Br I Nutr 1993; 69: 871–84.

16. Bechgaard H. Jespersen S. G[absorption of niacin in humans. J Pharm Sci 1977; 66: 871–2.

17. Beck MA. Nutritionally induced oxidative stress: effect on viral disease. Am I Clin Nutr 2000; 71: 1676S-81S.

18. Beck MA. Shi Q. Morris VC. Levander OA. Rapid genomic evolution of a non-virulent coxsackievirus B3 in selenium-deficient mice results in selection of identical virulent isolates. Nat Med 1995; 1: 433–6.

19. Beck WS. Cobalamin (Vitamin BI2). [n: Rucker RB. Suttie IW. McCormick DB. Machlin LJ, eds. Handbook of vitamins. New York: Marcel Dekker Inc. 2001: 463–512.

20. Bender DA. Daily doses of multivitamin tablets. BMI 2002;325: 173-4.

21. Bender DA. Effects of benserazide. carbidopa and isoniazid administration on tryptophan-nicotinamide nucleotide metabolism in the rat. BiochemPharmacol 1980;29:2099-104.

22. Bender DA. Non-nutritional uses of vitamin B6. Br I Nutr 1999;81: 7-20.

23. Benzie IF. Strain J). The ferric reducing ability of plasma (FRAP) as a measure of "antioxidant power": the FRAP assay. Anal Biochem 1996; 239: 70–6.

24. Berkner KL. The vitamin K-dependent carboxylase. J Nutr 2000; 130: 1877–80.

25. Berry RJ. Li Z. Erickson JD. Li S. Moore CA. Wang H. et al. Prevention of neural-tube defects with folic acid in China. China-U.S. Collaborative Project for Neural Tube Defect Prevention. N EnglI Med 1999; 341: 1485–90. Erratum in N Engl I Med 1999; 341:1864.

26. Bettendorff L. A non-cofactor role of thiamine derivatives in excitable cells? Arch PhysiolBiochem 1996;104: 745–51.

27. Beutler E. Blume KG. Kaplan IC. Lohr GW. Ramot B. Valentine WN. International Committee for Standardization in Haematology: recommended methods for red-cell enzyme analysis. Br I Haematol 1977; 35: 331–40.

28. Bieri IG. Evarts RP. Tocopherols and polyunsaturated fatty acids inhuman tissues. Am I Clin Nutr 1975; 28: 717–20.

29. Biesalski HK. Vitamin E requirements in parenteral nutrition. Gastroenterology 2009;137:S92–104.

30. Bingham SA. Welch AA. McTaggart A. Mulligan AA. Runswick SA. Luben R. et al. Nutritional methods in the European Prospective Investigation of Cancer in Norfolk. Public Health Nutr 2001; 4: 847–58.

31. Bjelakovic G. Nikolova D. Simonetti RG. Gluud e. Systematic review: primary and secondary prevention of gastrointesti-nal cancers with antioxidant supplements. Aliment Pharmacol Ther 2008; 28: 689–703.

32. Bor MV, Refsum H, Bisp MR, Bleie 0, Schneede I, Nordrehaug IE, et al. Plasma vitamin B6 vi tamers before and after oral vitamin B6 treatment: a randomized placebo-controlled study. Clin Chern 2003; 49: 155–61.

33. Bowman BB, McCormick DB, Rosenberg IH. Epithelial transport of water-soluble vitamins. Al1llU Rev Nutr 1989; 9: 187–99.

34. Brady J, Wilson L, McGregor L, Valente E, Orning L. Active B12: a rapid, automated assay for holotranscobalamin on the Abbott AxSYM analyzer. Clin Chem 2008; 54: 567–73.

35. Brattstrom L, Wilcken DE, Ohrvik J, Brudin L. Common methylenetetrahydrofolate reductase gene mutation leads to hyperhomocysteinemia but not to vascular disease: the result of a meta-analysis. Circulation 1998; 98: 2520–6.

36. Brigelius-Flohe R. Widened horizon of vitamin E research. Mol Nutr Food Res 2010; 54:581.

37. Brin M, Tai M, Ostashever AS, Kalinsky H. The effect of thiamine deficiency on the activity of erythrocyte hemolysate transketolase. J Nutr 1960; 71: 273–81.

38. Brown KH, Peerson 1M, Rivera J, Allen LH. Effect of supplemental zinc on the growth and serum zinc concentrations of prepubertal children: a meta-analysis of randomized controlled trials. Am I ClinNutr 2002; 75: 1062–71.

39. Buettner GR. The pecking order of free radicals and antioxidants: lipid peroxidation, alpha-tocopherol, and ascorbate. Arch BiochemBiophys 1993; 300: 535–43.

40. Burk RF, Hill KE, Motley AK. Selenoprotein metabolism and function: evidence for more than one function for selenoprotein P. I Nutr 2003;133:1517S-20S.

41. Burk RF, Norsworthy BK, Hill KE, Motley AK, Byrne DW. Effects of chemical form of selenium on plasma biomarkers in a high-dose human supplementation trial. Cancer Epidemiol Biomarkers Prev 2006; 15: 804–10.

42. Burk RF. Selenium: recent clinical advances. Curr Opin Gastroenterol 2001; 17: 162–6.

43. Burns CS, Aronoff-Spencer E, Legname G, Prusiner SB, Antholine WE, Gerfen GJ, et al. Copper coordination in the full-length, recombinant prion protein. Biochemistry 2003; 42: 6794–803.

44. Buzby GP, Mullen IL, Matthews DC, Hobbs CL, Rosato EF. Prognostic nutritional index in gastrointestinal surgery. Am I Surg 1980; 139: 160–7.

45. Calder PC, Albers R, Antoine 1M, Blum S, Bourdet-Sicard R, Ferns GA, et al. Inflammatory disease processes and interactions with nutrition. Br I Nutr 2009;101(Suppl1):SI-45.

46. Camblor M, De La Cuerda C, Breton I, Perez-Rus G, Alvarez S, Garcia P. Copper deficiency with pancytopenia due to enteral nutrition through jejunostomy. Clin Nutr 1997; 16: 129–31.

47. Capo-Chichi CD, Gueant IL, Feillet F, Namour F, Vidailhet M. Analysis of riboflavin and riboflavin cofactor levels in plasma by high-performance liquid chromatography. I Chromatogr B Biomed Sci Appl 2000; 739: 219–24.

48. Carlisle EM. Silicon as an essential trace element in animal nutrition. In: Evered D, O'Connor M, eds. Silicon bio-chemistry. Chichester: lohn Wiley, 1986: 123–39.

49. Carlson GL, Williams N, Barber D, et al. Biotin deficiency complicating long-term total parenteral nutrition in an adult patient. ClinNutr 1995; 14: 186–90.

50. Carmel R. Measuring and interpreting holo-transcobalamin (holo-transcobalamin II). ClinChern 2002; 48: 407–9.

51. Carmel R. Subtle and atypical cobalamin deficiency states. Am I HematoI 1990; 34: 108–14.

52. Carr A, Frei B. Does vitamin C act as a pro-oxidant under physiological conditions? FASEB I 1999; 13: 1007–24.

53. Chytil F, McCormick DB. Vitamins and coenzyme: methods in enzymology. Orlando, Fla: Academic Press Inc, 1986: Part H.

54. Cipriano C, Tesei S, Malavolta M, Giacconi R, Muti E, Costarelli L, et al. Accumulation of cells with short telomeres is associated with impaired zinc homeostasis and inflammation in old hypertensive participants. J Gerontol A Bioi Sci Med Sci 2009; 64: 745–51.

55. Cohen HJ, Brown MR, Hamilton D, Lyons-Patterson), Avissar N, Liegey P. Glutathione peroxidase and selenium deficiency in patients receiving home parenteral nutrition: time course for development of deficiency and repletion of enzyme activity in plasma and blood cells. Am J ClinNutr 1989; 49: 132–9.

56. Combs GE Biotin: the vitamins: fundamental aspects in nutrition and health. San Diego, Calif: Academic Press, 1992: 350–65.

57. Cook NR, Albert CM, Gaziano JM, Zaharris E, MacFadyen), Danielson E, et al. A randomized factorial trial of vitamins C and E and beta carotene in the secondary prevention of cardiovascular events in women: results from the Women's Antioxidant Cardiovascular Study. Arch Intern Med 2007; 167: 1610–8.

58. Cravo ML, Gloria LM, Selhub), Nadeau MR, Camilo ME, Resende MP, et al. Hyperhomocysteinemia in chronic alcoholism: correlation with folate, vitamin B-12, and vitamin B-6 status. Am J Clin Nutr 1996; 63: 220–4.

59. Dancis J, Lehanka J, Levitz M. Placental transport of riboflavin: differential rates of uptake at the maternal and fetal surfaces of the perfused human placenta. Am J Obstet GynecoI 1988; 158: 204–10.

60. Davis RE. Clinical chemistry of vitamin B12. Adv Clin Chem 1985; 24: 163–216.

61. Delves HT. Atomic absorption spectroscopy in clinical analysis. Ann Clin Biochem 1987; 24(Pt 6): 529–51.

62. DePaola DP. Nutrition in relation to dental medicine. In: Shils ME, Olson JA, Shihe M, Ross AC, eds. Modern nutrition in health and disease. Baltimore, Md: Williams and Wilkins, 1999: 1099–124.

63. Deutsch JC, Kolhouse JE Ascorbate and dehydroascorbate measurements in aqueous solutions and plasma determined by gas chromatography-mass spectrometry. Anal Chem 1993; 65: 321–6.

64. Devlin AM, Ling EH, Peerson JM, et al. Glutamate carboxypeptidase II: a polymorphism associated with lower levels of serum folate and hyperhomocysteinemia. Hum Mol Genet 2000; 9: 2837–44.

65. Devoto G, Gallo F, Marchello C, Racchi 0, Garbarini R, Bonassi S, et al. Prealbumin serum concentrations as a useful tool in the assessment of malnutrition in hospitalized patients. Clin Chem 2006;52: 2281–5.

66. Devrian TA. The physiological effects of dietary boron. Crit Rev Food Sci Nutr 2003; 43: 219–31.

67. Elia M, Crozier C, Neale G. Mineral metabolism during short-term starvation in man. Clin Chim Acta 1984; 139: 37–45.

68. Environmental health criteria: copper. Geneva, Switzerland: World Health Organization (WHO), 1998.

69. Evans We. Thiaminases and their effect on animals. In: Munson PL, Glover I, Diczfalusy E, Olson RE, eds. Vitamins and hormones. New York: Academic Press Inc, 1975: 467–504.

70. Farrell PM, Bieri IG, Fratantoni IF, Wood RE, di Sant'Agnese PA. The occurrence and effects of human vitamin E deficiency: a study in patients with cystic fibrosis. I Clin Invest 1977; 60: 233–41.

71. Fatemi N, Sarkar B. Molecular mechanism of copper transport in Wilson disease. Environ Health Perspect 2002; 110 (Suppl 5): 695–8.

72. Fenech M. Micronutrients and genomic stability: a new paradigm for recommended dietary allowances (RDAs). Food Chern Toxicol 2002; 40: 1113–7.

73. Fenton WA, Rosenberg LE. Disorders of proprionate and methylmalonate metabolism. In: Scriver CS, Beaudet AL, Sly WS, Valle D, eds. The metabolic and molecular basis of inherited disease. New York: McGraw-Hill, 1995: 1423–49.

74. Fenton WA, Rosenberg LE. Inherited disorders of cobalamins transport and metabolism. In: Scriver CR, Beaudet AL, Sly WS, Valle DR, eds. The metabolic and molecular bases of inherited disease. New York: McGraw-Hill, 1995: 3129–49.

75. Ferenci P, Caca K, Loudianos G, Mieli- Vergani G, Tanner S, Sternlieb I, et al. Diagnosis and phenotypic classification of Wilson disease. Liver 2003; 23: 139–42.

76. Ferland G. Vitamin K. In: Bowman BA, Russell RA, eds. Present knowledge in nutrition. Washington, DC: ILSI Press, 2001: 164–72.

77. Fernandez-Peralta AM, Daimiel L, Nejda N, Iglesias D, Medina Arana V, Gonzalez-Aguilera) J. Association of polymorph isms MTHFR C677T and A1298C with risk of colorectal cancer, genetic and epigenetic characteristic of tumors, and response to chemotherapy. Int I Colorectal Dis 2010; 25: 141–51.

78. Feskanich D, Weber P, Willett WC, Rockett H, Booth SL, Colditz GA. Vitamin K intake and hip fractures in women: a prospective study. Am I ClinNutr 1999;69:74-9.

79. Fleming IC, Tartaglini E, Steinkamp MP, Schorderet DF, Cohen N, Neufeld EI. The gene mutated in thiamine-responsive anaemia with diabetes and deafness (TRMA) encodes a functional thiamine transporter. Nat Genet 1999; 22: 305–8.

80. Floridi A, Pupita M, Palmerini CA, Fini C, Alberti FA. Thiamine pyrophosphate determination in whole blood and erythrocytes by high performance liquid chromatography. Int I Vitam Nutr Res 1984; 54: 165–71.

81. Food and Agriculture Organisation, World Health Organisation. Ioint FAO/WHO expert consultation on human vitamin and mineral requirements. Bangkok, Thailand: FAO/WHO, 1998.

82. Food and Nutrition Board. Dietary reference intakes for calcium, phosphorus, magnesium, vitamin D, and fluoride. Washington, DC: National Academy Press, 1999.

83. Food and Nutrition Board. Dietary reference intakes for thiamin, riboflavin, niacin, vitamin B6, folate, vitamin B12, pantothenic acid, biotin, and choline. Washington, DC: National Academy Press, 1998.

84. Food and Nutrition Board. Dietary reference intakes for vitamin C, vitamin E, selenium, and carotenoids. Washington, DC: National Academy Press, 2000.

85. Fredrich W. Thiamine. Vitamins. Berlin: de Gruyter, 1988: 341–94.

86. Frei B, Stocker R, England L, Ames BN. Ascorbate: the most effective antioxidant in human blood plasma. Adv Exp Med Bioi 1990; 264: 155–63.

87. French RJ, lones PI. Role of vanadium in nutrition: metabolism, essentiality and dietary considerations. Life Sci 1993; 52: 339–46.

88. Fritz 1, Said H, Harris C, et al. A new sensitive assay for plasma riboflavin using high performance liquid chromatography. I Am Coil Nutr 1987; 6: 454.

89. Fry PC, Fox HM, Tao HG. Metabolic response to a pantothenic acid deficient diet in humans. I NutrSciVitaminol (Tokyo) 1976;22: 339-46.

90. Fu CS, Swendseid ME, lacob RA, McKee RW. Biochemical markers for assessment of niacin status in young men: levels of erythrocyte niacin coenzymes and plasma tryptophan. I Nutr 1989; 1l9: 1949–55.

91. Fuhrman MP, Herrmann V, Masidonski P, Eby C. Pancyto-penia after removal of copper from total parenteral nutrition. IPEN I Parenter Enteral Nutr 2000; 24: 361–6.

92. Fujita M, Itakura T, Takagi Y, Okada A. Copper deficiency during total parenteral nutrition: clinical analysis of three cases. IPEN I Parenter Enteral Nutr 1989;13:421-5.

93. Fuller NI, Elia M. Inadequacy of urinary urea for estimating nitrogen balance. Ann ClinBiochem 1990;27(Pt 5):510-1.

94. Gaffney D, Fell GS, O'Reilly DS. ACP Best Practice No. 163. Wilson's disease: acute and presymptomatic laboratory diagnosis and monitoring. I Clin Pat hoI 2000; 53: 807–12.

95. Gale CR, Martyn CN, Winter PD, Cooper C. Vitamin C and risk of death from stroke and coronary heart disease in cohort of elderly people. BMI 1995; 310: 1563–6.

96. Galloway P, McMillan DC, Sattar N. Effect of the inflammatory response on trace element and vitamin status. Ann Clin Biochem 2000; 37(Pt 3): 289–97.

97. Hellborg R, Skog G. Accelerator mass spectrometry. Mass Spectrom Rev 2008; 27: 398–427.

98. HelphingstineCj, Bistrian BR. New Food and Drug Administration requirements for inclusion of vitamin K in adult parenteral multivitamins. jPEN j Parenter Enteral Nutr 2003; 27: 220–4.

99. Hermann J. Arquitt A, StoeckerBj. Effect of chromium supplementation on plasma lipids. apolipoproteins and glucose in elderly subjects. Nutr Res 1994; 14: 671–4.

100. Herrmann W, Obeid R, Schorr H, Geisel j. The usefulness of holotranscobalamin in predicting vitamin B12 status in different clinical settings. Curr Drug Metab 2005; 6: 47–53.

101. Herrmann W, Schorr H, Obeid R, Geisel j. Vitamin B-12 status. particularly holotranscobalamin II and methy-lmalonic acid concentrations, and hyperhomocysteinemia in vegetarians. Am j Clin Nutr 2003; 78: 131–6.

102. Heyssel RM. Bozian RC, Darby Wj, Bell Me. Vitamin B12 turnover in man: the assimilation of vitamin B12 from natural foodstuff by man and estimates of minimal daily dietary requirements. Am j ClinNutr 1966; 18: 176–84.

103. Higden j. An evidence-based approach to vitamins and minerals. New York/Stuttgart: Thieme, 2003.

104. Hill CH, Matrone G. Chemical parameters in the study of in vivo and in vitro interactions of transition elements. Fed Proc 1970; 29: 1474–81.

105. Kafritsa Y. Fell J. Long S. Bynevelt M. Taylor W. Milia P. Long-term outcome of brain manganese deposition in patients on home parenteral nutrition. Arch Dis Child 1998; 79: 263–5.

106. Kaler SG. Metabolic and molecular bases of Menkes disease and occipital horn syndrome. Pediatr Dev PathoI 1998; 1: 85–98.

107. Kallner A. Hartmann D. Hornig D. Steady-state turnover and body pool of ascorbic acid in man. Am J Clin Nutr 1979; 32: 530–9.

108. Kang JH. Cook NR. Manson JE. Buring JE. Albert CM. Grodstein F. Vitamin E. vitamin C. beta carotene. and cognitive function among women with or at risk of cardio-vascular disease: the Women's Antioxidant and Cardiovas-cular Study. Circulation 2009; 119: 2772–80.

109. Kanyo ZF. Scolnick LR. Ash DE. Christianson Ow. Structure of a unique binuclear manganese cluster in arginase. Nature 1996;383: 554-7.

110. Kaplan JH. Lutsenko S. Copper transport in mammalian cells: special care for a metal with special needs. J BioiChem 2009;284:25461-5.

111. Kappus H. Diplock AT. Tolerance and safety of vitamin E: a toxicological position report. Free RadicBioi Med 1992; 13: 55–74.

112. Kathman JV. Kies C. Pantothentic acid status of free living adolescents and young adults. Nutr Res 1984;4:245-50.

113. Kelleher BP. Broin SO. Microbiological assay for vitamin12 performed in 96-well microtitre plates. J ClinPathol 1991;44:592-5.

114. Kiihrle J. Gartner R. Selenium and thyroid. Best Pract Res Clin Endocrinol Metab 2009; 23: 815–27.

115. King JC. KeenCI.. Zinc. In: Shils ME. Olson JA. Shihe M. Ross AC. eds. Modern nutrition in health and disease. Baltimore. Md: Williams and Wilkins. 1999: 223–39.

116. Klein EA. Lippman SM. Thompson 1M. Goodman PJ. Albanes D. Taylor PRo et al. The selenium and vitamin E cancer prevention trial. World J UroI 2003; 21: 21–7.

117. Klevay LM. Trace element and mineral nutrition in ischemic heart disease. In: Bogden JD. Klevay LM. eds. Clinical nutrition of the essential trace elements and minerals. Totowa. NJ: Humana Press. 2000: 251–71.

118. Knasmuller S. Nersesyan A. Misik M. Gerner C. Mikulits W. Ehrlich V. et al. Use of conventional and -omics based methods for health claims of dietary antioxidants: a critical overview. Br J Nutr 2008; 99 (E Suppll):ES3-52.

119. Knoblock E. Hodr R. Janda J. Herzmann J. Houdkova V. Spectrofluorimetricmicromethod for determining riboflavin in the blood of newborn babies and their mothers. Int J VitamNutr Res 1979; 49: 144–51.

120. Konigsberger LC. Konigsberger E. May PM. Hefter GT. Complexation of iron(III) and iron(I1) by citrate: implications for iron speciation in blood plasma. J InorgBiochem 2000; 78: 175–84.

121. Konstantinides FN. Nitrogen balance studies in clinical nutrition. NutrClinPract 1992; 7: 231–8.

122. Kordas K, Stoltzfus RJ. New evidence of iron and zinc interplay at the enterocyte and neural tissues. J Nutr 2004; 134: 1295–8.

123. Krasinski SO. Russell RM. Furie BC. Kruger SF. Jacques PF. Furie B. TIle prevalence of vitamin K deficiency in chronic gastrointestinal disorders. Am J Clin Nutr 1985; 41: 639–43.

124. Krumdieck CL. Fukushima K. Fukushima T. Shiota T. Butterworth CE Jr. A long-term study of the excretion of folate and pterins in a human subject after ingestion of 14C folic acid. with observations on the effect of diphenyl-hydantoin administration. Am J Clin Nutr 1978; 31: 88–93.

125. Mason JB. Intestinal transport of monoglutamyl folates in mammalian systems. In: Picciano MF, Stokstad ELR, Gregory JF, eds. Folic acid metabolism in health and disease. New York: Wiley-Liss, [990: 47–64.

126. Massey V. The chemical and biological versatility of riboflavin. Biochem Soc Trans 2000; 28: 283–96.

127. Matherly LH, Goldman Di. Membrane transport of folates. Vitam Horm 2003; 66: 403–56.

128. May TW, Wiedmeyer RH. A table of polyatomic inter-ferences in ICP-MS. Atomic Spectroscopy 1998; 19: 150–5.

129. Mayne ST. Beta-carotene, carotenoids, and disease preven-tion in humans. FASEB J 1996; 10: 690–701.

130. McCall KA, Huang C, Fierke CA. Function and mechanism of zinc metalloenzymes. J Nutr 2000;130:1437S-46S.

131. McCormick DB, Snell BA. Pyridoxal phosphokinases: Ii. Effect of inhibitors. J BioI Chem 1961; 236: 2085–8.

132. McCormick DB, Wright LD. Vitamins and coenzyme: methods in enzymology. New York: Academic Press Inc, 1980: part F.

133. McCormick DB. Biochemistry of coenzymes. In: Meyers RA, ed. Encyclopedia of molecular biology and molecular medicine. New York: Wiley- VCH, 1996: 396–406.

134. McCormick DB. Biochemistry of coenzymes: pantothenic acid. In: Meyers RA, ed. Encyclopedia of molecular biology and molecular medicine. New York: Wiley-VC, 1996: 390–395.

135. McCormick DB. Biochemistry of coenzymes: pyridoxine B6. In: Meyers RA, ed. Encyclopedia of molecular biology and molecular medicine. New York: Wiley-VCH, 1996: 396–406.

136. McCormick DB. Riboflavin. In: Shils ME, Olson JA, Shihe M, Ross AC, eds. Modern nutrition in health and disease. Baltimore, Md: Williams and Wilkins, 1999: 391–9.

137. McCormick DB. Vitamin B6. In: Bowman BA, Russell RA, eds. Present knowledge in nutrition. Washington, DC: ILSI Press, 200 I : 207–13.

138. McMahon RJ. Biotin in metabolism and molecular biology. Annu Rev Nutr 2002; 22: 221–39.

139. Mehansho H, Henderson LM. Transport and accumulation of pyridoxine and pyridoxal by erythrocytes. J BioIChem 1980; 255: 11901–7.

140. Melhus H, Michaelsson K, Kindmark A, Bergstrom R, Holmberg L, Mallmin H, et al. Excessive dietary intake of vitamin A is associated with reduced bone mineral density and increased risk for hip fracture. Ann Intern Med 1998; 129: 770–8.

141. Mendel RR. Cell biology of molybdenum. Biofactors 2009; 35: 429–34.

142. Mertz W. Chromium research from a distance: from 1959 to 1980. J Am Coll Nutr 1998; 17: 544–7.

143. Mertz W. Trace minerals and atherosclerosis. Fed Proc 1982; 41: 2807–12.

144. Mertz W. Use and misuse of balance studies. J Nutr 1987; 117: 1811–3.

145. Meurs H, Maarsingh H, Zaagsma J. Arginase and asthma: novel insights into nitric oxide homeostasis and airway hyperresponsiveness. Trends Pharmacol Sci 2003; 24: 450–5.

146. Mewies M, McIntire WS, Scrutton NS. Covalent attachment of flavin adenine dinucleotide (FAD) and flavin mono-nucleotide (FMN) to enzymes: the current state of affairs. Protein Sci 1998; 7: 7–20.

147. Meydani M. Vitamin E. Lancet 1995; 345: 170–5.

148. Midttun 0, Hustad S, Schneede J, Vollset SE, Ueland PM. Plasma vitamin B-6 forms and their relation to trans-sulfuration metabolites in a large, population-based study. Am J ClinNutr 2007; 86: 131–8.

149. Millart H, Lamiable D. Determination of pyridoxal 5'-phos-phate in human serum by reversed phase high performance liquid chromatography combined with spectrofluorimetric detection of 4-pyridoxic acid 5'-phosphate as a derivative. Analyst, 1989; 114: 1225–8.

150. Miller Jw, Rogers LM, Rucker RB. Pantothentic acid. In: Bowman BA, Russell RA, eds. Present knowledge in nutrition. Washington, DC: ILSI Press, 2001: 253–60.

151. Miller NJ, Johnston JD, Collis CS, Rice-Evans e. Serum total antioxidant activity after myocardial infarction. Ann Clin Biochem1997; 34 (Pt 1): 85–90.

152. Mrochek JE, Jolley RL, Young DS, Turner WJ. Metabolic response of humans to ingestion of nicotinic acid and nicotinamide. Clin Chern 1976; 22: 1821–7.

153. Muller DP, Lloyd JK. Effect of large oral doses of vitamin E on the neurological sequelae of patients with abetalipoprot-einemia. Ann N Y Acad Sci 1982; 393: 133–44.

154. Muller T, Koppikar S, Taylor RM, Carragher F, Schlenck B, Heinz- Erian P, et al. Re-evaluation of the penicillamine challenge test in the diagnosis of Wilson's disease in children. J Hepatol 2007; 47: 270–6.

155. Muller T, Muller W, Feichtinger H. Idiopathic copper toxicosis. Am J Clin Nutr 1998; 67: 1082S-6S.

156. Munday R, Smith BL, Munday CM. Effects of butylated-hydroxyanisole and dicumarol on the toxicity of menadione to rats. ChernBioi Interact 1998; 108: 155–70.

157. Musilkova J, Kriegerbeckova K, Krusek J, Kovar J. Specific binding to plasma membrane is the first step in the uptake of non-transferrin iron by cultured cells. Biochim Biophys Acta 1998; 1369: 103–8.

158. Naito E, Ito M, Yokota I, Saijo T, Matsuda J, Ogawa Y, et al. Thiamine responsive pyruvate dehydrogenase deficiency in two patients caused by a point mutation (F205L and L216F) within the thiamine pyrophosphate binding region. Biochim Biophys Acta 2002; 1588: 79–84.

159. Nakasaki H, Ohta M, Soeda J, et al. Clinical and biochemical aspects of thiamine treatment for metabolic acidosis during total parenteral nutrition. Nutrition 1997;13: 110–7.

160. Napoli JL. A gene knockout corroborates the integral function of cellular retinol-binding protein in retinoid metabolism. Nutr Rev 2000; 58: 230–6.

161. National Research Council. Recommended dietary allowances, 10th edition. Washington, DC: National Academy of Sciences, 1989.

162. Neal RA. Vitamin deficiencies: thiamin. In: Hansen RG, Munro HN, eds. National Institute of Health Proceedings of Workshop on Problems of Assessment and Alleviation of Malnutrition in the United States, 1970, Nashville, Tenn.

163. Nelsestuen GL, Shah AM, Harvey SB. Vitamin K-dependent proteins. VitamHorm 2000; 58: 355–89.

164. Omenn GS, Goodman GE, Thornquist MD, Balmes J, Cullen MR, Glass A, et al. Effects of a combination of beta carotene and vitamin A on lung cancer and cardiovascular disease. N Engl J Med 1996; 334: 1150–5.

165. Ono J, Harada K, Kodaka R, Sakurai K, Tajiri H, Takagi Y, et al. Manganese deposition in the brain during long-term total parenteral nutrition. JPEN J Parenter Enteral Nutr 1995; 19: 310–2.

166. Ordonez YN, Bontes-Byron M, Blanco-Gonsolaz E, Paz-Jimenrez J, Tejerina-Lobo JM, Pena-Lopez JM, et al. Metal release in patients with total hip arthroplasty by DF-1CP-MS and their association with serum proteins. J Anal Atom Spectros 2009; 24: 1037–43.

167. Ottaway JM, Halls DJ. Determination of manganese in biological materials. Pure Appl Chern 1986; 1307–16.

168. Owen WE, Roberts WL. Comparison of five automated serum and whole blood folate assays. Am J Clin Pathol 2003; 120: 121–6.

169. Palmiter RD. Protection against zinc toxicity by metallothionein and zinc transporter 1. Proc Natl AcadSci USA 2004; 101: 4918–23.

170. Pan Q, Kleer CG, van Golen KL, et al. Copper deficiency induced by tetrathiomolybdate suppresses tumor growth and angiogenesis. Cancer Res 2002; 62: 4854–9.

171. Plesofsky-Vig N. Pantothentic acid. In: Shils ME, Olson JA, Shihe M, Ross AC, eds. Modern nutrition in health and disease. Baltimore, Md: Williams and Wilkins, 1999: 423–32.

172. Podmore !D, Griffiths HR, Herbert KE, et al. Vitamin C exhibits pro-oxidant properties. Nature 1998; 392: 559.

173. Pogribny I, Yi P, James S). A sensitive new method for rapid detection of abnormal methylation patterns in global DNA and within CpG islands. Biochem Biophys Res Commun 1999; 262: 624–8.

174. Powers H, Hill MH, Welfare M, et al. Responses of biomarkers of folate and riboflavin status to folate and riboflavin supplementation in healthy and colorectal polyp patients (the FAB2 Study). Cancer Epidemiol Biomarkers Prev 2007; 16: 2128–35.

175. Prasad AS, Mantzoros CS, Beck FVY,Hess)VY,Brewer G). Zinc status and serum testosterone levels of healthy adults. Nutrition 1996; 12: 344–8.

176. Prasad AS. Effects of zinc deficiency on immune functions.) Trace Elements Exp Med 2000; 13: 1–20.

177. Prasad AS. Zinc deficiency in patients with sickle cell disease. Am Clin Nutr 2002; 75:181-2.

178. Prasad PO, Ganapathy V. Structure and function of mammalian sodium-dependent multivitamin transporter. Curr Opin Clin Nutr Metab Care 2000;3:263-6.

179. Prentice AM, Bates C, Prentice A, Welch SG, Williams K, McGregor IA. The influence of G-6-PD activity on the response of erythrocyte glutathione reductase to riboflavin deficiency. Int)Vitam Nutr Res 1981;51:211-5.

180. Prior RL, Cao G. In vivo total antioxidant capacity: comparison of different analytical methods. Free Radic Bioi Med 1999; 27: 1173–81.

181. Puxty A, Haskew AE, Ratcliffe G, McMurray. Changes in erythrocyte transketolase activity and the thiamine pyrophosphate effect during storage of blood. Ann Clin Biochem 1985; 22(Pt 4): 423–7.

182. Quasim T, McMillan DC, Vasilaki A, et al. The relationship between plasma and red cell B-vitamin concentrations in critically-ill patients. Clin Nutr 2005; 24: 956–60.

183. Rahman MM, Vermund SH, Wahed MA, Fuchs Gj, Baqui AH, Alvarez)0. Simultaneous zinc and vitamin A supplementation in Bangladeshi children: randomised double blind controlled trial. BM) 200 I ; 323: 314–8.

184. Rahman MM, Wahed MA, Fuchs G), Baqui AH, Alvarez) 0. Synergistic effect of zinc and vitamin A on the biochemical indexes of vitamin A nutrition in children. Am)ClinNutr 2002; 75: 92–8.

185. Raiten OJ, Fisher KD. Assessment of folate methodology used in the Third National Health and Nutrition Examination Survey (NHANES III, 1988-1994).) Nutr 1995; 125:137IS-98S.

186. Rayman MP. The importance of selenium to human health. Lancet 2000; 356: 233–41.

187. Reeder R, Schoonen MAA, Lanzirotti A. Metal speciation in bio accessibility and bioavailability. Rev Miner Geochem 2006; 64: 59–113.

188. Refsum H, Smith AD. Homocysteine, B vitamins, and cardiovascular disease. N Engl Med 2006; 355: 207–11.

189. Reiss Genetics of molybdenum cofactor deficiency. Hum Genet 2000; 106: 157–63.

190. Reiss I, Johnson L. Mutations in the molybdenum cofactor biosynthetic genes MOCSI, MOCS2, and GEPH. Hum Mutat 2003; 21: 569–76.

191. Reynolds RD. Nationwide assay of vitamin B6 in human plasma by different methods. Fed Proc 1983; 42:665.

192. Ricciarelli R, Zingg JM, Azzi A. The 80th anniversary of vitamin beyond its antioxidant properties. Bioi Chern 2002; 383: 457–65.

193. Rindi G, Laforenza U. Thiamine intestinal transport and related issues: recent aspects. Proc Soc Exp Bioi Med 2000; 224: 246–55.

194. Rink L, Haase H. Zinc homeostasis and immunity. Trends Immunol 2007; 28: 1–4.

195. US population: NHANES II. 1976-1980. Am J ClinNutr 1990; 52: 707–16.

196. Verseick, Cornelis R. Normal levels of trace elements in human blood plasma or serum. Anal ChimActa 1980; 116: 217–54.

197. Versieck J, Cornelis R. Trace element in human plasma or serum. Boca Raton, Fla: CRC Press, 1989.

198. Vogel T, Li- Youcef N, Kaltenbach G, et al. Vitamin B12, folate and cognitive functions: a systematic and critical review of the literature. lnt I ClinPract 2009; 63: 1061–7.

199. Vuilleumier IP, Keck E. Fluorimetric assay of vitamin C in biological materials, using a centrifugal analyser with fluorescence attachment. I Micronutr Anal 1989; 5: 25–34.

200. Wald NJ, Law MR, Morris JK, Wald DS. Quantifying the effect of folic acid. Lancet 2001; 358: 2069–73.

201. Whitehead VM. Poly gamma glutamyl metabolites of folic acid inhuman liver. Lancet 1973; 1: 743–5.

202. Wiegand VW, Hartmann S, Hummler H. Safety of vitamin A: recent results. Int VitamNutr Res 1998; 68: 411–6.

203. Wilfond BS, Farrell PM, Laxova A, Mischler E. Severe hemolytic anemia associated with vitamin E deficiency in infants with cystic fibrosis: implications for neonatal screening. Clin Pediatr 1994; 33: 2–7.

204. Wilson)0. Disorders of vitamins: deficiency, excess, and errors of metabolism. In: Petersdorf RG, Adams RD, Braunwald E, et aI, eds. Harrison's principles of internal medicine. New York: McGraw-HillBook Company, 1991.

205. Wilson IX. The physiological role of dehydro ascorbic acid. FEBS Lett 2002; 527: 5–9.

206. Wolf B, Heard GS. Biotinidase deficiency. In: Barness L, Oski F, eds. Advances in pediatrics. Chicago: Medical Book Publishers, 1991: 1–21.

207. World Health Organisation. The global prevalence of vitamin A deficiency. 1995. Geneva. Micronutrient Series document WHO/NUT/95.3.

208. Wyse BW, Wittwer C, Hansen RG. Radioimmunoassay for pantothenic acid in blood and other tissues. Clin Chern 1979; 25: 108–10.

209. Yanik M, Vural H, Kocyigit A, Tutkun H, Zoroglu SS, Herken H, et al. Is the arginine-nitric oxide pathway involved in the pathogenesis ofschizophrenia? Neuropsychobiology 2003; 47: 61–5.

210. Ye Z, Song H. Antioxidant vitamin intake and the risk of coronary heart disease: meta-analysis of cohort studies. Eur Cardio vasc Prev Rehabil 2008; 15: 26–34.

211. Yoshida K, Kawano N, Yoshiike M, Yoshida M, Iwamoto T, Morisawa M. Physiological roles of semenogelin I and zinc in sperm motility and semen coagulation on ejaculation in humans. Mol Hum Reprod 2008; 14: 151–6.

212. Young IS, Woodside IV. Folate and homocysteine. Curr Opin Clin Nutr Metab Care 2000; 3: 427–32.

213. Zaman Z, Fielden P, Frost PG. Simultaneous determination of vitamins A and E and carotenoids in plasma by reversed-phase HPLC in elderly and younger subjects. ClinChern 1993; 39: 2229–34.

214. Zempleni. Biotin: present knowledge in nutrition. In: Bowman BA, Russell RA, eds. Present knowledge in nutrition. Washington, DC:ILSI Press, 2001.

19

Trace and Toxic Elements

INTRODUCTION

Almost half of the elements listed in the periodic table have been found in the human body. An element is considered **essential** if a deficiency impairs a biochemical or functional process, and replacement of the element corrects this impairment. Decreased intake, impaired absorption, increased excretion, and genetic abnormalities are all examples of conditions that could result in deficiency of one or several trace elements. The World Health Organization (WHO) has established the dietary requirement for nutrients as the smallest amount of the nutrient needed to maintain optimal function and health. Any element that is not considered essential is classified as **nonessential**. Nonessential trace elements are of medical interest primarily because many of them are toxic.

The trace and toxic elements included in this chapter all have biochemical importance, whether minor or major. The essential trace elements are often associated with an enzyme (**metalloenzyme**) or another protein (**metalloprotein**) as a cofactor. Deficiencies typically impair one or more biochemical functions and excess concentrations are associated with at least some degree of toxicity. Although trace elements, such as copper, and zinc, are found in milligram per liter or parts per million concentrations, ultratrace elements, such as selenium, chromium, and manganese, are found in microgram per liter or parts per billion concentrations.

Trace elements are naturally occurring, homogeneous, inorganic substance required in humans in amounts less than 100 mg/day. The human body needs a number of minerals in trace (milligram) quantities. These include iron, copper and zinc. Other minerals are required in ultratrace (microgram) amounts. These are chromium, manganese, fluoride, iodide, cobalt, selenium, silicon, arsenic, boron, and vanadium. Trace elements are vital for human body to maintain normal yet complex physiological functions related to body's growth and development.

TRACE ELEMENTS HOMEOSTASIS

Most aspects of intermediary metabolism require essential trace elements in the form of metalloenzymes that have a number of catalytic properties. Specific metalloproteins are required for the transport and safe storage of very reactive metal ions such as Fe^{3+} or Cu^{2+}.

Homeostatic controls are required to regulate the supply of essential trace elements to tissue cells in the face of varying dietary intakes. These involve regulation of intestinal absorption, specific transport systems in peripheral blood, uptake and storage mechanisms in tissue, and control of excretion.

The principal excretory route for some important trace metals (Zn, Cu) is in feces, both by regulation of initial absorption and by resecretion into the intestinal tract in bile and other intestinal fluids. In essence, if zinc homeostasis is used as an example, it can be seen that the more the intake, the greater the overall excretion associated with increasing overall element retention.

For the halides (iodide and fluoride), excess intake is excreted primarily in urine. For others (Se, Mo, and Cr), urinary output is also important. Loss of trace elements by other routes, such as through hair and/or nails, by skin celled squamation, and in sweat, is generally minor; published studies have reported such measured losses. Similarly, seminal fluid zinc loss could be important in specialized studies. Combinations of poor dietary supply, intestinal malabsorption caused by the antagonistic effects of other trace elements, and blockage of uptake by substances, such as phytate together with increased excretory losses as a result of disease, injury, and infection can result in overt, symptomatic trace element deficiency disease. Liver disease, inflammatory bowel disease, and renal disease will affect trace element absorption and excretion to a variable extent and may cause an acquired deficiency disease.

Catabolic responses to injury, infection, and malignant disease can result in increased essential trace element losses in feces and in urine; burn injury causes extensive loss in exudates through the damaged skin. If postsurgical patients, especially those with short bowel syndrome, require prolonged periods of nasogastric tube feeding or intravenous (IV) feeding and are treated with nutrient regimens lacking sufficient inorganic micronutrients, they will develop symptomatic deficiency disease.

COPPER

Copper (Cu) is a relatively soft yet tough metal with excellent electrical and heat conducting properties. Copper is widely distributed in nature both in its elemental form and in compounds. Copper forms alloys with zinc (brass), tin (bronze), and nickel (cupronickel, widely used in coins). Copper is an essential trace element found in four oxidation states, Cu(0), Cu(1+), Cu(2+), and Cu(3+), with Cu(2+) the most stable of all oxidation states. Copper is an important cofactor for several metalloenzymes and is critical for the reduction of iron in heme synthesis.

ABSORPTION, TRANSPORT, AND EXCRETION

The copper content in the normal human adult is 50–120 mg. Copper is distributed through the body with the highest concentrations found in liver, brain, heart, and kidneys.

Hepatic copper accounts for about 10% of the total copper in the body. Copper is also found in the cornea, spleen, intestine, and lung. The amount of copper absorbed from the intestine is 50–80% of ingested copper. The average daily intake is approximately 10 mg or more of copper. The exact mechanisms by which copper is absorbed and transported by the intestine are unknown, but an active transport mechanism at low concentrations and passive diffusion at high concentrations have been proposed. Copper is transported to the liver and bounds to albumin, transcuprein, and low-molecular-weight components in the portal system. In the liver, copper is incorporated into ceruloplasmin for distribution throughout the body. Ceruloplasmin is an α2-globulin, and each 132,000 Da molecular weight molecule contains six atoms of copper. In a normal physiological state, 98%

of copper excretion is through the bile, with copper losses in the urine and sweat comprising approximately 2% of dietary intake. Menstrual losses of copper are minor.

Health Effects

Copper is a component of several metalloenzymes, including ceruloplasmin, cytochrome C oxidase, super oxidedismutase, tyrosinase, metallothionein, dopamine hydroxylase, lysyl oxidase, clotting factor V, and an unknown enzyme that cross-links keratin in hair.

Acquired Copper Deficiency

If the genetic mechanisms controlling copper metabolism are normal, dietary deficiency rarely causes clinically significant copper deficiency. Causes include severe childhood protein deficiency, persistent infantile diarrhea (usually associated with a diet limited to milk), severe malabsorption (as in sprue or cystic fibrosis), gastric surgery (where vitamin B12 deficiency may also be present) and excessive zinc intake. Deficiency may cause neutropenia, impaired bone calcification, myelopathy, neuropathy, and hypochromic anemia not responsive to iron supplements. Diagnosis is based on low serum levels of copper and ceruloplasmin, although these tests are not always reliable. Treatment is directed at the cause, and copper 1.5–3 mg/day by mouth (usually as copper sulfate) is given.

INHERITED COPPER DEFICIENCY

Menkes Syndrome

Inherited copper deficiency occurs in male infants who inherit a mutant X-linked gene. Incidence is about 1 in 100,000 to 250,000 live births. Copper is deficient in the liver, serum, and essential copper proteins, including cytochrome-c oxidase, ceruloplasmin, and lysyl oxidase.

Signs and Symptoms

Symptoms of inherited copper deficiency are severe intellectual disability, vomiting, diarrhea, protein-losing enteropathy, hypopigmentation, bone changes, and arterial rupture; the hair is sparse, steely, or kinky. Most affected children die by age of 10 year.

Diagnosis

Diagnosis of inherited copper deficiency is based on low copper and ceruloplasmin levels in serum. Because early diagnosis and treatment seem to result in a better prognosis, the disorder is ideally detected before the age of 2 weeks. However, diagnostic accuracy of these tests is limited. Thus, other tests are being developed.

Treatment

Parenteral copper is usually given as copper histidine 250 μg SC twice a day to age 1 year, then 250 μg SC once a day until age 3 years; monitoring of kidney function is essential during treatment.

Despite early treatment, many children have abnormal neurodevelopment.

Acquired Copper Toxicity

Acquired copper toxicity can result from ingesting or absorbing excess copper (e.g. from ingesting an acidic food or beverage that has had prolonged contact with a copper container). Self-limited gastroenteritis with nausea, vomiting, and diarrhea may occur. More severe toxicity results from ingestion (usually with suicidal intent) of gram quantities of a copper salt (e.g. copper sulfate) or from absorption of large amounts through the skin (e.g. if compresses saturated with a solution of a copper salt are applied to large areas of burned skin). Hemolytic anemia and anuria can result and may be fatal.

Indian childhood cirrhosis, non-Indian childhood cirrhosis, and idiopathic copper toxicity are probably identical disorders in which excess copper causes cirrhosis. All appear to be caused by ingesting milk that has been boiled or stored in corroded copper or brass vessels. Studies suggest that idiopathic copper toxicity may develop only in infants with an unknown genetic defect. Diagnosis usually requires liver biopsy, which may show Mallory hyalin bodies.

Treatment of Acquired Copper Toxicity

For copper toxicity due to ingesting grams of copper, prompt gastric lavage is done. Copper toxicity that causes complications such as hemolytic anemia, anuria, or hepatotoxicity is also treated with either oral penicillamine 250 mg q 6 h to 750 mg q 12 h (1000–1500 mg/day in 2–4 doses) or dimercaprol 3–5 mg/kg IM q 4 h for 2 days, then q 4–6 h (chelation therapy). If used early, hemodialysis may be effective. Occasionally, copper toxicity is fatal despite treatment.

Laboratory Evaluation

Copper is measured by flame atomic absorption spectroscopy (AAS), inductively coupled plasma mass spectrometry (ICP-MS), inductively coupled plasma atomic emission spectroscopy (ICP-AES), and anodic stripping voltammetry (ASV). Serum copper and urine copper are used to monitor for nutritional adequacy and subacute management of copper toxicity. Direct measurement of free copper and ceruloplasmin in serum is used to screen for Wilson disease.

WILSON DISEASE

Wilson disease results in accumulation of copper in the liver and other organs. Hepatic or Neurologic symptoms develop. Diagnosis is based on a low serum ceruloplasmin level, high urinary excretion of copper, and sometimes liver biopsy results. Treatment consists of a low-copper diet and drugs, such as penicillamine or trientine.

Wilson disease is a disorder of copper metabolism that affects men and women; about 1 person in 30,000 has the disorder. Affected people are homozygous for the mutant recessive gene, located on chromosome 13. Heterozygous carriers, who constitute about 1.1% of the population, are asymptomatic.

Pathophysiology

The genetic defect in Wilson disease impairs copper transport. The impaired transport decreases copper secretion into the bile, thus causing the copper overload and resultant accumulation in the liver, which begins at birth. The impaired transport also interferes with incorporation of copper into the copper protein ceruloplasmin, thus decreasing serum levels of ceruloplasmin.

Hepatic fibrosis develops, ultimately causing cirrhosis. Copper diffuses out of the liver into the blood, then into other tissues. It is most destructive to the brain, but also damages the kidneys and reproductive organs and causes hemolytic anemia. Some copper is deposited around the rim of the cornea and edge of the iris, causing Kayser-Fleischer rings. The rings appear to encircle the iris.

Signs and Symptoms

Symptoms of Wilson disease usually develop between ages 5 and 35, but can develop from age 2–72 years. In almost half of patients, particularly adolescents, the first symptom is hepatitis which may develop at any time. In about 40% of patients, particularly young adults, the first symptoms reflect CNS involvement. Motor deficits are common, including any combination of tremors, dystonia, dysarthria, dysphagia, chorea, drooling, and incoordination. Sometimes, the CNS symptoms are

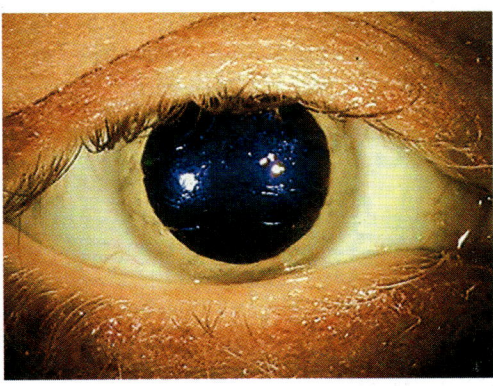

Fig. 19.1: Kayser-Fleischer rings or crescents

cognitive or psychiatric abnormalities. In 5–10% of patients, the first symptom is incidentally noted gold or greenish gold Kayser–Fleischer rings or crescents (due to copper deposits in the cornea) (Fig. 19.1), amenorrhea or repeated miscarriages, or hematuria.

Diagnosis

If Wilson disease is suspected, slit-lamp examination for Kayser–Fleischer rings is required, and serum ceruloplasmin and copper levels and 24 hours urinary copper excretion are measured. Transaminase levels are also often measured; high levels are consistent with the diagnosis.

Kayser–Fleischer Rings

These rings plus typical motor neurologic abnormalities or a decrease in ceruloplasmin are nearly pathognomonic for Wilson disease. Rarely, these rings occur in other liver disorders (e.g. biliary atresia, primary biliary cirrhosis), but ceruloplasmin levels should be unaffected.

Ceruloplasmin

Serum ceruloplasmin (normally 20–35 mg/dL) is usually low in Wilson disease but can be normal. It can also be low in heterozygous carriers and those with other liver disorders (e.g., viral hepatitis, drug- or alcohol-induced liver disease). A low ceruloplasmin level in a patient with a Kayser–Fleischer ring is diagnostic. Also, a level of <5 mg/dL is highly suggestive regardless of clinical findings.

Serum Copper

Serum copper levels may be high, normal, or low.

Urinary Copper Excretion

In Wilson disease, 24 hours urinary copper excretion (normally, ≤30 mg/day) is usually >100 µg/day. If serum ceruloplasmin is low and urinary copper excretion is high, diagnosis is clear. If levels are equivocal, measuring urinary copper excretion after penicillamine is given (penicillamine provocation test) may confirm the diagnosis; this test is not usually done in adults because cutoff values are not well-established.

Liver Biopsy

In unclear cases (e.g. elevated transaminases, no Kayser-Fleischer rings, indeterminate values for ceruloplasmin and urinary copper), the diagnosis is made by doing a liver biopsy to measure hepatic copper concentration. However, false-negative results may occur because of a sampling error (due to large variations in copper concentrations in the liver) or fulminant hepatitis (causing necrosis that releases large amounts of copper).

Screening for Wilson Disease

Because early treatment is most effective, screening is indicated for anyone who has a sibling, cousin, or parent with Wilson disease. Screening consists of a slit-lamp examination and measurement of transaminase levels, serum copper and ceruloplasmin, and 24 hours urine copper excretion. If any results are abnormal, liver biopsy is done to measure hepatic copper concentration. Infants should not be tested until after age 1 year because ceruloplasmin levels are low during the first few months of life. Children < 6 years with normal test results should be retested 5–10 years later. Genetic testing is under investigation.

Treatment

Continual, lifelong treatment of Wilson disease is mandatory regardless of whether symptoms are present. A low-copper diet (e.g. avoiding beef liver, cashews, black-eyed peas, vegetable juice, shellfish, mushrooms, and cocoa) and use of penicillamine, trientine, and sometimes oral zinc can prevent copper from accumulating. Copper content in drinking water should be checked, and people should be advised not to take any vitamin or mineral supplements containing copper.

Penicillamine is the most commonly used chelating drug but has considerable toxicity (e.g. fever, rash, neutropenia, thrombocytopenia, and proteinuria). Cross-reactivity may occur in people with penicillin allergy. Patients >5 years are given oral doses of 62.5 mg q 6 h to 250 mg q 12 h (250–500 mg/day in 2–4 doses) and slowly increased to a maximum of 250 mg q 6 h to 750 mg q 12 h (1000–1500 mg/day in 2–4 doses). Younger children are given 10 mg/kg twice a day or 6.7 mg/kg 3 times a day (20 mg/kg/day) by mouth. Pyridoxine 25 mg by mouth once a day is given with penicillamine. Occasionally, use of penicillamine is associated with worsening neurologic symptoms.

Trientine hydrochloride is an alternative treatment to penicillamine. Doses are 375–750 mg by mouth twice a day or 250–500 mg by mouth 3 times a day (750–1500 mg/day).

Zinc acetate 50 mg by mouth 3 times a day can reduce intestinal copper absorption, thus preventing re-accumulation of copper in patients who cannot tolerate penicillamine or trientine or who have neurologic symptoms that do not respond to the other drugs. Poor long-term adherence to drug therapy is common. After 1–5 years of therapy, lower dose maintenance drug therapy can be considered. Regular follow-up care with an expert in liver disease is recommended. Liver transplantation may be lifesaving for patients who have Wilson disease and fulminant hepatic failure or severe hepatic insufficiency refractory to drugs.

ZINC

Zinc (Zn) is a bluish white, lustrous metal that is stable in dry air and becomes covered with a white coating when exposed to moisture. Zinc is used in a production of alloys, especially brass (with copper), in galvanizing steel, in die casting, in paints, in skin lotions, as treatment for Wilson disease, and in many over-the-counter medications. Zinc is an essential trace element and deficiency is common throughout life, especially in individuals that do not ingest meat.

Absorption, Transport, and Excretion

The body content in a normal individual varies substantially with age and is predominantly distributed in the muscle (60%) and skeleton (30%). The remaining 10% is distributed in various other tissues with highest concentrations found in the eyes, prostate, and hair. Zinc absorption mainly occurs in the small intestine and especially in the jejunum. Factors increasing zinc absorption include the presence of animal proteins and amino acids in a meal, intake of calcium, and unsaturated fatty acids. Conversely, factors decreasing zinc absorption include the intake of iron, taking zinc on empty stomach, presence of copper at high levels, and age. In blood, the absorbed zinc is distributed between RBCs (80%), plasma (17%), and white blood cells (3%). 73 In normal dietary circumstances, about 90% of zinc is excreted in feces.

Health Effects

Zinc is second only to iron in importance as an essential trace element. The main biochemical role of zinc is seen in its influence on the activity of more than 300 enzymes in classes such as oxidoreductases, transferases, hydrolases, leases, isomerases, and lipases. As a result of the importance of zinc for the structure, regulation, and catalytic action of various enzymes, zinc is indirectly involved in the synthesis and metabolism of DNA Andrea, the synthesis and metabolism of proteins, the metabolism of glucose and cholesterol, membrane structure maintenance, insulin function, and growth factor affects. Chronic oral zinc supplementation interferes with copper absorption and may cause copper deficiency forming the basis for using zinc to treat Wilson disease.

Zinc Deficiency

Dietary deficiency is unlikely in healthy persons. Secondary zinc deficiency can develop in some patients with hepatic insufficiency, patients taking diuretics, patients with diabetes mellitus, sickle cell disease, chronic kidney disease, chronic alcoholism, or malabsorption.

patients with stressful conditions (e.g. sepsis, burns, head injury), and elderly institutionalized and home bound patients (common).

Maternal zinc deficiency may cause fetal malformations and low birth weight. Zinc deficiency in children causes impaired growth and impaired taste (hypogeusia). Other signs and symptoms in children include delayed sexual maturation and hypogonadism. In children or adults, symptoms include hypogonadism, alopecia, impaired immunity, anorexia, dermatitis, night blindness, anemia, lethargy, and impaired wound healing.

Zinc deficiency should be suspected in undernourished patients with typical symptoms or signs. However, because many of the signs and symptoms are nonspecific, clinical diagnosis of mild zinc deficiency is difficult. Laboratory diagnosis is also difficult. Low albumin levels, common in zinc deficiency, make serum zinc levels difficult to interpret; diagnosis usually requires the combination of low levels of zinc in serum and increased urinary zinc excretion. If available, isotope studies can measure zinc status more accurately. Treatment consists of elemental zinc 15–120 mg by mouth once a day until signs and symptoms resolve.

Acrodermatitis enteropathica a rare, once fatal autosomal recessive disorder (Fig. 19.2), causes malabsorption of zinc. Psoriasiform dermatitis develops around the eyes, nose, and mouth; on the buttocks; and in an acral distribution. The disorder also causes hair loss, paronychia, impaired immunity, recurrent infection, impaired growth, and diarrhea. Signs and symptoms usually develop after infants are weaned from breast milk. In such cases, doctors suspect the diagnosis. If correct, zinc sulfate 30–150 mg/day by mouth usually results in complete remission.

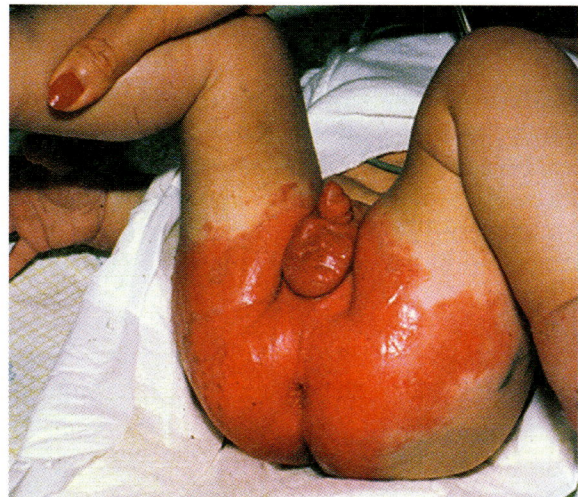

Fig. 19.2: Psoriasiform dermatitis has progressed to local erythroderma

Zinc Toxicity

The recommended upper limit for zinc intake is 40 mg/day. Toxicity is rare. Ingesting doses of elemental zinc ranging from 100–150 mg/day for prolonged periods interferes with copper metabolism and causes low blood copper levels, RBC microcytosis, neutropenia, and impaired immunity; higher doses should be given only for short periods of time and the patient followed closely.

Ingesting larger amounts (200–800 mg/day), usually by consuming acidic food or drink from a galvanized (zinc-coated) container, can cause anorexia, vomiting, and diarrhea. Chronic toxicity may result in copper deficiency and may cause nerve damage.

Metal fume fever, also called brass-founders' ague or zinc shakes, is caused by inhaling industrial zinc oxide fumes; it results in fever, dyspnea, nausea, fatigue, and myalgias. Symptom onset is usually 4–12 hours after exposure. Symptoms usually resolve after 12–24 hours in a zinc-free environment.

Diagnosis

Diagnosis of zinc toxicity is usually based on the time course and a history of exposure.

Treatment

Treatment of zinc toxicity consists of eliminating exposure to zinc; no antidotes are available.

Laboratory Evaluation

Zinc is measured by flame atomic absorption spectrometer (FAAS), inductively coupled plasma atomic emission spectroscopy (ICP-AES), and inductively coupled plasma mass spectrometry. Low urine zinc levels in the presence of low serum zinc levels usually confirm zinc deficiency. Low serum zinc in an apparently healthy (nonstressed and nonseptic) patient who has normal serum albumin levels can be used as evidence of zinc deficiency, especially if urine zinc levels are also low. Normal serum zinc cannot be interpreted as evidence of normal zinc stores. Zinc concentration in RBCs is approximately 10 times that in serum. Copper status should be monitored inpatients undergoing long-term zinc therapy.

SELENIUM

Selenium (Se) is a naturally occurring metalloid with many chemical and physical properties similar to those of sulfur. Selenium is an essential trace element and a major constituent of 40 minerals and a minor constituent of 37 others. Most processed selenium is used in the electronics industry; however, other uses include nutritional supplements, pigments, pesticides, rubber production, antidandruff shampoos, and fungicides.

Absorption, Transport, and Excretion

Selenium is well absorbed from the gastrointestinal tract (~50%). Selenium exposure occurs primarily from food but can be found in drinking water, usually in the form of inorganic sodium selenate or sodium selenite. Selenium homeostasis is largely achieved by excretion via urine and feces. Other routes of elimination include sweat and, at very high intakes, exhalation of volatile forms of selenium.

Health Effects

In the 1930s, selenium was considered a toxic element; but later in 1940s it was declared as an essential element; and since the 1960s and especially the 1970s, it has been viewed as an anticarcinogen. Glutathione peroxidase (in the form of selenocysteine) is part of the cellular antioxidant defense system against free radicals. Selenium is also involved in the metabolism of thyroid hormones (e.g. deiodinase enzymes and thioredoxin reductase).

Selenium Deficiency

Selenium deficiency predisposes patients to Keshan disease, an endemic viral cardiomyopathy affecting primarily children and young women. This cardiomyopathy can be prevented but not cured by sodium selenite supplements of 50 µg/day by mouth. Patients receiving long-term total parenteral nutrition (TPN) have developed selenium deficiency with muscle pain and tenderness that responded to a selenomethionine supplement. Selenium deficiency may contribute synergistically with iodine deficiency to the development of goiter and hypothyroidism.

Diagnosis

Diagnosis of selenium deficiency is made clinically or sometimes by measuring glutathione peroxidase activity or plasma selenium, but neither of these tests is readily available.

Treatment

Treatment of selenium deficiency consists of sodium selenite 100 µg/day by mouth.

Selenium Toxicity

At high doses (>900 µg/day), selenium causes toxicity. Manifestations include hair loss, abnormal nails, dermatitis, peripheral neuropathy, nausea, diarrhea, fatigue, irritability, and a garlic odor of the breath. Toxic levels of plasma selenium are not well defined.

Trace and Toxic Elements

Laboratory Evaluation

Selenium is most often determined by ICP-MS or graphite furnace atomic absorption spectroscopy (GFAAS). The determination of urinary and blood selenium is a useful measure of selenium status.

CHROMIUM

Chromium (Cr), from the Greek word chroma 'color', makes rubies red and emeralds green. Chromium is the 21st most abundant element in the earth's crust and is used in the manufacturing of stainless steel. Occupational exposure to chromium occurs in wood treatment, stainless steel welding, chrome plating, the leather tanning industry, and the use of lead chromate or strontium chromate paints. Chromium exists in two main valency states: trivalent and hexavalent.

Absorption, Transport, and Excretion

Cr(6+) is better absorbed and much more toxic than Cr(3+). Both transferrin and albumin are involved in chromium absorption and transport. Transferrin binds the newly absorbed chromium at site B, while albumin acts as an acceptor and transporter of chromium if the transferrin sites are saturated. Other plasma proteins, including β- and γ-globulins and lipoproteins, bind chromium.

Health Effects

Cr(3+) is an essential dietary element and plays a role in maintaining normal metabolism of glucose, fat, and cholesterol. The estimated safe and adequate daily intake of chromium for adults is in the range of 50–200 μg/d, although data are insufficient to establish a recommended daily allowance.

Dietary chromium deficiency is relatively uncommon and most cases occur in persons with specific clinical situations such as total parenteral nutrition, diabetes, and malnutrition. Chromium deficiency is characterized by glucose intolerance, glycosuria, hypercholesterolemia, decreased longevity, decreased sperm counts, and impaired fertility. Cr(6+) compounds are powerful oxidizing agents and are more toxic systemically than Cr(3+) compounds, given similar amounts and solubilities. At physiological pH, Cr(6+) forms CrO_4^{2-} and readily passes through cell membranes due to its similarity to essential phosphate and sulfate oxyanions. Intracellularly, Cr(6+) is reduced to reactive intermediates, producing free radicals and oxidizing deoxyribonucleic acid (DNA), both potentially inducing cell death. Severe dermatitis and skin ulcers can result from contact with Cr(6+) salts. Up to 20% of chromium workers develop contact dermatitis. Allergic dermatitis with eczema has been reported in printers, cement workers, metal workers, painters, and leather tanners.

Data suggest that a Cr(3+) protein complex is responsible for the allergic reaction. When inhaled, Cr(6+) is a respiratory tract irritant, resulting in airway irritation, airway obstruction, and possibly lung cancer. The target organ of inhaled chromium is the lung; the kidneys, liver, skin, and immune system may also be affected. Low-dose, chronic chromium exposure typically results only in transient renal effects. Elevated urinary β2-microglobulin levels (an indicator of renal tubular damage) have been found in chrome platers, and higher levels have generally been observed in younger persons exposed to higher Cr(6+) concentrations.

Chromium Deficiency

Four patients receiving long-term TPN developed possible chromium deficiency, with glucose intolerance, weight loss, ataxia, and peripheral neuropathy. Symptoms resolved in 3 who were given trivalent chromium 150–250 mg.

Chromium Toxicity

High doses of trivalent chromium given parenterally cause skin irritation, but lower doses given orally are not toxic. Exposure to hexavalent chromium (CrO_3) in the workplace may irritate the skin, lungs, and gastrointestinal (GI) tract and may cause perforation of the nasal septum and lung carcinoma.

Laboratory Evaluation

Chromium may be determined by GFAAS, instrumental neutron activation analysis (INAA), or ICP-MS. Plasma, serum, and urine do not indicate the total body status of the individual, whereas urine levels may be useful for metabolic studies. In the setting of suspected failure of metal-on-metal (MoM) hip implants that use a cobalt–chrome alloy femoral head, serum is the preferred specimen type for both chromium and cobalt analysis.

MANGANESE

Manganese (Mn) is found in over 250 minerals, of which 15 have commercial importance. Nearly all the elemental manganese is used in the production of the alloy ferromanganese widely used in steel production. Other uses of elemental manganese include a scavenger role in copper and aluminum alloys and in a production of dry cell batteries. Various manganese compounds are widely used in fertilizers, animal feeds, pharmaceutical products, dyes, paint dryers, catalysts, and wood preservatives and in production of glass and ceramics.

Absorption, Transport, and Excretion

Roughly 2–15% of dietary manganese is absorbed in the small intestine. Dietary factors that affect manganese absorption include iron, calcium, phosphates, and fiber. Manganese absorption is age dependent, with infants retaining higher levels of manganese than adults do. Manganese is a normal component in tissue with the highest levels found in fat and bone. Though accumulation of manganese in the healthy population has not been observed, chronic liver disease or other types of liver dysfunction can reduce manganese elimination and promote accumulation in various regions of the brain. Manganese elimination occurs predominately through the bile.

Health Effects

Manganese is biochemically essential as a constituent of metalloenzymes and as an enzyme activator. Manganese containing enzymes include arginase, pyruvate carboxylase, and manganese superoxide dismutase in the mitochondria. Manganese-activated enzymes include hydrolases, kinases, decarboxylases, and transferases. Many of these activations are not specific to manganese and other metal ions (magnesium, iron, or copper) can replace manganese as an activator and mask the effects of manganese deficiency.

Manganese Deficiency

Low levels of manganese have been associated with epilepsy, hip abnormalities, joint disease, congenital malformation, heart and bone problems, and stunted growth in children.

Manganese Toxicity

Manganese toxicity causes nausea, vomiting, headache, disorientation, memory loss, anxiety, and compulsive laughing or crying. Chronic manganese toxicity resembles Parkinson's disease with akinesia, rigidity, tremors, and mask-like faces. A clinical condition named locura manganic a (manganese madness) was described in Chilean manganese miners with acute manganese aerosol intoxication.

Laboratory Evaluation

Manganese is measured by ICP-MS and GFAAS. Urine manganese is used in conjunction with serum manganese to evaluate possible toxicity or deficiency.

IODINE

Iodine (I) occurs in the environment and in the diet primarily as iodide. In adults, about 80% of the iodide absorbed is trapped by the thyroid gland. Most environmental iodine occurs in seawater as iodide; a small amount enters the atmosphere and, through rain, enters ground water and soil near the sea.

Absorption, Transport, and Excretion

Iodine can be bound to amino acids, or it can be free, usually in the form of iodate or iodide ions. Iodide is the easiest form to absorb, so most of the bound iodine and iodate is converted to iodide by glutathione. The iodide ions are easily absorbed through the walls of the digestive tract in the stomach and small intestine. After it's absorbed, most of it concentrates in the thyroid gland. Some of it also accumulates in the ovaries, skin, and salivary, gastric and mammary glands.

Health Effect

People living far from the sea and at higher altitudes are at particular risk of deficiency. Fortifying table salt with iodide (typically 70 µg/g) helps ensure adequate intake (150 µg/day). Requirements are higher for pregnant (220 µg/day) and lactating (290 µg/day) women.

Iodine Deficiency

Iodine deficiency is rare in areas where iodized salt is used but common worldwide. Iodine deficiency develops when iodide intake is <20 µg/day.

Signs and Symptoms

In mild or moderate iodine deficiency, the thyroid gland, influenced by thyroid-stimulating hormone (TSH), hypertrophies to concentrate iodide in itself, resulting in colloid goiter. Usually, patients remain euthyroid; however, severe iodine deficiency in adults may cause hypothyroidism (endemic myxedema). It can decrease fertility and increase risk of stillbirth, spontaneous abortion, and prenatal and infant mortality.

Severe maternal iodine deficiency retards fetal growth and brain development, sometimes resulting in birth defects, and, in infants, causes cretinism, which may include intellectual disability, deaf-mutism, difficulty walking, short stature, and sometimes hypothyroidism.

Diagnosis

Diagnosis of iodine deficiency in adults and children is usually based on thyroid function, examination for goiter, and imaging tests identifying abnormalities in thyroid function and structure. All neonates should be screened by measuring the TSH level.

Treatment

Infants with iodine deficiency are given levothyroxine 3 µg/kg by mouth once a day for a week plus iodide 50–90 µg by mouth once a day for several weeks to quickly restore a euthyroid state. Children are treated with iodide 90–120 µg once a day. Adults are given iodide 150 µg once a day. Iodine deficiency can also be treated by giving levothyroxine. Serum TSH levels are monitored in all patients until the levels are normal (i.e. <5 µIU/mL).

Iodine Toxicity

Chronic toxicity may develop when intake is >1.1 mg/day. Most people who ingest excess amounts of iodine remain euthyroid. Some people who ingest excess amounts of iodine, particularly those who were previously deficient, develop hyperthyroidism (Jod-Basedow phenomenon). Paradoxically, excess uptake of iodine by the thyroid may inhibit thyroid hormone synthesis (called Wolff–Chaikoff effect). Thus, iodine toxicity can eventually cause iodide goiter, hypothyroidism, or myxedema.

Very large amounts of iodide may cause a brassy taste in the mouth, increased salivation, GI irritation, and acneiform skin lesions. Patients frequently exposed to large amounts of radiographic contrast dyes or the drug amiodarone also need to have their thyroid function monitored.

Diagnosis

Diagnosis of iodine toxicity is usually based on results of thyroid function testing and imaging, which are correlated with clinical data. Iodine excretion may be more specific but is not usually measured.

Treatment

Treatment of iodine toxicity consists of correcting thyroid abnormalities and, if intake is excessive, dietary modification.

MOLYBDENUM

Molybdenum (Mo) is a hard, silvery white metal occurring naturally as molybdenite, wulfenite, and powellite. Most molybdenum is used for the production of alloys, as well as catalysts, corrosion inhibitors, flame retardants, smoked pressants, lubricants, and molybdenum blue pigments. Molybdenum is an essential trace element with the importance of molybdenum-containing organic compounds in biological systems identified over 80 years ago.

Absorption, Transport, and Excretion

Between 25% and 80% of ingested molybdenum is absorbed predominately in the stomach and small intestine, with the majority of absorbed molybdenum retained in the liver, skeleton, and kidney. In blood, molybdenum is extensively bound to α2-macroglobulin and RBC membranes. Molybdenum can cross the placental barrier, and increased intake of molybdenum in the diet of the mother can increase its level in the liver of the neonate.

Health Effects

Molybdenum is vital to human health through its inclusion in at least three enzymes: xanthine oxidase, aldehyde oxidase, and sulfite oxidase. The active site of these enzymes binds molybdenum in the form of a cofactor molybdopterin.

Molybdenum Deficiency

Dietary molybdenum deficiency is rare with a single case reported because of total parenteral nutrition in a man with Crohn's disease. Molybdenum cofactor deficiency is a recessively inherited error of metabolism due to a lack of functional molybdopterin. The symptoms include seizures, anterior lens dislocation, decreased brain weight, and usually death prior to 1 year of age.

Molybdenum Toxicity

Molybdenum toxicity is rarely reported, as there are few known cases of human exposure to excess molybdenum. High dietary and occupational exposures to molybdenum have been linked to elevated uric acid in blood and an increased incidence of gout. Molybdenum is rapidly eliminated in both urine and bile, with urine excretion predominating when intake is high.

Laboratory Evaluation

Molybdenum levels are measured by ICP-MS and GFAAS. Blood levels are less than 60 µg/L.

FLUORIDE

Fluoride (Fl) is the most widely used of the 'pharmacologically beneficial trace elements' in the area of public health. Dental caries has been described as the last major epidemic of preventable bacterial disease, and dental decay leads to tooth loss, nutritional problems, and systemic infection.

Health Effect

Many studies over the past 50 years have established that addition of fluoride to drinking water reduces the incidence of tooth decay. Clinical studies from 1950–1980 in 20 different countries found that adding fluoride to community water supplies, within the interval 0.7–1.2 mg/L, reduced the incidence of caries by 40–50% in primary (infant) teeth and by 50–60% in permanent teeth. The subject is controversial, and 'mass medication with fluoride has been opposed. Reviews of the benefits and risks associated with the use of fluoride are available. Fluoride supplementation of salt, sugar, and milk has been used in areas where fluoride is not added to water supplies.

Absorption, Transport, and Excretion

Fluoride ions are absorbed from both the stomach and the small intestine. Soluble salts are efficiently absorbed, and a peak increase of fluoride occurs in blood plasma within

1 hour of ingestion. Ions are rapidly cleared from plasma into tissue in exchange with anions, such as hydroxyl, citrate, and carbonate. At least 95% of the 2.6 g of total body fluoride is located in bones and teeth. Almost 90% of excess fluoride is excreted in urine.

Fluoride Deficiency

Fluoride deficiency can lead to tooth decay (Fig. 19.3) and possibly osteoporosis. Consuming enough fluoride can make tooth decay less likely and may strengthen bones. The addition of fluoride (fluoridation) to drinking water that is low in fluoride or the use of fluoride supplements significantly reduces the risk of tooth decay. In areas where drinking water is not fluoridated, children may be given fluoride by mouth.

Fluoride Toxicity

Dental fluorosis, the mottling of enamel in the erupting teeth of children, is now estimated to affect around 20% of the population. This can be a disfiguring condition, and it occurs in a greater proportion of children than initially expected. This is possibly due to ingestion of fluoride-containing tooth paste by children. It is suggested that 'pediatric' toothpastes with lower fluoride content should be made available in areas where fluoridation of the water supply exists.

Occupational exposure to inhaled fluoride dusts among cryolite workers during aluminum refining has resulted in severe bone abnormalities, but safety equipment now limits such exposure. No cases of skeletal fluorosis are attributed to the use of controlled fluoridation of water supplies. However, skeletal fluorosis may occur in areas of the world where naturally occurring drinking water has high concentrations of fluoride. It is thought that exposure to fluoride intakes of 10–25 mg/d for 10 years or longer may result in skeletal fluorosis, but other nutritional factors may make these populations more susceptible. Numerous diverse adverse effects have been attributed to water fluoridation. Investigators have found no convincing evidence of increased rates of cancer, heart disease, kidney disease, liver disease, presenile dementia, birth defects, or Down syndrome.

Laboratory Evaluation

Laboratory analysis of drinking water may be required to assess possible fluoride excess in natural well waters, and may also be necessary during incidents of failure of the equipment used to treat drinking water. Determination of fluoride in urine can be used to assess exposure to different sources of fluoride. For drinking water and urine, direct determination using a fluoride-specific electrode is employed. For food, feces, and tissue, prior separation of fluoride from the sample matrix is required, using a Con way diffusion procedure. The combination of the fluoride electrode with flow injection has allowed the use of a rapid and sensitive method for serum and urine fluoride analysis. Concentrations of fluoride in body fluids and tissue vary widely, depending on the fluoride content of drinking water and input from diet, toothpaste, and mouth rinses. For urine, a guideline interval is 10.5–168 µmol/L.

ALUMINUM

Aluminum (Al) is a crystalline silver-white ductile metal. Aluminum is the most abundant metal in the earth's crust (~8%). It is always found combined with other elements, such as oxygen, silicon, and fluorine. Aluminum as the metal is obtained from aluminum-containing minerals. Due to its good conductivity of heat and electricity, ease of welding, tensile strength, light weight, and corrosion-resistant oxide coat, aluminum is applicable to a wide variety of industrial and household uses. Aluminum is used for beverage cans, pots and pans, airplanes, siding and roofing, and foil. Aluminum is often mixed with small amounts of other metals to form aluminum alloys, which are stronger and harder than aluminum alone. Aluminum compounds have many different uses, for example, as alums in water treatment and alumina in abrasives and furnace linings. They are also found in consumer products, such as antacids, astringents, buffered aspirin, food additives, cosmetics, and anti-perspirants.

Absorption, Transport, and Excretion

The average adult in the United States ingests about 7–9 mg aluminum per day in their food. The human organism can absorb aluminum and its compounds orally, by inhaling, and parenterally. There is no indication of dermal absorption. Approximately, 1.5–2% of inhaled and 0.01–5% of ingested aluminum is absorbed. The absorption efficiency is dependent on

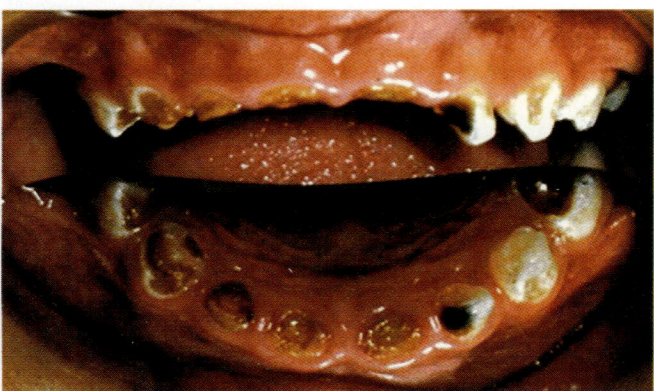

Fig. 19.3: Tooth decay due to fluoride deficiency

chemical form, particle size (inhalation), and concurrent dietary exposure to chelators, such as citric acid or lactic acid. After a relatively quick uptake of aluminum into the intestinal walls, its passage into the blood is much slower. In plasma, aluminum is bound to carrier proteins such as transferrin. Aluminum binds to various ligands in the blood and distributes to every organ, with highest concentrations ultimately found in bone (~50% of the body burden) and lung tissues (~25% of the body burden). Aluminum levels in lungs increase with age. Urine accounts for 95% of aluminum excretion with 2% eliminated in the bile.

Health Effects

The mechanism by which aluminum applies its toxicity is not well understood, though aluminum has been shown to interfere with a variety of enzymatic processes, and administration of aluminum to experimental animals is known to produce encephalopathy similar to that seen in Alzheimer disease in man. Although, aluminum-containing over-the-counter oral products are considered safe in healthy individuals at recommended doses, some adverse effects have been observed following long-term use in some individuals. Workers who breathe large amounts of aluminum dusts can have lung problems, such as coughing or changes that show up in chest X-rays.

Aluminum Toxicity

Signs and symptoms of aluminum toxicity include encephalopathy [stuttering, gait disturbance, myoclonic jerks, seizures, coma, and abnormal electroencephalography (EEG)]; osteomalacia or aplastic bone disease (painful spontaneous fractures, hypercalcemia, and tumorous calcinosis); proximal myopathy; increased risk of infection; microcyticanemia; and increased left ventricular mass and decreased myocardial function. Aluminum toxicity occurs in people with renal insufficiencies who are treated by dialysis with aluminum contaminated solutions or oral agents that contain aluminum. The clinical manifestations of aluminum toxicity include anemia, bone disease, and progressive dementia with increased concentrations of aluminum in the brain. Prolonged intravenous feeding of preterm infants with solutions containing aluminum is associated with impaired neurologic development.

Laboratory Evaluation

Aluminum is primarily measured using ICP-MS or graphite furnace atomic absorption spectrophotometry (GFAAS). Accurate measurements are often complicated by the increased risk of environmental contamination of specimens. Urine and serum levels are useful in determining toxic exposures, monitoring exposure over time, and monitoring chelation therapy.

ARSENIC

Arsenic (As) is a ubiquitous element displaying both metallic and non-metallic properties. Its content in the earth's crust is estimated at 1.5–2.0 mg/kg. For most people, food is the largest source of arsenic exposure (about 25–50 µg/d), with lower amounts coming from drinking water and air. Anthropogenic sources of arsenic (production of metals, burning of coil, fossil fuels, timber and its use in agriculture) release 3 times more of arsenic than natural sources. The main current use of arsenic is as a wood preservative. Other current and past uses of arsenic include pesticides, pigments, poison gases, ammunition manufacturing, semiconductor processing, and medicines.

Absorption, Transport, and Excretion

The main routes of exposure are ingestion of arsenic containing foods, water, and beverages or inhalation of contaminated air; however, arsenic toxicity is a complex topic. Organic forms of arsenic, such as arsenocholine and arsenobetaine are commonly found in fish and seafood, are considered relatively non-toxic, and are cleared rapidly (1–2 day). Inorganic species of arsenic are highly toxic and occur naturally in rocks, soil, and groundwater. They are also found in many synthetic products, poisons, and industrial processes. Methylated species are intermediate in toxicity and arise primarily from metabolism of inorganic species, but small amounts may arise directly from food. Organic methylated arsenic compounds, such as monomethyl arsonic acid (MMA) and dimethyl arsenic acid (DMA) are formed by hepatic metabolism of As (3+) and As (5+). The methylated inorganic forms are considered less toxic than As (3+) and As (5+); however, they are eliminated slowly (1–3 weeks). The Biological Exposure Index established for the sum of inorganic and methylated metabolites of arsenic in urine is 35 µg/L. However, clinical symptoms may not be evident at 35 µg/L.

Health Effects

The relation of clinical signs and symptoms to arsenic exposure depends on the duration and extent of the exposure to inorganic and methylated species of arsenic, as well as the underlying clinical status of the patient.

Arsenic Toxicity

For acute arsenic exposure, the symptoms may include gastrointestinal (nausea, emesis, abdominal pain, and rice water diarrhea), bone marrow (pancytopenia, anemia, and basophilic stippling), cardiovascular (ECG changes), central nervous system (encephalopathy and polyneuropathy), renal (renal insufficiency and renal failure), and hepatic (hepatitis) systems. For chronic arsenic exposure, systems and symptoms may include dermatologic (Mees' lines, hyperkeratosis, hyperpigmentation, and alopecia), hepatic (cirrhosis and hepatomegaly), cardiovascular [hypertension and peripheral vascular disease (PVD)], central nervous system ('socks and glove' neuropathy and tremor), and malignancies (squamous cell, hepatocellular, skin, bladder, lung, and adrenal carcinomas). Chronic arsenic exposure has been shown to cause Blackfoot disease, a severe form of PVD which leads to gangrenous changes. The white powder of arsenic trioxide is odorless, tasteless, and one of the most common poisons in human history. Doses of 0.01–0.05 g produce toxic symptoms.

The lethal dose is reported to be between 0.12 g and 0.3 g; however, recoveries from higher doses have been reported. Immediate treatment of expected exposure consists of lavage and use of activated charcoal to reduce arsenic absorption. The most effective antidotes for arsenic poisoning are the following chelating agents: Dimercaprol, penicillamine, and succimer. In 2000 arsenic trioxide was approved by United States Food and Drug Administration (FDA) for the treatment of acute promyelocytic leukemia.

Laboratory Evaluation

Arsenic is primarily measured using ICP-MS, GFAAS, or HG-AAS. In most cases, arsenic is best detected by urine due to the short half-life of arsenic in blood. When arsenic speciation is desired [typically following a high total urine arsenic value reported by ICP-MS or atomic absorption (AA], as eparation method is employed either online or off-lineprior to elemental analysis.

CADMIUM

Cadmium (Cd) is a soft, bluish-white metal, which is easily cut with a knife. Principal industrial uses of cadmium include manufacture of pigments and batteries, as well as in the metal-plating and plastics industries. The burning of fossil fuels such as coal and oil and the incineration of municipal waste materials constitute the largest sources of airborne cadmium exposure, along with zinc, lead, and copper smelters in some locations.

Absorption, Transport, and Excretion

Based on renal function (development of proteinuria), the reference dose for cadmium in drinking water is 0.0005 mg/kg/day and the dose for dietary exposure to cadmium is 0.001 mg/kg/day. Absorption of cadmium is higher in females than in males due to differences in iron stores. The absorption of inhaled cadmium in air is 10–50% with gastrointestinal absorption of cadmium estimated to be 5%. The absorption of cadmium in cigarette smoke is 10–50% and smokers of tobacco products have about twice the cadmium abundance in their bodies as nonsmokers. For nonsmokers, the primary exposure to cadmium is through ingested food. About 90% of ingested cadmium is excreted in the feces due to the low absorbance of cadmium from the gut.

Health Effects

Cadmium has no known role in normal human physiology.

Cadmium Toxicity

Ingestion of high amounts of cadmium may lead to a rapid onset with severe nausea, vomiting, and abdominal pain. Renal dysfunction is a common presentation for chronic cadmium exposure, often resulting in slow-onset proteinuria. Acute effects of inhalation of fumes containing cadmium include respiratory distress due to chemical pneumonitis and edema and can cause death. Breathing of cadmium vapors can also result in nasal epithelial damage and lung damage similar to emphysema. Cadmium exposure can affect the liver, bone, immune, blood, and nervous systems. Ethylenediaminetetraacetic acid (EDTA) can be used as a chelating agent in cadmium poisoning as a chelating agent in cadmium poisoning.

Laboratory Evaluation

Cadmium is usually quantified by GFAAS and ICP-MS; ICP-AES is also used. In blood, cadmium is found mostly (70%) in the RBCs. Cadmium in blood reflects the average uptake during the past few months and can be used for monitoring purposes, but does not accurately reflect a recent exposure. Urinary excretion is about 0.001% and 0.01% of the body burden per 24 hours. At low exposure, urine cadmium reflects the total accumulation.

LEAD

Metallic lead (Pb) is soft, bluish white, highly malleable, and ductile. It is a poor conductor of electricity and heat and is resistant to corrosion. Lead is widely distributed in the earth's crust and the main lead ores are galena, cerrusite, and anglesite. Lead is used in the production of storage batteries, ammunition, solder, and foils. Tetraethyl lead was once used extensively as an additive in gasoline (petrol) for its ability to increase the fuel's octane rating and is present in many paints manufactured before 1970. The manufacture of lead-based household paints was banned in the United States in 1972, but is still used in paints intended for nondomestic use. Toxic concentrations of lead can be found in areas adjacent to homes painted with lead-based paints and around highways, where it has accumulated from the past use of leaded gasoline. In recent years, there have been massive recalls of toys and costume jewelry produced in China, due to concerns over elevated lead content. Lead plays no known role in normal human physiology.

Absorption, Transport, and Excretion

Exposure to lead is primarily respiratory or gastro-intestinal. Inhalation results in 30–40% of absorption efficiency. Gut absorption depends on a variety of factors, including age and nutritional status, with enhanced gastrointestinal absorption occurring in children younger than 6 years of age. Certain substances, such as iron, calcium, magnesium, alcohol, and fat, may weaken lead absorption while low dietary zinc, ascorbic acid, and citric acid can enhance the absorption of lead. About 99% of absorbed lead is taken up by erythrocytes where it interferes with heme synthesis. Lead distributes to soft tissues, such as liver, kidneys, and brain, with the skeletal lead concentrations containing greater than 90% of the body burden of lead. Absorbed lead is excreted primarily in urine (76%) and feces (16%), and the remaining 8% is excreted in hair, sweat, nails, and others.

Health Effects

The clinical presentation of lead toxicity is variable.

Lead Toxicity

In children, obvious symptoms are usually seen at blood levels of 60 µg/dL or higher with 45 µg/dL as the typical threshold for acute, clinical intervention. Intelligence quotient (IQ) declines are seen in children with blood lead levels (BLLs) of 10 µg/dL or higher. Other central nervous system symptoms of lead toxicity in children may include clumsiness, gait abnormalities, headache, behavioral changes, seizures, and severe cognitive and behavioral problems.

Gastrointestinal symptoms include abdominal pain, constipation, and colic. Other conditions may include acute nephropathy and anemia. In adults, the following symptoms may be observed: peripheral neuropathies, motor weakness, chronic renal insufficiency and systolic hypertension, and anemia.

Lead exposure primarily arises in two settings: childhood exposure, usually through paint chips, and adult occupational exposure in the smelting, mining, ammunitions, soldering, plumbing, ceramic glazing, and construction industries. Other sources include lead-glazed ceramics and certain Asian herbal remedies.

Laboratory Evaluation

The most common specimen type is whole venous blood, the result of which is commonly referred to as the BLL. This is preferred over plasma and serum as circulating lead is predominantly associated with RBCs. Elevated lead levels in capillary blood specimens should be confirmed with a venous specimen to avoid the potential contribution of external contamination. Urine lead may be useful for detecting recent exposures to lead or to monitor chelation therapy. Other testing, such as plasma aminolevulinic acid, whole blood zinc protoporphyrin, and free erythrocyte protoporphyrin, may be useful for screening in occupational exposures. Non invasive measurements of lead in bone may be available radio-graphically. Removal of further lead exposure and parental education are essential parts to the management for patients with elevated BLLs.

Inductively coupled plasma mass spectrometry is a preferred method of analysis, although ICP-AES and GFAAS are also used.

MERCURY

Mercury (Hg), also called quicksilver, is a heavy, silvery metal. Along with bromine, mercury is one of only two elements that are liquid at room temperature and pressure. There are three naturally occurring oxidation states of mercury: Hg(0), Hg(1+), and Hg(2+). Organic mercury refers to various forms of mercury bound to a carbon atom, with mercury usually in the +2 oxidation state.

Mercury is released to the atmosphere as a product of the natural degassing of rock (30,000 tons/year) and through various human activities (20,000 tons/year). Mercury is used in dental amalgams, electronic switches, germicides, fungicides, and fluorescent light bulbs. The use of mercury in medicine has greatly declined in all respects; however, mercury compounds are found in some over-the-counter drugs, including topical anti-septics, stimulant laxatives, diaper-rash ointment, eyedrops, and nasal sprays. Mercury is widely used in the production of eye cosmetics, especially mascara.

Absorption, Transport, and Excretion

Routes of exposure include (1) inhalation, primarily as elemental mercury vapor but occasionally as dimethyl mercury; (2) ingestion of $HgCl_2$ and mercury-containing foods, such as predatory fish species; (3) cutaneous absorption of methyl mercury (MeHg) through the skin and even through latex gloves; (4) injection of relatively inert liquid mercury and mercury-containing tattoo pigments; and (5) dental amalgams. Inhaled mercury vapor is retained in the lungs to about 80%, whereas liquid metallic mercury passes through the gastrointestinal tract largely unabsorbed.

Mercury enters the food chain primarily by volcanic activity and man-made sources, such as coal combustion and smelting. Most of the dietary intake comes from consumption of meat and fish products, with estimates of dietary intake varying based upon geographical location and dietary sources. The kidney is the major storage organ after elemental or inorganic mercury exposure. MeHg is efficiently absorbed from the gastrointestinal tract, and distribution to tissues, including the brain, appears complete in 48 hours. Movement of MeHg across the blood–brain barrier appears to be dependent on coupling with the amino acid cysteine.

There is relatively little bioaccumulation of inorganic and elemental mercury. Half-lives vary according to the route of exposure and form of mercury, from 5 days in blood for phenylmercury to 90 days in urine for chronic exposure to inorganic mercury. Normally, the highest accumulation of mercury is in the kidney, liver, spleen, and brain. Mercury can accumulate in pituitary and thyroid glands, the pancreas, and the reproductive organs. The bulk of mercury accumulated in the body is eliminated in approximately 60 days; however, organic forms of mercury can accumulate in brain and may take up to several years to be eliminated. Fecal and urinary excretions are the main elimination routes for inorganic and organic mercury. A special form of elimination is the transfer of mercury from the fetus through the placenta.

Health Effects

Mercury has no known function in normal human physiology.

Mercury Toxicity

Toxicities have been observed following inhalation, ingestion, and dermal absorption of mercury compounds. Mercurial salts were historically used as diuretics, topical disinfectants, and laxatives before mercury toxicity was well understood. Since the 1930s, some vaccines contained the preservative thimerosal, a mercury-containing compound metabolized into ethylmercury. Although it was widely speculated that this mercury-based preservative can cause or trigger autism in children, scientific studies showed no evidence supporting any such link. Nevertheless, thimerosal has been removed from or reduced to trace amounts in all vaccines recommended for children of 6 years and younger, with the exception of the inactivated influenza vaccine. Organic mercury and elemental mercury vapor are toxic to both the central and peripheral nervous systems. Mercury attacks the central nervous system well before a victim shows symptoms.

Elemental mercury readily vaporizes, and its inhalation can produce harmful effects on the nervous, digestive, and immune systems and the lungs and kidneys. The inorganic salts of mercury can affect the skin, eyes, gastrointestinal tract, and kidneys. The toxicity of mercury is primarily through reaction with protein sulfhydryl groups melanocyte-stimulating hormone (MSH), resulting in dysfunction and inactivation. Liquid elemental mercury is poorly absorbed and relatively nontoxic but elemental mercury vapor is highly absorbed and is highly toxic. Inorganic, ionized forms of mercury are toxic. Further bioconversion to an alkyl mercury, such as MeHg, yields a very toxic species of mercury that is highly selective for lipid-rich mediums such as the brain.

Mercury intoxication can manifest in many signs and symptoms that affect several organ systems, including headache, tremor, impaired coordination, abdominal cramps, diarrhea, dermatitis, polyneuropathy, proteinuria, and hepatic dysfunction. Because many of these are relatively nonspecific signs and symptoms, laboratory testing provides a key role in assessing mercury intoxication.

Laboratory Evaluation

Mercury is usually determined as total mercury levels in blood and urine without regard to chemical form. Analytical methods include ICP-MS and **cold vapor AAS**.

Trace Elements Methods and Instrumentation

For many years, the most commonly used instrumentation for trace and toxic metal analysis has been the **atomic absorption (AA)** spectrometer, either with flame atomic absorption spectroscopy or flame less (i.e. graphite furnace atomic absorption spectroscopy) atomization. **Atomic emission** spectrometry is also useful for some elements, particularly if used in the form of inductively coupled plasma atomic emission spectroscopy for atomization and excitation. Recently, **inductively coupled plasma** mass spectrometry is becoming more widely used because of its sensitivity, wide range of elements covered, and relative freedom from interferences. No single technique is best for all purposes. A summary of the relative advantages and disadvantages of the main techniques is given in Table 19.1.

Sample Collection and Processing

Specimens for the analysis of trace elements must be collected with scrupulous attention to details, such as anticoagulant, collection apparatus, and specimen type (urine, serum, plasma, or blood). Because of the low

Table 19.1	Relative advantages and disadvantages of main techniques for elemental analysis			
	Flame AA	**GFAA**	**ICP-AES**	**ICP-MS**
Sensitivity	Moderate	Excellent	Moderate	Excellent
Selectivity	Excellent	Good	Poor	Good
Elemental coverage	Moderate	Good	Good	Excellent
Speed for one analyte	Fast	Slow	Fast	Fast
Multi-element capabilities	No	No	Yes	Yes
Initial cost of instrument	Low	Moderate	Moderate	High
Cost of consumables	Very low	Very high	Low	Moderate
Ease of operation	Excellent	Poor	Moderate	Moderate

concentration in biologic specimens and the ubiquitous presence in the environment, extraordinary measures are required to prevent contamination of the specimen. This includes using special sampling and collection devices, specially cleaned glassware, and water and reagents of high purity. The selection of needles, evacuated blood collection tubes, anticoagulants and other additives, water and other reagents, pipettes, and sample cups must be carefully evaluated for use in trace and ultratrace analyses. In addition, the laboratory environment must be carefully controlled.

Recommended measures include placing the trace elements laboratory in a separate room incorporating rigorous contamination control features, such as sticky mats at doors, nonshedding ceiling tiles, carefully controlled air flow to minimize particulate contamination, disposable booties worn over shoes, and particle monitoring equipment. Many useful measures are borrowed from those employed in semiconductor clean rooms.

Atomic Emission Spectroscopy

The simplified principle of the atomic emission spectroscopy (AES) instruments is presented in Fig. 19.4. The three most important components of atomic emission spectrophotometer are: (1) a source, in which the sample is atomized at a sufficient temperature to produce an excited-state species. Those species will emit radiation upon relaxation back to the ground state. (2) A wavelength selecting device (monochromator), for the spectral dispersion of the radiation and separation of the analytical line from other radiation. (3) A detector permitting measurement of radiation intensity.

A liquid sample, containing element(s) of interest, is converted into an aerosol and delivered into the source, where it receives energy sufficient to emit radiation. The intensity of the emitted radiation is correlated to the concentration of an analyte and is the basis for quantitation. The most commonly used sources in AES are flame and inductively coupled plasma (ICP). Flames are capable of producing temperatures up to 3,000 K.

Typical fuel gases include hydrogen and acetylene, while oxidant gases include air, oxygen, and nitrous oxide. The gases are combined in a specially designed mixing chamber. A sample is also introduced into the mixing chamber using a nebulizer that converts liquid into a fine spray. The mixing chamber and burner assembly are shown in Fig. 19.5. The same assembly can be used for AA instrumentation.

In AES, both atomic and ionic excited states can be produced (depending on the element and the source),

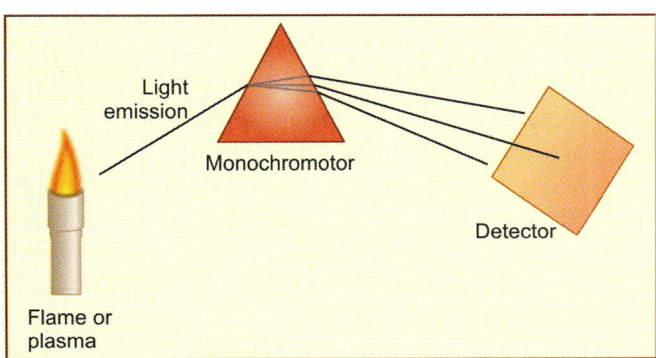

Fig. 19.4: Simplified schematic of AES

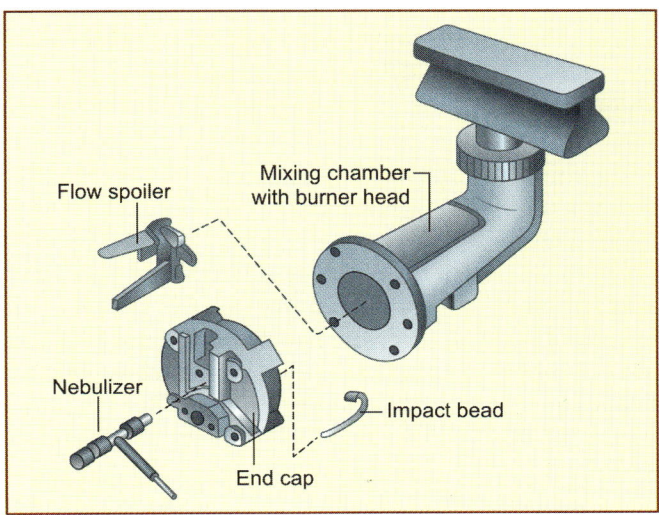

Fig. 19.5: Mixing chamber burner for flame AA

which leads to the production of complicated emission spectra. The 'emission spectrum' of an element is composed of a series of very narrow peaks (sometimes known as 'lines'), with each line at a different wavelength and each line matched to a specific transition.

Each element has its own characteristic emission spectrum. For example, sodium can be detected by tuning the monochromator to a wavelength of 589 nm. Ideally, each emission line of a given element would be distinct from all other emission lines of other elements. However, there are many cases where emission lines from distinct elements overlap resulting in interferences. The choice of interference-free wavelength (atomic or ionic line) may be challenging. While there are several possible wavelengths for a given element, wavelengths producing suitable analytical performance, such as limit of quantitation, freedom from interferences, and robustness, are selected.

The first detectors in AES used photographic film. Contemporary AES instruments feature photomultiplier tubes or array-based detector systems.

Atomic Absorption Spectroscopy

Atomic absorption spectroscopy is an analytical procedure for the quantitative determination of elements through the absorption of optical radiation by free atoms in the gas phase. The spectra of the atoms are line spectra that are specific for the absorbing elements.

Absorption is governed by the Beer-Lambert law

$$A = -\log_{10}(I_1/I_0)\, \varepsilon\, L C_g$$

where A is the absorbance of the sample, I_0 is the incident light intensity, I_1 is the transmitted light intensity, ε is the molar absorptivity of the target analyte for the wavelength being used, L is the path length, and C_g is the gas-phase concentration of the target analyte. Under some simplifying assumptions, this equation takes the form

$$A = KC$$

where K is a constant determined by calibration and C is the solution-phase concentration of the analyte.

The four most important components of AA spectrophotometer are (1) radiation (light) source, which emits the spectrum of the analyte element, (2) atomizer, in which the atoms of the element of interest in the sample are formed, (3) monochromator for the spectral dispersion of the radiation and separation of the analytical line from other radiation, and (4) detector permitting measurement of radiation intensity. The simplified principle of the AAS instruments is presented in Fig. 19.6.

Typical radiation sources for AAS are hollow cathode lamps (HCLs) and electrodeless discharge lamps (EDLs). The HCL contains a quantity of the target element in the

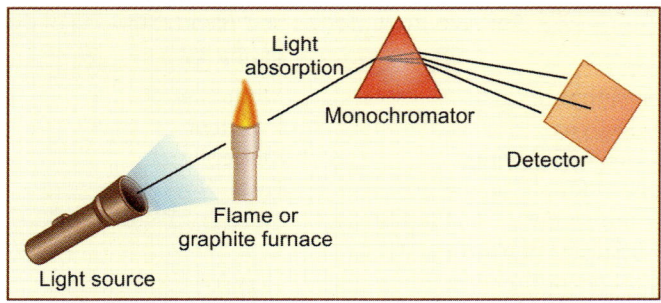

Fig. 19.6: Simplified schematic of AAS instrumentation

form of a hollow cylinder. During operation, a small quantity of the target element is vaporized, and some of the gas-phase atoms of the target element become electronically excited and emit photons with the right wavelength to be absorbed by atoms of the target element in the atomizer. While HCLs are an ideal source for determining most elements by AA, for volatile elements the use of EDLs is recommended. The most common sources in AAS are FAAS and GFAAS (also called flame less or electrothermal AAS).

The graphite tubes are the most commonly used atomizers in flame less AAS. Tubes are made of high-purity polycrystalline electrographite and coated with pyrolytic graphite and can be heated to a high temperature by an electrical current. A small aliquot (usually 20 μL) of liquid sample is placed in the tube at the ambient temperature.

The heating program (specifying the temperatures and times) is designed to first dry the sample, then pyrolyze, vaporize, and atomize the sample, followed by a cleaning step.

Selenium, cadmium, and lead are often measured by GFAAS. GFAAS allows for measurements of both liquid and solid samples. A common problem in GFAAS is that analyte volatility depends on the molecular form of the analyte and the sample matrix. To overcome this limitation, chemical modifiers (palladium nitrate, magnesium nitrate, or a mixture of both) are frequently added to samples, calibrators, and controls.

INDUCTIVELY COUPLED PLASMA MASS SPECTROMETRY

Inductively coupled plasma mass spectrometry is a state-of-the-art analytical technique for elemental analysis. The term *plasma* in ICP refers to an ionized gas (typically argon), in which a certain proportion of electrons are free. Like other mass spectrometers, the ICP-MS measures the **mass-to-charge ratio** [molecular mass divided by ionic charge (m/z)] of selected analyte ions and includes the following components—(1) an ion source, (2) a mass analyzer, and (3) an ion detector. A simplified schematic of an ICP-MS (Fig. 19.7).

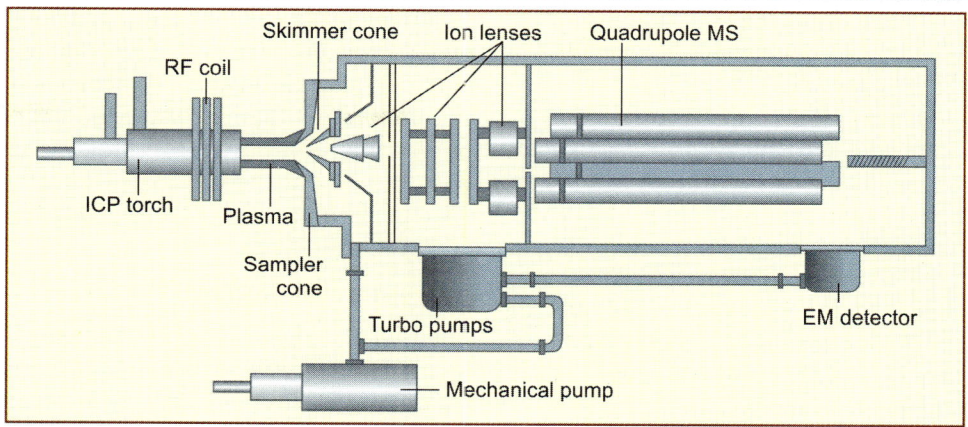

Fig. 19.7: Simplified schematic of ICP-MS instrumentation. ICP, inductively coupled plasma; RF, radio frequency; MS, mass spectrometer

The argon plasma induced by commercial ICP instruments (both ICP-AES and ICP-MS) generates temperatures ranging from 6,000–10,000 K and serves several purposes. First, it dries and then vaporizes the droplets produced by the nebulizer. This step is followed by atomization of any molecular species. Finally, atoms are thermally ionized, at which point they are ready for introduction into the mass spectrometer.

Nearly, all ICP torches consist of three concentric quartz tubes surrounded by a coil carrying radio-frequency (RF) power. The middle tube of the torch carries the argon (Ar) that forms the plasma.

Quantitative analysis for clinical samples is best performed with the use of an internal standard. All patient samples, calibrators, and controls are diluted with an internal standard, usually a solution of an uncommon element such as yttrium. Rather than using the raw signal level of the target elements as the basis for quantitation, the signal for each of the target elements is divided by the signal of the internal standard to give signal ratios (i.e. normalized intensities).

Quadrupole Mass Spectrometers

The typical mass spectrometer used for ICP-MS is a quadrupole mass spectrometer. The analyzer consists of four parallel conducting rods arranged in a square array. Applying RF and constant direct current (DC) voltages to the rods, the instrument can be tuned, so that only ions of a specific m/z ratio can pass through the device to reach the detector. This type of instrument tends to be relatively simple to use and maintain, but the resolution (the ability to discriminate between closely spaced m/z values) is limited, being able to well resolve peaks separated by one m/z unit but not able to resolve peaks separated by a small fraction of an m/z unit.

High-Resolution Mass Spectrometers

Other ICP-MS instruments incorporate high-resolution mass spectrometers. These are usually 'double focusing

sector field' instruments. Such instruments separate ions of different m/z values via deflection in a magnetic field, with ions of greater m/z being deflected to a lesser degree than those of lower m/z. The magnetic field is adjusted to allow only ions of a selected m/z to reach the detection system at any given point in time.

A second device known as an electrostatic analyzer corrects for certain non-ideal effects, allowing the instrument to achieve high resolution. Commercially available high resolution

ICP-MS instruments are capable of a resolution of 10,000 (10% valley). This is enough to resolve, e.g. 75As+ from 75ArCl+, both nominally 75 m/z units, but which differ by 1×10^3 units when viewed at high resolution. However, magnetic sector instruments are not able to resolve elemental isobaric interferences, such as 115Sn/115In and 40Ca/40Ar, which would require resolution much higher than 10,000.

INTERFERENCES

In general, the interferences in elemental analysis are classified as spectroscopic or non-spectroscopic.

Spectroscopic Analysis

Spectral interferences generally result from a spectral overlap with the spectrum of the target analyte. For example, in AA certain molecular species may have broad absorption spectra that may overlap the line spectra of the elements of interest, leading to false elevations of the target element concentrations. A much less common occurrence would be for the absorption spectrum of one element to overlap with that of another.

Various strategies are used to deal with spectral interferences in AAS. A continuum source background correct or may be included in the instrument design at the cost of some instrument complication. Another alternative is Zeeman background correction, which relies on shifting the atomic spectral lines by the application of a magnetic field. In ICP-MS, spectral interferences include polyatomic species whose m/z may overlap m/z of the target analyte.

For example, $^{56}ArO^+$ has the same nominal m/z as $^{56}Fe^+$. The argon oxide ion, which can be a significant component of plasma generated by an ICP torch, can potentially interfere with iron analysis by ICP-MS. Another well-known polyatomic interference is argon chloride ion $^{75}(ArCl)^+$ on determination of $^{75}As^+$.

Several approaches are used to deal with polyatomic interferences in ICP-MS. One applies algebraic equations, together with relative isotopic abundance information, to mathematically correct for interferences.

Another approach interposes a reaction cell or collision cell between the main ion lenses and the mass analyzer. A small amount of a gas, such as helium or ammonia introduced into the cell removes interferences, either by chemical reaction or by an energy filtering process, using the fact that polyatomic species, with their larger collisional cross sections, lose energy faster than atomic ions.

High-resolution mass spectrometers provide a third way to remove interferences as discussed in an earlier section. A second source of spectral interferences in ICP-MS arises from nearby elements in the periodic table. For example, tin (Sn) and cadmium (Cd) both have isotopes at 114 Da (atomic mass unit), so they could potentially interfere with each other if the instrument is set to measure 114 m/z. This can usually be handled by using a different isotope for the analysis. For example, cadmium also has an isotope at 111 Da that is free from isobaric elemental interferences.

A third source of spectral interferences in ICP-MS comes from doubly charged ions. For example, $^{136}Ba^{2+}$ appears at the same m/z as $^{68}Zn^+$ (136/2 equals 68/1).

These are relatively uncommon and can usually be avoided, such as by choosing a different isotope for analysis or tuning the torch to reduce multiply charged ions.

Non-spectroscopic Analysis

Matrix interferences involve the bulk physical properties of the sample to be analyzed. The aqueous samples may behave differently than organic and biological specimens, depending upon the technology used and the analyte of interest. The properties of significance are viscosity, presence of easily ionized elements, and presence of carbon. Matrix matching of the calibrators, controls, and specimens helps to overcome matrix interferences.

Dilution of the specimens helps minimize matrix effect, but it is only applicable to certain analytical techniques and to the determination of analytes with higher concentrations. Anything that could interfere with atomization of the sample could be classified as a non-spectral interference.

For example, in AA, a flame may not be hot enough for efficient atomization. Difference in sample viscosity between standards and unknown samples, resulting in differing rates of sample introduction, is another example of a non-spectral interference. In AES, anything that would prevent the efficient excitation or emission of spectral lines used for the analysis would constitute a non-spectral interference.

ELEMENTAL SPECIATION

The toxicity of elements may depend on their chemical forms. For example, arsenobetaine is a relatively nontoxic form of arsenic. Methylated forms of arsenic are intermediate in toxicity, and inorganic arsenic, such as As(V) and As(III), are highly toxic. In the medical evaluation of patients, it can be important to know whether an elevated arsenic level is due to relatively innocuous forms, such as arsenobetaine, perhaps from a seafood meal ingested up to 3 days before the specimen collection, or by dangerous forms such as inorganic arsenic. In addition, the concentrations of methylated forms may be useful information for monitoring recovery from toxic exposure. The methodologies for elemental analysis discussed in previous sections are generally not capable of specifying the chemical form of the target elements.

The so-called hyphenated techniques allow for speciation determinations. In a hyphenated analysis, the combination of two or more complementary analytical techniques is used to measure the specific form of an analyte. A classic example of this approach is liquid chromatography (LC-ICP-MS). The sample is injected into a liquid chromatograph which separates the different chemical forms of the analyte producing a characteristic retention time. Concurrently, the eluting sample is continuously analyzed by a mass spectrometer.

The retention time partially identifies the analytes, and the mass spectrometer further identifies the element. In some cases, AA may substitute for mass spectrometry (MS) in elemental speciation schemes. Methods for elemental speciation are becoming more common, especially in Europe. Despite clinical matrices being among the most difficult for speciation, several applications are reported; some among them are as follows:

- Arsenic speciation in urine by LC-ICP-MS and HG-GFAAS
- Copper in urine by size exclusion chromatography (SEC)-ICP-MS
- Copper in red blood cells by SEC-ICP MS
- Lead in blood by gas chromatography (GC)-GFAAS
- Selenium in serum by SEC-GFAAS
- Zinc in urine by anion exchange chromatography ICP-MS

Alternative Analytical Techniques

Voltammetric methods, such as anodic stripping voltammetry (ASV) and adsorptive stripping voltammetry, can be used in determination of selected metals and are the basis for some point-of-care devices. Ion chromatography can be used for the determination of copper, iron, and zinc in blood, serum, and plasma and for the determination of zinc in urine. Gas chromatography–mass spectrometry is capable of determination of cadmium, chromium, cobalt, copper, lead, and selenium in urine, copper in serum, and lead in blood. The methods accommodating direct analysis of solid samples, for instance, laser ablation ICP-MS (LA-ICPMS), are gaining recognition for selected clinical applications.

BIBLIOGRAPHY

1. Alfrey A. Aluminum. In: Mertz W, Underwood EJ, eds. Trace Elements in Human and Animal Nutrition. St. Louis, MO: Academic Press; 1986: 399–413.

2. Anghileri LJ. Iron, intracellular calcium ion, lipid peroxidation and carcino-genesis. Anticancer Res. 1995; 15(4): 1395–1400.

3. Anke M, Giel M. Molybdenum. In: Seiler H, Sigel A, Sigel H, eds. Handbook on Metals in Clinical and Analytical Chemistry. New York, NY: Marcel Dekker; 1994; 495–501.

4. Anke M. Arsenic. In: Mertz W, Underwood EJ, eds. Trace Elements in Human and Animal Nutrition. St. Louis, MO: Academic Press; 1986: 347–372.

5. Ashwood E. Clinical Testing. New York, NY: ARUP Laboratories; 2004: 101–102.

6. Bales CW, Steinman LC, Freeland-Graves JH, et al. The effect of age on plasma zinc uptake and taste acuity. Am J Clin Nutr. 1986; 44(5): 664–669.

7. Baselt R. In: Baselt R, ed. Disposition of Toxic Drugs and Chemicals in Man. Seal Beach, CA: Biomedical Publications; 2004: 39–41.

8. Beard JL, Dawson H, Piñero DJ. Iron metabolism: a comprehensive review. Nutr Rev. 1996; 54(10): 295-317.

9. Berlin M, Zalups R, Fowler B. Mercury. In: Nordberg G, et al. eds. Handbook on the Toxicology of Metals. Amsterdam; Boston, MA: Academic Press; 2007: 675–729.

10. Boffetta P, Nyberg F. Contribution of environmental factors to cancer risk. Br Med Bull. 2003;68:71-94.

11. Christensen J, Kristiansen J. Lead. In: Seiler H, Sigel A, Sigel H, eds. Handbook on Metals in Clinical and Analytical Chemistry. New York, NY: Marcel Dekker; 1994:425-440.

12. Cunnane SC. Maternal essential fatty acid supplementation increases zinc absorption in neonatal rats: relevance to the defect in zinc absorption in acrodermatitis enteropathica. Pediatr Res. 1982; 16(8): 599–603.

13. Donaldson J. The physiopathologic significance of manganese in brain: its relation to schizophrenia and neurodegenerative disorders. Neurotoxicology. 1987; 8(3): 451–462.

14. Drash G. Mercury. In: Seiler H, Sigel A, Sigel H, eds. Handbook on Metals in Clinical and Analytical Chemistry. New York, NY: Marcel Dekker; 1994: 479–493.

15. Ellingsen D, Horn N, Aaseth J. Copper. In: Nordberg G, et al. eds. Handbook on the Toxicology of Metals. Amsterdam; Boston, MA: Academic Press; 2007: 529–546.

16. Fisher GL. Function and homeostasis of copper and zinc in mammals. Sci Tot Environ. 1975;4(4): 373–412.

17. Fowler B, Chou C-HS, Jones R, et al. Arsenic. In: Nordberg G, et al. eds. Handbook on the Toxicology of Metals. Amsterdam; Boston, MA: Academic Press; 2007: 367–406.

18. Gladyshev VN, Jeang KT, Stadtman TC. Selenocysteine, identified as the penultimate C-terminal residue in human T-cell thioredoxin reductase, corresponds to TGA in the human placental gene. Proc Natl Acad Sci U S A. 1996; 93(12): 6146–6151.

19. Goyer R, Klaassen CD, Waalkes MP. Nervous system. In: Goyer R, Klaassen CD, Waalkes MP, eds. Metal Toxicology. San Diego, CA: Academic Press; 1995:199-235.

20. Hambridge K, Casey C, Krebs N. Zinc. In: Mertz W, Underwood EJ, eds. Trace Elements in Human and Animal Nutrition. St. Louis, MO: Academic Press; 1986: 1–137.

21. Herber RFM. Cadmium. In: Seiler HG, et al. eds. Handbook on Metals in Clinical and Analytical Chemistry. New York, NY: Marcel Dekker; 1994: 283–297.

22. Herbert V, Shaw S, Jayatilleke E. Vitamin C-driven free radical generation from iron. J Nutr. 1996;126(4 suppl):1213S-1220S.

23. Herold DA, Fitzgerald RL. Chromium. In: Seiler H, Sigel A, Sigel H, eds. Handbook on Metals in Clinical and Analytical Chemistry. New York, NY: Marcel Dekker; 1994: 321–332.

24. Higgins T, Beutler E, Doumas B. Hemoglobin, iron, and bilirubin. In: Burtis CA, Ashwood ER, Bruns DE, eds. Tietz Textbook of Clinical Chemistry and Molecular Diagnostics. Philadelphia, PA: WB Saunders; 2006: 1165–1208.

25. Högberg J, Alexander J. Selenium. In: Nordberg G, et al. eds. Handbook on the Toxicology of Metals. Amsterdam; Boston, MA: Academic Press; 2007: 783–807.

26. Holstege CP, Heavy metals. In: Holstege CP, Borloz MP, Benner JP, eds. Toxicology Recall. Baltimore, MD: Lippincott William & Wilkins; 2009: 256–310.

27. Iffland R. Arsenic. In: Seiler H, Sigel A, Sigel H, eds. Handbook on Metals in Clinical and Analytical Chemistry. New York, NY: Marcel Dekker; 1994: 237–253.

28. Jacobs DS, DeMott WR, Oxley DK. Jacobs &DeMott Laboratory Test Handbook. 5th ed. Lexi-Comp's Clinical Reference Library. Hudson, OH: Lexi-Comp; 2001:1031.

29. Kaiser J. State Court to rule on manganese fume claims. Science (New York, NY). 2003;300(5621):927.

30. Kamimura T, Miyamoto T, Harada M, et al. Advances in therapies for acute promyelocytic leukemia. Cancer Sci. 2011; 102(11): 1929–1937.

31. Langård S, Costa M. Chromium. In: Nordberg G, et al. eds. Handbook on the Toxicology of Metals. Amsterdam; Boston, MA: Academic Press; 2007: 487–510.

32. Levander O. Selenium. In: Mertz W, Underwood EJ, eds. Trace Elements in Human and Animal Nutrition. St. Louis, MO: Academic Press; 1986: 209–279.

33. Lönnderdal B. Iron-zinc-copper interactions. In: Micronutrient Interactions. Impact on Child Health and Nutrition. Washington, DC: International Life Sciences Institute; 1996: 3–10.

34. Magee R, James B. Selenium. In: Seiler H, Sigel A, Sigel H, eds. Handbook on Metals in Clinical and Analytical Chemistry. New York, NY: Marcel Dekker; 1994: 551–562.

35. May T, Wiedmeyer R. A table of polyatomic interferences in ICP-MS. Atom Spectrosc. 1998;19(5): 150–155.

36. McCord JM. Iron, free radicals, and oxidative injury. SeminHematol. 1998; 35(1): 5–12.

37. McMillin GA, Travis JJ, Hunt JW. Direct measurement of free copper in serum or plasma ultrafiltrate. Am J ClinPathol. 2009; 131(2): 160–165.

38. Meneghini R. Iron homeostasis, oxidative stress, and DNA damage. Free Rad Biol Med. 1997; 23(5): 783–792.

39. Moyer T, Burritt M, Butz J. Toxic metals. In: Burtis CA, Ashwood ER, Bruns DE, eds. Tietz Textbook of Clinical Chemistry and Molecular Diagnostics. Philadelphia, PA: Elsevier Saunders; 2006: 1377–1378.

40. Nordberg G, Nogawa K, Nordberg M, et al. Cadmium. In: Nordberg G, et al. eds. Handbook on the Toxicology of Metals. Amsterdam; Boston, MA: Academic Press; 2007: 445–486.

41. Offenbacher EG, Pi-Sunyer FX. Chromium in human nutrition. Ann Rev Nutr. 1988; 8: 543–563.

42. Pais I, Jones JB. The Handbook of Trace Elements. Boca Raton, FL: St. Lucie Press; 1997:xv, 223.

43. Porter W, Moyer T. Clinical toxicology. In: Burtis CA, Ashwood ER, eds. Tietz Fundamentals of Clinical Chemistry. Philadelphia, PA: WB Saunders; 2006: 427–456.

44. Rodushkin I, Odman F, Branth S, et al. Multi-elemental analysis of whole blood by high resolution inductively coupled plasma mass spectrometry. Fresenius Chem. 1999; 364 SRC: 338–346.

45. Rossi E. Hepcidin—the iron regulatory hormone. Clin Biochem Rev. 2005; 26(3): 47–49.

46. Sandstrom B, Arvidsson B, Cederblad A, et al. Zinc absorption from composite meals.I.The significance of wheat extraction rate, zinc, calcium, and protein content in meals based on bread. Am J ClinNutr. 1980;33(4): 739–745.

47. Sandstrom B, Cederblad A. Zinc absorption from composite meals. II. Influence of the main protein source. Am J ClinNutr. 1980; 33(8): 1778–1783.

48. Sandström B, Davidsson L, Cederblad A, et al. Oral iron, dietary ligands and zinc absorption. J Nutr. 1985; 115(3): 411–414.

49. Šaric´ M, Lucchini R. Manganese. In: Nordberg G, et al. eds. Handbook on the Toxicology of Metals. Amsterdam; Boston, MA: Academic Press; 2007: 645–674.

50. Sarkar B. Copper. In: Seiler HG, Sigel A, Sigel H, eds. Handbook on Metals in Clinical and Analytical Chemistry. New York, NY: Marcel Dekker; 1994: 339–347.

51. Schaller K, Letzel S, Angerer J. Aluminum. In: Seiler H, Sigel A, Sigel H, eds. Handbook on Metals in Clinical and Analytical Chemistry. New York, NY: Marcel Dekker; 1994: 217–226.

52. Schwartz CJ, Valente AJ, Sprague EA, et al. The pathogenesis of atherosclerosis: an overview. ClinCardiol. 1991;14 (2 suppl 1): I1-I16.

53. Shenkin A, Baines M, Lyon T. Vitamins and trace elements. In: Burtis CA, Ashwood ER, Bruns DE, eds. Tietz Textbook of Clinical Chemistry and Molecular Diagnostics. Philadelphia, PA: Elsevier Saunders; 2006: 1075–1164.

54. Sjögren B, Iregren A, Elinder C, et al. Aluminum. In: Nordberg G, et al. eds. Handbook on the Toxicology of Metals. Amsterdam; Boston, MA: Academic Press; 2007: 339–352.

55. Skerfving S, Bergdahl I. Lead. In: Nordberg G, et al. eds. Handbook on the Toxicology of Metals. Amsterdam; Boston, MA: Academic Press; 2007: 599–643.

56. Smith C, Mitchinson MJ, Aruoma OI, et al. Stimulation of lipid peroxidation and hydroxyl-radical generation by the contents of human atherosclerotic lesions. Biochem J. 1992; 286(pt 3): 901–905.

57. Smith MA, Perry G. Free radical damage, iron, and Alzheimer's disease. J Neurol Sci. 1995;134(suppl): 92–94.

58. Sobin C, Parisi N, Schaub T, et al. A Bland–Altman comparison of the Lead Care® System and inductively coupled plasma mass spectrometry for detecting low-level lead in child whole blood samples. J Med Toxicol. 2011; 7(1): 24–32.

59. Solomons NW. Biological availability of zinc in humans. Am J ClinNutr. 1982;35(5): 1048–1075.

60. Solomons NW. Competitive interaction of iron and zinc in the diet: consequences for human nutrition. J Nutr. 1986; 116(6): 927–935.

61. Thomas R. Practical Guide to ICP-MS: A Tutorial for Beginners. 2nd ed. Practical Spectroscopy. Boca Raton, FL: CRC Press; 2008:xxv, 347.

62. Thunus L, Lejeune R. Zinc. In: Seiler H, Sigel A, Sigel H, eds. Handbook on Metals in Clinical and Analytical Chemistry. New York, NY: Marcel Dekker; 1994: 667–674.

63. Tofaletti JG. Trace elements. In: Bishop ML, Fody EP, Schoeff LE, eds. Clinical Chemistry: Principles, Procedures, Correlations. Philadelphia, PA: Lippincott Williams & Wilkins; 2004: 403–423.

64. Turnlund J, Friberg L. Molybdenum. In: Nordberg G, et al. eds. Handbook on the Toxicology of Metals. Amsterdam; Boston, MA: Academic Press; 2007: 731–741.

65. Vaughan M, Horlick G. Correction procedures for rare earth analysis in inductively coupled plasma-mass spectrometry. Appl Spectrosc 1990; 44: 587–593.

66. Walter LR, Marel E, Harbury R, et al. Distribution of chromium and cobalt ions in various blood fractions after resurfacing hip arthroplasty. J Arthroplasty. 2008; 23(6): 814–821.

67. Weinberg ED. Cellular iron metabolism in health and disease. Drug Metab Rev. 1990; 22(5): 531–579.

20

Toxicology of Specific Agents

INTRODUCTION

Toxicology is the study of poisons, or, more comprehensively, the identification and quantification of adverse outcomes associated with exposures to physical agents, chemical substances and other conditions. As such, toxicology draws upon most of the basic biological sciences, medical disciplines, epidemiology and some areas of chemistry and physics for information, research designs and methods. Toxicology ranges from basic research investigations on the mechanism of action of toxic agents through the development and interpretation of standard tests characterizing the toxic properties of agents.

In drug overdose, it is essential to identify the responsible agent to ensure appropriate treatment. In a similar manner, identification of drug abuse in non-overdose situations provides a rationale for the treatment of addiction. For these reasons, testing for drugs of abuse is commonly done. This typically involves screening of a single urine specimen for many substances by qualitative screening procedures. In most instances, this procedure only detects recent drug use; therefore, with abstinence of relatively short duration, many abusing patients may not be identified. In addition, a positive drug screen cannot discriminate between single casual use and chronic abuse. Identification of chronic abuse usually involves several positive test results in conjunction with clinical evaluation. In a similar manner, a positive drug screen does not determine the time frame or dose of the drug taken. Drug abuse or overdose can occur with prescription, over-the-counter, or illicit drugs. The focus of this discussion is on substances with addictive potential. Testing for drug abuse has become commonplace in professional, industrial, and athletic settings.

The potential punitive measures associated with this testing may involve or result in civil or criminal litigation. Therefore, the laboratory must ensure that data are legally admissible and defendable. This requires the use of analytic methods that have been validated as accurate and precise. It also requires documentation of specimen security. Protocols and procedures must be established that prevent and detect specimen adulteration and that may prevent drug detection. Measurement of urinary temperature, pH, specific gravity, and creatinine is commonly done to ensure that these specimens have not been diluted or treated with substances that may interfere with testing. Specimen collection should be monitored and a chain of custody established to guard against specimen exchange.

Testing for drugs of abuse can be done by several methods. A two-tiered approach of screening and confirmation is usually used. Screening procedures should be simple, rapid, inexpensive, and capable of being automated. They are often referred to as spot tests. In general, screening procedures have good analytic sensitivity with marginal specificity; a negative result can rule out an analyte with a reasonable degree of certainty.

These methods usually detect classes of drugs based on similarities in chemical configuration. This allows the detection of parent compounds and congeners that have similar effects. Considering that many designer drugs are modified forms of established drugs of abuse, these methods increase the scope of the screening process.

A drawback to this type of analysis is that it may also detect chemically related substances that have no or low abuse potential; therefore, interpretation of positive test results requires integration of clinical context and further testing. Confirmation testing uses methods that have high sensitivity and specificity; many of these tests provide quantitative as well as qualitative information. Confirmatory testing requires the use of a method different from that used in the screening procedure. Gas chromatography mass spectrophotometry (GC–MS) is the reference method for confirmation of most analytes.

There are several general analytic procedures commonly used for the analysis of drugs of abuse. Chromogenic reactions, the generation of a colored product usually by a chemical reaction, are occasionally used as screening procedures. Immunoassay-based procedures are widely used as both screening and confirmatory assays. In general, immunoassays offer a high degree of sensitivity and are easily automated. A wide variety of chromatography techniques are used for the qualitative identification and quantitation of drugs. Thin-layer chromatography is an inexpensive method for the screening of many drugs and has the advantage that no instrumentation is required. GC and liquid chromatography (LC) allow complex mixtures of drugs to be separated and quantitated. These methods are generally labor intensive and not well suited to screening. Many drugs have the potential for abuse. Trends in drug abuse vary geographically and between different socioeconomic groups. For a clinical laboratory to provide an effective service requires knowledge of the drug or drug groups likely to be found within the patient population it serves.

AGENTS THAT CAUSE CELLULAR HYPOXIA

Carbon monoxide (CO) and methemoglobin-forming agents interfere with oxygen transport, resulting in cellular hypoxia. Cyanide interferes with oxygen use and therefore, causes an apparent cellular hypoxia.

CARBON MONOXIDE

Carbon monoxide is a colorless, odorless, and tasteless gas that is a product of incomplete combustion of carbonaceous material. Common exogenous sources of carbon monoxide include cigarette smoke, gasoline engines, and improperly ventilated home heating units. Small amounts of carbon monoxide are produced endogenously in the metabolic conversion of heme to biliverdin. This endogenous production of carbon monoxide is accelerated in hemolytic anemias.

Toxic Effects

When inhaled, carbon monoxide combines tightly with the heme Fe^{2+} of hemoglobin to form carboxyhemoglobin. The binding affinity of hemoglobin for carbon monoxide is about 250 times greater than that for oxygen. Therefore, high concentrations of carboxyhemoglobin limit the oxygen content of blood. Moreover, the binding of carbon monoxide to a hemoglobin subunit increases the oxygen affinity for the remaining subunits in the hemoglobin tetramer. Thus, at a given tissue pO2 value, less oxygen dissociates from hemoglobin when carbon monoxide is also bound, shifting the hemoglobin-oxygen dissociation curve to the left. Consequently, carbon monoxide not only decreases the oxygen content of blood, it also decreases oxygen availability to tissue, thereby producing a greater degree of tissue hypoxia than would result from an equivalent reduction in oxyhemoglobin due to hypoxia alone. Carbon monoxide may also bind to other heme proteins, such as myoglobin and mitochondrial cytochrome oxidase mitochondrial cytochrome c oxidase subunit 3; this may limit oxygen use when tissue pO2 is very low.

The toxic effects of carbon monoxide are a result of hypoxia. Organs with high oxygen demand, such as heart and brain, are most sensitive to hypoxia and thus account for the major clinical sequelae of carbon monoxide poisoning. It must be emphasized that the carboxyhemoglobin concentration, although helpful in diagnosis, does not always correlate with the clinical findings or prognosis. Factors other than carboxyhemoglobin concentration that contribute to toxicity include length of exposure, metabolic activity, and underlying disease, especially cardiac or cerebrovascular disease.

Moreover, low carboxyhemoglobin concentrations relative to the severity of poisoning may be observed if the patient was removed from the carbon monoxide-contaminated environment several hours before blood sampling.

An insidious effect of carbon monoxide poisoning is the delayed development of neuropsychiatric sequelae, which may include personality changes, motor disturbances, and memory impairment. These manifestations do not correlate with the length of exposure or with the maximum blood carboxyhemoglobin concentration.

Treatment for carbon monoxide poisoning involves removal of the individual from the contaminated area and administration of oxygen. The half-life (t1/2) of carboxyhemoglobin in the body is variable, and attempts to determine the exact elimination t1/2 for CO based on the inhaled oxygen concentration have not been validated. Hyperbaric oxygen therapy for CO is highly debated, and current position papers have found no evidence to support its use.

ANALYTICAL METHODS

Carbon monoxide may be released from hemoglobin and then measured by GC, or it may be determined indirectly as carboxyhemoglobin by spectrophotometry.

Gas chromatographic methods are accurate and precise even for very low concentrations of carbon monoxide. Spectrophotometric methods are rapid, convenient, accurate, and precise, except at very low concentrations of carboxyhemoglobin (<2–3%). Gas chromatographic methods measure the carbon monoxide content of blood. When blood is treated with potassium ferricyanide, carboxyhemoglobin is converted to methemoglobin, and carbon monoxide is released into the gas phase. Measurement of the released carbon monoxide may be performed by GC using a molecular sieve column and a thermal conductivity detector. A lower detection limit is achieved by incorporating a reducing catalyst (e.g. nickel) between the GC column and the detector to convert carbon monoxide to methane. The methane may then be detected with a flame ionization detector. A very low detection limit may be achieved with the use of a heated mercuric oxide reaction chamber between the GC column and an ultraviolet light detector. As carbon monoxide elutes from the column, it reacts with mercuric oxide to form mercury gas, which has a high molar absorptivity at 254 nm. In practice, the carbon monoxide binding capacity is also determined after an aliquot of the blood specimen is treated with carbon monoxide to saturate the hemoglobin. The results are then expressed as percent of carboxyhemoglobin:

$$\% \, HbCO = \frac{CO_{content}}{CO_{capacity}} \times 100$$

Gas chromatography methods are accurate and precise and are considered to be reference procedures. Normal values for carboxyhemoglobin in rural nonsmokers are about 0.5%; for urban nonsmokers, 1–2%; and for smokers, 5–6%. Values may be increased by about 3% in cases of hemolytic anemia.

Spectrophotometric methods rely on the characteristic spectral absorption properties of carboxyhemoglobin. Among several such methods, the most popular are based on automated, multi-wavelength measurements of several hemoglobin species. These methods are rapid and convenient for the determination of carboxyhemoglobin and other hemoglobin species. Spectrophotometric methods generally compare favorably with gas chromatographic procedures at carboxyhemoglobin concentrations greater than 2–3%, but their precision is poor below these concentrations. Therefore, they are sufficiently accurate and precise for measurement of carbon monoxide after exogenous exposure, but are too insensitive to detect the increased endogenous production of carbon monoxide that occurs in hemolytic anemia. Fetal hemoglobin has slightly different spectral properties than adult hemoglobin. Consequently, falsely high carboxy hemoglobin values of 4–7% may occur when blood from neonates is measured by some spectrophotometric methods utilizing fewer wavelengths. Moreover, erroneous results may occur with lipemic specimens, with bilirubin, and in the presence of methylene blue.

CYANIDE

Cyanide is a chemical group that consists of one atom of carbon bound to one atom of nitrogen by three molecular bonds (C=N). Inorganic cyanides (also known as cyanide salts) contain cyanide in the anion form (CN⁻) and are used in numerous industries, such as metallurgy, photographic developing, plastic manufacturing, fumigation, and mining.

Organic compounds that have a cyano group bonded to an alkyl residue are called nitriles. For example, methyl cyanide is also known as acetonitrile (CH_3CN). Hydrogen cyanide (HCN) is a colorless gas at standard temperature and pressure with a reported bitter odor. Cyanogen gas, a dimer of cyanide, reacts with water and breaks down into the cyanide anion.

Many plants, such as *Manihot spp.* (cassava), *Unum spp.*, *Lotus* spp., *Prunus* spp., *Sorghum* spp., and *Phaseolus* spp., contain cyanogenic glycosides. Iatrogenic cyanide poisoning may occur during use of nitroprusside as a vasodilator given to reduce blood pressure and after load. Each nitroprusside molecule contains five cyanide molecules, which are slowly released in vivo. If endogenous sulfate stores are depleted, as in the malnourished or postoperative patient, cyanide may accumulate even with therapeutic nitroprusside infusion rates (2–10 μg/kg/min).

Toxic Effects

Hydrocyanic acid binds to hemoglobin. The hydrocyanic acid bound in the erythrocyte is in equilibrium with free hydrocyanic acid in the serum at a ratio of 10:1. Cyanide in serum readily crosses all biological membranes and avidly binds to heme iron (Fe^{3+}) in the cytochrome a-a3 complex within mitochondria. When bound to cytochrome a-a3′ cyanide is a competitive inhibitor that causes decoupling of oxidative phosphorylation. Patients exposed to toxic concentrations of cyanide exhibit rapid onset of symptoms typical of cellular hypoxia-flushing, headache, tachypnea, dizziness, and respiratory depression, which progress rapidly to coma, seizures, complete heart block, and death if the dose is sufficiently large.

Hydroxycobalamin or the cyanide antidote kit should be administered as soon as cyanide poisoning is suspected. Hydroxocobalamin, a vitamin B12 precursor, is a metalloprotein with a central cobalt atom that complexes cyanide, forming cyanocobalamin (vitamin B12).

Cyanocobalamin is eliminated in the urine or releases the cyanide moiety at a rate sufficient to allow detoxification by rhodanese. The cyanide antidote kit contains amyl nitrite, sodium nitrite, and sodium thiosulfate. Thiosulfate donates the sulfur atoms necessary for rhodanese-mediated cyanide biotransformation to thiocyanate. The mechanism of nitrite is less clear. The traditional rationale relies on the ability of nitrite to generate methemoglobin. Because cyanide has a higher affinity for methemoglobin than for cytochrome a3, cytochrome oxidase function is restored.

Analytical Methods

Following microdiffusion, whole blood CN^- is measured by photometric analysis or by head space gas chromatography. With the spectrophotometric method, a sealed, two-well microdiffusion cell is used to separate hydrocyanic acid from blood by mixing a sample of whole blood with strong acid in a sealed chamber and allowing the hydrocyanic acid gas generated to be absorbed into a strong base located in another part of the sealed chamber. One well of the cell contains the blood specimen and strong acid (unmixed until the cell is sealed), and the other well contains a strong base to absorb the hydrocyanic acid gas. After the hydrocyanic acid is collected in the aqueous base medium, pyridine, barbituric acid, and chloramine-T are added to generate a red complex, with the intensity of the color proportional to the concentration of CN^-. A good quality spectrophotometer is required to measure the absorbance.

METHEMOGLOBIN-FORMING AGENTS

The heme iron in hemoglobin is normally present in the ferrous state (Fe^{2+}). When oxidized to the ferric state (Fe^{3+}), methemoglobin is formed, and this form of hemoglobin cannot bind oxygen (Fig. 20.1). The principal physiologic system that maintains hemoglobin iron in the reduced state is nicotinamide adenine dinucleotide (NADH)-methemoglobin reductase. The NADH for this enzyme is supplied by normal glycolysis (Embden-Meyerhof pathway).

A minor pathway for methemoglobin reduction involves nicotinamide adenine dinucleotide phosphate (NADPH)-methemoglobin reductase, and the NADP for this enzyme reaction is derived from the hexose-monophosphate shunt. Congenital methemoglobinemia may result from a deficiency of NADH-methemoglobin reductase or, more rarely, from hemoglobin variants (hemoglobin M), in which heme iron is both more susceptible to oxidation and more resistant to reduction by the methemoglobin reductase system.

Toxic Effects

An acquired (toxic) methemoglobinemia may be caused by various drugs and chemicals (Table 20.1). The normal percentage of methemoglobin is <1.5% of total hemoglobin. In otherwise healthy individuals, methemoglobin percentages up to 20%, may cause slate-gray cutaneous discoloration, cyanosis, and chocolate-brown blood. Percentages between 20% and 50% may cause dyspnea, exercise intolerance, fatigue, weakness, and syncope. More severe symptoms of dysrhythmias, seizures, metabolic acidosis, and coma are associated with methemoglobin percentages of 50–70%, and >70% may be lethal. All of these symptoms are a consequence of hypoxia associated with the diminished O_2 content of the blood, and with a decreased O_2 dissociation from hemoglobin species in which some, but not all, subunits contain heme iron in the ferric state (i.e. shift of

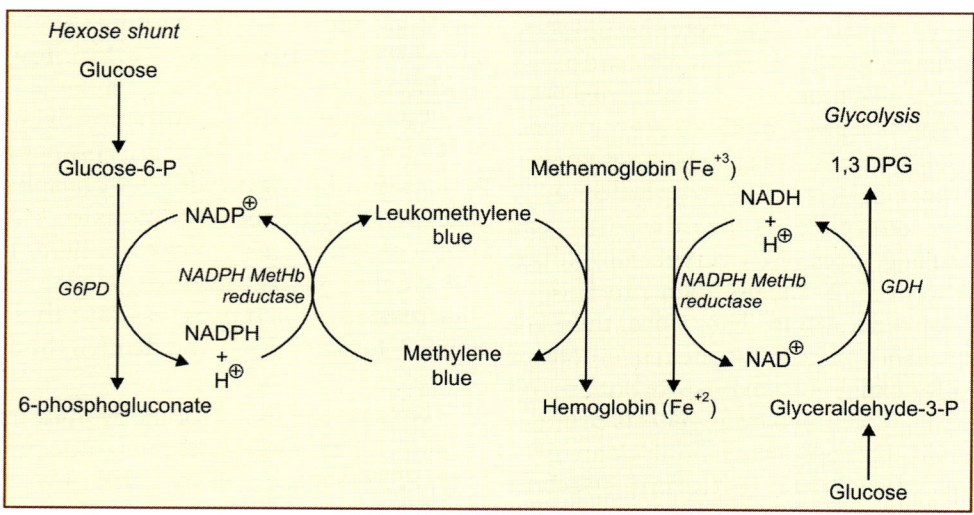

Fig. 20.1: Enzymatic pathways for methemoglobin reduction

Table 20.1	Examples of acquired causes of methemoglobinemia	
Drugs		**Chemical agents**
Amyl nitrite		Aniline
Benzocaine		Amyl nitrite
Chloroquine		Butyl nitrite
Dapsone		Chlorobenzene
Nitroglycerin		Naphthalene
Phenacetin		Nitrates
Phenazopyridine		Nitrites
Primaquine		Nitrophenol
Sulfonamides		Nitrous oxide

dissociation curve to the left). The pO2 is normal in these patients, and therefore, is the calculated hemoglobin oxygen saturation. Thus, a normal pO2 in a cyanotic patient is a significant indication for the possible presence of methemoglobinemia.

Specific therapy for toxic methemoglobinemia involves the administration of methylene blue, which acts as an electron transfer agent in the NADPH methemoglobin reductase reaction, thereby increasing the activity of this system several fold. Methylene blue and sulfhemoglobin cause spectral interference in the measurement of methemoglobin with some co-oximeters.

Analytical Methods

Methemoglobin is measured in blood manually, or by automated multi-wavelength measurements with a co-oximeter. Methemoglobin interferes with the noninvasive pulse oximetry method, measuring the absorbance of light at 660 nm (oxyhemoglobin) and 940 nm (deoxyhemoglobin). Because methemoglobin is not stable at room temperature, specimens should be kept on ice or refrigerated but not frozen. The stability of methemoglobin at 4°C has not been well studied. Some sources indicate significant decreases in methemoglobin concentration after 4–8 hours, whereas others report little or no change after 24 hours. Freezing results in an increase in methemoglobin concentration.

ALCOHOLS OF TOXICOLOGIC INTEREST

Several alcohols are toxic and medically important. They include ethanol, methanol, isopropanol, acetone, and ethylene glycol.

ETHANOL

Ethanol is the most widely used and often abused chemical substance. Consequently, measurement of ethanol is one of the more frequently performed tests in the toxicology laboratory. Although, less frequently encountered, it is important to include methanol, isopropanol, acetone (a metabolite of isopropanol), and ethylene glycol in a test battery for alcohols for proper evaluation of the acutely intoxicated patient. The principal pharmacologic action of ethanol is central nervous system (CNS) depression. CNS effects vary depending on the blood ethanol concentration (Table 20.2), but are also heavily influenced by an individual's tolerance. Symptoms vary from euphoria

Table 20.2	Stages of acute alcoholic influence/intoxication	
Blood alcohol concentration, g/ 100 mL or mg/dL	**Influence**	**Clinical signs/symptoms**
0.01–0.05	Subclinical	Influence/Effects not apparent or obvious, behavior nearly normal by ordinary observation, impairment detectable by special tests
0.03–0.12	Euphoria	Mild euphoria, sociability, talkativeness, increased self-confidence; decreased inhibitions, diminution of attention, judgment, and control, some sensorimotor impairment, slowed information processing, loss of efficiency in finer performance tests, impairment of perception, memory
0.09–0.25	Excitement	Emotional instability; loss of critical judgment comprehension, decreased sensory response; increased reaction time, reduced visual acuity, peripheral vision, and glare recovery, sensorimotor incoordination; impaired balance, drowsiness
0.18–0.30	Confusion	Disorientation, mental confusion; dizziness, exaggerated emotional states (fear, rage, grief, etc.), disturbances of vision (diplopia, etc.) and of perception of color, form, motion, dimensions increased pain threshold increased muscular incoordination: staggering gait; slurred speech, apathy lethargy
0.25–0.40	Stupor	General inertia; approaching loss of motor functions, markedly decreased response to stimuli, marked muscular incoordination; inability to stand or walk, vomiting; incontinence of urine and feces, impaired consciousness; sleep or stupor
0.35–0.50	Coma	Complete unconsciousness; coma; anesthesia, depressed or abolished reflexes, subnormal temperature, impairment of circulation and respiration, possible death
0.45 +	Death	Death from respiratory arrest

and decreased inhibitions, to increased disorientation and incoordination, and then to coma and death. A blood alcohol concentration of 80 mg/dL (0.08%) has been established as the per se limit for operation of a motor vehicle in most countries.

Because of many factors, not all individuals experience the same degree of CNS dysfunction at similar blood alcohol concentrations. Moreover, the CNS actions of ethanol are more pronounced when the blood ethanol concentration is increasing (absorptive phase) than when it is declining (elimination phase), in part because of the phenomenon of acute tolerance. In addition, heavy alcohol use leads to a more chronic form of tolerance. When consumed with other CNS depressant drugs, ethanol exerts a potentiation or synergistic depressant effect. This can occur at relatively low alcohol concentrations, and numerous deaths have resulted from combined ethanol and drug ingestion.

The pharmacologic mechanisms for the CNS depressant actions of ethanol are complex and incompletely understood, but probably involve both enhancement of major inhibitory neurons and impairment of excitatory neurons. The principal CNS inhibitory neuronal system is mediated by the neurotransmitter γ-aminobutyric acid (GABA). When GABA binds to its postsynaptic receptor subtype GABA$_A$, this oligomeric ion-gated complex 'opens' to allow inward flux of Cl, leading to membrane hyperpolarization and subsequent decreased electrical response. This GABA-mediated inhibitory response is enhanced by ethanol and sedative, hypnotic, and anesthetic agents, including barbiturates, benzodiazepines, and volatile anesthetics. Neuronal nicotinic acetylcholine receptors also may be prominent molecular targets of alcohol. Both enhancement and inhibition of nicotinic acetylcholine receptor function have been reported depending on receptor subunit concentration and the concentrations of ethanol tested. Ethanol also inhibits the function of the N-methyl-D-aspartate (NMDA)-and kainate-receptor subtypes; AMPA receptors are largely resistant to alcohol.

The aforementioned chronic tolerance to ethanol is considered to be mediated by ethanol-induced increased responsiveness and upregulation in the synthesis of NMDA receptors, attained by concomitant down regulation and desensitization through phosphorylation of GABAA and glutamate receptors. Largely because of these adaptive changes, abrupt withdrawal from chronic, heavy ethanol use leads to a physical abstinence syndrome that has prominent features of CNS excitation. Included among these withdrawal symptoms are anxiety, irritability, insomnia, muscle tremor and cramps, seizures, hallucinations, and increased temperature, blood pressure, and heart rate.

Ethanol is metabolized principally by liver alcohol dehydrogenase to acetaldehyde, which is subsequently oxidized to acetic acid by aldehyde dehydrogenase (Fig. 20.2). The rate of elimination of ethanol from blood approximates a zero order process. This rate varies among individuals, averaging about 15 mg/dL/h for males and 18 mg/dL/h for females. At both low (<20 mg/dL) and high (>300 mg/dL) ethanol concentrations, elimination becomes more nearly first-order; it is accelerated at high concentrations. The elimination rate is also influenced by drinking practices (e.g. alcoholics have increased elimination rates caused by enzyme induction). Ethanol is a teratogen, and alcohol consumption during pregnancy can result in the birth of a baby with fetal alcohol spectrum disorder (FASD). FASD is an umbrella term that describes the variety of effects that can occur in an individual whose mother drank alcohol during pregnancy. These effects may include physical, mental, behavioral, and/or learning disabilities with possible lifelong implications and are 100% preventable when a woman completely abstains from alcohol during her pregnancy.

METHANOL

Methanol is used as a solvent in several commercial products, as a constituent of antifreeze and window cleaning fluids, and as a component of canned fuel. It may be consumed intentionally by alcoholics as an ethanol substitute or accidentally when present as a contaminant in illegal whiskey.

Accidental ingestions have occurred in children. The CNS effects of methanol are substantially less severe than those of ethanol. Methanol is oxidized by liver alcohol dehydrogenase (at about one-tenth the rate of ethanol) to formaldehyde. Formaldehyde in turn is rapidly

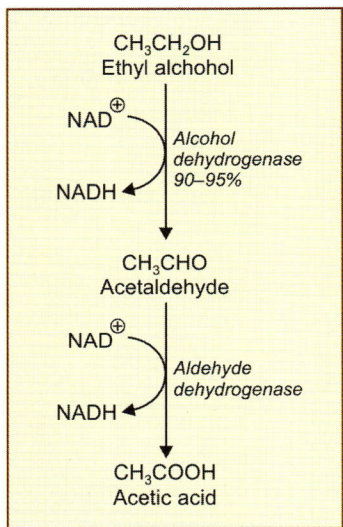

Fig. 20.2: Metabolism of ethanol

oxidized by aldehyde dehydrogenase to formic acid, which may cause serious acidosis and optic neuropathy, resulting in blindness or death. Serum formate concentrations correlate better with the degree of acidosis and the severity of CNS and ocular toxicity than do serum methanol concentrations. Therefore, some investigators recommend the measurement of serum formate to assess the severity of toxicity and to guide appropriate therapy in cases of methanol ingestion. The mainstay of therapy for methanol toxicity includes the administration of ethanol or fomepizole as a competitive alcohol dehydrogenase inhibitor, either folate or folinic acid, and dialysis.

ISOPROPANOL AND ACETONE

Isopropanol is readily available to the general population as a 70% aqueous solution for use as rubbing alcohol. It has about twice the CNS depressant action as ethanol, but it is not as toxic as methanol. Isopropanol has a short t1/2 of 2.5–3.0 hours, as it is rapidly metabolized by alcohol dehydrogenase to acetone, which is eliminated much more slowly (t1/2 > 3–6 hours). Therefore, concentrations of acetone in serum often exceed those of isopropanol during the elimination phase following isopropanol ingestion. Acetone has CNS depressant activity similar to that of ethanol, and because of its longer t1/2, it may prolong the apparent CNS effects of isopropanol. Supportive care is the mainstay of treatment, with rare reports of dialysis in severe intoxication.

ETHYLENE GLYCOL

Ethylene glycol, present in antifreeze products, may be ingested accidentally or for the purpose of inebriation or suicide. Ethylene glycol itself is relatively nontoxic, and its initial CNS effects resemble those of ethanol. However, metabolism of ethylene glycol by alcohol dehydrogenase (ADH) results in the formation of numerous acid metabolites, including lactate, oxalic acid and glycolic acid. These acid metabolites are responsible for much of the toxicity of ethylene glycol. Serum concentrations associated with death from ethylene glycol ingestion have been observed to vary from 0.06–4.3 g/L, highlighting the lack of correlation between ethylene glycol concentration and severity of toxicity. It is thus impossible to define a serum ethylene glycol concentration associated with a high probability of death. The serum concentration of glycolic acid correlates more closely with clinical symptoms and mortality than does the concentration of ethylene glycol. Because of the rapid elimination of ethylene glycol (t1/2 > 2–5 hours), its serum concentration may be low or undetectable at a time when glycolic acid remains elevated, Thus, the determination of ethylene glycol and glycolic acid provides useful clinical and confirmatory analytical information in cases of ethylene glycol ingestion. The mainstay of therapy for ethylene glycol toxicity includes administration of ethanol or fomepizole as a competitive alcohol dehydrogenase inhibitor and dialysis.

Analysis of Ethanol

Serum, plasma, and whole blood are suitable blood-related specimens for the determination of ethanol. The venipuncture site should be cleansed with an alcohol-free disinfectant, such as aqueous benzalkonium chloride.

Serum/Plasma and Blood Ethanol

Alcohol distributes into the aqueous compartments of blood; because the water content of serum is greater than that of whole blood, higher alcohol concentrations are obtained with serum as compared with whole blood. Experimentally, the serum-to-whole blood ethanol ratio is 1.18 (1.10–1.35) and varies slightly with hematocrit. Therefore, laboratories that perform alcohol determinations should make clear the choice of specimen. Because of the volatile nature of alcohols, specimens should be kept capped to avoid evaporative loss. Blood may be stored, when properly sealed, for 14 days at room temperature or at 4°C, with or without preservative. For longer storage or for nonsterile postmortem specimens, sodium fluoride should be used as a preservative to prevent a decrease or occasionally an increase (via fermentation) in ethanol concentration.

To measure ethanol in serum/plasma, enzymatic analysis is the method of choice for many laboratories. In this method, ethanol is measured by oxidation to acetaldehyde with NAD, a reaction catalyzed by ADH. With this reaction, the formation of NADH, measured at 340 nm, is proportional to the amount of ethanol in the specimen:

$$\text{Ethanol} + \text{NAD} \xrightarrow{\text{ADH}} \text{Acetaldehyde} + \text{NADH}$$

Under most assay conditions, ADH is reasonably specific for ethanol, with interferences by isopropanol, acetone, methanol, and ethylene glycol of typically <1%. However, spuriously increased results for ethanol have been described in the presence of high concentrations of lactate dehydrogenase (LDH) and lactate. This phenomenon is a result of the production of NADH by LDH:

$$\text{Lactate} + \text{NAD} \xrightarrow{\text{LDH}} \text{Pyruvate} + \text{NADH}$$

Serum or plasma is the most common specimen for ethanol analysis by ADH methods; this method also performs well with urine or oral fluid, although in some methods, whole blood may be used directly or a precipitation step may be required before analysis to avoid interference from hemoglobin. Results from these methods generally compare closely with those from gas chromatographic methods.

ESTIMATION OF BLOOD ALCOHOL

During the early part of the twentieth century, Dr Erik MP Widmark, a Swedish physician, did much of the foundational research regarding alcohol pharmacokinetics in the human body. In addition, he developed an algebraic equation that allows one to estimate the amount of alcohol consumed by an individual or the associated blood alcohol concentration when the values of the other variables are given:

$$N = W.\rho.\ [C_t + \beta.t]/(d.Z)$$

N = number of drinks
W = body weight (kg)
ρ = volume of distribution (L/kg) (0.68 for males, 0.55 for females)
C_t = blood alcohol concentration (kg/L)
b = rate of ethanol elimination (0.15 g/L/h)
t = time since first drink (h)
d = specific gravity of alcohol (0.8)
Z = amount of ethanol alcohol per drink (L) (15 mL of ethanol in a standard drink)

Typically, one wants to calculate the amount of ethanol consumed or the associated ethanol concentration. Note that it may be necessary to convert the units from those more commonly reported. It is important to remember that this formula is applicable only after completion of alcohol absorption, and when equilibrium has been reached between blood and body tissue.

Frequently the time since the first drink is unknown; the formula can be modified to estimate the number of drinks in an individual's system at the time of the test.

$$N = W.\rho.\ [C_t]/(d.Z)$$

The rate of elimination in the average person is commonly estimated at 0.015 g/100 mL/h (range, 0.010–0.030 g/100 mL/h). Retrograde extrapolation is an estimation of a subject's alcohol concentration at a prior time, derived from a blood alcohol concentration measured at a later time. This process may be applied when certain assumptions are made concerning absorption rates, elimination rates, and patterns of alcohol consumption, including drinking duration and volume consumed. Unfortunately, to be forensically useful and scientifically valid, such extrapolations may require facts about the person and that person's alcohol consumption, as well as related information that often is not available. Consequently, significant legal debate surrounds the validity and accuracy of retrograde extrapolation.

Breath Ethanol

The fundamental principle for use of breath analysis is that alcohol in capillary alveolar blood rapidly equilibrates with alveolar air in a ratio of approximately 2100:1(blood:breath). This blood-to-breath ratio may actually be closer to 2300:1 but in any case is variable. The lower blood-to-breath ratio will predict a slightly lower than actual blood alcohol concentration; its use therefore is not prejudicial. To alleviate confusion and uncertainty surrounding the conversion from breath to blood alcohol concentration, the traffic laws in many countries specify per se limits for blood and/or breath. Before breath alcohol analysis, a deprivation period of 15 minutes is required to allow for clearance of any residual alcohol that may have been present in the mouth (e.g. very recent drinking, use of alcohol-containing mouthwash, vomiting of alcohol-rich gastric fluid). Duplicate tests, performed 5–10 minutes apart and within 20 mg/dL (0.02%) are used as an additional safeguard against mouth alcohol contamination.

During the period of active alcohol absorption, generally 30–60 minutes depending on a variety of factors, and before peak blood alcohol concentration is obtained, the alcohol concentration in arterial blood will be initially higher than that in peripheral venous blood, and the converse is true in the postabsorptive phase. Because end-expiratory air equilibrates with pulmonary alveolar/capillary blood, the breath alcohol concentration more closely reflects that of arterial alcohol; however, the difference between arterial and venous blood is within the analytical error of most assays.

Determination of ethanol in expired air requires specialized breath alcohol analyzers. Several commercial evidential breath alcohol measurement devices are available. Principles of measurement used in such analyzers include (1) infrared absorption spectrometry (most common), (2) dichromate sulfuric acid oxidation-reduction (photometric), (3) GC (flame ionization or thermal conductivity detection), (4) electrochemical oxidation (fuel cell), and (5) metal oxide semiconductor sensors. Breath alcohol devices also may be used for the medical evaluation of patients at the point of care (e.g. emergency department).

Oral Fluid Ethanol

Because oral fluid (saliva) may be easily and non-invasively collected, interest is growing in its use for ethanol measurements and for the detection of drugs of abuse, but it is not a frequently used sample for ethanol determinations.

Urine Ethanol

Urine has been used as an alternative, less invasive specimen for the determination of alcohol use. During the postabsorptive phase following alcohol ingestion, the concentration of alcohol in urine is roughly 1.3 times that in blood. However, the use of urine alcohol measurements to estimate blood concentrations is discouraged because the ratio of 1.3 is highly variable, and, perhaps more important, the urine alcohol concentration may better reflect an average of the blood alcohol concentration during the period in which urine is collected in the bladder. The detection of alcohol in urine represents ingestion of alcohol within the previous 8–12 hours.

ETHYL GLUCURONIDE

Ethyl glucuronide (EtG) is a phase II metabolite of ethanol formed through the UDP glucuronosyl transferase-catalyzed conjugation of ethanol with glucuronic acid. Because of its long urinary elimination time, its specificity for ethanol exposure, and the low detection limits of assays, the use of EtG has been proposed as a marker of recent ethanol intake in a variety of clinical and legal settings, including medical monitoring for relapse, emergency department patient evaluation, postmortem assessment, and transportation accident investigation. However, challenges associated with factors, such as establishing appropriate cutoff concentrations capable of distinguishing between drinking and no beverage sources of ethanol exposure, no uniform laboratory reporting limits, sample stability, and microbial activity substantially complicate accurate interpretation of results.

ANALYSIS OF VOLATILE ALCOHOLS (METHANOL, ISOPROPANOL, AND ACETONE)

Methanol poisoning can be lethal if not recognized early. Unfortunately, in some instances, a latent period can be as long as 12–24 hours before toxicity is recognized, making laboratory identification of this poisoning critical. Development of gas chromatographic methods for volatiles in 1964 was a significant step in the recognition and treatment of this very toxic alcohol.

Flame ionization GC remains the most common method for the detection and quantitation of volatile alcohols in biological samples. Not only does it distinguish between ethanol, methanol, isopropanol, and acetone, but also it has the capability to measure concentrations as low as 10 mg/dL (0.01%).

Specimens are prepared by a variety of methods; the two most common are direct injection and head space analysis. Direct injection involves injection of a sample prepared by diluting it with an aqueous solution of internal standard. Repeated injection of biological aqueous matrix into the GC will cause buildup on the injector and front of the analytical column, requiring frequent maintenance and column replacement.

This can be alleviated by the use of head space injection. The volatility of the alcohols is used to separate them from the matrix. Specifically, the 'Gas Law' states that at a given temperature, the amount of volatile substance in the air space above the liquid-head space-is proportional to the concentration of the volatile alcohol in the solution. Therefore, the sample in the head space allows calculation of the concentration in the specimen.

Head space gas chromatographic analysis is another excellent method for the measurement of methanol, isopropanol, acetone, and ethanol. In addition, an adaptation of this technique may be used to measure formate, the toxic metabolite of methanol, after esterification to methyl formate. Conversely, direct injection GC is the method of choice for ethylene glycol, because it has a higher boiling point and is not as amenable to head space analysis. A modification of the GC procedure has the potential of combining both toxic alcohols in a single gas liquid chromatography (GLC) analysis. Methods that simultaneously measure ethylene glycol and glycolic acid have the advantage of being free from interference by propylene glycol (a diluent for parenteral drugs) or 2, 3-butanediol (may be present in serum from some alcoholics). Similar techniques are used to measure volatile alcohols in blood, serum, oral fluid, urine, other clinical specimens, and postmortem specimens (e.g. vitreous fluid, skeletal muscle).

Drugs of Abuse

Drug use and abuse are widespread in society, and public awareness has been heightened as to their impact on public safety and on lost productivity in industry. To resolve these issues, governmental, industrial, educational, and sports agencies are increasingly requiring drug testing of prospective and existing employees, students, and participants in professional and amateur athletics. Moreover, drug abuse during pregnancy is a matter of concern, both medically and socially. Testing for drugs of abuse may be a medical requirement for (1) organ transplantation candidates, (2) pain management clinics, (3) drug abuse treatment programs, and (4) psychiatric programs. Drug testing for these purposes represents a significant activity for toxicology laboratories.

Testing for drugs of abuse usually involves testing a single urine specimen for various drugs. It should be noted, however, that a single urine drug test detects only fairly recent drug use and it does not differentiate casual use from chronic drug abuse. The latter requires sequential drug testing and clinical evaluation. Moreover, urine drug testing alone cannot determine the degree of impairment, the dose of drug taken, or the exact time of use.

Drug testing results for nonmedical purposes may provide the sole evidence for punitive action or denial of individual rights. Therefore, this testing should be considered a forensic toxicology activity, requiring the highest standards of analytical methods, specimen security, and documentation. Moreover, laboratories engaged in this testing should be appropriately certified or recognized by forensic urine drug testing laboratory.

Several techniques are used by persons attempting to mask or adulterate drugs to avoid detection. These tactics may include the exchange of urine from a drug-free individual or dilution of the urine specimen by excessive consumption of water, use of a diuretic, or simple addition of water to the specimen to reduce drug concentrations to below cutoff limits. Also, readily available adulterants, such as detergent, bleach, salt, alkali, ammonia, tetrahydrozoline, or acid, maybe added to the specimen after collection in an attempt to interfere with immunoassay screening procedures. Other more sophisticated adulterants specifically marketed to avoid drug detection include glutaraldehyde (urine aid; clear choice), nitrite, chromate, and a combination of peroxide and peroxidase. These adulterants also interfere with immunoassays to variable degrees, and the oxidizing agents (nitrite, chromate, and peroxide/peroxidase) may result in destruction of morphine, codeine, and the principal metabolite resulting from marijuana use, thus interfering with their GC-mass spectrometry (MS) confirmation and with immunoassays.

Direct observation of urine collection is the most stringent means to guard against specimen exchange or adulteration. However, an individual's right to privacy and dignity must be weighed against the need for the highest degree of certainty of specimen integrity. Alternative measures to prevent specimen adulteration include (1) limitations on clothing or other personal belongings allowed in the specimen collection area, (2) addition of coloring agent to toilet water, and (3) inactivation of the hot water tap. In addition, several validity checks for specimen integrity may be made at the collection site and at the testing site. Validity testing criteria have been established by the department of health and human services (DHHS) for the drug testing program mandated for the United States Federal Employees. According to these criteria, the specimen must be examined for unusual color, odor, foaming, or precipitate, and its temperature should be 90–100 °F (32–38°C) when determined within 4 minutes of collection. A specimen is reported as dilute when the specific gravity is >1.0010 but <1.0030 and the creatinine is >2 mg/dL but ≤20 mg/dL. A substituted specimen is defined by a specific gravity ≤1.0010 or ≥1.0200 and a creatinine <2 mg/dL. Adulterated urine has pH<3 or ≥11 or nitrite >500 µg/mL (much lower concentrations occur with some urinary tract infections), or may be confirmed if a specific adulterant is detected and confirmed. A specimen is invalid if the pH is ≥3 and <4.5 or ≥9 and <11, if the creatinine and specific gravity are inconsistent, if nitrite is >200 and <500 µg/mL, or if the presence of other adulterants is suspected. In such cases, the urine specimen is rejected and generally is not tested for drugs. The finding of a substituted or an adulterated specimen is deemed equivalent to a refusal to test and would result in removal of the individual from safety-sensitive duties. Numerous commercial reagents for validity testing are available in both test strip and liquid forms.

Urine should be collected in tamper-proof specimencups, and a chain of custody maintained to identify all individuals involved in specimen collection, transfer, and testing.

Specimens that test positive should be stored frozen for a minimum of 1 year.

The most widely accepted method for drug confirmation is GC-MS. Liquid chromatography-tandem mass spectrometry is also used for rapid detection and confirmation of drugs of abuse. For confirmation, quantitative drug measurements are performed using selective ion monitoring with GC-MS.

The result may be reported as positive or negative relative to the cutoff value. However, the actual concentration may be helpful when morphine and codeine results are interpreted, and when individuals enrolled in drug treatment programs are monitored. In the latter case, subjects who test positive, but who have decreasing values on sequential testing may be judged abstinent, whereas those whose values suddenly increase are likely noncompliant. For this purpose, it is essential to normalize the drug concentration-to-urine creatinine concentration (nanograms of drug per milligram of creatinine). This will help compensate for fluctuations in absolute drug concentration related to physiologic variation in urine dilution or concentration.

Cannabinoids

Cannabinoids are a group of C21 compounds found in the marijuana plant *Cannabis sativa*. Cannabis is the most extensively abused drug in the world and it has been used as a medicinal and an illicit psychotropic agent for centuries. The main psychotropic effects are (1) euphoria, (2) distorted perceptions, (3) relaxation, and (4) a feeling of well-being.

Since 1996 cannabis was legalized for medical conditions such as glaucoma, chemotherapy-related nausea and vomiting, migraine, and anorexia. In 2005, the Gonzales vs. Raich ruling permitted the federal government to ban the nonmedical and medical use of cannabis.

Delta-9-tetrahydrocannabinol (THC), the primary psychoactive component of the *C. sativa* plant (Fig. 20.3),

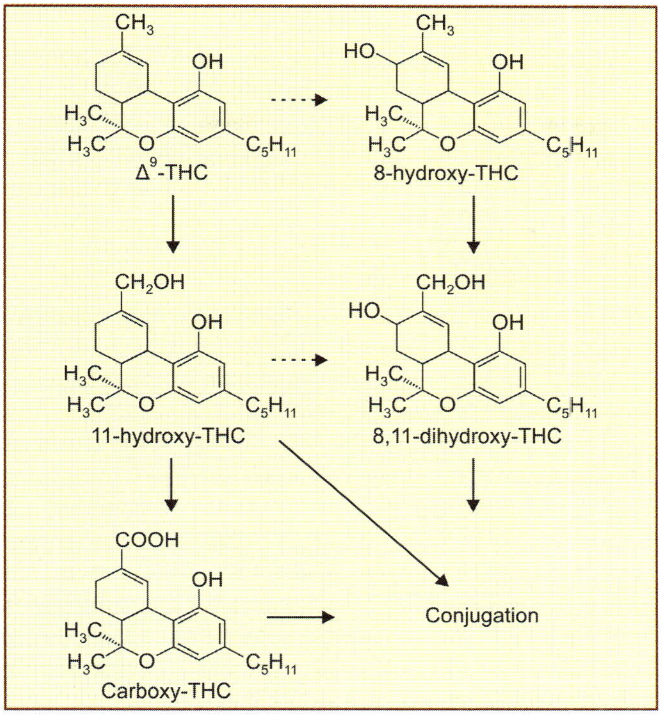

Fig. 20.3: Principal metabolic route for delta-9-tetrahydrocannabinol (THC) in humans

binds to endogenous cannabinoid receptors, CB1 (neuronal) and CB2 (immune cells). These transmembrane receptors are G-protein-coupled receptors that mediate signal transduction through inhibition of adenylate cyclase and calcium ions, and activation of potassium ion channels.

The distribution pattern of CB1 receptors in the CNS accounts for most of the clinical effects of THC, such as mood, memory, cognition, pain, and appetite. CB2 may regulate immune and inflammatory processes.

Delta-9-tetrahydrocannabinol is typically consumed by smoking the plant leaves, flower buds, and sometimes stems. THC also has been extracted from the glandular hairs of cannabis flowers and produced as a resin (hashish). Hashish is often a more potent form and has been mixed into foods, brewed as tea then ingested, or smoked. Hemp oil also has been extracted from cannabis seeds for use in soaps, body care products, and dietary supplements and is used because of its high essential fatty acid content, but negligible THC content.

PHARMACOLOGIC RESPONSE

When marijuana is smoked, THC rapidly diffuses into the plasma in seconds and is distributed multiphasically. First, it distributes to highly vascularized tissues in minutes because of its lipophilic nature. THC then is redistributed back into the bloodstream, undergoes hepatic metabolism, and slowly accumulates into less vascularized and fatty tissues. After cessation of marijuana smoking, THC and its metabolites are slowly released from fat stores.

The main psychotropic effects after inhalation of marijuana occur within minutes and persist for several hours. The peak plasma concentration of THC is dependent on the dose and occurs during the early acute phase (6–10 minutes). Numerous factors contribute to the variability in dose, such as (1) method of consumption, (2) depth of inhalation, (3) exposure frequency, and (4) cannabis potency.

Onset of clinical symptoms and peak plasma concentrations after oral ingestion of THC is slower (2–6 hours) than after inhalation, primarily as the result of first-pass hepatic clearance. The intensity of clinical effects described for smoked cannabis occurs during multiple phases: acute (0–60 minutes), post-acute (60–150 minutes), and residual (>150 minutes). THC blood concentrations accurately reflect clinical psychotropic effects observed during the early postacute phase after smoking cannabis. Therefore, plasma concentrations of THC can be monitored to discriminate between intoxication and prior use of cannabis. The ratio of THC to II-nor-delta-9-tetrahydrocannabinol-9-carboxylicacid (THC-COOH) metabolite has been used to estimate the time of exposure to marijuana.

This approach may be useful in naive users, but is unreliable in chronic abusers of marijuana. Although marijuana is the most frequently used illicit drug, it does have some limited legitimate medicinal use. Dronabinol (Marinol) contains synthetic THC and is used to treat anorexia and nausea in patients with acquired immunodeficiency syndrome (AIDS) and those with nausea and vomiting associated with chemotherapy, or asthma and glaucoma. Measurement in urine of the principle THC metabolite THC-COOH, present in cannabis but not in dronabinol, has been proposed as a means to distinguishingestion of marijuana from ingestion of marinol.

Analytical Methods

An immunoassay method is typically used to screen for potential cannabinoid use in workplace drug testing, athlete drug testing, and clinical specimens. A presumptive positive sample should be confirmed by quantitative GC-MS. Confirmation of quantitative concentrations of the parent compound, THC, is typically reserved for forensic samples.

Screening

Legitimate concern has been raised concerning the potential for false-positive results from dietary sources and 'passive inhalation' of sufficient side stream-marijuana smoke from nearby users, resulting in a positive urine cannabinoid test. Hemp seeds and oil are produced from the same *C. sativa* plant that is harvested for drug use. Hemp has been used to make soaps, lotions, rope, and clothing, and as an ingredient in a wide variety of food products.

As a precaution against passive inhalations resulting in a positive test, some laboratories screen for urine cannabinoids at a cutoff concentration of 100 ng/mL THC-COOH equivalents.

THC is metabolized by CYP2D6 liver enzymes to greater than 100 metabolites. The main active metabolite, 11-hydroxydelta-9-THC, is further oxidized to the most abundant inactive THC-COOH (Fig. 20.3). Immunoassay screens have been designed to detect cannabis use in urine samples using antibody reagents developed against the inactive THC-COOH metabolite; these reagents cross-react with numerous other THC metabolites. Therefore, the presence of multiple cannabinoid metabolites in a patient specimen will have an additive effect in immunoscreen analyses. Quantitative results based on these metabolites are 1.5–8 times greater than the actual concentration of THC-COOH as determined by GC-MS. Therefore, immunoassay results are interpreted as THC-COOH equivalents. The National Institution Drug Abuse guidelines specify that a 50 ng/mL cutoff should be used for immunoscreen. A positive result from a urine cannabinoid screen or confirmation does not indicate intoxication or degree of exposure.

The window of detection for the urine concentration of THC-COOH varies among casual (2–7 days) and chronic abusers (up to 73 days) of marijuana and is dose dependent. Variables affecting the duration of detection include (1) dose, (2) frequency of exposure, (3) route of exposure, (4) body composition, (5) fluid excretion, and (6) method of detection. Therefore, monitoring of abstinence is particularly challenging. Dilution of urine due to normal biological fluctuations (hydration) or ingested adulterants has caused a negative result one day and a positive on the next. To correct for hydration fluctuations, urine concentrations of THC-COOH per milligram creatinine are normalized for monitoring individuals who are resuming cannabis use. Using these normalized THC-COOH: creatinine concentrations, a ratio is calculated by comparing any normalized urine specimen (U2) with a previously collected normalized urine specimen (U1). 'New use' is defined as a U2/U1 ratio of ≥0.5–1.5 collected from urine specimens taken more than 12 hours. apart and containing THC-COOH concentrations >15 ng/mL. Using the 1.5 cutoff rate results in decreased false positives, but increased false-negative decisions.

Confirmation

A positive screening result for THC obtained by immunoassay is confirmed by GC-MS analysis of the urine specimen. In the United States, the division of workplace programs (DWP) in SAMHSA set the cutoff for confirming the presence of TCH-COOH metabolite at 15 ng/mL (GC-MS).

Opiates (Opioids)

The term opioid describes a wide range of compounds encompassing the natural and semisynthetic opiates-essentially variations on the structure of morphine and fully synthetic opioids with minimal structural homology to the natural alkaloids (Fig. 20.4). The defining characteristic of this class of drugs is its morphine-like ant nociceptive activity stemming from interaction with opioid receptors, which play a major role in pain perception. Other compounds that are somewhat loosely referred to as 'opioids' include receptor antagonists and mixed agonist/antagonists, as well as other opium-derived alkaloids, such as papaverine that are not known to bind opioid receptors.

Pharmacologic Response

For pain management, opioid therapy is a mainstay in treating acute needs, such as postsurgical analgesia, and in relieving moderate to severe chronic pain. In the latter case, opioids are well accepted in the setting of cancer-related pain, but the propriety and effectiveness of their use in nonmalignant chronic pain are controversial. Most opioids have both substantial addictive capacity and potentially life-threatening side-effects; thus the benefits of their use in non-end-stage patients must be carefully weighed against the chance of rather serious consequences. In addition, the development of tolerance and the risk of prescription diversion complicate even further the process of monitoring long-term opioid therapy for compliance and efficacy.

The hallmark of opioids is their ability to interact with the family of opioid receptors that are variably distributed throughout the body; opioid receptor agonists typically produce analgesia, and antagonists block this response. The biochemistry of opioid receptor binding, regulation, a signaling is complex and has been reviewed in detail elsewhere. A general overview is presented here. The classical opioid receptors are divided into the mu, delta, and kappa (μ, δ, and κ, or MOR, DOR, and KOR, respectively) subfamilies, which exhibit consider able over lap in ligand specificity and downstream signaling. A related protein, the ORL-1/nociceptin receptor, has also been described as an opioid receptor, although its characterization lags behind that of the other receptors. Finally, the sigma receptor family will interact with some

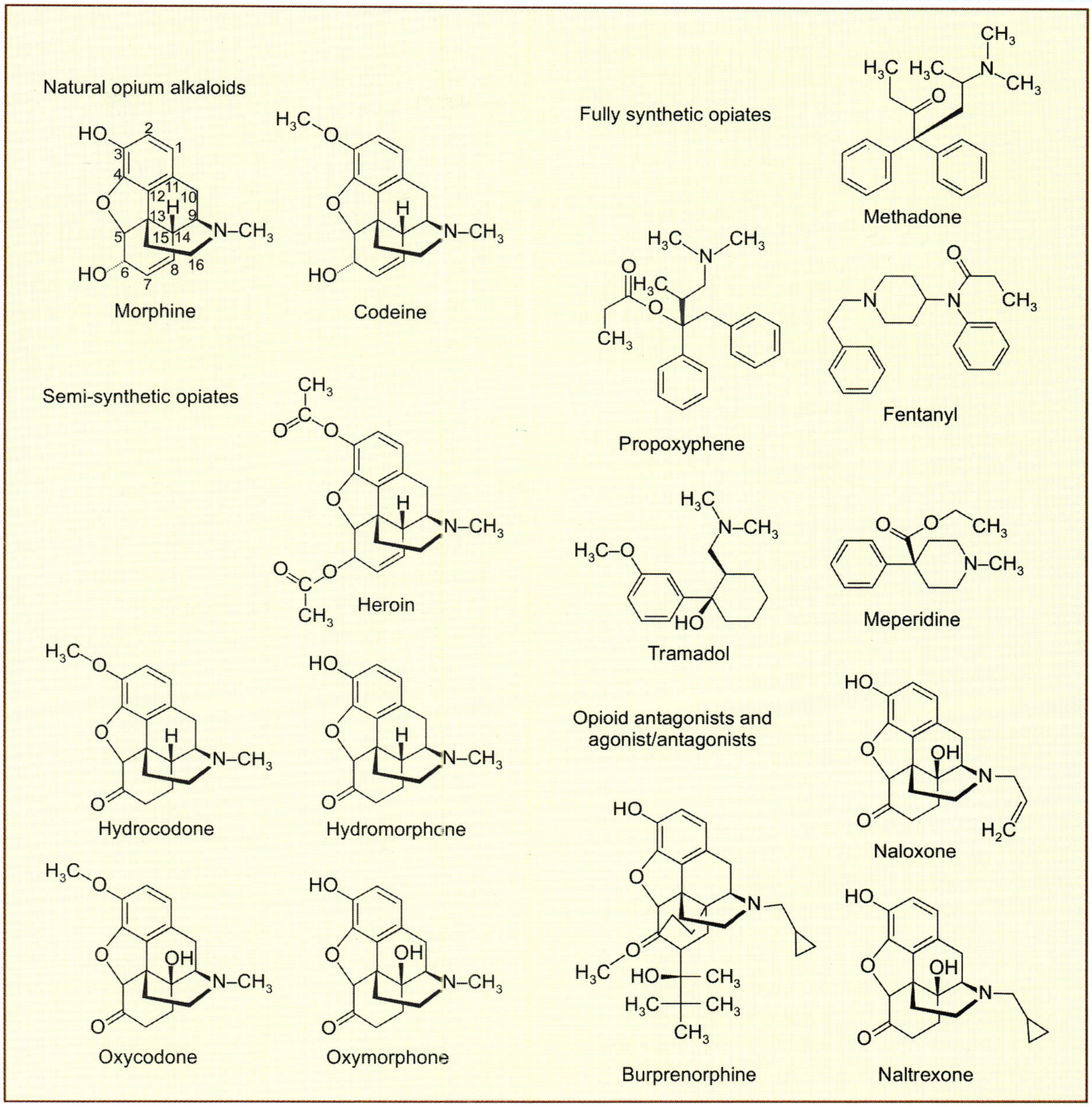

Fig. 20.4: Structure of common opioids

opioids but produces very different physiologic responses, including cardiac excitation and tachypnea; sigma receptors are now considered to be completely distinct from the classical opioid receptors.

Opioids also have preferential or selective binding to one or more of the different receptor classes. It is possible for a compound to stimulate one opioid receptor subtype while inhibiting another, as with mixed agonist/antagonist compounds. The effect of ligand binding varies between receptor classes, morphine-like analgesia is thought to be mediated primarily through stimulation of MOR, although compounds with preferential binding to DOR or KOR also produce analgesia. Other classical sequelae of opioid treatment are also attributable to MOR,

including sedation and inhibition of respiratory function and gastrointestinal transit. In contrast, neither DOR nor KOR is thought to affect respiration; DOR agonists do not produce sedation or reduce gastrointestinal motility, KOR and its endogenous ligand dynorphin are implicated in response to addiction to numerous drugs, such as opioids; KOR gene polymorphisms have been linked to susceptibility to alcohol dependence, supporting a role for this receptor in addictive behavior.

In addition to undesirable side effects, a major concern in long-term opioid therapy is the development of tolerance. Tolerant individuals may require many-fold increases in dose to achieve the same concentration of analgesia, which can greatly complicate interpretation of serum results and establishment of a therapeutic window. Tolerance to a particular opioid is thought to be a consequence of altered regulation of the opioid receptor(s) to which that compound binds; for this reason, cross-tolerance can occur when multiple drugs interact with the same receptor.

In addition, several of the enzymes involved in opioid metabolism (see later) display substrate-dependent alterations inactivity, although substrate inhibition and induction represent different phenomena than tolerance, the clinical effect can be similar and may necessitate modification of the therapeutic regimen.

The metabolism of opioids is varied, but numerous biotransformations are common to these drugs. Several of the most commonly used opiates are formed in vivo by metabolism of other compounds, as is seen with codeine demethylation resulting in conversion to morphine. This interconversion is a frequent source of confusion and must be considered when the results of opiate screens are interpreted; specific details will be outlined later for key opioids with active metabolites. One of the more important CYP (cytochromes P) enzyme, CYP2D6, is particularly notable for its role in variable clinical response to opioids; it will be discussed in greater detail in a later section. Many additional CYP enzymes are involved in opioid metabolism, including CYP3A and CYP2C isoforms, among others. It is important to note that several of these enzymes are subject to substrate inhibition and/or induction. Substrate-dependent changes in metabolic activity are affected by other drugs, herbal supplements, or endogenous compounds that are substrates of the same enzyme.

Types

Types of opiates include natural opium alkaloids, semisynthetic opiates, fully synthetic opioids, and opioid antagonists and mixed agonist/antagonists.

Natural Opium Alkaloids

Morphine and codeine are examples of natural opiates. The juice and seeds of the poppy plant are their primary source.

Source

Opium is obtained from the unripe seed capsules of the poppy plant, *Papaver sornniferum.* The milky juice is dried and powdered to make powdered opium, which contains several alkaloids. Only a few-morphine, codeine, and papaverine have clinical usefulness. These alkaloids are divided into two distinct chemical classes: phenanthrenes and benzylisoquinolines. The principal phenanthrenes are morphine (10% of opium), codeine (0.5%), and thebaine (0.2%).

The principal benzylisoquinolines are papaverine (1%), which is a smooth muscle relaxant and noscapine (6%). Poppy seeds contain morphine and to a lesser extent codeine. Ingestion of bakery products containing poppyseeds leads to excretion of morphine (and codeine) inurine. Because of first-pass metabolism, no pharmacologic effect is experienced from poppy seed ingestion. Consumption of large amounts has been known to result in urinemorphine concentrations up to 2000 ng/mL for a period of 6–12 hours after ingestion. In practice, it is obvious that caution is required when the results of a positive urine test for morphine and codeine are interpreted.

MORPHINE

The archetypical opiate, morphine, is used as the basis of comparison for relative characterizations of the opioid class. Morphine interacts primarily with MOR to mediate its effects, but it also shows some affinity for KOR. Its major metabolites are glucuronide conjugates, including inactive morphine-3-glucuronide (M3G; approximately 60%), active morphine-6-glucuronide (M6G; approximately 10%), and a small amount of morphine-3,6-diglucuronide. Free hydroxyl groups, such as the 3- and 6-hydroxy moieties of morphine, are frequently glucuronidated by enzymes of the uridinediphosphate glucuronyl transferase (UGT) family.

Uridine diphosphate-glucuronosyl transferase 2B7 is the isoform primarily responsible for morphine glucuronidation in humans; other UGT enzymes, such as UGT1A1 and UGT1A8 metabolize morphine *in vitro*, but their relevance *in vivo* remains uncertain. Most morphine glucuronides are excreted in the feces, where substantial enterohepatic circulation of conjugated and intestinallyde conjugated morphine occurs. The detection time for morphineis usually 48 hours, but this varies with individual differences in metabolism excretion and route and frequency of use.

With long-term administration and when morphine concentrations are high, a minor fraction is converted to hydromorphone (up to 2.5% of the urine morphine concentration).

Morphine-6-glucuronide has greater MOR agonist activity than morphine and appears to contribute less to unwanted side-effects. However, the relative importance of morphine and M6G in analgesia and adverse responses remains controversial. The elimination half-life for glucuronides is longer than for morphine. Therefore, glucuronides accumulatein serum to greater concentrations than morphine, and in patients with renal insufficiency, morphine glucuronides are thought to significantly contribute to opioid toxicity, as patients are unable to excrete the water-soluble metabolites.

CODEINE

Codeine is one of the most frequently prescribed opiates in the world because of its anti-tussive and analgesic properties; it is frequently combined with non-opiate-analgesic agents, such as aspirin and acetaminophen. Therefore, detection of salicylate or acetaminophen along with codeine in the urine of patients who display an opiate toxidrome should lead to the measurement of salicylate or acetaminophen in serum to assess its toxicity. Alternatively, empirical quantitative serum acetaminophen and salicylate determinations are appropriate for patients with the opioid toxidrome. Codeine has only about one-tenth the analgesic potency of morphine and shows poor affinity for MOR, with only a fraction of the pain-relieving capacity of morphine; therefore, it is generally considered a prodrug. Analgesia is attributed to the small fraction <10% of codeine converted to morphine by CYP2D6 via O-demethylation, although some studies suggest that the predominant (approximately 80%) metabolite, codeine-6-glucuronide, may be capable of mediating CNS effects independently of morphine. Both codeine and morphine may be detected in urine following codeine ingestion; however, after 30 hours only morphine may be detectable. Codeine is also converted to an inactive metabolite, norcodeine (10%), and long-term high-dose administration leads to metabolism to the active compound hydrocodone (up to 11% of the urine codeine concentration). During the early phase of excretion, codeine and conjugates predominate, but after this time, morphine conjugates are the major product. Approximately, 3 days after codeine use, morphine and its conjugates are the only metabolites detected.

SEMISYNTHETIC OPIATES

Heroin, hydrocodone, hydromorphone, oxycodone, and oxymorphone are examples of semisynthetic opiates.

HEROIN

Heroin is a synthetic opiate that is made from morphine and is also called diacetylmorphine or diamorphine; it has an analgesic potency 2–3 times that of morphine because of its better penetration across the blood-brain barrier. Heroin is no longer legally produced in the United States, but it is still used elsewhere for fast-acting analgesia. The two acetyl groups enhance CNS distribution, providing a rapid effect when first-pass metabolism is bypassed (e.g. intravenous administration). Heroin itself is rarely found in body fluids because of its extremely short half-life (2–6 minutes). The metabolite, 6-acetylmorphine, is hydrolyzed to morphine, and although it has a longer half-life (6–25 minutes), it is detectable in urine only for about 8 hours after administration. Both 6-acetylmorphine and morphine are pharmacologically active, with 6-monoacetylmorphine (6-MAM) being 4–6 times more potent than morphine. Other than the presence of its unique metabolite 6-MAM, which is definitive for heroin use, the metabolic profile of heroin resembles that of morphine. Given that acetyl codeine is a common contaminant of heroin, both morphine and low concentrations of codeine are frequently detected in urine following heroin use.

HYDROCODONE

Hydromorphone has about 6 times the potency and greater oral bioavailability than codeine, but it is thought to be more toxic than codeine. Hydrocodone is O-demethylated to hydromorphone, N-demethylated to formnorhydrocodone, and C6-keto-reduced to form approximately equal amounts of 6-β- and 6-β-hydrocol. Similar to codeine, hydrocodone is metabolized by CYP2D6 to an active metabolite (hydromorphone) and therefore may be subject to pharmacogenetic variability in patients with abnormal CYP2D6 activity.

It has been suggested that most of the pharmacologic effects of hydrocodone actually result from the hydromorphone formed during metabolism. However, studies are somewhat contradictory. Hydrocodone may provide effective pain relief even in the absence of CYP2D6 mediated conversion to hydromorphone. It remains unclear whether this is due primarily to the activity of hydrocodone itself or to that of other active metabolites.

HYDROMORPHONE

Oral hydromorphone is 5–7 times more potent than morphine. Though, it is used as an analgesic in its own right with potency somewhat higher than hydrocodone, hydromorphone is also an active metabolite of hydrocodone. Similar to morphine, not only hydromorphone is metabolized in large part to a 3-glucuronide by UGT2B7, but also to a lesser extent by UGT1A3. Hydromorphone lacks a free hydroxyl group at the 6-position, thus there is no metabolite analogous to M6G. Metabolites of hydromorphone-dihydromorphine and dihydroisomorphine, have demonstrated pharmacologic activity, but their contribution may be minimal because of the small amount formed.

OXYCODONE

Oxycodone is a potent analgesic with high oral bioavailability that is frequently formulated in combination with aspirin or acetaminophen. Therefore, the detection of salicylate or acetaminophen along with oxycodone in the urine of patients who display an opiate toxidrome should lead to measurement of serum salicylate or acetaminophen concentration to assess toxicity. No combination oxycodone is also available in immediate- and extended-release dosage forms. The latter (Oxy Contin®) is a very effective oral analgesic for patients with chronic pain (e.g. cancer patients). The pills may be chewed, crushed, snorted, or solubilized for IV injection to permit immediate availability of the entire dose, which is intended for extended release over a 12-hour period.

OXYMORPHONE

Oxymorphone provides potent analgesia with minimal interaction with CYP enzymes, although it is also a substrate for CYP2C9 and CYP3A4. The majority of oxymorphone is metabolized by UGT2B7 to the 3-glucuronide; a minor metabolite, 6-hydroxyoxymorphone, is an active analgesic with a steady-state area under the curve (AUC) similar to the parent compound. Oxymorphone is a metabolite of oxycodone that is formed via CYP2D6.

FULLY SYNTHETIC OPIOIDS

Fentanyl, meperidine, methadone, propoxyphene, and tramadol are examples of fully synthetic opioids.

FENTANYL

Fentanyl is alipophilic drug with numerous routes of administration that is used in applications ranging from anesthesia to rapid management of breakthrough pain. Fentanyl provides the structural backbone for a number of related, ultra-shortacting opioids, including remi-fentanil and sufentanil. Norfentanyl, the primary metabolite, is generated by CYP3A and is inactive; the high potency of fentanyl and the clinical insignificance of its metabolites make it a preferred analgesic for patients with major organ failure. Transdermal fentanyl patches are used for longer-term administration and are gaining popularity among drug abusers, although nonstandard application of the patch (e.g. chewing, extraction) carries substantial risk for overdose.

MEPERIDINE

Originally synthesized as an anticholinergic, meperidine has analgesic potency comparable with or somewhat lower than that of morphine. One major metabolite, normeperidine, also has analgesic activity; normeperidine is thought to be responsible for the serotonergic toxicity of meperidine, particularly in patients receiving concomitant monoamine oxidase inhibitors. Meperidine use has declined in recent years in favor of alternatives such as fentanyl.

METHADONE

A relatively long-acting opiate, methad one is used both for analgesia and in the treatment of opioid addiction. It is thought to provide (1) milder withdrawal, (2) somewhat lower potential for abuse, and (3) reduced exposure to the risks of illicit intravenous drug use. Methadone has affinity for both MOR and DOR, the latter of which may explain its apparent utility in patients whose pain no longer responds to other opioids. Substantial inter-individual and intraindividual variability in metabolism and elimination has been noted; both urine pH and seemingly self-inducible metabolism substantially influence the pharmacokinetics of this compound, as do commonly coadministered drugs such as benzodiazepines and antiretrovirals.

Although a large fraction of methadone is excreted unchanged, measurement of a metabolite such as 2-ethylidene-1,5-dimethyl-3,3-diphenylpyrrolidine in the setting of addiction treatment provides evidence for patient compliance rather than an exogenously spiked sample. EDDP excretion is less pH dependent than is clearance of the parent drug. Use of the methadone/EDDP ratio to assess compliance has been suggested, but is complicated by the pharmacokinetic variability already described.

PROPOXYPHENE

A relatively weak analgesic, propoxyphene is less potent than codeine but carries the significant risk of atypical adverse effects such as cardiac arrhythmia and seizure. The incidence of such negative responses is particularly high in the elderly.

TRAMADOL

Unlike the majority of opioid agonists, tramadol has low abuse potential and therefore is unscheduled. It has low affinity for opioid receptors and mediates analgesia through opioid-independent regulation of neurotransmitter uptake; however, its main active metabolite (O-desmethyltramadol, or M1) is a potent opioid receptor agonist.

These mechanisms are thought to work synergistically to provide greater total pain relief than the sum of each individual component. Metabolism to M1 occurs via CYP2D6; thus opioid-like effects are subject to genetic variability, as with codeine. However, because of its effects on neurotransmission, tramadol has the potential to cause serotonergic toxicity even in patients lacking CYP2D6. Infect, several synthetic phenylpiperidine opioids (tramadol, methadone, dextromethorphan, and propoxyphene) have been associated with increased risk of serotonin toxicity caused by weak reuptake inhibition of monoamines when used in combination with serotonin reuptake inhibitors, monoamine oxidase inhibitors, and amphetamine-type stimulants.

OPIOID ANTAGONISTS AND MIXED AGONIST/ANTAGONISTS

These clinically useful compounds produce very different physiologic responses, depending on the situation. For example, in opioid-naive patients, mixed agonist/antagonists (MAAs) provide MOR-mediated analgesia with less risk of an adverse reaction, but the same dose in an opioid tolerant patient may precipitate immediate withdrawal. In medical usage, coadministration of low-dose antagonists or MAAs alleviates minor opioid-induced side effects and appears useful in preventing opioid tolerance. In opioid addiction treatment, the addition of a low-dose antagonist to maintenance therapy seems to minimize subjective 'feel good' effects without substantially worsening withdrawal symptoms. Buprenorphine, naloxone, and naltrexone are examples of opioid antagonists and mixed agonist/antagonists.

BUPRENORPHINE

A semisynthetic derivative of the Baine, buprenorphine is a MOR partial agonist and a KOR antagonist. Low doses provide analgesia through MOR activation, but unlike full agonists, pain relief has a maximal threshold or ceiling effect. Buprenorphine is available as sublingual tablets (with or without naloxone) for the treatment of opioid dependence. Buprenorphine is metabolized via N-dealkylation by CYP3A4 to the active compound, norbuprenorphine, both of which can be further conjugated to inactive glucuronides by UGT1A1. CYP3A4 and UGT1A1 are subject to environmental and genetic variability, although the effects of these factors on buprenorphine are not well characterized. The drug is eliminated primarily in feces, with only a small amount in urine, and is usually detectable for 1–3 days.

NALOXONE

The prototypical opioid antagonist naloxone binds nonspecifically to all three receptor types, with the greatest effect at MOR and the least effect at DOR. Its efficacy is much greater by intravenous administration as compared with oral and sublingual routes. This characteristic is advantageous in deterring misuse of prescribed opioids; oral or sublingual opioid/naloxone formulations provide the desired benefit when taken properly, but when diverted for intravenous use cause opioid antagonism and may precipitate withdrawal. Naloxone is commonly used in comatose patients as a therapeutic and diagnostic agent. The standard dosage regimen is 0.4 mg/mL administered slowly, preferably intravenously, with the dose increased until the desired end point is achieved, namely, restoration of respiratory function, ability to protect the airway, and improved level of consciousness. Naloxone has been known to precipitate profound withdrawal symptoms in opioid-dependent patients. Its clinical efficacy lasts for as little as 45 minutes. Therefore, patients are at risk for recurrence of narcotic effect. This is particularly true for patients exposed to opioids with long elimination half-lives, such as methadone and sustained-release opioid products. Patients should be observed for resedation for at least 4 hours after reversal with naloxone. Because naloxone is via the kidney eliminated, patients with renal dysfunction may have delayed resedation past the 4 hours and should therefore be observed for a longer period of time. Naltrexone. Commonly used for the treatment of alcoholism, naltrexone is a potent antagonist of all three opioid receptors. Its combined formulation with opioid agonists is less common than are naloxone/opioid combinations; however, the greater oral bioavailability of naltrexone suggests that it may be useful in applications where poor oral delivery limits the utility of naloxone.

Analytical Methods

Many different immunoassay methods are used to screen for opiates. Gas chromatography with mass spectroscopic detection (GC-MS) is the technique of choice for confirmation of a positive screening test.

Screening Assays

Given their relatively rapid turnaround time and ability to identify several opiates, immunoassays are the methods of choice to screen urine samples for their opiate content. For clinical application, a cutoff of 300 ng/mL morphine (or morphine equivalents) is commonly used to distinguish negative from positive urine specimens, whereas a cut off of 2000 ng/mL is mandated by SAMHSA for workplace drug screening. Antibodies in opiate abuse screens commonly target morphine, because commercial immunoassay development has largely been driven by detection of illicit heroin use. Wide variability in cross-reactivity to other congeners has been noted; thus some opiates or opioids (Fig. 20.4) with high abuse potential, such as oxycodone are often poorly detected. To address this problem, several immunoassays are commercially available for individual synthetic opioids, such as fentanyl. Finally, analytical interferences are also a problem with opiate immunoassays.

Other general opiate screening methods are available, including thin-layer chromatography, but these techniques are more labor intensive and may not provide adequate turnaround time for stat or emergency testing. In this setting, point-of-care devices are being used more frequently.

In pain management programs, urine drug testing is often used to monitor compliance, diversion, or substitution for prescribed drugs. Based on the results of such tests, an individual may be dismissed from the program. It is important for drug-testing laboratories to communicate relevant aspects of the metabolic interconversion of opiates to physicians responsible for these programs. Monitoring compliance for oxycodone in pain management programs is problematic because of the low cross-reactivity of oxycodone in most opiate immunoassays. In this instance, a false-negative opiate immunoassay test may lead to an accusation of oxycodone diversion. Direct determination of oxycodone by a confirmatory method (GC-MS, LC-MS, and LC-MS-MS), is more appropriate to monitor compliance for this drug.

Confirmation Testing

For compound-specific confirmation assays, GC with mass spectroscopic detection (GC-MS) has historically been considered the method of choice. Analysis of specific opioids is typically performed using GC or LC. GC generally results in longer run times and is often incompatible with larger metabolites, such as glucuronide conjugates. LC systems require large quantities of organic solvents and are not considered acceptable for federal testing. A wide variety of detectors are available for both GC and LC; MS or tandem MS is often preferred for the structural and mass specific information provided. Analytical and technical considerations are discussed in detail later.

SAMPLE PREPARATION AND EXTRACTION

The matrix and rationale for opioid testing influence the choice of method. Analysis of urine requires hydrolysis to recover glucuronide- or sulfate-conjugated metabolites of various opioids. Hydrolysis is performed by acidification (e.g. concentrated hydrochloric acid at 115–120 DC for 15 minutes) or by enzymatic treatment with β-glucuronidase alone or in combination with arylsulfatase. Acid hydrolysis is simpler and more rapid, and typically provides greater recovery than enzymatic methods, although a few studies have shown better recovery of some analytes with glucuronidase. Acidification, however, destroys the metabolite 6-MAM, preventing conclusive determination of heroin use; it also partially degrades morphine. For this reason, drugs of-abuse testing for opiates typically employs enzymatic hydrolysis, regardless of its generally poorer analytical performance. Serum analysis is performed with or without a hydrolysis step; if a hydrolysis step is included, results reflect the sum of parent drug and metabolites, that is, 'total' drug concentration.

For detection of illicit drug use, total concentrations are typically sufficient. However, omitting hydrolysis to preserve conjugated metabolites can be useful, e.g. when both the parent and the metabolite are active compounds, as with morphine and M6G. Methods of analysis from serum or urine were initially developed using liquid-liquid extraction (LLE), although solid-phase extraction (SPE) now often preferred.

Some methods do not derivatize prior to GC analysis, but this typically results in poor chromatographic properties. Although, the number of derivatizing agents described in the literature is relatively limited, great variability in experimental conditions has been noted.

Gas Chromatography

Several GC-MS methods have been developed to quantitate various combinations of morphine. Other opiates, and their metabolites from extracts of human-urine. GC-MS is considered the reference method for determination of most natural and semisynthetic opiates, particularly in forensic settings, although other detectors are available and have been used for GC applications. Various GC-MS methods have been described for the identification and determination of opiates. Some investigators use chemicalionization, electron impact mode is more common. The GC is typically equipped with a 12- or 15-m fused-silica capillary column with a polar stationary phase of cross-linked dimethyl silicone, phenyl methyl silicone, or 95% dimethyl 5% polysiloxane. Because of structural similarities between many opiates, particularly natural and semisynthetic opiates, assays must be evaluated for interference from metabolites and congeners. The degree of overlap is such that the fragmentation patterns of various opioids can resemble one another greatly, as is seen with the mass spectra of the trimethylsilane (TMS) derivatives of hydromorphone, morphine, and norcodeine. Chromatographic resolution of these compounds must be carefully optimized to provide reliable characterization, particularly because many structurally related opiates are commercially available and are part of the same metabolic pathways. Although, acetyl derivatives have the advantage of being stable for up to 72 hours when stored at room temperature in ethyl acetate, incomplete derivatization may occur when acetyl-donating agents are used. Both morphine and 6-MAM are converted to diacetylmorphine (heroin); thus acetyl derivatization does not permit distinction between morphine, 6-MAM, and heroin. In addition to diacetylmorphine, a small amount of 3-monoacetyl-morphine (3-MAM) is formed by acetylating agents; although clinically insignificant, 3-MAM shares the m/z 285 ion with deuterated (d3) d3-acetylcodeine and interferes with analysis of these compounds.

In contrast to acetylating agents, TMS creates single derivatives for most opiates, although TMS derivatives are sensitive to moisture. Several analytical interferences are associated with TMS: codeine and norcodeine derivatives coelute on gas chromatography, while 6-MAM produces an additional peak that coelutes with morphine and increases with room temperature storage. Like TMS, pentafluoropropionic anhydride (PFP) derivatives are moisture-sensitive; however, no breakdown products are detected after storage for 24 hours. The addition of pentafluoropropanol (PFPOH) improves the yield of PFP derivatives and allows morphine and 6-MAM to be clearly distinguished.

Liquid Chromatography

Despite the long-standing role of GC in opiate analysis, LC methods are common and are often analytically advantageous. One notable example is that LC provides the ability to analyze glucuronide-conjugated metabolites as well as parent compounds. In addition, LC methods are able to measure polar metabolites without prior derivatization, and on-column extraction is possible with some LC systems. As with GC, a variety of detectors are available for LC. For example, HPLC methods for opioid analysis have been described using fluorescence (FD), ultraviolet visible (UV), electrochemical (EC), and diode array detection (DAD), alone and in various combinations. In addition, several analytical methods for morphine and its glucuronide metabolites exist for LC-MS or LC-MS-MS with different MS interfaces.

Analytical methods also include common opioids such as methadone or buprenorphine, or other non-opioid drugs of abuse such as cocaine, amphetamines, and lysergic acid diethylamide (LSD). For TDM testing, several reports have focused on quantitation of multiple opioids used therapeutically (e.g. in palliative care). For example, in one study, an LC-MS-MS method was developed that was capable of measuring 11 opioids and 5 metabolites, namely, buprenorphine, codeine, fentanyl, hydromorphone, methadone, morphine, oxycodone, oxymorphone, piritramide, tilidine, and tramadol, with the metabolites bisnortilidine, morphine glucuronides, norfentanyl, and nortilidine. In another study, a combination screening and confirmation method was developed that could be used to identify fentanyl, alfentanil, remifentanil, and sufentanil and their respective N-dealkylated or de-esterified metabolites by LC-MS-MS. Metabolite profiling is another growing area in TDM testing, especially for compounds with known active metabolites such as tramadol.

DRUGS OF ABUSE RELATED TO THE SYMPATHOMIMETIC SYNDROME

Several stimulants and hallucinogens chemically related tophenylethylamine are referred to collectively as amphetamine type stimulants (ATSs). They are considered to be sympathomimetic drugs, meaning that they mimic endogenous transmitters in the sympathetic nervous system. Other drugs related to the sympathomimetric syndrome include cocaine and LSD.

COCAINE

Cocaine is an alkaloid found in *Erythroxylon coca*, which grows principally in the northern South American Andes and to a lesser extent in India, Africa, and Java. In clinical medicine, it is used mainly for local anesthesia and vasoconstriction in nasal surgery, and to dilate pupils in ophthalmology.

Sigmund Freud famously proposed its use to treat depression and alcohol dependence, but the realities of cocaine addiction quickly brought this idea to an end. Cocaine abuse has a long history and is rooted in the drug culture in the United States. Cocaine is still one of the most common illicit drugs of abuse.

Cocaine is sold in two forms: a hydrochloride salt (powder) and a free-base product known as 'crack'. The hydrochloride salt form of cocaine is administered by nasal insufflation ('snorting') or, less frequently, intravenously.

'Crack' is a free-base form that has not been neutralized by an acid to make the hydrochloride salt. It comes as a rock crystal that is heated and its vapors smoked. The term refers to the crackling sound heard when it is heated. It should be noted that the use of 'crack' cocaine is not to be confused with 'free-basing,' which is a process in which the user purifies cocaine HCl by mixing an aqueous solution of cocaine with baking soda or ammonia and adding diethyl ether, thereby extracting the free form of the drug into the organic solvent, which is then evaporated to dryness. The drug can then be smoked. However, because of the extremely flammable nature of diethyl ether, and therefore the risk of igniting any remaining ether, 'free-basing' is no longer commonly practiced.

Chemically, cocaine is methylbenzoylecognine (COC), an ester of benzoic acid and the amino alcohol (methylecognine) that contains a tropine moiety. Its metabolism is complex (Fig. 20.5) and occurs via both nonenzymatic hydrolysis and enzymatic transformation in the plasma and liver, where it is rapidly metabolized to benzoylecgonine (BE) and ecogonine methyl ester, both of which are inactive. COC contains two ester moieties; the alkyl ester is hydrolyzed to its major metabolite BE via spontaneous hydrolysis at physiologic and alkaline pH. It has been shown that COC is also hydrolyzed to BE by liver carboxylesterases. BE is considered to be a pharmacologically inactive metabolite, but because its half-life is longer than that of COC, it is the most commonly monitored analyte in urine for determination of COC use.

Benzoylecgonine is further metabolized, to minor metabolites, such as m-hydroxybenzoylecgonine (m-HOBE) and p-hydroxybenzoylecgonine (p-HOBE). Of these, m-HOBE has been shown to be an important metabolite in the meconium of cocaine-exposed babies. Positive BE results in urine are sometimes challenged in legal and administrative proceedings on the grounds that the presence of BE is due to the addition of COC to the urine sample with subsequent *in vitro* hydrolysis to BE. However, m-HOBE is believed to arise exclusively via in vivo metabolism; therefore, its presence confirms COC use. Additionally, in adults, m-HOBE has a longer half-life and has the potential to be detected for longer periods of time than BE; it has been useful in the clinical management of patients because it expands the detection window. It should be noted that coca ethylene possesses the same CNS stimulatory activity as cocaine in experimental animals. Norcocaine (NC) is an N-demethylated metabolite of COC produced by liver cytochrome P450; it is of clinical interest because of its conversion into hepatotoxic metabolites. NC is subsequently metabolized to hydroxylnorcocaine and then to norcocaine-nitroxide. Although, the mechanism for hepatotoxicity is not well understood, it appears to be related to one or more of the N-oxidative metabolites. In animals, these metabolites have been reported to inhibit mitochondrial respiration leading to ATP depletion and subsequent cell death. Norcocaine concentrations have been shown to be present in greater concentrations in cholinesterase-deficient subjects and in simultaneous cocaine and ethanol users.

Anhydroecgonine methyl ester (AEME; methyl ecgonidine) has been identified as a unique COC metabolite after smoked COC ('crack') administration. Anhydroecgonine ethyl ester (AEEE; ethyl ecgonidine) has been identified in COC smokers who also use ethyl alcohol.

PHARMACOLOGIC RESPONSE

Cocaine has cardiovascular effects and is a potent CNS stimulant that elicits a state of increased alertness and euphoria with actions similar to those of amphetamine but of shorter duration. These CNS effects are thought to be largely associated with the ability of cocaine to block dopamine reuptake at nerve synapses, thereby prolonging the action of dopamine in the CNS. It is this response that leads to recreational abuse of cocaine.

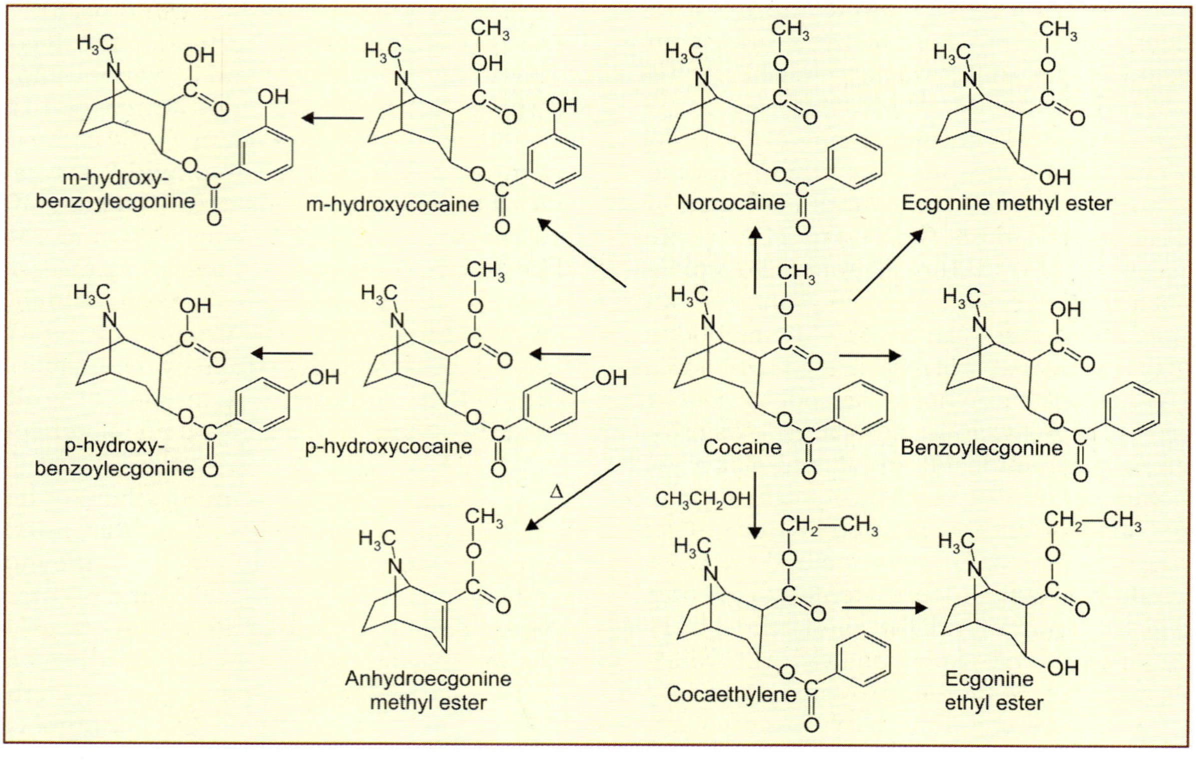

Fig. 20.5: Metabolism of cocaine

Cocaine also blocks the reuptake of norepinephrine at presynaptic nerve terminals; this produces a sympathomimetic response (including an increase in blood pressure, heart rate, and body temperature). Cocaine is effective as a local anesthetic and vasoconstrictor of mucous membranes and therefore is used clinically for nasal surgery, rhinoplasty, and emergency nasotracheal intubation. The CNS and cardiovascular effects of cocaine exhibit acute tolerance; its effects are more pronounced when the concentration of cocaine in blood is increasing than when it is at a similar but decreasing concentration. Thus, a clockwise hysteresis is observed when the blood concentration of cocaine is plotted against its CNS or cardiovascular effects over time. This phenomenon mitigates against attempts to correlate isolated blood concentration values with psychomotor effects. Because rate of change is probably more significant than absolute concentration, the psychomotor stimulant effects of cocaine are dependent both on dose and on route of administration, with IV administration and smoking resulting in the most rapid rates of increase in concentration.

Acute cocaine toxicity produces a sympathomimetic response that may result in (1) mydriasis, (2) diaphoresis, (3) hyperactive bowel sounds, (4) tachycardia, (5) hypertension, (6) hyperthermia, (7) hyperactivity, (8) agitation, (9) seizures, or (10) coma. Sudden death due to cardiotoxicity may occur following cocaine use. Death may also occur following the sequential development of hyperthermia, agitated delirium, and respiratory arrest. Excited delirium and extreme physical activity may lead to rhabdomyolysis, acute renal failure, and disseminated intravascular coagulopathy. COC is frequently used with other drugs, most commonly ethanol. In simultaneous COC and ethanol use, liver methyl esterase catalyzes the conversion of COC to BE and the transesterification of COC to CE in the presence of ethyl alcohol. This reaction occurs about 3.5 times faster than hydrolysis to BE. COC administered with ethanol produced greater euphoria and enhanced perception of well being relative to COC. CE appears to be equipotent to cocaine with regard to dopamine transporter affinity but is less potent than cocaine pharmacologically. As a consequence, large amounts of COC and ethanol may be ingested, placing users at greater risk for toxicity than if either drug were used alone. The elimination half-life for cocaethylene is longer than that for cocaine. This longer elimination half-life may contribute to the toxicity of cocaethylene. Additionally, with simultaneous administration of COC and ethanol, the production of NC may be increased, along with the potential for toxicity. It has been suggested that simultaneous COC and ethanol use carries an 18–25-fold increase in risk for immediate death over COC alone.

Analytical Methods

The elimination half-life for cocaine varies from 0.5–1.5 hours, for ecgonine methyl ester from 3–4 hours, and for benzoylecgonine from 4–7 hours. The principal urinary metabolites are benzoylecgonine and ecgonine methyl ester. Only small amounts of cocaine are excreted in urine. The elimination half-life for cocaethylene is 2.5–6 hours, which is considerably longer than that for cocaine. This longer elimination half-life may contribute to the toxicity of cocaethylene. BE excretion is detectable for 1–3 days following cocaine use. However, for chronic heavy cocaine users, the detection time may extend to 10–22 days following the last dose, apparently because of tissue storage of cocaine. Ordinarily, cocaine may be detected in urine by chromatographic methods for only about 8–12 hours after use, but in heavy chronic users, this detection period may last 4–5 days. These facts should be considered when the results of urine drug testing for individuals in drug treatment programs are interpreted. A positive urine drug test for benzoylecgonine beyond 3 days after the last dose does not necessarily indicate continued use. For such purposes, it is better to monitor quantitatively the urinary excretion of benzoylecgonine, normalized to creatinine, over time. Drug abstinence would be indicated by decreasing urinary excretion of cocaine metabolites.

However, creatinine normalization may not always reliably indicate reuse. The initial screening test for cocaine (BE) is typically immunoassay. For confirmation of a presumptive positive, BE is quantified by GC-MS.

Screening

The half-life of cocaine is 0.5–1.5 hours, of ecgonine methyl ester 3–4 hours, and of BE 4–7 hours.

Thus, BE is the analyte of choice in screening for cocaine use. The initial screening test for BE is typically immunoassay, and screening immunoassays frequently apply a 300 ng/mL cutoff.

Confirmation

Most confirmation assays offer quantification of both parent drug and metabolite. Numerous methods have been described for the measurement of COC and various metabolites. GC techniques for analysis of COC and its metabolites require derivatization, especially of polar metabolites. Early detection techniques have included flame ion detection (FID), EC, and nitrogen-phosphorous detector (NPD). GC-MS is the method of choice for many laboratories. Some methods have included not only COC and BE, but also clinically and forensically relevant secondary metabolites, such as m-HOBE, CE, NC, AEME, and AEEE. The use of LC-based separation techniques that detect COC, BE, and CE has been described previously, including LC-UV detection, as well as LC-DAD. LC-MS-MS methods have also been described, including COC, BE, and m-HOBE, along with other relevant secondary metabolites such as CE, NC, AEME, and AEEE. Reports have suggested that AEME is not a truly unique indicator of smoked cocaine use, because it has been reported to be produced in the injector port of a GC high temperatures. However, less than 1% generation of AEME occurs if the injector port of the GC is maintained at 250°C. In an LC method, high temperatures are not present in the injector or in any other part of the LC; therefore, AEME is not generated, and its presence identifies a smoked route of COC use.

BIBLIOGRAPHY

1. Aabakken L, Johansen KS, Rydningen EB, Bredesen JE, Ovrebo S, Jacobsen D. Osmolal and anion gaps in patients admitted to an emergency medical department. Hum Exp Toxicol 1994; 13: 131–4.

2. Aalberg L, DeRuiter, Noggle FT, et al. Chromatographic and mass spectral methods of identification for the side-chain and ring regioisomers of methylenedioxy methamphetamine. J Chromatogr Sci 2000; 38: 329–37.

3. Abou-Donia MB, Lapadula DM. Mechanisms of organophosphorus ester-induced delayed neurotoxicity: type I and type II. Annu Rev Pharmacol Toxicol 1990; 30: 405–40.

4. Adamowicz P, Kala M. Date-rape drugs scene in Poland. Przegl Lek 2005; 62: 572-5.

5. Agency for Toxic Substance and Disease Registry: Medical Management Guidelines for Mercury. Atlanta: Division of Toxicology, Centers for Disease Control and Prevention, 2004.

6. Agency WA-D. The prohibited list. Geneva, Switzerland: International Organization for Standardization, 2009.

7. Agurell S, Halldin M, Lindgren JE, Ohlsson A, Widman M, Gillespie H, et al. Pharmacokinetics and metabolism of delta I-tetrahydrocannabinol and other cannabinoids with emphasis on man. Pharmacol Rev 1986;38:21-43.

8. Ahanya SN, Lakshmanan J, Morgan BL, Ross MG. Meconium passage in utero: mechanisms, consequences, and management. Obstet Gynecol Surv 2005; 60: 45–56; quiz 73-4.

9. AI-Asmari AI, Anderson RA. Method for quantification of opioids and their metabolites in autopsy blood by liquid chromatography tandem mass spectrometry. J Anal Toxicol 2007; 31: 394–408.

10. Aldridge WN. Some properties of specific cholinesterase with particular reference to the mechanism of inhibition by diethyl p-nitrophenyl thiophosphate (E 605) and analogues. Biochem J 1950; 46: 451–60.

11. Allen MJ. Procedures for transportation workplace drug testing programs. Fed Reg 1989; 54: 49854–84.

12. Allen RM, Young SJ. Phencyclidine-induced psychosis. Am J Psychiatry 1978; 135: 1081–4.

13. Alozie SO, Martin BR, Harris LS, Dewey WL. 3H-Delta-9-tetrahydrocannabinol, 3H-cannabinol and 3H-cannabidiol: penetration and regional distribution in rat brain. Pharmacol Biochem Behav 1980;12:217-21.

14. Ambre n, Belknap SM, Nelson), Ruo 1'1, Shin SG, Atkinson AJ Jr. Acute tolerance to cocaine in humans. Clin Pharmacol Ther 1988; 44: 1–8.

15. American Academy of Clinical Toxicology; European Association of Poisons Centres and Clinical Toxicologists. Position statement and practice guidelines on the use of multi-dose activated charcoal in the treatment of acute poisoning. J Toxicol Clin Toxicol 1999; 37: 731–51.

16. American College of Obstetricians and Gynecologists. Committee opinion no. 422: at-risk drinking and illicit drug use: ethical issues in obstetric and gynecologic practice. Obstet Gynecol 2008;112: 1449–60.

17. Amin J, Weiss DS. GABAA receptor needs two homologous domains of the â-subunit for activation by GABA but not by pentobarbital. Nature 1993; 366: 565–9.

18. Anderson IB, Kim SY, Dyer JE, Burkhardt CB, 1knoian JC, Walsh MJ, et al. Trends in gamma-hydroxybutyrate (GHB) and related drug intoxication: 1999 to 2003. Ann Emerg Med 2006; 47: 177–83.

19. Anderson RJ, Potts DE, Gabow PA, Rumack BH, Schrier RW. Unrecognized adult salicylate intoxication. Ann Intern Med 1976; 85: 745–8.

20. Anderson WHo Therapeutic drugs II: antidepressants. In: Levine 13, ed. Principles of forensic toxicology, 2nd edition. Washington, DC: AACC Press, 2003: 297–314.

21. Andrews P. Cocaethylene toxicity. J Addict Dis 1997; 16: 75–84.

22. Andrinolo D, Michea LF, Lagos N. Toxic effects, pharmacokinetics and clearance of saxitoxin, a component of paralytic shellfish poison (PSP), in cats. Toxicon 1999; 37: 447–64.

23. Anonymous. Ambien CR (zolpidem tartrate extended-release) prescribing information. Bridgewater, NJ: Sanofi-Aventis US LLC, January 2008a.

24. Anonymous. An overview of club drugs, Drug Intelligence Brief, DEA, February 2000.

25. Araki Y. Nitrogenous substances in saliva. I. Protein and non-protein nitrogens. J pn J Physiol 1951; 2:69–78.

26. Arch JR, Ainsworth AT, Cawthorne MA, Piercy V, Sennitt MV, Thody VE, et al. Atypical β-adrenoceptor on brown adipocytes as target for anti-obesity drugs. Nature 1984; 309: 163–5.

27. Ariano RE, Kassum DA, Aronson KJ. Comparison of sedative recovery time after midazolam versus diazepam administration. Crit Care Med 1994; 22: 1492–6.

28. Arima H, Sobue K, So M, Morishima T, Ando H, Katsuya H. Transient and reversible parkinsonism after acute organophosphate poisoning. J Toxicol Clin Toxicol 2003; 41: 67–70.

29. Armstrong SC, Cozza KL. Pharmacokinetic drug interactions of morphine, codeine, and their derivatives: theory and clinical reality, part I. Psychosomatics 2003; 44: 167–71.

30. Armstrong SC, Cozza KL. Pharmacokinetic drug interactions of morphine, codeine, and their derivatives: theory and clinical reality, part II. Psychosomatics 2003; 44: 515–20.

31. Arndt PA, Kumpel 13M. Blood doping in athletes-detection of allogeneic blood transfusions by flow cytofluorometry. Am J Hematol 2008; 83: 657–67.

32. Ashbourne JF, Olson KR, Khayam-Bashi H. Value of rapid screening for acetaminophen in all patients with intentional drug overdose. Ann Emerg Med 1989; 18: 1035–8.

33. Babu KM, Ferm RP. Hallucinogens. In: Goldfrank LR, Flomenbaum NE, Hoffman RS, Howland MA, Lewin NA, Nelson L, eds. Goldfrank's toxicologic emergencies, 8th edition. New York, NY: McGraw- Hill, 2006: 1202– I 1.

34. Bach MV, Coutts RT, Baker GB. Involvement of CYP2D6 in the in vitro metabolism of amphetamine, two N-alkylamphetamines and their 4-methoxylated derivatives. Xenobiotica 1999; 29: 719–32.

35. Badcock NR, O'Reilly DA. False-positive EMIT-ST ethanol screen with post-mortem infant plasma. Clin Chem 1992; 38: 434.

36. Baden LR, Horowitz G, Jacoby H, Eliopoulos GM. Quinolones and false-positive urine screening for opiates by immunoassay technology. JAMA 2001; 286: 3115–9.

37. Bailey RB, Jones SR. Chronic salicylate intoxication: a common cause of morbidity in the elderly. J Am Geriatr Soc 1989; 37: 556–61.

38. Baker AM, Johnson DG, Levisky JA, Hearn WL, Moore KA, Levine B, et al. Fatal diphenhydramine intoxication in infants. J Forensic Sci 2003; 48: 425–8.

39. Baldessarini R), Tarazi FI. Pharmacotherapy of psychosis and mania (Chapter 18). In: Brunton LL, Lazo JS, Parker KL, eds. Goodman and Gilman's the pharmacological basis of therapeutics, 1I th edition. New York, NY: McGraw-Hill, 2006

40. Baldessarini R. Drug therapy of depression and anxiety disorders (Chapter 17). In: Brunton LL, Lazo JS, Parker KL, eds. Goodman & Gilman's the pharmacological basis of therapeutics, 11th edition. New York, NY: McGraw-Hill, 2006.

41. Bamigbade TA, Davidson C, Langford RM, et. al. Actions of tramadol, its enantiomers and principal metabolite, O-desmethyltramadol, on serotonin (5-HT) efflux and uptake in the rat dorsal raphe nucleus. Br J Anaesth 1997; 79: 352–6.

42. Banerji S, Anderson lB. Abuse of Coricidin HBP cough and cold tablets: episodes recorded by a poison center. Am J Health Syst Pharm 2001; 58: 1811–4.

43. Barbour AD. GC/MS analysis of propylated barbiturates. J Anal Toxicol 1991; 15: 214-5.

44. Bardin PG, van Eeden SF, Moolman JA, Foden AP, Joubert JR. Organophosphate and carbamate poisoning. Arch Intern Med 1994; 154:1433-41.

45. Barkin RL, Barkin S), Barkin DS. Propoxyphene (dextro-propoxyphene): a critical review of a weak opioid analgesic that should remain in antiquity. Am J Ther 2006; 13: 534–42.

46. Barrett C, Good C, Moore C: Comparison of point-cf-collection screening of drugs of abuse in oral fluid with a laboratory-based urine screen. Forensic Sci Int 2001; 122: 163–166.

47. Barrueto F Jr, et al: Cardioactive steroid poisoning from an herbal cleansing preparation. Ann Emerg Med 2003; 41: 396–399.

48. Bartlett R. Carbon monoxide poisoning. In: Haddad l., Shannon M, Winchester J, eds. Clinical management of poisoning and drug overdose, 3rd edition. Philadelphia, Pa: WB Saunders, 1998: 885–98.

49. Baselt RC Acetone. In: Baselt RC, ed. Disposition of toxic drugs and chemical in man, 8th edition. Foster City, Calif: Biomedical Publications, 2008: 15-7.

50. Baselt RC Amphetamine. In: Baselt RC, ed. Disposition of toxic drugs and chemical in man, 8th edition. Foster City, Calif: Biomedical Publications, 2008:83-6.

51. Baselt RC Carbon monoxide. In: Baselt RC, ed. Disposition of toxic drugs and chemical in man, 8th edition. Foster City, Calif: Biomedical Publications, 2008.

52. Baselt RC Codeine. In: Baselt RC, ed. Disposition of toxic drugs and chemical in man, 8th edition. Foster City, Calif: Biomedical Publications, 2008: 355–60.

53. Baselt RC Ephedrine. In: Baselt RC, ed. Disposition of toxic drugs and chemical in man, 8th edition. Foster City, Calif: Biomedical Publications, 2008: 542–4.

54. Baselt RC Ethanol. In: Baselt RC, ed. Disposition of toxic drugs and chemical in man, 8th edition. Foster City, Calif: Biomedical Publications, 2008: 561–5.

55. Baselt RC Ethylene glycol. In: Baselt RC, ed. Disposition of toxic drugs and chemical in man, 8th edition. Foster City, Calif: Biomedical Publications, 2008: 578–82.

56. Baselt RC Flunitrazepam. In: Baselt RC, ed. Disposition of toxic drugs and chemical in man, 8th edition. Foster City, Calif: Biomedical Publications, 2008: 633–5.

57. Baselt RC Heroin. In: Baselt RC, ed. Disposition of toxic drugs and chemical in man, 8th edition. Foster City, Calif: Biomedical Publications, 2008: 730–5.

58. Baselt RC Hydrocodone. In: Baselt RC, ed. Disposition of toxic drugs and chemical in man, 8th edition. Foster City, Calif: Biomedical Publications, 2008: 745–6.

59. Baselt RC Hydromorphone. In: Baselt RC, ed. Disposition of toxic drugs and chemical in man, 8th edition. Foster City, Calif: Biomedical Publications, 2008: 750–2.

60. Baselt RC In: Baselt RC, ed. Disposition of toxic drugs and chemical in man, 8th edition. Foster City, Calif: Biomedical Publications, 2008.

61. Baselt RC Isopropanol. In: Baselt RC, ed. Disposition of toxic drugs and chemical in man, 8th edition. Foster City, Calif: Biomedical Publications, 2008: 789–91.

62. Baselt RC Methadone. In: Baselt RC, ed. Disposition of toxic drugs and chemical in man, 8th edition. Foster City, Calif: Biomedical Publications, 2008: 941–5.

63. Baselt RC Methylenedioxyethylamphetamine. In: Baselt RC, ed. Disposition of toxic drugs and chemical in man, 8th edition. Foster City, Calif: Biomedical Publications, 2008: 995–6.

64. Baselt RC Methylphenidate. In: Baselt RC, ed. Disposition of toxic drugs and chemical in man, 8th edition. Foster City, Calif: Biomedical Publications, 2008: 1008–11.

65. Baselt RC Oxycodone. In: Baselt RC, ed. Disposition of toxic drugs and chemical in man, 8th edition. Foster City, Calif: Biomedical Publications, 2008: 1166–8.

66. Baselt RC Phenylpropanolamine. In: Baselt RC, ed. Disposition of toxic drugs and chemical in man, 8th edition. Foster City, Calif: Biomedical Publications, 2008: 1252–4.

67. Baselt RC Pseudoephedrine. In: Baselt RC, ed. Disposition of toxic drugs and chemical in man, 8th edition. Foster City, Calif: Biomedical Publications, 2008: 1344–6.

68. Bass R. The antipsychotic drugs. In: Haddad 1., Shannon M, Winchester J, eds. Clinical management of poisoning and drug overdose, 3rd edition. Philadelphia, Pa: WB Saunders, 1998:780-93.

69. Baumgartner AM, Jones PF, Baumgartner WA, Black CT. Radioimmunoassay of hair for determining opiate-abuse histories. J Nucl Med 1979; 20: 748–52.

70. Baumgartner WA, Hill V. Hair analysis for drugs of abuse: decontamination issues. In: Sunshine I, ed. Recent developments in therapeutic drug monitoring and clinical toxicology, New York: Marcel Dekker Inc, 1992: 577–97.

71. Bayer MJ, McKay C Advances in poison management. Clin Chem 1996;42: 136 1–6.

72. Bearer CF, l.ee S, Salvator AE, Minnes S, Swick A, Yamashita T, Singer l.T. Ethyllinoleate in meconium: a biomarker for prenatal ethanol exposure. Alcohol Clin Exp Res 1999; 23: 487--93.

73. Beckett AH, Rowland M. Urinary excretion of methylamphetamine in man. Nature 1965; 206: 1260–1.

74. Beers MH, Berkow RB: The Merck Manual of Diagnosis and Therapy, ed 17. Rahway, NJ: Merck & Co., 1999.

75. Bell R, Taylor EH, Ackerman B, Pappas AA. Interpretation of urine quantitative II-nor-delta-9 tetrahydrocannabinol-9-carboxylic acid to determine abstinence from marijuana smoking. J Toxicol Clin Toxicol 1989;27: 109–15.

76. Bengtsson F: Therapeutic drug monitoring of psychotropic drugs: TDM "nouveau". Ther Drug Monit 2004; 26:145–151.

77. Bermejo AM, Ramos I, Fernandez P, l.opez-Rivadulla M, Cruz A, Chiarotti M, et al. Morphine determination by gas chromatography/ mass spectroscopy in human vitreous humor and comparison with radioimmunoassay. J Anal Toxicol 1992; 16: 372–4.

78. Bernard S, Neville KA, Nguyen AT, Flockhart DA. Interethnic differences in genetic polymorphisms of CYP2D6 in the U.S. population: clinical implications. The Oncologist 2006; II: 126–35.

79. Bernasconi R, Mathivet P, Bischoff S, Marescaux C Gammahydroxybutyric acid: an endogenous neuromodulator with abuse potential? Trends Pharmacol Sci 1999; 20: 135–41.

80. Bertholf Rl., Bazooband A, Mansouri V, et al. False-positive acetaminophen results in a hyperbilirubinemic patient. Clin Chem 2003; 49: 695–8.

81. Bizovi K, Smilkstein M. Acetaminophen. In: Goldfrank l., Flomenbaum N, l.ewin N, Howland M, Hoffman R, Nelson l., eds. Goldfrank's toxicologic emergencies, 7th edition. New York, NY: McGraw-Hill, 2002: 480–501.

82. Blanchet M, Bru G, Guerret M, Bromet-Petit M, Bromet N. Routine determination of morphine, morphine 3-β-D-glucuronide and morphine 6-β-D-glucuronide in human serum by liquid chromatography coupled to electrospray mass spectrometry. J Chromatogr A 1999; 854: 93–108.

83. Blanke R, Decker W. Analysis of toxic substances. In: Tietz N, ed. Textbook of clinical chemistry, 1st edition. Philadelphia, Pa: WB Saunders, 1986: 1670–744.

84. Boehnert MT, l.ovejoy FH Jr. Value of the QRS duration versus the serum drug level in predicting seizures and ventricular arrhythmias after an acute overdose of tricyclic antidepressants. N Engl J Med 1985; 313: 474–9.

85. Boess F, Ndikum-Moffor FM, Boelsterli UA, Roberts SM. Effects of cocaine and its oxidative metabolites on mitochondrial respiration and generation of reactive oxygen species. Biochem Pharmacol 2000; 60: 615–23.

86. Bogusz M, Pach J, Stasko W. Comparative studies on the rate of ethanol elimination in acute poisoning and in controlled conditions. J Forensic Sci 1977; 22: 446–51.

87. Bogusz M, Wu M. Standardized HPl.C/DAD system, based on retention indices and spectral library, applicable for systematic toxicological screening. J Anal Toxicol 1991; 15: 188–97.

88. Bogusz MJ. Liquid chromatography-mass spectrometry as a routine method in forensic sciences: a proof of maturity. J Chromatogr 2000; 748: 3–19.

89. Bourland JA, et al: Quantitation of cocaine, benzoylecgonine, cocaethylene, methylecgonine, and norcocaine in human hair by positive ion chemical ionization (PICI) gas chromatography-tandem mass spectrometry. J Anal Toxicol 2000; 24: 489–495.

90. Cannon DJ: Toxicology of heavy metals, parts 1 & 2. TDM/Tox In-Service Training and Continuing Education 13(2): 7–11; 13(3): 9–13, 1991.

91. Cham BE, et al: Simultaneous liquid-chromatographic quantitation of salicylic acid, salicyluric acid and gentisic acid in plasma. Clin Chem 1979; 25: 1420–1425.

92. Chunying C, et al: Increased oxidative DNA damage, as assessed by urinary 8-hydroxy- 2'-deoxyguanosine concentrations, and serum redox status in persons exposed to mercury. Clin Chem 2005; 51:759–767.

93. Colbert DL. Drug abuse screening with immunoassays: unexpected cross-reactivities and other pitfalls. Br j Biomed Sci 1994; 51: 136–46.

94. Combie J, Blake j\N, Nugent TE, Tobin T. Morphine glucuronide hydrolysis: superiority of β-glucuronidase from Patella vulgata. Clin Chem 1982; 28: 83–6.

95. Concheiro M, de Castro A, Lopez-Rivadulla M, et al Determination of drugs of abuse and their metabolites in human plasma by liquid chromatography-mass spectrometry: an application to 156 road fatalities. j Chromatogr B Analyt Technol Biomed Life Sci 2006; 832: 81–9.

96. Cone EJ, Darwin WD, Buchwald WE Assay for codeine, morphine and ten potential urinary metabolites by gas chromatography-mass fragmentography. j Chromatogr 1983; 275: 307–18.

97. Cone Ej, Darwin WD. Simultaneous determination of hydromorphone, hydrocodone and their 6α- and 6β-hydroxy metabolites in urine using selected ion recording with methane chemical ionization. Biomed Mass Spectrom 1978; 5: 291.

98. Cone EJ, Heit HA, Caplan YH, et al. Evidence of morphine metabolism to hydromorphone in pain patients chronically treated with morphine. j Anal Toxicol 2006;30: 1–5.

99. Cone EJ, Hillsgrove M, Darwin WD. Simultaneous measurement of cocaine, cocaethylene, their metabolites, and "crack" pyrolysis products by gas chromatography-mass spectrometry. Clin Chem 1994; 40: 1299–305.

100. Cone Ej, Hillsgrove Mj, jenkins Aj, Keenan RM, Darwin WD. Sweat testing for heroin, cocaine, and metabolites. j Anal Toxicol 1994; 18: 298–305.

101. Cone Ej, Lange R, Darwin WD. In vivo adulteration: excess fluid ingestion causes false-negative marijuana and cocaine urine test results. j Anal Toxicol 1998; 22: 460–73.

102. Cone Ej, Oyler J, Darwin WD. Cocaine disposition in saliva following intravenous, intranasal, and smoked administration. j Anal Toxicol 1997; 2 I : 465–75.

103. Cone Ej. Mechanisms of drug incorporation into hair. 1her Drug Monit 1996; 18: 438–43.

104. Cone Ej. Saliva testing for drugs of abuse. Ann N Y Acad Sci 1993; 694: 91–127.

105. Contin M, et al: Levetiracetam therapeutic monitoring in patients with epilepsy: effect of concomitant antiepileptic drugs. Ther Drug Monit 2004; 26: 375–379.

106. Contopoulos-Ioannidis DG, et al: Extended-interval aminoglycoside administration for children: a meta-analysis. Pediatrics 2004; 114:e111–e118.

107. Crouch DJ, et al: A field evaluation of five on-site drug-testing devices. J Anal Toxicol 2002; 26: 493–499.

108. Gowda RM, Cohen RA, Khan IA: Toad venom poisoning: resemblance to digoxin toxicity and therapeutic implications. Heart 2003; 89:e14.

109. Gupta A, et al: A case of nondigitalis cardiac glycoside toxicity. Ther Drug Monit 1997; 19: 711–714.

110. Hardman JG, et al (eds): Goodman & Gilman's The Pharmacological Basis of Therapeutics, ed 10. New York: McGraw-Hill, 2001.

111. Inter-Organization Programme for the Sound Management of Chemicals: Elemental Mercury and Inorganic Mercury Compounds. Geneva: World Health Organization. 2003.

112. Jaffe AM, Gephardt D, Courtemanche L: Poisoning due to ingestion of Veratrum viride (false hellebore). J Emerg Med 1990; 8: 161–167.

113. Jolley ME, et al: Fluorescent polarization immunoassay: an automated system for therapeutic drug determination. Clin Chem 1981; 27: 1575–1579.

114. Kintz P, Samyn N: Use of alternative specimens: drugs of abuse in saliva and doping agents in hair. Ther Drug Monit 2002; 24: 239–246.

115. Koda-Kimble MA, Young LY: Applied Therapeutics: The Clinical Use of Drugs, ed 7.

116. Kolbrich EA, et al: Cozart RapiScan Oral Fluid Drug Testing System: an evaluation of sensitivity, specificity, and efficiency for cocaine detection compared with ELISA and GC-MS following controlled cocaine administration. J Anal Toxicol 2003; 27: 407–411.

117. Luzzi VI, et al: Analytic performance of immunoassays for drugs of abuse below established cutoff values. Clin Chem 2004; 50: 717–722.

118. Lyon AW, Whitley C, Eintracht SL: Analytic evaluation and application of a novel spectrophotometric serum lithium method to a rapid response laboratory. Ther Drug Monit 2004; 26: 98–101.

119. McEvoy GK: AHFS Drug Information 2003. Bethesda, MD: American Society of Health-System Pharmacists, 2003.

120. Members of the German Study Group on Pediatric Renal Transplantion: Cyclosporin A absorption profiles in pediatric renal transplant recipients predict the risk of acute rejection. Ther Drug Monit 2004; 26: 415–424.

121. Nordgren HK, Beck O: Multicomponent screening for drugs of abuse: direct analysis of urine by LC-MS-MS. Ther Drug Monit 2004; 26: 90–97.

122. Orsay EM, et al: The impaired driver: hospital and police detection of alcohol and other drugs of abuse in motor vehicle crashes. Ann Emerg Med 1995; 25: 430–431.

123. Paterson S, et al: Qualitative screening for drugs of abuse in hair using GC-MS. J Anal Toxicol 2001; 25: 203–208.

124. Philadelphia: Lippincott, Williams & Wilkins, 2001.

125. Phillips JE, et al: Signify ER Drug Screen Test evaluation: comparison to Triage Drug of Abuse Panel plus tricyclic antidepressants. Clin Chim Acta 2003; 328: 31–38.

126. Quattrocchi F, et al: Effect of serum separator blood collection tubes on drug concentrations. Ther Drug Monit 1983; 5:359.

127. Rich SA, Libera JM, Locke RJ: Treatment of foxglove extract poisoning with digoxin specific Fab fragments. Ann Emerg Med 1993; 22: 1904–1907.

128. Slaughter RL, Schneider PJ, Visconti JA: Appropriateness of the use of serum digoxin and digitoxin assays. Am J Hosp Pharm. 1978; 35: 1376–1379.

129. Smith TW: Digitalis toxicity: epidemiology and clinical use of serum concentration measurements. Am J Med 1975; 58: 470–476..

130. Steinhoff BJ, et al: The ideal characteristics of antiepileptic therapy: an overview of old and new AEDs. Acta Neurol Scand 2003; 107: 87–95.

131. Sunshine I, Jatlow PI. Methology for Analytical Toxicology, vol 2. Boca Raton, FL: CRC Press, 1982.

132. Taylor PJ: Therapeutic drug monitoring of immunosuppressant drugs by highperformance liquid chromatography-mass spectrometry. Ther Drug Monit 2004; 26: 215–219.

133. Verstraete AG: Detection times of drugs of abuse in blood, urine, and oral fluid. Ther Drug Monit 2004; 26: 200–205.

21

The Porphyrias and Other Disorders of Porphyrin Metabolism

INTRODUCTION

The porphyrias are a group of uncommon, inherited disorders of heme biosynthesis. Each porphyria results from a partial deficiency of one of the enzymes of the pathway converting δ-aminolevulinate (ALA) to heme or, in one rare disorder, an increase in activity of the rate controlling enzyme of erythroid heme synthesis. Each functional abnormality is associated with a specific pattern of overproduction, accumulation, and excretion of the intermediates of the pathway. These intermediates are excreted in excessive amounts in urine, feces, or both. The clinical consequences depend on the nature of the heme precursors that accumulate. In the acute porphyrias, excess porphyrin precursors [ALA and porphobilinogen (PBG)] are associated with potentially fatal acute neurovisceral attacks that often are provoked by (1) various commonly prescribed drugs, (2) hormonal factors, (3) alcohol, (4) starvation, (5) stress, or (6) infection. In the nonacute porphyrias, and in those acute porphyrias in which both acute neurovisceral attacks and skin lesions occur, accumulation of porphyrins results in photosensitization of sun-exposed skin. Diagnosis depends on laboratory investigation to demonstrate the pattern of heme precursor accumulation specific for each type of porphyria and requires examination of appropriate specimens for the key metabolites using adequately sensitive and specific methods. Technical advances in the field of molecular genetics have made it possible to investigate all porphyrias at the molecular level. Although rarely essential for diagnosis of symptomatic cases, DNA analysis is now the method of choice for the investigation of families with porphyria and continues to provide new information about the pathology of these disorders. Abnormalities of porphyrin excretion and accumulation also occur in a wide variety of other disorders that are collectively far more common than the porphyrias. Recognition of these secondary porphyrin disorders is important to avoid diagnostic errors.

CHEMISTRY OF PORPHYRINS

The porphyrins found in nature are all compounds in which the side-chains are substituted for the eight hydrogen atoms found in the four **pyrrole** rings that make up porphyrin (Fig. 21.1). Because of the wide variety of substitutions, many porphyrins have been described in nature. The pigment chlorophyll is a magnesium porphyrin and is essential for plants to use light energy to synthesize carbohydrates. Four basic isomers may exist for every porphyrin compound; however, only type I and type III occur in nature. The difference between type I and

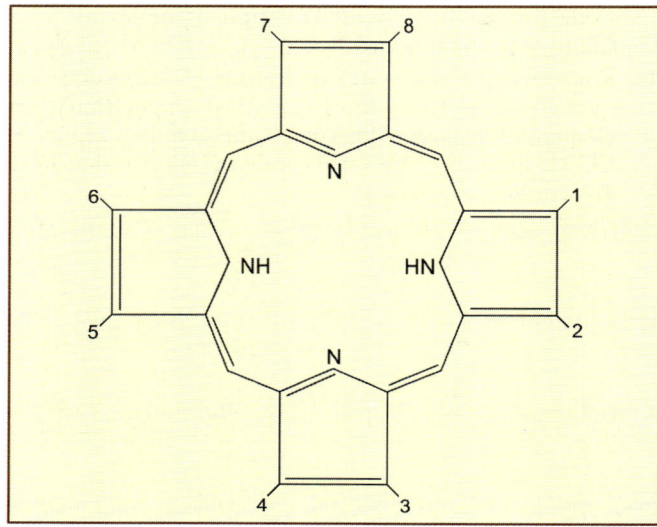

Fig. 21.1: Basic structure of porphyrins

type III isomers is in the arrangement of side-chains. Only type III isomers form heme; however, in some disorders, the functionless type I isomers may be present in excess in the tissue. Porphyrins are stable compounds, red-violet to red-brown in color, that fluoresce red when excited by light near 400 nm. Only three porphyrin compounds are clinically significant in humans: protoporphyrin (PROTO), uroporphyrin (URO), and coproporphyrin (COPRO). Their presence in excess in biologic fluids is a clinical sign of abnormal heme synthesis. The three compounds have different solubility properties and different degrees of ionization determined by the addition of various carboxyl groups to the basic porphyrin structure. This allows for separate assays of each. URO is excreted primarily in the urine, PROTO in the feces, and COPRO in either, depending on the rate of formation of the urine and its pH.

The reduced forms of porphyrins are termed **porphyrinogens,** the functional form of the compound that must be used in heme synthesis. Porphyrinogens are highly unstable and colorless and do not fluoresce, which makes them more difficult to analyze. With light, oxygen, or oxidizing agents, porphyrinogens are readily oxidized to the corresponding porphyrin form. Therefore, the porphyrin form is routinely analyzed in clinical laboratories as a result of the increased stability and ease of detection by various common clinical laboratory systems.

PORPHYRIN SYNTHESIS

All cells contain hemoproteins and can synthesize heme; however, the bone marrow and liver are the mainsites. The series of irreversible reactions is shown in Fig. 21.2. Some steps occur in the mitochondria of the cell and some steps occur in the cytoplasm. The transport of substrates across the mitochondrial membrane is a complex process and a potential point for interruptions in heme synthesis.

Control of the rate of heme synthesis in the cells of the liver is achieved largely through regulation of the enzyme δ aminolevulinic acid synthase (ALAS).

The main mechanism is repression of synthesis of new enzyme. A negative feedback mechanism exists in which increases in the pool of hepatic heme diminish the production of ALAS. Conversely, ALAS production is increased with a depletion of heme. The size of the regulatory heme pool may be affected by the requirement for hemoproteins in the liver. Drugs and other compounds appear to induce ALAS production via several different mechanisms, but all result in a depletion of the regulatory heme pool. Therefore, the rate of heme synthesis is flexible and can change rapidly in response to a wide variety of external stimuli. In bone marrow erythrocytes, other enzymes in the pathway and the rate of cellular iron uptake seem to control the rate of heme synthesis.

PORPHYRIA DISORDERS

Porphyrias result from genetic or acquired deficiencies of enzymes of the heme biosynthetic pathway. These deficiencies allow heme precursors to accumulate, causing toxicity. Porphyrias are defined by the specific enzyme deficiency. Two major clinical manifestations occur, i.e. neurovisceral abnormalities (the acute porphyrias) and cutaneous photosensitivity (the cutaneous porphyrias).

Heme, an iron-containing pigment, is an essential cofactor of numerous hemoproteins. Virtually, all cells of the human body require and synthesize heme. However, most heme is synthesized in the bone marrow (by erythroblasts and reticulocytes) and is incorporated into hemoglobin. The liver is the second most active site of heme synthesis, most of which is incorporated into cytochrome P-450 enzymes. Heme synthesis requires

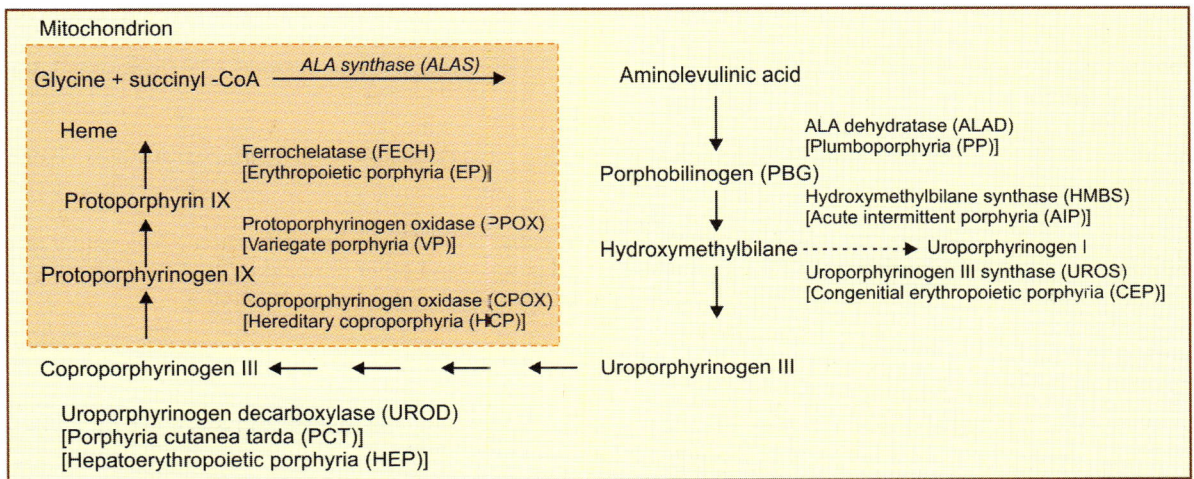

Fig. 21.2: Synthesis of heme. Brackets indicate diseases associated with enzyme deficiencies

eight enzymes (Table 21.1). These enzymes produce and transform molecular species called porphyrins (and their precursors); accumulation of these substances causes the clinical manifestations of the porphyrias.

Etiology

With the exception of the sporadic type of porphyria cutanea tarda (PCT), the porphyrias are inherited diseases. Autosomal dominant (AD) inheritance is most common. In the AD porphyrias, homozygous or compound heterozygous states (i.e. two separate heterozygous mutations, one in each allele of the same gene in the same patient) may be incompatible with life, typically causing fetal death. Disease penetrance in heterozygotes varies; thus, clinically expressed disease is less common than genetic prevalence. The two most common porphyrias,

PCT and acute intermittent porphyria (AIP), are AD (20% of PCT is AD). The prevalence of PCT is about 1/10,000. The prevalence of the causative genetic mutation for AIP is about 1/1500, but because penetrance is low, the prevalence of clinical disease is also about 1/10,000. Prevalence of both PCT and AIP varies widely among regions and ethnic groups. In the autosomal recessive porphyrias, only homozygous or compound heterozygous states cause disease. Erythropoietic protoporphyria, the third most common porphyria, is autosomal recessive. X-linked inheritance occurs in one of the porphyrias, X-linked protoporphyria.

Pathophysiology

Porphyrias result from a deficiency of any of the last seven enzymes of the heme biosynthetic pathway or from

Table 21.1	Substrates and enzymes of the heme biosynthetic pathway and the diseases associated with their deficiency			
Substrate/Enzyme*	Porphyria	Neurovisceral symptoms	Cutaneous symptoms	Inheritance
Glycine + Succinyl CoA Erythroid specific δ aminolevulinic acid synthase-2 (ALAS 2)†	X-linked protoporphyria (due to increased enzyme activity)†	No	Phenotypically similar to EPP	X-linked
δ aminolevulinic acid δ aminolevulinic acid dehydratase (ALAD)	ALAD-deficient porphyria	Yes	No	Autosomal recessive
Porphobilinogen Porphobilinogen deaminase	Acute intermittent porphyria	Yes	No	Autosomal dominant
Hydroxymethylbilane Uroporphyrinogen III cosynthase	Congenital erythropoietic porphyria	No	Severe, mutilating skin disease	Autosomal recessive
Uroporphyrinogen III Uroporphyrinogen decarboxylase	Porphyria cutanea tarda	No	Fragile skin, blisters	Two variants: • Autosomal dominant (20–25% of cases) • Without known genetic correlate (sporadic, 75–80%)
	Hepatoerythropoietic porphyria	No	Severe blistering	Autosomal recessive
Coproporphyrinogen III Coproporphyrinogen oxidase	Hereditary coproporphyria	Yes	Fragile skin, blisters	Autosomal dominant
Protoporphyrinogen IX Protoporphyrinogen oxidase	Variegate porphyria	Yes	Fragile skin, blisters	Autosomal dominant
Protoporphyrin IX† Ferrochelatase	Erythropoietic protoporphyria (EPP)	No, except in patients with severe hepato-biliary pathology	Skin pain, lichenification and other minor skin changes, but no blistering	Autosomal recessive
Heme (final product incorporated in various heme proteins)	—	—	—	—

*Listed are successive intermediates in the heme biosynthetic pathway, beginning with glycine and succinyl CoA and ending with heme. Deficiency of an enzyme causes buildup of precursor compounds.

†X-linked protoporphyria results from gain-of-function mutations that increase the activity of ALAS 2, causing accumulation of protoporphyrin. Decreased activity of ALAS 2 causes a sideroblastic anemia.

increased activity of the first enzyme in the pathway, ALA synthase-2 (ALAS 2). (Deficiency of ALAS 2 causes sideroblastic anemia rather than porphyria.) Single genes encode each enzyme; any of numerous possible mutations can alter the levels and/or the activity of the enzyme encoded by that gene. When an enzyme of heme synthesis is deficient or defective, its substrate and any other heme precursors normally modified by that enzyme may accumulate in bone marrow, liver, skin, or other tissues and have toxic effects. These precursors may appear in excess in the blood and be excreted in urine, bile, or stool.

Although, porphyrias are most precisely defined according to the deficient enzyme, classification by major clinical features (phenotype) is often useful. Thus, porphyrias are usually divided into two classes:

Acute porphyrias manifest as intermittent attacks of abdominal, mental, and neurologic symptoms. They are typically triggered by drugs, cyclic hormonal activity in young women, and other exogenous factors. Cutaneous porphyrias tend to cause continuous or intermittent symptoms involving cutaneous photosensitivity. Some acute porphyrias (hereditary coproporphyria, variegate porphyria) may also have cutaneous manifestations. Because of variable penetrance in heterozygous porphyrias, clinically expressed disease is less common than genetic prevalence (Table 21.2).

Urine discoloration (red or reddish brown) may occur in the symptomatic phase of all porphyrias except erythropoietic protoporphyria (EPP) and ALA dehydratase (ALAD)-deficiency porphyria. Discoloration results from oxidation of the porphyrinogens, the porphyrin precursor PBG, or both. Sometimes the color develops after the urine has stood in light for about 30 minutes, allowing time for nonenzymatic oxidation. In the acute porphyrias, except in ALAD-deficiency porphyria, about 1 in 3 heterozygotes (more frequently in females than males) also have increased urinary excretion of PBG (and urine discoloration) during the latent phase.

Diagnosis

Patients with symptoms suggesting porphyria are screened by blood or urine tests for porphyrins or the porphyrin precursors PBG and ALA (Table 21.3). Abnormal results on screening are confirmed by further testing.

Table 21.2	Major features of the two most common porphyrias			
Porphyria	Presenting symptoms	Exacerbating factors	Most important screening tests*	Treatment
Acute intermittent porphyria	Neurovisceral (intermittent, acute)	Drugs (mostly cytochrome P-450 inducers) Fasting Alcohol ingestion Organic solvents Infections Stress	Urinary PBG	Glucose Heme
Porphyria cutanea tarda	Blistering skin lesions (chronic)	Iron Alcohol ingestion Estrogens Hepatitis C virus Halogenated hydrocarbons	Urinary or plasma porphyrins	Phlebotomy Low-dose chloroquine or hydroxychloroquine

*In symptomatic phase. PBG, porphobilinogen.

Table 21.3	Screening for porphyrias	
Testing	In patients with acute neurovisceral symptoms	In patients with photosensitivity
Screening	Urinary PBG (semiquantitative, random urine sample)	Plasma porphyrins*
Confirmation (when screening test results are significantly abnormal)	Urinary ALA and PBG (quantitative) Fecal and urinary porphyrins RBC PBG deaminase Plasma porphyrins*	RBC porphyrins Urinary ALA, PBG, and porphyrins (quantitative) Fecal porphyrins Plasma porphyrins*

*The preferred method is by direct fluorescent spectrophotometry.
Urinary and fecal porphyrins are fractionated only if the total is increased.
Results are corrected according to urine creatinine level.
ALA, δ aminolevulinic acid; PBG, porphobilinogen.

Asymptomatic patients, including suspected carriers and people who are between attacks, are evaluated similarly. However, the tests are less sensitive in these circumstances; measurement of RBC or WBC enzyme activity is considerably more sensitive. Genetic analysis is highly accurate and preferentially used within families when the mutation is known. Prenatal testing (involving amniocentesis or chorionic villus sampling) is possible but rarely indicated.

Secondary Porphyrinuria

Several diseases unrelated to porphyrias may involve increased urinary excretion of porphyrins; this phenomenon is described as secondary porphyrinuria.

Hematologic disorders, hepatobiliary diseases, and toxins (e.g. alcohol, benzene, and lead) can cause elevated urinary coproporphyrin excretion. Elevated coproporphyrin excretion in the urine can occur in any hepatobiliary disorder because bile is one of the routes of porphyrin excretion. Uroporphyrin may also be elevated in patients with hepatobiliary disorders. Protoporphyrin is not excreted in urine because it is water insoluble.

Some patients present with abdominal pain and neurologic symptoms mimicking acute porphyrias. Urinary ALA and PBG are typically not elevated in these diseases, and normal levels help distinguish secondary porphyrinuria from acute porphyrias. However, some patients with lead poisoning can have elevated urinary ALA levels. Blood lead levels should be measured in such patients. If urinary ALA and PBG are normal or only slightly increased, measurement of urinary total porphyrins and high-performance liquid chromatography profiles of these porphyrins are helpful for differential diagnosis of acute porphyric syndromes.

ACUTE PORPHYRIAS

Acute porphyrias result from deficiency of certain enzymes in the heme biosynthetic pathway, resulting in accumulation of heme precursors that cause intermittent attacks of abdominal pain and neurologic symptoms.

Acute porphyrias include, acute intermittent porphyria (AIP), variegate porphyria (VP), hereditary coproporphyria (HCP), and δ aminolevulinic acid dehydratase (ALAD)–deficiency porphyria (exceedingly rare). Patients with VP and HCP, with or without neurovisceral symptoms, may develop bullous eruptions especially on the hands, forearms, face, neck, or other areas of the skin exposed to sunlight.

Among heterozygotes, acute porphyrias are rarely expressed clinically before puberty; after puberty, they are expressed in only about 2–4%. Among homozygotes and compound heterozygotes, onset typically is in childhood, and symptoms are often severe.

Precipitating Factors

Many precipitating factors exist, typically accelerating heme biosynthesis above the catalytic capacity of the defective enzyme. Accumulation of the porphyrin precursors porphobilinogen and δ aminolevulinic acid, or in the case of ALAD-deficiency porphyria, ALA alone, results.

Attacks probably result from several, sometimes unidentifiable, factors. Identified precipitating factors include (1) hormonal changes in women, (2) drugs, (3) low-calorie, low-carbohydrate diets, (4) alcohol, (5) exposure to organic solvents, (6) infections and other illnesses, (7) surgery, and (8) emotional stress.

Hormonal factors are important. Women are more prone to attacks than men, particularly during periods of hormonal change (e.g. luteal phase of the menstrual cycle, during oral contraceptive use, during early weeks of gestation, in the immediate postpartum period). Nevertheless, pregnancy is not contraindicated.

Other factors include drugs (including barbiturates, hydantoins, other antiepileptic drugs, and sulfonamide antibiotic (Table 21.4) and reproductive hormones (progesterone and related steroids), particularly those that induce hepatic ALA synthase and cytochrome P-450 enzymes. Attacks usually occur within 24 hours after exposure to a precipitating drug. Exposure to sunlight precipitates cutaneous symptoms in VP and HCP.

Table 21.4	Drugs and porphyria*		
Category/Disorder treated	**Unsafe**	**Safe**	**Probably safe**
Analgesic	Dextropropoxyphene	Aspirin	Atropine
	Diclofenac	Buprenorphine	Dexibuprofen
	Meprobamate	Caffeine	Fentanyl
	Propoxyphene	Codeine	Hydromorphone
	Tramadol	Morphine	Ketobemidone
		Propofol	Ketoprofen
			Naproxen

Contd.

Table 21.4	Drugs and porphyria* *(Contd.)*		
Category/Disorder treated	**Unsafe**	**Safe**	**Probably safe**
Anesthetic (local)	Lidocaine	Bupivacaine	Articaine
Anesthetic (premedication, induction, or maintenance)	Barbiturates	Atropine	Alfentanil
		Morphine	Desflurane
		Propofol	Droperidol
			Fentanyl
			Isoflurane
			Remifentanil
			Scopolamine
			Sufentanil
Antidepressant	—	Lithium	Fluoxetine
Antidiarrheal	—	Active carbon	—
		Loperamide	
Antiemetic	—	Chlorpromazine	Granisetron
			Ondansetron
			Scopolamine
			Tropisetron[†]
Anticonvulsant	Barbiturates	—	Clonazepam
	Carbamazepine		Diazepam (active seizure)
	Diones (paramethadione, trimethadione)		Gabapentin
	Felbamate		Levetiracetam
	Lamotrigine		Topiramate
	Mephenytoin		Vigabatrin
	Phenytoin		
	Primidone		
	Succinimides (ethosuximide, methsuximide)		
	Valproate		
Antihyperglycemic	Sulfonylureas	Acarbose	—
		Insulin	
		Metformin	
Anti-infective	Chloramphenicol	Acyclovir	Amphotericin B
	Clindamycin	Amikacin	Azithromycin
	Erythromycin	Amoxicillin	Bacampicillin[†]
	Indinavir	Amoxicillin with a	Cephalosporins
	Ketoconazole	β-lactamase inhibitor	Ciprofloxacin
	Mecillinam	Ampicillin	Didanosine
	Nitrofurantoin	Cloxacillin[†]	Ethambutol
	Pivampicillin	Dicloxacillin	Ertapenem
	Pivmecillinam	Fusidic acid	Famciclovir
	Rifampin	Ganciclovir	Flucytosine
	Ritonavir	Gentamicin	Foscarnet
	Sulfonamides	Immune globulin	Fosfomycin
	Trimethoprim	Immune sera	Imipenem/Cilastatin
		Methenaminehippurate	Levofloxacin
		Netilmicin	Meropenem
		Oseltamivir	Moxifloxacin
		Penicillin G	Norfloxacin
		Penicillin V	Ofloxacin
		Piperacillin	Piperacillin with
		Teicoplanin	tazobactam
		Tobramycin	Ribavirin
		Vaccines	
		Valacyclovir	
		Vancomycin	
		Zanamivir	

Contd.

Table 21.4   Drugs and porphyria* (Contd.)

Category/Disorder treated	Unsafe	Safe	Probably safe
Anti-inflammatory or antirheumatic	—	Hyaluronic acid Penicillamine Salicylates	Abacavir Dexibuprofen Ibuprofen Ketoprofen Lamivudine Lornoxicam Naproxen Piroxicam Tenofovir disoproxil fumarate Tenoxicam Zalcitabine
Anxiolytic, sedative-hypnotic, or antipsychotic	Ethchlorvynol Glutethimide Hydroxyzine Meprobamate	Chlorpromazine Droperidol Fluoxetine Fluphenazine Haloperidol Levomepromazine Prochlorperazine Propiomazine	Alprazolam Clozapine Dixyrazine Eszopiclone Lorazepam Olanzapine Oxazepam Perphenazine Triazolam
Cardiovascular disorders	Dihydralazine[†] Ergoloidmesylate Hydralazine Lidocaine Methyldopa Nifedipine Spironolactone	Amiloride β-Blockers Cholestyramine Colestipol Digitalis glycosides Diltiazem Enalapril Epinephrine Heparins Lisinopril Losartan Niacin Organic nitrates	Adenosine Amrinone Bendroflumethiazide Bezafibrate Bumetanide Digoxin Dobutamine Dopamine Dopexamine Doxazosin Ethacrynic acid Etilefrine Fenofibrate Furosemide Hydrochlorothiazide Milrinone Phenylephrine Prostaglandins Quinidine
Hormones	Danazol Progesterone Synthetic progestins	Nonreproductive hormones, including glucocorticoids	Natural estrogens
Laxatives	—	Bisacodyl Cascara sagrada Dietary fiber Lactitol Lactulose Lauryl sulfate Psyllium seed Senna glycosides Sodium docusate Sodium picosulfate Sorbitol	—

Contd.

Table 21.4	Drugs and porphyria* *(Contd.)*		
Category/Disorder treated	**Unsafe**	**Safe**	**Probably safe**
Migraines	Ergots	—	—
Muscle relaxants	Carisoprodol Orphenadrine	Atracurium Cisatracurium Mivacurium Pancuronium Rocuronium Succinylcholine (suxamethonium) Vecuronium	Baclofen
Osteoporosis	—	Bisphosphonates Calcium supplements	—
Peptic ulcers	—	Alginic acid Ca-containing antacids Cimetidine Mg-containing antacids Sucralfate	Famotidine Misoprostol Nizatidine Ranitidine
Respiratory disorders	Clemastine Dimenhydrinate	Albuterol (salbutamol) Alimemazine Codeine Corticosteroids Dipalmitoyl phosphatidylcholine Dornase α Ephedrine Ethylmorphine Ipratropium Phenylpropanolamine Phospholipid surfactant	Bambuterol Cromolyn Desloratadine Fenoterol[†] Fexofenadine Formoterol Levocabastine Lidocaine (solution for gargling) Loratadine Mizolastine Oxymetazoline Salmeterol Terbutaline Tiotropium

*The classification of the drugs in the list is based on a combination of clinical observations, case reports in the literature, and theoretical considerations derived from the structure and metabolism of the substances. However, clinical observations may in many cases be unreliable. Also, the biochemical and molecular-biologic models for the activation of the disease are incomplete. This list is meant as guidance only and is neither complete nor applicable to all patients. Drugs must always be used cautiously in people who carry genes for acute porphyria. For questions about specific drugs.

Signs and Symptoms

Signs and symptoms of acute porphyrias involve the nervous system, abdomen, or both (neurovisceral). Attacks develop over hours or days and can last up to several weeks. Most gene carriers experience no, or only a few, attacks during their lifetime. Others experience recurrent symptoms. In women, recurrent attacks often coincide with the luteal phase of the menstrual cycle.

The Acute Porphyric Attack

Constipation, fatigue, irritability, and insomnia typically precede an acute attack. The most common symptoms of an attack are abdominal pain and vomiting. The pain may be excruciating and is disproportionate to abdominal tenderness or other physical signs. Abdominal manifestations may result from effects on visceral nerves or from local vasoconstrictive ischemia. Because there is no inflammation, the abdomen is not tender and there are no peritoneal signs. Temperature and WBC count are normal or only slightly increased. Bowel distention may develop as a result of paralytic ileus. The urine is red or reddish brown and positive for PBG during an attack.

All components of the peripheral nervous system and the CNS may be involved. Motor neuropathy is common with severe and prolonged attacks. Muscle weakness usually begins in the extremities but can involve any motor neuron or cranial nerve and proceed to tetraplegia. Bulbar involvement can cause respiratory failure.

Central nervous system involvement may cause seizures or mental disturbances (e.g. apathy, depression, agitation, frank psychosis, hallucinations). Seizures, psychotic behavior, and hallucinations may be due to or exacerbated by hyponatremia or hypomagnesemia, which can also contribute to cardiac arrhythmias. Hyponatremia may occur during an acute attack due to excessive vasopressin [antidiuretic hormone (ADH)] release and/or administration of hypotonic IV solutions (5% or 10% dextrose in water), a standard therapy for acute attacks.

Excess catecholamines generally cause restlessness and tachycardia. Rarely, catecholamine-induced arrhythmias cause sudden death. Labile hypertension with transiently high BP may cause vascular changes progressing to irreversible hypertension if untreated. Renal failure in acute porphyria is multifactorial; acute hypertension (possibly leading to chronic hypertension) is likely a main precipitating factor.

Subacute or Subchronic Symptoms

Some patients have prolonged symptoms of lesser intensity (e.g. obstipation, fatigue, headache, back or thigh pain, paresthesia, tachycardia, dyspnea, insomnia, depression, anxiety or other disturbances of mood, seizures).

Skin Symptoms in Variegate Porphyria and Hereditary Coproporphyria

Fragile skin and bullous eruptions may develop on sun-exposed areas, even in the absence of neurovisceral symptoms. Often patients are not aware of the connection to sun exposure. Cutaneous manifestations are identical to those of porphyria cutanea tarda; lesions typically occur on the dorsal aspects of the hands and forearms, the face, ears, and neck.

Late Manifestations of Acute Porphyrias

Motor involvement during acute attacks may lead to persistent muscle weakness and muscle atrophy between attacks. Cirrhosis, hepatocellular carcinoma, systemic arterial hypertension, and renal impairment become more common after middle age in AIP and possibly also in VP and HCP, especially in patients with previous porphyric attacks.

Diagnosis

Acute Attack

Misdiagnosis is common because the acute attack is confused with other causes of acute abdomen (sometimes leading to unnecessary surgery) or with a primary neurologic or mental disorder. However, in patients previously diagnosed as gene carriers or who have a positive family history, porphyria should be suspected.

Still, even in known gene carriers, other causes must be considered.

Red or reddish brown urine, not present before onset of symptoms, is a cardinal sign and is present during full-blown attacks. A urine specimen should be examined in patients with abdominal pain of unknown cause, especially if severe constipation, vomiting, tachycardia, muscle weakness, bulbar involvement, or mental symptoms occur.

If porphyria is suspected, the urine is analyzed for PBG using a rapid qualitative or semiquantitative determination. A positive result or high clinical suspicion necessitates quantitative ALA and PBG measurements preferentially obtained from the same specimen. PBG and ALA levels >5 times normal indicate an acute porphyric attack unless patients are gene carriers in whom porphyrin precursor excretion occurs at similar levels even during the latent phase of the disorder.

If urinary PBG and ALA levels are normal, an alternative diagnosis must be considered. Measurement of urinary total porphyrins and high-performance liquid chromatography profiles of these porphyrins are helpful. Elevated urinary ALA and coproporphyrin with normal or slightly increased PBG suggests lead poisoning, ALAD-deficiency porphyria, or hereditary tyrosinemia type 1. Analysis of a 24 hours urine specimen is not necessary. Instead, a random urine specimen is used, and PBG and ALA levels are corrected for dilution by relating to the creatinine level of the sample. Electrolytes and Mg should be measured. Hyponatremia may be present because of excessive vomiting or diarrhea after hypotonic fluid replacement or because of the syndrome of inappropriate antidiuretic hormone secretion (SIADH).

Determination of Acute Porphyria Type

Because treatment does not depend on the type of acute porphyria, identification of the specific type is valuable mainly for finding gene carriers among relatives. When the type and mutation are already known from previous testing of relatives, the diagnosis is clear but may be confirmed by gene analysis. Activity of the enzymes ALAD and PBGD in the red blood cells is readily measurable and can be helpful for establishing the diagnosis in ALAD-deficiency porphyria and acute intermittent porphyria, respectively. RBC-PBG deaminase levels that are about 50% of normal suggest AIP. If there is no family history to guide the diagnosis, the different forms of acute porphyria are distinguished by characteristic patterns of porphyrin (and precursor) accumulation and excretion in plasma, urine, and stool. When urinalysis reveals increased levels of ALA and PBG, fecal porphyrins may be measured. Fecal porphyrins are usually normal or minimally increased in AIP but elevated in HCP and VP. Often, these markers are not present in the quiescent phase of the disorder. Plasma fluorescence emission after excitation with Soret band of light (approximately 410 nm) can be used to differentiate HCP and VP, which have different peak emissions.

Family Studies in Acute Porphyrias

Children of a gene carrier for an autosomal dominant form of acute porphyria (AIP, HCP, and VP) have a 50% risk of inheriting the disorder. In contrast, children of patients with ALAD-deficiency porphyria (autosomal recessive inheritance) are obligate carriers but are very unlikely to develop clinical disease. Because early diagnosis followed by counseling reduces the risk of morbidity, children in affected families should be tested before the onset of puberty. Genetic testing is used if the mutation has been identified in the index case. If not, pertinent RBC or WBC enzyme levels are measured. Gene analysis can be used for in utero diagnosis (using amniocentesis or chorionic villus sampling) but is seldom indicated because of the favorable outlook for most gene carriers.

Prognosis

Advances in medical care and self-care have improved the prognosis of acute porphyrias for symptomatic patients. Still, some patients develop recurrent crises or progressive disease with permanent paralysis or renal failure. Also, frequent need for opioids analgesics may give rise to opioid dependence.

Treatment

Treatment of the acute attack is identical for all the acute porphyrias. Possible triggers (e.g. excessive alcohol use, drugs) are identified and eliminated. Unless the attack is mild, patients are hospitalized in a darkened, quiet, private room. Heart rate, BP, and fluid and electrolyte balance are monitored. Neurologic status, bladder function, muscle and tendon function, respiratory function, and O_2 saturation are continuously monitored. Symptoms (e.g. pain, vomiting) are treated with nonporphyrinogenic drugs as needed (Table 21.4).

Dextrose 300–500 g daily down-regulates hepatic ALA synthase (ALAS1) and relieves symptoms. Dextrose can be given by mouth if patients are not vomiting; otherwise, it is given IV. The usual regimen is 3 L of 10% dextrose solution, given by a central venous catheter over 24 hours (125 mL/h). However, to avoid overhydration with consequent hyponatremia, 1 L of 50% dextrose solution can be used instead.

Intravenous heme is more effective than dextrose and should be given immediately in severe attacks, electrolyte imbalance, or muscle weakness. Heme usually resolves symptoms in 3–4 days. If heme therapy is delayed, nerve damage is more severe and recovery is slower and possibly incomplete. The dose is 3–4 mg/kg IV once a day for 4 days. An alternative is heme arginate, which is given at the same dose, except that it is diluted in 5% dextrose or half-normal or quarter-normal saline. Hematin and heme arginate may cause venous thrombosis and/or thrombophlebitis. Risk of these adverse events appears to be lower if the heme is administered bound to human serum albumin. Such binding also decreases the rate of development of hematin aggregates. Thus, most authorities recommend administration of hematin or heme arginate with human serum albumin.

Recurrent Attacks

In patients with severe recurrent attacks, who are at risk of renal damage or permanent neurologic damage, liver transplantation is an option. Successful liver transplantation leads to permanent cure of all acute porphyrias other than ALAD-deficiency porphyria. Patients with acute porphyrias should not serve as liver donors even though their liver may appear structurally normal (i.e. no cirrhosis) because recipients have developed acute porphyric syndromes; such an outcome helped establish that the acute porphyrias are hepatic disorders. Renal transplantation, with or without simultaneous liver exchange, should be considered in patients with active disease and terminal renal failure because there is considerable risk that nerve damage will progress at the start of dialysis.

Prevention

Diets for obesity should provide gradual weight loss and be adopted only during periods of remission. Carriers of VP or HCP should minimize sun exposure; sunscreens that block only ultraviolet B-light are ineffective, but opaque zinc oxide or titanium dioxide preparations are beneficial.

A high-carbohydrate diet may decrease the risk of acute attacks. Some patients can sometimes treat mild acute attacks by increasing their intake of dextrose or glucose. Prolonged use should be avoided in order to decrease risk of obesity and dental caries.

Patients who experience recurrent and predictable attacks (typically women with attacks related to the menstrual cycle) may benefit from prophylactic heme therapy given shortly before the expected onset. There is no standardized regimen; a specialist should be consulted. Frequent premenstrual attacks in some women are aborted by administration of a gonadotropin-releasing hormone agonist plus low-dose estrogen. Low-dose oral contraceptives are sometimes used successfully, but the progestin component is likely to exacerbate the porphyria.

To prevent renal damage, chronic hypertension should be treated aggressively (using safe drugs). Patients with evidence of impaired renal function are referred to a nephrologist. Recent anecdotal experience indicates that tolvaptan, an ADH blocker, is helpful in the management of hyponatremia during acute attacks.

The incidence of hepatocellular cancer is high among carriers of acute porphyria, especially in patients with active disease. Patients who are >50, should undergo yearly or twice yearly surveillance, including liver screening with ultrasonography. Early intervention can be curative and increases life expectancy.

CUTANEOUS PORPHYRIAS

In all cutaneous porphyrias except EPP and X-linked protoporphyria (XLPP), cutaneous photosensitivity manifests as fragile skin and bullous eruptions. Skin changes generally occur on sun-exposed areas (e.g. face, neck, dorsal aspects of hands and forearms) or traumatized skin. The cutaneous reaction is insidious, and often patients are unaware of the connection to sun exposure. In contrast, the photosensitivity in EPP and XLPP occurs within minutes or hours after sun exposure, manifesting as a burning pain that persists for hours, without any blistering and often without any objective signs on the skin. However, swelling and erythema may occur. Chronic liver disorders are common in cutaneous porphyrias.

The cutaneous porphyrias are all accompanied by elevated total plasma porphyrins, and are specifically diagnosed by measurements of porphyrins in RBCs, plasma, urine, and stool, as well as by genetic or enzyme analysis. Treatment involves avoidance of sunlight, measures to protect the skin, and sometimes other treatments directed according to the specific diagnosis.

Porphyria Cutanea Tarda

Porphyria cutanea tarda is a comparatively common hepatic porphyria affecting mainly the skin. Liver disease is also common. PCT is due to an acquired or inherited deficiency in the activity of hepatic uroporphyrinogen decarboxylase, an enzyme in the heme biosynthetic pathway (Table 21.1). Porphyrins accumulate, particularly when there is increased oxidative stress in the hepatocytes, which is usually due to increased hepatic iron, but which may also be due to alcohol, smoking, estrogens, or hepatitis C or HIV infection. Symptoms include fragile, easily blistered skin, mainly on sun-exposed areas. Diagnosis is by porphyrin analysis of urine and stool. Differentiation from the acute, cutaneous porphyrias hereditary coproporphyria and variegate porphyria is important. Treatment includes iron depletion by phlebotomy and enhancing porphyrin excretion by treatment with low dose chloroquine or hydroxychloroquine. Prevention is by avoidance of sunlight, alcohol, smoking, estrogens, and iron-containing drugs and successful treatment of any concomitant hepatitis C and HIV infections.

Pathophysiology

Porphyria cutanea tarda results from hepatic deficiency of uroporphyrinogen decarboxylase (Table 21.1). Porphyrins accumulate in the liver and are transported to the skin, where they cause photosensitivity. The partial (approximately 50%) deficiency in UROD activity in heterozygous patients itself is not sufficient to cause biochemical or clinical features of PCT; additional factors (e.g. elevated hepatic iron, alcohol use, halogenated hydrocarbon exposure, hepatitis C virus or HIV infection) are required to cause the >75% decrease in hepatic UROD activity needed for features of PCT to manifest. These factors increase the oxidation of uroporphyrinogens and other porphyrinogens to the corresponding porphyrins and also help form inhibitors of UROD. The drugs that commonly trigger acute porphyria (Table 21.4) do not trigger PCT.

Liver disease is common in PCT and may be due partly to porphyrin accumulation, chronic hepatitis C infection, concomitant hemosiderosis, or excess alcohol ingestion. Cirrhosis occurs in ≤35% of patients, and hepatocellular carcinoma occurs in 7–24% (more common among middle-aged men).

There are two main types of PCT: type 1 (acquired or sporadic) and type 2 (hereditary or familial). Type 1 accounts for 75–80% of cases and type 2 for 20–25%. Type 3 accounts for <1% of cases.

In **type 1 PCT,** decarboxylase deficiency is restricted to the liver and no genetic predisposition is present. It usually manifests in middle age or later.

In **type 2 PCT,** decarboxylase deficiency is inherited in an autosomal dominant fashion with limited penetrance. Deficiency occurs in all cells, including RBCs. It may develop earlier than type 1, occasionally in childhood. The partial (approximately 50%) deficiency in UROD activity in heterozygous patients itself is not sufficient to cause biochemical or clinical features of PCT; additional factors (e.g. elevated hepatic iron, alcohol use, halogenated hydrocarbon exposure, hepatitis C virus or HIV infection) are required to cause the >75% decrease in hepatic UROD activity needed for features of PCT to manifest. These factors increase the oxidation of uroporphyrinogens and other porphyrinogens to the corresponding porphyrins and also help form inhibitors of UROD. Hepatoerythropoietic porphyria (Table 21.5), which features profound UROD deficiency, is very rare

Table 21.5 | Some less common porphyrias

Description	Signs and symptoms	Diagnosis	Treatment
Congenital erythropoietic porphyria (Günther disease)			
Severe deficiency of uroporphyrinogen III cosynthase (UROS)	In utero or shortly after birth: Severe cases manifesting as nonimmune hydrops Soon after birth: Skin blistering, hemolytic anemia, hyperbilirubinemia, red urine, dark diapers that show a red fluorescence under UV light Phototherapy for hyperbilirubinemia leads to severe skin blistering In adulthood: Facial disfiguration, increased hair growth, corneal scarring (possibly severe), hemolytic anemia, splenomegaly, erythrodontia, deposition of porphyrins in bone, bone demineralization (possibly substantial)	Porphyrins in plasma, urine, and stool elevated to levels higher than those in other porphyrias uroporphyrin I and coproporphyrin I the predominant porphyrins in urine and stool: Urinary ALA and PBG virtually normal Can be confirmed by low RBC UROS activity (<10%), but test not readily available Genetic analysis of UROS gene, which reveals homozygous or compound heterozygous mutations on chromosome 10 (most common mutation is C73R) For in utero diagnosis: Measurement of amniotic porphyrins or genetic analysis	Avoidance of sunlight (including lights for treating neonatal hyperbilirubinemia) Use of sun-protective clothing Avoidance of skin trauma Prompt treatment of secondary bacterial infections to help prevent scarring Splenectomy possibly beneficial for patients with hemolytic anemia Repeated RBC transfusions and hydroxyurea to keep bone marrow porphyrin production low; deferoxamine for transfusion-related iron overload Bone marrow transplantation potentially curative
Hepatoerythropoietic porphyria			
Severe deficiency of uroporphyrinogen decarboxylase (UROD)	Skin blistering Red urine Anemia	Elevated isocoproporphyrin in stool and urine Elevated zinc protoporphyrin in RBCs (to differentiate from PCT) Confirmed by very low RBC UROD activity Genetic analysis of UROD gene, which reveals homozygous or compound heterozygous mutations	Avoidance of sunlight Phlebotomy possibly beneficial to patients with milder cases Treatment of severe disease similar to that of congenital erythropoietic porphyria
Dual porphyria			
Disorders resulting from deficiencies of >1 enzyme of the heme biosynthetic pathway	Clinical and biochemical manifestations of both disorders In acute porphyrias: Neurovisceral symptoms triggered by porphyrogenic agents In cutaneous porphyrias: Hypersensitivity to sunlight with blistering and fragile skin	Porphyrin and porphyrin precursor excretion patterns Confirmed by family history and enzyme analyses	In acute porphyrias: Avoidance of triggering agents In cutaneous porphyrias: Skin protection and avoidance of sunlight

ALA, δ aminolevulinic acid; PBG, porphobilinogen; PCT, porphyria cutanea tarda; UV, ultraviolet.

and is often regarded as an autosomal recessive form of type 2 PCT.

Type 3 PCT, which is very rare, is hereditary but without any defect in the UROD gene; a defect in another, unidentified gene appears to be the cause.

Types 1 and 2 are the major forms of the disease. They have the same precipitants, symptoms, and treatment. Overall prevalence may be on the order of 1/10,000 but is probably higher in people exposed to halogenated aromatic hydrocarbons or other precipitants of the disease.

PSEUDOPORPHYRIA

Renal failure, ultraviolet absorption (UVA) and certain drugs can cause PCT-like symptoms without elevated porphyrin levels (pseudoporphyria). Commonly implicated drugs are furosemide, tetracyclines, sulfonamides, and naproxen and other NSAIDs.

Because porphyrins are poorly dialyzed, some patients receiving long-term hemodialysis develop a skin condition that resembles PCT; this condition is termed pseudoporphyria of end-stage renal disease.

Signs and Symptoms

Patients with PCT present with fragile skin, mainly on sun-exposed areas. Phototoxicity is delayed; patients do not always connect sun exposure with symptoms. Spontaneously or after minor trauma, tense bullae develop. Some bullae are hemorrhagic. Accompanying erosions and ulcers may develop secondary infection; they heal slowly, leaving atrophic scars. Sun exposure occasionally leads to erythema, edema, or itching, (Fig. 21.3). Hyperemic conjunctivitis may develop, but other mucosal sites are not affected. Areas of hypopigmentation or hyperpigmentation may develop, as may facial hypertrichosis and pseudosclerodermoid changes.

Diagnosis

In otherwise healthy patients, fragile skin and blister formation suggest PCT. Differentiation from acute porphyrias with cutaneous symptoms (variegate porphyria and hereditary coproporphyria) is important because in patients with variegate porphyria and hereditary coproporphyria, the erroneous prescription of porphyrogenic drugs may trigger the severe neurovisceral symptoms of the acute porphyrias. Previous unexplained neurologic symptoms or abdominal pain may suggest an acute porphyria. A history of exposure to chemicals that can cause pseudoporphyria should be sought.

Although all porphyrias that cause skin lesions are accompanied by elevated plasma porphyrins, elevated urinary uroporphyrin and heptacarboxyl porphyrin and fecal isocoproporphyrin indicate PCT. Urine levels of porphyrin precursor porphobilinogen is normal in PCT. Urinary δ aminolevulinic acid may be slightly increased (<3 times the upper limit of normal). RBC activity of UROD is normal in type 1 and type 3 PCT but decreased (by approximately 50%) in type 2.

All patients with PCT should be tested for hepatitis C and HIV infections. They should also be tested for iron overload with serum iron and ferritin levels, and total iron-binding capacity; if results suggest iron overload, genetic testing for hereditary hemochromatosis is done.

Treatment

The treatment is monitored by determinations of serum ferritin (if iron reduction therapy is used) and urinary porphyrin excretion every other or every third month until full remission.

Iron removal by therapeutic phlebotomy is usually effective. A unit of blood is removed every week or two. When serum ferritin falls slightly below normal, phlebotomy is stopped. Usually, 6–10 sessions are needed. Urine and plasma porphyrins fall gradually with treatment, lagging behind but paralleling the fall in ferritin. The skin eventually becomes normal. After remission, further phlebotomy is needed only if there is a recurrence.

Low-dose chloroquine or hydroxychloroquine 100–125 mg by mouth twice a week removes excess porphyrins from the liver and perhaps other tissues by increasing the excretion rate. Higher doses can cause transient liver damage and worsening of porphyria. When remission is achieved, the regimen is stopped.

Chloroquine and hydroxychloroquine are not effective in advanced renal disease, and phlebotomy is usually contraindicated because of underlying anemia. However, recombinant erythropoietin mobilizes excess iron and resolves the anemia enough to permit phlebotomy. In end-stage renal disease, deferoxamine is an adjunct to phlebotomy for reduction of hepatic iron, the complexed iron being removed during dialysis. Dialyzers with ultra-permeable membranes and extra high blood flow rates are needed.

Patients with overt PCT and hepatitis C infection should be evaluated for treatment with pegylated interferon α-2a, ribavirin, and an antiviral drug (telaprevir, boceprevir). Previous iron depletion augments the response to antiviral therapy.

Children with symptomatic PCT are treated with small-volume phlebotomies or oral chloroquine; dosage is determined by body weight.

Skin symptoms occurring during pregnancy are treated with phlebotomy. In refractory cases, low-dose chloroquine can be added; no teratogenic effects have

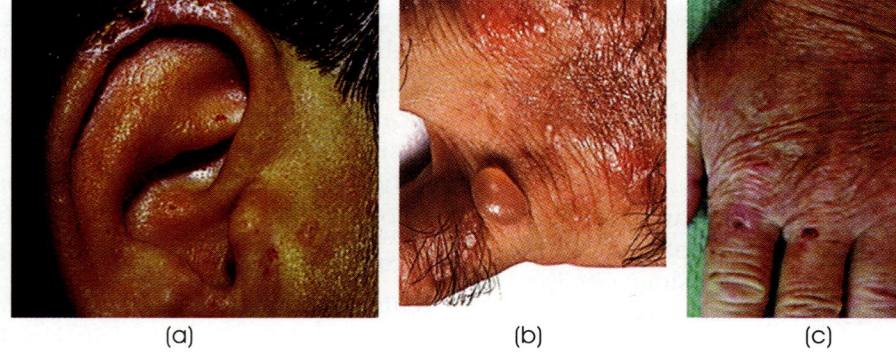

(a)   (b)   (c)

Fig. 21.3: (a) Porphyria cutanea tarda affects predominantly sun-exposed areas including the earlobes in this patient; (b) Erythema, bullae, and milia over the dorsum of the hand of a man with porphyria cutanea tarda; (c) Atrophic scars have developed after rupture of bullae. Some bullae are hemorrhagic

been recognized. Depending on degree of hemodilution and iron depletion, the skin symptoms usually abate as pregnancy advances. Postmenopausal estrogen supplementation is interrupted during treatment for PCT; stopping estrogens often induces remission.

Prevention

Patients should avoid sun exposure; hats and clothing protect best, as do zinc or titanium oxide sunscreens. Typical sunscreens that block UV light are ineffective, but UV radiation-absorbing sunscreens, such as those containing dibenzylmethanes, may help somewhat. Alcohol ingestion should be avoided permanently, but estrogen supplementation can usually be resumed safely after a disease remission.

ERYTHROPOIETIC PROTOPORPHYRIA AND X-LINKED PROTOPORPHYRIA

Erythropoietic protoporphyria is due to an inherited deficiency in the activity of the enzyme ferrochelatase, and X-linked protoporphyria is due to an inherited increase in the activity of δ aminolevulinic acid synthase-2; both enzymes are in the heme biosynthetic pathway (Table 21.1). EPP and XLPP are nearly identical clinically. They typically manifest in infancy with burning or itching skin pain after even short exposure to sunlight. Gallstones are common later in life, and chronic liver disease occurs in about 10%. Diagnosis is based on symptoms and increased levels of protoporphyrin in RBCs and plasma. Prevention is by avoidance of triggers (e.g. sunlight, alcohol, and fasting) and perhaps use of oral β-carotene. Acute skin symptoms can be alleviated by cold baths or wet towels, analgesics, and topical and/or oral corticosteroids. Patients with liver failure may need liver transplantation, but liver transplantation is not curative because the predominant source of excess protoporphyrin production is the bone marrow. Because XLPP is so similar to EPP, it is sometimes regarded as a variant of EPP.

Etiology

EPP, which comprises about 90% of EPP phenotypic presentations results from inherited deficiency of the enzyme ferrochelatase (FECH). The inheritance pattern is autosomal recessive; thus, clinical manifestations occur only in people with two defective FECH alleles, or more commonly, one defective and one low-expressing wild-type allele.

XLPP, which comprises the remaining 10% of cases, results from gain-of-function mutations that increase the activity of erythroid-specific δ-aminolevulinate synthase (ALAS2) in the bone marrow; the inheritance is X-linked.

The phenotype of heterozygous females can vary from asymptomatic that of affected males.

Prevalence of EPP phenotype is about 1/75,000. Protoporphyrin accumulates in bone marrow and RBCs, enters the plasma, and is deposited in the skin or excreted by the liver into bile. About 10% of patients develop chronic liver disease; a few of these patients develop cirrhosis, which may progress to liver failure. A more common complication is pigment gallstones due to heavy protoporphyrin excretion.

Signs and Symptoms

Symptom severity varies greatly, even among patients within a single family. Most patients develop symptoms in early childhood. Brief exposure to sunlight can cause severe pain, burning, erythema, and edema of the exposed skin. Usually, an infant or young child cries for hours after even short exposure to sun. Sometimes skin swelling and erythema may be subtle or absent, and EPP and XLPP may go undiagnosed longer than any other of the porphyrias. Crusting may develop around the lips and on the back of the hands after prolonged sun exposure. However, blistering and scarring, as are typical in porphyria cutanea tarda, hereditary coproporphyria, and congenital erythropoietic porphyria, do not occur. If skin protection is chronically neglected, rough, thickened, and leathery skin (lichenification) may develop, especially over the knuckles. Linear perioral furrows (carp mouth) may develop. Patients with XLPP tend to have more severe photosensitivity and liver disease than those with EPP.

If unrecognized, EPP and XLPP may cause psychosocial problems because children inexplicably refuse to go outdoors. The fear or anticipation of pain may be so distressing that children become nervous, tense, aggressive, or even develop feelings of detachment from the surroundings or suicidal thoughts.

Diagnosis

EPP or XLPP should be suspected in children and adults with painful cutaneous photosensitivity who experience no blisters or scarring. Gallstones in children should prompt testing for EPP and XLPP. Family history is usually negative.

The diagnosis is confirmed by finding increased RBC and plasma protoporphyrin levels. RBC protoporphyrin should also be fractionated to determine the proportions of metal-free and zinc protoporphyrin. In EPP, the proportion of RBC protoporphyrin that is metal-free is almost always >85%. The presence of >15% zinc protoporphyrin suggests XLPP. If measured, plasma coproporphyrin and urinary porphyrin levels are normal.

Stool protoporphyrin may be elevated, but coproporphyrin level is normal.

Potential carriers among relatives can be identified by showing increased RBC protoporphyrin and by genetic testing if a mutation has been identified in the index case.

Treatment

Patients should avoid sun exposure; protective clothing, hats and light-opaque titanium dioxide or zinc oxide containing sunscreens should be used. Oral β-carotene, an antioxidant, reduces photosensitivity. However, patient adherence with β-carotene is often poor because it is not very effective in controlling symptoms and also causes orange skin pigmentation. β-carotene dose depends on patient s age (Table 21.6). Other drugs that also may decrease photosensitivity include cysteine, an antioxidant, and afamelanotide, a synthetic analog of melanocyte stimulating hormone. Afamelanotide is currently available in parts of the European Union. Drugs that trigger acute porphyrias need not be avoided.

Acute skin symptoms can be alleviated by cold baths or wet towels, analgesics, and topical and/or oral corticosteroids. Symptoms can take up to a week to resolve. If these measures are ineffective (e.g. patients have increasing photosensitivity, rising porphyrin levels, progressive jaundice), giving hematin and/or RBC hypertransfusion (i.e. to above-normal Hb levels) may reduce protoporphyrin overproduction. Administration of bile acids may facilitate biliary excretion of protoporphyrin. Oral cholestyramine or charcoal have been used to interrupt the enterohepatic circulation of protoporphyrin and increase fecal excretion.

Patients who develop decompensated end stage liver disease require liver transplantation. However, liver transplantation does not correct the underlying metabolic defect and EPP hepatopathy often develops in the transplanted liver. Bone marrow transplant is curative for EPP but is not routinely done because the risk typically outweighs the benefits. Patients should be protected from operating lights during liver transplantation or other prolonged surgery to avoid serious phototoxic injury to internal organs. Light sources should be covered with commercially available filters that block wavelengths approximately 380–420 nm. Endoscopy, laparoscopy, and brief (<1.5 h) abdominal surgery do not usually cause phototoxic damage.

Regular physician-patient consultations that provide information, discussion, and opportunities for genetic counseling together with physical checkups are important. Liver function and RBC and plasma protoporphyrin levels should be checked annually. Patients with abnormal liver function test results should be evaluated by a hepatologist; a liver biopsy may be needed to stage the degree of fibrosis. Patients with known chronic liver disease should undergo screening ultrasonography every 6 months to check for hepatocellular carcinoma. Vitamin D levels should be checked because deficiency is common (patients tend to avoid sun exposure); supplements are given if levels are low. All EPP patients should be vaccinated against hepatitis A and hepatitis B and advised to avoid alcohol.

LABORATORY DIAGNOSIS OF PORPHYRIA

Specimen Collection and Stability

For porphyrin analysis, all samples must be protected from light, as urinary porphyrin concentrations have been observed to decrease by up to 50%, if kept in the light for 24 hours. Urinary porphyrins and PBG are best analyzed in fresh, random (10–20 mL) samples collected without preservative.

Very dilute urine (creatinine <2 mmol/L) is unsuitable for analysis. Urine often is of normal color in the non-acute porphyrias, except in CEP, when it is usually red, occasionally to such an extent that it is mistaken for hematuria. During an acute attack, urine may be a red-brown color because of the presence of uroporphyrin and other pigments formed by the non-enzymatic polymerization of PBG.

Twenty-four-hour urine collections (1) offer little advantage, (2) delay diagnosis, and (3) increase the risk of losses during the collection period. PBG and porphyrins are stable in urine in the dark at 4°C for up to 48 hours, and for at least a month at −20°C. Specimens for ALA estimation should be promptly refrigerated. Urine specimens have been stored at 4°C in the dark for at least 2 weeks without significant loss of ALA, and frozen specimens are stable for weeks. Whereas PBG is more stable around pH 8–9, ALA is more stable around pH 3–4, although more acidic environments notably reduce ALA stability.

About 5–10 g wet weight of feces is adequate for porphyrin measurements. Diagnostically, important changes in concentration are unlikely to occur within 36 hours at room temperature, and samples are stable for

Table 21.6	Doses of β-carotene in erythropoietic protoporphyria	
Patient age (years)	**Dose (oral)**
1–4	60–90 mg once/day
5–8	90–120 mg once/day
9–12	120–150 mg once/day
13–16	150–180 mg once/day
>16	Up to 300 mg once/day*

*To maintain serum levels of 11–15 μmol/L.

many months at –20°C. Blood, anticoagulated with ethylene diaminetetra acetic acid (EDTA), shows no loss of protoporphyrin for up to 8 days at room temperature and for at least 8 weeks at 4°C in the dark.

External Quality Assessment

Comparison of analyses between specialist laboratories has revealed differences in analytical quality that may influence their ability to diagnose and monitor porphyria. External quality assessment (EQA) and internal quality control are therefore essential to secure acceptable analytical quality for constituents used for these purposes. EQA schemes for the more common analyses are available in some countries and may accept participants from other countries.

METHODS FOR PORPHYRIN PRECURSORS

The water-soluble metabolites, PBG and ALA, are excreted by the kidney and usually are measured in the urine in the clinical laboratory. Both have been measured in plasma by high-performance liquid chromatography (HPLC)-mass spectrometry and fluorometric enzyme assays.

Porphobilinogen

Most methods for PBG are based on the reaction of Ehrlich' sreagent (dimethylaminobenzaldehyde in acidic solution) with the α-methene carbon of the pyrrole ring to form a colored product variously described as 'rose red' or 'magenta'; which has a characteristic absorption spectrum with a peak at 553 nm and a shoulder at 540 nm. Porphyrins do not contain any (α-methene hydrogens and so do not react. Some other substances in urine may react with the reagent to give red products, notably urobilinogen, may inhibit the reaction, or are pigmented themselves and so mask the red chromogen. All need to be removed. This is best achieved by ion-exchange chromatography, but methods for accurate quantification of PBG based on this procedure are time-consuming.

Qualitative screening tests in which urine is reacted directly with Ehrlich's reagent and is assessed visually for the formation of red chromogen (e.g., the Watson-Schwartzand Hoeschtests) are convenient but have been criticized for poor detection limits and interferences, even when solvent extraction has been used to separate the PBG-Ehrlich compound from the urobilinogen-Ehrlich complex.

The Mauzerall-Granick method has been modified in attempts to produce an alternative that is acceptable for screening purposes. Buttery and Stuare avoided the use of columns by employing batch-wise treatment with resin, and visually compared the final color with that of a surrogate calibrator. Blake and colleagues eliminated the centrifugation steps by using resin-filled syringes with detachable filters and compared the final color with a variety of artificial calibrators.

These modifications reduced the time taken to perform the test to 10 minutes and produced a semiquantitative result. A commercial kit based on Blake's method is available and has been found to be more analytically sensitive and specific for initial screening than the qualitative solvent extraction procedures. The modification used resin-filled nylon sacs instead of columns.

If a qualitative or semiquantitative screening test is used, it is essential to include appropriate controls and to confirm all positive test results using a specific quantitative method. The procedure described uses commercially available ion exchange columns, but some laboratories may prefer to prepare an ion-exchange resin themselves. PBG in the resin eluate reacts with Ehrlich's reagent to form a colored product that is scanned in a spectrometer. Reference intervals are given in Table 21.7. Scanning the spectrum of the product is

Table 21.7	Adult reference intervals	
Specimen	**Analyte**	**Reference interval**
Urine	Porphobilinogen	<10 µmol/L
	Total porphyrin	<1.5 µmol/mmol creatinine
	Uroporphyrin	20–320 nmol/L
	Heptacarboxylate porphyrin	<35 nmol/mmol creatinine
	Coproporphyrin–I	0.8–3.1 nmol/mmol creatinine 9
	Coproporphyrin–III	<0.9 nmol/mmol creatinine
	% Coproporphyrin–III*	1.2–5.7 nmol/mmol creatinine
		4.8–23.8 nmol/mmol creatinine 68–86
Feces	Total porphyrin	10–200 nmol/g dry wt
	Coproporphyrin-I	1.1–5.5 nmol/g feces
	Coproporphyrin–III	0.2–2.5 nmol/g feces
	Coproporphyrin-III/I ratio	0.3–1.4
	Total dicarboxylate porphyrin	0.5–12.8 nmol/g feces 9
Erythrocytes	Total porphyrin	0.4–1. 7 µmol/L erythrocytes

*Percentage of total coproporphyrin.

essential if interferences are to be identified. Imipenem, e.g. often gives a peak at 580 nm with Ehrlich's reagent. The coefficient of variation at the cutoff of 9 µmol/L is approximately ±10%, but the method is less precise at lower concentrations. Urinary PBG that is raised at least 2–3 times the upper reference limit is diagnostic of an acute porphyria, but it is important that individual laboratories determine a cut point above which further investigation is required.

δ Aminolevulinic acid

It is possible to measure ALA directly, but it is more usually converted into an Ehrlich's-reacting pyrrole through condensation with a reagent, such as acetyl acetone after separation from PBG by two-stage anion-exchange chromatography. A method for measurement of PBG and ALA, based on that of Mauzerall and Granick, is available commercially (Bio-Rad Laboratories, Hercules, Calif). A photometric method has been proposed for more rapid testing. Compared with PBG procedures, interferences are more common with ALA. For example, the acetylacetone derivatization step forms a compound with penicillin that reacts with Ehrlich's reagent.

ANALYSIS OF PORPHYRINS IN URINE AND FECES

Methods for porphyrin fractionation are complex and time consuming and are not available in every laboratory. Consequently, simple qualitative screening tests are often used to differentiate the majority of specimens that do not require further investigation from the few that justify fractionation of the individual porphyrins. Screening tests in which extracts of urine or feces are examined visually for typical red-pink fluorescence of porphyrins are not sensitive analytically and should not be used. Methods based on spectrophotometric scanning of acidified urine or fecal extracts for the presence of the Soret band are recommended and yield semiquantitative information. Quantitative fluorometric methods are also available.

All methods for the fractionation of porphyrins are based on the different solubilities of individual porphyrins caused by their different β-substituents and, to a lesser extent, on the substituent order around the macrocycle. Methods include (1) differential extraction with solvents, (2) paper and thin layer chromatography, and (3) HPLC. Solvent extraction methods should not be used because they yield only limited and sometimes misleading information. Reversed-phase HPLC, the current method of choice, separates all porphyrins of clinical interest, including isomers and metal chelates, without the need for prior methylation. Spectrophotometric or fluorometric detection has been used; the latter method is more sensitive and specific.

Semiquantitative Method for Total Porphyrin in Urine

This simple method for total urine porphyrins uses scanning spectrometry. A typical spectrum is shown in Figure 21.4. Reference values are given in Table 21.7. This method is reproducible but is only semiquantitative. The detection limit depends on the amount of background absorbance, but concentrations of approximately 50 nmol/L should be detected in urine of normal color. Ideally, concentrations should be expressed as a ratio to creatinine concentration to correct for urine concentration. Very occasionally, urine contains substances that produce very high background absorbance, making identification of any peak in the 400-nm region difficult. Such samples require analysis by alternative methods, such as HPLC. Increased concentrations require further investigation to identify individual porphyrins; porphyria should not be diagnosed on the basis of increased total porphyrin alone.

Semiquantitative Method for Total Porphyrin in Feces

This simple method for total fecal porphyrins uses scanning spectrometry after extraction. Reference values are given in Table 21.7. The expression of concentration on a dry weight basis corrects for the moisture content of feces. Total fecal porphyrin determined by this method, unlike most of those based on solvent extraction, includes uroporphyrin. Very occasionally, feces contain substances that produce very high background absorbance, making identification of any peak in the 400-nm

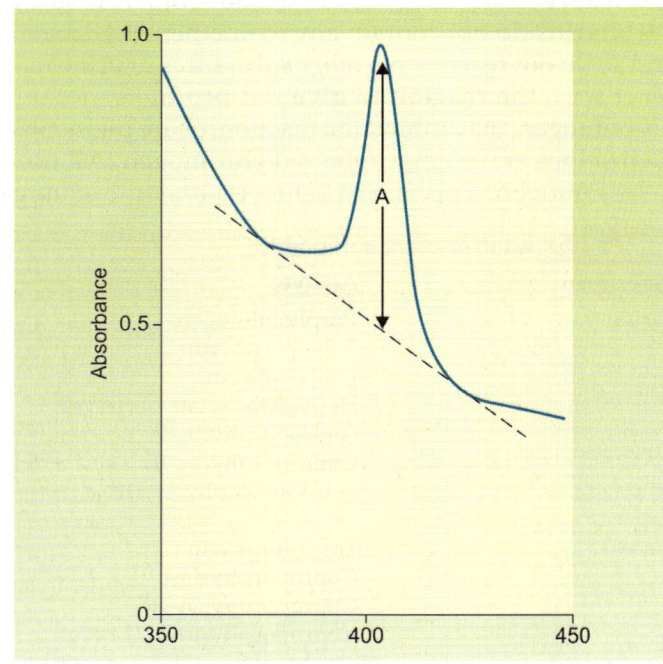

Fig. 21.4: Absorption spectrum of acidified urine showing the procedure for measurement of corrected absorbance (A) of the porphyrin peak

region difficult. Such samples require analysis by alternative methods, such as HPLC. Increased total fecal porphyrin concentration requires further investigation by fractionation, identification, and quantification of individual porphyrins using a technique, such as reversed-phase HPLC, which resolves coproporphyrin-I and -III isomers. Porphyria should never be diagnosed on the basis of raised total fecal porphyrin alone.

HPLC FRACTIONATION OF PORPHYRINS IN URINE AND FECES

This method for fractionation of urinary and fecal porphyrins uses sample preparation, HPLC separation, and fluorometric detection. Samples are assayed with and without addition of calibrator to assist with fluorometric peak identification. Figure 21.5 shows typical profiles from patients with various types of porphyria. For diagnostic purposes, quantification of individual porphyrins is rarely necessary, particularly if the concentrations are clearly elevated. Table 21.8 shows expected findings in the various types of porphyria, and reference values for individual porphyrin fractions are given in Table 21.7. Considerable variation is evident in the reference values quoted in the literature, probably as a consequence of difficulties in calibration.

The extraction method for fecal porphyrins results in some interference with the chromatography caused by dissolution of a proportion of the diethyl ether in the aqueous phase. As a result, an extra peak elutes just before the uroporphyrin position. This peak contains any uroporphyrin in the sample, up to 50% of the heptacarboxylate porphyrins, and smaller quantities of hexacarboxylate and pentacarboxylate porphyrins.

METHODS FOR BLOOD PORPHYRINS

The methods described later require a spectrofluorometer with a red-sensitive photomultiplier. If such equipment is not available locally, samples should be referred to a specialized laboratory. Erythrocyte and plasma measurements are rarely required for the urgent assessment of acutely ill patients.

Determination of Erythrocyte Total Porphyrin

This method for erythrocyte total porphyrin uses double extraction and fluorometry. Reference intervals are given in Table 21.7. Total erythrocyte porphyrin concentrations are increased in (1) EPP, (2) congenital erythropoietic porphyria (CEP), (3) the rare homozygous variants of the autosomal dominant porphyrias, (4) iron deficiency, (5) hemolytic anemia, (6) some other forms of anemia, and (7) lead poisoning.

A total porphyrin concentration within the reference interval excludes EPP. Distinction between EPP and other causes of increased erythrocyte total porphyrin

concentration requires differentiation between protoporphyrin and its zinc chelate, because the acidic condition of this assay dissociates the zinc chelate and provides only a measure of total porphyrin.

Qualitative Determination of Zinc-protoporphyrin and Protoporphyrin

This qualitative method for zinc protoporphyrin (ZPP) and protoporphyrin uses extraction and fluorometry. Emission peaks for ZPP and free protoporphyrin are 587 nm and 630 nm, respectively. In EPP, the concentration of free protoporphyrin greatly exceeds that of ZPP, except in the 2% of patients with X-linked dominant protoporphyria (XLDPP) in whom ZPP concentration may constitute up to 60% of the greatly increased

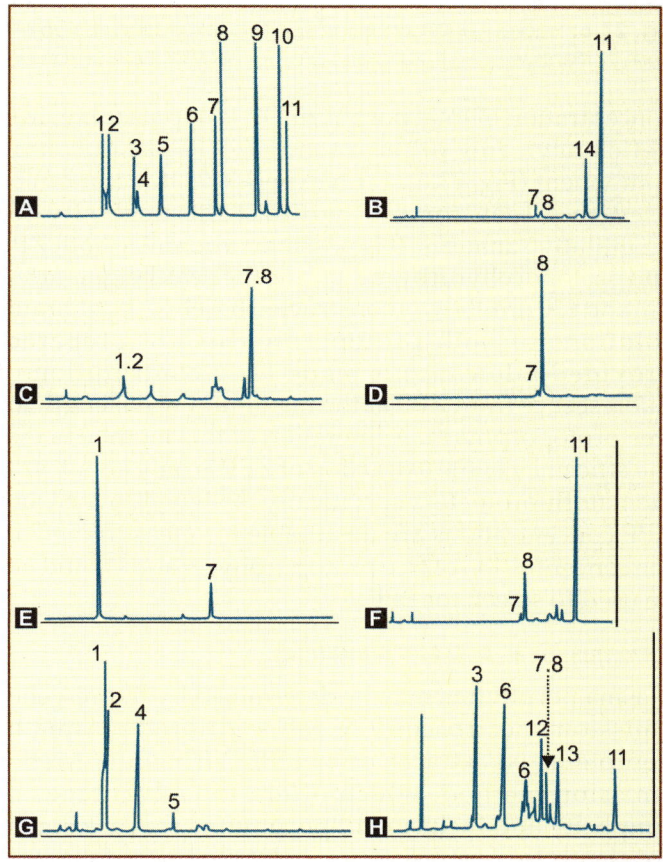

Fig. 21.5: Representative high-performance liquid chromatography (HPLC) chromatograms for (A) working standard, (B) normal feces, (C) normal urine, (D) feces-hereditary coproporphyria, (E) urine-congenital erythropoietic porphyria, (F) feces-variegate porphyria, (G) urine-porphyria cutanea tarda, and (H) feces porphyria cutanea tarda chromatographic conditions. Peaks are (I) uroporphyrin-I, (2) uroporphyrin-III, (3) heptacarboxylate porphyrin-I, (4) heptacarboxylate porphyrin-III, (5) hexacarboxylate porphyrin, (6) pentacarboxylate porphyrin, (7) coproporphyrin-I, (8) coproporphyrin-III, (9) deuteroporphyrin-IX, (10) mesoporphyrin-IX, (II) protoporphyrin-IX, (12) hydroxyisocoproporphyrin, (13) isocoproporphyrin, and (14) pemptoporphyrin-IX

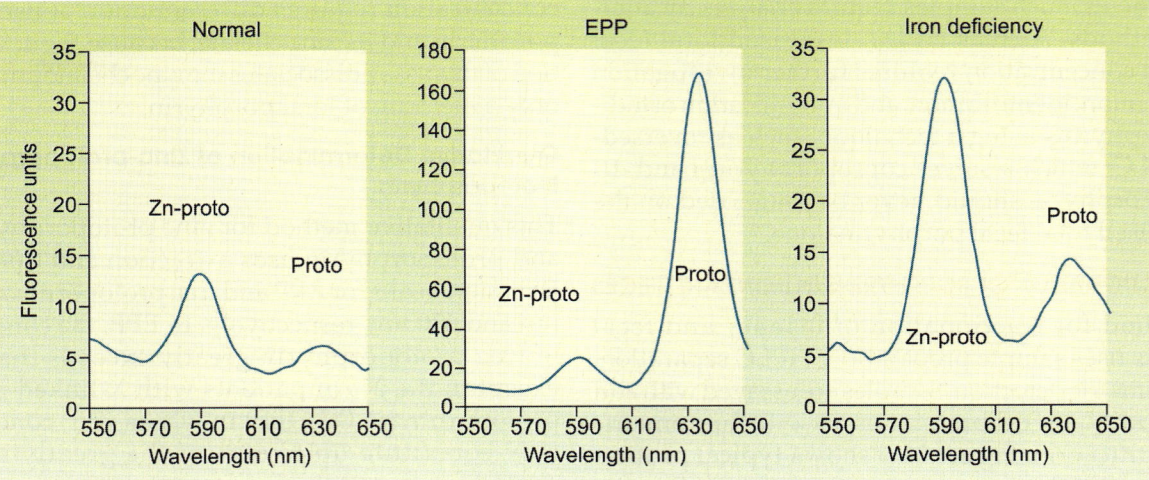

Fig. 21.6: Fluorescence emission spectra (excitation at 405 nm) of ethanolic extracts of erythrocytes from a normal individual and from patients with erythropoietic protoporphyria (EPP) or iron deficiency. Note that different scales are used

concentration of total porphyrin. In lead poisoning, iron deficiency, and other anemias, ZPP is the main component (Fig. 21.6). With experience, this test can be used to screen for EPP without the necessity for quantitative analysis. It is possible to quantify both ZPP and protoporphyrin by measuring the peak heights at 587 nm and 630 nm above a constructed baseline, if calibrator solutions of both protoporphyrins are prepared, provided allowance is made for a contribution of fluorescence from ZPP at the maximum wavelength for free protoporphyrin. A limitation of this method is that the efficiency of the extraction of ZPP is only about 50%. Hematofluorometers specifically designed to measure ZPP concentrations are unsuitable for measurement of the concentration of free protoporphyrin and should not be used to screen for EPP.

ANALYSIS OF PLASMA PORPHYRINS

Plasma porphyrins may be determined by fluorescence emission spectroscopy of saline-diluted plasma or deproteinized extracts, or by HPLC. The fluorescence emission method, which offers the advantages of simplicity and inclusion of porphyrins that are bound covalently to plasma proteins, is detailed in the following sections.

Fluorescence Emission Spectroscopy of Plasma Porphyrins

This method determines the fluorescence emission spectrum of saline-diluted plasma excited at 405 nm. Figure 21.7 shows typical fluorescence emission maximum wavelengths for various porphyrias. In VP, the plasma contains porphyrin covalently bound to protein with a fluorescence emission maximum at 624–628 nm. In other porphyrias, porphyrin is noncovalently bound

to albumin and hemopexin. In freshly separated plasma, protoporphyrin has a fluorescence emission peak around 632 nm. If separation is delayed, binding to globin released from red cells decreases the peak toward 626 nm. Apart from porphyrias (Table 21.8), the plasma porphyrin concentration may be increased in conditions in which porphyrin excretion is impaired, such as renal failure and cholestasis.

Enzyme Measurements

Assay of individual enzymes of the heme biosynthetic pathway is rarely required for the assessment of patients with symptoms of porphyria. However, measurement of enzyme activities is useful for family studies when it is

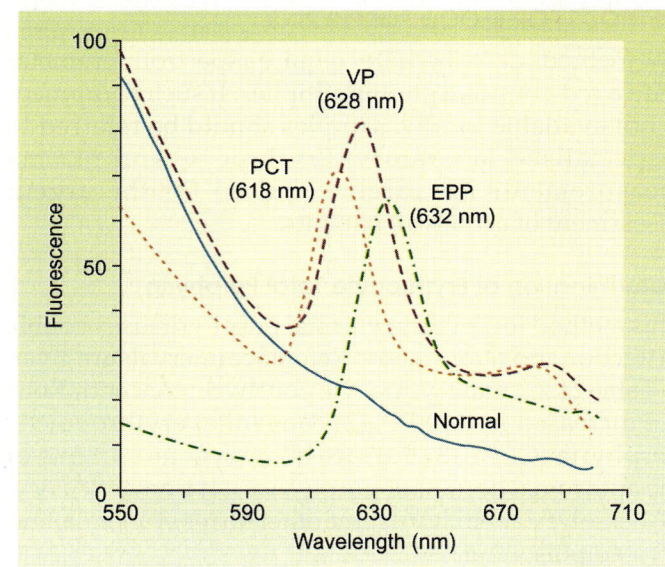

Fig. 21.7: Fluorescence emission spectra (excitation, 405 nm) of dilutions in phosphate-buffered saline (PBS) of plasma from a normal individual and from patients with various porphyrias

Table 21.8	The porphyrias: patterns of overproduction of heme precursors during clinically overt phase of disease				
Porphyria	Urine PBG/ALA	Urine porphyrins	Fecal porphyrins	Erythrocyte porphyrins	Plasma fluorescence emission peak
ADP	ALA	COPRO-III	Not increased	ZPP	—
AIP	PBG>ALA	Mainly uroporphyrin from PBG	Normal or Increased[a] COPRO-I/ III ratio normal	Not increased	615–622 nm[b]
CEP	Not increased	URO-I, COPRO-I	COPRO-I	ZPP, PROTO, COPRO-I, URO-I	615–620 nm
PCT	Not increased	URO, HEPTA[c]	ISOCOPRO, HEPTA	Not increased	615–622 nm
HCP	PBG>ALA[d]	COPRO-III, uroporphyrin from PBG	COPRO-III COPRO- III/I ratio increased	Not increased	615–622 nm[b]
VP	PBG>ALA[d]	COPRO-III, uroporphyrin from PBG	PROTO-IX >COPRO-III[e], X-porphyrin	Not increased	624–628 nm
EPP (FECH-deficient)	Not increased	Not increased	±PROTO[f]	PROTO	626–634 nm[g]
EPP (XLDPP)	Not increased	Not increased	PROTO	PROTO, ZPP[h]	626–634 nm

[a]Slight increase only unless uroporphyrin is present. [b]Not always increased during acute attack. [c]Other methylcarboxylate-substituted porphyrins are increased to a smaller extent; uroporphyrin is a mixture of type I and III isomers; heptacarboxylate porphyrin is mainly type III. [d]PBG and ALA may be normal when only skin lesions are present. [e]Coproporphyrin-III/1 ratio may be increased, but increase is usually less than in overt HCP. [f]Not increased in about 40% of patients. [g]Protoporphyrin bound to globin (if hemolysis is seen in the sample) has a peak at 626 to 628 nm. [h]Zn-protoporphyrin 20 to 60% of total protoporphyrin.

not possible to identify the individual mutation, or when DNA analysis is not available, and for the identification of uncommon subtypes, such as non-erythroid AIP and 'homozygous' forms of autosomal dominant porphyrias. Erythrocytes are a convenient source of cytoplasmic enzymes [ALAD, hydroxymethylbilane synthase (HMBS), uroporphyrinogen III synthase (UROS), and UROD, but assay of the mitochondrial enzymes coproporphyrinogen oxidase (CPO), protoporphyrinogen oxidase (PPOX), and FECH] requires nucleated cells such as lymphocytes, Epstein-Barr virus (EBV)-transformed lymphoblasts, or cultured fibroblasts. Assays for enzymes that use porphyrinogens as substrates are difficult because the substrate (1) is unstable; (2) has to be prepared fresh, and, particularly with protoporphyrinogen; (3) undergoes nonenzymatic oxidation during the assay. However, erythrocyte HMBS measurement is relatively straightforward and is the most widely used of these enzyme assays.

Assay of Erythrocyte Hydroxymethylbilane Synthase Activity

The enzymatic assay measures the rate of formation of porphyrinogens from PBG by hemolyzed erythrocytes. The reference interval [mean ±2 standard deviations (SD)] is 20–42 nmol uroporphyrin per milliliter of erythrocytes per minute at 37°C. Measurement of erythrocyte HMBS activity discriminates between individuals with AIP and their unaffected relatives, with

a likelihood ratio of 3.4. Although, activities are usually below the reference interval in AIP, some overlap is noted between activities in AIP and healthy individuals, and activities are within the reference interval in the uncommon nonerythroid form. In addition, erythrocyte HMBS activity declines sharply with erythrocyte age and is markedly influenced by the proportions of reticulocytes and young cells in peripheral blood. Therefore, HMBS assay should not be used for pre symptomatic diagnosis of AIP in patients who (1) are hematologically abnormal, (2) have received a recent blood transfusion, or (3) are younger than 1 year old. Activity may increase in acutely ill patients, e.g. during an acute attack of porphyria, and may also be increased or decreased in disorders other than porphyria, including liver disease and chronic alcohol abuse. In France, the prevalence of abnormally low HMBS activities in the general population is about 1 in 800.

BIBLIOGRAPHY

1. Aarsand AK, Boman H, Sandberg S. Familial and sporadic porphyria cutanea tarda: characterization and diagnostic strategies. Clin Chem. 2009;55:795-803.
2. Allen KR, Whatley SD, Degg TJ, Barth JH. Hereditary coproporphyria: comparison of molecular and biochemical investigations in a large family. J Inherit Metab Dis 2005; 28: 779–85.
3. Anderson KE, Sassa S, Bishop DF, Desnick RJ. Disorders of heme biosynthesis: X-linked sideroblastic anemia and the porphyrias. Scriver CR, Beaudet AL, Sly WS, Valle D, eds.

The metabolic and molecular basis of inherited disease, 8th edition. New York: McGraw- Hill, 2000: 2961–3062.

4. Anstey AV, Hift RJ. Liver disease in erythropoietic proto porphyria: insights and implications for management. Postgrad Med J 2007; 83: 739–48.

5. Astner I, Schulze JO, van den Heuvel J, Jahn D, Schubert WD, Heinz DW. Crystal structure of 5-amino!evulinate synthase, the first enzyme of heme biosynthesis, and its link to XLSA in humans. EMBO J 2005; 24: 3166–77.

6. Badenas C, To-Figueras J, Phillips JD, Warby CA, Munoz C, Herrero C. Identification and characterization of novel uroporphyrinogen decarboxylase gene mutations in a large series of porphyria cutanea tarda patients and relatives. Clin Genet 2009; 75: 346–53.

7. Battersby AR, Fookes CJ, Matcham GW, McDonald E. Biosynthesis of the pigments of life: formation of the macro-cycle. Nature 1980; 285: 17–21.

8. Berk PD, Rodkey FL, Blaschke TF, et al. Comparison of plasma bilirubin turnover and carbon monoxide production in man. J Lab Clin Med 1974; 83: 29–36.

9. Beukeveld GJ, Wolthers BG, van Saene n, de Haan TH, de Ruyter-Buitenhuis LW, van Saene RH. Patterns of porphyrin excretion in feces as determined by liquid chromatography: reference values and the effect of tlora suppression. Clin Chem 1987; 33: 2164–70.

10. Blake D, McManus J, Cronin V, Ratnaike S. Fecal copro-porphyrin isomers in hereditary coproporphyria. Clin Chem 1992; 38: 96–100.

11. Blake D, Poulos V, Rossi R. Diagnosis of porphyria-recom-mended methods for peripheral laboratories. Clin Biochem Rev 1992; 13(Suppl I): S 1–24.

12. Bonkovsky HL, Barnard GE Diagnosis of porphyric syn-dromes: a practical approach in the era of molecular biology. Semin Liver Dis 1998; 18: 57–65.

13. Bottomley SS. Sideroblastic anemias. In: Greer JP, Foerster J, Lukens JN, Rogers GM, Paraskevas F, Glader BE, eds. Wintrobe's clinical hematology. Philadelphia: Lippincott Williams & Wilkins, 2004: 1012–33.

14. Brodie MJ, Moore MR, Thompson GG, Goldberg A. The treatment of acute intermittent porphyria with laevulose. Clin Sci Mol Med 1977; 53: 365–71.

15. Bulaj ZJ, Phillips JD, Ajioka RS, Franklin MR, Griffen LM, Guinee DJ, et al. Hemochromatosis genes and other factors contributing to the pathogenesis of porphyria cutanea tarda. Blood 2000; 95: 1565–71.

16. Burnham BE The chemistry of porphyrins. Semin Haematol 1968; 5: 296–322.

17. Buttery JE, Stuart S, Panall PRo An improved direct method for the measurement of urinary o-δ Aminolevulinic acid. Clin Biochem 1995; 28: 477–80.

18. Buttery JE, Stuart S. Measurement of porphobilinogen in urine by a simple resin method with use of a surrogate standard. Clin Chem 1991; 37: 2133–6.

19. Chen W, Dailey HA, Paw BH. Ferrochelatase forms an oligomeric complex with mitoferrin-1 and Abcb 10 for erythroid heme biosynthesis. Blood 2010; 116: 628–30.

20. Corradi HR, Corrigall AV, Boix E, Mohan CG, Sturrock ED, Meissner PN, et al. Crystal structure of protoporphyrinogen

oxidase from Myxococ Cllsxanthus and its complex with the inhibitor acifluorfen. J BioIC
hem 2006; 281: 386 25–33.

21. Cox TM. Protoporphyria. In: Kadish KM, Smith KM, Guilard R, eds. The porphyrin handbook. Volume 14. Medical aspects of porphyrias. Amsterdam: Academic Press, 2003: 121–50.

22. Dailey HA. Enzymes of heme biosynthesis. J BioIInorgChem 1997; 2: 411–7.

23. De Rooij FW, Edixhoven A, Wilson JHP. Porphyria: a diagnostic approach. In: Kadish KM, Smith KM, Gui[ard R, eds. The porphyrin handbook. Volume 14. Medical aspects of porphyrias. Amsterdam: Academic Press, 2003: 211–46.

24. Deacon AC, Elder GH. ACP best practice no. 165: front line tests for the investigation of suspected porphyria. J Clin PathoI 2001; 54: 500–7.

25. Deacon AC, Ledden JA. Limitations of solvent fractionation techniques for urinary and faecal porphyrins. Ann Clin Biochem 1998; 35: 314–6.

26. Deacon AC, Peters TJ. Identification of acute porphyria: evaluation of a commercial screening test for porpho-bilinogen. Ann Clin Biochem 1998; 35: 726–32.

27. Deacon AC. Performance of screening tests for porphyria. Ann Clin Biochem 1998; 25: 392–7.

28. Desnick RJ, Aplin KH. Congenital erythropoietic porphyria: advances in pathogenesis and treatment. Br J Haematol 2002; 117: 779–95.

29. Di Pierro E, Besana V, Moriondo V, Brancaleoni V, Tavazzi D, Casalgrandi G, et al. A large deletion on chromosome 11 in acute intermittent porphyria. Blood Cells Mol Dis 2006; 37: 50–4.

30. Doss MO, Stauch T, Gross U, Renz M, Akagi R, Doss-Frank M, et al. The third case of Doss porphyria (delta-amino-levulinic acid dehydratase deficiency) in Germany. J Inherit Metab Dis 2004; 27: 529–36.

31. Dowman JK, Gunson BK, Newsome PN, Bramhall S, Badminton MN Liver transplantation from donors with acute intermittent porphyria. Ann Intern Med. 2011; 154(8): 571–2.

32. Egger NG, Goeger DE, Payne DA, Miskovsky EP, Weinman SA, Anderson KE. Porphyria cutanea tarda: multiplicity of risk factors including HFE mutations, hepatitis C, and inherited

33. Egger NG, Goeger DE, Payne DA, Miskovsky EP, Weinman SA, Anderson KE. Porphyria cutanea tarda: multiplicity of risk factors including HFE mutations, hepatitis C, and inherited uroporphyrinogen decarboxylase deficiency. Dig Dis Sci 2002; 47: 419–26.

34. Elder GH, Gouya L, Whatley SO, Puy H, Badminton MN, Deybach J-Co The molecular genetics of erythropoietic protoporphyria. Cell Mol Bioi (Noisy-ie-grand) 2009; 15: 118–26.

35. Elder GH, Hift RJ. Treatment of acute porphyria. Hosp Med 2001; 62: 422–8.

36. Elder GH. Hepatic porphyrias in children. J Inherit Metab Dis 1997; 20: 237–46.

37. Elder GH. Porphyria cutanea tarda and related disorders. In: Kadish KM, Smith KM, Guilard R. eds. The porphyrin handbook. Volume 14. Medical aspects of porphyrias. Amsterdam: Academic Press, 2003: 67–92.

38. Erskine PT, Senior A, Awan SJ, Lambert R, Lewis G, Tickle IJ, et al. X-ray structure of 5-aminolaevulinate dehydratase, a hybrid aldolase. Nat StructBioi 1997; 4: I 025–31.

39. Felitsyn N, McLeod C, Shroads AL, Stacpoole PW, Notterpek L. The heme precursor delta aminolevulinate blocks peripheral myelin formation. J Neurochem 2008; 106: 2068–79.

40. Fontanellas A, Coronel F, Santos)L, Herrero JA, Moran MJ, Guerra P, et al. Heme biosynthesis in uremic patients on CAPO or hemodialysis. Kidney Int 1994; 45: 220–3.

41. Fritsch C, Boisen K, Ruzicka T, Goerz G. Congenital erythropoietic porphyria. J Am Acad Dermatol 1997; 36: 594–610.

42. Garden JS, Mitchell DG, Jackson KW. Improved ethanol extraction procedure for determining zinc protoporphyrin in whole blood. Clin Chern 1977; 23: 264–9.

43. Ged C, Moreau-Gaudry F, Richard E, Robert-Richard E, de Verneuil H. Congenital erythropoietic porphyria: mutation update and correlations between genotype and phenotype. Cell Mol Bioi (Noisy-Ie-grand) 2009; 55: 53–60.

44. Ged C, OzallaO, Herrero C, Lecha M, Mendez M, de Verneuil H, et al. Description of a new mutation in hepatoerythropoietic porphyria and prenatal exclusion of a homozygous fetus. Arch DermatoI 2002; 138: 957–60.

45. Gibbs NK, Traynor N, Ferguson J. Biochemical diagnosis of the cutaneous porphyrias: five years experience of plasma spectrofluorimetry. Br J Dermatol 1995; 135 (Suppl45):18.

46. Gibson GE, McGinnity E, McGrath PM, Carmody M, Walshe J, Donohoe J, et al. Cutaneous abnormalities and metabolic disturbance of porphyrins in patients on maintenance dialysis. Clin Exp Dermatol 1997; 22: 124–7.

47. Gill R, Kolstoe SE, Mohammed F, AID-Bass A, Mosely JE, Sarwar M, et al. Structure of human porphobilinogen deaminase at 2.8 A: the molecular basis of acute intermittent porphyria. Biochem J 2009; 420: 17–25.

48. Glynne P, Deacon AC, Goldsmith O, Pusey C, Clutterbuck E. Bullous dermatoses in end-stage renal failure: porphyria or pseudoporphyria? Am J Kidney Dis 1999;34:155-60.

49. Goodwin RG, Kell WJ, Laidler P, Long Cc, Whatley SO, McKinley M, et al. Photosensitivity and acute liver injury in myeloproliferative disorder secondary to late-onset protoporphyria caused by deletion of a ferrochelatase gene in hematopoietic cells. Blood 2006;107: 60–2.

50. Gorchein A. Testing for porphobilinogen in urine. ClinChem 2002; 48:564-6.

51. Gouya L, Martin-Schmitt C, Robreau A-M, Austerlitz F, Da Silva V, Brun P, et al. Contribution of a single-nucleotide polymorphism to the genetic predisposition for erythropoietic protoporphyria. Am J Hum Genet 2006; 78: 2–14.

52. Gouya L, Puy H, Robreau AM, Lamoril J, Da Silva V, Grandchamp B, et al. The penetrance of autosomal dominant erythropoietic protoporphyria is modulated by expression of wild type FECH. Nat Genet 2002; 30: 23–7.

53. Guernsey DL, Jiang H, Campagna DR, et al. Mutations in mitochondrial carrier family gene SLC25A38 cause non-syndromic autosomal recessive congenital sideroblastic anemia. Nat Genet 2009; 41: 651–3.

54. Handschin C, Lin J, Rhee J, Peyer AK, Chin S, Wu FH, et al. Nutritional regulation of hepatic heme biosynthesis and porphyria through PGC-I u. Cell 2005; 122: 505–15.

55. Hart 0, Piomelli S. Simultaneous quantitation of zinc protoporphyrin and free protoporphyrin in erythrocytes by acetone extraction. Clin Chern 1981; 27: 220–2.

56. Hift R, Meissner P. Miscellaneous abnormalities in porphyrin production and disposal. In: Kadish KM, Smith KM, Guilard R, eds. The porphyrin handbook. Volume 14. Medical aspects of porphyrias. Amsterdam: Academic Press, 2003: 15 I–68.

57. Hift RJ, Davidson BP, van der Hooft C, Meissner OM, Meissner PN. Plasma fluorescence scanning and fecal porphyrin analysis for the diagnosis of variegate porphyria: precise determination of sensitivity and specificity with detection of protoporphyrinogen oxidase mutations as a reference standard. Clin Chern 2004; 50: 915–23.

58. Hift RJ, Meissner 0, Meissner PN. A systematic study of the clinical and biochemical expression of variegate porphyria in a large South African family. Br J Dermatol 2004; 151: 465–71.

59. Hift RJ, Meissner PN. An analysis of 112 acute porphyric attacks in Cape Town, South Africa. Medicine 2005; 84: 48–60.

60. Hindmarsh JT, Oliveras L, Greenway DC. Plasma porphyrins in the porphyrias. Clin Chem 1999; 45: 1070–6.

61. Holme SA, Anstey AV, Finlay AY, Elder GH, Badminton MN. Erythropoietic proto porphyria in the United Kingdom: clinical features and effect on quality of life. Br J Dermatol 2006; 155: 574–81.

62. Holme SA, Whatley SO, Roberts AG, Anstey AV, Elder GH, Ead RD, et al. Seasonal palmar keratoderma in erythropoietic protoporphyria indicates autosomal recessive inheritance. J Invest Dermatol 2009; 129: 599–605.

63. Holme SA, Worwood M, Anstey AV, Elder GH, Badminton MN. Erythropoiesis and iron metabolism in dominant erythropoietic protoporphyria. Blood 2007; 110: 4108–10.

64. Kauppinen R, Fraunberg M. Molecular and biochemical studies of acute intermittent porphyria in 196 patients and their families. Clin Chern 2002; 48: 1891–900.

65. Kaya AH, Plewinska M, Wong OM, Desnick RJ, Wetmur JG. Human delta-aminolaevulinate dehydratase (ALAD) gene: structure and alternative splicing of the erythroid and housekeeping mRNAs. Genomics 1994;19: 242–8.

66. Kean RW, Deacon AC, Delves HT, Moreton JA, Frost PG. Indian herbal remedies for diabetes as a cause of lead poisoning. Postgrad Med J 1994; 70: 113–4.

67. Kolluri S, Sadlon TJ, May BK, et al. Haem repression of the housekeeping 5-ä Aminolevulinic acid synthase gene in the hepatoma cell line LMH. Biochem J 2005; 392: 173–80.

68. Kontos A, Ozog 0, Bichakjian C, Lim HW. Congenital erythropoietic porphyria associated with myelodysplasia presenting in a 72-year old man: report of a case and review of the literature. Br J Dermatol 2003; 148: 160–4.

69. Kornfield JM, Ullman Ww. Penicillin interference with the determination of o-δ Aminolevulinic acid. ClinChimActa 1973; 46: 187–90.

70. Koskelo P, Muller-Eberhard U. Interaction of porphyrins with proteins. Semin Hematol 1977; 14: 221–6.

71. Kostrewska E, Gregor A. Increased activity of porphobilinogen deaminase in erythrocytes during attacks of acute intermittent porphyria. Ann Clin Res 1986; 18: 195–8.

72. Labbe RF, Rettmer RL. Zinc protoporphyrin: a product of irondeficient erythropoiesis. SeminHematol 1989; 26: 40–6.

73. Lamon J, With T, Redeker A. The Hoesch test: bedside screening for urinary PBG inpatients with suspected porphyria. Clin Chern 1974; 20: 1438–40.

74. Lamoril J, Puy H, Gouya L, Rosipal R, Da Silva V, Grand champ B, et aI. Neonatal hemolytic anemia due to inherited harderoporphyria: clinical characteristics and molecular basis. Blood 1998; 91: 1453–7.

75. Lee JS, Anvret M. Identification of the most common mutation within the porphobilinogen deaminase gene in Swedish patients with acute intermittent porphyria. Proc Natl Acad Sci USA 1991; 88: 10912–5.

76. Lee OS, Flachsova E, Bodmirova M, Demeier B, Martasek P, Raman CS. Structural basis of hereditary coproporphyria. Proc Natl Acad Sci USA 2005; 102: 14232–7.

77. Lim CK, Peters TJ. Urine and faecal porphyrin profiles by reversedphase high-performance liquid chromatography in the porphyrias. Clin Chim Acta 1984; 139: 55–63.

78. Luo J, Lim CK. Order of uroporphyrinogen-lll decarboxylations on incubation of porphobilinogen and uroporphyrinogen-lll with erythrocyte uroporphyrinogen decarboxylase. Biochem J 1993; 289: 519–23.

79. Maruno M, Furuyama K, Akagi R, Horie Y, Meguro K, Garbaczewski L, et al. Highly heterogeneous nature of delta-aminolevulinate dehydratase (ALAD) deficiencies in ALAD porphyria. Blood 2001; 97: 972–8.

80. Matthews MA, Schubert HL, Whitby FG, Alexander KJ, Schadick K, Bergonia HA, et al. Crystal structure of human uroporphyrinogen III synthase. EMBO J 2001; 21: 5832–9.

81. Mauzerall D, Granick S. The occurrence and determination of delta-δ Aminolevulinic acid and porphobilinogen in urine. J Bioi Chern 1956; 219: 435–46.

82. May BK, Dogra SC, Sadlon TJ, et al. Molecular regulation of heme biosynthesis in higher vertebrates. Prog Nucleic Acid Res Mol Bioi 1995; 51: 1–51.

83. McColl KE, Goldberg A. Abnormal porphyrin metabolism in diseases other than porphyria. Clin Hematol 1980; 9: 427–45.

84. McColl KE, Thompson GC, Moore MR, Goldbert A. Acute alcohol ingestion and haem biosynthesis in healthy subjects. Eur J Clin Invest 1980; 10: 107–12.

85. Meissner P, Adams P, Kirsch R. Allosteric inhibition of human lymphoblast and purified PBG-deaminase by protoporphyrinogen and coproporphyrinogen. J Clin Invest 1991; 91: 1436–44.

86. Merritt JE, Loening KL. Nomenclature of tetrapyrroles. Eur J Biochem 1982; 108: 1–30.

87. Meyer VA, Schuurmans MM, Lindberg RL. Acute porphyrias: pathogenesis of neurological manifestations. Semin Liver Dis 1998; 18: 43–52.

88. Millward LM, Kelly P, Deacon A, Senior V, Peters TJ. Self-rated psychosocial consequences and quality of life in the acute porphyrias. J Inherit Metab Dis 2001; 24: 733–47.

89. Minder EI, Schneider- Yin X, Steurer J, Bachmann LM. A systematic review of treatment options for dermal photosensitivity in erythropoietic protoporphyria. Cell Mol Bioi (Noisy-Ie-grand) 2009; 55: 84–97.

90. Nordmann Y, Puy H, Da Silva V, Simonin S, Robreau AM, Bonaiti C, et al. Acute intermittent porphyria: prevalence of mutations in the porphobilinogen deaminase gene in blood donors in France. J Intern Med 1997; 242: 213–7.

91. O'Reilly K, Snape J, Moore MR. Porphyria cutanea tarda resulting from primary hepatocellular carcinoma. Clin Exp Dermatol 1988; 13: 44–8.

92. Parker M, Corrigall AV, Hift RJ, Meissner PN. Molecular characterisation of erythropoietic protoporphyria in South Africa. Br J Dermatol 2008; 159: 182–91.

93. Phillips JD, Bergonia HA, Reilly CA, Franklin MR, Kushner JP. A porphomethene inhibitor of uroporphyrinogen decarboxylase causes porphyria cutanea tarda. Proc Natl AcadSci V S A 2007; 104: 5079–84.

94. Phillips JD, SteensmaDr, Pulsipher MA, Spangrude GJ, Kushner JP. Congenital erythropoietic porphyria due to a mutation in GATA1: the first trans-acting mutation causative for a human porphyria. Blood 2007; 109: 2618–21.

95. Phillips JD, Warby CA, Whitby FG, Kushner JP, Hill CP. Substrate shuttling between active sites of uroporphyrinogen decarboxylase is not required to generate coproporphyrinogen. J Mol Bioi 2009; 389: 306–14.

96. Piomelli S. Free erythrocyte porphyrin in the detection of undue absorption of lead and of iron deficiency. ClinChem 1977; 23: 264–9.

97. Pischik E, Kauppinen R. Neurological manifestations of acute intermittent porphyria. Ce1J Mol Bioi (Noisy-Ie-grand) 2009; 55: 72–83.

98. Pischik E, Kazakov V, Kauppinen R. Is screening for urinary porphobilinogen useful among patients with acute polyneuropathy or encephalopathy? J Neurol 2008; 255: 974–9.

99. Poh-Fitzpatrick MB. A plasma fluorescence marker for variegate porphyria. Arch Dermatol 1980; 116: 543–7.

100. Poh-Fitzpatrick ME. Clinical features of the porphyrias. ClinDermatol 1998; 16: 25 I–64.

101. Ponka P. Tissue-specific regulation of iron metabolism and heme synthesis: distinct control mechanisms in erythroid cells. Blood 1997;89: 1–25.

102. Puy H, Gouya L, Deybach J-C Porphyrias. Lancet 2010; 375: 924–37.

103. Rank JM, Pascual-Leone A, Payne W, Glock M, Freese D, Sharp H, et al. Hematin therapy for the neurologic crisis of tyrosinemia. J Pediatr 1991; 118: 136–9.

104. Robert-Richard E, Moreau-Gaudry F, Lalanne M, et al. Effective gene therapy of mice with congenital erythropoietic porphyria is facilitated by a survival advantage of corrected erythroid cells. Am J Hum Genet 2008; 82: 113–24.

105. Roels H, Lauwerys R, Buchet JP, Berlin A, Smeets J. Comparison of four methods for determination of ä Aminolevulinic acid in urine, and evaluation of critical factors. Clin Chern 1974; 20: 753–60.

106. Rose IS, Young GP, St John DJ, et al. Effect of ingestion of hemoproteins on fecal excretion of hemes and porphyrins. Clin Chern 1989; 35: 2290–6.

107. Rossi E, Attwood PV, Garcia-Webb P. Inhibition of human lymphocyte coproporphyrinogen oxidase activity by metals, bilirubin and haemin. Biochim Biophys Acta 1992; 1135: 262–8.

108. Rossi E. Increased fecal porphyrins in acute intermittent porphyria. Clin Chern 1999; 45: 281–3.

109. Sardh E, Harper P, Andersson DE, Floderus Y. Plasma porphobilinogen as a sensitive biomarker to monitor the clinical and therapeutic course of acute intermittent porphyria attacks. Eur J Intern Med 2009; 20: 201–7.

110. Sarkany RE. The management of porphyria cutanea tarda. ClinExp DermatoI 2001; 26: 225–32.

111. Schoenfeld N, Mamet R, Leibovici L, Lanir A. Alcohol-induced changes in urinary δ Aminolevulinic acid and porphyrins: unrelated to liver disease. Alcohol 1996; 13: 59–63.

112. Schreiber WE, Jamani A, Pudek MR. Screening tests for porphobilinogen are insensitive. Am J Clin Pat hci 1989; 92: 644–9.

113. Schultz I), Chen C, Paw BH, Hamza I. Iron and porphyrin trafficking in heme biogenesis. J Bioi Chern 2010; 285: 267 53–9.

114. Seth AK, Badminton MN, Mirza D, Russell S, Elias E. Liver transplantation for porphyria: who, when, and how? Liver Transpl 2007; 13: 1219–27.

115. Seubert S, Seubert A, Rumpf KW, Kiffe H. A porphyria cutanea tarda-like distribution pattern of porphyrins in plasma, hemodialysate, hemofiltrate, and urine of patients on chronic hemodialysis. J Invest Dermatol 1985; 85: 107–9.

116. Verneuil H, de Ged C, Moreau-Gaudry F. Congenital erythropoietic porphyria. In: Kadish KM, Smith KM, Guilard R, eds. The porphyrin handbook. Volume 14. Medical aspects of porphyrias. Amsterdam: Academic Press, 2003: 43–66.

117. Verstraeten L, Ledoux MC, Moos B, Callebaut B, Cornu G, Hassoun A. Interference of Tienam in the colorimetric determination of 5-δ Aminolevulinic acid and porphobilinogen in serum and urine. ClinChem 1992; 38: 2557–8.

118. Warren Mj, Scott AI. Tetrapyrrole assembly and modification into the ligands of biologically functional cofactors. Trends Biochem Sci 1990; 15: 486–91.

119. Watson Cj, Schwartz S. A simple test for urinary porphobilinogen. Proc Soc Exp Bioi 1941; 47: 393–4.

120. Wetmur IG, Kaya AH, Plewinska M, Desnick RI. Molecular characterization of the human aminolaevulinate dehydratase 2 (ALAD2) allele: implications for molecular screening of individuals for genetic susceptibility to lead poisoning. Am I Hum Genet 1991 ;49: 757–63.

121. Whatley SO, Ducamp S, Gouya L, Grandchamp B, Beaumont C, Badminton MN, et al. C-terminal deletions in the ALAS2 gene lead to gain of function and cause X-linked dominant protoporphyria without anemia or iron overload. Am J Hum Genet 2008; 83: 408–14.

122. Whatley SO, Mason NG, Holme SA, Anstey AV, Elder GH, Badminton MN. Gene dosage analysis identifies large deletions of the FECH gene in 10% of families with erythropoietic protoporphyria. I Invest Dermatol 2007; 127: 2790–4.

123. Whatley SO, Mason NG, Holme SA, Anstey AV, Elder GH, Badminton MN. Molecular epidemiology of erythropoietic protoporphyria in the United Kingdom. Br I DermatoI 2010; 162: 642–6.

124. Whatley SO, Mason NG, Woolf JR, Newcombe RG, Elder GH, Badminton MN. Diagnostic strategies for autosomal dominant acute porphyrias: retrospective analysis of 467 unrelated patients referred for mutational analysis of the HMBS, CPOX, or PPOX gene. Clin Chem 2009; 55: 1406–14.

125. Whitby FG, Phillips JD, Kushner JP, Hill CPo Crystal structure of human uroporphyrinogen decarboxylase. EMBO J 1998; 17: 2463–71.

126. Wiederholt T, Poblete-Gutierrez P, Gardlo K, Goerz G, Boisen K, Merk HF, et al. Identification of mutations in the uroporphyrinogen III cosynthase gene in German patients with congenital erythropoietic porphyria. Physiol Res 2006;55(Suppl 2):S85-92.

127. Woods JS, Miller HD. Quantitative measurement of porphyrins in biological tissues and evaluation of tissue porphyrins during toxicant exposures. Fundam Appl Toxicol 1993; 21: 291–7.

128. Wright OJ, Lim CK. Simultaneous determination of hydroxymethylbilane synthase and uroporphyrinogen-Ill synthase in erythrocytes by HPLC Biochem J 1983; 213: 85–8.

129. Wu CK, Dailey HA, Rose JP, Burden A, Sellers VM, Wang BC The 2.0 A structure of human ferrochelatase, the terminal enzyme of heme biosynthesis. Nat StructBioi 2000: 8: 156–60.

22

Inherited Disorders of Metabolism and Newborn Screening

INTRODUCTION

Most inherited disorders of metabolism (also called inborn errors of metabolism) are caused by mutations in genes that code for enzymes; enzyme deficiency or inactivity leads to accumulation of substrate precursors or metabolites or to deficiencies of the enzyme's products. Hundreds of disorders exist, and although most inherited disorders of metabolism are extremely rare individually, collectively they are not rare. The disorders are typically grouped by the affected substrate (e.g. carbohydrates, amino acids, and fatty acids).

Most states routinely do neonatal screening of all newborns for specific inherited disorders of metabolism and other conditions, including phenylketonuria, tyrosinemia, biokinetics deficiency, homo cystinuria, maple syrup urine disease, and galactosemia. Many states have an expanded screening program that covers many more inherited disorders of metabolism, including disorders of fatty acid oxidation and other organic acidemias.

CLINICAL PRESENTATION

Most inherited disorders of metabolism are rare, and therefore their diagnosis requires a high index of suspicion. Timely diagnosis leads to early treatment and may help avoid acute and chronic complications, developmental compromise, and even death.

Evaluation

Symptoms and signs tend to be nonspecific and are more often caused by something other than an inherited disorder of metabolism (e.g. infection); these more likely causes should also be investigated.

HISTORY AND PHYSICAL EXAMINATION

Disorders manifesting in the neonatal period tend to be more serious; manifestations of many of the disorders typically include lethargy, poor feeding, vomiting, and seizures. Disorders that manifest later tend to affect growth and development, but vomiting, seizures, and weakness may also appear.

Growth delay suggests decreased anabolism or increased catabolism and may be due to decreased availability of energy-generating substrates [e.g. in glycogen storage disease (GSD)] or inefficient energy or protein use (e.g. in organic acidemias or urea cycle defects).

Developmental delay may reflect chronic energy deficit in the brain (e.g. oxidative phosphorylation defects), decreased supply of needed carbohydrates that are non-energy substrates for the brain [e.g., lack of uridine-5'-diphosphate-galactose (UDP-galactose) in untreated galactosemia], or chronic amino acid deficit in the brain (e.g. tyrosine deficiency in phenyl-ketonuria).

Neuromuscular symptoms, such as seizures, muscle weakness, hypotonia, myoclonus, muscle pain, strokes, or coma, may suggest acute energy deficit in the brain (e.g. hypoglycemic seizures in GSD type I, strokes in mitochondrial oxidative phosphorylation defects) or muscle (e.g. muscle weakness in muscle forms of GSD). Neuromuscular symptoms may also reflect accumulation of toxic compounds in the brain (e.g. hyperammonemic coma in urea cycle defects) or tissue breakdown (e.g. rhabdomyolysis and myoglobinuria in patients with long-chain hydroxyacyl dehydrogenase deficiency or muscle forms of GSD).

Congenital brain malformation may reflect decreased availability of energy (e.g. decreased ATP output in pyruvate dehydrogenase deficiency) or critical precursors (e.g. decreased cholesterol in 7-dehydrocholestrol reductase deficiency or Smith-Lemli-Opitz syndrome) during fetal development.

Autonomic symptoms can result from hypoglycemia caused by increased glucose consumption or decreased glucose production (e.g. vomiting, diaphoresis, pallor, and tachycardia in GSD or hereditary fructose intolerance) or from metabolic acidosis (e.g. vomiting and Kussmaul respirations in organic acidemias). Some conditions cause both (i.e. in propionic acidemia, accumulation of acyl-CoAs causes metabolic acidosis and inhibits gluconeogenesis, thus causing hypoglycemia).

Nonphysiologic jaundice after the neonatal period usually reflects intrinsic hepatic disease, especially when accompanied by elevation of liver enzymes, but may be due to inherited disorders of metabolism (e.g. untreated galactosemia, hereditary fructose intolerance, tyrosinemia type I).

Unusual odors in body fluids reflect accumulation of specific compounds (e.g. sweaty feet odor in isovaleric acidemia, smoky-sweet odor in maple syrup urine disease, mousy or musty odor in phenylketonuria, boiled cabbage odor in tyrosinemia).

Change in urine color on exposure to air occurs in some disorders (e.g. darkish brown in alkaptonuria, purplish brown in porphyria). Organomegaly may reflect a failure in substrate degradation resulting in substrate accumulation within the organ cells (e.g. hepatomegaly in hepatic forms of GSD and many lysosomal storage diseases, cardiomegaly in GSD type II). Eye changes include cataracts in galactokinase deficiency or classic galactosemia, and ophthalmoplegia and retinal degeneration in oxidative phosphorylation defects.

Testing

When an inherited disorder of metabolism is suspected, evaluation begins with a review of neonatal screening test results and ordering of basic metabolic screening tests, which typically include the following: glucose, electrolytes, complete blood count (CBC) and peripheral smear, liver function tests, ammonia levels, serum amino acid levels, urinalysis, and urine organic acids.

Glucose measurement detects hypoglycemia or hyperglycemia; measurement may have to be timed relative to meals (e.g. fasting hypoglycemia in GSD).

Electrolyte measurement detects metabolic acidosis and presence or absence of an anion gap; metabolic acidosis may need to be corroborated by ABG measurement. Non-anion gap acidosis occurs in inherited disorders of metabolism that cause renal tubular damage (e.g. galactosemia, tyrosinemia type I). Anion gap acidosis occurs in inherited disorders of metabolism in which accumulation of titratable acids is typical, such as methylmalonic and propionic acidemias; it can also be caused by lactic acidosis (e.g. in pyruvate decarboxylase deficiency or mitochondrial oxidative phosphorylation defects). When the anion gap is elevated, lactate and pyruvate levels should be obtained. An increase in the lactate-pyruvate ratio distinguishes oxidative phosphorylation defects from disorders of pyruvate metabolism, in which the lactate-pyruvate ratio remains normal.

CBC and peripheral smear detect hemolysis caused by RBC energy deficits or WBC defects (e.g. in some pentose phosphate pathway disorders and GSD type Ib) and cytopenia caused by metabolite accumulation (e.g. neutropenia in propionic acidemia due to propionyl CoA accumulation).

Liver function tests detect hepatocellular damage, dysfunction, or both (e.g. in untreated galactosemia, hereditary fructose intolerance, or tyrosinemia type I). Ammonia levels are elevated in urea cycle defects, organic acidemias, and fatty acid oxidation defects. Urinalysis detects ketonuria (present in some GSDs and many organic acidemias); absence of ketones in the presence of acidosis suggests a fatty acid oxidation defect.

More specific tests may be indicated when >1 of the previously described simple screening tests support an inherited disorder of metabolism. Carbohydrate metabolites, mucopolysaccharides, and amino and organic acids can be measured directly by chromatography and mass spectrometry. Quantitative plasma amino acid tests should include a plasma acylcarnitine profile. Urine organic acid tests should include a urine acylglycine profile.

Confirmatory tests may also include biopsy (e.g. liver biopsy to distinguish hepatic forms of GSDs from other disorders associated with hepatomegaly, muscle biopsy to detect ragged red fibers in mitochondrial myopathy); enzyme studies (e.g. using blood and skin cells to diagnose lysosomal storage diseases); and DNA studies, which identify gene mutations that cause disease. DNA testing can be done on almost all cells (except RBCs and platelets), thus avoiding the need for tissue biopsies; however, sensitivity for any given disease is often suboptimal because not all mutations that cause disease have been characterized.

Challenge testing is used judiciously to detect symptoms, signs, or measurable biochemical abnormalities not detectable in the normal state. The need for challenge testing has diminished with the availability of highly sensitive metabolite detection methods, but it is still occasionally used. Examples include fasting tests (e.g. to provoke hypoglycemia in hepatic forms of GSD); provocative tests [e.g. fructose challenge to trigger symptoms in hereditary fructose intolerance, glucagon challenge in hepatic forms of GSD (failure to observe hyperglycemia suggests disease)]; and physiologic challenge (e.g. exercise stress testing to elicit lactic acid production and other deformities in muscle forms of GSD). Challenge tests are often associated with an element of risk, so they must be done under well-controlled conditions with a clear plan for reversing symptoms and signs.

Prenatal Diagnosis

Despite constant progress in medical treatment, several inherited disorders of metabolism result in severe morbidity and inevitable mortality early in life. Most of the disorders are inherited as autosomal recessive traits; therefore the recurrence risk in subsequent pregnancies of the same couple is 25%. Genetic counseling of parents consists of a balanced assessment of (1) familial risk factors (parental consanguinity and ethnic origin), (2) risk of pregnancy loss as a consequence of the sampling procedure [0.5–1% by chorionic villus sampling (CVS), 0.5% by amniocentesis], (3) risk of maternal complications, (4) clinical validity of the prenatal test, (5) the burden of the disease, and (6) variable phenotypic expression of the disease even within the same family.

Methods used for prenatal diagnosis of inherited disorders of metabolism have different requirements in terms of timing, sample collection, and options for independent confirmation. CVS is performed at 10–13 weeks gestational age, has a higher risk of fetal loss as compared with classic amniocentesis, and might not provide accurate results because of possible contamination with maternal tissue. Alternatively, certain enzymes, such as those of the glycine cleavage pathway defective in glycine encephalopathy, are expressed only in cells of chorionic villi, rendering this procedure the only possibility when DNA testing is not possible. Amniocentesis is performed later in pregnancy (14–20 weeks) and provides both amniocytes and amniotic fluid to be used for independent and complementary diagnostic methods. Reliance on separate tests based on independent methods performed by laboratories with adequate prior experience is strongly encouraged to avoid incorrect or inconclusive results. In some inherited disorders of metabolism (e.g. organic acidemias), amniotic fluid is tested for the presence or absence of specific metabolites, in addition to providing amniocytes for enzyme assay, DNA analysis, or both. The combination of at least two independent tests (e.g. enzyme assay +DNA; metabolite analysis + enzyme or

DNA) enhances confidence in establishing a prenatal diagnosis. Before entertaining a prenatal diagnosis, one should ensure that the proband (individual first brought to medical attention in whom the diagnosis was established) related to the index case has a diagnosis confirmed by traditional methods, including enzymology when appropriate. If DNA analysis is considered, mutations of the index case should be known and confirmed as causative of the disease. Major advantages of direct metabolite analysis in amniotic fluid include independence from tissue expression and rapid turnaround time. However, analysis of direct metabolites in amniotic fluid has been reported for only a very limited number of diseases.

Newborn Screening

Newborn screening is a public health activity aimed at early identification of conditions for which timely intervention is expected to result in elimination or reduction of morbidity, mortality, and disabilities. It is an important and effective component of preventive medicine. Originally instituted in the 1960s for the early detection of phenylketonuria (PKU), the number of diseases screened for in the newborn period has dramatically increased with the introduction of mass spectrometry (MS/MS) multiplex analyses of acylcarnitine and amino acid profiles.

Inclusion of inherited disorders of metabolism as a whole in newborn screening panels has been controversial, because with few exceptions, their incidence, natural history, and prospective screening experience, as well as the effectiveness of treatment, have not yet been defined. However, implementation of this expanded screening allows collection of these data leading to a better understanding of these diseases. The complexity of the interpretation of MS/MS newborn screening results has prompted the development of algorithms for proper confirmatory testing and differential diagnosis of all detectable inherited disorders of metabolism.

Although, metabolic disorders identified by MS/MS represent the largest group of diseases identifiable by newborn screening, other inherited disorders of metabolism and endocrine and hematologic disorders (such as galactosemia, biokinetics deficiency, cystic fibrosis, congenital hypothyroidism, congenital adrenal hyperplasia, and hemoglobinopathies) are identifiable through more traditional screening methods (e.g. enzyme assays, immunoassays, and electrophoresis). Advances in therapeutic interventions for inherited disorders of metabolism are continuously expanding the role of newborn screening. Newborn screening does not identify all metabolic disorders, and some patients can be missed by newborn screening. Therefore, a symptomatic patient, at any age, should be investigated despite normal newborn screening results.

Postmortem Screening

Among inherited disorders of metabolism, fatty acid oxidation (FAO) disorders are those recognized more often after the diagnosis of an affected sibling or as a cause of sudden death. Early reports attributed up to 5% of cases of sudden death in children younger than 5 years to FAO/ and mounting evidence indicates that some of these disorders can cause mortality in adults as well. The postmortem evaluation of unexpected death, independent of age, especially when evidence of acute illness or infection is found, should consider FAO as a cause. This is accomplished by analysis of acylcarnitines in blood and bile spots (Fig. 22.1).

Blood and bile are collected on filter paper identical to the cards used for newborn screening; once properly dried they are shipped to the laboratory at room temperature. In cases with a higher index of suspicion, an effort should be made to collect and freeze a specimen of liver and to collect a skin biopsy for establishing the fibroblast culture to be used, if needed, to confirm a diagnosis. Although, fatty infiltration of the liver and/or other organs (e.g. heart, muscle, and kidneys) is a common observation in FAO disorders, the finding of macroscopic steatosis should not be used as the only criterion in deciding whether to investigate a possible underlying FAO disorder during postmortem evaluation of a case of sudden death. Sudden death from cardiac arrhythmia can be the only finding in fatty acid oxidation defects, and the absence of obvious physical findings on autopsy does not exclude this, especially in adults. In cases of sudden infant death, if parental permission to

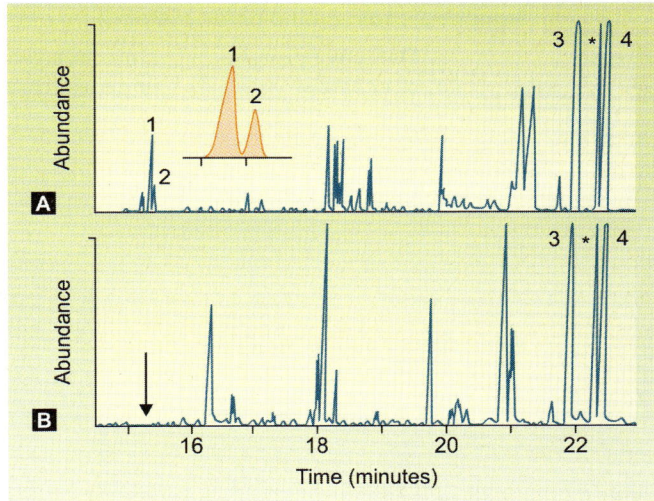

Fig. 22.1: Partial urine organic acid profiles. (A) Profile of acutely ill patient. Peaks I and 2 are derivatives of succinylacetone. (B) Reference profile of 15 month old patient. Note* marks the peak of internal standard

perform an autopsy is not granted, any leftover specimens or unused portions of blood spots collected for newborn screening, if still available, could be useful samples in obtaining a diagnosis.

AMINO ACID AND ORGANIC ACID METABOLISM DISORDERS

Branched-chain Amino Acid Disorders

Valine, leucine, and isoleucine are branched-chain amino acids; deficiency of enzymes involved in their metabolism leads to accumulation of organic acids with severe metabolic acidosis. There are numerous disorders of branched-chain amino acid metabolism (Table 22.1) as well as many other amino acid and organic acid metabolism disorders.

Table 22.1	Branched-chain amino acid* metabolism disorders		
Disease	**Defective proteins or enzymes**	**Defective gene or genes (chromosomal location)**	**Comments**
Maple syrup urine disease, or branched-chain ketoaciduria	Branched-chain α-keto acid dehydrogenase complex (BCKD)		Biochemical profile: Elevated plasma valine, leucine, isoleucine, and alloisoleucine
Type IA	BCKD E1α component	BCKDHA (19q13)[†]	Clinical features (molecular forms do not correlate with clinical forms except that a high percentage of type II mutations are associated with thiamin responsiveness):
Type IB	BCKD E1β component	BCKDHB (6p22–p21)[†]	
Type II	BCKD E2 component	DBT (1p31)[†]	
Type III	BCKD E3 component	DLD (7q31–q32)[†]	In classic form, hypertonia, seizures, coma, death
			In intermediate form, intellectual disability, neurologic symptoms, full-blown picture developing with stress
			In intermittent form, symptoms only with stress (e.g. fever, infection)

Contd.

Table 22.1	Branched-chain amino acid* metabolism disorders *(Contd.)*		
Disease	**Defective proteins or enzymes**	**Defective gene or genes (chromosomal location)**	**Comments**
			In thiamin-responsive form, features similar to mild intermediate form
			In E3 subunit deficient form, features similar to intermediate form but accompanied by severe lactic acidosis because E3 is needed for pyruvate dehydrogenase and α-ketoglutarate dehydrogenase
			Acute treatment: Peritoneal dialysis, hemodialysis, or both; aggressive nutrition management, including protein restriction, high-dose glucose, insulin, and special hyperalimentation; close monitoring for cerebral edema and acute pancreatitis
			Chronic treatment: Dietary branched-chain amino acid restriction, thiamin supplementation as needed
			Emergency plan for acute illness, which may provoke a metabolic crisis
			Liver transplantation
Propionic acidemia	Propionyl-CoA carboxylase		Biochemical profile: Elevated plasma glycine, urine methyl citrate, 3-hydroxypropionate, propionylglycine, and tiglylglycine
Type I	α-subunit	PCCA (13q32)[†]	
Type II	β-subunit	PCCB (3q21-q22)[†]	Clinical features: Hypotonia, vomiting, lethargy, coma, ketoacidosis, hypoglycemia, hyperammonemia, bone marrow suppression, growth delay, intellectual disability, physical disability
			Treatment: During acute episodes, high-dose glucose and aggressive fluid resuscitation, protein restriction
			For extreme hyperammonemia, may need hemodialysis or peritoneal dialysis.
			For long-term management, controlled intake of threonine, valine, isoleucine, and methionine; carnitine supplementation; biotin for responsive patients (see also multiple carboxylase deficiency and biotinidase deficiency, below)
			Intermittent courses of antibiotics considered for reduction of propionic acid load from intestinal bacteria
			Emergency plan for acute illness, which may provoke a metabolic crisis
Multiple carboxylase deficiency	Holocarboxylase synthetase	HLCS (21q22.1)[†]	Biochemical profile: Same as for propionic acidemia, but also elevated lactate and 3-methylcrotonate
			Clinical features: Skin rash, alopecia, seizures, hypotonia, developmental delay, ketoacidosis, defective T- and B-cell immunity, hearing loss
			Treatment: Biotin, carnitine
Biotinidase deficiency	Biotinidase	BTD (3p25)[†]	Similar to multiple carboxylase deficiency
Methylmalonic acidemia	Methylmalonyl-CoA mutase Mut0 (no enzyme activity)	MUT (6p21)[†]	Biochemical profile: Elevated plasma glycine; increased urine methylmalonate, 3-hydroxypropionate, methylcitrate, and tiglylglycine

Contd.

Table 22.1 Branched-chain amino acid* metabolism disorders *(Contd.)*

Disease	Defective proteins or enzymes	Defective gene or genes (chromosomal location)	Comments
	Mut- (some residual enzyme activity)		Clinical features: Hypotonia, vomiting, lethargy, coma, ketoacidosis, hypoglycemia, hyperammonemia, bone marrow suppression, growth delay, intellectual disability, and physical disability
			Treatment: During acute episodes, high-dose glucose, aggressive fluid resuscitation, and protein restriction
			Close monitoring for stroke, renal failure, and acute pancreatitis
			For extreme hyperammonemia, may need hemodialysis or peritoneal dialysis
			For long-term management, controlled intake of threonine, valine, isoleucine, and methionine; carnitine supplementation; vitamin B12 for patients with mut- type
			Intermittent courses of antibiotics considered for reduction of propionic acid load from intestinal bacteria
			Emergency plan for acute illness, which may provoke a metabolic crisis
Methylmalonic acidemia	Mitochondrial cobalamin translocase	MMAA (4q31.1–q31.2)[†]	Biochemical profile: Similar to methylmalonic acidemia due to mutase deficiency
			Clinical features: Similar to methylmalonic acidemia due to mutase deficiency
			Treatment: Responsive to high-dose hydroxycobalamin
Methylmalonic acidemia	ATP:cob(1)alamin adenosyl transferase	MMMB (12q24)[†]	Biochemical profile: Similar to methylmalonic acidemia due to mutase deficiency
			Clinical features: Similar to methylmalonic acidemia due to mutase deficiency
			Treatment: Responsive to high-dose hydroxycobalamin
Methylmalonic acidemia-homocystinuria-megaloblastic anemia	Methylmalonyl-CoA mutase and methylene tetrahydrofolate: homocysteine methyltransferase	Genetically heterogeneous	Biochemical profile: Similar to methylmalonic acidemia cblA and cblB, but also homocystinemia, homocystinuria, low methionine, and high cystathionine; normal serum cobalamin
			Clinical features: Similar to cblA and cblB, but also megaloblastic anemia
			Treatment: Protein restriction, high-dose hydroxycobalamin
Methylmalonic acidemia-homocystinuria-megaloblastic anemia	Not determined	Genetically heterogeneous	Similar to methylmalonic acidemia cblC
Methylmalonic acidemia-homocystinuria-megaloblastic anemia	Defective lysosomal release of cobalamin	Genetically heterogeneous	Similar to methylmalonic acidemia cblC
Methylmalonic acidemia-homocystinuria-megaloblastic anemia	Intrinsic factor	GIF (11q13)[†]	Similar to methylmalonic acidemia cblC
Methylmalonic acidemia-homocystinuria-megaloblastic anemia	Cubilin (intrinsic factor receptor)	CUBN (10p12.1)[†]	Similar to methylmalonic acidemia cblC

Contd.

Table 22.1	Branched-chain amino acid* metabolism disorders (Contd.)		
Disease	**Defective proteins or enzymes**	**Defective gene or genes (chromosomal location)**	**Comments**
Methylmalonic acidemia-homocystinuria-megaloblastic anemia	Transcobalamin II	TC2 (22q11.2)[†]	Similar to methylmalonic acidemia cblC
Methylmalonic semialdehyde dehydrogenase deficiency with mild methylmalonic acidemia	Methylmalonic semialdehyde dehydrogenase (see also disorders of β- and γ-amino acids, below)	ALDH6A1 (14q24.1)	Biochemical profile: Moderate urine methylmalonate Clinical features: Developmental delay, seizures Treatment: No effective treatment
Methylmalonic acidemia-homocystinuria	Not determined	Genetically heterogeneous	Similar to methylmalonic acidemia cblA
Isovaleric acidemia	Isovaleryl-CoA dehydrogenase	IVD(15q14–q15)[†]	Biochemical profile:Isovaleryl glycine, 3-hydroxyisovalerate Clinical features: Characteristic sweaty feet odor, vomiting, lethargy, acidosis, intellectual disability, bone marrow suppression, hypoglycemia; ketoacidosis, hyperammonemia, neonatal death Treatment: Controlled leucine intake, glycine, carnitine
3-Methylcrotonyl-CoA carboxylase deficiency	3-Methylcrotonyl CoA carboxylase		Biochemical profile: Elevated 3-hydroxyisovalerate, 3-methylcrontylglycine, and 3-hydroxyisovalerylcarnitine
Type I	α-subunit	MCCC1 (3q25–q27)[†]	
Type II	β-subunit	MCCC2 (5q12–q13)[†]	Clinical features: Episodic vomiting, acidosis, hypoglycemia, hypotonia, intellectual disability, coma; sometimes asymptomatic intellectual disability Treatment: Controlled leucine intake (see also multiple carboxylase deficiency and biotinidase deficiency, above)
3-Methylglutaconic aciduria type I	3-methylglutaconyl-CoA hydratase	AUH (9)[†]	Biochemical profile: Elevated urine 3- methylglutaconate and 3-hydroxyisolvalerate Clinical features: Acidosis, hypotonia, hepatomegaly, speech delay Treatment: Carnitine; benefit of leucine restriction unclear
3-Methylglutaconic aciduria type II	Tafazzin	TAZ (Xq28)[†]	Biochemical profile: Elevated urine 3-methylglutaconate and 3-methylglutarate Clinical features: Myopathy, dilated cardiomyopathy, mitochondrial abnormality, neutropenia, developmental delay Treatment: Pantothenic acid
3-Methylglutaconic aciduria type III	Not determined	OPA3 (19q13)[†]	Biochemical profile: Elevated urine 3-methyl glutaconate and 3-methylglutarate Clinical features: Optic atrophy, ataxia, spasticity, choreiform movement Treatment: No effective treatment
3-Methylglutaconic aciduria type IV	Not determined	Not determined	Biochemical profile: Elevated urine 3-methylglutaconate and 3-methylglutarate Clinical features: Variable expression, growth and developmental delay, hypotonia, seizures, optic atrophy, deafness, cardiomyopathy, acidosis Treatment: No effective treatment

Contd.

Table 22.1	Branched-chain amino acid* metabolism disorders *(Contd.)*		
Disease	**Defective proteins or enzymes**	**Defective gene or genes (chromosomal location)**	**Comments**
3-hydroxy-3-methyl-glutaryl-CoA lyase deficiency	3-hydroxy-3-methylglutaryl-CoA lyase	HMGCL (1pter-p33)[†]	Biochemical profile: Elevated urine 3-hydroxy-3-methylglutarate, 3-methylglutaconate, and 3-hydroxyisovalerate; elevated plasma 3-methylglutarylcarnitine Clinical features: Reye-like syndrome, vomiting, hypotonia, acidosis, hypoglycemia, lethargy, hyperammonemia without ketosis Treatment: Restricted leucine intake, control of hypoglycemia
Mevalonic aciduria	Mevalonate kinase	MVK (12q24)[†]	Biochemical profile: Elevated creatine kinase, transaminase, leukotriene, and urinary mevalonic acid; decreased cholesterol Clinical features: In classic form, short stature, hypotonia, developmental delay, dysmorphic features, cataracts, vomiting, diarrhea, hepato-splenomegaly, arthralgia, lymphadenopathy, cerebral and cerebellar atrophy, anemia, thrombocytopenia, early death In hyper IgD form, recurrent febrile episodes, vomiting, diarrhea, arthralgia, abdominal pain, rash, splenomegaly, elevated serum IgD and IgA levels Treatment: No effective treatment; cortico-steroids during acute attacks possibly helpful
Mitochondrial acetoacetyl-CoA thiolase deficiency	Acetyl-CoA thiolase	ACAT1 (11q22.3–a23.1)[†]	Biochemical profile: Elevated urine 2-methyl-3-hydroxybutyrate and 2-methylacetoacetate, elevated plasma tiglylglycine Clinical features: Episodes of ketoacidosis, vomiting, diarrhea, coma, intellectual disability Treatment: Low-protein diet, controlled isoleucine intake
Isobutyryl-CoA dehydrogenase deficiency	Isobutyryl-CoA dehydrogenase	Not determined	Biochemical profile: Elevated C-4 carnitine, low free carnitine Clinical features: Anemia, cardiomyopathy Treatment: Carnitine
3-hydroxyisobutyryl-CoA deacylase deficiency	3-Hydroxyisobutyryl-CoA deacylase	Not determined	Biochemical profile: Elevated S-(2-carboxypropyl)-cysteine and S-(2-carboxypropyl)-cysteamine Clinical features: Growth and developmental delay, dysmorphic feature, vertebral anomaly, CNS malformations, death Treatment: No effective treatment
3-hydroxyisobutyric aciduria	3-hydroxyisobutyrate dehydrogenase	HIBADH (chromosomal location not determined)	Biochemical profile: Elevated urine 3-hydro-xyisobutyrate; in 50% patients, elevated lactate Clinical features: Dysmorphic features, CNS malformations, hypotonia, ketoacidosis Treatment: Low-protein diet, carnitine
2-methylbutyryl glycinuria	Short branched-chain acyl-CoA dehydrogenase	ACADSB (10q25–q26)[†]	Biochemical profile: Elevated urine 2-methylbutyrulglycine Clinical features: Hypotonia, muscular atrophy, lethargy, hypoglycemia, hypothermia Treatment: No effective treatment

Contd.

Table 22.1	Branched-chain amino acid* metabolism disorders (Contd.)		
Disease	**Defective proteins or enzymes**	**Defective gene or genes (chromosomal location)**	**Comments**
Ethylmalonic encephalopathy	Mitochondrial protein of undetermined function	ETHE1 (19q13.32)[†]	Biochemical profile: Elevated urine ethylmalonic and methylsuccinic acids, elevated serum lactate Clinical features: Retinopathy, acrocyanosis, diarrhea, petechiae, developmental delay, intellectual disability, extrapyramidal symptoms, ataxia, seizures, hyperintense lesions in the basal ganglia Treatment: No effective treatment
Malonic aciduria	Malonyl-CoA decarboxylase	MLYCD (16q24)[†]	Biochemical profile: Elevated lactate, malonate, methylmalonate, and malonylcarnitine Clinical features: Hypotonia, developmental delay, hypoglycemia, acidosis Treatment: No effective treatment; low-fat, high-carbohydrate diet Carnitine possibly helpful in some patients
Hypervalinemia or hyperisoleucine-hyperleucinemia	Mitochondrial branched-chain aminotransferase 2	BCAT2 (19q13)	Biochemical profile: Elevated urine and serum valine Clinical features: Growth retardation Treatment: Controlled valine intake

*The branched-chain amino acids are valine, leucine, and isoleucine.
[†]Gene has been identified, and molecular basis has been elucidated.

MAPLE SYRUP URINE DISEASE

This is a group of autosomal recessive disorders caused by deficiency of one or more subunits of a dehydrogenase active in the second step of branched-chain amino acid catabolism. Although quite rare, incidence is significant (perhaps 1/200 births) in Amish and Mennonite populations.

Clinical manifestations include body fluid odor that smells like maple syrup (particularly strong in cerumen) and overwhelming illness in the first days of life, beginning with vomiting and lethargy, and progressing to seizures, coma, and death if untreated. Patients with milder forms of the disease may manifest symptoms only during stress (e.g. infection, surgery).

Biochemical findings are profound ketonemia and acidemia. Diagnosis of maple syrup urine disease is by finding elevated plasma levels of branched-chain amino acids (particularly leucine).

Acutely, treatment of maple syrup urine disease with peritoneal dialysis or hemodialysis may be required, along with IV hydration and nutrition (including protein restriction and high-dose dextrose). Patients should be closely monitored for cerebral edema and acute pancreatitis. Long-term management is restriction of dietary branched-chain amino acids; however, small amounts are required for normal metabolic function. Thiamin is a cofactor for the decarboxylation, and some patients respond favorably to high-dose thiamin (up to 200 mg by mouth once a day). An emergency plan for how to manage acute illness, which may provoke a metabolic crisis, should be in place. Liver transplantation is curative.

Isovaleric Acidemia

The third step of leucine metabolism is the conversion of isovaleryl CoA to 3-methylcrotonyl CoA, a dehydrogenation step. Deficiency of this dehydrogenase results in isovaleric acidemia, also known as 'sweaty feet' syndrome, because accumulated isovaleric acid emits an odor that smells like sweat.

Clinical manifestations of the acute form occur in the first few days of life with poor feeding, vomiting, and respiratory distress as infants develop profound anion gap metabolic acidosis, hypoglycemia, and hyperammonemia. Bone marrow suppression often occurs. A chronic intermittent form may not manifest for several months or years.

Diagnosis of isovaleric acidemia is made by detecting elevated levels of isovaleric acid and its metabolites in blood or urine.

Acute treatment of isovaleric acidemia is with IV hydration and nutrition (including high-dose dextrose) and measures to increase renal isovaleric acid excretion by conjugation with glycine. If these measures are insufficient, exchange transfusion and peritoneal dialysis may be needed. Long-term treatment is with dietary leucine restriction and continuation of glycine and carnitine supplements. Prognosis is excellent with treatment.

PROPIONIC ACIDEMIA

Deficiency of propionyl CoA carboxylase, the enzyme responsible for metabolizing propionic acid to methylmalonate, causes propionic acid accumulation.

Illness begins in the first days or weeks of life with poor feeding, vomiting, and respiratory distress due to profound anion gap metabolic acidosis, hypoglycemia, and hyperammonemia. Seizures may occur, and bone marrow suppression is common. Physiologic stresses may trigger recurrent attacks. Survivors may have tubular nephropathies, intellectual disability, and neurologic abnormalities. Propionic acidemia can also be seen as part of multiple carboxylase deficiency, biotin deficiency, or biotinidase deficiency.

Diagnosis of propionic acidemia is suggested by elevated levels of propionic acid metabolites, including methylcitrate and tiglate and their glycine conjugates in blood and urine, and confirmed by measuring propionyl CoA carboxylase activity in WBCs or cultured fibroblasts.

Acute treatment of propionic acidemia is with IV hydration (including high-dose dextrose), nutrition, and protein restriction; carnitine may be helpful. If these measures are insufficient, peritoneal dialysis or hemodialysis may be needed. Long-term propionic acidemia treatment is dietary restriction of precursor amino acids and odd-chain fatty acids and possibly continuation of carnitine supplementation. A few patients respond to high-dose biotin because it is a cofactor for propionyl CoA and other carboxylases. Intermittent courses of antibiotics should be considered for reducing a proprionic acid load resulting from intestinal bacteria. An emergency plan for how to manage acute illness, which may provoke a metabolic crisis, should be in place.

METHYLMALONIC ACIDEMIA

This disorder is caused by deficiency of methylmalonyl CoA mutase, which converts methylmalonyl CoA (a product of the propionyl CoA carboxylation) into succinyl CoA. Adenosylcobalamin, a metabolite of vitamin B12, is a cofactor; its deficiency also may cause methylmalonic acidemia (and also homocystinuria and megaloblastic anemia). Methylmalonic acid accumulates. Age of onset, clinical manifestations, and treatment are similar to those of propionic acidemia except that cobalamin, instead of biotin, may be helpful for some patients.

METHIONINE METABOLISM DISORDERS

Number of defects in methionine metabolism lead to accumulation of homocysteine (and its dimer, homocystine) with adverse effects including thrombotic tendency, lens dislocation, and CNS and skeletal abnormalities.

There are numerous disorders of methionine and sulfur metabolism as well as many other amino acid and organic acid metabolism disorders (Table 22.2). Homocysteine is an intermediate in methionine metabolism; it is either remethylated to regenerate methionine or combined with serine in a series of trans

Table 22.2	Methionine and sulfur metabolism disorders		
Disease	Defective proteins or enzymes	Defective gene or genes (chromosomal location)	Comments
Homocystinuria	Cystathionine β-synthase	CBS (21q22.3)*	Biochemical profile: Methioninuria, homocystinuria Clinical features: Osteoporosis, scoliosis, fair complexion, ectopia lentis, progressive intellectual disability, thromboembolism Treatment: Pyridoxine, folate, betaine for unresponsive patients, low methionine diet with some L-cysteine supplementation
Methylenetetrahydrofolate reductase deficiency	Methylenetetrahydrofolate reductase	MTHFR (1p36.3)*	Biochemical profile: Low to normal plasma methionine, homocystinemia, homocystinuria Clinical features: Varies from asymptomatic to microcephaly, hypotonia, seizures, gait abnormality, and intellectual disability to apnea, coma, and death Treatment: Pyridoxine, folate (folic acid), hydroxycobalamin, methionine, betaine

Contd.

Table 22.2	Methionine and sulfur metabolism disorders (Contd.)		
Disease	**Defective proteins or enzymes**	**Defective gene or genes (chromosomal location)**	**Comments**
Methylmalonic acidemia-homocystinuria	Methionine synthase reductase	MTRR (5p15)*	Biochemical profile: Homocystinuria, homocystinemia, low plasma methionine, no methylmalonic aciduria, normal B12 and folate Clinical features: Feeding difficulty, growth failure, intellectual disability, ataxia, cerebral atrophy Treatment: Hydroxycobalamin, folate, L-methionine
Methylmalonic acidemia-homocystinuria	Methylene tetrahydrofolate homocysteine methyltransferase	MTR (1q43)*	Same as methylmalonic acidemia-homocystinuria cblE
Hypermethioninemia	Methionine adenosyl transferase I and III	MAT1A (10q22)*	Biochemical profile: Elevated plasma methionine Clinical features: Mainly asymptomatic, fetid breath Treatment: None needed
Cystathioninuria	γ-cystathionase	CTH (16)*	Biochemical profile: Cystathioninuria Clinical features: Usually normal; intellectual disability reported Treatment: Pyridoxine
Sulfite oxidase deficiency	Sulfite oxidase	SUOX (12q13)*	Biochemical profile: Elevated urine sulfite, thiosulfate, and S-sulfocysteine; decreased sulfate Clinical features: Developmental delay, ectopia lentis, eczema, delayed dentition, fine hair, hemiplegia, infantile hypotonia, hypertonia, seizures, choreoathetosis, ataxia, dystonia, death Treatment: No effective treatment
Molybdenum cofactor defect	MOCS1A and MOCS1B proteins Molybdopterin synthase Gephyrin	MCOS1 (14q24)* MCOS2 (6p21.3)* GEPH (5q21)*	Biochemical profile: Elevated urinary sulfite, thiosulfate, S-sulfocysteine, taurine, hypoxanthine, and xanthine; decreased sulfate and urate Clinical features: Not only similar to sulfite oxidase deficiency, but also urinary stones Treatment: No effective treatment Low sulfur diet possibly helpful in patients with milder symptoms

*Gene has been identified, and molecular basis has been elucidated.

sulfuration reactions to form cystathionine and then cysteine. Cysteine is then metabolized to sulfite, taurine, and glutathione. Various defects in remethylation or transsulfuration can cause homocysteine to accumulate, resulting in disease.

The first step in methionine metabolism is its conversion to adenosylmethionine; this conversion requires the enzyme methionine adenosyltransferase. Deficiency of this enzyme results in methionine elevation, which is not clinically significant except that it causes false-positive neonatal screening results for homocystinuria.

CLASSIC HOMOCYSTINURIA

This disorder is caused by an autosomal recessive deficiency of cystathionine β-synthase, which catalyzes cystathionine formation from homocysteine and serine. Homocysteine accumulates and dimerizes to form the disulfide homocystine, which is excreted in the urine. Because remethylation is intact, some of the additional homocysteine is converted to methionine, which accumulates in the blood. Excess homocysteine predisposes to thrombosis and has adverse effects on connective tissue (perhaps involving fibrillin), particularly the eyes and skeleton; adverse neurologic effects may be due to thrombosis or a direct effect. Arterial and venous thromboembolic phenomena can occur at any age. Many patients develop ectopia lentis (lens subluxation), intellectual disability, and osteoporosis. Patients can have a marfanoid habitus even though they are not usually tall.

Diagnosis of classic homocystinuria is by neonatal screening for elevated serum methionine; elevated total plasma homocysteine levels are confirmatory. Enzymatic assay in skin fibroblasts can also be done.

Treatment of classic homocystinuria is a low-methionine diet, combined with high-dose pyridoxine (a cystathionine synthetase cofactor) 100–500 mg by mouth once a day. Because about half of patients respond to high-dose pyridoxine alone, some clinicians do not restrict methionine intake in these patients. Betaine (trimethylglycine), which enhances remethylation, can also help lower homocysteine; dosage is 100–125 mg/kg by mouth bid. Folate 500–1000 µg once a day is also given. With early treatment, intellectual outcome is normal or near normal.

OTHER FORMS OF HOMOCYSTINURIA

Various defects in the remethylation process can result in homocystinuria. Defects include deficiencies of methionine synthase (MS) and MS reductase (MSR), delivery of methylcobalamin and adenosylcobalamin, and deficiency of methylenetetrahydrofolate reductase (MTHFR, which is required to generate the 5-methyl-tetrahydrofolate needed for the MS reaction). Because there is no methionine elevation in these forms of homocystinuria, they are not detected by neonatal screening.

Clinical manifestations are similar to other forms of homocystinuria. In addition, MS and MSR deficiencies are accompanied by neurologic deficits and megaloblastic anemia. Clinical manifestation of MTHFR deficiency is variable, including intellectual disability, psychosis, weakness, ataxia, and spasticity.

Diagnosis of MS and MSR deficiencies is suggested by homocystinuria and megaloblastic anemia and confirmed by DNA testing. Patients with cobalamin defects have megaloblastic anemia and methylmalonic acidemia. MTHFR deficiency is diagnosed by DNA testing.

Treatment is by replacement of hydroxycobalamin 1 mg IM once a day (for patients with MS, MSR, and cobalamin defects) and folate in supplementation similar to characteristic homocystinuria.

CYSTATHIONINURIA

This disorder is caused by deficiency of cystathionase, which converts cystathionine to cysteine. Cystathionine accumulation results in increased urinary excretion but no clinical symptoms.

SULFITE OXIDASE DEFICIENCY

Sulfite oxidase converts sulfite to sulfate in the last step of cysteine and methionine degradation; it requires a molybdenum cofactor. Deficiency of either the enzyme or the cofactor causes similar disease; inheritance for both is autosomal recessive. In its most severe form, clinical manifestations appear in neonates and include seizures, hypotonia, and myoclonus, progressing to early death. Patients with milder forms may present similarly to cerebral palsy and may have choreiform movements.

Diagnosis of sulfite oxidase deficiency is suggested by elevated urinary sulfite and confirmed by measuring enzyme levels in fibroblasts and cofactor levels in liver biopsy specimens. Treatment is supportive.

PHENYLKETONURIA

Phenylketonuria is a disorder of amino acid metabolism that causes a clinical syndrome of intellectual disability with cognitive and behavioral abnormalities caused by elevated serum phenylalanine. The primary cause is deficient phenylalanine hydroxylase activity. Diagnosis is by detecting high phenylalanine levels and normal or low tyrosine levels. Treatment is lifelong dietary phenylalanine restriction. Prognosis is excellent with treatment.

Phenylketonuria is most common among all white populations and relatively less common among Ashkenazi Jews, Chinese, and blacks. Inheritance is autosomal recessive; incidence is about 1/10,000 births among whites (Table 22.3).

Pathophysiology

Excess dietary phenylalanine (i.e. that not used for protein synthesis) is normally converted to tyrosine by phenylalanine hydroxylase; tetrahydrobiopterin (BH4) is an essential cofactor for this reaction. When one of several gene mutations results in deficiency or absence of phenylalanine hydroxylase, dietary phenylalanine accumulates; the brain is the main organ affected, possibly due to disturbance of myelination.

Some of the excess phenylalanine is metabolized to phenylketones, which are excreted in the urine, giving rise to the term phenylketonuria. The degree of enzyme deficiency, and hence severity of hyperphenylalaninemia, varies among patients depending on the specific mutation.

Variant Forms

Although nearly all cases (98–99%) of PKU result from phenylalanine hydroxylase deficiency, phenylalanine can also accumulate if BH4 is not synthesized because of deficiencies of dihydrobiopterin synthase or not regenerated because of deficiencies of dihydropteridine reductase. Additionally, because BH4 is also a cofactor for tyrosine hydroxylase, which is involved in the synthesis of dopamine and serotonin, BH4 deficiency alters synthesis of neurotransmitters, causing neurologic symptoms independently of phenylalanine accumulation.

Symptoms and Signs

Most children with phenylketonuria are normal at birth but develop symptoms and signs slowly over several months as phenylalanine accumulates. The hallmark of untreated PKU is severe intellectual disability. Children also manifest extreme hyperactivity, gait disturbance, and psychoses and often exhibit an unpleasant, mousy body odor caused by phenylacetic acid (a breakdown product of phenylalanine) in urine and sweat. Children also tend to have a lighter skin, hair, and eye color than unaffected family members, and some may develop a rash similar to infantile eczema.

Diagnosis

In many developed countries, all neonates are screened for phenylketonuria 24–48 hours after birth with one of several blood tests; abnormal results are confirmed by directly measuring phenylalanine levels. In classic PKU, neonates often have phenylalanine levels >20 mg/dL. Those with partial deficiencies typically have levels <8–10 mg/dL while on a normal diet (levels >6 mg/dL require treatment); distinction from classic PKU requires a liver phenylalanine hydroxylase activity assay showing activity between 5% and 15% of normal or a mutation analysis identifying mild mutations in the gene.

Tetrahydrobiopterin deficiency is distinguished from other forms of PKU by elevated concentrations of biopterin or neopterin in urine, blood, CSF, or all three; recognition is important, and the urine biopterin profile should be determined routinely at initial diagnosis because standard PKU treatment does not prevent neurologic damage.

Children in families with a positive family history can be diagnosed prenatally by using direct mutation studies after chorionic villus sampling or amniocentesis.

Prognosis

Adequate treatment begun in the first days of life prevents all manifestations of disease. Treatment begun after 2–3 years may be effective only in controlling the extreme hyperactivity and intractable seizures. Children born to mothers with poorly controlled PKU (i.e. they have high phenylalanine levels) during pregnancy are at high risk of microcephaly and developmental deficit.

Treatment

Treatment of phenylketonuria is lifelong dietary phenylalanine restriction. All natural protein contains about 4% phenylalanine. Therefore dietary staples include low-protein natural foods (e.g. fruits, vegetables, certain cereals), protein hydrolysates treated to remove phenylalanine, and phenylalanine-free elemental amino acid mixtures. Examples of commercially available phenylalanine-free products include XPhe products (PKU anamix for infants, XP maxamaid for children 1–8 years, XP maxamum for children >8 years); phenex-1 and phenex-2; phenyl-Free 1 and phenyl-free 2; PKU 1, PKU 2, and PKU 3; phenylAde (varieties); PKU lophlex LQ; and phlexy-10 (multiple formulations). Some phenylalanine is required for growth and metabolism; this requirement is met by measured quantities of natural protein from milk or low-protein foods.

Frequent monitoring of plasma phenylalanine levels is required; recommended targets are 120–240 μmol/L for children <12 years and between 120–600 μmol/L for children >12 years. Dietary planning and management need to be initiated in women of childbearing age before pregnancy to ensure a good outcome for the child. Tyrosine supplementation is increasingly used because it is an essential amino acid in patients with PKU. In addition, sapropterin is increasingly being used. For those with BH4 deficiency, treatment also includes tetrahydrobiopterin 1–5 mg/kg by mouth 3 times a day; levodopa, carbidopa, and 5-OH tryptophan; and folinic acid 10–20 mg by mouth once a day in cases of dihydropteridine reductase deficiency. However, treatment goals and approach are the same as those for PKU.

Tyrosine Metabolism Disorders

Tyrosine is an amino acid that is a precursor of several neurotransmitters (e.g. dopamine, norepinephrine, epinephrine), hormones (e.g. thyroxine), and melanin; deficiencies of enzymes involved in its metabolism lead to a variety of syndromes. There are numerous disorders of phenylalanine and tyrosine metabolism (Table 22.3).

TRANSIENT TYROSINEMIA OF THE NEWBORN

Transient immaturity of metabolic enzymes, particularly 4-hydroxyphenylpyruvic acid dioxygenase, sometimes leads to elevated plasma tyrosine levels (usually in premature infants, particularly those receiving high-protein diets); metabolites may show up on routine neonatal screening for phenylketonuria. Most infants are asymptomatic, but some have lethargy and poor feeding. Tyrosinemia is distinguished from PKU by elevated plasma tyrosine levels. Most cases resolve spontaneously.

Table 22.3	Phenylalanine and tyrosine metabolism disorders		
Disease	**Defective proteins or enzymes**	**Defective gene or genes (chromosomal location)**	**Comments**
Phenylketonuria (PKU), with classic and mild forms	Phenylalanine hydroxylase	PAH (12q24.1)*	Biochemical profile: Elevated plasma phenylalanine Clinical features: Intellectual disability, behavioral problems Treatment: Dietary phenylalanine restriction, tyrosine supplementation
Dihydropteridine reductase deficiency	Dihydropteridine reductase	QDPR (4p15.31)*	Biochemical profile: Elevated plasma phenylalanine, high urine biopterin, low plasma biopterin Clinical features: Similar to mild PKU, but if neurotransmitter deficiency is unrecognized, development of intellectual disability, seizures, and dystonia Treatment: Dietary phenylalanine restriction, tyrosine supplementation, folinic acid, neuro-transmitter replacement
Pterin-4α-carbinola-mine dehydratase deficiency	Pterin-4α-carbinolamine dehydratase	PCBD (10q22)*	Biochemical profile: Elevated plasma phenylalanine, high urine neopterin and primapterin, low plasma biopterin Clinical features: Similar to mild PKU, but if neurotransmitter deficiency is unrecognized, development of intellectual disability, seizures, and dystonia Treatment: Dietary phenylalanine restriction, tyrosine supplementation, neurotransmitter replacement
Biopterin synthesis deficiency	GTP-cyclohydrolase 6-Pyruvoyl-tetrahy-dropterin synthase Sepiapterin reductase	GCH1 (14q22)* PTS (11q22-q23)* SPR (2p14-p12)*	Biochemical profile: Elevated plasma phenylalanine, low urine biopterin, low (GCH) or high (PTS and SPR) urine neopterin Clinical features: Similar to mild PKU, but if neurotransmitter deficiency is unrecognized, development of intellectual disability, seizures, and dystonia Treatment: Tetrahydrobiopterin and neuro-transmitter supplementation
Tyrosinemia type I	Fumarylacetoacetate hydrolase	FAH (15q23-q25)*	Biochemical profile: Elevated plasma tyrosine, elevated plasma and urinary succinylacetone Clinical features: Cirrhosis, acute liver failure, peripheral neuropathy, Fanconi syndrome Treatment: Dietary phenylalanine, tyrosine, and methionine restriction; nitisinone; liver transplantation
Tyrosinemia type II	Tyrosine aminotransferase	TAT (16q22.1-q22.3)*	Biochemical profile: Elevated plasma tyrosine and phenylalanine Clinical features: Intellectual disability, palmo-plantar hyperkeratitis, corneal ulcers Treatment: Dietary phenylalanine and tyrosine restriction
Tyrosinemia type III	4-hydroxyphenyl-pyruvate dioxygenase	HPD (12q24-qter)*	Biochemical profile: Elevated plasma tyrosine, elevated urinary 4-hydroxyphenyl derivatives Clinical features:Developmental delay, seizures, ataxia Treatment: Dietary phenylalanine and tyrosine restriction, ascorbate supplementation

Contd.

Table 22.3	Phenylalanine and tyrosine metabolism disorders (Contd.)		
Disease	**Defective proteins or enzymes**	**Defective gene or genes (chromosomal location)**	**Comments**
Transient tyrosinemia of the newborn	4-hydroxyphenyl-pyruvate dioxygenase	Not genetic	Biochemical profile: Elevated plasma phenylalanine and tyrosine Clinical features: Usually occurring in premature infants; mostly asymptomatic Occasionally poor feeding and lethargy Treatment: Tyrosine restriction and ascorbate supplementation for symptomatic patients only
Hawkinsinuria	4-hydroxyphenyl-pyruvate dioxygenase complex	HPD (12q24-qter)*	Biochemical profile: Mild hypertyrosinemia, elevated urinary hawkinsin Clinical features: Failure to thrive, ketotic metabolic acidosis Treatment: Dietary phenylalanine and tyrosine restriction, ascorbate supplementation
Alkaptonuria	Homogentisate oxidase	HGD (3q21-q23)*	Biochemical profile: Elevated urine homogentisic acid Clinical features: Dark urine, ochronosis, arthritis Treatment: None; ascorbate supplementation to reduce pigmentation
Oculocutaneous albinism type I	Tyrosinase	TYR (11q21)*	Biochemical profile: No abnormality in plasma and urine amino acids, absent (IA) or decreased (IB) tyrosinase Clinical features: Absent (IA) or decreased (IB) pigment in skin, hair, iris, and retina; nystagmus; blindness; skin cancer Treatment: Protection of skin and eyes from actinic radiation

*Gene has been identified, and molecular basis has been elucidated.

Symptomatic patients should have dietary tyrosine restriction (2 g/kg/day) and be given vitamin C 200– 400 mg by mouth once a day.

Tyrosinemia Type I

This disorder is an autosomal recessive trait caused by deficiency of fumarylacetoacetate hydroxylase, an enzyme important for tyrosine metabolism. Disease may manifest as fulminant liver failure in the neonatal period or as indolent subclinical hepatitis, painful peripheral neuropathy, and renal tubular disorders (e.g. normal anion gap metabolic acidosis, hypophosphatemia, and vitamin D resistant rickets) in older infants and children. Children who do not die of associated liver failure in infancy, have a significant risk of developing liver cancer.

Diagnosis of tyrosinemia type I is suggested by elevated plasma levels of tyrosine; it is confirmed by a high level of succinylacetone in plasma or urine and by low fumarylacetoacetate hydroxylase activity in blood cells or liver biopsy specimens. Treatment with nitisinone is effective in acute episodes and slows progression. A diet low in phenylalanine and tyrosine is recommended. Liver transplantation is effective.

Tyrosinemia Type II

This rare autosomal recessive disorder is caused by tyrosine transaminase deficiency. Accumulation of tyrosine causes cutaneous and corneal ulcers. Secondary elevation of phenylalanine, though mild, may cause neuropsychiatric abnormalities if not treated.

Diagnosis of tyrosinemia type II is by elevation of tyrosine in plasma, absence of succinylacetone in plasma or urine, and measurement of decreased enzyme activity in liver biopsy. This disorder is easily treated with mild to moderate restriction of dietary phenylalanine and tyrosine.

ALKAPTONURIA

This rare autosomal recessive disorder is caused by homogentisic acid oxidase deficiency; homogentisic acid oxidation products accumulate in and darken skin, and crystals precipitate in joints. The condition is usually diagnosed in adults and causes dark skin pigmentation (ochronosis) and arthritis. Urine turns dark when exposed to air because of oxidation products of homogentisic acid. Diagnosis of alkaptonuria is by finding elevated urinary levels of homogentisic acid (>4–8 g/24 hours).

There is no effective treatment for alkaptonuria, but ascorbic acid 1 g by mouth once a day may diminish pigment deposition by increasing renal excretion of homogentisic acid.

OCULOCUTANEOUS ALBINISM

Tyrosinase deficiency results in absence of skin and retinal pigmentation, causing a much increased risk of skin cancer and considerable vision loss. Nystagmus is often present, and photophobia is common.

UREA CYCLE DISORDERS

Urea cycle disorders are characterized by hyperammonemia under catabolic or protein-loading conditions. There are many types of urea cycle and related disorders (Table 22.4). Primary urea cycle disorders (UCDs) include

carbamoyl phosphate synthase (CPS) deficiency, ornithine transcarbamylase (OTC) deficiency, argininosuccinate synthetase deficiency (citrullinemia), argininosuccinate lyase deficiency (argininosuccinic aciduria), and arginase deficiency (argininemia). In addition, N-acetylglutamate synthetase (NAGS) deficiency has been reported. The more 'proximal' the enzyme deficiency is, the more severe the hyperammonemia; thus, disease severity in descending order is NAGS deficiency, CPS deficiency, OTC deficiency, citrullinemia, argininosuccinic aciduria, and argininemia. Inheritance for all UCDs is autosomal recessive, except for OTC deficiency, which is X-linked.

Symptoms and Signs

Clinical manifestations range from mild (e.g. failure to thrive, intellectual disability, episodic hyperammonemia) to severe (e.g. altered mental status, coma, and death). Manifestations in females with OTC deficiency range from growth failure, developmental delay, psychiatric abnormalities, and episodic (especially postpartum)

Table 22.4	Urea cycle and related disorders		
Disease	**Defective proteins or enzymes**	**Defective gene or genes (chromosomal location)**	**Comments**
Ornithine-transcarbamoylase (OTC) deficiency	OTC	OTC (Xp21.1)*	Biochemical profile: Elevated ornithine and glutamine, decreased citrulline and arginine, markedly increased urine orotate
			Clinical features: In males, recurrent vomiting, irritability, lethargy, hyperammonemic coma, cerebral edema, spasticity, intellectual disability, seizures, death
			In female carriers, variable manifestations, ranging from growth delay, small stature, protein aversion, and postpartum hyperammonemia to symptoms as severe as those in males with the deficiency
			Treatment: Hemodialysis for emergent hyperammonemic crisis, Na benzoate, Na phenylacetate, Na phenylbutyrate, low-protein diet supplemented with essential amino acid mixture and arginine, citrulline, experimental attempts at gene therapy, liver transplantation (which is curative)
N-acetylglutamate synthetase deficiency	N-acetylglutamate synthetase	NAGS (17q21.31)	Biochemical profile: Similar to OTC deficiency except for normal to low urine orotate
			Clinical features: Similar to OTC deficiency except carriers are asymptomatic
			Treatment: Not only similar to OTC deficiency, but also N-carbamylglutamate supplementation
Carbamoyl phosphate synthetase (CPS) deficiency	Carbamoyl phosphate synthetase	CPS1 (2q35)*	Biochemical profile: Similar to OTC deficiency except for normal to low urine orotate
			Clinical features: Similar to OTC deficiency except carriers are asymptomatic
			Treatment: Na benzoate and arginine

Contd.

Table 22.4	Urea cycle and related disorders *(Contd.)*		
Disease	**Defective proteins or enzymes**	**Defective gene or genes (chromosomal location)**	**Comments**
Citrullinemia type I	Argininosuccinic acid synthetase	ASS (9q34)*	**Biochemical profile:** High plasma citrulline and glutamine, citrullinuria, orotic aciduria **Clinical features:** Episodic hyperammonemia, growth failure, protein aversion, lethargy, vomiting, coma, seizures, cerebral edema, developmental delay **Treatment:** Similar to that for OTC deficiency except citrulline supplementation is not recommended Liver transplantation
Citrullinemia type II	Citrin	SCL25A13 (7q21.3)*	**Biochemical profile:** Elevated plasma citrulline, methionine, galactose, and bilirubin **Clinical features:** With neonatal onset, cholestasis resolved by 3 months With adult onset, enuresis, delayed menarche, sleep reversal, vomiting, delusions, hallucinations, psychosis, coma **Treatment:** Liver transplantation; otherwise no clear treatment
Argininosuccinic aciduria	Argininosuccinate lyase	ASL (7cen-q11.2)*	**Biochemical profile:** Elevated plasma citrulline and glutamine, elevated urine argininosuccinate **Clinical features:** Episodic hyperammonemia, hepatic fibrosis, elevated liver enzymes, hepatomegaly, protein aversion, vomiting, seizures, intellectual disability, ataxia, lethargy, coma, trichorrhexis nodosa **Treatment:** Arginine supplementation
Argininemia	Arginase I	ARG1 (6q23)*	**Biochemical profile:** Elevated plasma arginine, diaminoaciduria (argininuria, lysinuria, cystinuria, ornithinuria), orotic aciduria, pyrimidinuria **Clinical features:** Growth and developmental delay, anorexia, vomiting, seizures, spasticity, irritability, hyperactivity, protein intolerance, hyperammonemia **Treatment:** Low-protein diet, benzoate, phenylacetate
Lysinuric protein intolerance	Dibasic amino acid transporter	SLC7A7 (14q11.2)*	**Biochemical profile:** Elevated urine lysine, ornithine, and arginine **Clinical features:** Protein intolerance, episodic hyperammonemia, growth and developmental delay, diarrhea, vomiting, hepatomegaly, cirrhosis, leucopenia, osteopenia, skeletal fragility, coma **Treatment:** Low-protein diet, citrulline
Hyperornithinemia, hyperammonemia, and homocitrullinemia	Mitochondrial ornithine translocase	SLC25A15 (13q14)*	**Biochemical profile:** Elevated plasma ornithine, homocitrullinemia **Clinical features:** Intellectual disability, progressive spastic paraparesis, episodic confusion, hyperammonemia, dyspraxia, seizures, vomiting, retinopathy, abnormal nerve conduction and evoked potentials, leukodystrophy **Treatment:** Lysine, ornithine, or citrulline supplementation

Contd.

Table 22.4 Urea cycle and related disorders *(Contd.)*

Disease	Defective proteins or enzymes	Defective gene or genes (chromosomal location)	Comments
Ornithinemia	Ornithine aminotransferase	OAT (10q26)*	Biochemical profile: Elevated plasma ornithine and urine ornithine, lysine, and arginine; low plasma lysine, glutamic acid, and glutamine Clinical features: Myopia, night blindness, blindness, progressive loss of peripheral vision, progressive gyrate atrophy of choroid and retina, mild proximal hypotonia, myopathy Treatment: Pyridoxine, low-arginine diet, lysine and α-aminoisobutyrate to increase renal loss of ornithine; proline or creatine supplementation
Hyperinsulinism-hyperammonemia syndrome	Hyperactivity of glutamate dehydrogenase	GLUD1 (10q23.3)*	Biochemical profile: Elevated urine α-ketoglutarate Clinical features: Seizures, recurrent hypoglycemia, hyperinsulinism, asymptomatic hyperammonemia Treatment: Prevention of hypoglycemia

*Gene has been identified, and molecular basis has been elucidated.

hyperammonemia to a phenotype similar to that of affected males (i.e. recurrent vomiting, irritability, lethargy, hyperammonemic coma, cerebral edema, spasticity, intellectual disability, seizures, death).

Diagnosis

Diagnosis of urea cycle disorders is based on amino acid profiles. For example, elevated ornithine indicates CPS deficiency or OTC deficiency, whereas elevated citrulline indicates citrullinemia. To distinguish between CPS deficiency and OTC deficiency, orotic acid measurement is helpful because accumulation of carbamoyl phosphate in OTC deficiency results in its alternative metabolism to orotic acid.

Treatment

Treatment of urea cycle disorders is dietary protein restriction that still provides adequate amino acids for growth, development, and normal protein turnover. Arginine has become a staple of treatment. It supplies adequate urea cycle intermediates to encourage the incorporation of more nitrogen moieties into urea cycle intermediates, each of which is readily excretable.

Arginine is also a positive regulator of acetylglutamate synthesis. Recent studies suggest that oral citrulline is more effective than arginine in patients with OTC deficiency. Additional treatment is with sodium benzoate, phenylbutyrate, or phenylacetate, which by conjugating glycine (sodium benzoate) and glutamine (phenylbutyrate and phenylacetate) provides a 'nitrogen sink.'

Despite these therapeutic advances, many UCDs remain difficult to treat, and liver transplantation is eventually required for many patients. Timing of liver transplantation is critical. Optimally, the infant should grow to an age when transplantation is less risky (>1 year), but it is important to not wait so long as to allow an intercurrent episode of hyperammonemia (often associated with illness) to cause irreparable harm to the CNS.

In addition, there are a number of other disorders of amino acid and organic acid metabolism, including those involving beta- and gamma-amino acids, the gamma-glutamyl cycle, glycine, histidine, lysine, proline and hydroxyproline, and miscellaneous other amino acid disorders (Tables 22.5–22.11).

Table 22.5 Beta-amino acid and gamma-amino acid disorders

Disease	Defective proteins or enzymes	Defective gene or genes (chromosomal location)	Comments
Hyper-β-alaninemia	β-alanine-α-ketoglutarate aminotransferase	Not determined	Biochemical profile: Elevated urinary β-alanine, taurine, γ-aminobutyrate (GABA), and β-aminoisobutyrate Clinical features: Seizures, somnolence, death Treatment: Pyridoxine

Contd.

Table 22.5   Beta-amino acid and gamma-amino acid disorders (Contd.)

Disease	Defective proteins or enzymes	Defective gene or genes (chromosomal location)	Comments
Methylmalonate/ malonate semialdehyde dehydrogenase deficiency with 3-amino and 3-hydroxy aciduria	Methylmalonate/malonate semialdehyde dehydrogenase	ALDH6A1 (14q24.3)*	Biochemical profile: Elevated 3-3-hydroxyisobutyrate 3-aminoisobutyrate, 3-hydroxypropionate β-alanine, and 2-ethyl-3-hydroxypropionate Clinical features: None to mild Treatment: Not determined
Methylmalonic semi-aldehyde dehydrogenase deficiency with mild methylmalonic acidemia	Methylmalonic semialdehyde dehydrogenase (see also branched-chain amino acid metabolism, above)	ALDH6A1 (14q24.1)	Biochemical profile: Moderately elevated urine methylmalonate Clinical features: Developmental delay, seizures Treatment: No effective treatment
Hyper-β-aminoiso-butyric aciduria	D(R)-3-aminoisobutyrate: pyruvate aminotransferase	Not determined	Biochemical profile: Elevated β-aminoisobutyric acid Clinical features: Benign Treatment: None needed
Pyridoxine dependency with seizures	Not determined	Specific gene not determined (5q31.2-q31.3)	Biochemical profile: Elevated CSF glutamate Clinical features: Seizure disorder refractory to conventional anticonvulsants, high-pitched cry, hypothermia, jitteriness, dystonia, hepatomegaly, hypotonia, dyspraxia, developmental delay Treatment: Pyridoxine
GABA-transaminase deficiency	4-aminobutyrate-α-keto-glutarate aminotransferase	ABAT (16p13.3)*	Biochemical profile: Elevated plasma and CSF GABA and β-alanine, elevated carnosine Clinical features: Accelerated linear growth, seizures, cerebellar hypoplasia, psychomotor delay, leukodystrophy, burst suppression EEG pattern Treatment: No known treatment
4-Hydroxybutyric aciduria	Succinic semialdehyde dehydrogenase	ALDH5A1 (6p22)*	Biochemical profile: Elevated urinary 4-hydroxybutyrate and glycine Clinical features: Psychomotor retardation, speech delay, hypotonia Treatment: Vigabatrin
Carnosinemia, homo-carnosinosis, or both	Carnosinase	Specific gene not determined (18q21.3)	Biochemical profile: In carnosinemia pheno-type, carnosinuria despite meat-free diet, elevated urine anserine after ingestion of food containing imidazole dipeptides, normal CSF In homocarnosinosis phenotype, elevated CSF homocarnosine, normal serum carnosine Clinical features: Usually benign; reported symptoms probably due to ascertainment bias Treatment: None needed

*Gene has been identified, and molecular basis has been elucidated.

Table 22.6   Gamma-glutamyl cycle disorders

Disease	Defective proteins or enzymes	Defective gene or genes (chromosomal location)	Comments
γ-glutamylcysteine synthetase deficiency	γ-glutamylcysteine synthetase	GGLC (6p12)*	Biochemical profile: Aminoaciduria, glutathione deficiency Clinical features: Hemolysis, spinocerebellar degeneration, peripheral neuropathy, myopathy Treatment: No clear treatment; avoidance of drugs that trigger hemolytic crisis in G6PD deficiency

Contd.

Table 22.6	Gamma-glutamyl cycle disorders *(Contd.)*		
Disease	**Defective proteins or enzymes**	**Defective gene or genes (chromosomal location)**	**Comments**
Pyroglutamic aciduria	Glutathione synthetase	GSS (20q11.2)*	Biochemical profile: Elevated urinary, plasma, and CSF 5-oxoproline; increased γ-glutamylcysteine; decreased glutathione level
			Clinical features: Hemolysis, ataxia, seizures, intellectual disability, spasticity, metabolic acidosis
			In mild form, no evidence of neurologic damage
			Treatment: Na bicarbonate or citrate, vitamins E and C, avoidance of drugs that trigger hemolytic crisis in G6PD deficiency
γ-glutamyltranspeptidase deficiency	γ-glutamyltranspeptidase	Specific gene not determined (22q11.1-q11.2)	Biochemical profile: Elevated plasma and urinary glutathione
			Clinical features: Intellectual disability
			Treatment: No specific treatment
5-oxoprolinase deficiency	5-oxoprolinase	Not determined	Biochemical profile: Elevated urinary 5-oxoproline
			Clinical features: Probably benign
			Treatment: None needed

*Gene has been identified, and molecular basis has been elucidated.

Table 22.7	Glycine metabolism disorders		
Disease	**Defective proteins or enzymes**	**Defective gene or genes (chromosomal location)**	**Comments**
Non-ketotic hyperglycinemia	Glycine cleavage enzyme system		Biochemical profile: Elevated plasma and CSF glycine
	P-protein	GLDC (9p22)*	Clinical features: In neonatal form, hypotonia, seizures, myoclonus, apnea, death
	H-protein	GCSH (16q23)*	In infantile and episodic forms, seizures, intellectual disability, episodic delirium, chorea, vertical gaze palsy
	T-protein	ATM (3p21)*	In late-onset form, progressive spastic diplegia, optic atrophy, but no cognitive impairment or seizures
	L-protein	Not determined	Treatment: No effective treatment; in some patients, temporary benefit from Na benzoate and dextromethorphan

*Gene has been identified, and molecular basis has been elucidated

Table 22.8	Histidine metabolism disorders		
Disease	**Defective proteins or enzymes**	**Defective gene or genes (chromosomal location)**	**Comments**
Histidinemia	Classic: l-histidine ammonia-lyase (liver and skin) Variant: l-histidine ammonia-lyase (liver only)	HAL (12q22-q23)*	Biochemical profile: Elevated plasma histidine
			Clinical features: Frequently benign; neurologic manifestations in some patients
			Treatment: Low-protein diet
			For symptomatic patients only, controlled histidine intake
Urocanic aciduria	Urocanase	Not determined	Biochemical profile: Elevated urine urocanic acid
			Clinical features: Probably benign
			Treatment: None needed

*Gene has been identified, and molecular basis has been elucidated.

Table 22.9	Lysine metabolism disorders		
Disease	**Defective proteins or enzymes**	**Defective gene or genes (chromosomal location)**	**Comments**
Hyperlysinemia	Lysine: α-ketoglutarate reductase	AASS (7q31.3)*	Biochemical profile: Hyperlysinemia Clinical features: Muscle weakness, seizures, mild anemia, intellectual disability, joint and muscular laxity, ectopia lentis; sometimes benign Treatment: Limited lysine intake
2-ketoadipic acidemia	2-ketoadipic dehydrogenase	Not determined	Biochemical profile: Elevated urine 2-ketoadipate, 2-aminoadipate, and 2-hydroxyadipate Clinical features: Benign Treatment: None needed
Glutaric acidemia type I	Glutaryl CoA dehydrogenase	(19q13.2)*	Biochemical profile: Elevated urinary glutaric acid and 2-hydroxyglytaric acid Clinical features: Dystonia, dyskinesia, degeneration of the caudate and putamen, frontotemporal atrophy, arachnoid cysts Treatment: Aggressive treatment of inter-current illness, carnitine, Protein, lysine, and tryptophan restriction possibly helpful
Saccharopinuria	α-aminoadipic semialdehyde-glutamate reductase	AASS (7q31.3)*	Biochemical profile: Elevated urine lysine, citrulline, histidine, and saccharopine Clinical features: Intellectual disability, spastic diplegia, short stature, EEG abnormality Treatment: No clear treatment

*Gene has been identified, and molecular basis has been elucidated.

Table 22.10	Proline and hydroxyproline metabolism disorders		
Disease	**Defective proteins or enzymes**	**Defective gene or genes (chromosomal location)**	**Comments**
Hyperprolinemia type I	Proline oxidase (proline dehydrogenase)	PRODH (22q11.2)*	Biochemical profile: Elevated plasma proline and urinary proline, hydroxyproline, and glycine Clinical features: Usually benign; hereditary nephritis, nerve deafness Treatment: None needed
Hyperprolinemia type II	δ1-pyrroline-5-carboxylate dehydrogenase	P5CDH (1p36)*	Biochemical profile: Elevated plasma proline and pyrroline-5-carboxylate (P5C); elevated urinary P5C, Δ1-pyrroline-5-carboxylate, proline, hydroxyproline, and glycine Clinical features: During childhood, seizures, intellectual disability During adulthood, benign Treatment: None needed
δ1-pyrroline-5-carboxylate synthetase deficiency	δ1-pyrroline-5-carboxylate synthetase	PYCS (10q24.3)*	Biochemical profile: Low plasma proline, citrulline, arginine, and ornithine Clinical features: Hyperammonemia, cataracts, intellectual disability, joint laxity Treatment: Avoidance of fasting
Hyperhydroxyprolinemia	4-hydroxyproline oxidase	Not determined	Biochemical profile: Hydroxyprolinemia Clinical features: Disease association not proven Treatment: None needed

Contd.

Table 22.10	Proline and hydroxyproline metabolism disorders *(Contd.)*		
Disease	**Defective proteins or enzymes**	**Defective gene or genes (chromosomal location)**	**Comments**
Prolidase deficiency (170100)	Prolidase	PEPD (19q12-q13.11)*	Biochemical profile: Amino acid profile normal in unhydrolyzed urine, but excessive proline and hydroxyproline in acid-hydrolyzed urine Clinical features: Skin ulcers, frequent infections, dysmorphic features, immunodeficiency, intellectual disability Treatment: Proline supplement, Mn++ and ascorbic acid, essential amino acids, blood transfusion (packed RBC), topical proline and glycine ointment

*Gene has been identified, and molecular basis has been elucidated.

Table 22.11	Miscellaneous amino acid and organic acid metabolism disorders		
Disease	**Defective proteins or enzymes**	**Defective gene or genes (chromosomal location)**	**Comments**
Sarcosinemia	Sarcosine dehydrogenase	Specific gene not determined (9q34)	Biochemical profile: Elevated plasma sarcosine Clinical features: Benign; intellectual disability reported Treatment: None needed
D-glyceric aciduria	D-glycerate kinase	Not determined	Biochemical profile: Elevated urinary D-glyceric acid Clinical features: Chronic acidosis, hypotonia, seizures, intellectual disability Treatment: Bicarbonate or Citrate for acidosis
Hartnup disease	System B(0) neutral amino acid transporter	SLC6A19 (5p15)*	Biochemical profile: Neutral aminoaciduria Clinical features: Atrophic glossitis, photodermatitis, intermittent ataxia, hypertonia, seizures, psychosis Treatment: Nicotinamide
Cystinuria	Renal dibasic amino acid transporter	—	Biochemical profile: Elevated urinary cystine, lysine, arginine, and ornithine
Type I	Heavy subunit	SLC3A1 (2p16.3)*	Clinical features: Nephrolithiasis, increased risk of impaired cerebral function
Types II and III	Light subunit	SLC7A9 (19q13.1)*	Treatment: Maintenance of fluid intake, bicarbonate or citrate, penicillamine or mercaptopropionylglycine
Iminoglycinuria	Renal transporter of proline, hydroxyproline, and glycine	Not determined	Biochemical profile: Elevated urinary proline, hydroxyproline, and glycine but normal plasma levels Clinical features: Probably benign Treatment: None needed
Guanidinoacetate methyltransferase deficiency	Guanidinoacetate methyltransferase	GAMT (19p13.3)*	Biochemical profile: Elevated guanidinoacetate, decreased creatine and phosphocreatine Clinical features: Developmental delay, hypotonia, extrapyramidal movements, seizures, autistic behavior Treatment: Creatine supplementation

*Gene has been identified, and molecular basis has been elucidated.

CARBOHYDRATE METABOLISM DISORDERS

Carbohydrate metabolism disorders are errors of metabolism that affect the catabolism and anabolism of carbohydrates. The inability to effectively use metabolites of carbohydrates accounts for the majority of these disorders. These disorders include deficiency of enzymes that metabolize fructose may be asymptomatic or cause hypoglycemia. Fructose is a monosaccharide that is present in high concentrations in fruit and honey and is a constituent of sucrose and sorbitol. Fructose metabolism disorders are one of the many carbohydrate metabolism disorders.

Fructose 1-phosphate Aldolase (Aldolase B) Deficiency

This deficiency causes the clinical syndrome of hereditary fructose intolerance. Inheritance is autosomal recessive; incidence is estimated at 1/20,000 births. Infants are healthy until they ingest fructose; fructose 1-phosphate then accumulates, causing hypoglycemia, nausea and vomiting, abdominal pain, sweating, tremors, confusion, lethargy, seizures, and coma. Prolonged ingestion may cause cirrhosis, mental deterioration, and proximal renal tubular acidosis with urinary loss of phosphate and glucose.

Diagnosis of fructose 1-phosphate aldolase deficiency is suggested by symptoms in relation to recent fructose intake and is confirmed by enzyme analysis of liver biopsy tissue or by induction of hypoglycemia by fructose infusion 200 mg/kg IV. Diagnosis and identification of heterozygous carriers of the mutated gene can also be made by direct DNA analysis. Short-term treatment of fructose 1-phosphate aldolase deficiency is glucose for hypoglycemia; long-term treatment is exclusion of dietary fructose, sucrose, and sorbitol. Many patients develop a natural aversion to fructose-containing food. Prognosis is excellent with treatment.

Fructokinase Deficiency

This deficiency causes benign elevation of blood and urine fructose levels (benign fructosuria). Inheritance is autosomal recessive; incidence is about 1/130,000 births. The condition is asymptomatic and diagnosed accidentally when a non-glucose reducing substance is detected in urine.

Deficiency of Fructose-1,6-biphosphatase

This deficiency compromises gluconeogenesis and results in fasting hypoglycemia, ketosis, and acidosis. This deficiency can be fatal in neonates. Inheritance is autosomal recessive; incidence is unknown. Febrile illness can trigger episodes. Acute treatment of fructose-1, 6-biphosphatase deficiency is oral or IV glucose. Tolerance to fasting generally increases with age.

GALACTOSEMIA

Galactosemia is a carbohydrate metabolism disorder caused by inherited deficiencies in enzymes that convert galactose to glucose. Symptoms and signs include hepatic and renal dysfunction, cognitive deficits, cataracts, and premature ovarian failure. Diagnosis is by enzyme analysis of RBCs. Treatment is dietary elimination of galactose. Physical prognosis is good with treatment, but cognitive and performance parameters are often subnormal. Galactose is found in dairy products, fruits, and vegetables. Autosomal recessive enzyme deficiencies cause three clinical syndromes.

Galactose-1-phosphate Uridyl Transferase Deficiency

This deficiency causes classic galactosemia. Incidence is 1/62,000 births; carrier frequency is 1/125. Infants become anorectic and jaundiced within a few days or weeks of consuming breast milk or lactose-containing formula. Vomiting, hepatomegaly, poor growth, lethargy, diarrhea, and septicemia (*Escherichia coli*) develop, as does renal dysfunction (e.g. proteinuria, aminoaciduria and Fanconi syndrome), leading to metabolic acidosis and edema. Hemolytic anemia may also occur. Without treatment, children remain short and develop cognitive, speech, gait, and balance deficits in their teenage years; many also have cataracts, osteomalacia (caused by hypercalciuria), and premature ovarian failure. Patients with the Duarte variant have a much milder phenotype.

Galactokinase Deficiency

Patients develop cataracts from production of galactitol, which osmotically damages lens fibers; idiopathic intracranial hypertension (pseudotumor cerebri) is rare. Incidence is 1/40,000 births.

Uridine Diphosphate Galactose 4-epimerase Deficiency

There are benign and severe phenotypes. Incidence of the benign form is 1/23,000 births in Japan; no incidence data are available for the more severe form. The benign form is restricted to RBCs and WBCs and causes no clinical abnormalities. The severe form causes a syndrome indistinguishable from classic galactosemia, although sometimes with hearing loss.

Diagnosis

Diagnosis of galactosemia is suggested clinically and supported by elevated galactose levels and the presence of reducing substances other than glucose (e.g. galactose, galactose 1-phosphate) in the urine; it is confirmed by enzyme analysis of RBCs, hepatic tissue, or both. Most states require routine neonatal screening for galactose-1-phosphate uridyl transferase deficiency.

Treatment

Treatment of galactosemia is elimination of all sources of galactose in the diet, most notably lactose, which is a source of galactose present in all dairy products, including milk-based infant formulas and a sweetener used in many foods. A lactose-free diet prevents acute toxicity and reverses some manifestations (e.g. cataracts) but may not prevent neurocognitive deficits. Many patients require supplemental calcium and vitamins. For patients with epimerase deficiency, some galactose intake is critical to ensure a supply of uridine-5'-diphosphate-galactose (UDP-galactose) for various metabolic processes.

GLYCOGEN STORAGE DISEASES

Glycogen storage diseases are carbohydrate metabolism disorders and are caused by deficiencies of enzymes involved in glycogen synthesis or breakdown; the deficiencies may occur in the liver or muscles and cause hypoglycemia or deposition of abnormal amounts or types of glycogen (or its intermediate metabolites) in tissues.

Inheritance for glycogen storage diseases (GSDs) is autosomal recessive except for GSD type VIII/IX, which is X-linked. Incidence is estimated at about 1/25,000 births, which may be an underestimate because milder subclinical forms may be undiagnosed. For a more complete listing of glycogen storage diseases (Table 22.12).

Age of onset, clinical manifestations, and severity vary by type, but symptoms and signs are most commonly those of hypoglycemia and myopathy.

Diagnosis of glycogen storage diseases is suspected by history, examination, and detection of glycogen and intermediate metabolites in tissues by MRI or biopsy. Diagnosis is confirmed by significant decrease of enzyme

Table 22.12	Glycogen storage diseases and disorders of gluconeogenesis		
Disease	**Defective proteins or enzymes**	**Defective gene or genes (chromosomal location)**	**Comments**
GSD I (Von Gierkem disease)			Most common type of GSD I: Ia (>80%)
Type Ia	Glucose-6-phosphatase	G6PC (17q21)*	Onset: Before 1 year
Type Ib	Glucose-6-phosphate translocase	G6PT1 (11q23)*	Clinical features: Before 1 year, severe hypoglycemia, lactic acidosis, and hepatomegaly; later,
Type Ic	Microsomal phosphate or pyrophosphate transporter	G6PT1 (11q23)*	hepatic adenomas, renomegaly with progressive renal insufficiency and hypertension, short
Type Id	Microsomal glucose transporter	Probably same as IC	stature, hypertriglyceridemia, hyperuricemia, platelet dysfunction with epistaxis, and anemia
			In type Ib, less severe but including neutropenia, neutrophil dysfunction with recurrent infections, and inflammatory bowel disease
			Treatment: Uncooked cornstarch 1.5–2.5 g/kg by mouth q 4–6 h or lactose-free formula with maltodextrin to maintain normoglycemia; nocturnal feedings (important); fructose and galactose restriction; for lactic acidosis, bicarbonate 0.25–0.5 mmol/kg 4 times a day; allopurinol to keep uric acid to <6.4 mg/dL; liver and kidney transplantation (may be successful)
			For type Ib patients with neutropenia, G-CSF
GSD II			Onset: Infancy, childhood, or adulthood;
Type IIa	Lysosomal acid α-glucosidase	GAA (17q25)*	residual enzyme activity in child and adult forms
Type IIb	Lysosomal membrane protein-2	LAMP2 (Xq24)*	Clinical features: In infantile form, cardiomyopathy with heart failure, severe hypotonia, macroglossia
			In juvenile and adult forms, skeletal myopathy with delayed motor development, progressive peripheral and respiratory muscle weakness
			In type IIb, intellectual disability
			Treatment: None known
			For cardiomyopathy, heart transplantation
GSD III			Frequency: IIIa, 85%; IIIb, 15%; IIIc and IIId, rare

Contd.

Table 22.12   Glycogen storage diseases and disorders of gluconeogenesis (Contd.)

Disease	Defective proteins or enzymes	Defective gene or genes (chromosomal location)	Comments
Types IIIa and IIIb	Debrancher enzyme (amyloglucosidase and oligoglucanotransferase)	AGL (1p21)*	Onset: Infancy or Childhood Clinical features: In type IIIa, liver and muscle involvement with features of type Ia and II
Type IIIc	Amyloglucosidase only		In type IIIb, only liver involvement plus features of type Ia
Type IIId	Oligoglucanotransferase only		In types IIIc and IIId, various features depending on tissue affected Treatment: Uncooked cornstarch and continuous feeding to maintain normoglycemia, high-protein diet to stimulate gluconeogenesis
GSD IV	Branching enzyme	GBE1 (3p12)*	Onset: Early infancy; rarely, the neonatal period, late childhood, or adulthood (manifesting as a variant non-progressive or a neuromuscular form) Clinical features: Hepatomegaly with progressive cirrhosis and hypoglycemia, esophageal varices, and ascites; splenomegaly; failure to thrive In neuromuscular forms, hypotonia and muscle atrophy Treatment: None known For cirrhosis, liver transplantation, which treats the primary disease as well
GSD V	Muscle phosphorylase	PYGM (11q13)*	Onset: Adolescence or early adulthood Clinical features: Exercise intolerance due to muscle cramps, rhabdomyolysis Treatment: Carbohydrate administration before exercise, high-protein diet
GSD VI	Liver phosphorylase	PYGL (14q21-q22)*	Frequency: Rare Onset: Early childhood Clinical features: Benign course with symptoms lessening with aging; growth retardation, hepatomegaly, hypoglycemia, hyperlipidemia, ketosis Treatment: None necessary
GSD VII	Phosphofructokinase	PFKM (12q13.3)*	Onset: Middle childhood Clinical features: Exercise intolerance due to muscle cramps, rhabdomyolysis, hemolysis Treatment: Nonspecific, avoidance of exercise
GSD VIII/IX		—	Onset: Heterogeneous
Type VIII/IXa:	X-linked phosphorylase kinase	PHKA2 (Xp22)*	Clinical features: Heterogeneous; hepatomegaly, growth retardation, muscle hypotonia, hypercholesterolemia
Type IXb	Liver and muscle phosphorylase kinase	PHKB (16q12-q13)*	Treatment: Nonspecific
Type IXc	Liver phosphorylase kinase	PHKG2 (16p12.1-p11.2)*	Onset: Variable but often after cessation of night-time feedings or intercurrent illness
Type IXd	Muscle phosphorylase kinase	PHKA1 (Xq13)*	Clinical features: Fasting hypoglycemia and ketosis, postprandial lactic acidosis
GSD O	Glycogen synthase	GYS2 (12p12)*	Treatment: Frequent protein-rich meals, uncooked cornstarch at bedtime
Fanconi-Bickel syndrome	Glucose transporter-2	GLUT2 (3q26)*	Onset: Infancy Clinical features: Failure to thrive, abdominal distention, hepatomegaly, renomegaly, mild fasting hypoglycemia and hyperlipidemia, glucose intolerance, renal Fanconi syndrome Treatment: Diet similar to that for diabetes, replacement of renally lost electrolytes, vitamin D

Contd.

Table 22.12	Glycogen storage diseases and disorders of gluconeogenesis *(Contd.)*		
Disease	Defective proteins or enzymes	Defective gene or genes (chromosomal location)	Comments
Fructose 1, 6-biphosphatase deficiency	Fructose 1, 6-biphosphatase	FBP1 (9q22)*	Onset: Infancy or early childhood Clinical features: Episodic hyperventilation, apnea, hypoglycemia, ketosis, or lactic acidosis; episodes provoked by fasting, febrile infection, or ingestion of fructose, sorbitol, or glycerol Treatment: Avoidance of fasting and fructose, sorbitol, and glycerol; uncooked cornstarch
Phosphoenolpyruvate carboxykinase deficiency	Phosphoenolpyruvate carboxykinase	PCK1 (20q13.31)*	Onset: Childhood Clinical features: Failure to thrive, hypotonia, hepatomegaly, lactic acidosis, hypoglycemia Treatment: Avoidance of fasting, uncooked cornstarch

*Gene has been identified, and molecular basis has been elucidated. G -CSF, granulocyte colony-stimulating factor; GSD, glycogen storage disease.

activity in liver (types I, III, VI, and VIII/IX), muscle (types IIb, III, VII, and VIII/IX), skin fibroblasts (types IIa and IV), or RBCs (type VII) or by lack of an increase in venous lactate with forearm activity/ischemia (types V and VII).

Prognosis and treatment of glycogen storage diseases vary by type, but treatment typically includes dietary supplementation with cornstarch to provide a sustained source of glucose for the hepatic forms of GSD and exercise avoidance for the muscle forms.

Defects in glycolysis (rare) may cause syndromes similar to GSDs. Deficiencies of phosphoglycerate kinase, phosphoglycerate mutase, and lactate dehydrogenase mimic the myopathies of GSD types V and VII; deficiencies of glucose transport protein 2 (Fanconi-Bickel syndrome) mimic the hepatopathy of other GSD types (e.g. I, III, IV, VI).

PYRUVATE METABOLISM DISORDERS

Inability to metabolize pyruvate causes lactic acidosis and a variety of CNS abnormalities. Pyruvate is an important substrate in carbohydrate metabolism. Pyruvate metabolism disorders are included among the carbohydrate metabolism disorders.

Pyruvate Dehydrogenase Deficiency

Pyruvate dehydrogenase is a multi-enzyme complex responsible for the generation of acetyl CoA from pyruvate for the Krebs cycle. Deficiency results in elevation of pyruvate and thus elevation of lactic acid levels. Inheritance is X-linked or autosomal recessive.

Clinical manifestations vary in severity but include lactic acidosis and CNS malformations and other postnatal changes, including cystic lesions of the cerebral cortex, brain stem, and basal ganglia; ataxia; and psychomotor retardation.

Diagnosis of pyruvate dehydrogenase deficiency is confirmed by enzyme analysis of skin fibroblasts, DNA testing, or both. There is no clearly effective treatment for pyruvate dehydrogenase deficiency, although a low-carbohydrate or ketogenic diet and dietary thiamin supplementation have been beneficial for some patients.

Pyruvate Carboxylase Deficiency

Pyruvate carboxylase is an enzyme important for gluconeogenesis from pyruvate and alanine generated in muscle. Deficiency may be primary, or secondary to deficiency of holocarboxylase synthetase, biotin, or biotinidase; inheritance for both is autosomal recessive, and both result in lactic acidosis.

Primary deficiency incidence is <1/250,000 births but may be higher in certain American Indian populations. Psychomotor retardation with seizures and spasticity are the major clinical manifestations. Laboratory abnormalities include hyperammonemia; lactic acidosis; ketoacidosis; elevated levels of plasma lysine, citrulline, alanine, and proline; and increased excretion of α-ketoglutarate. Secondary deficiency is clinically similar, with failure to thrive, seizures, and other organic aciduria.

Diagnosis of pyruvate carboxylase deficiency is confirmed by enzyme analysis of cultured skin fibroblasts or DNA analysis. There is no effective treatment for pyruvate carboxylase deficiency, but some patients with primary deficiency and all those with secondary deficiencies should be given biotin supplementation 5–20 mg by mouth once a day.

Other Carbohydrate Metabolism Disorders

Phosphoenolpyruvate carboxykinase deficiency impairs gluconeogenesis and results in symptoms and signs similar to the hepatic forms of glycogen storage disease but without hepatic glycogen accumulation.

Other deficiencies include those of glycolytic enzymes or enzymes in the pentose phosphate pathway. Common examples are pyruvate kinase deficiency (Embden-Meyerhof pathway defects) and glucose-6-phosphate dehydrogenase (G6PD) deficiency, both of which may result in hemolytic anemia. Wernicke-Korsakoff syndrome is caused by a partial deficiency of transketolase, which is an enzyme for the pentose phosphate pathway that requires thiamin as a cofactor.

FATTY ACID AND GLYCEROL METABOLISM DISORDERS

Fatty acids are the preferred energy source for the heart and an important energy source for skeletal muscle during prolonged exertion. Also, during fasting, the bulk of the body's energy needs must be supplied by fat metabolism. Using fat as an energy source requires catabolizing adipose tissue into free fatty acid and glycerol. The free fatty acid is metabolized in the liver and peripheral tissue via β-oxidation into acetyl CoA; the glycerol is used by the liver for triglyceride synthesis or for gluconeogenesis. Carnitine is required for long-chain fatty acid oxidation. Carnitine deficiencies can be primary or secondary. Secondary carnitine deficiency is a secondary biochemical feature of many organic acidemias and fatty acid oxidation defects.

There are a number of other disorders of fatty acid and glycerol metabolism, including those involving fatty acid transport and mitochondrial oxidation, glycerol, ketones, peroxisome biogenesis and very long-chain fatty acids. Other disorders of fat metabolism are listed in Tables 22.13 and 22.14.

Table 22.13	Ketone metabolism disorders		
Disease	Defective proteins or enzymes	Defective gene or genes (chromosomal location)	Comments
3-hydroxy-3-methylglutaryl-CoA synthase deficiency	3-hydroxy-3-methylglutaryl-CoA synthase	HMGCS2 (600234)	Biochemical profile: See below Clinical features: Episodic non-ketotic hypoglycemia Treatment: Avoidance of fasting
3-hydroxy-3-methylglutaryl-CoA lyase deficiency	Branched chain amino acid metabolism disorders (Table: 22.1)		
Succinyl-CoA 3-oxoacid-CoA transferase deficiency	Succinyl-CoA 3-oxoacid-CoA transferase	OXCT (5p13)*	Biochemical profile: Ketonuria Clinical features: Severe episodic ketoacidosis, vomiting, hyperventilation Treatment: Glucose during acute episode plus judicious use of bicarbonate, high-carbohydrate diet with some restriction of protein and fat
Mitochondrial acetoacetyl-CoA thiolase deficiency	Branched chain amino acid metabolism disorders (Table: 22.1)		
Cytoplasmic acetoacetyl-CoA thiolase deficiency	Cytoplasmic acetoacetyl-CoA thiolase	ACAT2 (6q25.3-q26)	Biochemical profile: Nonspecific Clinical features: Intellectual disability, hypotonia Treatment: Not established

*Gene has been identified, and molecular basis has been elucidated.

Table 22.14	Other fat metabolism disorders		
Disease	Defective proteins or enzymes	Defective gene or genes (chromosomal location)	Comments
Sjögren-Larsson syndrome	Fatty aldehyde dehydrogenase	ALDH3A2 (17p11.2)*	Biochemical profile: No readily detectable plasma or urinary abnormality Clinical features: Ichthyosis, intellectual disability, spastic diplegia or tetraplegia, retinopathy, seizures Treatment: Symptomatic; topical keratolytics or systemic retinoids, reduced long-chain fat and increased medium-chain triglycerides in diet

*Gene has been identified, and molecular basis has been elucidated.

BETA-OXIDATION CYCLE DISORDERS

In these processes, there are numerous inherited defects, which typically manifest during fasting with hypoglycemia and acidosis; some cause cardiomyopathy and muscle weakness. Beta-oxidation cycle disorders (Table 22.15) are among the fatty acid and glycerol metabolism disorders.

Acetyl CoA is generated from fatty acids through repeated beta-oxidation cycles. Sets of four enzymes (an acyl dehydrogenase, a hydratase, a hydroxyacyl

Table 22.15	Fatty acid transport and mitochondrial oxidation disorders		
Disease	**Defective proteins or enzymes**	**Defective gene or genes (chromosomal location)**	**Comments**
Systemic primary carnitine deficiency	Plasma membrane carnitine transport OCTN2	SLC22A5 (5q31.1)*	Biochemical profile: High urinary carnitine excretion despite very low plasma carnitine, absence of significant dicarboxylic aciduria Clinical features: Hypoketotic hypoglycemia, fasting intolerance with hypotonia, depressed CNS, apnea, seizures, dilated cardiomyopathy, developmental delay Treatment: L-carnitine
Long-chain fatty acid transport deficiency	—	—	Biochemical profile: Low to normal free carnitine; during acute episodes, elevated plasma C8–C18 acylcarnitine esters Clinical features: Episodic acute liver failure, hyperammonemia, encephalopathy Treatment: Liver transplantation
Carnitine palmitoyl transferase I (CPT-I) deficiency	CPT-I	CPT1A (11q13)*	Biochemical profile: Normal to elevated total and free plasma carnitine, no dicarboxylic aciduria Clinical features: Fasting intolerance, hypoketotic hypoglycemia, hepatomegaly, seizures, coma, elevated creatine kinase Treatment: Avoidance of fasting; frequent feeding; during acute episodes, high-dose glucose; replacement of long-chain dietary fat with medium-chain fat
Carnitine/Acylcarnitine translocase deficiency	Carnitine/Acylcarnitine translocase	SLC25A20 (3p21.31)*	Biochemical profile: Low total plasma carnitine, with most conjugated to long-chain fatty acids; elevated C16 carnitine ester Clinical features: In the neonatal form, fasting intolerance with hypoglycemic coma, vomiting, weakness, cardiomyopathy, arrhythmia, mild hyperammonemia In the mild form, recurrent hypoglycemia with no cardiac involvement Treatment: Avoidance of fasting; frequent feeding; if plasma level is low, carnitine; during acute episodes, high-dose glucose
Carnitine palmitoyl transferase II (CPT-II) deficiency	CPT-II	CPTII (1p32)*	Biochemical profile: Elevated C16 carnitine ester In the classical muscle form, carnitine usually normal In the severe form, low total plasma carnitine, with most conjugated to long-chain fatty acids Clinical features: In the classical muscle form, presentation in adulthood with episodic myoglobinuria and weakness after prolonged exercise, fasting, intercurrent illness, or stress In the severe form, presentation in neonatal period or infancy with hypoketotic hypoglycemia, cardiomyopathy, arrhythmia, hepatomegaly, coma, or seizures Treatment: Avoidance of fasting; frequent feeding; if plasma level is low, carnitine; during acute episodes, high-dose glucose

Contd.

Table 22.15 | **Fatty acid transport and mitochondrial oxidation disorders** *(Contd.)*

Disease	Defective proteins or enzymes	Defective gene or genes (chromosomal location)	Comments
Very long-chain acyl-CoA dehydrogenase (VLCAD) deficiency	VLCAD	ACADVL (17p12-p11.1)*	Biochemical profile: Elevated saturated and unsaturated C14–C18 acylcarnitine esters, elevated urinary C6–C14 dicarboxylic acids Clinical features: In the VLCAD-C type, arrhythmia, hypertrophic cardiomyopathy, sudden death In the VLCAD-H type, recurrent hypoketotic hypoglycemia, encephalopathy, mild acidosis, mild hepatomegaly, hyperammonemia, elevated liver enzymes Treatment: Avoidance of fasting; high-carbohydrate diet; carnitine; medium-chain triglycerides; during acute episodes, high-dose glucose
Long-chain 3-hydroxyacyl-CoA dehydrogenase (LCHAD) deficiency	LCHAD	HADHA (2p23)*	Biochemical profile: Elevated saturated and unsaturated C16–C18 acylcarnitine esters, elevated urinary C6–C14 3-hydroxydicarboxylic acids Clinical features: Fasting-induced hypoketotic hypoglycemia, exercise-induced rhabdomyolysis, cardiomyopathy, cholestatic liver disease, retinopathy, maternal HELLP syndrome Treatment: Avoidance of fasting; high-carbohydrate diet; carnitine; medium-chain triglycerides; during acute episodes, high-dose glucose For retinopathy, docosahexanoic acid possibly useful
Mitochondrial trifunctional protein (TFP) deficiency	Mitochondrial TFP α-subunit β-subunit	 HADHA (2p23)* HADHB (2p23)*	Biochemical profile: Similar to LCHAD deficiency Clinical features: Liver failure, cardiomyopathy, fasting hypoglycemia, myopathy, sudden death Treatment: Similar to that for LCHAD deficiency
Medium-chain acyl-CoA dehydrogenase (MCAD) deficiency	MCAD	ACADM (1p31)*	Biochemical profile: Elevated saturated and unsaturated C8–C10 acylcarnitine esters; elevated urinary C6–C10 dicarboxylic acids, suberylglycine, and hexanoylglycine; low free carnitine Clinical features: Episodic hypoketotic hypoglycemia after fasting, vomiting, hepatomegaly, lethargy, coma, acidosis, SIDS, Reye-like syndrome Treatment: Avoidance of fasting; frequent feeding, including bedtime snacks; high-carbohydrate diet; carnitine; during acute episodes, high-dose glucose
Short-chain acyl-CoA dehydrogenase (SCAD) deficiency	SCAD	ACADS (12q22-qter)*	Biochemical profile: In the neonatal form, intermittent ethylmalonic aciduria In the chronic form, low muscle carnitine Clinical features: In the neonatal form, neonatal acidosis, vomiting, growth and developmental delay In the chronic form, progressive myopathy Treatment: Avoidance of fasting

Contd.

Table 22.15	Fatty acid transport and mitochondrial oxidation disorders (Contd.)		
Disease	Defective proteins or enzymes	Defective gene or genes (chromosomal location)	Comments
Glutaric aciduria type II	Electron transfer flavoprotein (ETF)	—	Biochemical profile: Elevated urinary ethylmalonic, glutaric, 2-hydroxyglutaric, 3-hydroxyisovaleric, and C6–C10 dicarboxylic acids and isovalerylglycine; elevated glutaryl carnitine, isovalerylcarnitine, and straight-chain acylcarnitine esters of C4, C8, C10, C10:1, and C12 fatty acids; low serum carnitine; increased serum sarcosine
	α-subunit	ETFA (15q23-q25)*	
	β-subunit	ETFB (19q13.3)*	
	ETF: ubiquinone oxidoreductase (ETF:QO)	ETFDH (4q32-qter)*	
			Clinical features: Fasting hypoketotic hypoglycemia, acidosis, sudden death, CNS anomalies, myopathy, possibly liver and cardiac involvement
			Treatment: Avoidance of fasting; frequent feeding; carnitine; riboflavin; during acute episodes, high-dose glucose
Short-chain 3-hydroxyacyl-CoA dehydrogenase (SCHAD) deficiency	SCHAD	HADHSC (4q22-q26)	Biochemical profile: Ketotic C8–C14 3-hydroxydicarboxylic aciduria
			Clinical features: Recurrent myoglobinuria, ketonuria, hypoglycemia, encephalopathy, cardiomyopathy
			Treatment: Avoidance of fasting
Short/Medium-chain 3-hydroxyacyl-CoA dehydrogenase (S/MCHAD) deficiency	S/MCHAD	—	Biochemical profile: Marked elevation of MCHADs and acylcarnitines
			Clinical features: Liver failure, encephalopathy
			Treatment: Avoidance of fasting
Medium-chain 3-ketoacyl-CoA thiolase (MCKAT) deficiency	MCKAT		Biochemical profile: Lactic aciduria, ketosis, elevated urinary C4–C12 dicarboxylic aciduria (especially C10 and C12)
			Clinical features: Fasting intolerance, vomiting, dehydration, metabolic acidosis, liver dysfunction, rhabdomyolysis
			Treatment: Avoidance of fasting
2,4-dienoyl-CoA reductase deficiency	2,4-Dienoyl-CoA reductase	DECR1 (8q21.3)*	Biochemical profile: Hyperlysinemia, low plasma carnitine, 2-trans,4-cis decadienoylcarnitine in plasma and urine
			Clinical features: Neonatal hypotonia, respiratory acidosis
			Treatment: Not established

*Gene has been identified, and molecular basis has been elucidated. HELLP, hemolysis, elevated liver enzymes, and low platelet count.

dehydrogenase, and a lyase) specific for different chain lengths (very long chain, long chain, medium chain, and short chain) are required to catabolize a long-chain fatty acid completely. Inheritance for all fatty acid oxidation defects is autosomal recessive.

Medium-chain Acyl-CoA Dehydrogenase Deficiency

Medium-chain acyl-CoA dehydrogenase deficiency (MCADD) is the most common defect in the β-oxidation cycle and has been incorporated into expanded neonatal screening in many states.

Clinical manifestations typically begin after 2–3 months of age and usually follow fasting (as little as 12 hours). Patients have vomiting and lethargy that may progress rapidly to seizures, coma, and sometimes death [which can also appear as sudden infant death syndrome (SIDS)]. During attacks, patients have hypoglycemia, hyperammonemia, and unexpectedly low urinary and serum ketones. Metabolic acidosis is often present but may be a late manifestation.

Diagnosis of MCADD is by detecting medium-chain fatty acid conjugates of carnitine in plasma or glycine in urine or by detecting enzyme deficiency in cultured fibroblasts; however, DNA testing can confirm most cases.

Treatment of acute attacks is with 10% dextrose IV at 1.5 times the fluid maintenance rate; some clinicians also advocate carnitine supplementation during acute episodes. Prevention is a low-fat, high-carbohydrate diet and avoidance of prolonged fasting. Cornstarch therapy is often used to provide a margin of safety during overnight fasting.

Long-chain 3-hydroxyacyl-CoA Dehydrogenase Deficiency

Long-chain 3-hydroxyacyl-CoA dehydrogenase deficiency (LCHADD) is the second most common fatty acid oxidation defect. It shares many features of MCADD, but patients may also have cardiomyopathy; rhabdomyolysis, massive creatine kinase elevations, and myoglobinuria with muscle exertion; peripheral neuropathy; and abnormal liver function. Mothers with an LCHADD fetus often have HELLP syndrome (hemolysis, elevated liver function tests, and low platelet count) during pregnancy.

Diagnosis of LCHADD is based on the presence of excess long-chain hydroxy acids on organic acid analysis and on the presence of their carnitine conjugates in an acylcarnitine profile or glycine conjugates in an acylglycine profile. LCHADD can be confirmed by enzyme study in skin fibroblasts.

Treatment during acute exacerbations includes hydration, high-dose glucose, bed rest, urine alkalinization, and carnitine supplementation. Long-term treatment includes a high-carbohydrate diet, medium-chain triglyceride supplementation, and avoidance of fasting and strenuous exercise.

Very Long-chain Acyl-CoA Dehydrogenase Deficiency

Very long-chain acyl-CoA dehydrogenase deficiency (VLCADD) is similar to LCHADD, but is commonly associated with significant cardiomyopathy.

GLUTARIC ACIDEMIA TYPE II

A defect in the transfer of electrons from the coenzyme of fatty acyl dehydrogenases to the electronic transport chain affects reactions involving fatty acids of all chain lengths (multiple acyl-coA dehydrogenase deficiency); oxidation of several amino acids is also affected.

Clinical manifestations thus include fasting hypoglycemia, severe metabolic acidosis, and hyperammonemia.

Diagnosis of glutaric acidemia type II is by increased ethylmalonic, glutaric, 2- and 3-hydroxyglutaric, and other dicarboxylic acids in organic acid analysis, and glutaryl and isovaleryl and other acylcarnitines in tandem mass spectrometry studies. Enzyme deficiencies in skin fibroblasts can be confirmatory.

Treatment of glutaric acidemia type II is similar to that for MCADD, except that riboflavin may be effective in some patients.

GLYCEROL METABOLISM DISORDERS

Glycerol is converted to glycerol-3-phosphate by the hepatic enzyme glycerol kinase; deficiency results in episodic vomiting, lethargy, and hypotonia. Glycerol metabolism disorders (Table 22.16) are among the fatty acid and glycerol metabolism disorders. Glycerol kinase deficiency is X-linked; many patients with this deficiency also have a chromosomal deletion that extends beyond

Table 22.16	Glycerol metabolism disorders		
Disease	Defective proteins or enzymes	Defective gene or genes (chromosomal location)	Comments
Glycerol kinase deficiency	Glycerol kinase	GK (xp21.3-p21.2)* (Complex form: Deletion of the GK gene and contiguous genes including congenital adrenal hypoplasia, Duchenne muscular dystrophy, or both Juvenile and adult forms: Isolated GK gene mutation)	Biochemical profile: Hyperglycerolemia Clinical features: In the complex form, symptoms of the juvenile form, in addition to those due to the specific gene or genes deleted In the juvenile form, episodic vomiting, acidosis, hypotonia, CNS depression, Reye-like syndrome In the adult form, pseudohypertriglyceridemia Treatment: Low-fat diet, avoidance of prolonged fasting
Glycerol intolerance syndrome	—	—	Biochemical profile: Hypoglycemia, ketonuria, reports of decreased activity of fructose-1, 6-biphosphatase and increased sensitivity of this enzyme to the inhibition of glycerol-3-phosphate Clinical features: History of prematurity; after exposure to glycerol, hypoglycemia, lethargy, sweating, seizure, coma Treatment: Low-fat diet

*Gene has been identified, and molecular basis has been elucidated.

the glycerol kinase gene into the contiguous gene region, which contains the genes for congenital adrenal hypoplasia and Duchenne muscular dystrophy. Thus, patients with glycerol kinase deficiency may have one or more of these disease entities.

Symptoms of glycerol metabolism disorders begin at any age and are usually accompanied by acidosis, hypoglycemia, and elevated blood and urine levels of glycerol.

Diagnosis of glycerol metabolism disorders is by detecting an elevated level of glycerol in serum and urine and is confirmed by DNA analysis. Glycerol metabolism disorder treatment is with a low-fat diet, but glucocorticoid replacement is critical for patients with adrenal hypoplasia.

LYSOSOMAL STORAGE DISORDERS

Lysosomal enzymes break down macromolecules, either those from the cell itself (e.g. when cellular structural components are being recycled) or those acquired outside the cell. Inherited defects or deficiencies of lysosomal enzymes (or other lysosomal components) can result in accumulation of undegraded metabolites. Because there are numerous specific deficiencies, storage diseases are usually grouped biochemically by the accumulated metabolite. Subgroups include mucopolysaccharidoses, sphingolipidoses (lipidoses), and mucolipidoses.

The most important are the mucopolysaccharidoses and sphingolipidoses. Type 2 glycogenosis is a lysosomal storage disorder, but most glycogenoses are not. Because reticuloendothelial cells (e.g. in the spleen) are rich in lysosomes, reticuloendothelial tissues are involved in a number of lysosomal storage disorders, but, generally, tissues richest in the substrate are most affected. Thus, the brain, which is rich in gangliosides, is particularly affected by gangliosidoses, whereas mucopolysaccharidoses affect many tissues because mucopolysaccharides are present throughout the body.

MUCOPOLYSACCHARIDOSIS

Mucopolysaccharidosis (MPS) are inherited deficiencies of enzymes involved in glycosaminoglycan breakdown. Glycosaminoglycans (previously termed mucopolysaccharides) are polysaccharides abundant on cell surfaces and in extracellular matrix and structures. Enzyme deficiencies that prevent glycosaminoglycan breakdown cause accumulation of glycosaminoglycan fragments in lysosomes and cause extensive bone, soft tissue, and CNS changes. Inheritance is usually autosomal recessive (except for MPS type II).

Age at presentation, clinical manifestations, and severity vary by type (Table 22.17). Common manifestations include coarse facial features, neurodevelopmental delays and regression, joint contractures, organomegaly,

Table 22.17	Mucopolysaccharidosis		
Disease	Defective proteins or enzymes	Defective gene or genes (chromosomal location)	Comments
MPS I-H MPS I-S MPS I H/S	α-l-Iduronidase	IDUA (4p16.3)*	Onset: In I-H, first year In I-S, > 5 years In I-H/S, 3-8 years Urine metabolites: Dermatan sulfate, heparin sulfate Clinical features: Corneal clouding, stiff joints, contractures, dysostosis multiplex, coarse facies, coarse hair, macroglossia, organomegaly, intellectual disability with regression, valvular heart disease, hearing and vision impairment, inguinal and umbilical hernia, sleep apnea, hydrocephalus Treatment: Supportive care, enzyme replacement, stem cell or bone marrow transplantation
MPS II	Iduronate sulfate sulfatase	IDS (Xq28)*	Onset: 2–4 years Urine metabolites: Dermatan sulfate, heparin sulfate Clinical features: Similar to Hurler syndrome but milder and no corneal clouding In mild form, normal intelligence In severe form, progressive intellectual and physical disability, death before age 15 Treatment: Supportive care, stem cell or bone marrow transplantation

Contd.

Table 22.17	Mucopolysaccharidosis (Contd.)		
Disease	Defective proteins or enzymes	Defective gene or genes (chromosomal location)	Comments
MPS III			Onset: 2–6 years
Type III-A	Heparan-S-sulfate sulfamidase	SGSH (17q25.3)*	Urine metabolites: Heparin sulfate
Type III-B	N-acetyl-D-glucosaminidase	NAGLU (17q21)*	Clinical features: Similar to Hurler syndrome but with severe intellectual disability and mild somatic manifestations
Type III-C	Acetyl-CoA-glucosaminide N-acetyltransferase	(14)	
Type III-D	N-acetyl-glucosaminine-6-sulfate sulfatase	GNS (12q14)*	Treatment: Supportive care
MPS IV (Morquio syndrome)			Onset: 1–4 year
Type IV-A	Galactosamine-6-sulfate sulfatase	GALNS (16q24.3)*	Urine metabolites: Keratin sulfate; in IV-B, also chondroitin 6-sulfate
Type IV-B	β-galactosidase	GLB1 (Table 22.18)	Clinical features: Similar to Hurler syndrome but with severe bone changes including odontoid hypoplasia; possibly normal intelligence
			Treatment: Supportive care
			For type IV-A, enzyme replacement therapy with elosulfase alfa
MPS VI	N-acetyl galactosamine α-4-sulfate sulfatase (arylsulfatase B)	ARSB (5q11-q13)*	Onset: Variable but can be similar to Hurler syndrome
			Urine metabolites: Dermatan sulfate
			Clinical features: Similar to Hurler syndrome but normal intelligence
			Treatment: Supportive care
MPS VII	β-glucuronidase	GUSB (7q21.11)*	Onset: 1–4 years
			Urine metabolites: Dermatan sulfate, heparin sulfate, chondroitin 4-, 6-sulfate
			Clinical features: Similar to Hurler syndrome but greater variation in severity
			Treatment: Supportive care, stem cell or bone marrow transplantation
MPS IX	Hyaluronidase deficiency	HYAL1 (3p21.3-p21.2)*	Onset: 6 months
			Urine metabolites: None
			Clinical features: Bilateral soft-tissue periarticular masses, dysmorphic features, short stature, normal intelligence
			Treatment: Not established

*Gene has been identified, and molecular basis has been elucidated.

stiff hair, progressive respiratory insufficiency (caused by airway obstruction and sleep apnea), cardiac valvular disease, skeletal changes, and cervical vertebral subluxation.

Diagnosis of mucopolysaccharidoses is suggested by history, physical examination, and bone abnormalities (e.g., dysostosis multiplex) found during skeletal survey, and elevated total and fractionated urinary glycosaminoglycans. Diagnosis is confirmed by enzyme analysis of cultured fibroblasts (prenatal) or peripheral WBCs (postnatal). Additional testing is required to monitor organ-specific changes (e.g. echocardiography for valvular disease, audiometry for hearing changes).

Treatment of MPS type I (Hurler disease) is enzyme replacement with α-l-iduronidase, which effectively halts progression and reverses all non-CNS complications of the disease. Hematopoietic stem cell (HSC) transplantation has also been used. The combination of enzyme replacement and HSC transplantation is under study. For patients with MPS type IV-A (Morquio A syndrome), enzyme replacement with elosulfase alfa may improve functional status, including mobility.

SPHINGOLIPIDOSES

Sphingolipids are normal lipid components of cell membranes; they accumulate in lysosomes and cause extensive neuronal, bone, and other changes when enzyme deficiencies prevent their breakdown. Although incidence is low, carrier rate of some forms is high. There are many types of sphingolipidosis (Table 22.18); the most common sphingolipidosis is Gaucher disease; others sphingolipidoses include cholesteryl ester storage disease, Fabry disease, Krabbe disease, metachromatic leukodystrophy, Niemann-Pick disease, Sandhoff disease, Tay-Sachs disease, and Wolman disease.

Table 22.18	Sphingolipidosis		
Disease	Defective proteins or enzymes	Defective gene or genes (chromosomal location)	Comments
GM1 gangliosidosis, generalized Type I	Ganglioside β-galactosidase	GLB1 (3p21.33*; allelic to to MPS IVB)	— Type I onset: 0–6 months Urine metabolites: None Clinical features: Coarse facies; clear cornea, cherry-red macular spot, gingival hyperplasia, organomegaly, dysostosis multiplex, hypertrichosis, angiokeratoma corporis diffusum, cerebral degeneration; death in infancy Treatment: Supportive care
Type II (juvenile type)			Type II onset: 6–12 months Urine metabolites: None Clinical features: Gait disturbance, spasticity, dystonia, loss of psychomotor milestones, mild visceromegaly and bone abnormality Treatment: Supportive care
Type III (adult type)			Type III onset: 3–50 years Urine metabolites: None Clinical features: Angiokeratoma corporis diffusum, spondyloepiphyseal dysplasia, dysarthria, cerebellar dysfunction; no macular red spots or visceromegaly Treatment: Supportive care
GM2 gangliosidosis Type I (Tay-Sachs disease) Type II (Sandhoff disease) Type III (juvenile type)	β-hexosaminidase A β-hexosaminidase B β-hexosaminidase A	HEXA (15q23-q24)* HEXB (5q13)* —	Onset: In types I and II, 5–6 months In type III, 2–6 years Urine metabolites: None Clinical features:Doll-like facies; cherry-red retina; early blindness; exaggerated startle reflex; initial hypotonia followed by hypertonia; psychomotor retardation followed by regression, seizures, and impaired sweating; death by age 5 years In type I, increased frequency in Ashkenazi Jews Treatment: Supportive care
GM2 activator protein deficiency (Tay-Sachs disease AB variant, GM2A)	GM2 activator protein	GM2A (5q31.3-q33.1)*	Treatment: Supportive care, stem cell or bone marrow transplantation Same as that for GM2 types I and II
Niemann-Pick disease Type A	Sphingomyelinase	SMPD1 (11p15.4-p15.1)*	Onset:< 6 months Clinical features: Growth delay, cherry-red retina, frequent respiratory infections, hepatosplenomegaly, vomiting, constipation, osteoporosis, lymphadenopathy, hypotonia followed by spasticity, sea-blue histiocytes on tissue biopsies, large vacuolated foam cells in bone marrow (NP cells), death by age 3 years Treatment: Supportive care, stem cell or bone marrow transplantation

Contd.

Table 22.18	Sphingolipidosis *(Contd.)*		
Disease	**Defective proteins or enzymes**	**Defective gene or genes (chromosomal location)**	**Comments**
Type B			Onset: Variable
			Clinical features: Much milder symptoms, no neurologic involvement, survival to adulthood
			Increased frequency in ashkenazi Jews
			Treatment: Supportive care, stem cell or bone marrow transplantation
Gaucher disease Type I (adult or chronic form)	Glucosylceramide β-glucosidase	GBA (1q21)*	Onset: Childhood or adolescence
			Urine metabolites: None
			Clinical features: Hepatosplenomegaly, osteolytic lesions with bone pain, avascular necrosis of the femoral head, vertebral compression, thrombocytopenia, anemia
			Increased frequency in Ashkenazi Jews
			Treatment: Supportive care
			Splenectomy
			Enzyme replacement (eliglustat)
			Bone marrow or stem cell transplantation
Type II (infantile form)			Onset: Infancy
			Urine metabolites: None
			Clinical features: Infantile hydrops, hepatosplenomegaly, dysphagia, bone lesions, hypertonicity, pseudobulbar palsy, laryngeal spasm, ichthyosis, developmental delay, hypersplenism, death by age 2 years
			Treatment: Supportive care
Type III (juvenile form, Norrbottnian type)			Onset: 4–8 years
			Urine metabolites: None
			Clinical features: Similar to type II except milder, possible survival into adulthood
			Treatment: Supportive care
Farber disease (lipogranulomatosis)	Ceramidase	ASAH (8p22-p21.3)*	Onset: First weeks of life
			Urine metabolites: Ceramide
			Clinical features: Lipogranulomatosis, periarticular subcutaneous nodules, irritability, hoarse cry, psychomotor and growth delay, respiratory insufficiency, histiocytosis in multiple tissues, nephropathy, hepatosplenomegaly, cherry-red macular spot
			Milder variants sometimes divided into seaven subtypes according to severity
			Treatment: Supportive care
Fabry disease	Trihexosylceramide α-galactosidase	GLA (Xq22)*	Onset: Childhood or Adolescence
			Urine metabolites: Globosylceramide
			Clinical features: Painful crisis involving extremities and abdomen precipitated by stress, fatigue, or exercise; angiokeratoma; growth and pubertal delay; corneal dystrophy; renal failure; cardiomyopathy; MI and heart failure, hypertension; lymphedema; obstructive lung disease; strokes; seizures; death
			Generally, only males affected but occasionally females
			Treatment: Supportive care, enzyme replacement

Contd.

Table 22.18	Sphingolipidosis *(Contd.)*		
Disease	**Defective proteins or enzymes**	**Defective gene or genes (chromosomal location)**	**Comments**
Metachromatic leukodystrophy • Late infantile form • Juvenile form • Adult form • Pseudodeficiency form	Arylsulfatase A	ARSA (22q13.31)*	Onset: For late infantile form, 1–2 years For juvenile form, 4 years to puberty For adult form, any age after puberty Urine metabolites: Sulfatides Clinical features: Optic atrophy, gallbladder dysfunction, urinary incontinence, hypotonia, gait disturbance, hyporeflexia followed by hyperreflexia, bulbar palsies, ataxia, chorea, demyelination and developmental regression, increased CSF protein In adult form, also schizophrenia-like symptoms pseudodeficiency characterized by mild decrease in enzyme activity without neurologic degeneration Treatment: Supportive care, consideration of bone marrow or stem cell transplantation
Mucosulfatidosis (multiple sulfatase deficiency)	Sulfatase-modifying factor-1	SUMF1 (3p26)*	Onset: Infancy Urine metabolites: Sulfatides, mucopolysaccharides Clinical features: Similar to late infantile form of metachromatic leukodystrophy, plus ichthyosis and dysostosis multiplex Treatment: Supportive care
Krabbe disease • Infantile form • Late infantile form • Juvenile form • Adult form	Galactosylceramide β-galactosidase	GALC (14q31)*	Onset: In infantile form, 3–6 months In late infantile and juvenile forms, 15 months–17 years In adult form, variable Urine metabolites: None Clinical features: Growth delay, developmental delay followed by regression, deafness, blindness, vomiting, hyperirritability, hypersensitivity to stimuli, increased deep-tendon reflex, and spasticity; seizures; diffuse cerebral atrophy and demyelination; elevated CSF protein; peripheral neuropathy; episodic fever In adult form, mentation generally preserved Treatment: Supportive care, bone marrow or stem cell transplantation
Sphingolipid activator protein deficiencies			Onset: Infancy to early childhood Urine metabolites: Sulfatides
Prosaposin deficiency	Prosaposin	PSAP (10q22.1)*	Clinical features: In saposin B deficiency, features similar to those of metachromatic leukodystrophy
Saposin B deficiency (sulfatide activator deficiency)	Saposin B	PSAP (10q22.1)*	In saposin C deficiency, features similar to those of Gaucher disease type III
Saposin C deficiency (Gaucher activator deficiency)	Saposin C	PSAP (10q22.1)*	In prosaposin deficiency, features of saposin B and C deficiencies Treatment: Supportive care; consideration of bone marrow or stem cell transplantation; for features of Gaucher disease, consideration of enzyme replacement

*Gene has been identified, and molecular basis has been elucidated.
MPS, mucopolysaccharidosis.

CHOLESTERYL ESTER STORAGE DISEASE

Cholesteryl ester storage disease is less severe and may not manifest until later in life, even adulthood, at which time hepatomegaly may be detected; premature atherosclerosis, often severe, may develop.

Diagnosis is based on clinical features and detection of acid lipase deficiency in liver biopsy specimens or cultured skin fibroblasts, lymphocytes, or other tissues. Prenatal diagnosis is based on the absence of acid lipase activity in cultured chorionic villi. (Also see testing for suspected inherited disorders of metabolism.)

There is no proven treatment, but statins reduce plasma low-density lipoprotein (LDL) levels, and cholestyramine combined with a low-cholesterol diet has reportedly alleviated other signs.

FABRY DISEASE

Fabry disease is a sphingolipidosis, an inherited disorder of metabolism, caused by deficiency of α-galactosidase A, which causes angiokeratomas, acroparesthesias, corneal opacities, recurrent febrile episodes, and renal or heart failure. Fabry disease is an X-linked deficiency of the lysosomal enzyme α-galactosidase A, which is needed for normal trihexosylceramide catabolism. Glycolipid (globotriaosylceramide) accumulates in many tissues (e.g. vascular endothelium, lymph vessels, heart, and kidney).

Diagnosis in males is clinical, based on appearance of typical skin lesions (angiokeratomas) over the lower trunk and by characteristic features of peripheral neuropathy (causing recurrent burning pain in the extremities), corneal opacities, and recurrent febrile episodes. Death results from renal failure or cardiac or cerebral complications of hypertension or other vascular disease. Heterozygous females are usually asymptomatic but may have an attenuated form of disease often characterized by corneal opacities.

Diagnosis of Fabry disease is by assay of galactosidase activity prenatally in amniocytes or chorionic villi and postnatally in serum or WBCs.

Treatment of Fabry disease is enzyme replacement with recombinant α-galactosidase A (agalsidase beta) combined with supportive measures for fever and pain. Kidney transplantation is effective for treating renal failure.

GAUCHER DISEASE

Gaucher disease is a sphingolipidosis, an inherited disorder of metabolism, resulting from glucocerebrosidase deficiency, causing deposition of glucocerebroside and related compounds. Symptoms and signs vary by type but are most commonly. Glucocerebrosidase normally hydrolyzes glucocerebroside to glucose and ceramide. Genetic defects of the enzyme cause glucocerebroside accumulation in tissue macrophages through phagocytosis, forming Gaucher cells. Accumulation of Gaucher cells in the perivascular spaces in the brain causes gliosis in the neuronopathic forms. There are 3 types, which vary in epidemiology, enzyme activity, and manifestations.

Type I (non-neuronopathic) is most common (90% of all patients). Residual enzyme activity is highest. Ashkenazi Jews are at greatest risk; 1/12 is a carrier. Onset ranges from age 2 years to late adulthood. Symptoms and signs include splenohepatomegaly, bone disease (e.g. osteopenia, pain crises, and osteolytic lesions with fractures), growth failure, delayed puberty, ecchymoses, and pingueculae. Epistaxis and ecchymoses resulting from thrombocytopenia are common. X-rays show flaring of the ends of the long bones (Erlenmeyer flask deformity) and cortical thinning.

Type II (acute neuronopathic) is rarest, and residual enzyme activity in this type is lowest. Onset occurs during infancy. Symptoms and signs are progressive neurologic deterioration (e.g. rigidity, seizures) and death by age 2 years.

Type III (subacute neuronopathic) falls between types I and II in incidence, enzyme activity, and clinical severity. Onset occurs at any time during childhood. Clinical manifestations vary by subtype and include progressive dementia and ataxia (IIIa), bone and visceral involvement (IIIb), and supranuclear palsies with corneal opacities (IIIc). Patients who survive to adolescence may live for many years.

Diagnosis

Diagnosis of Gaucher disease is by enzyme analysis of WBCs. Carriers are detected, and types are distinguished by mutation analysis. Although, biopsy is unnecessary, Gaucher cells lipid-laden tissue macrophages in the liver, spleen, lymph nodes, bone marrow, or brain that have a wrinkled tissuepaper appearance; are diagnostic. DNA analysis is being done more and more frequently.

Treatment

Enzyme replacement with IV glucocerebrosidase is effective in types I and III; there is no treatment for type II. The enzyme is modified for efficient delivery to lysosomes. Patients receiving enzyme replacement require routine Hb and platelet monitoring, routine assessment of spleen and liver volume by CT or MRI, and routine assessment of bone disease by skeletal survey, dual-energy X-ray absorptiometry scanning, or MRI.

Miglustat (100 mg by mouth three times a day), a glucosylceramide synthase inhibitor, reduces glucocerebroside concentration (the substrate for glucocerebrosidase) and is an alternative for patients unable to receive enzyme replacement.

Eliglustat (84 mg by mouth once a day or bid), another glucosylceramide synthase inhibitor, also reduces glucocerebroside concentration.

Splenectomy may be helpful for patients with anemia, leukopenia, or thrombocytopenia or when spleen size causes discomfort. Patients with anemia may also need blood transfusions. Bone marrow transplantation or stem cell transplantation provides a definitive cure but is considered a last resort because of substantial morbidity and mortality.

KRABBE DISEASE

Krabbe disease is a sphingolipidosis, an inherited disorder of metabolism that causes intellectual disability, paralysis, blindness, deafness, and pseudobulbar palsy, progressing to death. Krabbe disease is caused by an autosomal recessive galactocerebroside β-galactosidase deficiency. It affects infants and is characterized by intellectual disability, paralysis, blindness, deafness, and pseudobulbar palsy, progressing to death.

Diagnosis of Krabbe disease is by detecting enzyme deficiency in WBCs or cultured skin fibroblasts. Because bone marrow transplantation effectively delays onset of symptoms, prenatal testing or neonatal screening is sometimes done.

METACHROMATIC LEUKODYSTROPHY

Metachromatic leukodystrophy is a sphingolipidosis, an inherited disorder of metabolism, caused by arylsulfatase A deficiency, which causes progressive paralysis and dementia resulting in death by age of 10 years. In metachromatic leukodystrophy, arylsulfatase A deficiency causes metachromatic lipids to accumulate in the white matter of the CNS, peripheral nerves, kidney, spleen, and other visceral organs; accumulation in the nervous system causes central and peripheral demyelination. Numerous mutations exist; patients vary in age at onset and speed of progression.

The infantile form is characterized by progressive paralysis and dementia usually beginning before age of 4 years and resulting in death about 5 years after onset of symptoms.

The juvenile form manifests between 4 years and 16 years of age with gait disturbance, intellectual impairment, and findings of peripheral neuropathy. Contrary to the infantile form, deep tendon reflexes are usually brisk. There is also a milder adult form.

Diagnosis of metachromatic leukodystrophy is suggested clinically and by findings of decreased nerve conduction velocity; it is confirmed by detecting enzyme deficiency in WBCs or cultured skin fibroblasts. There is no effective treatment for metachromatic leukodystrophy.

Tay-Sachs Disease and Sandhoff Disease

Tay-Sachs disease and Sandhoff disease are sphingolipidoses, inherited disorders of metabolism, caused by hexosaminidase deficiency that causes severe neurologic symptoms and early death.

Gangliosides are complex sphingolipids present in the brain. There are two major forms, GM1 (monosialotetrahexosylganglioside) and GM2, both of which may be involved in lysosomal storage disorders; there are two main types of GM2 gangliosidosis, each of which can be caused by numerous different mutations.

Tay-Sachs Disease

Deficiency of hexosaminidase A results in accumulation of GM2 in the brain. Inheritance is autosomal recessive; the most common mutations are carried by 1/27 normal adults of Eastern European (Ashkenazi) Jewish origin, although other mutations cluster in some French-Canadian and Cajun populations.

Children with Tay-Sachs disease start missing developmental milestones after age 6 months and develop progressive cognitive and motor deterioration resulting in seizures, intellectual disability, paralysis, and death by age 5 years. A cherry-red macular spot is common. Diagnosis of Tay-Sachs disease is clinical and can be confirmed by enzyme assay. In the absence of effective treatment, management is focused on screening adults of childbearing age in high-risk populations to identify carriers (by way of enzyme activity and mutation testing) combined with genetic counseling.

Sandhoff Disease

There is a combined hexosaminidase A and B deficiency. Clinical manifestations include progressive cerebral degeneration beginning at 6 months, accompanied by blindness, cherry-red macular spot, and hyperacusis. It is almost indistinguishable from Tay-Sachs disease in course, diagnosis, and management, except that there is visceral involvement (hepatomegaly and bone change) and no ethnic association.

PURINE AND PYRIMIDINE METABOLISM DISORDERS

Purines are key components of cellular energy systems (e.g. ATP, NAD), signaling (e.g. GTP, cAMP, cGMP), and, along with pyrimidines, RNA and DNA production. Purines and pyrimidines may be synthesized de novo or recycled by a salvage pathway from normal catabolism. The end product of complete catabolism of purines is uric acid.

Purine Catabolism Disorders

In addition to purine catabolism disorders, purine metabolism disorders (Table 22.19) include purine nucleotide synthesis disorders and purine salvage disorders.

Myoadenylate Deaminase Deficiency (or Muscle Adenosine Monophosphate Deaminase Deficiency)

The enzyme myoadenylate deaminase converts AMP to inosine and ammonia. Deficiency may be asymptomatic or it may cause exercise-induced myalgias or cramping; expression seems to be variable because, despite the high frequency of the mutant allele (10–14%), the frequency of the muscle phenotype is quite low in patients homozygous for the mutant allele. When symptomatic patients exercise, they do not accumulate ammonia or inosine monophosphate as do unaffected people; this is how the disorder is diagnosed.

Table 22.19 Purine metabolism disorders

Disease	Defective proteins or enzymes	Defective gene or genes (chromosomal location)	Comments
Ca pyrophosphate arthropathy	Increased nucleoside triphosphate pyrophosphohydrolase	ANKH (5p15.2-p14.1)*	Biochemical profile: Ca pyrophosphate dihydrate crystals in joints Clinical features: Recurrent episodes of mono-articular or multiarticular arthritis Treatment: No clear treatment
Lesch-Nyhan syndrome • Classic form • Variant form	Hypoxanthine-guanine phosphoribosyltransferase	HPRT (Xq26-q27.2)*	Biochemical profile: Hyperuricemia, hyperuricosuria Clinical features: Orange sandy crystals in diapers, growth failure, uric acid nephropathy and arthropathy, motor delay, hypotonia, self-injurious behavior, spasticity, hyperreflexia, extrapyramidal signs with choreoathetosis, dysarthria, dysphagia, developmental disabilities, megaloblastic anemia In variant form, no self-injurious behavior Treatment: Supportive care, protective measures, allopurinol, benzodiazepines, certain experimental approaches
Increased activity of phosphoribosylpyrophosphate synthetase	Phosphoribosylpyrophosphate synthetase	PRPS1 (Xq22-q24)*	Biochemical profile: Hyperuricemia Clinical features: Megaloblastic bone marrow, ataxia, hypotonia, hypertonia, psychomotor delay, polyneuropathy, cardiomyopathy, heart failure, uric acid nephropathy and arthropathy, diabetes mellitus, intracerebral calcification Treatment: Allopurinol, anti-inflammatory drugs, colchicines, probenecid, sulfinpyrazone
Phosphoribosylpyrophosphate synthetase deficiency	Phosphoribosylpyrophosphate synthetase	PRPS1 (Xq22-q24) PRPS2 (Xp22.3-p22.2)	Biochemical profile: Increased urinary orotate, hypouricemia Clinical features: Developmental disabilities, seizures with hypsarrhythmia, megaloblastic bone marrow Treatment: ACTH
Hereditary xanthinuria Type I Type II	Xanthine dehydrogenase Xanthine dehydrogenase and aldehyde oxidase	XDH (2p23-p22)*	Biochemical profile: Xanthinuria, hypouricemia, hypouricosuria Clinical features: Xanthine stones, nephropathy, myopathy Treatment: High fluid intake; low-purine diet
Adenine phosphoribosyltransferase deficiency Type I Type II	Adenine phosphoribosyltransferase No enzyme activity Residual enzyme activity	APRT (16q24.3)*	Biochemical profile: Urinary 2, 8-dihydroxyadenine Clinical features: Urolithiasis, nephropathy, round yellow-brown urine crystals Treatment: High fluid intake, low-purine diet, avoidance of dietary alkalis, renal transplantation

Contd.

Table 22.19	Purine metabolism disorders (Contd.)		
Disease	**Defective proteins or enzymes**	**Defective gene or genes (chromosomal location)**	**Comments**
Adenosine deaminase deficiency	Adenosine deaminase	ADA (20q13.11)*	Biochemical profile: Elevated serum adenosine and 2'-deoxyadenosine Clinical features: Growth failure, skeletal changes, recurrent infections, severe combined immunodeficiency, B-cell lymphoma, hemolytic anemia, idiopathic thrombocytopenia, hepatosplenomegaly, mesangial sclerosis Treatment: Supportive care, enzyme replacement, bone marrow or stem cell transplantation, experimental gene therapy
Increased adenosine deaminase	Adenosine deaminase	ADA	Biochemical profile: Mild hyperuricemia Clinical features: Hemolytic anemia with anisopoikilocytosis and stomatocytosis Treatment: Deoxycoformycin
Purine nucleoside phosphorylase deficiency	Purine nucleoside phosphorylase	NP (14q13.1)*	Biochemical profile: Hypouricemia; hypouricosuria; high serum inosine and guanine; high urinary inosine, 2'-deoxyinosine, and 2'-deodyguanosine Clinical features: Growth failure, cellular immunodeficiency, recurrent infections, hepatosplenomegaly, cerebral vasculitis, spastic diplegia, tetraparesis, ataxia, tremors, hypotonia, hypertonia, developmental disabilities, autoimmune hemolytic anemia, idiopathic thrombocytopenia, lymphoma, lymphosarcoma Treatment: Supportive care, stem cell transplantation
Myoadenylate deaminase deficiency	Myoadenylate deaminase	AMPD1 (1p21-p13)*	Biochemical profile: No specific change Clinical features: Neonatal weakness and hypotonia; exercise-induced weakness or cramping; after exercise, decreased purine release and low increase in serum ammonia (relative to lactate) Treatment: Ribose or xylitol
Adenylate kinase deficiency	Adenylate kinase	AK1 (9q34.1)*	Biochemical profile: No specific change Clinical features: Hemolytic anemia Treatment: Supportive care
Adenylosuccinate lyase deficiency • Type I (severe form) • Type II (mild form)	Adenylosuccinate lyase	ADSL (22Q13.1)*	Biochemical profile: Elevated succinyladenosine and succinylaminoimidazole carboxamide ribotides in body fluids Clinical features: Autism, severe psychomotor delay, seizures, growth delay, muscle wasting Treatment: Supportive care, adenine, and ribose

*Gene has been identified, and molecular basis has been elucidated.

Treatment of myoadenylate deaminase deficiency is exercise modulation as appropriate.

ADENOSINE DEAMINASE DEFICIENCY

Adenosine deaminase converts adenosine and deoxyadenosine to inosine and deoxyinosine, which are further broken down and excreted. Enzyme deficiency (from 1 of >60 known mutations) results in accumulation of adenosine, which is converted to its ribonucleotide and deoxyadenosine triphosphate forms by cellular kinases. The dATP increase results in inhibition of ribonucleotide reductase and underproduction of other deoxyribonucleotides. DNA replication is compromised as a result. Immune cells are especially sensitive to this defect;

adenosine deaminase deficiency causes one form of severe combined immunodeficiency. Diagnosis of adenosine deaminase deficiency is by low RBC and WBC enzyme activity.

Treatment of adenosine deaminase deficiency is by bone marrow or stem cell transplantation and enzyme replacement therapy. Somatic cell gene therapy is being evaluated as well.

PURINE NUCLEOSIDE PHOSPHORYLASE DEFICIENCY

This rare, autosomal recessive deficiency is characterized by immunodeficiency with severe T-cell dysfunction and often neurologic symptoms. Manifestations are lymphopenia, thymic deficiency, recurrent infections, and hypouricemia. Many patients have developmental delay, ataxia, or spasticity. Diagnosis of purine nucleoside phosphorylase deficiency is by low enzyme activity in RBCs. Treatment is with bone marrow or stem cell transplantation.

Xanthine Oxidase Deficiency

Xanthine oxidase is the enzyme that catalyzes uric acid production from xanthine and hypoxanthine. Deficiency causes buildup of xanthine, which may precipitate in the urine, causing symptomatic stones with hematuria, urinary colic, and UTIs.

Diagnosis of xanthine oxidase deficiency is by low serum uric acid and high urine and plasma hypoxanthine and xanthine. Enzyme determination requires liver or intestinal mucosal biopsy and is rarely indicated. Treatment of xanthine oxidase deficiency is high fluid intake to minimize likelihood of stone formation and allopurinol in some patients.

Purine Nucleotide Synthesis Disorders

Phosphoribosylpyrophosphate Synthetase Superactivity

This X-linked, recessive disorder causes purine overproduction. Excess purine is degraded, resulting in hyperuricemia and gout and neurologic and developmental abnormalities. Diagnosis of phosphoribosylpyrophosphate synthetase superactivity is by enzyme studies on RBCs and cultured skin fibroblasts. Phosphoribosylpyrophosphate synthetase superactivity treatment is with allopurinol and a low-purine diet.

Adenylosuccinase Deficiency

This autosomal recessive disorder causes profound intellectual disability, autistic behavior, and seizures. Diagnosis of adenylosuccinase deficiency is by identifying elevated levels of succinylaminoimidazole carboxamide riboside and succinyladenosine in CSF and urine. There is no effective treatment for adenylosuccinase deficiency.

Lesch-Nyhan Syndrome

This is a rare, X-linked, recessive disorder caused by deficiency of hypoxanthine-guanine phosphoribosyl transferase (HPRT); degree of deficiency (and hence manifestations) vary with the specific mutation. HPRT deficiency results in failure of the salvage pathway for hypoxanthine and guanine. These purines are instead degraded to uric acid. Additionally, a decrease in inositol monophosphate and guanosyl monophosphate leads to an increase in conversion of 5-phosphoribosyl-1-pyrophosphate (PRPP) to 5-phosphoribosylamine, which further exacerbates uric acid overproduction. Hyperuricemia predisposes to gout and its complications. Patients also have a number of cognitive and behavioral dysfunctions, etiology of which is unclear; they do not seem related to uric acid.

The disease usually manifests between 3 months and 12 months of age with the appearance of orange sandy precipitate (xanthine) in the urine; it progresses to CNS involvement with intellectual disability, spastic cerebral palsy, involuntary movements, and self-mutilating behavior (particularly biting). Later, chronic hyperuricemia causes symptoms of gout (e.g. urolithiasis, nephropathy, gouty arthritis, tophi).

Diagnosis of Lesch-Nyhan syndrome is suggested by the combination of dystonia, intellectual disability, and self-mutilation. Serum uric acid levels are usually elevated, but confirmation by HPRT enzyme assay is usually done.

CNS dysfunction has no known treatment; management is supportive. Self-mutilation may require physical restraint, dental extraction, and sometimes drug therapy; a variety of drugs has been used. Hyperuricemia is treated with a low-purine diet (e.g. avoiding organ meats, beans, sardines) and allopurinol, a xanthine oxidase inhibitor (the last enzyme in the purine catabolic pathway). Allopurinol prevents conversion of accumulated hypoxanthine to uric acid; because hypoxanthine is highly soluble, it is excreted.

Adenine Phosphoribosyltransferase Deficiency

This is a rare autosomal recessive disorder that results in the inability to salvage adenine for purine synthesis. Accumulated adenine is oxidized to 2, 8-dihyroxyadenine, which precipitates in the urinary tract, causing problems similar to those of uric acid nephropathy (e.g. renal colic, frequent infections, and, if diagnosed late, renal failure). Onset can occur at any age.

Diagnosis of adenine phosphoribosyl transferase deficiency is by detecting elevated levels of 2, 8-dihyroxyadenine, 8-hyroxyadenine, and adenine in urine and confirmed by enzyme assay; serum uric acid is normal.

Treatment of adenine phosphoribosyl transferase deficiency is with dietary purine restriction, high fluid intake, and avoidance of urine alkalinization. Allopurinol can prevent oxidation of adenine; renal transplantation may be needed for end-stage renal disease.

Pyrimidine Metabolism Disorders

Pyrimidines may be synthesized de novo or recycled by a salvage pathway from normal catabolism. The catabolism of pyrimidines produces citric acid cycle intermediates. There are several disorders of pyrimidine metabolism (Table 22.20).

URIDINE MONOPHOSPHATE SYNTHASE DEFICIENCY (HEREDITARY OROTIC ACIDURIA)

Uridine monophosphate is the enzyme that catalyzes orotate phosphoribosyl transferase and orotidine-5'-monophosphate decarboxylase reactions. With deficiency, orotic acid accumulates, causing clinical manifestations of megaloblastic anemia, orotic crystalluria and nephropathy, cardiac malformations, strabismus, and recurrent infections. Diagnosis of uridine monophosphate synthase deficiency is by enzyme assay in a variety of tissues. Treatment of uridine monophosphate synthase deficiency is with oral uridine supplementation.

Table 22.20	Pyrimidine metabolism disorders		
Disease	**Defective proteins or enzymes**	**Defective gene or genes (chromosomal location)**	**Comments**
Hereditary orotic aciduria			Biochemical profile: Elevated urinary orotate
Type I	UMP synthase (orotidine-5'-pyrophosphorylase and decarboxylase)	UMPS (3q13)*	Clinical features: Megaloblastic anemia, recurrent infections, cellular immunodeficiency, developmental disabilities
Type II	Orotidine-5'-decarboxylase	—	Treatment: Uridine, uridylic and cytidylic acid
Dihydropyrimidine dehydrogenase deficiency • Inborn error form • Pharmacogenetic form	Dihydropyrimidine dehydrogenase	DPYD (1p22)*	Biochemical profile: Elevated urinary uracil, thymine, and 5-hydroxymethyluracil Clinical features: In inborn error form, growth and developmental delay, seizures, spasticity, microcephaly In pharmacogenetic form, adverse reactions to 5-flurouracil, including myelosuppression, neurotoxicity, GI and skin symptoms, death Treatment: No specific treatment except for withdrawal of offending drug
Dihydropyrimidinuria	Dihydropyrimidinase	DPYS (8q22)*	Biochemical profile: Elevated urinary dihydrouracil and dihydrothymine Clinical features: Variable; feeding problems, seizures, lethargy, somnolence, metabolic acidosis Sometimes benign Treatment: Not established
β-ureido propionase deficiency	β-ureido propionase (β-alanine synthase)	UPB1 (22q11.2)	Biochemical profile: Elevated urinary ureidopropionate and ureidobutyrate Clinical features: Microcephaly, developmental delay, dystonia, scoliosis Treatment: Not established
Pyrimidine 5'-nucleotidase deficiency	5'-monophosphate hydrolase	NT5C3 (7p15-p14)*	Biochemical profile: No specific profile Clinical features: Hemolytic anemia, basophilic stippling Treatment: Supportive care
Activation-induced cytidine deaminase deficiency	Activation-induced cytidine deaminase	AICDA (12p13)*	Biochemical profile: High IgM, low to absent IgG and IgA Clinical features: Recurrent bacterial infections, defective Ig class switching Treatment: Control of infections

*Gene has been identified, and molecular basis has been elucidated.

Laboratory Diagnosis of Amino Acid Analysis by Ion-exchange Chromatography

Several methods have been used in the analysis of amino acids in biological fluids, such as plasma, urine, and cerebrospinal fluid. All involve chromatographic separation of amino acids with pre-column [high-performance liquid chromatography (HPLC), GC methods] or post-column (ion-exchange chromatography) derivatization, followed by detection by ultraviolet (UV), fluorescence, or mass spectrometry.

The gold standard for analysis of amino acids remains ion-exchange chromatography (IEC), even though recent workusing tandem mass spectrometry is showing promisingresults. The challenge with amino acid analysis includes theneed (1) to cover a wide dynamic range, (2) to have a verylow detection limit, and (3) to have a high upper limit of linearity. In addition to these analytical requirements, isomers need to be separated and quantified. With ion-exchange chromatography,the sample (plasma/urine/CSF) is deproteinized and injected onto an ion-exchange column (typically a lithium cation-exchange column). Amino acids are separated on the basis of their pKa by changing the pH and ionic strength of eluting buffers and the temperature of the column. Acidic amino acids are eluted first, followed by neutral then basic amino acids. After their elution from the column, amino acids are mixed with ninhydrin at 135°C to form a coloredad duct. The intensity of their absorbance is proportional tothe concentration of the amino acid. Absorbance is read at two different wavelengths: 570 nm (maximum absorbance for amino acids) and 440 nm (maximum absorbance for imino acids, such as proline and hydroxyproline). The concentration of amino acids is calculated using an internal standard and external calibration. Identification of individual amino acids relies on retention time, ratio of absorbance at the two wavelengths (440/570 nm), and, in case of doubt, spiking of the sample with a standard.

Plasma collected under fasting conditions is the specimen of choice. In infants and small children, the sample should be collected at least 2 hours after the last feeding. Collection of serum should be avoided because of artifacts deriving from the clotting process. Blood should be collected with an anticoagulant (lithium/sodium heparin) and immediately separated and frozen until the time of analysis. Storage of samples at inappropriate temperature, at room temperature, or refrigerated has been known to result in deamination of glutamine and binding of sulfur amino acids to protein. The concentration of most amino acids in red blood cells is very similar to their concentration in plasma; however, some amino acids (e.g. aspartic acid, taurine, and glutamic acid) are present at higher concentrations in red blood cells; therefore, hemolysis will result in an artificially increased concentration of those amino acids. In addition, red blood cells contain the enzyme arginase, which converts arginine to ornithine and urea.

Hemolysis may release this enzyme, resulting in decreased concentrations of arginine and increased concentrations of ornithine. Results of plasma amino acid analysis are usually expressed in micromoles/liter.

Urine amino acids are useful only in the investigation of disorders of amino acid transport (e.g. cystinuria, lysinuric protein intolerance, Hartnup disorder) or of prolidase deficiency.

A random urine sample, without preservative, is usually sufficient. Specific reabsorption studies may require a timed (24 hour) urine collection. The sample should be collected without preservative and kept refrigerated until the end of the collection. Urine samples, like plasma, should be frozen as soon as possible and kept frozen until analysis. Results are usually normalized to the concentration of creatinine in the specimen.

Analysis of cerebrospinal fluid amino acids is performed for very specific cases, such as in the diagnostic investigation of glycine encephalopathy (non-ketotic hyperglycinemia) and in disorders of serine metabolism. CSF should be collected while avoiding blood contamination; it should be frozen immediately and kept frozen until the time of analysis. Measurements of CSF amino acids are expressed in μm/L. Amino acid results, independent of specimen type, should be correlated with clinical status, diet, and medications.

Urine Organic Acid Analysis by Gas Chromatography/ Mass Spectrometry

The label organic acids includes metabolites of almost all pathways of intermediary metabolism and exogenous compounds. Organic acids analyzed by gas chromatography/mass spectrometry (GC/MS) are separated on the basis of their volatility and solubility in the stationary nonpolar liquid phase of the capillary gas chromatography column. Before GC/MS analysis is performed, organic acids must be (1) extracted, usually with an organic solvent; (2) converted to volatile trimethylsilyl (TMS) derivatives; and (3) dissolved in organic solvents. With this technique, the mass spectrometer is employed as a detector, thus allowing positive identification of organic acids both by retention time and by their characteristic fragmentation spectrum. A random urine specimen is routinely used for this analysis; however, the most informative samples for the diagnosis of inherited disorders of metabolism are collected during acute metabolic decompensation. Organic acid analysis in blood or CSF usually is not informative to establish a diagnosis. Their interpretation is challenging because hundreds of compounds will be present in a specimen.

Key factors in correct interpretation of results include (1) recognition of abnormal patterns and possible interferences due to dietary or medication artifacts, (2) knowledge about metabolic disorders and their presentation, and (3) information about the clinical status of patients.

PLASMA ACYLCARNITINE PROFILE

Acylcarnitines derive from conjugation of carnitine with acyl-CoA. Carnitine [3-hydroxy-4-(trimethylazaniumyl) butanoate] is a water-soluble molecule that is essential in the transfer of long-chain fatty acids inside mitochondria for beta-oxidation. In addition, carnitine binds acyl residues accumulating in several organic acidemias and in fatty acid oxidation disorders, to facilitate their excretion. In the presence of a metabolic block (organic acidemia or fatty acid oxidation disorder), specific acylcarnitines, derived from conjugation of carnitine with acyl-CoA upstream of the metabolic block, accumulate, producing a pattern that is characteristic for each disease or group of diseases, so acylcarnitine analysis plays an essential role in the diagnosis of metabolic disorders (Fig. 22.1). Such an analysis is usually performed by tandem mass spectrometry (MS/MS) with or without liquid chromatographic separation prior to MS/MS detection. Plasma/Serum is the biological fluid of choice, and whole blood spotted on filter paper is used for screening of newborns. Concentrations of acylcarnitines in plasma differ from concentrations in whole blood, especially for long-chain acylcarnitines. This is thought to be due to binding of long-chain acylcarnitines to the membranes of blood cells, resulting in reduced long-chain species in plasma. Plasma for analysis of acylcarnitines should be separated immediately after collection and kept frozen until analysis. Hemolysis has been known to result in elevated long-chain acylcarnitines, misleading the diagnosis. Storage of the sample at room temperature or even refrigerated may result in hydrolysis and, consequently, reduced concentrations of acylcarnitines. Urine acylcarnitine analysis is performed only in the diagnostic work-up of specific disorders, such as glutaric acidemia type I, and only if equivocal results are obtained with other tests.

Quantification of acylcarnitines is typically performed using stable isotope dilution. However, some deuterated internal standards are not available for all identified acylcarnitine species. Caution should be taken when acylcarnitine results from different laboratories are compared, because the values may change depending on the internal standards used.

BIBLIOGRAPHY

1. AI-Dirbashi OY, Abu-Amero KK, Alswaid AF, Hoffmann GF, AI-Qahtani K, Rashed MS. LC-MS/MS determination of dibasic amino acids for the diagnosis of cystinuria: application in a family affected by a novel splice-acceptor site mutation in the SLC7 A9 gene. j Inherit Metab Dis 2007; 30: 611.

2. Andresen BS, Dobrowolski SF, O'Reilly L, Muenzer j, McCandless SE, Frazier DM, et al. Medium-chain acyl-CoA dehydrogenase (MCAD) mutations identified by MS/MS-based prospective screening of newborns differ from those observed in patients with clinical symptoms: identification and characterization of a new, prevalent mutation that results in mild MCAD deficiency. Am j Hum Genet 2001; 68: 1408–18.

3. Andresen BS, Olpin S, PoorthuisBj, Scholte HR, Vianey-Saban C, Wanders R, et al. Clear correlation of genotype with disease phenotype in very-long-chain acyl-CoA dehydrogenase deficiency. Am j Hum Genet 1999; 64: 479–94.

4. Applegarth DA, Toone JR. Nonketotic hyperglycinemia (glycine encephalopathy): laboratory diagnosis. Mol Genet Metab 2001: 74: 139–46.

5. Bennett Mj, Rinaldo P. The metabolic autopsy comes of age. ClinChern 200 I ; 47: 1145–6.

6. Bhattacharya K, Khalili V, Wiley V, Carpenter K, Wilcken B. Newborn screening may fail to identify intermediate forms of maple syrup urine disease. j Inherit Metab Dis 2006;29:586.

7. Boles RG, Buck EA, Blitzer MG, Platt MS, Cowan TM, Martin SK, et al. Retrospective biochemical screening of fatty acid oxidation disorders in postmortem livers of 418 cases of sudden death in the first year of life. jPediatr 1998: 132: 924–33.

8. Boneh A, Andresen BS, Gregersen N, Ibrahim M, Tzanakos N, Peters H, et al. VLCAD deficiency: pitfalls in newborn screening and confirmation of diagnosis by mutation analysis. Mol Genet Metab 2006:88: 166–70.

9. BonnefontjP, Djouadi F, Prip-Buus Co Gobin S, Munnich A, Bastin j. Carnitine palmitoyltransferases I and 2: biochemical, molecular and medical aspects. Mol Aspects Med 2004; 25: 495–520.

10. Botkin JR. Research for newborn screening: developing a national framework. Pediatrics 2005; 116: 862–71.

11. Carpenter K, Pollitt Rj, Middleton B. Human liver long-chain 3-hydroxyacyl-coenzyme A dehydrogenase is a multifunctional membrane-bound beta-oxidation enzyme of mitochondria. BiochemBiophys Res Commun 1992; 183: 443–8.

12. Chace DH, DiPernajC, Mitchell BL, Sgroi B, Hofman LF, Naylor EW. Electrospray tandem mass spectrometry for analysis of acylcarnitines in dried postmortem blood specimens collected at autopsy from infants with unexplained cause of death. Clin Chern 2001; 47: 1166–82.

13. Chace DH, Kalas TA. A biochemical perspective on the use of tandem mass spectrometry for newborn screening and clinical testing. Clin Biochem 2005; 38: 296–309.

14. Chace DH, Lim T, Hansen CR, Adam BW, Hannon Who Quantification of malonylcarnitine in dried blood spots by use of MS/MS varies by stable isotope internal standard composition. Clin Chim Acta 2009: 402: 14–8.

15. Chuang DT, Chuang jL, Wynn RM. Lessons from genetic disorders of branched-chain amino acid metabolism. jNutr 2006: 136: 243S-9S.

16. Clarke R, Lewington S. Homocysteine and coronary heart disease. SeminVasc Med 2002; 2: 391–9.

17. Danner Dj, Doering CB. Human mutations affecting branched chain alpha-ketoacid dehydrogenase. Front Biosci 1998; 3: d517 -24.

18. Deodato F, Boenzi S, Santorelli FM, Dionisi- Vici C. Methylmalonic and propionic aciduria. Am j Med Genet C Semin Med Genet 2006;142C: 104–12.

19. Derks TG, Boer TS, van Assen A, Bos T, Ruiter J, Waterham HR, et al. Neonatal screening for medium-chain acyl-CoA dehydrogenase (MCAD) deficiency in The Netherlands: the importance of enzyme analysis to ascertain true MCAD deficiency. j Inherit Metab Dis 2008:31: 88–96.

20. Dinopoulos A, Matsubara Y, Kure S. Atypical variants of nonketotic hyperglycinemia. Mol Genet Metab 2005: 86: 61–9.

21. Echenne B, Roubertie A, Assmann B, Lutz T, PenzienjM, Thony B, et al. Sepiapterin reductase deficiency: clinical presentation and evaluation oflong-term therapy. Pediatr Neurol 2006: 35: 308–13.

22. Eskelin PM, Laitinen KA, Tyni TA. Elevated hydroxyacylcarnitines in a carrier of LCHAD deficiency during acute liver disease of pregnancy: a common feature of the pregnancy complication? Mol Genet Metab 20 I 0: 100: 204–6.

23. Fernhoff PM, Lubitz D, Danner DJ, Dembure PP, Schwartz HP, Hillman R, et al. Thiamine response in maple syrup urine disease. Pediatr Res 1985: 19: 1011–6.

24. Fingerhut R, Roschinger W, Muntau AC, Dame T, Kreischer J, Arnecke R, et al. Hepatic carnitine palmitoyltransferase I deficiency: acylcarnitine profiles in blood spots are highly specific. Clin Chern 2001: 47: 1763–8.

25. Finkelstein JD, Martin N. Homocysteine. Int J Biochem Cell Bioi 2000; 32: 385–9.

26. Gan-Schreier H, Kebbewar M, Fang-Hoffmann j, Wilrich j, Abdoh G, Ben-Omran T, et al. Newborn population screening for classic homocystinuria by determination of total homocysteine from Guthrie cards. jPediatr 2010; 156: 427–32.

27. Iafolla AK, Thompson RJ Jr, Roe CR. Medium-chain acyl-coenzyme A dehydrogenase deficiency: clinical course in 120 affected children. J Pediatr 1994; 124: 409–15.

28. Jethva R, Bennett MJ, VockIey J. Short-chain acyl-coenzyme A dehydrogenase deficiency. Mol Genet Metab 2008; 95: 195–200.

29. Kaspar H, Dettmer K, Chan Q, Daniels S, Nimkar S, Daviglus ML, et al. Urinary amino acid analysis: a comparison of iTRAQ-LC-MS/MS, GC-MS, and amino acid analyzer. J Chromatogr B Analyt Technol Biomed Life Sci 2009; 877: 1838–46.

30. Kikuchi G, Motokawa Y, Yoshida T, Hiraga K. Glycine cleavage system: reaction mechanism, physiological significance, and hyperglycinemia. Proc JpnAcadSer B Phys Bioi Sci 2008; 84: 246–63.

31. Koch R, Hanley W, Levy H, Matalon K, Matalon R, Rouse B, et al. The Maternal Phenylketonuria International Study: 1984-2002. Pediatrics 2003; 112: 1523–9.

32. Lang TF. Adult presentations of medium-chain acyl-CoA dehydrogenase deficiency (MCADD). J Inherit Metab Dis 2009; 32: 675–83.

33. Liu A, Johnson Ow, Pasquali M. Addition of formic acid improves acetonitrile extraction of dicarboxylic acylcarnitines. Clin Chim Acta 2009; 404: 169–70.

34. Liu A, Kushnir MM, Roberts WL, Pasquali M. Solid phase extraction procedure for urinary organic acid analysis by gas chromatography mass spectrometry. J Chromatogr B Analyt Technol Biomed Life Sci 2004; 806: 283–7.

35. Liu A, Pasquali M. Acidified acetonitrile and methanol extractions for quantitative analysis of acylcarnitines in plasma by stable isotope dilution tandem mass spectrometry. J Chromatogr B AnalytTechnol Biomed Life Sci 2005; 827: 193–8.

36. Longo N, Amat di San Filippo C, Pasquali M. Disorders of carnitine transport and the carnitine cycle. Am J Med Genet C Semin Med Genet 2006; 142C: 77–85.

37. Longo N. Disordersofbiopterin metabolism. J Inherit Metab Dis 2009;32:333-42.

38. Longo N. Mitochondrial encephalopathy. NeurolClin 2003; 21: 817–31.

39. Lund AM, Joensen F, Hougaard OM, Jensen LK, Christensen E, Christensen M, et al. Carnitine transporter and holocarboxylase synthetase deficiencies in The Faroe Islands. J Inherit Metab Dis 2007;30:341-9.

40. Matern O, Tortorelli S, Oglesbee 0, Gavrilov 0, Rinaldo P. Reduction of the false-positive rate in newborn screening by implementation of MS/MS-based second-tier tests: the Mayo Clinic experience (2004-2007). I Inherit Metab Dis 2007; 30: 585–92.

41. Morton DH, Strauss KA, Robinson DL, Puffenberger EG, Kelley RI. Diagnosis and treatment of maple syrup disease: a study of 36 patients. Pediatrics 2002; 109: 999–1008.

42. Nassogne MC, Heron B, Touati G, Rabier O, Saudubray JM. Urea cycle defects: management and outcome. J Inherit Metab Dis 2005; 28: 407–14.

43. Orendac M, Zeman J, Stabler SP, Allen RH, Kraus JP, Bodamer O, et al. Homocystinuria due to cystathionine beta-synthase deficiency: novel biochemical findings and treatment efficacy. J Inherit Metab Dis 2003; 26: 761–73.

44. Palmieri F. Diseases caused by defects of mitochondrial carriers: a review. BiochimBiophysActa 2008;1777: 564–78.

45. Ravn K, Chloupkova M, Christensen E, Brandt NJ, Simonsen H, Kraus JP, et al. High incidence of propionic acidemia in greenland is due to a prevalent mutation, 1540insCCC, in the gene for the beta-subunit of propionyl CoA carboxylase. Am J Hum Genet 2000;67:203-6.

46. Rinaldo P, Matern 0, Bennett MJ. Fatty acid oxidation disorders. Annu Rev Physiol 2002; 64: 477–502.

47. Rinaldo P, Studinski AL, Matern D. Prenatal diagnosis of disorders of fatty acid transport and mitochondrial oxidation. PrenatDiagn 2001; 21: 52–4.

48. Smith W, Kishnani PS, Lee B, Singh RH, Rhead WI, Sniderman King L, et al. Urea cycle disorders: clinical

presentation outside the newborn period. Crit Care Clin 2005;21:S9-17.

49. Souri M, Aoyama T, Orii K, Yamaguchi S, Hashimoto T. Mutation analysis of very-long-chain acyl-coenzyme A dehydrogenase (VLCAD) deficiency: identification and characterization of mutant VLCAD cDNAs from four patients. Am I Hum Genet 1996;58:97-106.

50. Spiekerkoetter U, Sun B, Khuchua Z, Bennett MJ, Strauss AW. Molecular and phenotypic heterogeneity in mitochondrial trifunctional protein deficiency due to beta-subunit mutations. Hum Mutat 2003; 21: 598–607.

51. Steegers- Theunissen RP, Boers GH, Trijbels F/, Eskes TK. Neural-tube defects and derangement of homocysteine metabolism. N Engll Med 1991; 324: 199–200.

52. Strauss AW, Bennett MJ, Rinaldo P, Sims HF, O'Brien LK, Zhao Y, et al. Inherited long-chain 3-hydroxyacyl-CoA dehydrogenase deficiency and a fetal-maternal interaction cause maternal liver disease and other pregnancy complications. Semin Perinatol 1999; 23: 100–12.

53. Tiranti V, D:Adamo P, Briem E, Ferrari G, Mineri R, Lamantea E, et al. Ethylmalonic encephalopathy is caused by mutations in ETHEl, a gene encoding a mitochondrial matrix protein. Am I Hum Genet 2004; 74: 239–52.

54. Tiranti V, Viscomi C, Hildebrandt T, Di Meo I, Mineri R. Tiveron C, et al. Loss of ETHEl, a mitochondrial dioxygenase.

causes fatal sulfide toxicity in ethylmalonic encephalopathy. Nat Med 2009; 15: 200–5.

55. Tortorelli S, Hahn SH, Cowan TM, Brewster TG, Rinaldo P, Matern D. The urinary excretion of glutarylcarnitine is an informative tool in the biochemical diagnosis of glutaric acidemia type I. Mol Genet Metab 2005; 84: 137–43.

56. van Maldegem BT, Duran M, Wanders RJ, Niezen-Koning KE, Hogeveen M, Ijlst L, et al. Clinical, biochemical, and genetic heterogeneity in short-chain acyl-coenzyme A dehydrogenase deficiency. JAM A 2006; 296: 943–52.

57. Vockley J, Ensenauer R. Isovaleric acidemia: new aspects of genetic and phenotypic heterogeneity. Am J Med Genet C Semin Med Genet 2006; 142C: 95–1 03

58. Waddell L, Wiley V, Carpenter K, Bennetts B, Angel L, Andresen BS, et al. Medium-chain acyl-CoA dehydrogenase deficiency: genotypebiochemical phenotype correlations. Mol Genet Metab 2006; 87: 32–9.

59. Waterval WA, Scheijen) L, Ortmans-Ploemen MM, Habets-van der PoelCD, Bierau). Quantitative UPLC- MS/MS analysis of underivatised amino acids in body fluids is a reliable tool for the diagnosis and follow-up of patients with inborn errors of metabolism. Clin Chim Acta 2009; 407: 36–42.

60. Woontner M, Goodman SI. Chromatographic analysis of amino and organic acids in physiological fluids to detect inborn errors of metabolism. CurrProtoc Hum Genet 2006; Chapter 17: Unit 172: I– I 9.

23

Analytic Techniques and Instrumentation

INTRODUCTION

Instrumentation is the mainstay of clinical chemistry. Of all departments in the clinical laboratory, clinical chemistry is the most automated and dependent upon large-volume automated instrumentation. Automated instrumentation employs the same chemistry reactions used in manual biochemistry and general chemistry laboratories. Automation is able to achieve more precise and accurate results than manual methods due to more reliable control of volumes, timing, and analysis.

The majority of techniques fall into one of the four basic disciplines within the field of analytic chemistry; spectrometry [including spectrophotometry, atomic absorption, and mass spectrometry (MS)]; luminescence (including fluorescence and chemiluminescence); electroanalytic methods (including electrophoresis, potentiometry, and amperometry); and chromatography (including gas, liquid, and thin layer). Due to the rapid growth and increased utilization in clinical laboratories, chromatography and MS.

SPECTROPHOTOMETRY

The instruments that measure electromagnetic radiation have several concepts and components in common. Shared instrumental components are discussed in some detail in a later section. Photometric instruments measure light intensity without consideration of wavelength. Most instruments today use filters (photometers), prisms, or gratings (spectrometers) to select (isolate) an arrow range of the incident wavelength. Radiant energy that passes through an object will be partially reflected, absorbed, and transmitted.

Electromagnetic radiation is described as photons of energy traveling in waves. The relationship between wavelength and energy E is described by Planck's formula:

$$E = h\nu$$

where h is a constant (6.62×10^{-27} erg sec), known as Planck's constant, and ν is frequency. Because the frequency of a wave is inversely proportional to the wavelength, it follows that the energy of electromagnetic radiation is inversely proportional to wavelength. Figure 23.1A shows this relationship; electromagnetic radiation includes a spectrum of energy from short wavelength, highly energetic gamma rays and X-rays on the left to long-wavelength radio frequencies on the right (Fig. 23.1B). Visible light falls in between, with the color violet at 400 nm and red at 700 nm wavelengths being the approximate limits of the visible spectrum.

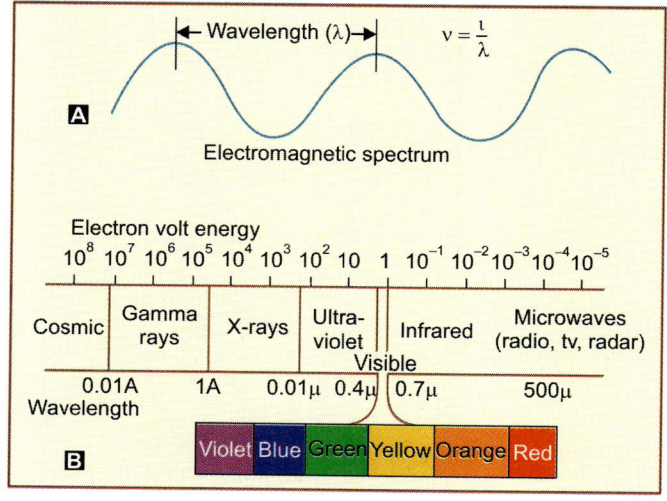

Fig. 23.1: Electromagnetic radiation; relationship of energy and wavelength

The instruments discussed in this section measure either absorption or emission of radiant energy to determine the concentration of atoms or molecules. The two phenomena, absorption and emission, are closely related. For a ray of electromagnetic radiation to be absorbed, it must have the same frequency as a rotational or vibrational frequency in the atom or molecule that it strikes. Levels of energy that are absorbed move in discrete steps, and any particular type of molecule or atom will absorb only certain energies and not others. When energy is absorbed, valence electrons move to an orbital with a higher energy level. Following energy absorption, the excited electron will fall back to the ground state by emitting a discrete amount of energy in the form of a characteristic wavelength of radiant energy.

Absorption or emission of energy by atoms results in a line spectrum. Because of the relative complexity of molecules, they absorb or emit a bank of energy over a large region. Light emitted by incandescent solids (tungsten or deuterium) is in a continuum. The three types of spectra are shown in Figure 23.2.

BEER'S LAW

The relationship between absorption of light by a solution and the concentration of that solution has been described by Beer and others. Beer's law states that the concentration of a substance is directly proportional to the amount of light absorbed or inversely proportional to the logarithm of the transmitted light. Percent transmittance (% T) and absorbance (A) are related photometric terms that are explained in this section.

Figure 23.3A shows a beam of monochromatic light entering a solution; some of the light is absorbed. The remainder passes through, strikes a light detector, and is converted to an electric signal. Percent transmittance is the ratio of the radiant energy transmitted (T) divided by the radiant energy incident on the sample (I). All light absorbed or blocked results in 0% T. A level of 100% T is obtained if no light is absorbed. In practice, the solvent without the constituent of interest is placed in the light path (Fig. 23.3B). Most of the light is transmitted, but a

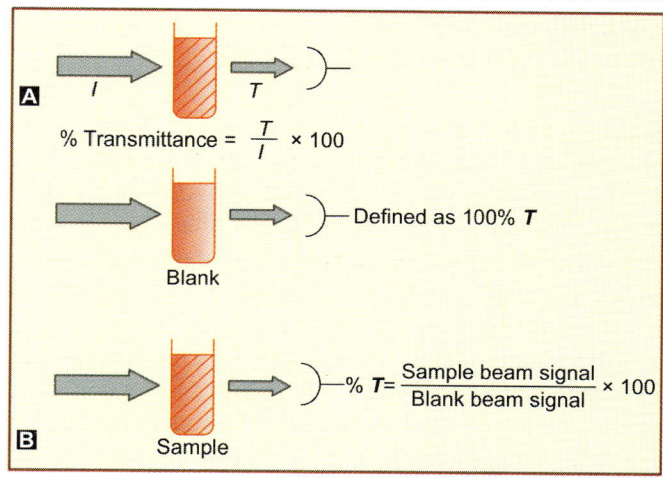

Fig. 23.3: Percent transmittance (% T)

small amount is absorbed by the solvent and cuvette or is reflected away from the detector.

The electrical readout of the instrument is set arbitrarily at 100% T, while the light is passing through a 'blank' or reference. The sample containing absorbing molecules to be measured is placed in the light path. The difference in amount of light transmitted by the blank and that transmitted by the sample is due only to the presence of the compound being measured. The % T measured by commercial spectrophotometers is the ratio of the sample transmitted beam divided by the blank transmitted beam.

Equal thicknesses of an absorbing material will absorb a constant fraction of the energy incident upon the layers. For example, in a tube containing layers of solution (Fig. 23.4A), the first layer transmits 70% of the light incident upon it. The second layer will, in turn, transmit 70% of the light incident upon it. Thus, 70% of 70% (49%) is transmitted by the second layer. The third layer transmits 70% of 49%, or 34% of the original light. Continuing on, successive layers transmit 24% and 17%, respectively. The %T values, when plotted on linear graph paper, yield the curve (Fig. 23.4B). Considering each equal layer as many monomolecular layers, we can translate layers of material to concentration. If semilog graph paper is used to plot the same figures, a straight line is obtained (Fig. 23.4C), indicating that, as concentration increases, % T decreases in a logarithmic manner. Absorbance A is the amount of light absorbed. It cannot be measured directly by a spectrophotometer but rather is mathematically derived from % T as follows:

$$\%T = I/I_0 \times 100$$

where I_0 is the incident light and I is the transmitted light.

Absorbance is defined as follows:

$$A = -\log(I/I_0) = \log(100\%) - \log \%T$$
$$= 2 - \log \%T$$

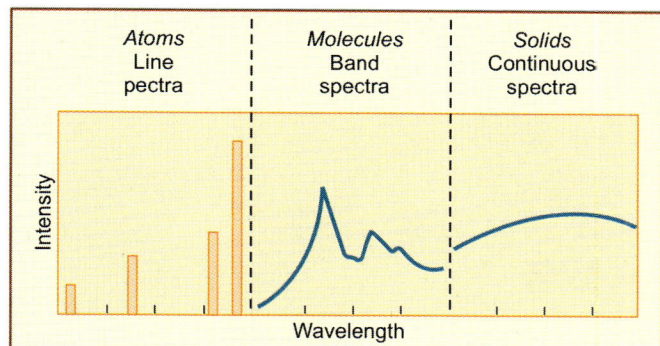

Fig. 23.2: Characteristic absorption or emission spectra

According to Beer's law, absorbance is directly proportional to concentration (Fig. 23.4D):

$$A = e \times b \times c$$

where e = molar absorptivity, the fraction of a specific wavelength of light absorbed by a given type of molecule; b is the length of light path through the solution; and c is the concentration of absorbing molecules.

Absorptivity depends on the molecular structure and the way in which the absorbing molecules react with different energies. For any particular molecular type, absorptivity changes as wavelength of radiation changes. The amount of light absorbed at a particular wavelength depends on the molecules and ion types present and may vary with concentration, pH, or temperature. Because the path length and molar absorptivity are constant for a given wavelength,

$$A \sim c$$

Unknown concentrations are determined from a calibration curve that plots absorbance at a specific wavelength versus concentration for standards of known concentration. For calibration curves that are linear and have a zero y-intercept, unknown concentrations can be determined from a single calibrator. Not all calibration curves result in straight lines. Deviations from linearity are typically observed at high absorbances. The stray light within an instrument will ultimately limit the maximum absorbance that a spectrophotometer can achieve, typically 2.0 absorbance units.

SPECTROPHOTOMETRIC INSTRUMENTS

A spectrophotometer is used to measure the light transmitted by a solution to determine the concentration of the light-absorbing substance in the solution. Illustration of the basic components of a single beam spectrophotometer is shown in Figure 23.5.

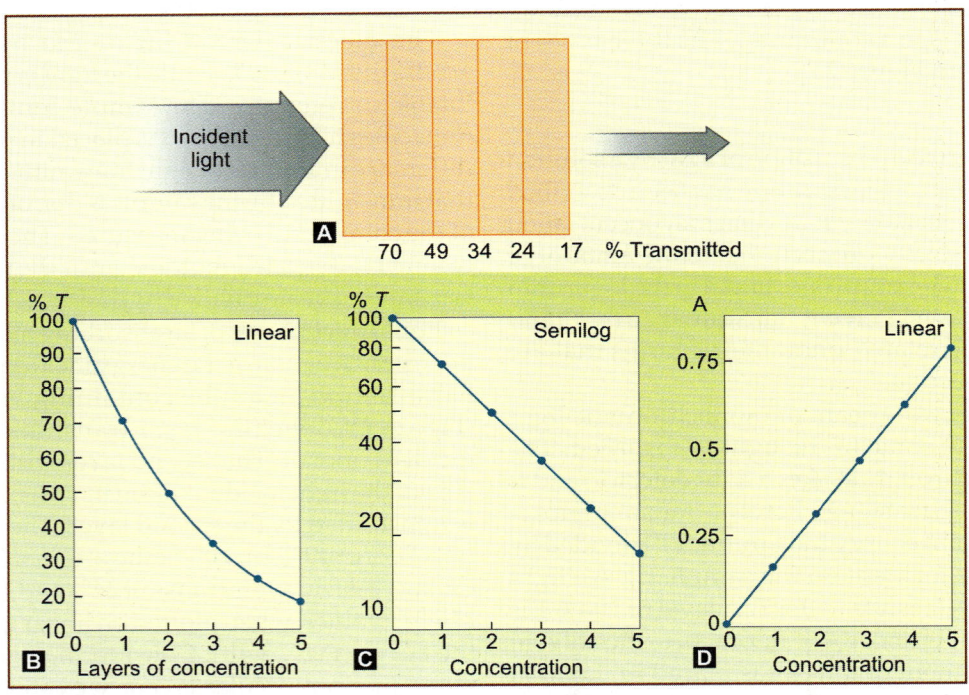

Fig. 23.4: (A) Percent of original incident light transmitted by equal layers of light-absorbing solution. (B) Percent *T* vs. concentration on linear graph paper. (C) Percent *T* vs. concentration on semilog graph paper. (D) *A* vs. concentration on linear graph paper

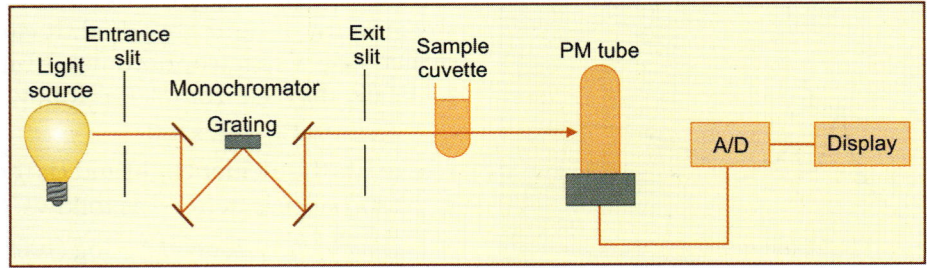

Fig. 23.5: Single-beam spectrophotometer

COMPONENTS OF A SPECTROPHOTOMETER

Light Source

The most common source of light for work in the visible and near-infrared regions is the incandescent tungsten or tungsten-iodide lamp. Only about 15% of radiant energy emitted falls in the visible region, with most emitted as near-infrared. Often, a heat-absorbing filter is inserted between the lamp and the sample to absorb the infrared radiation. The lamps most commonly used for ultraviolet (UV) work are the deuterium discharge lamp and the mercury arc lamp. Deuterium provides continuous emission down to 165 nm. Low-pressure mercury lamps emit a sharp line spectrum, with both UV and visible lines. Medium and high-pressure mercury lamps emit a continuum from UV to the mid-visible region. The most important factors for a light source are range, spectral distribution within the range, the source of radiant production, stability of the radiant energy, and temperature.

Monochromators

Isolation of individual wavelengths of light is an important and necessary function of a monochromator. The degree of wavelength isolation is a function of the type of device used and the width of entrance and exit slits. The band pass of a monochromator defines the range of wavelengths transmitted and is calculated as width at more than half the maximum transmittance (Fig. 23.6).

Numerous devices are used for obtaining monochromatic light. The least expensive are colored glass filters. These filters usually pass a relatively wide band of radiant energy and have a low transmittance of the selected wavelength. Although not precise, they are simple, inexpensive, and useful. Interference filters produce monochromatic light based on the principle of constructive interference of waves. Two pieces of glass, each mirrored on one side, are separated by a transparent spacer that is precisely one-half the desired wavelength. Light waves enter one side of the filter and are reflected at the second surface. Wavelengths that are twice the space between the two glass surfaces will reflect back and forth, reinforcing others of the same wavelengths and finally passing on through. Other wavelengths will cancel out because of phase differences (destructive interference). Because interference filters also transmit multiples of the desired wavelengths, they require accessory filters to eliminate these harmonic wavelengths. Interference filters can be constructed to pass a very narrow range of wavelengths with good efficiency. The prism is another type of monochromator. A narrow beam of light focused on a prism is refracted as it enters the more dense glass. Short wavelengths are refracted more than long wavelengths, resulting in dispersion of white light into a continuous spectrum. The prism can be rotated, allowing only the desired wavelength to pass through an exit slit.

Diffraction gratings are most commonly used as monochromators. A diffraction grating consists of many parallel grooves (15,000 or 30,000 per inch) etched onto a polished surface. Diffraction, the separation of light into component wavelengths, is based on the principle that wavelengths bend as they pass a sharp corner. The degree of bending depends on the wavelength. As the wavelengths move past the corners, wave fronts are formed. Those that are in phase reinforce one another, whereas those not in phase cancel out and disappear. This results in complete spectra. Gratings with very fine line rulings produce a widely dispersed spectrum. They produce linear spectra, called orders, in both directions from the entrance slit. Because the multiple spectra have a tendency to cause stray light problems, accessory filters are used.

Sample Cell

The next component of the basic spectrophotometer is the sample cell or cuvette, which may be round or square. The light path must be kept constant to have absorbance proportional to concentration. This is easily checked by preparing a colored solution to read midscale when using the wavelength of maximum absorption. Fill each cuvette to be tested, take readings, and save those that match within an acceptable tolerance (e.g. $\pm 0.25\%$ T).

Because it is difficult to manufacture round tubes with uniform diameters, they should be etched to indicate the position for use. Cuvettes are sold in matched sets. Square cuvettes have plane-parallel optical surfaces and a constant light path. They have an advantage over round cuvettes in that there is less error from the lens effect,

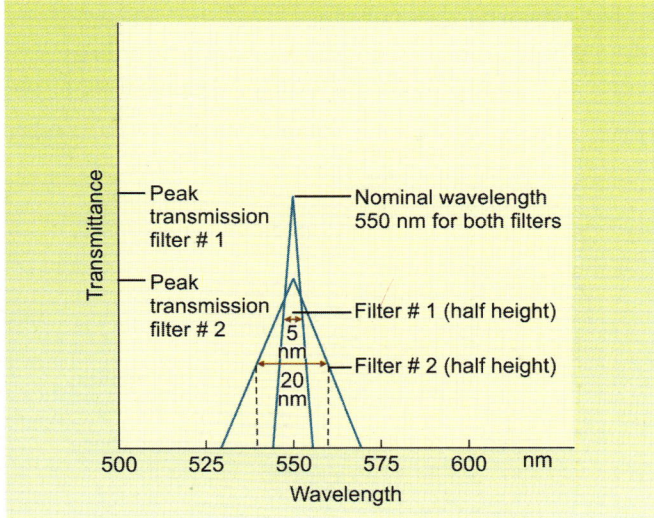

Fig. 23.6: Spectral transmittance of two monochromators with band pass at half height of 5 and 20 nm

orientation in the spectrophotometer, and refraction. Cuvettes with scratched optical surfaces scatter light and should be discarded. Inexpensive glass cuvettes can be used for applications in the visible range, but they absorb light in the UV region. Quartz cuvettes must, therefore, be used for applications requiring UV radiation.

PHOTODETECTORS

The purpose of the detector is to convert the transmitted radiant energy into an equivalent amount of electrical energy. The least expensive of the devices is known as a barrier-layer cell, or photocell. The photocell is composed of a film of light-sensitive material, frequently selenium, on a plate of iron. Over the light-sensitive material is a thin, transparent layer of silver. When exposed to light, electrons in the light-sensitive material are excited and released to flow to the highly conductive silver. In comparison with the silver, a moderate resistance opposes the electron flow toward the iron, forming a hypothetical barrier to flow in that direction. Consequently, this cell generates its own electromotive force, which can be measured. The produced current is proportional to the incident radiation. Photocells require no external voltage source but rely on internal electron transfer to produce a current in an external circuit. Because of their low internal resistance, the output of electrical energy is not easily amplified. Consequently, this type of detector is used mainly in filter photometers with a wide band pass, producing a fairly high level of illumination, so that there is no need to amplify the signal. The photocell is inexpensive and durable; however, it is temperature sensitive and nonlinear at very low and very high levels of illumination.

A phototube (Fig. 23.7) is similar to a barrier-layer cell in that it has photosensitive material that gives off electrons when light energy strikes it. It differs in that an outside voltage is required for operation. Phototubes contain a negatively charged cathode and a positively charged anode enclosed in a glass case. The cathode is composed of a material (e.g. rubidium or lithium) that acts as a resistor in the dark but emits electrons when exposed to light. The emitted electrons jump over to the positively charged anode, where they are collected and return through an external, measurable circuit.

The cathode usually has a large surface area. Varying the cathode material changes the wavelength at which the phototube gives its highest response. The photocurrent is linear, with the intensity of the light striking the cathode as long as the voltage between the cathode and the anode remains constant. A vacuum within the tubes avoids scattering of the photoelectrons by collision with gas molecules.

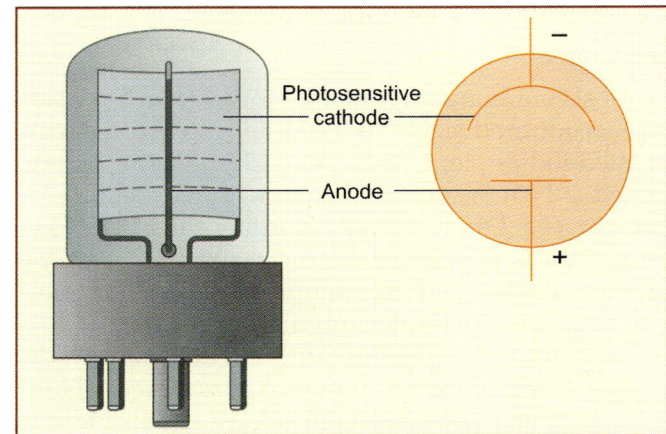

Fig. 23.7: Schematic phototube drawing

The third major type of light detector is the photo-multiplier (PM) tube, which detects and amplifies radiant energy; the incident light strikes the coated cathode, emitting electrons (Fig. 23.8). The electrons are attracted to a series of anodes, known as dynodes, each having a successively higher positive voltage. These dynodes are of a material that gives off many secondary electrons when hit by single electrons. Initial electron emission at the cathode triggers a multiple cascade of electrons within the PM tube itself. Because of this amplification, the PM tube is 200 times more sensitive than the phototube. PM tubes are used in instruments designed to be extremely sensitive to very low light levels and light flashes of very short duration. The accumulation of electrons striking the anode produces a current signal, measured in amperes, that is proportional to the initial intensity of the light. The analog signal is converted first to a voltage and then to a digital signal through the use of an analog-to-digital converter. Digital signals are processed electronically to produce absorbance readings.

In a photodiode, absorption of radiant energy by a reverse-biased pn-junction diode (pn, positive-negative)

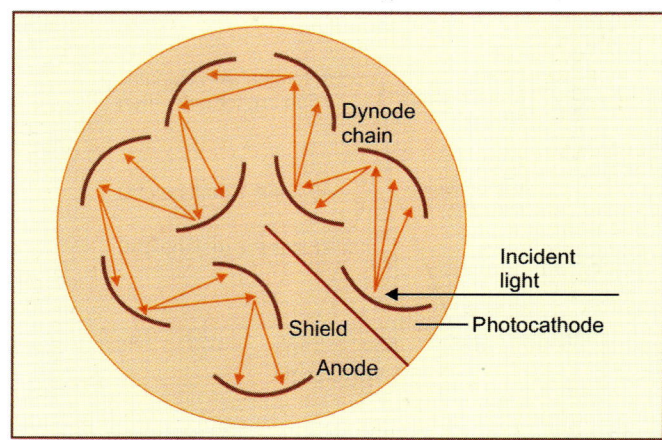

Fig. 23.8: Dynode chain in a photomultiplier

produces a photocurrent that is proportional to the incident radiant power. Although, photodiodes are not as sensitive as PM tubes because of the lack of internal amplification, their excellent linearity (6–7 decades of radiant power), speed, and small size make them useful in applications where light levels are adequate. Photodiodearray (PDA) detectors are available in integrated circuits containing 256–2,048 photodiodes in a linear arrangement (Fig. 23.9). Each photodiode responds to a specific wavelength, and as a result, a complete UV/visible spectrum can be obtained in less than 1 second. Resolution is 1–2 nm and depends on the number of discrete elements. In spectrophotometers using PDA detectors, the grating is positioned after the sample cuvette and disperses the transmitted radiation on to the PDA detector (Fig. 23.9).

For single-beam spectrophotometers, the absorbance reading from the sample must be blanked using an appropriate reference solution that does not contain the compound of interest. Double-beam spectrophotometers permit automatic correction of sample and reference absorbance (Fig. 23.10). Because the intensities of light sources vary as a function of wavelength, double-beam spectrophotometers are necessary when the absorption spectrum for a sample is to be obtained. Computerized, continuous zeroing, single-beam spectrophotometers have replaced most double-beams pectrophotometers.

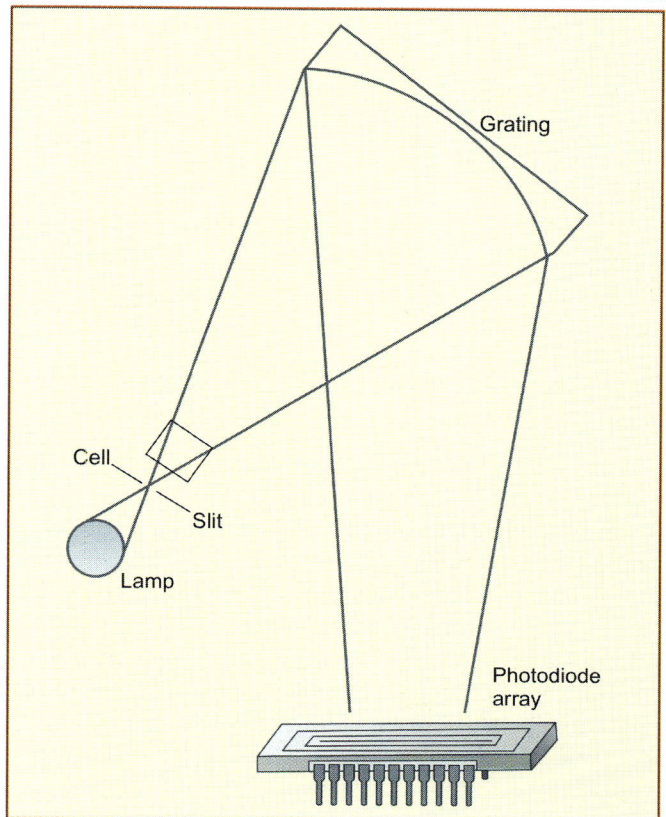

Fig. 23.9: Photodiode array spectrophotometer illustrating the placement of the sample cuvette before the monochromator

ATOMIC ABSORPTION SPECTROPHOTOMETER

The atomic absorption spectrophotometer is used to measure concentration by detecting the absorption of electromagnetic radiation by atoms rather than by molecules. The basic components are shown in Fig. 23.11. The usual light source, known as a hollow-cathode lamp, consists of an evacuated gas-tight chamber containing an anode, a cylindrical cathode, and an inert gas, such as helium or argon. When voltage is applied, the filler gas is ionized. Ions attracted to the cathode collide with the metal, knock atoms off, and cause the metal atoms to be excited. When they return to the ground state, light energy is emitted that is characteristic of the metal in the cathode. Generally, a separate lamp is required for each metal (e.g. a copper hollow-cathode lamp is used to measure Cu). Electrodeless discharge lamps are a relatively new light source for atomic absorption spectrophotometers. A bulb is filled with argon and the element to be tested. A radio frequency generator around the bulb supplies the energy to excite the element, causing a characteristic mission spectrum of the element. The analyzed sample must contain the reduced metal in the atomic vaporized state. Commonly, this is done by using the heat of a flame to break the chemical bonds and form free, unexcited atoms. The flame is the sample cell in this instrument, rather than a cuvette. There are various

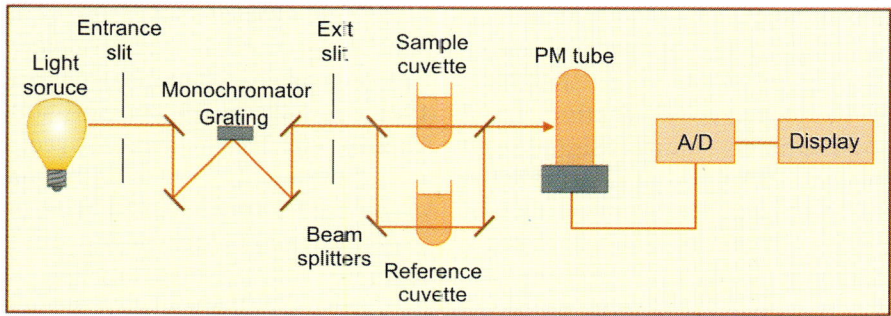

Fig. 23.10: Double-beam spectrophotometer

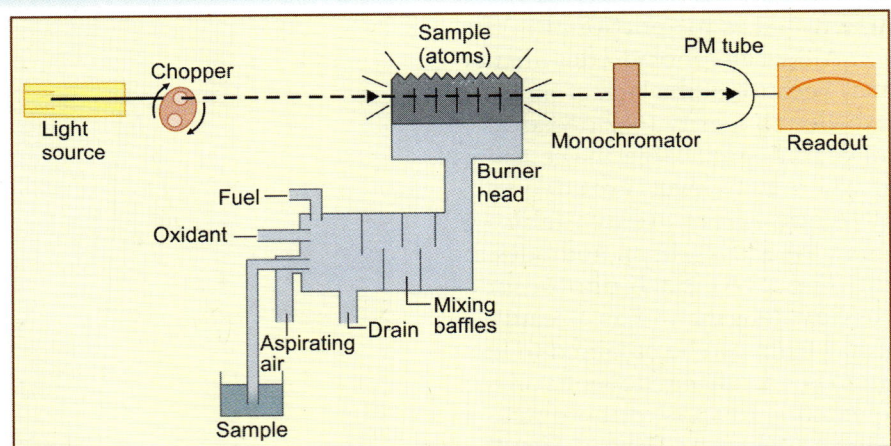

Fig. 23.11: Single-beam atomic absorption spectrophotometer; basic components

designs; however, the most common burner is the premix long-path burner. The sample, in solution, is aspirated as a spray into a chamber, where it is mixed with air and fuel. This mixture passes through baffles, where large drops fall and are drained off. Only fine droplets reach the flame. The burner is a long, narrow slit, to permit a longer path length for absorption of incident radiation. Light from the hollow-cathode lamp passes through the sample of ground state atoms in the flame.

The amount of light absorbed is proportional to the concentration. When a ground state atom absorbs light energy, an excited atom is produced. The excited atom then returns to the ground state, emitting light of the same energy as it absorbed. The flame sample thus contains a dynamic population of ground state and excited atoms, both absorbing and emitting radiant energy. The emitted energy from the flame will go in all directions and it will be a steady emission. Because the purpose of the instrument is to measure the amount of light absorbed, the light detector must be able to distinguish between the light beam emitted by the hollow-cathode lamp and that emitted by excited atoms in the flame.

To do this, the hollow-cathode light beam is modulated by inserting a mechanical rotating chopper between the light and the flame or by pulsing the electric supply to the lamp. Because the light beam being absorbed enters the sample in pulses, the transmitted light will also be in pulses. There will be less light in the transmitted pulses because part of it will be absorbed. There are, therefore, two light signals from the flame; an alternating signal from the hollow-cathode lamp and a direct signal from the flame emission. The measuring circuit is tuned to the modulated frequency. Interference from the constant flame emission is electronically eliminated by accepting only the pulsed signal from the hollow cathode. The monochromator is used to isolate the desired emission line from other lamp emission lines. In addition, it serves

to protect the photodetector from excessive light emanating from flame emissions. A PM tube is the usual light detector.

Flame less atomic absorption requires an instrument modification that uses an electric furnace to break chemical bonds (electrothermal atomization). A tiny graphite cylinder holds the sample, either liquid or solid. An electric current passes through the cylinder walls, evaporates the solvent, ashes the sample, and, finally, heats the unit to incandescence to atomize the sample. This instrument, like the spectrophotometer, is used to determine the amount of light absorbed. Again, Beer's law is used for calculating concentration. A major problem is that background correction is considerably more necessary and critical for electrothermal techniques than for flame-based atomic absorption methods. Currently, the most common approach uses a deuterium lamp as a secondary source and measures the difference between the two absorbance signals. However, there has also been extensive development of background correction techniques based on the Zeeman effect. The presence of an intense static magnetic field will cause the wavelength of the emitted radiation to split into several components. This shift in wavelength is the Zeeman effect.

Atomic absorption spectrophotometry is sensitive and precise. It is routinely used to measure concentration of trace metals that are not easily excited. It is generally more sensitive than flame emission because the vast majority of atoms produced in the usual propane or air acetylene flame remain in the ground state available for light absorption. It is accurate, precise, and specific. One disadvantage, however, is the inability of the flame to dissociate samples into free atoms. For example, phosphate may interfere with calcium analysis by formation of calcium phosphate. This may be overcome by adding cations that compete with calcium for phosphate.

Routinely, lanthanum or strontium is added to samples to form stable complexes with phosphate. Another possible problem is the ionization of atoms following dissociation by the flame, which can be decreased by reducing the flame temperature. Matrix interference, due to the enhancement of light absorption by atoms in organic solvents or formation of solid droplets as the solvent evaporates in the flame, can be another source of error.

This interference may be overcome by pretreatment of the sample by extraction. Recently, inductively coupled plasma (ICP) has been used to increase sensitivity for atomic emission. The torch, an argon plasma maintained by the interaction of a radio frequency field and an ionized argon gas, is reported to have used temperatures between 5,500 K and 8,000 K. Complete atomization of elements is thought to occur at these temperatures. Use of ICP as a source is recommended for determinations involving refractory elements such as uranium, zirconium, and boron. ICP with MS detection is the most sensitive and specific assay technique for all elements on the periodic chart. Atomic absorption spectrophotometry is used less frequently because of this newer technology.

FLAME PHOTOMETRY

The flame emission photometer, which measures light emitted by excited atoms, was widely used to determine concentration of Na^+, K^+, or Li^+. With the development of ion-selective electrodes (ISEs) for these analytes, flame photometers are no longer routinely used in clinical chemistry laboratories.

Fluorometry

As seen with the spectrophotometer, light entering a solution may pass mainly through or may be absorbed partly or entirely, depending on the concentration and the wavelength entering that particular solution. Whenever absorption occurs, there is a transfer of energy to the medium. Each molecular type possesses a series of electronic energy levels and can pass from a lower energy level to a higher energy level only by absorbing an integral unit (quantum) of light that is equal in energy to the difference between the two energy states. There are additional energy levels owing to rotation or vibration of molecular parts. The excited state lasts about 10–5 seconds before the electron loses energy and returns to the ground state. Energy is lost by collision, heat loss, transfer to other molecules, and emission of radiant energy. Because the molecules are excited by absorption of radiant energy and lose energy by multiple interactions, the radiant energy emitted is less than the absorbed energy. The difference between the maximum

wavelengths, excitation, and emitted fluorescence is called Stokes shift. Both excitation (absorption) and fluorescence (emission) energies are characteristic for a given molecular type; for example the absorption and fluorescence spectra of quinine in 0.1 N sulfuric acid (Fig. 23.12). The dashed line on the left shows the short-wavelength excitation energy that is maximally absorbed, whereas the solid line on the right is the longer wavelength (less energy) fluorescent spectrum.

BASIC INSTRUMENTATION

Filter fluorometers measure the concentrations of solutions that contain fluorescing molecules (Fig. 23.13). The source emits short-wavelength high-energy excitation light. A mechanical attenuator controls light intensity. The primary filter, placed between the radiation source and the sample, selects the wavelength that is best

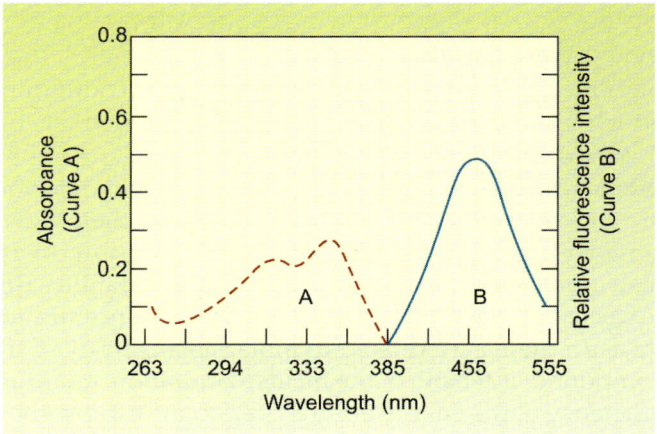

Fig. 23.12: Absorption and fluorescence spectra of quinine in 0.1 N sulfuric acid. (Adapted from Coiner D. Basic Concepts in Laboratory Instrumentation)

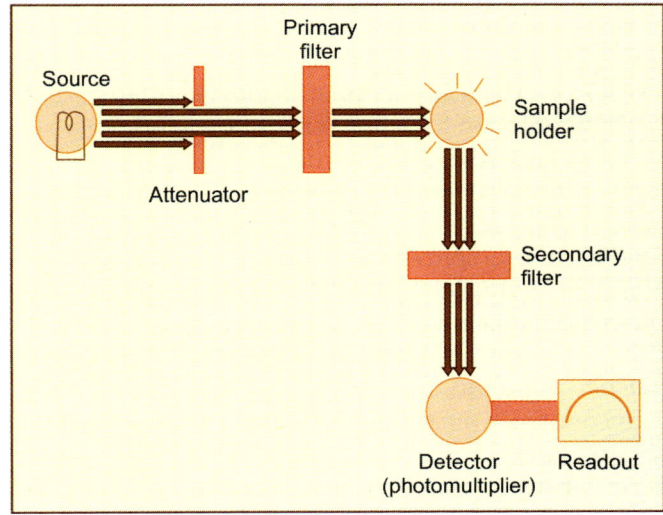

Fig. 23.13: Basic filter fluorometer

absorbed by the solution to be measured. The fluorescing sample in the cuvette emits radiant energy in all directions. The detector (placed at right angles to the sample cell) and a secondary filter that passes the longer wavelengths of fluorescent light prevent incident light from striking the photodetector. The electrical output of the photodetector is proportional to the intensity of fluorescent energy. In spectrofluorometers, the filters are replaced by prisms or grating monochromators.

Gas discharge lamps (mercury and xenon arc) are the most frequently used sources of excitation radiant energy. Incandescent tungsten lamps are seldom used because they release little energy in the UV region. Mercury vapor lamps are commonly used in filter fluorometers. Mercury emits a characteristic line spectrum. Resonance lines at 365–366 nm are commonly used. Energy at wavelengths other than the resonance lines is provided by coating the inner surface of the lamp with a material that absorbs the 254 nm mercury radiation and emits a broad band of longer wavelengths. Most spectrofluorometers use a high-pressure xenon lamp. Xenon has a good continuum, which is necessary for determining the excitation spectra.

Monochromator fluorometers use grating, prisms, or filters for isolation of incident radiation. Light detectors are almost exclusively PM tubes because of their higher sensitivity to low light intensities. Double-beam instruments are used to compensate for instability due to electric power fluctuation. Fluorescence concentration measurements are related to molar absorptivity of the compound, intensity of the incident radiation, quantum efficiency of the energy emitted per quantum absorbed, and length of the light path. In dilute solutions with instrument parameters held constant, fluorescence is directly proportional to concentration. Generally, a linear response will be obtained until the concentration of the fluorescent species is so high that the sample begins to absorb significant amounts of excitation light. A curve demonstrating on linearity as concentration increases (Fig. 23.14). The solution must absorb less than 5% of the exciting radiation for a linear response to occur.

As with all quantitative measurements, a standard curve must be prepared to demonstrate that the concentration used falls in a linear range. In fluorescence polarization, radiant energy is polarized in a single plane. When the sample (fluorophore) is excited, it emits polarized light along the same plane as the incident light if the fluorophore does not rotate in solution (i.e. it is attached or bound to a large molecule).

In contrast, a small molecule emits depolarized light because it will rotate out of the plane of polarization during its excitation lifetime. This technique is widely used for the detection of therapeutic and abused drugs.

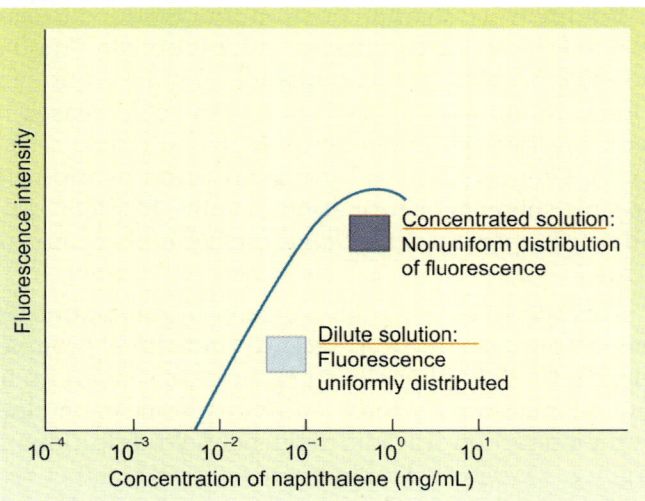

Fig. 23.14: Dependence of fluorescence on the concentration of fluorophore

In the procedure, the sample analyte is allowed to compete with a fluorophore-labeled analyte for a limited antibody to the analyte. The lower the concentration of the sample analyte, the higher the macromolecular antibody analyte fluorophore formed and the lower the depolarization of the radiant light.

ADVANTAGES AND DISADVANTAGES OF FLUOROMETRY

Fluorometry has two advantages over conventional spectrophotometry: specificity and sensitivity. Fluorometry increases specificity by selecting the optimal wavelength for both absorption and fluorescence, rather than just the absorption wavelength seen with spectrophotometry. Fluorometry is approximately 1,000 times more sensitive than most spectrophotometric methods. One reason is because the emitted radiation is measured directly; it can be increased simply by increasing the intensity of the exciting radiant energy. In addition, fluorescence measures the amount of light intensity present over a zero background. In absorbance, however, the quantity of the absorbed light is measured indirectly as the difference between the transmitted beams. At low concentrations, the small difference between 100% T and the transmitted beam is difficult to measure accurately and precisely, limiting the sensitivity.

The biggest disadvantage is that fluorescence is very sensitive to environmental changes. Changes in pH affect availability of electrons, and temperature changes the probability of loss of energy by collision rather than fluorescence. Contaminating chemicals or a change of solvents may change the structure. UV light used for excitation can cause photochemical changes. Any decrease in fluorescence resulting from any of these possibilities is known as quenching. Because so many factors may change the intensity or spectra of fluorescence, extreme care is mandatory in analytic technique and instrument maintenance.

CHEMILUMINESCENCE

In chemiluminescence reactions, part of the chemical energy generated produces excited intermediates that decay to a ground state with the emission of photons. The emitted radiation is measured with a PM tube, and the signal is related to analyte concentration.

Chemiluminescence is different from fluorescence in that no excitation radiation is required and no monochromators are needed because the chemiluminescence arises from one species. Most importantly, chemiluminescence reactions are oxidation reactions of luminol, acridinium esters, and dioxetanes characterized by a rapid increase in intensity of emitted light followed by a gradual decay. Usually, the signal is taken as the integral of the entire peak. Enhanced chemiluminescence techniques increase the chemiluminescence efficiency by including an enhancer system in the reaction of a chemiluminescent agent with an enzyme. The time course for the light intensity is much longer (60 minutes) than that for conventional chemiluminescent reactions, which last for about 30 seconds (Fig. 23.15). Advantages of chemiluminescence assays include subpicomolar detection limits, speed (with flash-type reactions, light is only measured for 10 seconds), ease of use (most assays are one-step procedures), and simple instrumentation. The main disadvantage is that impurities can cause a background signal that degrades the sensitivity and specificity.

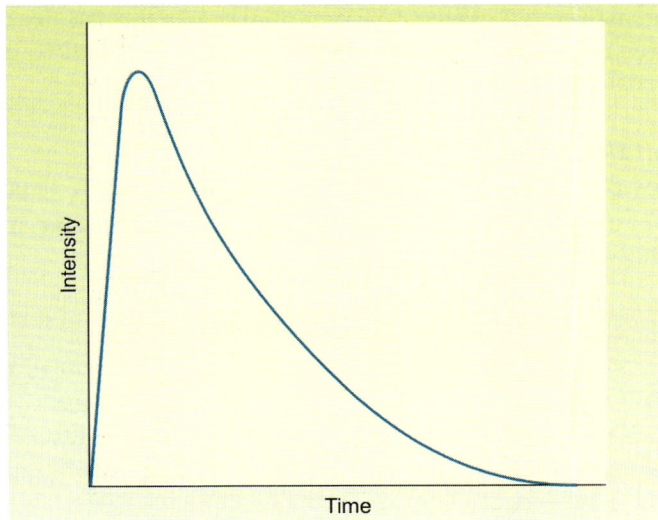

Fig. 23.15: Representative intensity vs. time curve for a transient chemiluminescence signal

TURBIDITY AND NEPHELOMETRY

Turbidimetric measurements are made with a spectrophotometer to determine the concentration of particulate matter in a sample. The amount of light blocked by a suspension of particles depends not only on concentration but also on size. Because particles tend to aggregate and settle out of suspension, sample handling becomes critical. Instrument operation is the same as for any spectrophotometer. Nephelometry is similar, except that light scattered by the small particles is measured at an angle to the beam incident on the cuvette. The below illustrate demonstrates two possible optical arrangements for a nephelometer (Fig. 23.16). Light scattering depends on wavelength and particle size. For macromolecules with a size close to or larger than the wavelength of incident light, sensitivity is increased by measuring the forward light scatter. Instruments are available with detectors placed at various forward angles, as well as at 90° to the incident light. Monochromatic light obtains uniform scatter and minimizes sample heating. Certain instruments use light amplification by stimulated emission of radiation (laser) as a source of monochromatic light; however, any monochromator may be used. Measuring light scatter at an angle other than at 180° in turbidimetry minimizes error from colored solutions and increases sensitivity. Because both the methods depend on particle size, some instruments quantitate initial change in light scatter rather than total scatter. Reagents must be free of any particles, and cuvettes must be free of any scratches.

Laser Applications

Laser is based on the interaction of radiant energy with suitably excited atoms or molecules. The interaction leads to stimulated emission of radiation. The wavelength, direction of propagation, phase, and plane of polarization of the emitted light are the same as those of the incident radiation. Laser light is polarized and coherent and has narrow spectral width and small cross sectional area with low divergence. The radiant emission can be very

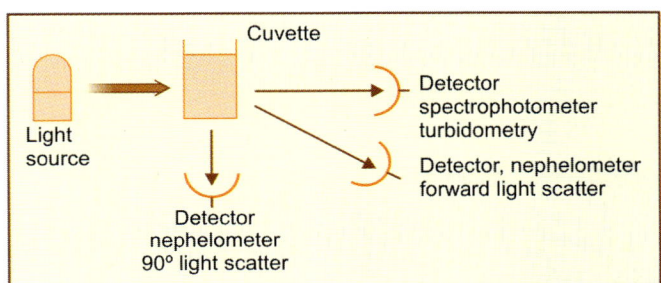

Fig. 23.16: Nephelometer vs. spectrophotometer; optical arrangements

powerful and either continuous or pulsating. Laser light can serve as the source of incident energy in a spectrometer or nephelometer. Some lasers produce bandwidths of a few kilohertz in both the visible and infrared regions, making these applications about 3–6 orders more sensitive than conventional spectrometers. Laser spectrometry can also be used for the determination of structure and identification of samples, as well as for diagnosis. Quantitation of samples depends on the spectrometer used. An example of the clinical application of laser is the Coulter counter, which is used for differential analysis of white blood cells.

Electrochemistry

Many types of electrochemical analyses are used in the clinical laboratory, including potentiometry, amperometry, coulometry, and polarography. The two basic electrochemical cells involved in these analyses are galvanic and electrolytic cells.

GALVANIC AND ELECTROLYTIC CELLS

An electrochemical cell can be set up by two half-cells and a salt bridge, which can be a piece of filter paper saturated with electrolytes. Instead of two beakers as shown, the electrodes can be immersed in a single, large beaker containing a salt solution (Fig. 23.17). In such a setup, the solution serves as the salt bridge. In a galvanic cell, as the electrodes are connected, there is spontaneous flow of electrons from the electrode with the lower electron affinity (oxidation; e.g. silver).

These electrons pass through the external meter to the cathode (reduction), where OH^- ions are liberated. This reaction continues until one of the chemical components is depleted, at which point, the cell is 'dead' and cannot produce electrical energy to the external meter. Current may be forced to flow through the dead cell only by applying an external electromotive force E. This is called an electrolytic cell. In short, a galvanic cell can be built from an electrolytic cell. When the external E is turned off,

accumulated products at the electrodes will spontaneously produce current in the opposite direction of the electrolytic cell.

Half-cells

It is impossible to measure the electrochemical activity of one half-cell; two reactions must be coupled and one reaction compared with the other. To rate half-cell reactions, a specific electrode reaction is arbitrarily assigned 0.00 V. Every other reaction coupled with this arbitrary zero reaction is either positive or negative, depending on the relative affinity for electrons. The electrode defined as 0.00 V is the standard hydrogen electrode: H_2 gas at 1 atmosphere (atm). The hydrogen gas in contact with H^+ in solution develops a potential. The hydrogen electrode coupled with a zinc half-cell is cathodic, with the reaction:

$$2H^+ + 2e^- \rightarrow H_2$$

Because H_2 has a greater affinity than Zn for electrons. Cu, however, has a greater affinity than H_2 for electrons, and thus the anodic reaction:

$$H_2 \rightarrow 2H^+ + 2e^-$$

Occurs when coupled to the Cu-electrode half-cell. The potential generated by the hydrogen-gas electrode is used to rate the electrode potential of metals in 1 mol/L solution. Reduction potentials for certain metals are shown in Table 23.1. A hydrogen electrode is used to determine the accuracy of reference and indicator electrodes, the stability of standard solutions, and the potentials of liquid junctions.

Ion-selective Electrodes

Potentiometric methods of analysis involve the direct measurement of electrical potential due to the activity of free ions. Ion-selective electrodes are designed to be sensitive toward individual ions.

pH Electrodes

An ISE universally used in the clinical laboratory is the pH electrode; the basic components of a pH meter are shown in Figure 23.18.

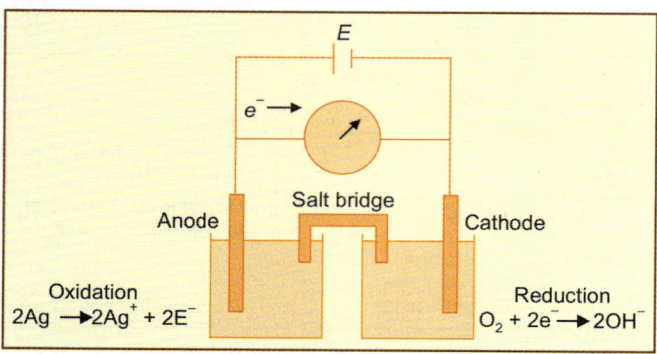

Fig. 23.17: Electrochemical cell

Table 23.1	Standard reduction potentials	
		Potential, V
$Zn^{2+} + 2e^- \leftrightarrow Z$		−0.7628
$Cr^{2+} + 2e^- \leftrightarrow Cr$		−0.913
$Ni^{2+} + 2e^- \leftrightarrow Ni$		−0.257
$2H^+ + 2e^- \leftrightarrow H_2$		0.000
$Cu^{2+} + 2e^- \leftrightarrow Cu$		0.3419
$Ag+ + e^- \leftrightarrow Ag$		0.7996

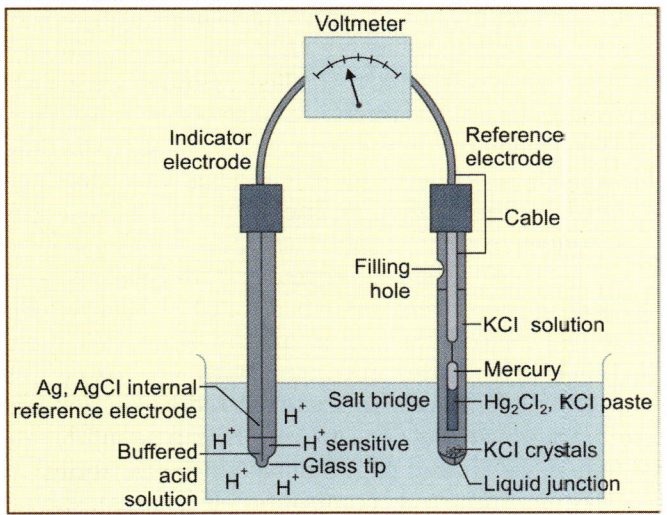

Fig. 23.18: Necessary components of a pH meter

INDICATOR ELECTRODE

The pH electrode consists of a silver wire coated with AgCl, immersed into an internal solution of 0.1 mmol/L HCl, and placed into a tube containing a special glass membrane tip. This membrane is only sensitive to hydrogen ions (H^+). Glass membranes that are selectively sensitive to H^+ consist of specific quantities of lithium, cesium, lanthanum, barium, or aluminum oxides in silicate. When the pH electrode is placed into the test solution, movement of H^+ near the tip of the electrode produces a potential difference between the internal solution and the test solution, which is measured as pH and read by a voltmeter. The combination pH electrode also contains a built-in reference electrode, either Ag/AgCl or calomel (Hg/Hg_2Cl_2) immersed in a solution of saturated KCl.

The specially formulated glass continually dissolves from the surface. The present concept of the selective mechanism that causes the formation of electromotive force at the glass surface is that an ion-exchange process is involved. Cationic exchange occurs only in the gel layer there is no penetration of H^+ through the glass. Although, the glass is constantly dissolving, the process is slow, and the glass tip generally lasts for several years. pH electrodes are highly selective for H^+; however, other cations in high concentration interfere, the most common of which is sodium. Electrode manufacturers should list the concentration of interfering cations that may cause error in pH determinations.

Reference Electrode

The reference electrode commonly used is the calomel electrode. Calomel, a paste of predominantly mercurous chloride, is in direct contact with metallic mercury in an electrolyte solution of potassium chloride. As long as the electrolyte concentration and the temperature remain constant, a stable voltage is generated at the interface of the mercury and its salt. A cable connected to the mercury leads to the voltmeter. The filling hole is needed for adding potassium chloride solution. A tiny opening at the bottom is required for completion of electric contact between the reference and indicator electrodes. The liquid junction consists of a fiber or ceramic plug that allows a small flow of electrolyte filling solution. Construction varies, but all reference electrodes must generate a stable electrical potential. Reference electrodes generally consist of a metal and its salt in contact with a solution containing the same anion. Mercury/Mercurous chloride, as in this example, is a frequently used reference electrode; the disadvantage is that it is slow to reach a new stable voltage following temperature change and it is unstable above 80°C. Ag/AgCl is another common reference electrode. It can be used at high temperatures, up to 275°C, and the AgCl-coated Ag wire makes a more compact electrode than that of mercury. In measurements in which chloride contamination must be avoided, a mercury sulfate and potassium sulfate reference electrode may be used.

LIQUID JUNCTIONS

Electrical connection between the indicator and reference electrodes is achieved by allowing a slow flow of electrolyte from the tip of the reference electrode. A junction potential is always set up at the boundary between two dissimilar solutions because of positive and negative ions diffusing across the boundary at unequal rates. The resultant junction potential may increase or decrease the potential of the reference electrode. Therefore, it is important that the junction potential be kept to a minimum reproducible value when the reference electrode is in solution. KCl is a commonly used filling solution because K^+ and Cl^- have nearly the same mobilities. When KCl is used as the filling solution for Ag/AgCl electrodes, the addition of AgCl is required to prevent dissolution of the AgCl salt. One way of producing a lower junction potential is to mix K^+, Na^+, NO_3^-, and Cl^- in appropriate ratios.

Readout Meter

Electromotive force produced by the reference and indicator electrodes is in the millivolt range. Zero potential for the cell indicates that each electrode half-cell is generating the same voltage, assuming there is no liquid junction potential. The isopotential is that potential at which a temperature change has no effect on the response of the electrical cell. Manufacturers generally achieve this by making the midscale (pH 7.0) correspond to 0 V at all temperatures. They use an internal buffer whose pH changes due to temperature compensate for the changes in the internal and external reference electrodes.

Nernst Equation

The electromotive force generated because of H⁺ at the glass tip is described by Nernst equation, which is shown in a simplified form:

$$\varepsilon = \Delta pH \times \frac{RT \ln 10}{F} \times \Delta PH \times 0.059\,V$$

where e is the electromotive force of the cell, F is the Faraday constant (96,500 C/mol), R is the molar gas constant, and T is temperature, in Kelvin. As the temperature increases, H⁺ activity increases and the potential generated increases. Most pH meters have a temperature compensation knob that amplifies the millivolt response when the meter is on pH function. pH units on the meter scale are usually printed for use at room temperature. On the voltmeter, 59.16 is read as 1 pH unit change. The temperature compensation changes the millivolt response to compensate for changes due to temperature from 54.2 at 0°C to 66.10 at 60°C. However, most pH meters are manufactured for greatest accuracy in the 10–60°C range.

Calibration

The steps necessary to standardize a pH meter are fairly straightforward. First, balance the system with the electrodes in a buffer with a 7.0 pH. The balance or intercept control shifts the entire slope (Fig. 23.19). Next, replace the buffer with one of a different pH. If the meter does not register the correct pH, amplification of the response changes the slope to match that predicted by Nernst equation. If the instrument does not have as lope control, the temperature compensator performs the same function.

pH Combination Electrode

The most commonly used pH electrode has both the indicator and reference electrodes combined in one small probe, which is convenient when small samples are tested. It consists of an Ag/AgCl internal reference electrode sealed in a narrow glass cylinder with a pH-sensitive glass tip. The reference electrode is an Ag/AgCl wire wrapped around the indicator electrode. The outer glass envelope is filled with KCl and has a tiny pore near the tip of the liquid junction. The solution to be measured must completely cover the glass tip; examples of other ISEs (Fig. 23.20). The reference electrode, electrometer, and calibration system described for pH measurements are applicable to all ISEs. There are three major ISE types: inert metal electrodes in contact with a redox couple, metal electrodes that participate in a redox reaction, and membrane electrodes. The membrane can be solid material (e.g. glass), liquid (e.g. ion-exchange electrodes), or special membrane (e.g. compound electrodes), such as gas-sensing and enzyme electrodes.

The standard hydrogen electrode is an example of an inert metal electrode. The Ag/AgCl electrode is an example of the second type; the electrode process produces an electrical potential proportional to chloride ion (Cl⁻) activity:

$$AgCl + e^- \rightarrow Ag^+ + Cl^-$$

When Cl⁻ is held constant, the electrode is used as a reference electrode. The electrode in contact with varying Cl⁻ concentrations is used as an indicator electrode to measure Cl⁻ concentration. The H⁺ sensitive gel layer of the glass pH electrode is considered a membrane. A change in the glass formulation makes the membrane more sensitive to sodium ions (Na⁺) than to H⁺, creating a sodium ISE. Other solid-state membranes consist of either a single crystal or fine crystals immobilized in an inert matrix, such as silicone rubber. Conduction depends on a vacancy defect mechanism, and the crystals are formulated to be selective for a particular size, shape, and change for example, F⁻-selective electrodes of LaF3, Cl⁻-sensitive electrodes with AgCl crystals, and AgBr electrodes for the detection of Br⁻.

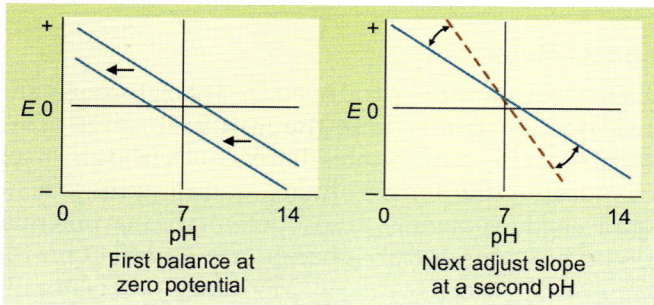

Fig. 23.19: pH meter calibration

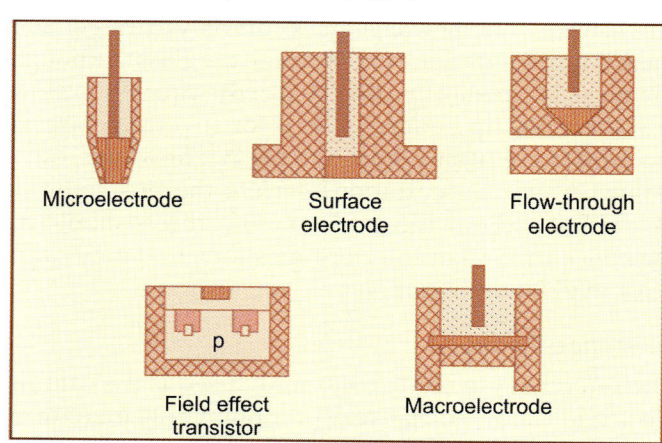

Fig. 23.20: Other examples of ion-selective electrodes

The calcium ISE is a liquid membrane electrode. Anion-selective carrier, such as dioctylphenyl phosphonate dissolved in an inert water-insoluble solvent, diffuses through a porous membrane. Because the solvent is insoluble in water, the test sample cannot cross the membrane, but calcium ions (Ca^{2+}) are exchanged. The Ag/AgCl internal reference in a filling solution of $CaCl_2$ is in contact with the carrier by means of the membrane. Potassium-selective liquid membranes use the antibiotic valinomycin as the ion-selective carrier. Valinomycin membranes show great selectivity for K^+. Liquid membrane electrodes are recharged every few months to replace the liquid ion exchanger membrane and the porous membrane.

GAS-SENSING ELECTRODES

Gas electrodes are similar to pH glass electrodes but are designed to detect specific gases (e.g. CO_2 and NH_3) in solutions and are usually separated from the solution by a thin, gas-permeable hydrophobic membrane. Figure 23.21 shows a schematic illustration of the pCO_2 electrode. The membrane in contact with the solution is permeable only to CO_2, which diffuses into a thin film of sodium bicarbonate solution. The pH of the bicarbonate solution is changed as follows:

$$CO_2 + H_2O \leftrightarrow H_2CO_3 \leftrightarrow H^+ + HCO_3^-$$

The change in pH of the HCO_3^- is detected by a pH electrode. The pCO_2 electrode is widely used in clinical laboratories as a component of instruments for measuring serum electrolytes and blood gases. In the NH_3 gas electrode, the bicarbonate solution is replaced by ammonium chloride solution, and the membrane is permeable only to NH_3 gas. As in the pCO_2 electrode, NH_3 changes the pH of NH_4Cl as follows:

$$NH_3 + H_2O \leftrightarrow NH_4^+ + OH^-$$

The amount of OH^- produced varies linearly with the log of the partial pressure of NH_3 in the sample. Other gas-sensing electrodes function on the basis of an amperometric principle; that is measurement of the current flowing through an electrochemical cell at a constant applied electrical potential to the electrodes. Examples are the determination of pO_2, glucose, and peroxidase.

The chemical reactions of the pO_2 electrode (Clark electrode), an electrochemical cell with a platinum cathode and an Ag/AgCl anode (Fig. 23.17). The electrical potential at the cathode is set to -0.65 V and will not conduct current without oxygen in the sample. The membrane is permeable to oxygen, which diffuses through to the platinum cathode. Current passes through the cell and is proportional to the pO_2 in the test sample.

Glucose determination is based on the reduction in pO_2 during glucose oxidase reaction with glucose and oxygen. Unlike the pCO_2 electrode, the peroxidase electrode has a polarized platinum anode and its potential is set to $+0.6$ V. Current flows through the system when peroxide is oxidized at the anode as follows:

$$H_2O_2 \rightarrow 2H^+ + 2e^- + O_2$$

ENZYME ELECTRODES

The various ISEs may be covered by immobilized enzymes that can catalyze a specific chemical reaction. Selection of the ISE is determined by the reaction product of the immobilized enzyme. Examples include urease, which is used for the detection of urea, and glucose oxidase, which is used for glucose detection. A urea electrode must have an ISE that is selective for NH_4^+ or NH_3, whereas glucose oxidase is used in combination with a pH electrode.

Coulometric Chloridometers and Anodic Stripping Voltammetry

Chloride ISEs have largely replaced coulometric titrations for the determination of chloride in body fluids. Anodic stripping voltammetry was widely used for the analysis of lead and is best measured by electrothermal (graphite furnace) atomic absorption spectroscopy or, preferably, ICP-MS.

Electrophoresis

Electrophoresis is the migration of charged solutes or particles in an electrical field. Iontophoresis refers to the migration of small ions, whereas zone electrophoresis is the migration of charged macromolecules in a porous support medium such as paper, cellulose acetate, or agarose gel film. An electrophoretogram is the result of zone electrophoresis and consists of sharply separated zones of a macromolecule. In a clinical laboratory, the macromolecules of interest are proteins in serum, urine, cerebrospinal fluid (CSF), and other biologic body fluids and erythrocytes and tissue.

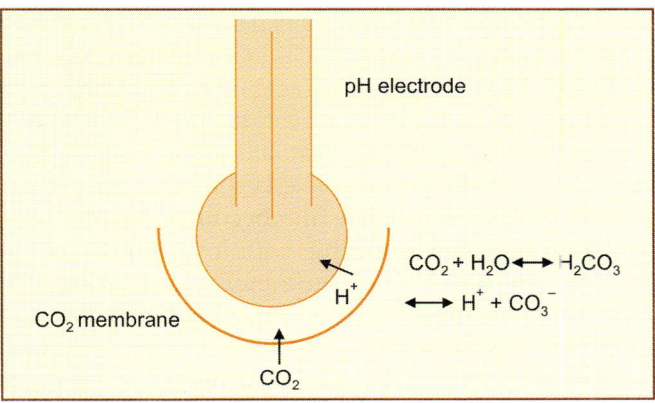

Fig. 23.21: The pCO_2 electrode

Electrophoresis consists of five components: the driving force (electrical power), the support medium, the buffer, the sample, and the detecting system. A typical electrophoretic apparatus is shown in Figure 23.22. Charged particles migrate toward the opposite charged electrode. The velocity of migration is controlled by the net charge of the particle, the size and shape of the particle, the strength of the electric field, chemical and physical properties of the supporting medium, and the electrophoretic temperature.

The rate of mobility of the molecule (μ) is given by:

$$\mu = \frac{Q}{K} \leftrightarrow r \leftrightarrow n$$

where Q is net charge of the particle, K is a constant, r is the ionic radius of the particle, and n is the viscosity of the buffer. From the equation, the rate of migration is directly proportional to the net charge of the particle and inversely proportional to its size and the viscosity of the buffer.

Procedure

The sample is soaked in hydrated support for approximately 5 minutes. The support is put into the electrophoresis chamber, which was previously filled with the buffer. Sufficient buffer must be added to the chamber to maintain contact with the support. Electrophoresis is carried out by applying a constant voltage or constant current for a specific time. The support is then removed and placed in a fixative or rapidly dried to prevent diffusion of the sample. This is followed by staining the zones with an appropriate dye. The uptake of dye by the sample is proportional to sample concentration. After excess dye is washed away, the supporting medium may need to be placed in a clearing agent. Otherwise, it is completely dried.

Power Supply

Power supplies operating at either constant current or constant voltage are available commercially. In electrophoresis, heat is produced when current flows through a medium that has resistance, resulting in an increase in thermal agitation of the dissolved solute (ions) and leading to a decrease in resistance and an increase in current. The increase leads to increases in heat and evaporation of water from the buffer, increasing the ionic concentration of the buffer and subsequent further increases in the current. The migration rate can be kept constant by using a power supply with constant current. This is true because, as electrophoresis progresses, a decrease in resistance as a result of heat produced also decreases the voltage.

Buffers

Two buffer properties that affect the charge of ampholytes are pH and ionic strength. The ions carry the applied electric current and allow the buffer to maintain constant pH during electrophoresis. An ampholyte is a molecule, such as protein, having a net charge either positive or negative. If the buffer is more acidic than the isoelectric point (pI) of the ampholyte, it binds H^+, becomes positively charged, and migrates toward the cathode. If the buffer is more basic than the pI, the ampholyte loses H^+, becomes negatively charged, and migrates toward the anode. A particle without a net charge will not migrate, remaining at the point of application. During electrophoresis, ions cluster around a migrating particle. The higher the ionic concentration, the higher the size of the ionic cloud and the lower the mobility of the particle. Greater ionic strength produces sharper protein-band separation but leads to increased heat production. This may cause denaturation of heat-labile proteins. Consequently, the optimal buffer concentration should be determined for any electrophoretic system. Generally, the most widely used buffers are made of monovalent ions because their ionic strength and molality are equal.

Support Materials
Cellulose Acetate

Paper electrophoresis use has been replaced by cellulose acetate or agarose gel in clinical laboratories. Cellulose is acetylated to form cellulose acetate by treating it with acetic anhydride. Cellulose acetate, a dry, brittle film composed of about 80% airspace, is produced commercially. When the film is soaked in buffer, the air spaces fill with electrolyte and the film becomes pliable. After electrophoresis and staining, cellulose acetate can be made transparent for densitometer quantitation. The dried transparent film can be stored for long periods. Cellulose acetate prepared to reduce electroendosmosis is available commercially. Cellulose acetate is also used in isoelectric focusing.

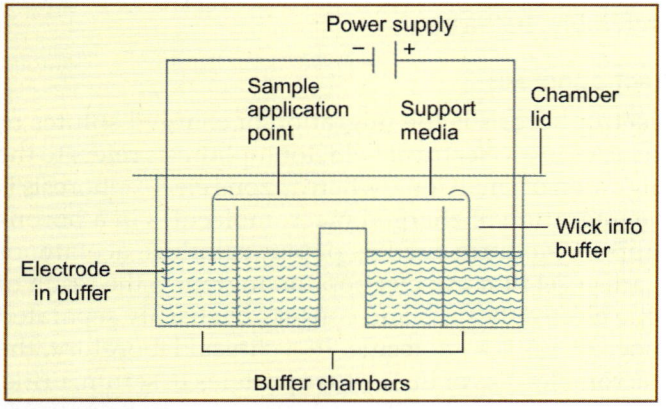

Fig. 23.22: Electrophoresis apparatus; basic components

Agarose Gel

Agarose gel is another widely used supporting medium. Used as a purified fraction of agar, it is neutral and, therefore, does not produce electroendosmosis. After electrophoresis and staining, it is detained (cleared), dried, and scanned with a densitometer. The dried gel can be stored indefinitely. Agarose gel electrophoresis requires small amounts of sample (approximately 2 mL); it does not bind protein and, therefore, migration is not affected.

Polyacrylamide Gel

Polyacrylamide gel electrophoresis involves separation of protein on the basis of charge and molecular size. Layers of gel with different pore sizes are used. The gel is prepared before electrophoresis in a tube-shaped electrophoresis cell. The small-pore separation gel is at the bottom, followed by a large-pore spacer gel and, finally, another large-pore gel containing the sample. Each layer of gel is allowed to form a gelatin before the next gel is poured over it. At the start of electrophoresis, the protein molecules move freely through the spacer gel to its boundary with the separation gel, which slows their movement. This allows for concentration of the sample before separation by the small-pore gel. Polyacrylamide gel electrophoresis separates serum proteins into 20 or more fractions rather than the usual 5 fractions separated by cellulose acetate or agarose. It is widely used to study individual proteins (e.g. isoenzymes).

Starch Gel

Starch gel electrophoresis separates proteins on the basis of surface charge and molecular size, as does poly-acrylamide gel. The procedure is not widely used because of technical difficulty in preparing the gel.

Treatment and Application of Sample

Serum contains a high concentration of protein, especially albumin, and therefore, serum specimens are routinely diluted with buffer before electrophoresis. In contrast, urine and CSF are usually concentrated. Hemoglobin hemolysate is used without further concentration. Generally, preparation of a sample is done according to the suggestion of the manufacturer of the electrophoretic supplies. Cellulose acetate and agarose gel electrophoresis require approximately 2–5 mL of sample. These are the most common routine electrophoreses performed in clinical laboratories. Because most commercially manufactured plates come with a thin plastic template that has small slots through which samples are applied, overloading of agarose gel with sample is not a frequent problem. After serum is allowed to diffuse into the gel for approximately 5 minutes, the template is blotted to remove excess serum before being removed from the gel surface. Sample is applied to cellulose acetate with a twin-wire applicator designed to transfer a small amount.

Detection and Quantitation

Separated protein fractions are stained to reveal their locations. Different stains come with different plates from different manufacturers. The simplest way to accomplish detection is visualization under UV light, whereas densitometry is the most common and reliable way for quantitation. Most densitometers will automatically integrate the area under a peak, and the result is printed as percentage of the total. A schematic illustration of a densitometer is shown in Figure 23.23.

Electroendosmosis

The movement of buffer ions and solvent relative to the fixed support is called endosmosis or electroendosmosis. Support media, such as paper, cellulose acetate, and agar gel, take on a negative charge from adsorption of hydroxyl ions. When current is applied to the electrophoresis system, the hydroxyl ions remain fixed while the free positive ions move toward the cathode. The ions are highly hydrated, resulting in net cathodic movement of solvent. Molecules that are nearly neutral are swept toward the cathode with the solvent. Support media such as agarose and acrylamide gel are essentially neutral, eliminating electroendosmosis. The position of proteins in any electrophoresis separation depends not only on the nature of the protein but also on all other technical variables.

Isoelectric Focusing

Isoelectric focusing is a modification of electrophoresis. Charged proteins migrate through a support medium that has a continuous pH gradient. Individual proteins move in the electric field until they reach a pH equal to their isoelectric point, at which point they have no charge and cease to move.

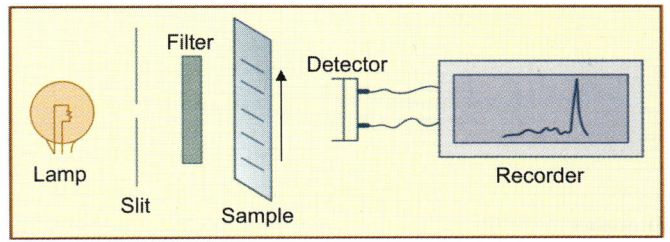

Fig. 23.23: Densitometer; basic components

Capillary Electrophoresis

In capillary electrophoresis (CE), separation is performed in narrow-bore fused silica capillaries (inner diameter 25–75 μm). Usually, the capillaries are only filled with buffer, although gel media can also be used (Fig. 23.24). Initially, the capillary is filled with buffer and then the sample is loaded; applying an electric field performs the separation. Detection can be made near the other end of the capillary directly through the capillary wall.

A Fundamental CE Concept is the Electro-osmotic Flow

Electro-osmotic flow (EOF), is the bulk flow of liquid toward the cathode upon application of an electric field and it is superimposed on electrophoretic migration. EOF controls the amount of time solutes remain in the capillary. Cations migrate fastest because both EOF and electrophoretic attraction are toward the cathode; neutral molecules are all carried by the EOF, but are not separated from each other; and anions move slowest because, although they are carried to the cathode by the EOF, they are attracted to the anode and repelled by the cathode (Fig. 23.25). Widely used for monitoring separated analytes, UV-visible detection is performed directly on the capillary; however, sensitivity is poor because of the small dimensions of the capillary, resulting in a short path length. Fluorescence, laser-induced fluorescence, and chemiluminescence detection can be used for higher sensitivity.

CE has been used for the separation, quantitation, and determination of molecular weights of proteins and peptides; for the analysis of polymerase chain reaction products; and for the analysis of inorganic ions, organic acids, pharmaceuticals, optical isomers, and drugs of abuse in serum and urine. While traditionally serum protein electrophoresis for the diagnosis of plasma cell dyscrasias has been performed using polyacrylamide gel

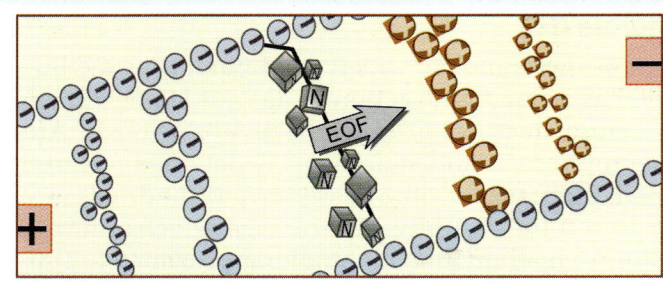

Fig. 23.25: Differential solute migration superimposed on electro-osmotic flow in capillary zone electrophoresis

electrophoresis, CE has now become widely used for this analysis due to its faster run time and its relative automation.

Two Dimensional Electrophoresis

This electrophoresis assay combines two different electrophoresis dimensions to separate proteins from complex matrices such as serum or tissue. In the first dimension, proteins are resolved according to their isoelectric points, using immobilized pH gradients. Commercial gradients are available in a variety of pH ranges. In the second dimension, proteins are separated according to their relative size (molecular weight), using sodium dodecyl sulfate polyacrylamide gel electrophoresis (Fig. 23.26). Gels can be run under denaturing or non-denaturing conditions (e.g. for the maintenance of enzyme activity) and visualized by a variety of techniques, including the use of colorimetric dyes (e.g. Coomassie blue or silver stain) and radiographic,

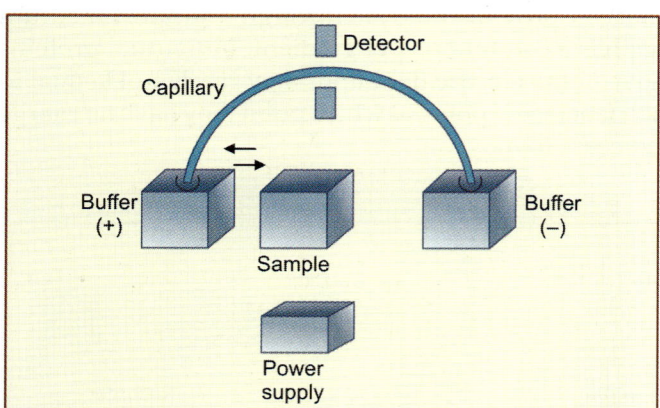

Fig. 23.24: Schematic of capillary electrophoresis instrumentation. Sample is loaded on the capillary by replacing the anode buffer reservoir with the sample reservoir

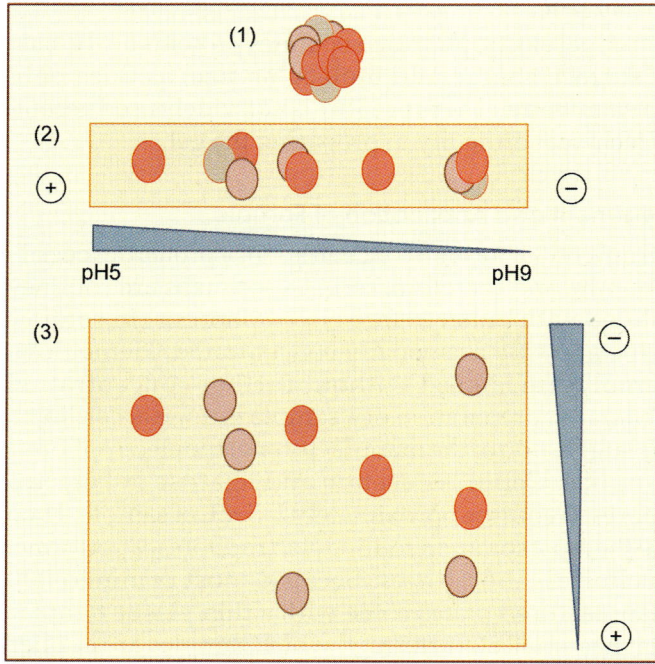

Fig. 23.26: Two dimensional electrophoresis

fluorometric, or chemiluminescence of appropriately labeled polypeptides. These latter techniques are considerably more sensitive than the colorimetric dyes.

OSMOMETRY

An osmometer is used to measure the concentration of solute particles in a solution. The mathematic definition is:

$$\text{Osmolality} = j \times n \times C$$

where j is the osmotic coefficient, n is the number of dissociable particles (ions) per molecule in the solution, and C is the concentration in moles per kilogram of solvent.

The osmotic coefficient is an experimentally derived factor to correct for the fact that some of the molecules, even in a highly dissociated compound, exist as molecules rather than as ions. The four physical properties of a solution that change with variations in the number of dissolved particles in the solvent are osmotic pressure, vapor pressure, boiling point, and freezing point. Osmometers measure osmolality indirectly by measuring one of these colligative properties, which change proportionally with osmotic pressure. Osmometers in clinical use measure either freezing pointde pression or vapor pressure depression; results are expressed in milliosmolal per kilogram (mOsm/kg) units.

Freezing Point Osmometer

The basic components of a freezing point osmometer is shown in Figure 23.27; the sample in a small tube is lowered into a chamber with cold refrigerant circulating from a cooling unit. A thermistor is immersed in the sample. To measure temperature, a wire is used to gently stir the sample until it is cooled to several degrees below its freezing point. It is possible to cool water to as low as −40°C and still have liquid water, provided nocrystals or particulate matter is present. This is referred to as a supercooled solution. Vigorous agitation when the sample is supercooled results in rapid freezing.

Freezing can also be started by 'seeding' a supercooled solution with crystals. When the supercooled solution starts to freeze as a result of the rapid stirring, a slush is formed and the solution actually warms to its freezing point temperature. The slush, an equilibrium of liquid and ice crystals, will remain at the freezing point temperature until the sample freezes solid and drops below its freezing point. Impurities in a solvent will lower the temperature at which freezing or melting occurs by reducing the bonding forces between solvent molecules, so that the molecules break away from each other and exist as a fluid at a lower temperature. The decrease in the freezing point temperature is proportional to the number of dissolved particles present. The thermistor is a material that has less resistance when the temperature increases. The readout uses a Wheatstone bridge circuit that detects temperature change as proportional to change in thermistor resistance. Freezing point depression is proportional to the number of solute particles. Standards of known concentration are used to calibrate the instruments in mOsm/kg.

AUTOMATION OF SPECIMEN PREPARATION

Specimen Delivery

Automated methods are often used to deliver specimens to the laboratory instead of the historic method (courier service). These include (1) pneumatic tube systems, (2) electric track vehicles, and (3) mobile robots.

Pneumatic Tube Systems

Pneumatic tube systems provide rapid specimen transportation and are reliable when installed as point-to-point services (Fig. 23.28). However, when switching mechanisms are introduced to allow carriers the bullet - shaped containers used to hold specimens (Fig. 23.29) to be sent to various locations, mechanical problems may occur and may cause misrouting of carriers. In addition, close attention to the design of the pneumatic tube system is necessary to prevent hemolysis of the specimen.

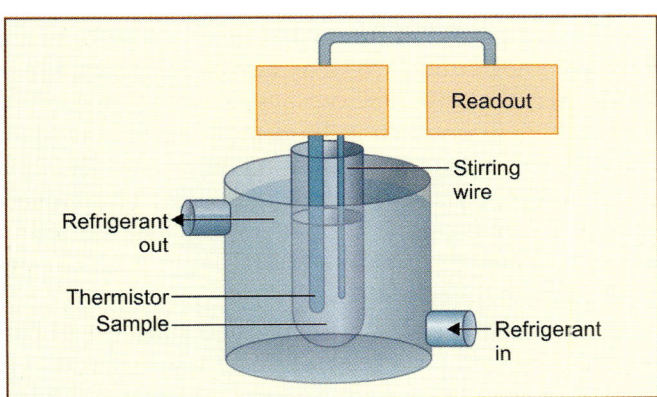

Fig. 23.27: Freezing point osmometer

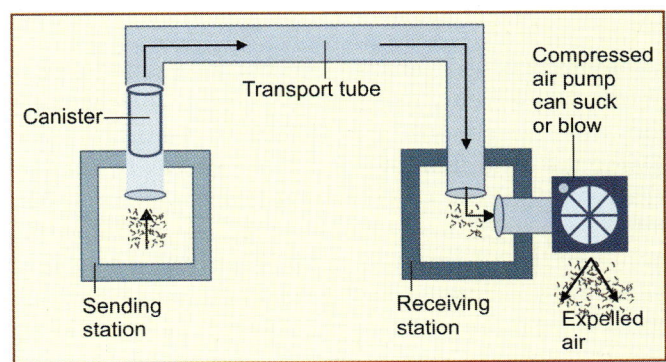

Fig. 23.28: Pneumatic tube systems

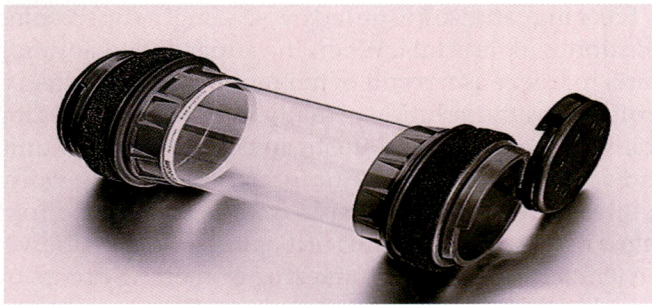

Fig. 23.29: Bullet shaped container

Avoidance of sudden accelerations and decelerations and the use of proper packing material inside the carriers will minimize hemolysis.

Electric Track Vehicles

Electric track vehicles have a larger carrying capacity than pneumatic tube systems and do not have problems with damaging specimens by acceleration and/or deceleration forces. Some systems maintain the carrier in an upright position with the use of a gimbal (a device that permits a body to incline freely in any direction or suspends it, so it will remain level when its support is tipped), enabling the carrier to move both vertically and horizontally on an installed electric track. The containers can hold dry ice or refrigerated gel packs with specimens if desired. They are especially useful in quickly transporting specimens between floors or between laboratory locations that are some distance from each other, by making use of the space in the ceiling plenum above the laboratory.

A primary disadvantage is the cost of moving the track and loading/unloading stations if the laboratory is expanding or moving; in addition, the stations may be larger than the pneumatic tube stations. If the station is not located directly in the central laboratory (centralized testing; core laboratory), additional staff may be necessary to unload the carts and transport the specimens to their final destination, and the electric track system may not achieve its desired goal of rapid specimen transport.

MOBILE ROBOTS

Automated guided vehicles (AGVs), also called mobile robots, have been used successfully to transport laboratory specimens both within the laboratory and outside the central laboratory. They are easily adapted to carry various sizes and shapes of specimen containers and are reprogrammable with changes in laboratory geometry. In addition, in a busy laboratory setting, delivery of specimens to laboratory benches by a mobile robot can be more frequent than human pickup and has been shown to be cost-effective. Inexpensive models follow a line on the floor, whereas others have more sophisticated guidance systems. Their limitations include the need to batch specimens for greater efficiency and, in most cases, the requirement for laboratory personnel to place specimens onto or remove specimens from the mobile robot at each stopping place. Some mobile robots have been integrated with robotic systems that automate loading and unloading of specimens; others initiate an audible or visual signal of their arrival at a specified station so that employees are able to load or unload the specimens being transported.

Specimen Loading and Aspiration

In most situations, the specimen for automatic analysis is serum or plasma. Many analyzers directly sample serum from primary collection tubes of various sizes. With such analyzers, the collection tubes most frequently used contain separator material that forms a barrier between serum or plasma and cells. Many analyzers also sample from cups or tubes filled with serum transferred from the original specimen tubes. Often the design of the sampling cup is unique for a particular analyzer. Each cup should be designed to minimize dead volume, i.e. the excess serum that must be present in a cup to permit aspiration of the full volume required for testing. Cups must be made of inert material, so they do not interact with the analytes being measured. Specimen cups also should be disposable to minimize cost and contamination, and their shape should, even without a cap, minimize evaporation by minimizing the surface area of sample exposed to the air. Specimens may undergo other forms of degradation in addition to evaporation. For example, specimens that contain thermolabile constituents may undergo degradation of such analytes if held at ambient temperatures. Other constituents, such as bilirubin, are photolabile. Thermolability is minimized when both specimens and calibrators are held in a refrigerated loading zone. Photodegradation is reduced by the use of semi-opaque cups and placement of smoke- or orange-colored plastic covers over the specimen cups.

The loading zone of an analyzer is the area in which specimens are held in the instrument before they are analyzed. The holding area may be a circular tray, a rack or series of racks built into a cassette, or a serpentine chain of containers into which individual tubes are inserted. When specimens are not identified automatically, they must be presented to the sampling device in the correct sequence, as specified by a loading list. The sampling mechanism determines the exact volume of sample removed from the specimen.

For most analyzers, specimens for a subsequent run may be prepared on a separate tray while one run is already in progress. This process permits machine operation and human actions to proceed in parallel for optimal efficiency. In some analyzers, specimens may be added continuously by the operator as they become available. A desirable feature of any automated analyzer is the ability to insert new specimens ahead of specimens already in place in the loading zone. This feature allows the timely analysis of a specimen with a high medical priority. When specimen identification is machine-read, it is possible for the operator to easily reposition specimens in the loading zone. When specimen identification is tied to a loading list, however, insertion or repositioning of specimens must be accompanied by revision of the loading list.

Transmission of infectious diseases by automated equipment is a concern in clinical laboratories. The method of transmission by equipment is primarily through splatter of serum or blood during the acquisition of samples from rapidly moving specimen probes. The use of level sensors, which restrict the penetration of sample probes into specimens, and provision of software for smoother motion control greatly reduce splatter. Because the potential for contamination exists when the stoppers of primary containers are opened or 'popped' to decant serum into specimen cups, several firms have developed closed-container sampling systems for use in their automated hematology and chemistry analyzers. In these systems, the specimen probe passes through a hollow needle that initially penetrates the primary container's rubber stopper. This configuration prevents damage or plugging of the specimen probe while allowing the level sensor (used to reduce carry over and to detect short samples) to remain active. After the specimen probe is withdrawn, the outer hollow needle is also withdrawn, so the stopper reseals and no specimen escapes. Closed-container sampling is used widely in hematology analyzers.

Sample Pretreatment

Automation of analytical procedures requires the capability to remove proteins and other interferents from some specimens to ensure the specificity of an analytical method. Dialysis, column chromatography, and filtration have been used for this purpose.

SAMPLE INTRODUCTION AND INTERNAL TRANSPORT

The method used to introduce the sample into the analyzer and its subsequent transport within the analyzer is the major difference between continuous-flow and discrete systems. In continuous-flow systems, the sample is aspirated through the sample probe into a stream of flowing liquid, whereby it is transported to analytical stations in the instrument. In discrete analysis, the sample is aspirated into the sample probe and then is delivered, often with reagent, through the same orifice into a

reaction cup or other container. Carryover is a potential problem with both types of systems. Technic on instruments corporation pioneered the use of peristaltic pumps and plastic tubing to advance the sample and reagents in continuous-flow analysis. Peristaltic pumps trap a 'slug' of fluid between two rollers that occlude the tubing. As the rollers travel over the tubing, the trapped fluid is pushed forward and, as the leading roller lifts from the tubing, is added to the fluid beyond it. The peristaltic pump still is used in some hematology analyzers and analyzers with ion-selective electrodes, as well as for wash systems.

Discrete Processing Systems

Positive-liquid displacement pipettes are used for sampling in most discrete automated systems in which specimens, calibrators, and controls are delivered by a single pipette to the next stage in the analytical process. A positive-displacement pipette may be designed for one of two operational modes: (1) to dispense only aspirated sample into the reaction receptacle, or (2) to flush out sample together with diluent. Both systems use a plastic or glass syringe with a plunger, the tip of which usually is made of Teflon.

Pipettes may be categorized as (1) fixed-, (2) variable, or (3) selectable-volume. Selectable-volume pipettes allow the selection of a limited number of predetermined volumes. Pipettes with unlimited or selectable volumes are used in systems that allow many different applications, whereas fixed-volume pipettes usually are used for samples and reagents in instruments dedicated to the performance of only a small variety of tests.

Carryover

Carryover is defined as the transfer of a quantity of analyte or reagent from one specimen reaction into a subsequent one. Because it erroneously affects analytical results from the subsequent reaction, carryover should be minimized or eliminated. In discrete systems with disposable reaction vessels and measuring cuvettes, carryover is caused by the pipetting system. In instruments with reusable cuvettes or flow cells, carryover may also arise from incomplete cleaning of the cuvettes or flow cells between assays.

Most manufacturers of discrete systems reduce sample-to-sample carryover by using disposable pipette tips or by incorporating wash stations for the sample probe that flush the internal and external surfaces of the probe with copious amounts of diluent. An adequate ratio of flush and rinse to specimen volume controls carryover in many cases to acceptable values. Appropriate choice of sample probe material, geometry, and surface conditions also influences carryover. Some systems wipe the outside of the sample probe to prevent transfer of a portion of the previous specimen into the next specimen cup. Use of disposable sample probe tips allows complete elimination of contamination of one sample by another inside the probe, as well as the carryover of one specimen into the specimen in the next cup, because a new pipette tip is used for each pipetting. In practice, the reduction of sample-to-sample carryover is a more stringent requirement for automated analyzers that perform immunoassays in which some analytes (e.g. human chorionic gonadotropin) have a wide range of concentrations.

Some systems use extra steps, such as additional washes, or an additional washing device to reduce carryover for selected tests to acceptable limits. Because extra steps reduce overall throughput, additional rinsing functions are initiated (by computer operator selection) only for assays with a large analytical measurement range. Sample-to-sample carryover can be detected by the preparation of two sample pools, one having a very high analyte concentration (H), the other having a low concentration(L). By running sequences of tests, such as HHHLLLHHLLHHLL, if sample-to-sample carryover is present, higher results will be noted in the low-concentration sample analyses that immediately follow a high-concentration sample analysis.

Reagent-to-reagent carryover also can occur on discrete systems that use a common reagent probe for pipetting all reagents; its minimization or elimination requires use of the same approaches just described for sample-to-sample carryover. Detection of reagent-to-reagent carryover can be difficult for end-users and usually requires the involvement of the instrument vendor. Users should be aware that the introduction of third party reagents in 'open' channels on otherwise closed systems may introduce problems with reagent-to-reagent carryover. Consultation with the system manufacturer is advised to determine how to test for and minimize such carryover.

REAGENT HANDLING AND STORAGE

Many automated systems use liquid reagents stored in plastic or glass containers. For those analyzers in which a working inventory is maintained in the system, the volumes of reagents stored depend on the number of tests to be performed without operator intervention. For many analyzers in which specimens are not processed continuously, reagents are stored in laboratory refrigerators and are introduced into the instruments as required. In larger systems, sections of the reagent storage compartments are maintained at 4–10°C. Some systems

use reagents or antibodies that have been immobilized in a reaction coil or chamber to allow their repetitive use in a chemical reaction. Other systems use enzymes immobilized on membranes coupled to sensing electrodes. The reaction products then are measured by the sensing device. Only a buffer is required as a diluent and a wash solution; thus the membrane has an extended life, which lowers the cost of each test.

Reagent Identification

Labels on reagent containers include information, such as (1) reagent identification, (2) volume of the contents or the number of tests for which the contents of the containers are to be used, (3) expiration date, and (4) lot number. Many reagent containers now carry bar codes that contain some or all of this information, and the manufacturer is able to retrieve any pertinent information when necessary. Other advantages of using reagent bar codes include (1) facilitation of inventory management, (2) ability to insert reagent containers in random sequence, and (3) ability to automatically dispense a particular volume of liquid reagent. Furthermore, when a bar code reader is coupled with a level sensing system on the reagent probe, it alerts the operator as to whether a sufficient quantity of reagent exists to complete a workload. A bar code on a reagent container may also contain information about (multiple) calibrators, such as the definition of a calibration curve algorithm and values of curve constants defined at the time of reagent manufacture. Accompanying calibrator materials provided in their own bar code tubes at the time of manufacture ensure that calibration functions are integrated properly into the analysis.

Open Versus Closed Systems

Automated analyzers are classified as 'open' or 'closed' in an open analyzer, the operator is able to change the parameters related to an analysis and to prepare 'in-house' reagents or use reagents from a variety of suppliers. Such analyzers usually have considerable flexibility and adapt readily to new methods and analytes. A closed-system analyzer is one in which reagents and calibrators are provided only by the manufacturer and other reagents or methods cannot be used.

Reagent Delivery

Liquid reagents are acquired and delivered to mixing and reaction chambers by pumps (through tubes) or by positive displacement syringe devices. In those analyzers in which more than one reagent is acquired and dispensed by the same syringe, washing or flushing of the probe is essential to prevent reagent carryover.

Chemical Reaction Phase

Sample and reagents react in the chemical reaction phase. Factors that are important in this phase include (1) vessel in which the reaction occurs; (2) cuvette in which the reaction is monitored; (3) timing of the reaction(s); (4) mixing and transport of reactants; (5) thermal conditioning of fluids; and (6) for some immunoassay systems, separation of bound and unbound fractions.

Type of Reaction Vessel and Cuvette

In continuous-flow systems, each specimen passes through the same continuous stream and is subjected to the same analytical reactions as every other specimen and at the same rate. In such systems, the reaction occurs in the flow-through component. In discrete systems, each specimen in a batch has its own physical and chemical space, separate from every other specimen. Discrete analyzers use individual (disposable or reusable) reaction vessels transported through the system after sample and reagent have been dispensed, or they use a stationary reaction chamber.

Reaction vessels are reused in many instruments. The time before reusable cuvette/reaction vessels must be replaced depends on their composition and the washing mechanisms used. Some manufacturers have computer algorithms that automatically control when individual cuvette/reaction vessels are discarded, depending on how many assays and what types of assays have been performed in a given cuvette.

Mixing of Reactants

Various techniques are used to mix reactants. In a discrete system, these include (1) forceful dispensing; (2) magnetic stirring; (3) vigorous lateral displacement; (4) physical stirring; and (5) vigorous lateral displacement. Dry reagent systems obviate the need for mixing because the serum completely interacts with the dry chemicals as it flows through the matrix of the reaction unit. However, regardless of the technique used, mixing is a difficult process to automate and one that can contribute to reaction-to-reaction carryover among reused components.

Thermal Regulation

Thermal regulation requires the establishment of a controlled temperature environment in close contact with the reaction container and efficient heat transfer from the environment to the reaction mixture. Various technologies have been used for temperature regulation, including airbaths, water baths, and piezoelectric devices.

BARCODING

A major advance in the automation of specimen identification in the clinical laboratory is the incorporation of barcoding technology into analytical systems. A barcoding system consists of a barcode printer and a barcode reader, or scanner. One- and two-dimensional barcoding systems are available. A one-dimensional barcode is an array of rectangular bars and spaces arranged in a predetermined pattern according to unambiguous rules to represent elements of data referred to as characters. A barcode is transferred and affixed to an object by a barcode label that carries the barcode and, optionally, other noncoded readable information. Symbology is the term used to describe the rules specifying the way data are encoded into the bars and spaces. The width of the bars and spaces, as well as the number of each, is determined by a specification for that symbology. Different combinations of bars and spaces represent different characters. When a barcode scanner is passed over the barcode, the light beam from the scanner is absorbed by the dark bars and is not reflected; the beam is reflected by the light spaces. A photocell detector in the scanner receives the reflected light and converts that light into an electrical signal that then is digitized. A one dimensional barcode is 'vertically redundant' in that the same information is repeated vertically-the heights of the bars can be truncated without any loss of information. In practice, vertical redundancy allows a symbol with printing defects, such as spots or voids, to be read.

In practice, a barcode label (often generated by the laboratory information system and bearing the sample accession number) is placed onto the specimen container and is subsequently 'read' by one or more bar code readers placed at key positions in the analytical sequence. The resultant identifying and ancillary information then is transferred to and processed by the system software. Initiating barcode identification at a patient's bedside ensures greater integrity of the specimen's identity in an analyzer. Systems to transfer information concerning a patient's identity to blood tubes at the patient's bedside have been introduced in many hospitals, and several companies are now offering these systems.

Unequivocal positive identification of each specimen is achieved in analyzers with barcode readers. Advantages of the use of barcode labels include the following:

1. Elimination of work lists for the system,
2. Avoidance of mistakes made in the placement of tubes in the analyzer or during sampling,
3. Avoidance of the need for analysis of specimens in a defined sequence, and
4. Decrease in identification errors.

Examples of types of barcodes that are used in chemistry analyzers are shown in Figure 23.30.

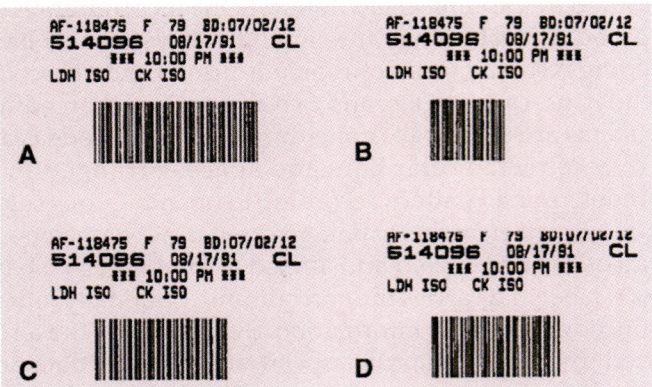

Fig. 23.30: Examples of barcodes used in chemistry analyzers containing the same information. (A) Code 39. (B) Code I 2/5. (C) Code 128B. (D) Codbar

Chromatography

Chromatography refers to the group of techniques used to separate complex mixtures on the basis of different physical interactions between the individual compounds and the stationary phase of the system. The basic components in any chromatographic technique are the mobile phase (gas or liquid), which carries the complex mixture (sample); the stationary phase (solid or liquid), through which the mobile phase flows; the column holding the stationary phase; and the separated components (eluate).

MODES OF SEPARATION

Adsorption

Adsorption chromatography, also known as liquid-solid chromatography, is based on the competition between the sample and the mobile phase for adsorptive sites on the solid stationary phase. There is an equilibrium of solute molecules being adsorbed to the solid surface and desorbed and dissolved in the mobile phase. The molecules that are most soluble in the mobile phase move fastest; the least soluble move slowest. Thus, a mixture is typically separated into classes according to polar functional groups. The stationary phase can be acidic polar (e.g. silica gel), basic polar (e.g. alumina), or nonpolar (e.g. charcoal). The mobile phase can be a single solvent or a mixture of two or more solvents, depending on the analytes to be desorbed. Liquid-solid chromatography is not widely used in clinical laboratories because of technical problems with the preparation of a stationary phase that has homogeneous distribution of absorption sites.

Partition

Partition chromatography is also referred to as liquid-liquid chromatography. Separation of solute is based on relative solubility in an organic (nonpolar) solvent and an aqueous (polar) solvent. In its simplest form, partition (extraction) is performed in a separatory funnel. Molecules containing polar and nonpolar groups in an aqueous solution are added to an immiscible organic solvent. After vigorous shaking, the two phases are allowed to separate. Polar molecules remain in the aqueous solvent; nonpolar molecules are extracted in the organic solvent. This results in the partitioning of the solute molecules into two separate phases.

The ratio of the concentration of the solute in the two liquids is known as the partition coefficient:

$$K = \frac{\text{Solute in stationary phase}}{\text{Solute in mobile phase}}$$

Modern partition chromatography uses pseudoliquid stationary phases that are chemically bonded to the support or high-molecular-weight polymers that are insoluble in the mobile phase. Partition systems are considered normal phase when the mobile solvent is less polar than the stationary solvent and reverse phase when the mobile solvent is more polar. Partition chromatography is applicable to any substance that may be distributed between two liquid phases. Because ionic compounds are generally soluble only in water, partition chromatography works best with nonionic compounds.

STERIC EXCLUSION

Steric exclusion, a variation of liquid-solid chromatography, is used to separate solute molecules on the basis of size and shape. The chromatographic column is packed with porous material (Fig. 23.31).

A sample containing different-sized molecules moves down the column dissolved in the mobile solvent. Small molecules enter the pores in the packing and are

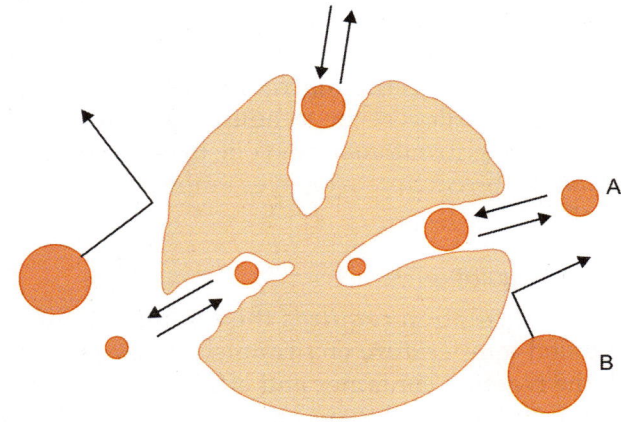

Fig. 23.31: Pictorial concept of steric exclusion chromatography. Separation of sample components by their ability to permeate pore structure of column-packing material. Smaller molecules A, permeating the interstitial pores; large excluded molecules B.

momentarily trapped. Large molecules are excluded from the small pores and so move quickly between the particles. Intermediate-sized molecules are partially restricted from entering the pores and, therefore, move through the column at an intermediate rate that is between those of the large and small molecules. Early methods used hydrophilic beads of cross-linked dextran, poly-acrylamide, or agarose, which formed a gel when soaked in water. This method was termed gel filtration. A similar separation process using hydrophobic gel beads of polystyrene with a non-aqueous mobile phase was called gel permeation chromatography. Current porous packing uses rigid inorganic materials such as silica or glass. The term steric exclusion includes all these variations. Pore size is controlled by the manufacturer, and packing materials can be purchased with different pore sizes, depending on the size of the molecules being separated.

Ion-Exchange Chromatography

In ion-exchange chromatography, solute mixtures are separated by virtue of the magnitude and charge of ionic species. The stationary phase is a resin, consisting of large polymers of substituted benzene, silicates, or cellulose derivatives, with charged functional groups. The resin is insoluble in water, and the functional groups are immobilized as side-chains on resin beads that are used to fill the chromatographic column. Figure 23.32A shows a resin with sulfonate functional groups. H^+ ions are loosely held and free to react. This is an example of a cation-exchange resin. When a cation, such as Na^+ comes in contact with these functional groups, an equilibrium is formed, following the law of mass action. Because there are many sulfonate groups, Na^+ is effectively and completely removed from solution. The Na^+ concentrated on the resin column can be eluted from the resin by pouring acid through the column, driving the equilibrium to the left. Anion-exchange resins are made with exchangeable hydroxyl ions such as the diethyla-mine functional group (Fig. 23.32B). They are used like cation exchange resins, except that hydroxyl ions are exchanged for anions. The example shows Cl^- in sample solution exchanged for OH^- from the resin functional group. Anion and cation resins mixed together (mixed-bed resin) are used to deionize water. The displaced protons and hydroxy lions combine to form water. Ionic functional groups other than the illustrated examples are used for specific analytic applications. Ion-exchange chromatography is used to remove interfering substances from a solution, to concentrate dilute ion solutions, and to separate mixtures of charged molecules, such as amino acids. Changing pH and ionic concentration of the mobile phase allow separation of mixtures of organic and inorganic ions.

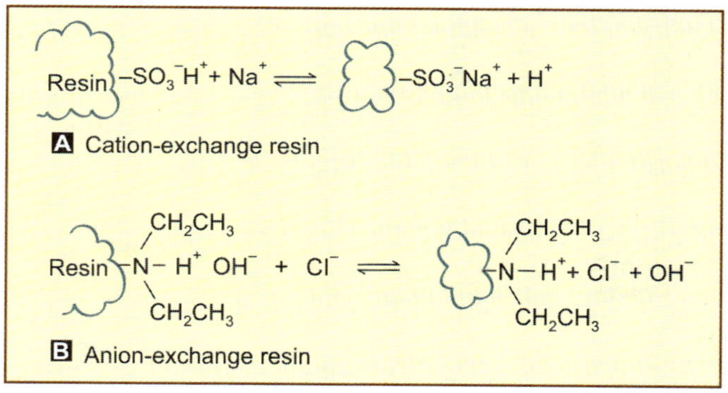

Fig. 23.32: Chemical equilibrium of ion-exchange resins. (A) Cation-exchange resin. (B) Anion-exchange resin

CHROMATOGRAPHIC PROCEDURES

Thin-layer Chromatography

Thin-layer chromatography (TLC) is a variant of column chromatography. A thin layer of sorbent, such as alumina, silica gel, cellulose, or cross-linked dextran, is uniformly coated on a glass or plastic plate. Each sample to be analyzed is applied as a spot near one edge of the plate (Fig. 23.33). The mobile phase (solvent) is usually placed in a closed container until the atmosphere is saturated with solvent vapor. One edge of the plate is placed in the solvent, as shown. The solvent migrates up the thin layer by capillary action, dissolving and carrying sample molecules. Separation can be achieved by any of the four processes previously described, depending on the sorbent (thin layer) and solvent chosen. After the solvent reaches a predetermined height, the plate is removed and dried. Sample components are identified by comparison with standards on the same plate. The distance a component migrates, compared with the distance the solvent front moves, is called the retention factor, Rf:

$$Rf = \frac{\text{Distance leading edge of component moves}}{\text{Total distance solvent front moves}}$$

Each sample component Rf is compared with the Rf of standards. Using (Fig. 23.33) as an example, standard A has an Rf value of 0.4, standard B has an Rf value of 0.6, and standard C has an Rf value of 0.8. The first unknown contains A and C, because the Rf values are the same. This ratio is valid only for separations run under identical conditions. Because Rf values may overlap for some components, further identifying information is obtained by spraying different stains on the dried plate and comparing colors of the standards. TLC is most commonly used as a semi-quantitative screening test. Technique refinement has resulted in the development of semi-automated equipment and the ability to quantitate separated compounds. For example, sample applicators apply precise amounts of sample extracts in concise areas. Plates prepared with uniform sorbent

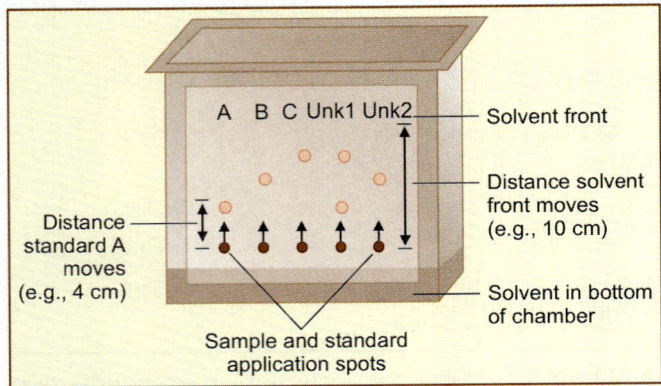

Fig. 23.33: Thin-layer chromatography plate in chromatographic chamber

thickness, finer particles, and new solvent systems have resulted in the technique of high-performance thin-layer chromatography (HPTLC). Absorbance of each developed spot is measured using a densitometer, and the concentration is calculated by comparison with a reference standard chromatographed under identical conditions.

HIGH-PERFORMANCE LIQUID CHROMATOGRAPHY

Modern high-performance liquid chromatography (HPLC) uses pressure for fast separations, controlled temperature, in-line detectors, and gradient elution techniques (Fig. 23.34).

Pumps

A pump forces the mobile phase through the column at a much greater velocity than that accomplished by gravity flow columns and includes pneumatic, syringe, reciprocating, or hydraulic amplifier pumps. The most widely used pump today is the mechanical reciprocating pump, which is used as a multihead pump with two or more reciprocating pistons. During pumping, the pistons operate out of phase (180° for two heads, 120° for three heads) to provide constant flow. Pneumatic pumps are used for preoperative purposes; hydraulic amplifier pumps are no longer commonly used.

Columns

The stationary phase is packed into long stainless steel columns. HPLC is usually run at ambient temperatures, although columns can be put in an oven and heated to enhance the rate of partition. Fine, uniform column packing results in much less band broadening, but requires pressure to force the mobile phase through. The packing can also be pellicular (an inert core with a porous layer), inert and small particles, or macroporous particles. The most common material used for column packing is silica gel. It is very stable and can be used in different ways. It can be used as solid packing in liquid-solid chromatography or coated with a solvent, which serves as the stationary phase (liquid-liquid). As a result of the short lifetime of coated particles, molecules of the mobile-phase liquid are now bonded to the surface of silica particles.

Reversed-phase HPLC is now popular; the stationary phase is nonpolar molecules (e.g. octadecyl C-18 hydrocarbon) bonded to silica gel particles. For this type of column packing, the mobile phase commonly used is acetonitrile, methanol, water, or any combination of solvents. A reversed-phase column can be used to separate-ionic, nonionic, and ionizable samples. A buffer is used to produce the desired ionic characteristics and pH for separation of the analyte. Column packings vary in size (3–20 mm), using smaller particles mostly for analytic separations and larger ones for preparative separations.

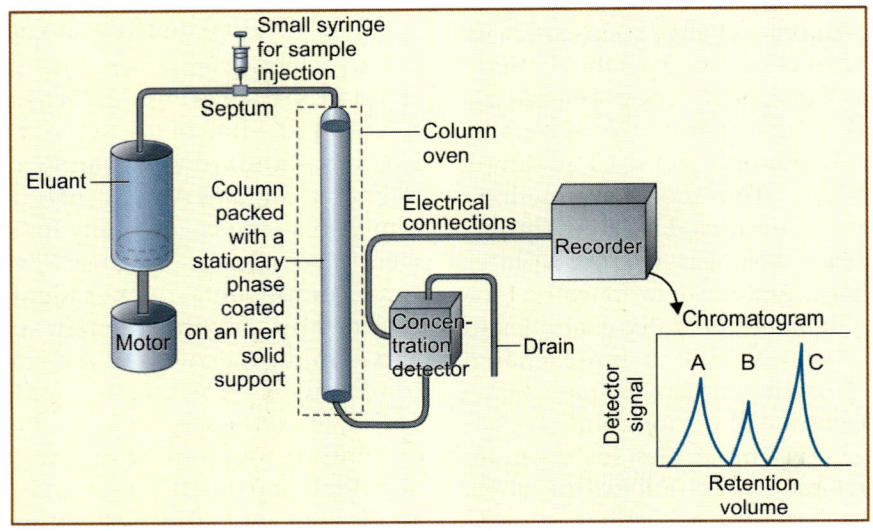

Fig. 23.34: High-performance liquid chromatography basic components

SAMPLE INJECTORS

A small syringe can be used to introduce the sample into the path of the mobile phase that carries it into the column (Fig. 23.34). The best and most widely used method, however, is the loop injector. The sample is introduced into a fixed-volume loop. When the loop is switched, the sample is placed in the path of the flowing mobile phase and flushed onto the column. Loop injectors have high reproducibility and are used at high pressures. Many HPLC instruments have loop injectors that can be programmed for automatic injection of samples. When the sample size is less than the volume of the loop, the syringe containing the sample is often filled with the mobile phase to the volume of the loop before filling the loop. This prevents the possibility of air being forced through the column because such a practice may reduce the lifetime of the column-packing material.

Detectors

Modern HPLC detectors monitor the eluate as it leaves the column and, ideally, produce an electronic signal proportional to the concentration of each separated component. Spectrophotometers that detect absorbances of visible or UV light are most commonly used. Photodiode array (PDA) and other rapid scanning detectors are also used for spectral comparisons and compound identification and purity. These detectors have been used for drug analysis in urine. Obtaining a UV scan of a compound as it elutes from a column can provide important information as to its identity. Unknowns can be compared against library spectra in a similar manner to MS. Unlike gas chromatography/MS, which requires volatilization of targeted compounds, liquid chromatography (LC)/PDA enables direct injection of aqueous urine samples. Because many biologic substances fluoresce strongly, fluorescence detectors are also used, involving the same principles discussed in the section on spectrophotometric measurements. Another common HPLC detector is the amperometric or electrochemical detector, which measures current produced when the analyte of interest is either oxidized or reduced at some fixed potential set between a pair of electrodes.

Recorders

The recorder is used to record detector signal versus the time the mobile phase passed through the instrument, starting from the time of sample injection. The graph is called a chromatogram (Fig. 23.35). The retention time is used to identify compounds when compared with standard retention times run under identical conditions. Peak area is proportional to concentration of the compounds that produced the peaks.

When the elution strength of the mobile phase is constant throughout the separation, it is called isocratic elution. For samples containing compounds of widely differing relative compositions, the choice of solvent is a

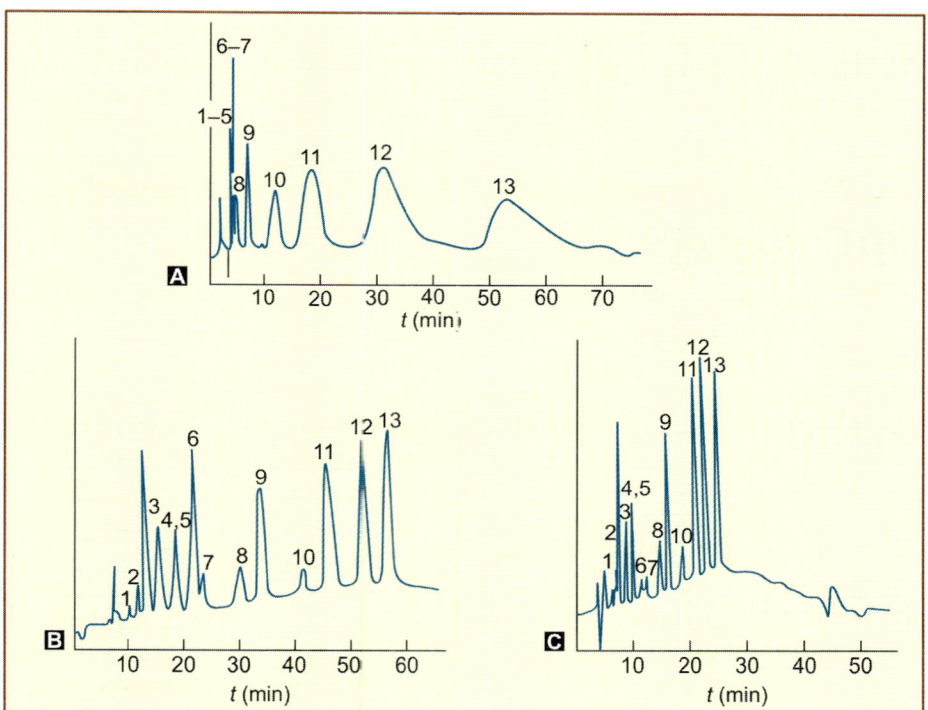

Fig. 23.35: Chromatograms. (A) Isocratic ion-exchange separation mobile phase contains 0.055 mol/L NaNO$_3$. (B) Gradient elution mobile phase gradient from 0.01–0.1 mol/L NaNO$_3$ at 2% per min. (C) Gradient elution 5% per minute

compromise. Early eluting compounds may have retention times close to zero, producing a poor separation (resolution), as shown in figure 23.35A. Basic compounds often have low retention times because C-18 columns cannot tolerate high pH mobile phases. The addition of cation-pairing reagents to the mobile phase (e.g. octanesulfonic acid) can result in better retention of negatively charged compounds onto the column. The late-eluting compounds may have long retention times, producing broad bands resulting in decreased sensitivity. In some cases, certain components of a sample may have such a great affinity for the stationary phase that they do not elute at all. Gradient elution is an HPLC technique that can be used to overcome this problem. The composition of the mobile phase is varied to provide a continual increase in the solvent strength of the mobile phase entering the column (Fig. 23.35B). The same gradient elution can be performed with a faster change in concentration of the mobile phase (Fig. 23.35C).

GAS CHROMATOGRAPHY

Gas chromatography is used to separate mixtures of compounds that are volatile or can be made volatile. GC may be gas solid chromatography, with a solid stationary phase, or gas-liquid chromatography (GLC), with a nonvolatile liquid stationary phase. GLC is commonly used in clinical laboratories. Figure 23.36 illustrates the basic components of a GC system. The setup is similar to HPLC, except that the mobile phase is a gas and samples are partitioned between a gaseous mobile phase and a liquid stationary phase. The carrier gas can be nitrogen, helium, or argon. The selection of a carrier gas is determined by the detector used in the instrument. The instrument can be operated at a constant temperature or programmed to run at different temperatures if a sample has components with different volatilities. This is analogous to gradient elution described for HPLC. The sample, which is injected through a septum, must be injected as a gas or the temperature of the injection port must be above the boiling point of the components, so that they vaporize upon injection. Sample vapor is swept through the column partially as a gas and partially dissolved in the liquid phase. Volatile compounds that are present mainly in the gas phase will have a low partition coefficient and will move quickly through the column. Compounds with higher boiling points will move slowly through the column. The effluent passes through a detector that produces an electric signal proportional to the concentration of the volatile components. As in HPLC, the chromatogram is used both to identify the compounds by the retention time and to determine their concentration by the area under the peak.

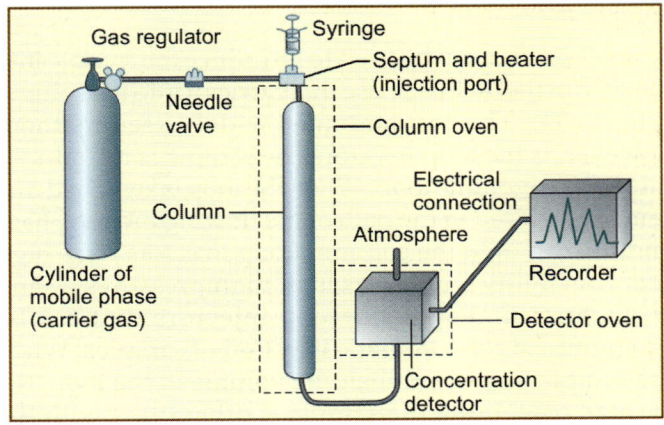

Fig. 23.36: Gas-liquid chromatography basic components

Columns

Gas-liquid chromatography columns are generally made of glass or stainless steel and are available in a variety of coil configurations and sizes. Packed columns are filled with inert particles such as diatomaceous earth or porous polymer or glass beads coated with a nonvolatile liquid (stationary) phase. These columns are usually 1/8 to 1/4 inch wide and 3–12 feet long. Capillary wall-coated open tubular columns have inside diameters in the range of 0.25 to 0.50 mm and are up to 60 m long. The liquid layer is coated on the walls of the column. A solid support coated with a liquid stationary phase may in turn be coated on column walls. The liquid stationary phase must be nonvolatile at the temperatures used, must be thermally stable, and must not react chemically with the solutes to be separated. The stationary phase is termed nonselective when separation is primarily based on relative volatility of the compounds. Selective liquid phases are used to separate polar compounds based on relative polarity (as in liquid-liquid chromatography).

Detectors

Although there are many types of detectors, only thermal conductivity (TC) and flame ionization detectors are discussed because they are the most stable (Fig. 23.37). TC detectors contain wires (filaments) that change electrical resistance with change in temperature. The filaments form opposite arms of a Wheatstone bridge and are heated electrically to raise their temperature. Helium, which has a high TC, is usually the carrier gas. Carrier gas from the reference column flows steadily across one filament, cooling it slightly. Carrier gas and separated compounds from the sample column flow across the other filament. The sample components usually have a lower TC, increasing the temperature and resistance of the sample filament. The change in resistance results in an unbalanced bridge circuit. The electrical change is

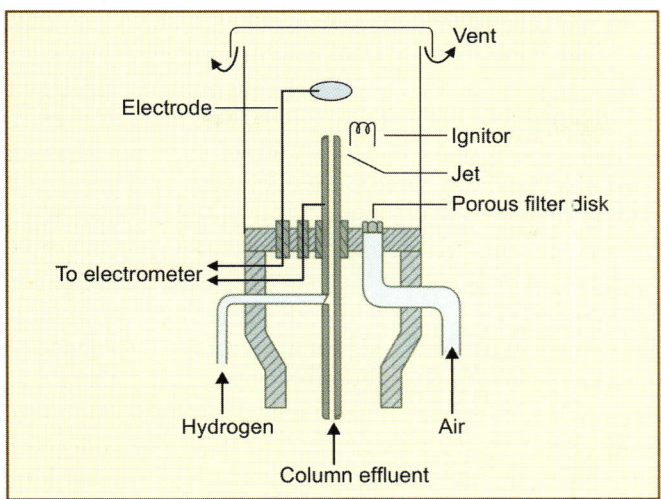

Fig. 23.37: Schematic diagram of a flame ionization detector

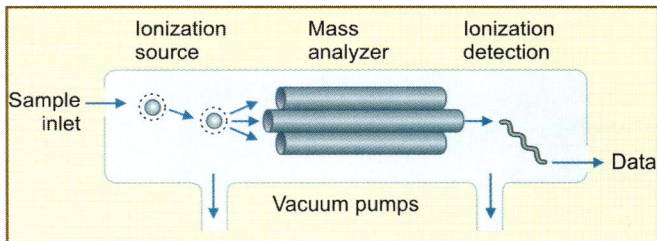

Fig. 23.38: The components of a mass spectrometer. In this case, the ionization source pictured is electrospray ionization and the mass analyzer is a quadrupole

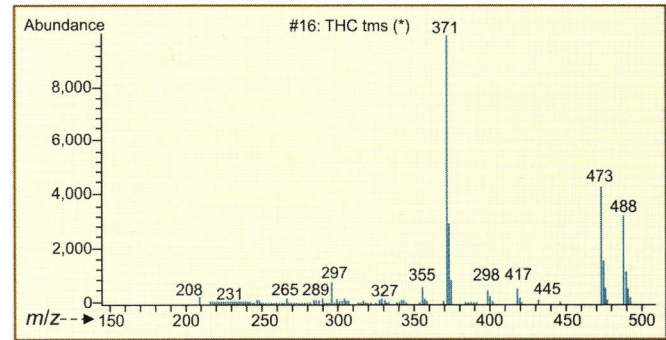

Fig. 23.39: Mass spectrum of the trimethylsilane derivative of Δ9-carboxytetrahydrocannabinol

amplified and fed to the recorder. The electrical change is proportional to the concentration of the analyte.

Flame ionization detectors are widely used in the clinical laboratory. They are more sensitive than TC detectors. The column effluent is fed into a small hydrogen flame burning in excess air or atmospheric oxygen. The flame jet and a collector electrode around the flame have opposite potentials. As the sample burns, ions form and move to the charged collector. Thus, a current proportional to the concentration of the ions is formed and fed to the recorder.

Mass Spectrometry

Definitive identification of samples eluting from GC or HPLC columns is possible when an MS is used as a detector. The coupled techniques, GC/MS and LC/MS, have powerful analytic capabilities with widespread clinical applications. The sample in an MS is first volatilized and then ionized to form charged molecular ions and fragments that are separated according to their mass-to-charge (m/z) ratio; the sample is then measured by a detector, which gives the intensity of the ion current for each species. These steps take place in the four basic components that are standard in all MSs: the sample inlet, ionization source, mass analyzer, and ion detector (Fig. 23.38). Ultimately, molecule identification is based on the formation of characteristic fragments. Figure 23.9 illustrates the mass spectrum of Δ9-carboxy tetrahydrocannabinol, a metabolite of marijuana.

Sample Introduction and Ionization

Direct infusion is commonly used to interface a GC or LC with an MS; however, the challenge of introducing a liquid sample from an LC column into an MS was a significant barrier until recent technological advances in ionization techniques.

ELECTRON IONIZATION

The most common form of ionization used in GC/MS is electron ionization (EI). This method requires a source of electrons in the form of a filament to which an electric potential is applied, typically at 70 eV. The molecules in the source are bombarded with high-energy electrons, resulting in the formation of charged molecular ions and fragments. Molecules break down into characteristic fragments according to their molecular structure (Fig. 23.40). The ions formed and their relative proportions are reproducible and can be used for qualitative identification of the compound. Since most instruments use the same 70 eV potential, the fragmentation of molecules on different days and different instruments is remarkably similar, allowing the comparison of unknown spectra to spectra in a published reference library.

Atmospheric Pressure Ionization

Unlike EI in GC/MS, most LC/MS ionization techniques are conducted at atmospheric pressure. As such, the ion source of this type of instrument is not included in the high-vacuum region of the instrument. Two types of ionization for LC/MS will be discussed here, i.e. electrospray ionization (ESI) and atmospheric pressure chemical ionization (APCI), while matrix-assisted laser desorption ionization (MALDI) and surface-enhanced

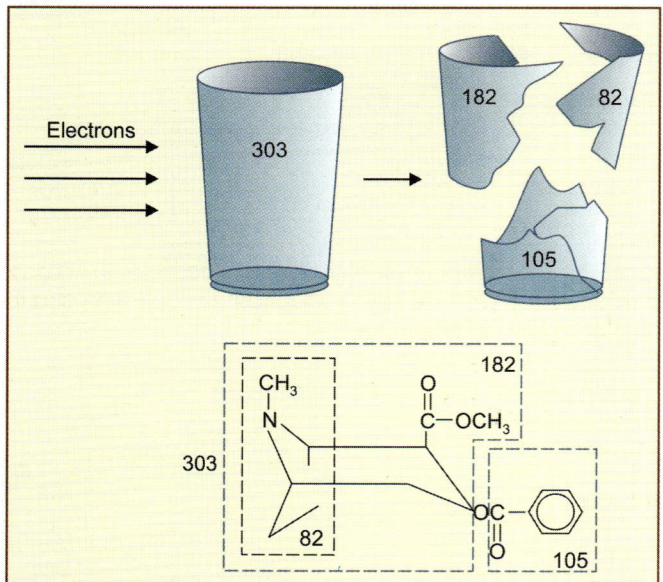

Fig. 23.40: Electron bombardment breaks cocaine into fragments, with number and size quantified. Unlike the illustrative glass tumbler, the result of mass fragmentation of cocaine or other chemical compounds is both predictable and reproducible, especially with electron ionization.

laser desorption ionization (SELDI) will be discussed later in the section on proteomics. ESI and APCI also differ from EI in that they are 'soft' ionization techniques that leave the molecular ion largely intact in the source. Many LC/MS techniques employ technologies after the source, in the mass analyzer, to fragment molecules and generate the daughter or fragment ions used in identification. However, ionization techniques used in LC/MS produce fragments and therefore mass spectra that are somewhat less reproducible between instruments than EI used in GC/MS. This may prove to limit the utility of reference library spectra produced in other instruments.

Electrospray Ionization

Thanks to its wide mass range and high sensitivity, ESI can be applied to a wide range of biological macro-molecules in addition to small molecules and has become the most common ionization source for LC/MS. ESI involves passing the LC effluent through a capillary to which a voltage has been applied. The energy is transferred to the solvent droplets, which become charged. Evaporation of the solvent through heat and gas causes the droplets to decrease in size, which increases the charge density on the surface. Eventually, the Coulombic repulsion of like charges leads to the ejection of ions from the droplet (Fig. 23.41). The individually charged molecules are drawn into the MS for mass analysis. ESI is adept at forming singly charged small molecules, but larger molecules can also be ionized using this method. Larger molecules such as proteins become multiply charged in ESI, and since MSs measure the m/z, even these large molecules can be observed in an instrument with a relatively small mass range (Fig. 23.42).

ATMOSPHERIC PRESSURE CHEMICAL IONIZATION

Another important ionization source is APCI, which is similar to ESI in that the liquid from LC is introduced directly into the ionization source. However, the droplets are not charged and the source contains a heated vaporizer to allow rapid de-solvation of the drops. A high voltage is applied to a corona discharge needle, which emits a cloud of electrons to ionize compounds after they a reconverted to the gas phase.

Mass Analyzer

The actual measuring of the m/z occurs when the gas phase ions pass into the mass analyzer. Mass analyzers generate electric fields that can manipulate the charged molecules to sort them according to their m/z.

Quadrupole

A diagram of a quadrupole MS is shown in Figure 23.43. The quadrupole is the most common mass analyzer in use today. The electric field on the two sets of diagonally

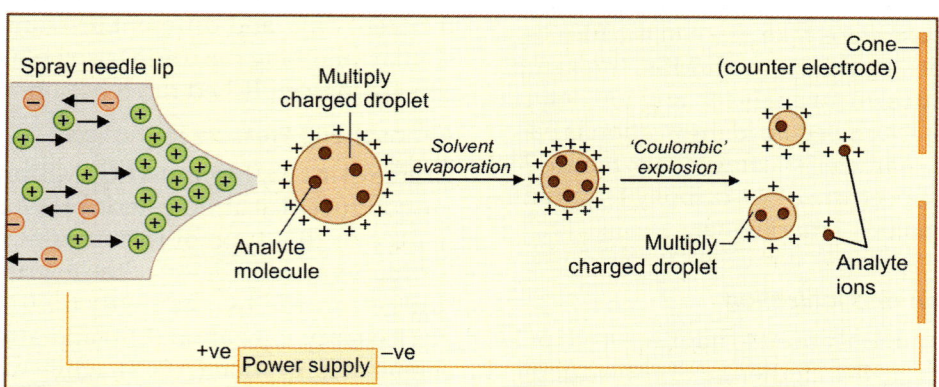

Fig. 23.41: Diagram of electrospray ionization, the most common ionization source for liquid chromatography/mass spectrometry

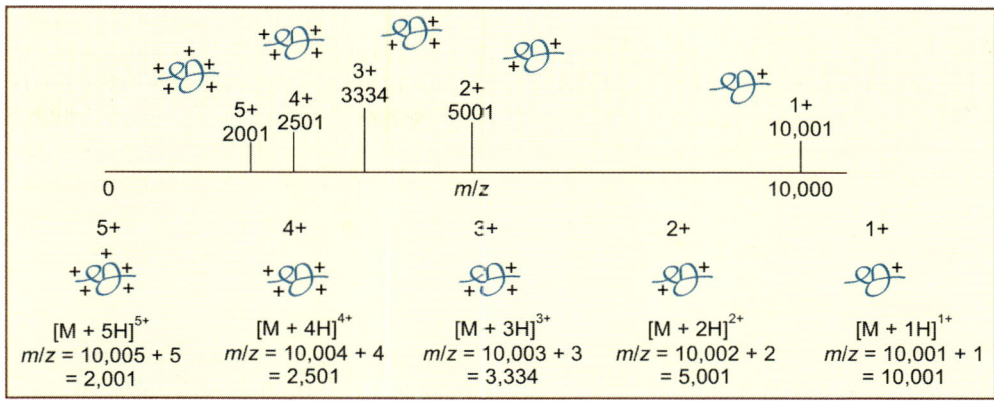

Fig. 23.42: A theoretical protein with a molecular weight of 10,000 can be multiply charged, which will generate numerous peaks. A mass spectrometer with a relatively small mass range can still detect the multiply charged ions since the m/z is reduced

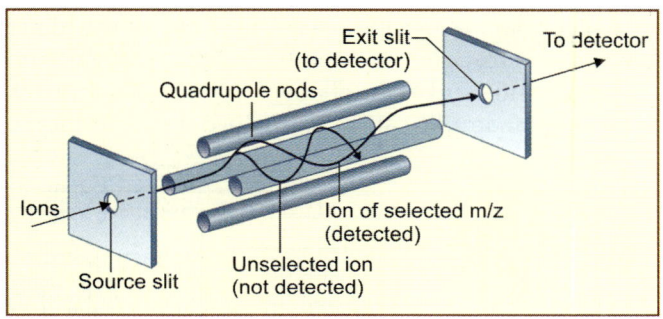

Fig. 23.43: Single quadrupole mass spectrometer

opposed rods allows only ions of a single selected m/z value to pass through the analyzer to the detector. All other ions are deflected into the rods. The rods can be scanned from low to high mass to allow ions of increasing mass to form stable sinusoidal orbits and traverse the filtering sector. This technique will generate a full scan mass spectrum. Alternatively, specific masses can be selected to monitor a few target analytes. This technique is called selected ion monitoring (SIM) and it allows for a longer dwell time (time spent monitoring a single ion) and therefore higher sensitivity. A full scan provides more information than SIM since ions not specifically selected in SIM are not detected. Therefore, a full scan would be preferable for general unknown screening while SIM analysis is more suitable for target compound analysis.

Ion Trap

The ion trap can be thought of as a modified quadrupole. A linear ion trap employs a stopping potential on the end electrodes to confine ions along the two-dimensional axis of the quadrupoles. In a three dimensional ion trap, the four rods, instead of being arranged parallel to each other, form a three-dimensional sphere in which ions are 'trapped'. In all ion traps, after a period of accumulation, the electric field adjusts to selectively destabilize the trapped ions, which are mass-selectively ejected from the

cavity to the detector based on their m/z. The unique feature of ion trap MSs is that they trap and store ions generated over time, effectively concentrating the ions of interest and yielding a greater sensitivity.

TANDEM MASS SPECTROMETRY

Tandem MSs (GC/MS/MS and LC/MS/MS) can be used for greater selectivity and lower detection limits. A common form of MS/MS is to link three quadrupoles in series; such an instrument is referred to as a triple quad (Fig. 23.44). Generally, each quadrupole has a separate function. Following an appropriate ionization method, the first quadrupole (Q1) is used to scan across a preset m/z range and select an ion of interest. The second quadrupole (Q2) functions as a collision cell. In a process called collision-induced dissociation, the ions are accelerated to high kinetic energy and allowed to collide with neutral gas molecules (usually nitrogen, helium, or argon) to fragment the ions. The single ion that passed through the first analyzer is called the precursor (or parent) ion, while the ions formed during fragmentation of the precursor ions are called product (or daughter) ions. The third quadrupole (Q3) serves to analyze the product

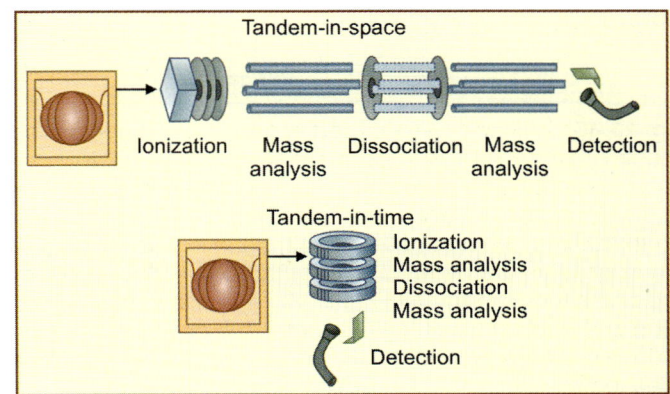

Fig. 23.44: Triple quadrupole mass spectrometer

ions generated in Q2. This last quadrupole can be set to scan all of the product ions to produce a full product ion scanor to selectively allow one or more of these product ions through to the detector in a process called selected reaction monitoring. Various scanning modes commonly usedin a triple quad Fig. 23.45. In some triple quad instruments, the third quadrupole can also functionas a linear ion trap to add further sensitivity to MS/MS.

HIGH-RESOLUTION MASS SPECTROSCOPY

Newer technologies utilizing high-resolution mass spectrometers based on time-of-flight (TOF) or Orbitrap (thermo fisher) technologies have gained popularity in recent years. These instruments can measure large numbers of analytes simultaneously in complex biological matrices and have been particularly useful for drug screening applications. Compared with traditional or 'nominal resolution' mass spectrometers that determine masses to –0.5 Da, high-resolution instruments, such as TOF and Orbitrap mass spectrometers operate at resolutions that allow the exact mass of an unknown compound to be calculated to ~0.001–0.0001 Da. The resolution of a mass spectrometer is defined as the mass of a given compound divided by the width of the corresponding peak and is commonly designated by the term full width at half maximum (FWHM) (Fig. 23.46A). TOF mass spectrometers achieve resolutions of 10,000–50,000 FWHM utilizing the principle that given the same kinetic energy, lighter ions travel faster than heavier ions. By measuring the time it takes an ion to traverse the flight

tube and hit the detector, the m/z ratio can be calculated (Fig. 23.46B). Orbitrap mass spectrometers operate on a different principle. With Orbitrap instruments, ions are injected tangentially to the electric field between the outer barrel-like electrode and the inner spindle-like electrode and the stable orbit achieved is proportional to the m/z value (Fig. 23.46C). Orbitrap mass spectrometers can achieve 100,000–250,000 FWHM.

Detector

The most common means of detecting ions employs an electron multiplier (Fig. 23.47). In this detector, a series of dynodes with increasing potentials are linked. When ions strike the first dynode surface, electrons are emitted. These electrons are attracted to the next dynode where more secondary electrons are emitted due to the higher potential of subsequent dynodes. A cascade of electrons is formed by the end of the chain of dynodes, resulting in overall signal amplification on the order of 1 million or greater.

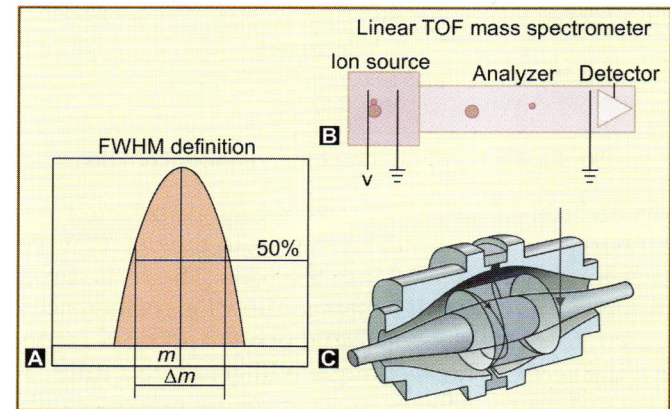

Fig. 23.46: (A) Pictorial representation of the full width at half maximum (FWHM) definition of mass resolution. Reprinted with permission from Thermo Fisher Scientific. (B) Diagram of the principle of time-of-flight (TOF) mass spectrometers. Reprinted with permission. (C) Diagram of Orbitrap mass spectrometry

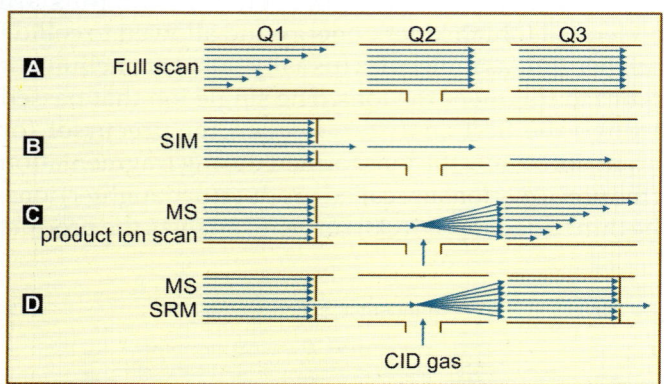

Fig. 23.45: Scanning modes used in a triple quadrupole mass spectrometer. (A) Full scan mass spectrometry (MS) detects all ions. (B) Selected ion monitoring (SIM) detects ions of one selected m/z. (C) Product ion scans select ions of one m/z in Q1 to pass on to Q2, the collision cell, where the ion is fragmented. All ion fragments are allowed to pass through to the detector. (D) Selected reaction monitoring (SRM) is similar to the product ion scan, but only fragments of one selected m/z are allowed to pass on to the detector. Both (C) and (D) are examples of tandem mass spectrometry (MS/MS). CID, collision-induced dissociation

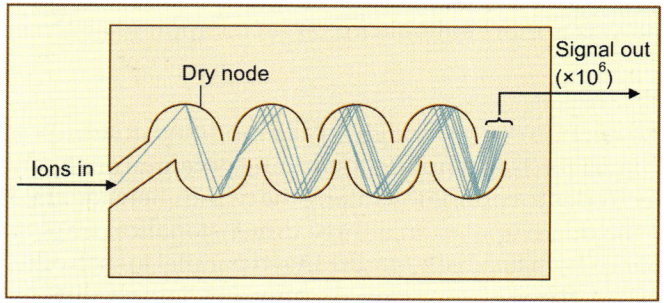

Fig. 23.47: Diagram of an electron multiplier detector in a mass spectrometer

BIBLIOGRAPHY

1. Bender GT. Chemical Instrumentation: A Laboratory Manual Based on Clinical Chemistry. Philadelphia, PA: WB Saunders; 1972.

2. Boyd j. Tech sight. Robotic laboratory automation. Science 2002; 295: 517-8.

3. Boyd jC, Felder RA. Preanalytical automation in the clinical laboratory. In: Ward-Cook KM, Lehmann CA, Schoetf LE, Williams RH, eds. Clinical diagnostic technology: the total testing process, volume I. The preanalytical phase. Washington, DC: AACC Press, 2002: 107–29.

4. Carbonnelle E, Mesquita C, Bille E, et al. MALDI-TOF mass spectrometry tools for bacterial identification in clinical microbiology laboratory. ClinBiochem. 2011; 44: 104–109.

5. Clinical and Laboratory Standards Institute. Autoverification of clinical laboratory test results. CLSI Approved Standard AUTOIO-A. Wayne, Pa: Clinical and Laboratory Standards Institute, 2006.

6. Clinical and Laboratory Standards Institute. Laboratory automation: specimen container/specimen carrier. CLSI Approved Standard AUTOOI-A. Wayne, Pa: Clinical and Laboratory Standards Institute, 2000.

7. Clinical and Laboratory Standards Institute. Laboratory automation: electromechanical interfaces. CLSI Approved Standard AUT005-A. Wayne, Pa: Clinical and Laboratory Standards Institute, 2001.

8. Clinical and Laboratory Standards Institute. Laboratory automation: communications with automated clinical laboratory systems, instruments, devices, and information systems. CLSI Approved Standard AUT003-A2. Wayne, Pa: Clinical and Laboratory Standards Institute, 2009.

9. Constantin E, Schnell A. Mass Spectrometry. New York, NY: Ellis Horwood; 1990.

10. Hawker CD, Garr SB, Hamilton LT, Penrose JR, Ashwood ER, Weiss RL. Automated transport and sorting system in a large reference laboratory. Part I: Evaluation of needs and alternatives and development of a plan. Clin Chern 2002; 48: 1751–60.

11. Hawker CD, Roberts WL, Garr SB, Hamilton LT, Penrose jR, Ashwood ER, et al. Automated transport and sorting system in a large reference laboratory. Part 2: Implementation of the system and performance measures over three years. Clin Chern 2002; 48: 1761–67.

12. Horváth C. High Performance Liquid Chromatography, Advances and Perspectives. New York, NY: Academic Press; 1980.

13. Jiwan JL, Wallemacq P, Hérent MF. HPLC-high resolution mass spectrometry in clinical laboratory? ClinBiochem. 2011; 44: 136–147.

14. Jurk H. Thin-Layer Chromatography. Reagents and Detection Methods, Vol. 1a. Weinheim: Verlagsgesellschaft; 1990.

15. Karasek FW, Clement RE. Basic Gas Chromatography: Mass Spectrometry. New York, NY: Elsevier; 1988.

16. Kebarle E, Liang T. From ions in solution to ions in the gas phase. Anal Chem. 1993; 65:972A.

17. Levine B. Principles of Forensic Toxicology. Washington, DC: AACC Press; 2006.

18. Melanson SEF, Lindeman NI, jarolim P. Selecting automation for the clinical chemistry laboratory. Arch Pathol Lab Med 2007; 131: 1063–9.

19. Michael L. Bishop. Clinical Chemistry: Principles, Techniques, and Correlations, 7thedition. Philadelphia, Wolters Kluwer/Lippincott Williams & Wilkins, 2013.

20. Middleton S, Mountain P. Process control and on-line optimization. In: Kost GJ. ed. Handbook of clinical automation, robotics, and optimization. New York: john Wiley & Sons, 1996: 515–40.

21. Paegel BM, Blazej RG, Mathies RA. Microfluidic devices for DNA sequencing: sample preparation and electrophoretic analysis. Curr Opin BiotechnoI 2003; 14: 42–50.

22. Parris NA. Instrumental Liquid Chromatography: A Practical Manual on High Performance Liquid Chromatographic Methods. New York,NY: Elsevier; 1976.

23. Price CP, Newman DJ, eds. Principles and practice of immunoassay, 2nd edition. New York: Stockton Press, 1997.

24. Sasaki M, Kageoka T, Ogura K, Kataoka H, Ueta T, Sugihara S. Total laboratory automation in japan: past, present, and the future. ClinChimActa 1998;278: 217–27.

25. Shayanfar N, Tobler U, von Eckardstein A, Bestmann L. Automated urinalysis: first experiences and a comparison between the Iris iQ200 urine microscopy system, the Sysmex UF-I00 flow cytometer and manual microscopic particle counting. ClinChern Lab Med 2007; 45: 1251–6.

26. Shen Y, Wu BL. Microarray-based genomic DNA profiling technologies in clinical molecular diagnostics. ClinChern 2009; 55: 659–69.

27. Siuzdak, G. The Expanding Role of Mass Spectrometry in Biotechnology. San Diego, CA: MCC Press; 2006.

28. Voelkerding KV, Dames SA, DurtschijD. Next-generation sequencing: from basic research to diagnostics. ClinChern 2009; 55: 641–58.

29. Walter B: Dry reagent chemistries in clinical analysis. Anal Chern 1983; 55: 498A-514B.

30. Wild D, ed. The immunoassay handbook, 3rd edition. San Diego, Calif: Elsevier, 2005.

24

Point-of-Care Testing

INTRODUCTION

Point-of-care testing (POCT) presents some of the most controversial and difficult laboratory management challenges. This chapter identifies how management of POCT differs from other types of laboratory testing. It describes cost factors in POCT and approaches for analysis of the costs of testing. One of the key initial steps in the management of POCT is the development of institutional goals. In developing the management structure for POCT, there are political issues that central administration and departmental leaders need to sort out. These include issues what department and who will direct testing, institutional priorities for POCT, and how costs and revenues will be assigned. The chapter explains how to operate a POCT program and to ensure the quality of testing. An important part of deciding whether a point-of-care test should be adopted is assessing its potential clinical impact. The chapter explains the challenges of implementing POCT in developing countries and the clinical benefit of POCT. One of the greatest challenges and a key to making POCT work is training and assurance of the competency of staff. The challenges of conducting quality POCT in developed countries with established hospital infrastructures are magnified when performed in the context of a developing country or rural setting. The chapter discusses how technological advances are driving change in the scope of POCT. Ongoing advances in the microfabrication of devices and in nanotechnology provide the promise of substantial future technological change and further reduction in the size of POCT devices.

Point-of-care testing is increasingly being used not only in the emergency department, operating rooms, and intensive care units (ICUs), but also in the clinics, physician offices, nursing homes, pediatric units, pharmacies, counseling centers, and ambulances. Advances in medical, analytical, and engineering technologies in the last two decades led to the appearance of a large number of portable measurement devices for a variety of the different analytes. These include tests for electrolytes, glucose, hemoglobin A1c, urinalysis, pregnancy, drugs of abuse, therapeutic drug monitoring, occult blood, blood gases, coagulation tests, enzymes, and cardiac markers. POCT is also available for infectious diseases, such as HIV, gonorrhea, syphilis, streptococcus, influenza, fungal infections, and tuberculosis. Improving clinical and process outcomes has the potential to reduce errors and wastage of resources while also reducing the cost of care and increasing societal gain. This argument can be applied simply to the testing process (Fig. 24.1) or to the wider aspects of the whole patient journey. POCT offers several advantages compared with central laboratory testing (Table 24.1). The major advantage of POCT is faster delivery of results. POCT is designed to work with the flow of patient management and care physicians can order and perform the test and immediately make a medical decision. Smaller sample volume allows POCT use in neonatal and pediatric population and is ideal for those patients requiring frequent testing. The overall cost of patient care is arguably smaller due to improved patient work flows. Testing near the patient requires fewer steps than transporting a specimen to the laboratory, processing, aliquoting, testing, and communicating results back to clinical staff, all of which may reduce preanalytical and postanalytical laboratory-related errors. Portability of POCT allows for increased access to testing in a wider variety of sites, e.g. rural areas, accident sites, areas with limited infrastructure and personnel, and locations with

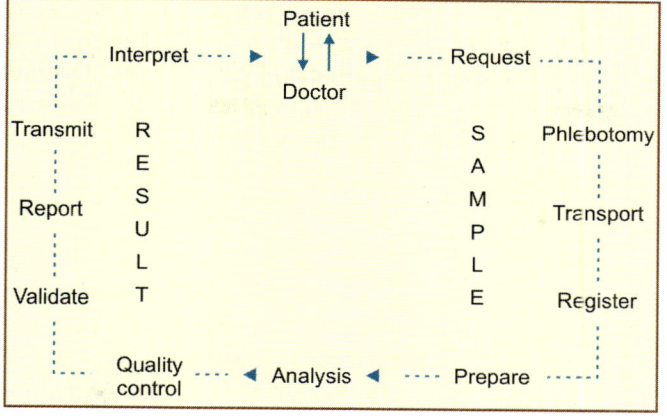

Fig. 24.1: Schematic representation of the key steps in requesting, delivering, and using a diagnostic test result

under served populations. One example of the latter is the use of a portable POCT to test for tuberculosis in the risk populations in low-income countries. Although. POCT offers many advantages, there are some negative aspects of POCT (Table 24.1). On a cost per test basis, POCT is more expensive than the cost of central laboratory testing as a result of the higher disposable and reagent costs of the POCT analyzers. End-users may be able to counterbalance these increased costs by gaining efficiencies in improved patient work flows.

Additionally, quality of results is a concern because POCT is usually performed by non-laboratory personnel who may include nurses, physicians, emergency medical technicians, pharmacists, medics, patients, and medical office assistants. End-users with multiple responsibilities and limited laboratory training may not appreciate the value of laboratory quality control (QC) in ensuring quality test results.

LABORATORY REGULATIONS

Accreditation

Accreditation of POCT should be part of the overall accreditation of laboratory medicine services, or indeed should be part of the accreditation of the full clinical service, as has been the case for several years in many countries, including the United States and the United Kingdom. Thus, the Clinical Laboratory Improvement Amendments of 1988 (CLIA) and the final rule on quality

Table 24.1	Potential advantages and disadvantages of POCT*
Advantages	**Disadvantages**
Convenience for both the attending physician/nurse and patient	POCT is significantly more expensive than the cost of central laboratory testing due to the higher disposable and reagent costs of the POCT analyzers
Reduced turnaround time for test results to expedite medical decision-making in operating rooms, emergency department, and intensive care units	Maintenance of quality control and quality assurance is difficult as anyone can run the analysis
Reduction in clinic visits, hospital admissions, and length of hospital stay due to faster laboratory services	Management of POCT is challenging—there are numerous operators to train, multiple sites to manage, and hundreds of POC tests to validate
Better patient management due to improved visibility and interaction with a patient	Preanalytic, analytic, and postanalytic issues are not recognized easily if tests are performed by untrained staff
Decreased manpower needs associated with test requesting and reporting, especially for patients necessitating tests several times a day (e.g. glucose determination)	Inter-individual variability in POCT results may be greater when compared with central laboratory testing
Fingerstick POCT is less traumatic for a patient as smaller sample volume is required	Difficulties with documentation of test results, billing, and regulatory compliance
Reduced risk of preanalytical errors due to absence of transporting a specimen to a core laboratory, processing, aliquoting, testing, and communicating results back to clinical staff. Reduced risk of sample deterioration	Proper integration of test result into the patient's electronic medical record may be more difficult
Improved patient outcome	Managing reagent supply and storage at multiple sites is problematic
Improved cost of overall patient care	Central laboratory test results and POCT results are not always comparable due to differences in specimen types, technology, interfering substances, etc.

Wide menu of POC analytes for specimens that do not require processing

Availability to a wider variety of sites (e.g. rural areas, areas with limited infrastructure/personnel, and sites with underserved populations)

*POCT, point-of-care testing.

systems requirements as specified in 2003 legislation in the United States stipulate that all POCT must meet certain minimum standards. In the United States, the Centers for Medicare and Medicaid Services, the Joint Commission on Accreditation of Health care Organizations, and the College of American Pathologists are responsible for inspecting sites, and each is committed to ensuring compliance with testing regulations for POCT. All laboratories performing POCT must be certified under one of the five types of CLIA certificates listed in Table 24.2.

The CLIA certificate must be appropriate for the testing that is performed in the laboratory (i.e. appropriate complexity). In addition to the federal program, state departments of public health or public organizations may apply for 'deemed' status, which allows these organizations to perform laboratory accreditation and inspections.

POCT Complexity

Tests are classified based on their complexity. The Food and Drug Administration (FDA) uses several criteria to assign complexity to any test, and the three categories are 'waived' tests, **moderate-complexity tests**, and **high complexity tests**. **Waived tests** are a category of tests defined by CLIA, such as dipstick tests, urine pregnancy tests, and blood glucose monitoring devices, which are subject to the lowest level of regulation and are cleared by the FDA for home uses. They employ methodologies that are as simple and accurate as to render the likelihood of erroneous results negligible and pose almost no risk of harm to the patient if the test is performed incorrectly. Laboratories performing non-waived tests (moderate-complexity tests and high complexity tests) must fulfill all the requirements for personnel qualifications, proficiency testing and inspections, quality assurance and QCs, and patient test management. The majority of POCT is moderate complexity. The fourth category of POCT is provider-performed microscopy procedures, or PPMPs, which is a subcategory of moderate-complexity testing. These tests involve the use of a microscope, limited to bright-field or phase-contrast microscopy. Generally, the specimens are labile and cannot survive transport to a clinical laboratory. Only licensed physicians, dentists, and midlevel practitioners may perform PPMP. There are usually no QC materials available for PPMP.

IMPLEMENTATION

Establishing Need

When establishing a POCT site, the approach and steps in the implementation will be different in nearly every case insofar as organizational characteristics, personnel competency, and financial situation of any given institution may vary greatly. However, there are some common guidelines to implementation that apply to nearly every case. Support of the organization must be present to evaluate the requests for POCT. Typically, a multidisciplinary committee consisting of laboratory staff, physician, nursing representatives, and hospital/laboratory administration is formed to create a structure for receiving and establishing criteria for approving requests for POCT. Before implementing a POCT service, an interdisciplinary committee should address the questions similar to those listed in Box 24.1. The decision to establish POCT program is made after justifying the clinical need, cost, and the analytic performance requirements. Other factors should also be considered, including space, any previous track record of regulatory compliance, personnel who will be performing the testing, and metrics to determine if the POCT implementation is successful.

POCT Policy and Accountability

Implementation of a POCT service requires a POCT policy that establishes all of the procedures required to ensure delivery of high-quality service, together with the responsibility and accountability of all staff associated with the POCT. This may be (1) part of the organization's total quality management system, (2) part of its clinical governance policy, and (3) required for accreditation purposes. The elements of a POCT policy are listed in (Box 24.2).

Table 24.2	Types of clinical laboratory improvement amendments certificates*
Certificate of waiver	Issued to a laboratory to perform only waived tests
Certificate of registration	Issued to a laboratory that enables the entity to conduct moderate or high-complexity laboratory testing or both until the entity is determined by survey to be in compliance with CLIA regulations
Certificate for PPMPs	Issued to a laboratory in which a physician, midlevel practitioner, or dentist performs no tests other than the microscopy procedures, permits the laboratory to also perform waived tests
Certificate of compliance	Issued to a laboratory after an inspection that finds the laboratory to be in compliance with all applicable CLIA requirements
Certificate of accreditation	Issued to a laboratory on the basis of the laboratory's accreditation by an accreditation organization approved by the health care finance administration

CLIA, Clinical Laboratory Improvement Amendments; POCT, point-of-care testing; PPMP, provider-performed microscopy procedure.
*Clinical Laboratory Improvement Act. How to obtain a CLIA certificate of waiver,
http://www.cms.gov/Regulations-and-Guidance/Legislation/CLIA/downloads//howobtaincertificateofwaiver.pdf

- Which test is required and in which specific area?
- What is the turnaround time required?
- How the service is currently provided and what are the problems?
- What is the expected annual test volume?
- What clinical question is being asked when requesting this test?
- What clinical decision is likely to be made and action to be taken upon receipt of the result?
- How will POCT increase patient satisfaction?
- Are personnel competent to perform the POCT?
- Are facilities available to perform the test and store equipment, reagents, and documentation?
- Will a change in practice be required?
- Can central laboratory deliver the required service?
- How do POCT cost, reference ranges, accuracy, and precision compare to similar tests in a laboratory?
- Are available POCT analyzers user-friendly?
- Can POCT analyzers interface with an LIS and a patient electronic medical record?
- Are both internal and external QC materials available?
- Does the company providing POCT analyzers and reagents offer a reliable support service?
- What clinical question is being asked when requesting this test?
- Is staff available to perform the test?
- Will you abide by the organization's POCT policy?
- Are there operational benefits to this POCT strategy?
- Are there economic benefits to this POCT strategy?
- Will a change in practice be required to deliver these benefits?
- Is it feasible to make the changes in practice that might be required?

Box 24.2: Elements of a point-of-care testing policy

Catalog information- review time	• Approved by • Original distribution • Related policies • Further information • Policy replaces
Introduction -background	• Definition • Accreditation of services • Audit of services
Laboratory services in the organization-location	• Logistics
Management of POCT- committee and accountability	• Policy on diagnostic testing • Officers • Committee members • Terms of reference • Responsibilities; meetings
Equipment and consumable procurement-criteria for procurement	• Process of procurement
Standard operating procedures	• Training and certification of staff-training • Certification; recertification
Quality control and quality assurance-procedures	• Documentation and review
Health and safety procedures bibliography	

POCT Implementation Protocol

After making the decision to implement POCT, the responsible party selects the method of choice and begins validation. Desirable characteristics of POCT analyzers include ease of use, method accuracy and comparability to main laboratory method, portability, durability, low maintenance, simple QC, QC lockout features, simple sample handling requirements, barcode patient and operator identification capabilities, and the ability to interface with a laboratory information system (LIS).

The manufacturer should aid in providing minimum acceptability requirements, instrument manuals, package inserts for reagents and QCs, materials safety data sheet, and training materials. Method validation should confirm the manufacturer's specifications and a procedure should be written for each test. This should not be simply a collection of materials obtained from a manufacturer; rather, these documents should aid in the development of an easy-to-follow, simple, and concise procedure. The procedure should include information on the principle of the method; personnel qualifications; specimen, reagents, supplies, and equipment requirements; QC and calibrations; patient testing procedure; reference ranges; reporting limits; and interfering substances if applicable. All required regulatory or certifying standards should be in place prior to initiating patient testing (Table 24.3).

Personnel Requirements

For a POC program with moderate-complexity tests, unlike for those POC with certificate of Waiver or certificate for PPMP, institutions are required to have a certain organizational and administrative structure where staff has established qualifications, competency, and experience.

The director of laboratory is usually a PhD scientist, or a MD physician with at least 5 years of experience directing a laboratory with updated continuing medical education credits, or a person with a bachelor's degree with 10 years' laboratory experience plus 5 years of supervising experience with updated continuing medical education credits. Responsibilities of a director are very broad and include policy making, ensuring compliance with regulatory standards, and administrative duties.

Importantly, the director is responsible for the analytic performance of all tests. The director must make technical decisions based on a constant monitoring of ongoing proficiency, accuracy, and precision. Such individuals should be a liaison between the clinicians, hospital administration, and laboratory personnel. Each laboratory performing moderate-complexity tests must have a technical and a clinical consultant. The technical

Table 24.3	Point-of-care checklist
1. Quality management	The POC program has a written QM program as well as organizational system setting forth levels of authority, responsibility, and accountability. There is a documented system to address unusual patient results or instrument troubleshooting. There is a written procedure for each POCT.
2. Specimen handling	There is a documented procedure describing methods for patient identification and preparation, as well as for specimen collection, accessioning, and preservation before testing. There is a procedure for entering POCT results into the permanent medical record of a patient. Reference intervals should be established.
3. Reagents	All reagents should be stored and labeled as recommended by the manufacturer.
4. Instruments and equipment	Equipment must be evaluated and scheduled for a regular maintenance.
5. Personnel	The director of the POCT program is a physician or a doctoral scientist. The testing personnel have adequate, specific training to ensure competence and this must be documented.
6. Quality control and calibration	Calibrations and quality controls are run at regular intervals (at least daily). Acceptable limits are defined for control procedures, and there are documented corrective actions when control results exceed defined acceptability limits. Upper and lower limits of the analytical measurement range (AMR) for each analyte are defined.
7. Safety	There is a program to assure that the safety of patients and health-care personnel is not compromised by POCT.

consultant is responsible for scientific over sight of the POCT, while the clinical consultant is required to provide clinical and medical advice. The director of a POCT program, the technical consultant, and the clinical consultant may be the same person. Even though, the implementation of the POCT program may be done differently depending on an institution, the entity responsible for quality management of the POCT program is always the laboratory. It is useful, therefore, for a laboratory to have a person supervising the POCT program, so a POCT coordinator (POCC) fulfills this role. Even though, a POCC does not monitor day-to-day activities of testing personnel, it is the responsibility of the POCC to coordinate POC patient testing and facilitate compliance with procedures and policies and regulatory requirements. The POCC develops a training program for testing personnel and ensures documentation of competency training. The POCC also oversees completion of proficiency testing programs, performs on-site review of patient testing, QC, and maintenance logs and reports problems and regulatory noncompliance to appropriate management personnel.

Even though the laboratory is responsible for the POCT policies and procedures, it is the clinical staff that does the actual testing. Fostering a partnership between the operators and laboratory will help solve problems that may arise during the testing process. In this decentralized testing model, the specifics of how training is performed, how competency records are maintained, and how reagents are ordered may be different for each institution. The laboratory should monitor POC areas and ensure consistent feedback is provided regarding compliance with any applicable regulations. However, before any testing is initiated, clarifying individual roles and expectations is key to the success of the program.

QUALITY MANAGEMENT

Accuracy Requirements

Understanding how accurate the results need to be in the context of how the test will be used clinically is important before any patient testing is initiated. Ideally, a POC test will provide equivalent results with those from the central laboratory. If this were the case, depending on a clinical situation, physicians would have an option to choose either test and achieve the same clinical outcome. Unfortunately, despite the ongoing harmonization and standardization efforts, currently, there are still accuracy and imprecision concerns with some POCT. The management group shall assist in evaluating and selecting POCT devices and systems. Performance criteria for POCT devices should include consideration of accuracy, precision, detection limits, and interferences. Practicability should also be considered. Due to complaints about glucose meter inaccuracy, the FDA is currently developing new standards for glucose meter accuracy.

QC and Proficiency Testing

The purpose of a quality management program is to ensure quality test results. A thorough validation should verify the analytical performance and any applicable limitations with the assay. Ongoing daily QC will alert the operator to any reagent or instrument issues. Some devices have both internal and external QC, both of which have distinctly different roles. Internal QC, which is also referred to as on board QC, internal checks, electronic QC, or intelligent QC, is performed at specific time intervals or at least daily. Internal QC ensures the electronics of the device are performing as expected or, if a manual test, the integrity of the device unit. Some instruments automate QC and/or calibration, which is helpful for regulatory compliance, but also ensures the instrument is ready to perform quality testing at all times.

Another important feature is to tie QC performance requirements to test availability. If QC has not been performed as required and is unsatisfactory, the instrument does not allow patient testing until corrective action has taken place. This is known as QC lockout. The entire testing process should be checked periodically according to the manufacturer and regulatory requirements by running an external QC. Here, a control sample is introduced to the test system in the same manner as a patient sample. Another form of external QC is proficiency testing where blind samples are sent to participating laboratories to perform testing. In the United States, results from one laboratory are compared with the results from the laboratories using the same method (peer group). Laboratories performing non-waived testing are not required to participate.

Quality management programs also need to ensure that the operators are competent to perform testing. After initial training, ongoing assessment of their performance is required. Careful control of personnel records is an important part of the quality management program and may be managed at the POCT site or directly by the laboratory. Some instruments will allow 'super-users' (supervisors, managers, or POCC) to track training renewal dates and to lockout operators whose training has expired. The greatest source of error in POCT is the preanalytical error. While the above features are necessary for any POCT program, it is more difficult to identify errors arising from poor specimen, e.g. sample contamination, dilution, circulating interference (lipemia, icterus, and hemolysis), and proper specimen source (arterial, venous, and fingerstick). For this reason, careful assessment of an area's compliance in proper specimen collection and handling is needed prior to implementing testing.

Preventing postanalytic errors in reporting can be achieved more reliably with **connectivity**. With the aid of barcodes, modern technology has improved patient identification and decreased transcription errors in many health-care applications. However, linear barcode identification methods are not fail-safe. Hospitals should work with laboratories, pharmacy, radiology, and admissions to standardize scanning and printing specifications across a system. Careful control of barcode scanning and printing equipment specifications will minimize the misidentification threat to patient safety.

Total-system POCT quality assurance is thus the combination of several QC mechanisms: (1) a mechanism to perform a thorough systems validation, (2) reliable, user-friendly POCT device, (3) training of POCT operators, (4) competency assessment of all individuals involved in POCT, (5) QC testing and monitoring, (6) proficiency testing, and (7) connectivity and barcoding technologies.

POC Applications

A wide variety of POCT devices can be loosely classified into the single-use, hand held devices, the bench top devices, and the wearable devices (Table 24.4). POCT devices are designed with a consideration for the operators who may have little to no laboratory training. Hand-held devices are getting smaller and more ergonomic with every generation. A variety of analytical principles used in a laboratory have also been implemented in POCT devices, including the following: (1) reflectance, (2) electrochemistry, electrical impedance, (3) light scattering/optical motion, (4) immunoturbidimetry, (5) lateral flow, flow-through, or solid phase immunoassays, (6) spectrophotometry, multiwavelength spectrophotometry, (7) fluorescence, time-resolved fluorescence, and (8) polymerase chain reaction.

Table 24.4	Types of POCT analyzers
Single-use, qualitative, or semiquantitative cartridge/strip tests	• Urine and blood chemistry • Infectious disease agents, cardiac markers, hCG
Single-use quantitative cartridge/strip tests with a reader device	• Glucose • Blood chemistry • Coagulation • Cardiac markers, drugs, C-reactive protein (CRP), allergy, fertility tests • Chlamydia • HbA1c, urine albumin • Blood chemistry • pH, blood gases, electrolytes, metabolites
Multiple-use quantitative cartridge/benchtop devices	• Hemoglobin species, bilirubin • pH, blood gases, electrolytes, metabolites • Cardiac markers, drugs, CRP • Complete blood count

Contemporary POCT analyzers are capable of delivering test results in less than a minute using a single-step protocol on a variety of unprocessed specimens, such as whole blood, cerebrospinal fluid, urine, and stool specimens. Ideally, the results of POCT should meet the analytical specifications that are 'fit-for-purpose' and should be comparable to those of the central laboratory.

Glucose testing is the highest volume POCT. These are devices with single-use cartridges or strips that use the reflectance or electrochemistry analytical principles for glucose measurement. Hemoglobin A1c testing is also rapidly increasing, although we are yet to see a device that measures both glucose and hemoglobin A1c. Both of these tests should not be used for a tight glucose control at bedside but rather employed as monitoring procedures because of the cases of hypoglycemia as well as cases of erroneous POCT measurements due to interfering substances. Mature POCT areas are measurements of urine and blood chemistry, coagulation testing, pH and blood gases, hemoglobin and bilirubin, and complete blood count. Other areas of POCT that are rapidly evolving are intraoperative immunoassay of parathyroid hormone, creatinine and cardiac markers in emergency departments, and infectious diseases (HIV).

INFORMATICS AND POCT

POCT devices require the same variety of informatic functions required by conventional laboratory analyzers. Primarily, these functions are associated with electronic transfer of data from analyzers to the LIS and ultimately into a patient's electronic medical record. This provides health care professionals with quick, accurate, and appropriate access to the patient's medical history and information. In reality, it is rare for POCT devices to be directly connected to the LIS, and they are usually connected via some sort of docking station and/or data management system (DM), which, in turn, is connected to the LIS (Fig. 24.2).

Informatic Requirements in POCT Devices

With advances in software and hardware capabilities, it is possible to considerably enhance the value and quality of the patient result with additional accompanying information. In the course of selecting a POCT device and its associated informatics, consideration should be given to devices that ensures that certain information items always accompany the patient result across the two interfaces. These obligatory information items include the following: (1) patient identifiers: medical record number or similar number and name, (2) sample identifiers or accession number, (3) date and time of specimen collection, (4) type of specimen, (5) test requested, (6) test result, (7) units to be attributed to the result if applicable, (8) date and time of analysis, (9) operator identifier, (10) device identifier, (11) error messages and action messages.

Other optional information items that operators may wish to transfer from the device to the DM and possibly to the LIS include (1) reference interval, if not generated by the LIS, (2) specific comments (e.g. error messages); (3) consumable material details (e.g. lot number and expiry date); (4) calibration information, including expiration date; (5) QC parameters; and (6) date and time of system alerts, such as 'low battery' and 'calibration due'.

Development of POCT Connectivity Standards

Although the importance of linking POCT devices to information systems and enhancing the value of the patient result is clear, problems have been associated with achieving this goal, primarily because of interfacing difficulties. These difficulties arose because specific vendor instruments and accompanying DM systems came with proprietary interfaces that rarely allowed devices from other vendors to be linked without significant cost. Because it is common for laboratories to

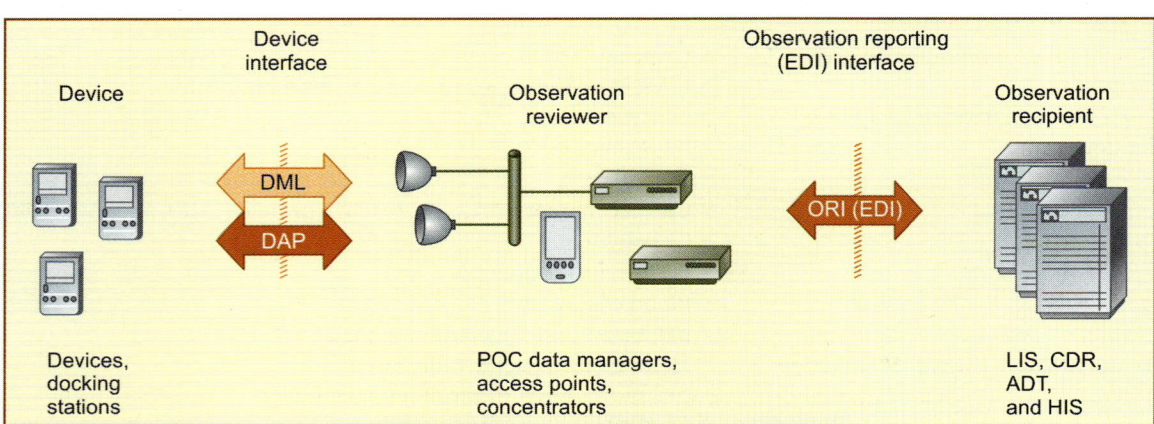

Fig. 24.2: Schematic diagram of the interfaces between point-of-care testing (POCT) devices and information systems

use POCT devices from multiple vendors, this lack of ability to connect different devices through a single DM led to many devices not being linked to any sort of information system. Consequently, patient results often did not get entered into the patient record, thus running the risk of duplicate testing, or they were entered manually with risk of transcription error.

At the time, it was thought that the development of a set of common universal 'plug and play' interfacing standards for incorporation into all POCT devices would address this problem. Such standards would ensure that POCT devices meet critical user requirements, such as (1) bidirectionality, (2) device connection commonality, (3) commercial software intraoperability, security; and (4) QC and/or regulatory compliance.

Accordingly, the Connectivity Industry Consortium (CIC) of more than 30 companies involved in the POCT industry designed a set of connectivity standards that incorporated the following features: (1) use of a proven architecture and notation, (2) use of existing standards and architectural patterns wherever possible, (3) focus on services that would enable software intraoperability and add value to overall functionality, and (4) reduction in the complexity of device communications.

Connectivity industry consortium connectivity standards are represented simply as the two interfaces between POCT devices and information systems (Fig. 24.2). The device interface passes patient results and QC information between the POCT instrument and devices, such as docking stations, concentrators, terminal servers, and point-of-care data managers. The latter have to be linked to a variety of information systems via the observation reporting interface or electronic data interface, for transmission of ordering information and patient results.

The initial connectivity standard was approved by the National Committee for Clinical Laboratory Standards in 2001, and a revised second edition was published in 2006. A POCT device that conforms to this standard should be able to communicate with DM and LIS systems, allowing exchange of data and information in a standardized format, irrespective of vendor or location.

Unfortunately, the uptake of POCT01-A2 has not been as rapid as was anticipated, and not all POCT device companies have adopted the standard. To promote awareness of the potential benefits that could be gained from a universal connectivity standard, CLSI published POCT02-A, 'An Implementation Guide of POCT01 for Health care Providers;' a document that provides in relatively nontechnical terms an explanation of connectivity and what users should look for in POCT01-compliant devices.

Benefits of Connectivity and Future Developments

One of the most important benefits of connectivity is to facilitate the transfer and capture of patient POCT and quality related data into permanent medical records. Other destinations for point-of-care data include the bedside monitors and clinical information systems that reside in critical care units. These systems integrate data from various sources, including vital signs and diagnostic results. In conjunction with clinical guidelines and expert systems, they can produce critical care maps used in the management of the critically ill patient. Integration of POCT data with other laboratory and clinical information is now commonly seen in disease management systems supporting the care of patients with chronic diseases, such as diabetes mellitus and hyperlipidemia. In the case of diabetes mellitus, the DM serves to maintain a record of blood glucose results and any other observations that the patient wishes to record, to bring to the attention of the clinician at the next clinic visit. This record is then used to help patients in the management of their own disease. In the case of hyperlipidemia, data may be fed into an algorithm together with other observations to calculate a risk score that is used by the patient and his or her clinician to identify lifestyle, dietary, and therapy changes, together with expected outcomes (e.g. reduced risk of cardiovascular disease). Linking POCT with decision support tools and associated treatment algorithms is seen as the future in a number of situations, including glycemic control in intensive care, management of diabetes, management of heart failure, and assistance with self-dosing for patients on anticoagulants.

Improvements in the quality management of POCT are also assisted by an ability to easily link devices to networks and to those who are ultimately responsible for the device. Most manufacturers of POCT devices now provide software to allow central laboratories to monitor their instruments in remote locations. In conjunction with network technology, remote control software not only allows monitoring of the performance of the device, it also enables those responsible for the instrument to carry out some service procedures or even to shut the instrument down completely if required. Such software can manage a large number of devices that may be geographically dispersed, and, by reducing the necessity to physically visit each device, its use can result in significant staff savings.

Informatic-related features for the future include greater adoption of the POCT01-A2 standard. Although, one can appreciate that some device vendors may prefer to always retain their proprietary interfaces rather than open their systems to competitor devices, there remains a call by users for more universal connectivity.

A randomized controlled trial of POCT in general practice in Australia was ground breaking in many respects, but it did not include the use of any form of comprehensive data management or informatics, partly because the devices used were obtained from multiple vendors, and it was impossible to easily interface them to a single data management system. A second important demand for the future is wireless connectivity, which would provide many management benefits, particularly for those devices used in conjunction with docking stations.

EQUIPMENT PROCUREMENT AND EVALUATION

Equipment procurement and evaluation involve first identifying candidate POCT equipment having the prerequisite analytical and operational capabilities to meet the clinical requirements of a POCT service. Performance requirements should then be established and compared with the performance characteristics of these devices (obtained from the manufacturer or assessed as part of the procurement exercise). These characteristics include parameters, such as accuracy, precision, specificity for the analyte, turnaround time (TAT), calibration frequency, potential interferents, calibrator and reagent stability, lot-to-lot variation for reagents and calibrators, and QC requirements. In addition, operational requirements have to be identified, and the potential for operator error (e.g. effects of delayed addition of the sample and use of an incorrect sample volume) determined.

Independent validation of these analytical and operational characteristics can be obtained from (1) published evaluations performed by agencies, such as the Medicine and Health care Products Regulatory Agency (MHRA) in the United Kingdom; (2) Norwegian Quality Improvement of Primary Care Laboratories; and (3) reports in the peer reviewed literature. When performance data are reviewed, particular attention should be paid to the precision and accuracy of measurement, including concordance between results from the POCT device and the routine laboratory method, because patients are likely to be managed using both analytical systems.

An economic assessment of the equipment, including the costs of consumables and servicing, should also be completed. Any comparison of costs with the laboratory service will highlight only the cost per test, which, as stated earlier, will not give an accurate assessment of the cost-effectiveness of using the system. However, it is helpful at this point to obtain a good assessment of the relative staff costs associated with different systems, because these are likely to be key features in the decision-making process.

After comparison data have been obtained, tabulated, and interpreted, a POCT device is selected if the assessment has indicated value in using such an approach. It is recommended that the laboratory professional should then conduct a short evaluation of the equipment to gain familiarization with the system. This evaluation will help to determine the content of the training program that will be used, as well as a troubleshooting protocol. Such an evaluation should document the concordance between results generated with the device and those provided by the laboratory. All of this information should then be recorded in a logbook associated with the equipment. In addition, the organization may wish to undertake some form of safety check, give the device some form of local code, and enter the code into the local equipment register.

TRAINING AND CERTIFICATION OF OPERATORS

The confidence of the clinician, the health care provider, and the patient in results generated by a POCT device depends heavily on the robustness of the instrument and the competence of the operator, assuming that it has already been shown to meet the analytical requirements of the clinical setting. Many of the agencies involved in the regulation of health care delivery now require that all personnel associated with the delivery of diagnostic results demonstrate their competence through a process of regulation, and this applies equally to POCT personnel.

The elements of a training program are listed in Box 24.3. In practice, such a program is tailored to suit the needs of the individual and the organization. These may include formal presentation to groups, or on a one-to-one basis, self-directed learning using agreed documentation, or computer-aided learning. For example, several of the current models of blood gas and electrolyte analyzers have on board computer-aided training modules.

Whatever the training strategy employed, it is important to document satisfactory completion of training, and that the individual has been tested and found competent with a combination of questions concerned with understanding and practical demonstration of the skills gained. The latter can be achieved by performing tests on a series of QC materials and repeat testing of samples that have been analyzed recently (parallel testing). Finally, the operator should be observed on a minimum of three occasions throughout the procedure involved in the POCT. Competence on a long-term basis is maintained through regular practice of skills and continuing education; it is important to build these features into any education and training program. Regular review of performance in QC and quality assurance programs will provide a means of overseeing

Box 24.3: Main elements of a POCT training program

1. Understanding the context of the test-pathophysiologic context
   - Clinical requirement for the test
   - Action taken on basis of result
   - Nature of test and method used
2. Patient preparation required-relevance of diurnal variation
   - Relevance of drug therapy
3. Sample requirement and specimen collection
4. Preparation of analytical device-machine and/or consumables
5. Performance of test
6. Performance of quality control
7. Documentation of test result and quality control result
8. Reporting of test result to appropriate personnel
9. Interpretation of result and sources of advice
10. Health and safety issues (e.g. disposal of sample and test device, cleaning of machine and test area)

the competence of operators. However, this is not always sufficient, particularly when operators are employed on irregular shifts or may not always be called upon to perform POCT. In this latter situation, it may be necessary to create specific arrangements for individuals to undertake tests on QC material. The error log may highlight when problems area rising. However, the most important thing is to encourage an open approach to the assessment of competence, so that operators themselves can seek help if they believe that problems are occurring. Such an open approach should be supported with audit and performance review meetings where problems are aired and developments discussed. Regular assessment of competence should be built into a formal program for recertification that will be a requirement of most accreditation programs.

POCT end-users Competency

All staff are trained and evaluated for competency on each POCT they perform. When new test methodology or instrumentation is instituted, employees are retrained and reevaluated. The POCT coordinator and department supervisors will develop a program for competency assessment and acceptability standards based on the training protocol, procedure manual, and department policies. Supervisors will evaluate common group deficiencies, review current policies and procedures, and take corrective action to improve performance.

Waived competency (1) competence for waived testing is assessed at the time of orientation and annually thereafter, (2) competency for waived testing is assessed using at least two of the following methods per person per test; performance of a test on a blind specimen, periodic observation of routine work by the supervisor or qualified designee, monitoring of each user's quality control performance, use of a written test specific to the test assessed, and (3) this competency is documented and place in employee personnel file.

Non-waived competency (1) competency for non-waived testing is accessed initially and at 6 months post-training and annually thereafter, (2) competency assessment includes direct observations of routine patient test performance, including patient preparation, if applicable, and specimen collection, handling, processing, and testing, monitoring, recording, and reporting of test results, review of intermediate test results or work sheets, quality control, proficiency testing, and preventive maintenance performance, direct observation of performance of instrument maintenance function checks and calibration, test performance as defined by laboratory policy (for example, testing previously analyzed specimens, internal blind testing samples, external proficiency, or testing samples), problem-solving skills as appropriate to the job, and (3) this competency is documented and place in employee personnel file.

MAINTENANCE AND INVENTORY CONTROL

Implementation and maintenance of a POCT service require that a supply of devices (both instrumentation and consumables) be maintained at all times, and that this is supported by a formal program. This approach may be taken for larger bench top systems within a large organization; however, similar arrangements (e.g. rapid replacement of faulty units) can be achieved for smaller organizations (e.g. a physician's office laboratory) through an appropriate arrangement with the supplier. In the case of consumables, the key points in this process are to (1) adhere to recommended storage conditions for reagents, calibrators, and controls, (2) be aware of the stated shelf life of consumables, and (3) ensure that stocks are released in time for any preanalytical preparation to be accommodated (e.g. thawing). When multiple sites are using the same materials, a central purchasing, supply, and inventory control system should be put in place-not only to gain benefit from bulk purchasing, but also to ensure that individual systems are not supplied unknowingly with different batches of consumables.

Complexity in the maintenance of reusable devices will vary from system to system, but clear guidelines will be available from the manufacturer and should be adhered to rigorously. Issues that usually require particular vigilance include expiration dates, bio-contamination, electrical safety, maintenance of optics, and inadvertent use of inappropriate consumables.

DOCUMENTATION

Documentation of all aspects of a POCT service has been a major issue for many years, compounded by the fact that the storage of data in laboratory and hospital information systems has often been limited and inconsistent. Thus, it is critically important to keep an accurate record of the test request, the result, and the action taken as an absolute minimum.

Although, the last point may be seen as beyond the scope of the laboratory, the incidence of errors in laboratory medicine that have been attributed to preanalytical and postanalytical phases suggests that the laboratory should play a more integrated role in the whole care process. Some of the issues concerning documentation are now being resolved with the advent of the electronic patient record, electronic requesting, and better connectivity of POCT instrumentation to information systems.

Documentation should extend from the standard operating procedure(s) for the POCT systems to records of training and certification of operators, reagents, calibrator and control inventory, verification of performance of devices and shipments of consumables, and QC and external quality assurance, together with error logs and any corrective action taken.

Future of POCT

The health care environment is changing so rapidly, the change process shows no sign of slowing down. In fact, all aspects of this field are moving equally fast: technology, automation, robotics, informatics, economics, etc. It is no wonder that POCT is moving rapidly ahead, as one of the major approaches to solving what seems to be the major challenge; the three key drivers for expansion of POCT services in the future will be (1) changes in the way health care is provided, (2) patients' needs and expectations, and (3) technological innovations. We also observed that trends in the way that clinical care is being delivered are completely opposite to those in which diagnostic testing services are moving. Christensen and coworkers suggested that POCT and information technologies (namely, connectivity, the electronic patient record, and decision support systems) provide some of the key technologies to enable a disruptive solution to the provision of health care, namely, offering solutions to the problems that many health systems face today by radically changing the way that care is organized and delivered. Patient expectations are increasing and will drive the trend toward a more patient-focused style of care, with fewer clinic visits, shorter waiting times, and an expectation of better care.

POCT has been shown to be capable of shorter 'lengths of stay' and, in many cases, improved health outcomes. As health service decision makers (both purchasers and providers) realize that it is possible to achieve lower 'costs per patient episode' with the use of POCT, more effort will be put into this testing modality. So what will facilitate this revolution?

The answer lies in new technology in terms of the development of new delivery platforms and the discovery of new markers with the use of new business models and value networks. Considerable efforts are being made to develop and manufacture miniaturized analytical devices that will enable faster analytical times to be achieved, with smaller sample requirements. Several examples in the field of micro-fabricated devices have been shown to meet these aspirations. In the future, continued technological advances will result in even smaller devices that can be tailored for a large number of analytes and that are very simple to operate.

Non-invasive testing remains the 'holy grail' for POCT, and over the past two decades, evidence has suggested some success in this area. Most work has been performed on a range of imaging techniques that seek a signature of the molecule of interest (e.g. glucose) from among the many signatures of the extracellular and tissue matrices. Alternative approaches have sought to access the extracellular fluid space or to sample extracellular fluid directly.

Areas of testing that are showing significant progress include (1) testing for infectious agents using molecular based techniques, (2) testing for predisposition to disease, and (3) assessing an individual's response profile toward a new drug. In all three scenarios, the key to having a POCT is the need for early decision making to implement therapy (or lifestyle change), together with the need for patient counseling. The technology is clearly available to detect any form of biological entity at the point-of-care, including very rapid analysis of deoxyribonucleic acid (DNA) from saliva samples. However, many ethical issues surround analysis for genetic predisposition and tests for certain infectious diseases. These developments not withstanding, evidence also indicates that POCT is being used increasingly in the management of long-term conditions, probably the area where the greatest volume of testing is focused.

If one accepts that patient empowerment is a key development in health care for the future, self-testing is likely to increase. This is an area that is well established for blood glucose and is increasingly used in the management of oral anticoagulation therapy. As emphasis slowly moves toward health promotion and well ness monitoring, issues of access to testing will become significant drivers of the use of diagnostic tests. Perhaps the most interesting aspect of patient empowerment, however, is the fact that it changes the relationship between the patient and the health professional. It could be argued that in the not too distant future, the patient will not be expected to make an appointment or to travel to see the health professional, but rather will expect better access and convenience.

As with any change, most people at first resist POCT. This attitude has significantly changed in the last few years, but there still are those who would rather ignore it than consider it. You need to manage POCT, not resist it. Maintaining the status quo is not a strategy for survival in laboratory medicine today nor it will suffice for the future.

BIBLIOGRAPHY

1. Antmann EM, Grudzien C, Sachs DB. Evaluation of a rapid bedside assay for detection of serum cardiac troponin T. JAMA 1995; 273: 1279–82.

2. Apple FS, Christenson RH, Valdes R, Wu AHB, Andriak AJ, Duh SH, et al. Simultaneous rapid measurement of whole blood myoglobin, creatine kinase MB, and cardiac troponin I by the Triage Cardiac Panel for detection of myocardial infarction. Clin Chem 1999; 273: 1279–82.

3. Ashby JP, ed. The patient and de centralised testing. Lancaster, UK: MTP Press Ltd, 1988.

4. Bailey TM. A practicum on making point-of-care testing work. Am Clin Lab.1997;16(1):10-11. 14. Seamonds B. Conference report: medical, economic, andregulatory factors affecting point-of-care testing. Clin Chim Acta. 1996; 249: 1–19.

5. Baum jM, Monhaut NM, Parker DR, Price CP o Improving the quality of self-monitoring blood glucose measurement: a study in reducing calibration errors. Diabetes TechnolTher 2006; 8: 347–57.

6. Belanger AC. Point-of-care testing: the JCAHO perspective. Med Lab Obs. June 1994: 46–49.

7. Bender GT. Chemical Instrumentation: A Laboratory Manual Based on Clinical Chemistry. Philadelphia, PA: WB Saunders; 1972.

8. Beneteau-Burnat B, Bocque MC, Lorin A, Martin C, Vaubourdolle M. Evaluation of the blood gas analyzer Gem PREMIER 3000. ClinChem Lab Med 2004; 42: 96–101.

9. Beneteau-Burnat B, Pernet P, Pilon A, Latour D, Goujon S, Feuillu A, et al. Evaluation of the GEM Premier 4000: a compact blood gas CO-oximeter and electrolyte analyzer for point-of-care and laboratory testing. ClinChem Lab Med 2008; 46: 271–9.

10. Bingham D, Kendall J, Clancy M. The portable laboratory an evaluation of the accuracy and reproducibility of I-STAT Ann ClinBiochem 1999; 36: 66–71.

11. Boehme CC, Nabeta P, Hillemann D, et al. Rapid molecular detection of tuberculosis and rifampin resistance N Engl J Med. 2010; 363: 1005–1015.

12. Bonnar j, Flynn A, Freundl G, Kirkman R, Royston R, Snowden R. Personal hormone monitoring for contraception. Brit j Fam Planning 1999; 24: 128–34.

13. BorgardjP, Szymanowicz A, Pellae I, Szmidt-Adjide V, Rota M. Determination of total bilirubin in whole blood from neonates: results from a French multicenter study. ClinChem Lab Med 2006; 44: 1103–10.

14. Boyd JC, Bruns DE. Quality specifications for glucose meters: assessment by simulation modeling of errors in insulin dose. Clin Chem. February 2001; 47(2): 209–214.

15. Boyd jC, Bruns DE. Quality specifications for glucose meters:assessment by simulation modeling of errors in insulin dose. Clin Chem 2001; 47: 209–14.

16. BrunellejA, Degtiarov AM, Moran RF, Race LA. Simultaneous measurement of total hemoglobin and its derivatives in blood using CO-oximeters: analytical principles; their application in selecting analytical wavelengths and reference methods; a comparison of the results and the choices made. Scand j Clin Lab Invest 1996; 56(Suppl 224): 47–69.

17. Bubner TK, Lawrence CO, Gialamas A, Yelland LN, Ryan P, Wilson KJ, et al. Effectiveness of point-of-care testing for therapeutic control of chronic conditions: results from the PoCT in General PracticeTrial. Med j Aust 2009; 190: 624–6.

18. Buechler KF, Moi S, Noar B, McGrath D, Villela j, Clancy M, et al. Simultaneous detection of seven drugs of abuse by the triage panel for drugs of abuse. Clin Chem 1992; 38: 1678–84.

19. Bullock DG. Quality control and quality assurance. In: Price CP, St john A, Hicks jH, eds. Point-of-care testing. Washington DC: AACC Press, 2004: 137–45.

20. Burnett D. A practical guide to accreditation in laboratory medicine. London: ACB Venture Publications, 2002: 1–314.

21. Burnett D. Accreditation and point-of-care testing. Ann Clin Biochem 2000; 37: 241–3.

22. CAP Commission on Laboratory Accreditation, Laboratory Accreditation Program. Point-of-Care Testing Checklist. Northfield, IL: CAP; April 2012.

23. Carlson DA. Point of care testing: regulation and accreditation. Clin Lab Sci. 1996; 9(5): 298–302.

24. Castro HJ, Oropello JM, Halpern N. Point-of-care testing in the intensive care unit: theintensive care physician's perspective. Am J Clin Pathol. 1995; 104(4) suppl 1: S95–S99.

25. Cembrowski GS, Tran DV, Slater-MacLean L, Chin D, Gibney RT, Jacka M. Could susceptibility to low hematocrit interference have compromised the results of the NICE-SUGAR trial? Clin Chem. July 2010; 56(7): 1193–1195.

26. Chapin KC, Blake P, Wilson CD. Performance characteristics and utilization of rapid antigen test, DNA probe, and culture for detection of group A streptococci in an acute care clinic. J Clin Microbiol 2002; 40: 4207–10.

27. Chin HL, Krall MA. Successful implementation of a comprehensive computer-based patient record system in Kaiser Permanente Northwest: strategy and experience. Eff Clin Pract 1998; I: 51–60.

28. Christensen CM, Grossman jH, Hwang j. The innovator's prescription: a disruptive solution to health care. New York: McGraw Hill, 2009: 1–44I.

29. Clinical Laboratory Standards Institute. Implementation guide of POCTOI for healthcare providers: approved guideline. CLSI Document POCT02-A. Wayne, Pa: CLSI, 2008.

30. Clinical Laboratory Standards Institute. Point-of-care connectivity: approved standard, 2nd edition. CLSI Document POCTOI-A2.Wayne, Pa: CLSI, 2006.

31. Clinical Laboratory Standards Institute. Point-of-care in vitro diagnostic (IVD) testing: approved guidelines, 2nd edition. CLSI Document POCT4-A2. Wayne, Pa: CLSI, 2006.

32. Clinical Laboratory Standards Institute. Quality management for unit-use testing: approved guideline. CLSI Document EPI8-A.Volume 22 Number 28 Wayne, Pa: CLSI, 2002.

33. Clinical Laboratory Standards Institute. Selection criteria for point of care testing devices. CLSI Document POCT09-A. Wayne, Pa: CLSI, 2010.

34. College of American Pathologists. Information (e.g., drugs of abuse testing program). Available at: www.cap.org (accessed on April 14, 2011).

35. Collinson PO, john C, Lynch S, Rao A, Canepa-Anson R, Carson E,et al. A prospective randomized controlled trial of point-of-care testing on the coronary care unit. Ann ClinBiochem 2004; 41: 397–404.

36. Crook M. Handbook of Near-Patient Testing. London: Greenwich Medical Media Limited; 1999: 1–116.

37. Davis G. Microfabricated sensors and the commercial development of the i-Stat" point-of-care system. In: Ramsay G, ed. Commercial biosensors. New York: john Wiley & Sons, 1998: 47–76.

38. D'CostaEj, Higgins IJ, Turner AP. Quinoprotein glucose dehydrogenase and its application in an amperometric glucose sensor. Biosensors 1986; 2: 71–87.

39. Dickinson KJ, Troxler M, Homer- Vanniasinkam S. The surgical application of point-of-care haemostasis and platelet function testing. Br j Surg 2008; 95: 1317–30.

40. D'Orazio P. Biosensors in clinical chemistry. ClinChimActa 2003; 334: 41–69.

41. Ehrmeyer SS, Laessig RH. Regulation, accreditation and education for point-of-care testing. In: Kost G, ed. Principles and practice of point-of-care testing. Philadelphia: Lippincott Williams and Wilkins, 2002: 434–43.

42. Erickson KA, Wilding P. Evaluation of a novel point-of-care system: the I-Stat portable clinical analyzer. ClinChem 1993; 39: 283–7.

43. Farhat SE, Finn S, Chua R, Smith B, Simor AE, George P, et al. Rapid detection of infectious mononucleosis-associated heterophile antibodies by a novel immunochromatographic assay and a latex agglutination test. J Clin Microbiol 1993; 31: 1597–600.

44. Fermann GJ, Suyama J. Point of care testing in the emergency department. J Emerg Med 2002; 22: 393–404.

45. Fleisher M, Schwartz MK. Automated approaches to rapid-response testing: acomparative evaluation of point-of-care and centralized laboratory testing. Am J ClinPathol. 1995; 104(4)suppl 1: S18–S25.

46. Harrison JR, Bevan J, Furth EE, Metz DC. Accu Stat whole blood finger stick test for Helicobacter pylori infection: a reliable screening method. J Clin GastroenteroI 1998; 27: 50–3.

47. Hedberg P, Wennecke G. A preliminary evaluation of the AQT90FLEX TnI immunoassay. ClinChem Lab Med 2009; 47: 376–8.

48. Heneghan C, Alonso-Coello P, Garcia-Alamino JM, Perera R, MeatsE, Glasziou P. Self-monitoring of oral anticoagulation: a systematic review and meta-analysis. Lancet 2006; 367: 404–11.

49. Heslop L, Howard A, Fernando J, Rothfield A, Wallace L. Wireless communications in acute health-care. J Telemed Telecare 2003; 9: 187–93.

50. Hillier SC, Flower SE, Frost CG, Jenkins ATA, Keay R, BravenH,et al. An electrochemical gene detection assay utilising T7 exonuclease activity on complementary probe-target oligonucleotide sequences. ElectrochemComm 2004; 6: 1227–32.

51. Hirst D, St. John A. Keeping the spotlight on quality from a distance. Accred Qual Assur 2000; 5; 9–13.

52. Hobbs FD, Delaney BC, Fitzmaurice DA, Wilson S, Hyde C), Thorpe GH, et al. A review of near patient testing in primary care. Health Technol Assess 1997; 1: 1–230.

53. Hoedemaekers CW, Klein Gunnewiek JM, Van der Hoeven JG. Point-of-care glucose measurement systems should be used with great caution in critically ill intensive care unit patients. Crit Care Med. January 2010; 38(1):339; author reply 339-340.

54. Holtzinger C, Szelag E, DuBois JA, Shirey TL, Presti S. Evaluation ofa new POCT bedside glucose meter and strip with hematocrit and interference corrections. Point of Care 2008; 7: 1–6.

55. Jacobs E, Hinson KA, Tolnai J, Simson E. Implementation, management and continuous quality improvement of point-of-care testing in an academic health care setting. ClinChim Acta 2001; 307: 49–59.

56. Jina A. A novel point-of-care prothrombin time monitoring system. Chest 2000; 118 (Suppl):2835.

57. Johnson RE, Newhall WJ, Papp JR, Knapp JS, Black CM, Gift TL,et al. Screening tests to detect Chlamydia trachomatis and Neisseria gonorrhoeae infections-2002. MMWR Recomm Rep 2002; 51: 1–38; quiz CEI-4.

58. Jones R, St. John A. Informatics in point-of-care testing. In: Price CP, St. John A, Hicks JM, eds. Point-of-care testing. Washington, DC: AACC Press, 2004:197-208.

59. Jurgens R, Elliott R. Rapid HIV screening at the point of care: legal and ethical issues. Can HIV AIDS Policy Law Newsl 2000; 5: 28–33.

60. Karon BS, McBane RD, Chaudhry R, Beyer LK, Santrach PJ. Accuracy of capillary whole blood international normalized ratio on the Coagu Chek S, CoaguChek XS, and i-STAT 1 point-of-care analyzers. Am J Clin Pat hoi 2008; 130: 88–92.

61. Keffer JH. Economic considerations of point-of-care testing. Am J Clin Pathol. 1995; 104(4) suppl 1: S107–S110.

62. Kendall J, Reeves B, Clancy M. Point of care testing: randomised, controlled trial of clinical outcome. BMJ 1998; 316: 1052–7.

63. Khalil OS. Spectroscopic and clinical aspects of noninvasive glucose measurements. ClinChem 1999; 45: 165–75.

64. Khandurina J, Guttman A. Bioanalysis in microfluidic devices. J Chromatogr A 2002; 943: 159–83.

65. Kohn LT, Corrigan JM, Donaldson MS, Eds. To err is human: building a safer health system. Institute of Medicine. Washington, DC: National Academies Press, 2000: 1–287.

66. Kost GJ, ed. Principles and practice of point-of-care testing. Philadelphia: Lippincott Williams & Wilkins, 2002: 1–654.

67. Kost GJ. Guidelines for point-of-care testing: improving patient outcomes. Am J Clin Pathol. 1995;104(4)suppl 1: S111-S127.

68. Kost GJ. Preventing medical errors in point-of-care testing: security, validation, safeguards, and connectivity. Arch Pathol Lab Med 2001; 125: 1307–15.

69. Kricka LJ, Thorpe GHG. Technology of handheld devices for point-of-care testing. In: Price CP, St. John A, Kricka LJ, eds. Point-of caretesting, 3rd edition. Washington, DC: AACC Press, 2010: 27–42

70. Kricka LJ. Microchips, microarrays, biochips, and nano chips: personal laboratories for the 21st century. ClinChimActa 2001; 307: 219–23.

71. Kricka LJ. Microchips: the hitchhiker's guide to analytical microchips. Washington: AACC Press, 2002: 1–94.

72. Kricka LJ. Point-of-care technologies for the future: technological innovations and hurdles to implementation. Point of Care 2009; 8: 42–5.

73. Lang HK. Point-of-care testing: friend or foe to medical technologists? Advance for Medical Laboratory Professionals. December 26, 1994: 18–19.

74. Lauks IR, inventor. Point-of-care in-vitro blood analysis system. U.S. Patent 6,845,327; January 18, 2005.

75. Lee-Lewandrowski E, Corboy D, Lewandrowski K, Sinclair J, McDermott S, Benzer Tl. Implementation of a point-of-care satellite laboratory in the emergency department of an academic medicalcenter: impact on test turnaround time and patient emergency department length of stay. Arch Pathol Lab Med 2003; 127: 456–60.

76. Lee-Lewandrowski E, Laposata M, Eschenbach K, et al. Utilization and cost analysis ofbedside capillary glucose testing in a large teaching hospital: implications for managingpoint of care testing. Am J Med. 1994; 97: 222–230.

77. Lehmann CA, Mintz N, Giacini JM. Impact of telehealth on heathcareutilization by congestive heart failure patients. Dis Manage Health Outcomes 2006; 14: 163–9.

78. Lewandrowski K. Three wishes for POCT testing: a compendium ofunmet needs from the perspective of practitioners in the field. Point of Care 2008; 7: 86–88.

79. Lindemans J, Hoefkens P, van Kessel AL, Bonnay M, KulpmannWR, vanSuijlen JD. Portable blood gas and electrolyte analyzer evaluated in a multi institutional study. Clin Chem 1999; 45: 111–17.

80. Lott JA, Johnson WR, Luke KE. Evaluation of an automated urine chemistry reagent-strip analyzer. J Clin Lab Anal 1995; 9: 212–17.

81. Magny E, Renard MF, Launay JM. Analytical evaluation of Rapidpoint400 blood gas analyzer. Ann BioIClin (Paris) 2001; 59: 622–8.

82. Mahoney JJ, Maguire P, Ellison JM, Cariski AT. Response to Cembrowski et al. regarding "Could susceptibility to low hematocrit interference have compromised the results of the NICESUGAR trial?" Clin Chem. October 2010; 56(10):1643; author reply 1643–1644.

83. Mass D. Consulting to physician office laboratories. In: Snyder JR, Wilkinson DS, eds. Management in Laboratory Medicine. 3rd ed. New York, NY: Lippincott; 1998: 443–450.

84. Mass D. Consulting to physician office laboratories. In: Snyder JR, Wilkinson DS, eds. Management in laboratory medicine, 3rd edition. New York: Lippincott, 1998: 443–50.

85. Michael L. Bishop. Clinical Chemistry: Principles, Techniques, and Correlations, 7th edition. Philadelphia, Wolters Kluwer/Lippincott Williams & Wilkins, 2013.

86. NICE-SUGAR Study Investigators, Finfer S, Chittock DR, et al. Intensive versus conventional glucose control in critically ill patients. N Engl J Med. 2009; 360: 1283–1297.

87. Niewenhaus) H, van Kasteel M. The role of consumer electronics in point-of-care testing. In: Price CP, St. John A, Kricka L), eds. Point-of-care testing, 3rd edition. Washington, DC: AACC Press, 2010: 97–106.

88. Norwegian Quality Improvement of Primary Care Laboratories. Available at: v,'ww.noklus.no (accessed on April 14, 2011).

89. Nosanchuk JS, Keefner R. Cost analysis of point-of-care laboratory testing in acommunity hospital. Am J ClinPathol. 1995; 103(2): 240–243.

90. Oberhardt BJ. Thrombosis and hemostasis testing at the point of care. Am J Clin Pathol.1995; 104(4) suppl 1: S72-S78.

91. Oliver G. On Bedside Testing. London: HK Lewis; 1884: 1–128.

92. Oliver NS, Toumazou C, Cass AE, Johnston DG. Glucose sensors: a review of current and emerging technology. Diabet Med 2009; 26: 197–210.

93. Oral Anticoagulation Monitoring Study Group. Point-of-care prothrombin time measurement for professional and patient self-testing use: a multicenter clinical experience. Am) Clin Pathol 2001; 115: 288–96.

94. Oral Anticoagulation Monitoring Study Group. Prothrombin measurement using a patient self-testing system. Am Clin Pat hoI 2001; 115: 280–7.

95. Osei-Bimpong A, Jury C, McLean R, Lewis SM. Point-of-care method for total white cell count: an evaluation of the HemoCue WBC device.Int) Lab Hematol 2009; 31: 657–64.

96. Parsons MP, Newman DJ, Newall RG, Price CPo Validation of a point-of-care assay for the urinary albumin: creatinine ratio. Clin Chem 1999; 45: 414–17.

97. Parvin CA, Lo SF, Deuser SM, et al. Impact of point-of-care testing on patients' length ofstay in a large emergency department. Clin Chem. 1996; 42(5): 711–717.

98. Phillips DL. Quality systems for unit-use testing devices. Clin Chem1997; 43: 893–6.

99. Plesch W, Wolf T, Breitenbeck N, Dikkeschei LD, Cervero A, PerezPL, et al. Results of the performance verification of the CoaguChekXS system. Thromb Res 2008; 123: 381–9.

100. Pope RM, Apps) M, Page MD, Allen K, Bodansky HJ. A novel devicefor the rapid in-clinic measurement of haemoglobin Ale. Diabet Med1993; 3: 260–3.

101. Price CP, St. John A, Kricka L), eds. Point-of-care testing: needs, opportunity and innovation, 3rd edition. Washington, DC: AACC Press, 2010: 1–582.

102. Price CP, St. John A. Point-of-care testing for managers and policymakers. Washington, DC: AACC Press, 2006: 1–120.

103. Price CP, Thorpe GH. Disposable analytical devices for point-of-care testing. In: Price CP, Hicks J M, eds. Point-of-care testing. Washington, DC: AACC Press, 1999: 19–40.

104. Price CP. Quality assurance of extra-laboratory analyses. In: Marks V, Alberti KG, eds. Clinical Biochemistry Nearer the Patient II. London: Bailliere Tindall; 1987: 166–178.

105. Price CPo Point of care testing: potential for tracking disease management outcomes. Dis Manage Health Outcomes 2002; 10: 749–61.

106. Price CPo Point-of-care testing. BM 2001; 322: 1285–8.

107. Price CPO Quality assurance of extra-laboratory analyses. In: Marks V, Alberti KG, eds. Clinical biochemistry nearer the patient II. London: Bailliere Tindall, 1987: 166–78.

108. Prisco D, Paniccia R. Point-of-care testing of hemostasis in cardiac surgery. Thromb J 2003; 1: 1–10.

109. Pugia M J, Lott J A, Clark LW, Parker DR, Wallace JF, Willis TW. Comparisons of urine dipsticks with quantitative methods for microalbuminuria. Eur J Clin Chem Clin Biochem 1997; 35: 693–700.

110. Raine CH. Self-monitored blood glucose: a common pitfall. Endo Pract 2003; 9: 137–9.

111. Rao LV, Ekberg BA, Connor D, Jakubiak F, Vallaro GM, Snyder M. Evaluation of a new point of care automated complete blood count(CBC) analyzer in various clinical settings. Clin Chim Acta 2008; 389: 120–5.

112. Rolinski B, Kuster H, Ugele B, Gruber R, Horn K. Total bilirubin measurement by photometry on a blood gas analyzer: potential for use in neonatal testing at the point of care. Clin Chem 2001; 47: 1845–7.

113. Scott MG. Faster is better-it's rarely that simple! ClinChem 2000; 46: 441–2.

114. Sirkin A, Jalloh T, Lee L. Selecting an accurate point-of-care testing system: clinical and technical issues and implications in neonatal blood glucose monitoring. Spec PediatrNurs 2002; 7: 104–12.

115. St John A, Davis TM, Goodall I, Townsend MA, Price C Po Nurse based evaluation of assays for glycated hemoglobin. Clin Chim Acta 2005; 365: 257–263.

116. St. Louis P. Status of point-of-care testing: promise, realities, and possibilities. Clin Biochem 2000; 33: 427–40.

117. Stephens E J. Developing open standards for point-of-care connectivity. IVD Technol 1999; 10: 22–5.

118. Storto Poe S, Case-Cromer DL. Nursing strategies for point-of-care testing. In: Kost G, ed. Principles and practice in point-of-care testing. Philadelphia: Lippincott Williams and Wilkins, 2002: 214–35.

119. Tamada A, Garg S, Jovanovic L, Pitzer KR, Fermi S, Potts RO. Noninvasive glucose monitoring: comprehensive clinical results. Cygnus Research Team. JAMA 1999; 282: 1839–44.

120. Tripodi A, Chantarangkul V, Mannucci P. Near-patient testing devices to monitor oral anticoagulant therapy. Br) Haematol 2001; 113: 847–52.

121. Tsai WW, Nash DB, Seamonds B, et al. Point-of-care versus central laboratory testing: an economic analysis in an academic medical center. Clin Ther. 1994; 16(5): 898–910.

122. Van den Berghe G, Wouters P, Weekers F, et al. Intensive insulin therapy in critically ill patients. N Engl J Med. November 2001; 345 (19): 1359–1367.

25

Clinical Chemistry and the Geriatric Patient

INTRODUCTION

Gerontology is the study of aging including biologic, sociologic, and psychologic changes, and **geriatrics** refers to medical care for the elderly, an age group that is not easy to define precisely. 'Older people' is sometimes preferred but is equally imprecise; >65 is the age often used, but most people do not need geriatrics expertise in their care until age 70 or 75.

The differentiation of 'normal' or 'healthy' aging versus the accumulation of multiple medical problems with age is an area of active research and debate. There are several analytical measurements that change when comparing a diseased individual to a healthy one, but because there are also a number of biochemical changes that occur as a consequence of normal aging, it can be difficult to differentiate between abnormal physiological changes and normal signs of aging in geriatric patients. Table 25.1 outlines some of the age-specific changes that occur in regard to certain chemistry analytes.

AGING

Aging refers to the inevitable, irreversible decline in organ function that occurs over time even in the absence of injury, illness, environmental risks, or poor lifestyle choices (e.g. unhealthy diet, lack of exercise, substance abuse). Initially, the changes in organ function do not affect baseline function; the first manifestations are a reduced capacity of each organ to maintain homeostasis under stress (e.g. illness, injury). The cardiovascular, renal, and central nervous systems are usually the most vulnerable (the weakest links).

Diseases interact with pure aging effects to cause geriatric-specific complications (now referred to as geriatric syndromes), particularly in the weak-link systems, even when those organs are not the primary ones affected by a disease. Typical examples are delirium complicating pneumonia or urinary tract infection (UTIs)

Table 25.1	Changes in selected clinical chemistry analytes with age		
Increase		**Decrease**	**Unchanged**
ANP			ACTH
ALP (females)		ADH	Calcium
Calcitonin		Albumin	Chloride
C-reactive protein			Cortisol
EPO		Aldosterone	Creatinine
Ferritin		Vitamin B12	HDL-C
Fibrinogen		LDL-C	Insulin
Folic acid		Cholesterol	Sodium
FSH		DHEA-S	Total T4
Free T4		Estrogen	pH or slight decrease
Gamma globulins		Ferritin	
Homocysteine		Growth hormone	
Insulin		IGF-1	
Lactate		PO2	
Parathyroid hormone		Progesterone	
Potassium		Testosterone	
TBG		T3	
TSH (slight)		Total protein	
Transferrin		Uric acid	
Triglycerides		Vitamin D	
GGT			

ANP, atrial natriuretic peptide; ACTH, adrenocorticotropic hormone; ADH, antidiuretic hormone; EPO, erythropoietin; HDL-C, high-density lipoprotein cholesterol; LDL-C, low-density lipoprotein cholesterol; FSH, follicle-stimulating hormone; DHEA-S, sulfated dehydroepiandrosterone; IGF-1, insulin-like growth factor-1; TBG, thyroid binding globulin; TSH, thyroid-stimulating hormone; GGT, γ-glutamyl transferase; T3, triiodothyronine.

and the falls, dizziness, syncope, urinary incontinence, and weight loss that often accompany many minor illnesses in the elderly. Aging organs are also more susceptible to injury, e.g. intracranial hemorrhage is more common and is triggered by less clinically important injury in the elderly. The effects of aging must be taken into account during diagnosis and treatment of the elderly. clinicians should not mistake pure aging for disease (e.g. slow information retrieval is not dementia), mistake disease for pure aging (e.g. ascribe debilitating arthritis, tremor, or dementia to old age), ignore the increased risk of adverse drug effects on weak-link systems stressed by illness, and forget that the elderly often have multiple underlying disorders (e.g. hyper-

tension, diabetes, and atherosclerosis) that accelerate the potential for harm. In addition, clinicians should be alert for diseases and problems that are much more common among the elderly (e.g. diastolic heart failure, Alzheimer disease, incontinence, and atrial fibrillation). This approach enables clinicians to better understand and manage the complexity of the diseases that often coexist in older patients.

GENERAL PHYSIOLOGIC CHANGES WITH AGING

Most age-related biologic functions peak before age 30 and gradually decline linearly thereafter (Table 25.2); the decline may be critical during stress, but it usually has little or no effect on daily activities. Therefore, disorders,

Table 25.2	Selected physiologic age-related changes	
Affected organ or system	**Physiologic change**	**Clinical manifestations**
Body composition	↓ Lean body mass ↓ Muscle mass ↓ Creatinine production ↓ Skeletal mass ↓ Total body water ↑ Percentage adipose tissue (until age 60, then ↓ until death)	Changes in drug levels (usually ↑) ↓ Strength Tendency toward dehydration
Cells	↑ DNA damage and ↓ DNA repair capacity ↓ Oxidative capacity Accelerated cell senescence ↑ Fibrosis Lipofuscin accumulation	↑ Cancer risk
CNS	↓ Number of dopamine receptors ↑ Alpha-adrenergic responses ↑ Muscarinic parasympathetic responses	Tendency toward Parkinsonian symptoms (e.g. ↑ muscle tone, ↓ arm swing)
Ears	Loss of high-frequency hearing	↓ Ability to recognize speech
Endocrine system	↑ Insulin resistance and glucose intolerance Menopause, ↓ estrogen and progesterone secretion ↓ Testosterone secretion ↓ Growth hormone secretion ↓ Vitamin D absorption and activation ↑ Incidence of thyroid abnormalities ↑ Bone mineral loss ↑ Secretion of ADH in response to osmolar stimuli	↑ Incidence of diabetes Vaginal dryness, dyspareunia ↓ Muscle mass ↓ Bone mass ↑ Fracture risk Changes in skin Tendency toward water intoxication
Eyes	↓ Lens flexibility ↑ Time for pupillary reflexes (constriction, dilation) ↑ Incidence of cataracts	Presbyopia ↑ Glare and difficulty adjusting to changes in lighting ↓ Visual acuity
GI tract	↓ Splanchnic blood flow ↑ Transit time	Tendency toward constipation and diarrhea
Heart	↓ Intrinsic heart rate and maximal heart rate Blunted baroreflex (less increase in heart rate in response to decrease in BP) ↓ Diastolic relaxation ↑ Atrioventricular conduction time ↑ Atrial and ventricular ectopy	Tendency toward syncope ↓ Ejection fraction ↑ Rates of atrial fibrillation ↑ Rates of diastolic dysfunction and diastolic heart failure

Contd.

Table 25.2	Selected physiologic age-related changes *(Contd.)*	
Affected organ or system	**Physiologic change**	**Clinical manifestations**
Immune system	↓ T-cell function ↓ B-cell function	Increased susceptibility to infections and possibly cancer ↓ Antibody response to immunization or infection but ↑ autoantibodies
Joints	Degeneration of cartilaginous tissues Fibrosis ↑ Glycosylation and cross-linking of collagen Loss of tissue elasticity	Tightening of joints Tendency toward osteoarthritis
Kidneys	↓ Renal blood flow ↓ Renal mass ↓ Glomerular filtration ↓ Renal tubular secretion and reabsorption ↓ Ability to excrete a free-water load	Changes in drug levels with ↑ risk of adverse drug effects Tendency toward dehydration
Liver	↓ Hepatic mass ↓ Hepatic blood flow ↓ Activity of CYP 450 enzyme system	Changes in drug levels
Nose	↓ Smell	↓ Taste and consequent ↓ appetite ↑ Likelihood (slightly) of nosebleeds
Peripheral nervous system	↓ Baroreflex responses ↓ Beta-adrenergic responsiveness and number of receptors ↓ Signal transduction ↓ Muscarinic parasympathetic responses Preserved alpha-adrenergic responses	Tendency toward syncope ↓ Response to beta-blockers Exaggerated response to anticholinergic drugs
Pulmonary system	↓ Vital capacity ↓ Lung elasticity (compliance) ↑ Residual volume ↓ FEV1 ↑ V/Q mismatch	↑ Likelihood of shortness of breath during vigorous exercise if people are normally sedentary or if exercise is done at high altitudes ↑ Risk of death due to pneumonia ↑ Risk of serious complications (e.g. respiratory failure) for patients with a pulmonary disorder
Vasculature	↓ Endothelin-dependent vasodilation ↑ Peripheral resistance	Tendency toward hypertension

↓ = decreased; ↑ = increased; FEV1= forced expiratory volume in 1 sec; V/Q =ventilation/perfusion.

rather than normal aging, are the primary cause of functional loss during old age. In many cases, the declines that occur with aging may be due at least partly to lifestyle, behavior, diet, and environment and thus can be modified. For example, aerobic exercise can prevent or partially reverse a decline in maximal exercise capacity, muscle strength, and glucose tolerance in healthy but sedentary older people.

Only about 10% of the elderly participate in regular physical activity for >30 minutes 5 times a week (a common recommendation). About 35–45% participate in minimal activity. The elderly tend to be less active than other age groups for many reasons, most commonly because disorders limit their physical activity.

The benefits of physical activity for the elderly are many and far exceed its risks (e.g. falls, torn ligaments, pulled muscles). Benefits include reduced mortality rates, even for smokers and the obese, preservation of skeletal muscle strength, aerobic capacity, and bone density, contributing to greater mobility and independence, reduced risk of obesity, prevention and treatment of cardiovascular disorders [including rehabilitation after myocardial infarction (MI)], diabetes, osteoporosis, colon cancer, and psychiatric disorders (especially mood disorders), prevention of falls and fall-related injuries by improving muscle strength, balance, coordination, joint function, and endurance, improved functional ability, opportunities for social interaction, enhanced sense of well-being, and possibly improved sleep quality. Physical activity is one of the few interventions that can restore physiologic capacity after it has been lost.

EVALUATION OF THE ELDERLY PATIENT

Evaluation of the elderly usually differs from a standard medical evaluation. For elderly patients, especially those who are very old or frail, history-taking and physical examination may have to be done at different times, and physical examination may require 2 sessions because patients become fatigued.

The elderly also have different, often more complicated health care problems, such as multiple disorders, which may require use of many drugs (sometimes called polypharmacy) and thus greater likelihood of a high-risk drug being prescribed. Diagnosis may be complicated, resulting in delayed, missed, or erroneous diagnoses leading to inappropriate use of drugs. Early detection of problems results in early intervention, which can prevent deterioration and improve quality of life, often through relatively minor, inexpensive interventions (e.g. lifestyle changes). Thus, some elderly patients, particularly the frail or chronically ill, are best evaluated using a comprehensive geriatric assessment, which includes evaluation of function and quality of life, best administered by an interdisciplinary team.

Multiple Disorders

On average, elderly patients have 6 diagnosable disorders, and the primary care physician is often unaware of some of them. A disorder in one organ system can weaken another system, exacerbating the deterioration of both and leading to disability, dependence, and, without intervention, death. Multiple disorders complicate diagnosis and treatment, and effects of the disorders are magnified by social disadvantage (e.g. isolation) and poverty (as patients outlive their resources and supportive peers) and by functional and financial problems. Clinicians should also pay particular attention to certain common geriatric symptoms (e.g. delirium, dizziness, syncope, falling, mobility problems, weight or appetite loss, and urinary incontinence) because they may result from disorders of multiple organ systems.

If patients have multiple disorders, treatments (e.g. bed rest, surgery, and drugs) must be well-integrated; treating one disorder without treating associated disorders may accelerate decline. Also, careful monitoring is needed to avoid iatrogenic consequences. For example, with complete bed rest, elderly patients can lose 1–3% of muscle mass and strength each day (causing sarcopenia), and effects of bed rest alone can ultimately result in death.

Missed or Delayed Diagnosis

Disorders that are common among the elderly are frequently missed, or the diagnosis is delayed. Clinicians should use the history, physical examination, and simple laboratory tests to actively screen elderly patients for disorders that occur only or commonly in the elderly (Table 25.3); when diagnosed early, these disorders can often be more easily treated. Early diagnosis frequently depends on the clinician's familiarity with the patient's behavior and history, including mental status.

Table 25.3	Disorders common among the elderly
Frequency	Disorders
Almost exclusive in the eldrely	Accidental hypothermia
	Normal-pressure hydrocephalus
	Urinary incontinence
	Diastolic heart failure
	Alzheimer disease
More common among the elderly than among other age groups	Atrial fibrillation
	Basal cell carcinoma
	Chronic lymphocytic leukemia
	Degenerative osteoarthritis
	Dementia
	Diabetic hyperosmolar nonketotic coma
	Falls
	Herpes zoster
	Hip fracture
	Monoclonal gammopathies
	Osteoporosis
	Parkinsonism
	Polymyalgia rheumatica
	Pressure ulcers
	Prostate cancer
	Stroke
Common among the elderly and treatable	Temporal arteritis (giant cell arteritis)
	Depression
	Diabetes mellitus
	Foot disorders interfering with mobility
	GI bleeding
	Hearing and vision abnormalities
	Heart failure
	Hypothyroidism
	Iron deficiency anemia
	Oral disorders interfering with eating
	Vitamin B12 deficiency

Commonly, the first signs of a physical disorder are behavioral, mental, or emotional. If clinicians are unaware of this possibility and attribute these signs to dementia, diagnosis and treatment can be delayed.

POLYPHARMACY

Prescription and over-the-counter (OTC) drug use should be reviewed frequently, particularly for drug interactions and use of drugs considered inappropriate for the elderly. When multiple drugs are used, electronic health record-based management is more efficient.

Care Giver Problems

Occasionally, problems of elderly patients are related to neglect or abuse by their care giver. Clinicians should consider the possibility of patient abuse and drug abuse by the care giver if circumstances and findings suggest it. Certain injury patterns or patient behaviors are particularly suggestive, including, frequent bruising, especially in difficult-to-reach areas (e.g. middle of the back), grip bruises of the upper arms, bruises of the genitals, peculiar burns, and unexplained fearfulness of a care giver in the patient.

History

Often, more time is needed to interview and evaluate elderly patients, partly because they may have characteristics that interfere with the evaluation. The following should be considered:

1. **Sensory deficits:** Dentures, eyeglasses, or hearing aids, if normally worn, should be worn to facilitate communication during the interview. Adequate lighting and elimination of visual or auditory distraction also helps

2. **Under reporting of symptoms:** Elderly patients may not report symptoms that they consider part of normal aging (e.g. dyspnea, hearing or vision deficits, memory problems, incontinence, gait disturbance, constipation, dizziness, and falls). However, no symptom should be attributed to normal aging unless a thorough evaluation is done and other possible causes have been eliminated

3. **Unusual manifestations of a disorder:** In the elderly, typical manifestations of a disorder may be absent. Instead, the elderly may present with nonspecific symptoms (e.g. fatigue, confusion, and weight loss)

4. **Functional decline as the only manifestation:** Disorders may manifest solely as functional decline. In such cases, standard questions may not apply

5. **Difficulty recalling:** Patients may not accurately remember past illnesses, hospitalizations, operations, and drug use; clinicians may have to obtain these data elsewhere (e.g. from family members, a home health aide, or medical records)

6. **Fear:** The elderly may be reluctant to report symptoms because they fear hospitalization, which they may associate with dying

7. **Age-related disorders and problems: Depression** (common among elderly who are vulnerable and sick), the cumulative losses of old age, and discomfort due to a disorder may make the elderly less apt to provide health-related information to clinicians. Patients with impaired cognition may have difficulty describing problems, impeding the physician's evaluation.

Interview

A clinician's knowledge of an elderly patient's everyday concerns, social circumstances, mental function, emotional state, and sense of well-being helps orient and guide the interview. Asking patients to describe a typical day elicits information about their quality of life and mental and physical function. This approach is especially useful during the first meeting. Patients should be given time to speak about things of personal importance. Clinicians should also ask whether patients have specific concerns, such as fear of falling. The resulting rapport can help the clinician communicate better with patients and their family members.

A mental status examination may be necessary early in the interview to determine the patient's reliability; this examination should be conducted tactfully, so that the patient does not become embarrassed, offended, or defensive. Routine screening for physical and psychologic disorders should be done annually, beginning at age 70.

Often, verbal and nonverbal clues (e.g. the way the story is told, tempo of speech, tone of voice, eye contact) can provide information, as for the following; **depression**— elderly patients may omit or deny symptoms of anxiety or depression but betray them by a lowered voice, subdued enthusiasm, or even tears, **physical and mental health**—what patients say about sleep and appetite may be revealing, and **weight gain or loss**—Clinicians should note any change in the fit of clothing or dentures.

Unless mental status is impaired, a patient should be interviewed alone to encourage the discussion of personal matters. Clinicians may also need to speak with a relative or care giver, who often gives a different perspective on function, mental status, and emotional state. These interviews may be done with the patient absent or present.

The clinician should ask the patient's permission before inviting a relative or care giver to be present and should explain that such interviews are routine. If the care giver is interviewed alone, the patient should be kept usefully occupied (e.g. filling out a standardized assessment questionnaire, being interviewed by another member of the interdisciplinary team).

If indicated, clinicians should consider the possibility of drug abuse by the patient and patient abuse by the care giver.

Medical History

When asking patients about their past medical history, a clinician should ask about disorders that used to be more common (e.g. rheumatic fever, poliomyelitis) and about outdated treatments [e.g. pneumothorax therapy for tuberculosis (TB), mercury for syphilis]. A history of immunizations (e.g. tetanus, influenza, and pneumococcus), adverse reactions to immunizations, and skin test results for TB is needed. If patients recall having surgery but do not remember the procedure or its purpose, surgical records should be obtained if possible.

Clinicians should ask questions designed to systematically review each body area or system (review of systems) to check for other disorders and common problems that patients may have forgotten to mention (Table 25.4).

Table 25.4	Clues to disorders in elderly patients	
Region or system	**Symptom**	**Possible causes**
Skin	Itching	Allergic reaction, cancer, dry skin, hyperthyroidism, jaundice, lice, scabies, uremia
Head	Headaches	Anxiety, cervical osteoarthritis, depression, giant cell arteritis, subdural hematoma, tumors
Eyes	Glare from lights at night	Cataracts, glaucoma
	Loss of central vision	Macular degeneration
	Loss of near vision (presbyopia)	Decreased accommodation of the lens
	Loss of peripheral vision	Glaucoma, retinal detachment, stroke
	Pain	Giant cell arteritis, glaucoma
Ears	Hearing loss	Acoustic neuroma, cerumen, foreign body in the external canal, ototoxicity due to use of drugs (e.g. aminoglycosides, aspirin, and furosemide), Paget disease, presbycusis, trauma due to noise, tumor of the cerebellopontine angle, viral infection
	Loss of high-frequency range	Presbycusis (usually caused by age-related changes in the cochlea)
Mouth	Burning mouth	Pernicious anemia, stomatitis
	Denture pain	Dentures that fit poorly, oral cancer
	Dry mouth (xerostomia)	Autoimmune disorders (e.g. RA, Sjögren syndrome, and SLE), dehydration, drugs (e.g. antidepressants including tricyclic antidepressants, antihistamines, antihypertensives, diuretics, psychoactive drugs), salivary gland damage due to infection or to radiation therapy for head and neck tumors
	Limited tongue motion	Oral cancer, stroke
	Loss of taste	Adrenal insufficiency, drugs (e.g. antihistamines, antidepressants), infection of the mouth or nose, nasopharyngeal tumor, radiation therapy, smoking, xerostomia
Throat	Dysphagia	Anxiety, cancer, esophageal stricture, foreign body, Schatzki ring, stroke, Zenker diverticulum
	Voice changes	Hypothyroidism, recurrent laryngeal nerve dysfunction, vocal cord tumor
Neck	Pain	Cervical arthritis, carotid or vertebral artery dissection, polymyalgia rheumatica
Chest	Dyspnea during exertion	Cancer, COPD, functional decline, heart failure, infection
	Paroxysmal nocturnal dyspnea	Gastroesophageal reflux, heart failure
	Pain	Angina pectoris, anxiety, aortic dissection, costochondritis, esophageal motility disorders, gastroesophageal reflux, herpes zoster, MI, myocarditis, pericarditis, pleural effusion, pleuritis, pneumonia, pneumothorax
GI	Constipation with no other symptoms	Colorectal cancer, dehydration, drugs (e.g. aluminum-containing antacids, anticholinergic drugs, iron supplements, opioids, tricyclic antidepressants), hypercalcemia (e.g. due to hyperparathyroidism), hypokalemia, hypothyroidism, inadequate exercise, laxative abuse, low-fiber diet
	Constipation with pain, vomiting, and intermittent diarrhea	Fecal impaction Bowel obstruction
	Fecal incontinence	Cerebral dysfunction, fecal impaction, rectal cancer, spinal cord lesions
	Lower abdominal pain (crampy, sudden onset)	Diverticulitis, gastroenteritis, ischemic colitis, obstruction
	Postprandial abdominal pain (2–3 h after eating, lasting 1–3 h)	Chronic intestinal ischemia
	Rectal bleeding	Colon angiodysplasia, colon cancer, diverticulosis, hemorrhoids, ischemic colitis

Contd.

Table 25.4	Clues to disorders in elderly patients *(Contd.)*	
Region or system	**Symptom**	**Possible causes**
GU	Frequency, dribbling, hesitancy, weak stream	Benign prostatic hyperplasia, constipation, drugs (e.g. anti-histamines, opioids), prostate cancer, urinary retention, UTI
	Dysuria with or without fever	Prostatitis, UTI
	Polyuria	Diabetes insipidus (decrease in ADH action), diabetes mellitus, diuretics
	Incontinence	Cystitis, functional decline, normal-pressure hydrocephalus, spinal cord dysfunction, stroke, urinary retention or overflow, UTI
Musculoskeletal	Back pain	Abdominal aortic aneurysm, compression fractures, infection, metastatic cancer, multiple myeloma, osteoarthritis, Paget disease, pyelonephritis, spinal stenosis
	Proximal muscle pain	Myopathies, polymyalgia rheumatica, use of statins
Extremities	Leg pain	Intermittent claudication, night cramps, osteoarthritis, radiculopathy (e.g. disk herniation, lumbar stenosis), restless legs syndrome
	Swollen ankles	Heart failure (if swelling is bilateral), hypoalbuminemia, renal insufficiency, venous insufficiency
Neurologic	Change in mental status with fever	Delirium, encephalitis, meningitis, sepsis
	Change in mental status without fever	Acute illness, cognitive dysfunction, fecal impaction, delirium, depression, drugs, paranoia, urinary retention
	Clumsiness in tasks requiring fine motor coordination (e.g. buttoning shirt)	Arthritis, Parkinsonism, spondylotic cervical myelopathy, intention tremor
	Excessive sweating during meals	Autonomic neuropathy
	Fall without loss of consciousness	Bradycardia, drop attack, neuropathy, orthostatic hypotension, postural instability, tachycardia, transient ischemic attack, vision impairment
	Hesitant gait with intention tremor	Parkinson disease
	Numbness with tingling in fingers	Carpal tunnel syndrome, peripheral neuropathy, spondylotic cervical myelopathy
	Sleep disturbances	Anxiety, circadian rhythm disturbances, depression, drugs, pain, Parkinsonism, periodic limb movement disorder, sleep apnea, urinary frequency
	Syncope	Aortic stenosis, cardiac arrhythmia, hypoglycemia, orthostatic hypotension (especially drug-related), seizure
	Transient interference with speech, muscle strength, sensation, or vision	Transient ischemic attack
	Tremor	Alcohol abuse, CNS disorder (e.g. cerebellar disorders, poststroke), essential tremor, hyperthyroidism, Parkinsonism

Drug History

The drug history should be recorded, and a copy should be given to patients or their care giver. It should contain, drugs used, dose, dosing schedule, prescriber, reason for prescribing the drugs, and precise nature of any drug allergies. All drugs used should be recorded, including, topical drugs (which may be absorbed systemically), OTC drugs (which can have serious consequences if overused and may interact with prescription drugs), dietary supplements, and medicinal herb preparations (because many can interact adversely with prescription and OTC drugs).

Patients or Family members should be asked to bring in all of the above drugs and supplements at the initial visit and periodically thereafter. Clinicians can make sure patients have the prescribed drugs, but possession of these drugs does not guarantee adherence. Counting the number of tablets in each vial during the first and subsequent visits may be necessary. If someone other than a patient administers the drugs, that person is interviewed. Patients should be asked to demonstrate their ability to read labels (often printed in small type), open containers (especially the child-resistant type), and recognize drugs. Patients should be advised not to put their drugs into one container.

Alcohol, tobacco, and recreational drug use history.

Patients who smoke should be counseled to stop and, if they continue, not to smoke in bed because the elderly are more likely to fall asleep while doing so. Patients should be checked for signs of alcohol use disorders, which are under diagnosed in the elderly. Such signs include confusion, anger, hostility, alcohol odor on the breath, impaired balance and gait, tremors, peripheral neuropathy, and nutritional deficiencies.

Nutrition History

Type, quantity, and frequency of food eaten are determined. Patients who eat ≤2 meals a day are at risk of undernutrition. The ability to eat (e.g. to chew and swallow) is evaluated. It may be impaired by xerostomia and/or dental problems, which are common among the elderly. Decreased taste or smell may reduce the pleasure of eating, so patients may eat less. Patients with decreased vision, arthritis, immobility, or tremors may have difficulty preparing meals and may injure or burn themselves when cooking. Patients who are worried about urinary incontinence may reduce their fluid intake; as a result, they may eat less food.

Mental Health History

Mental health problems may not be detected easily in elderly patients. Symptoms that may indicate a mental health disorder in younger patients (e.g. insomnia, changes in sleep patterns, constipation, cognitive dysfunction, anorexia, weight loss, fatigue, preoccupation with bodily functions, increased alcohol consumption) may have another cause in the elderly. Sadness, hopelessness, and crying episodes may indicate depression. Irritability may be the primary affective symptom of depression, or patients may present with cognitive dysfunction. Generalized anxiety is the most common mental disorder encountered in elderly patients and often is accompanied by depression.

Patients should be asked about delusions and hallucinations, past mental health care (including psychotherapy, institutionalization, and electroconvulsive therapy), use of psychoactive drugs, and recent changes in circumstances. Many circumstances (e.g. recent loss of a loved one, hearing loss, a change in residence or living situation, loss of independence) may contribute to depression. Patients' spiritual and religious preferences, including their personal interpretation of aging, declining health, and death, should be clarified.

PHYSICAL EXAMINATION

Observing patients and their movements (e.g. walking into the examination room, sitting in or rising from a chair, getting on and off an examination table, taking off or putting on socks and shoes) can provide valuable information about their function. Their personal hygiene (e.g. state of dress, cleanliness, and odor) may provide information about mental status and the ability to care for themselves.

If patients become fatigued, the physical examination may need to be stopped and continued at another visit. Elderly patients may require additional time to undress and transfer to the examining table; they should not be rushed. The examining table should be adjusted to a height that patients can easily access; a footstool facilitates mounting. Frail patients must not be left alone on the table. Portions of the examination may be more comfortable if patients sit in a chair.

Clinicians should describe the general appearance of patients (e.g. comfortable, restless, undernourished, inattentive, pale, dyspneic, and cyanotic). If they are examined at bedside, use of protective padding or a protective mattress, bedside rails (partial or full), restraints, a urinary catheter, or an adult diaper should be noted.

Vital Signs

Weight should be recorded at each visit. During measurement, patients with balance problems may need to grasp grab bars placed near or on the scale. Height is recorded annually to check for height loss due to osteoporosis. Temperature is recorded. Hypothermia can be missed if the thermometer cannot measure temperatures more than a few degrees lower than normal. Absence of fever does not exclude infection.

Pulses and BP are checked in both arms. Pulse is taken for 30 seconds, and any irregularity is noted. Because many factors can alter BP, BP is measured several times after patients have rested >5 minutes. BP may be overestimated in elderly patients because their arteries are stiff. This rare condition, called pseudohypertension, should be suspected if dizziness develops after antihypertensives are begun or doses are increased to treat persistently elevated systolic BP.

All elderly patients are checked for orthostatic hypotension because it is common. BP is measured with patients in the supine position, then after they have been standing for 3–5 minutes. If systolic BP falls ≥20 mmHg after patients stand, or any symptoms of hypotension are detected, orthostatic hypotension is diagnosed. Caution is required when testing hypovolemic patients. A normal respiratory rate in elderly patients may be as high as 25 breaths/min. A rate of >25 breaths/min may be the first sign of a lower respiratory tract infection, heart failure, or another disorder.

Skin

Initial observation includes color (normal rubor, pale, and cyanotic). Examination includes a search for premalignant and malignant lesions, tissue ischemia, and pressure ulcers. In the elderly, the following should be considered: (1) ecchymoses may occur readily when skin is traumatized, often on the forearm, because the dermis thins with aging, (2) uneven tanning may be normal because melanocytes are progressively lost with aging, (3) longitudinal ridges on the nails and absence of the crescent-shaped lunula are normal age-related findings, (4) nail plate fractures may occur because with aging, the nail plate thins, (5) black splinter hemorrhages in the middle or distal third of the fingernail are more likely to be due to trauma than to bacteremia, (6) a thickened, yellow toenail indicates onychomycosis, a fungal infection, (7) toenail borders that curve in and down indicate in grown toenail (onychocryptosis), (8) whitish nails that scale easily, sometimes with a pitted surface, indicate psoriasis, and (9) unexplained bruises may indicate abuse.

HEAD AND NECK

Face

Normal age-related findings may include the following: eyebrows that drop below the superior orbital rim, descent of the chin, loss of the angle between the submandibular line and neck, wrinkles, dry skin, and thick terminal hairs on the ears, nose, upper lip, and chin. The temporal arteries should be palpated for tenderness and thickening, which may indicate giant cell arteritis, suspicion of which requires immediate evaluation and treatment.

Nose

Progressive descent of the nasal tip is a normal age-related finding. It may cause the upper and lower lateral cartilage to separate, enlarging and lengthening the nose.

Eyes

Normal age-related findings include the following: loss of orbital fat: it may cause gradual sinking of the eye backward into the orbit (enophthalmos). Thus, enophthalmos is not necessarily a sign of dehydration in the elderly. enophthalmos is accompanied by deepening of the upper eyelid fold and slight obstruction of peripheral vision, pseudoptosis (decreased size of the palpebral aperture), entropion (inversion of lower eyelid margins), ectropion (eversion of lower eyelid margins), and arcus senilis (a white ring at the limbus). With aging, presbyopia develops; the lens becomes less elastic and less able to change shape when focusing on close objects. The eye examination should focus on testing visual acuity (e.g. using a snellen chart). Visual fields can be tested at the bedside by confrontation, i.e. patients are asked to stare at the examiner so that the examiner can determine differences between their and the examiner's visual field. However, such testing has low sensitivity for most visual disorders. Tonometry is occasionally done in primary care; however, it is usually done by ophthalmologists or optometrists as part of routine eye examinations or by ophthalmologists when a patient is referred to them because glaucoma is clinically suspected.

Ophthalmoscopy is done to check for cataracts, optic nerve or macular degeneration, and evidence of glaucoma, hypertension, or diabetes. Findings may be unremarkable unless a disorder is present because the retina's appearance usually does not change much with aging. In elderly patients, mild to moderate elevated intracranial pressure may not result in papilledema because cortical atrophy occurs with aging; papilledema is more likely when pressure is markedly increased. Areas of black pigment or hemorrhages in and around the macula indicate macular degeneration. For all elderly patients, an eye examination by an ophthalmologist or optometrist is recommended every 1–2 years because such an examination may be much more sensitive for certain common eye disorders (e.g. glaucoma, cataracts, and retinal disorders).

Ears

Tophi, a normal age-related finding, may be noted during inspection of the pinna. The external auditory canal is examined for cerumen, especially if a hearing problem is noted during the interview. If a patient wears a hearing aid, it is removed and examined. The ear mold and plastic tubing can become plugged with wax, or the battery may be dead, indicated by absence of a whistle (feedback) when the volume of the hearing aid is turned up.

To evaluate hearing, examiners, with their face out of the patient's view, whisper 3–6 random words or letters into each of the patient's ears. If a patient correctly repeats at least half of these words for each ear, hearing is considered functional for one-on-one conversations. Patients with presbycusis (age-related, gradual, bilateral, symmetric, and predominantly high-frequency hearing deficits) are more likely to report difficulty in understanding speech than in hearing sounds. Evaluation with a portable audioscope, if available, is also recommended because the testing sounds are standardized; thus, this evaluation can be useful when multiple providers are caring for a patient. Patients are asked whether hearing loss interferes with social, work, or family functioning, or they may be given the hearing handicap inventory for the elderly (HHIE), a self-assessment tool designed to determine the effects of hearing loss on the emotional and social adjustment of the elderly. If hearing loss interferes with functioning or if the HHIE score is positive, they are referred for formal audio logic testing.

Mouth

The mouth is examined for bleeding or swollen gums, loose or broken teeth, fungal infections, and signs of cancer (e.g. leukoplakia, erythroplakia, ulceration, mass). Findings may include darkened teeth due to extrinsic stains and less translucent enamel, which occur with aging, fissures in the mouth and tongue and a tongue that sticks to the buccal mucosa due to xerostomia, erythematous, edematous gingiva that bleeds easily usually indicating a gingival or periodontal disorder, and bad breath possibly indicating caries, periodontitis, another oral disorder, or sometimes a pulmonary disorder.

The dorsal and ventral surfaces of the tongue are examined. Common age-related changes include varicose veins on the ventral surface, benign migratory glossitis (geographic tongue), and atrophied papillae on the sides of the tongue. In edentulous patients, the tongue may enlarge to facilitate chewing; however, enlargement may also indicate amyloidosis or hypothyroidism. A smooth, painful tongue may indicate vitamin B12 deficiency.

Dentures should be removed before the mouth is examined. Dentures increase risk of oral candidiasis and resorption of the alveolar ridges. Inflammation of the palatal mucosa and ulcers of the alveolar ridges may result from poorly fitting dentures. The interior of the mouth is palpated. A swollen, firm, and tender parotid gland may indicate parotitis, particularly in dehydrated patients; pus may be expressed from Stensen duct when bacterial parotitis is present. The infecting organisms are often staphylococci. Painful, inflamed, fissured lesions at the lip commissures (angular cheilitis) may be noted in edentulous patients who do not wear dentures; these lesions are usually accompanied by a fungal infection.

Temporomandibular Joint

This joint should be evaluated for degeneration (osteoarthrosis), a common age-related change. The joint can degenerate as teeth are lost and compressive forces in the joint become excessive. Degeneration may be indicated by joint crepitus felt at the head of the condyle as patients lower and raise their jaw, by painful jaw movements, or by both.

Neck

The thyroid gland, which is located low in the neck of elderly people, often beneath the sternum, is examined for enlargement and nodules. Carotid bruits due to transmitted heart murmurs can be differentiated from those due to carotid artery stenosis by moving the stethoscope up the neck, a transmitted heart murmur becomes softer; the bruit of carotid artery stenosis becomes louder. Bruits due to carotid artery stenosis suggest systemic atherosclerosis. Whether asymptomatic patients with carotid bruits require evaluation or treatment for cerebrovascular disease is unclear.

The neck is checked for flexibility. Resistance to passive flexion, extension, and lateral rotation may indicate a cervical spine disorder. Resistance to flexion and extension can also occur in patients with meningitis, but unless meningitis is accompanied by a cervical spine disorder, the neck can be rotated passively from side to side without resistance.

Chest and Back

All areas of the lungs are examined by percussion and auscultation. Basilar rales may be heard in the lungs of healthy patients, but should disappear after patients take a few deep breaths. The extent of respiratory excursions (movement of the diaphragm and ability to expand the chest) should be noted. The back is examined for scoliosis and tenderness. Severe low back, hip, and leg pain with marked sacral tenderness may indicate spontaneous osteoporotic fractures of the sacrum, which can occur in elderly patients.

Breasts

In men and women, the breasts should be examined annually for irregularities and nodules. For women, self-examinations are sometimes recommended. Screening mammography is also recommended, especially for women who have a family history of breast cancer. If nipples are retracted, pressure should be applied around the nipples; pressure everts the nipples when retraction is due to aging, but not when it is due to an underlying lesion.

Heart

Heart size can usually be assessed by palpating the apex. However, displacement caused by kyphoscoliosis may make assessment difficult. Auscultation should be done systematically (rate, regularity, murmurs, clicks, and rubs). Unexplained and asymptomatic sinus bradycardia in apparently healthy elderly people may not be clinically important. An irregularly irregular rhythm suggests atrial fibrillation.

In elderly patients, a systolic murmur most commonly indicates **aortic valve sclerosis; typically**, this murmur is not hemodynamically significant, although risk of stroke may be increased. It peaks early during systole and is rarely heard in the carotid arteries. Rarely, sclerosis of the aortic valve progresses to hemodynamic significance and calcification; although infrequent, aortic valve sclerosis is now the most common lesion leading to symptomatic aortic stenosis and need for treatment. However, systolic murmurs may be due to other disorders, which should be identified; (1) **aortic valve stenosis**—this murmur, in contrast to that of usual aortic valve sclerosis, typically peaks later during systole, is transmitted to the carotid arteries, and is loud; the second heart sound is dampened, pulse pressure is narrow, and the carotid up stroke is slowed. However, in elderly patients, the murmur of aortic valve stenosis may be difficult to identify because it may be softer, a second heart sound is rarely audible, and narrow pulse pressures are uncommon. also, in many elderly patients with aortic valve stenosis, the carotid up stroke does not slow because vascular compliance is diminished, (2) **mitral regurgitation**—this murmur is usually loudest at the apex and radiates to the axilla, and (3) **hypertrophic obstructive cardiomyopathy**—this murmur intensifies when patients do a Valsalva maneuver.

Diastolic murmurs are abnormal in people of any age. Fourth heart sounds are common among elderly people without evidence of a cardiovascular disorder and are commonly absent among elderly people with evidence of a cardiovascular disorder. If new neurologic or cardiovascular symptoms develop in patients with a pacemaker, evaluation for variable heart sounds, murmurs, and pulses and for hypotension and heart failure is required. These symptoms and signs may be due to loss of atrioventricular synchrony.

Gastrointestinal System

The abdomen is palpated to check for weak abdominal muscles, which are common among elderly people and which may predispose to hernias. Most abdominal aortic aneurysms are palpable as a pulsatile mass; however, only their lateral width can be assessed during physical examination. In some patients (particularly thin ones), a normal aorta is palpable, but the vessel and pulsations do not extend laterally. Screening ultrasonography of the aorta is recommended for all older men who have ever smoked. The liver and spleen are palpated for enlargement. Frequency and quality of bowel sounds are checked, and the suprapubic area is percussed for tenderness, discomfort, and evidence of urinary retention.

The anorectal area is examined externally for fissures, hemorrhoids, and other lesions. Sensation and the anal wink reflex are tested. A digital rectal examination (DRE) to detect a mass, stricture, tenderness, or fecal impaction is done in men and women. Fecal occult blood testing is also done.

Male Genitourinary System

The prostate gland is palpated for nodules, tenderness, and consistency. Estimating prostate size by DRE is inaccurate, and size does not correlate with urethral obstruction; however, DRE provides a qualitative evaluation.

Female Reproductive System

Regular pelvic examinations, with a Papanicolaou (Pap) test every 2–3 years until age 65, are recommended. At age 65, testing can be stopped if results of the previous 2 consecutive tests were normal. If women ≥65 have not had regular Pap tests, they should have at least 2 negative tests, 1 years apart, before testing is stopped. Once Pap testing has been stopped, it is restarted only if new symptoms or signs of a possible disorder develop. If women have had a hysterectomy, Pap tests are required only if cervical tissue remains.

For bimanual pelvic examination, patients who lack hip mobility may lie on their left side. Postmenopausal reduction of estrogen leads to atrophy of the vaginal and urethral mucosa; the vaginal mucosa appears dry and lacks rugal folds. The ovaries should not be palpable 10 years after menopause; palpable ovaries suggest cancer. Patients should be examined for evidence of prolapse of the urethra, vagina, cervix, and uterus. They are asked to cough to check for urine leakage and intermittent prolapse.

Musculoskeletal System

Joints are examined for tenderness, swelling, subluxation, crepitus, warmth, redness, and other abnormalities, which may suggest a disorder; heberden nodes (bony over growths at the distal interphalangeal joints) or bouchard nodes (bony over growths at the proximal interphalangeal joints); osteoarthritis, subluxation of the metacarpophalangeal joints with ulnar deviation of the fingers; chronic rheumatoid arthritis (RA), and swan-neck deformity (hyperextension of the proximal inter-phalangeal joint with flexion of the distal interphalangeal joint) and boutonnière deformity (hyperextension of the distal interphalangeal joint with flexion of the proximal interphalangeal joint); RA. These deformities may interfere with functioning or usual activities. Active and passive range of joint motion should be determined. The presence of contractures should be noted. Variable resistance to passive manipulation of the extremities (gegenhalten) sometimes occurs with aging.

Feet

Diagnosis and treatment of foot problems, which become common with aging, help elderly people maintain their independence. Common age-related findings include hallux valgus, medial prominence of the first metatarsal head with lateral deviation and rotation of the big toe, and lateral deviation of the fifth metatarsal head. Hammer toe (hyperflexion of the proximal interphalangeal joint) and claw toe (hyperflexion of the proximal and distal interphalangeal toe joints) may interfere with functioning and daily activities. Toe deformities may result from years of wearing poorly fitting shoes or from RA, diabetes, or neurologic disorders (e.g. Charcot-Marie-Tooth disease). Occasionally, foot problems indicate other systemic disorders. Patients with foot problems should be referred to a podiatrist for regular evaluation and treatment.

Neurologic System

Neurologic examination for elderly patients is similar to that for any adult. However, non-neurologic disorders that are common among elderly people may complicate this examination. For example, visual and hearing deficits may impede evaluation of cranial nerves, and periarthritis (inflammation of tissues around a joint) in certain joints, especially shoulders and hips, may interfere with evaluation of motor function.

Signs detected during the examination must be considered in light of the patient's age, history, and other findings. Symmetric findings unaccompanied by functional loss and other neurologic symptoms and signs may be noted in elderly patients. Clinicians must decide whether these findings justify a detailed evaluation to check for a neurologic lesion. Patients should be reevaluated periodically for functional changes, asymmetry, and new symptoms.

CRANIAL NERVES

Elderly people often have small pupils; their pupillary light reflex may be sluggish, and their pupillary mitotic response to near vision may be diminished. Upward gaze and, to a lesser extent, downward gaze can be slightly limited. Eye movements, when tracking an examiner's finger during evaluation of visual fields, may appear jerky and irregular. Bell phenomenon (reflex upward movement of the eyes during closure) is sometimes absent. These changes occur normally with aging.

In many elderly people, sense of smell is diminished because they have fewer olfactory neurons, have had numerous upper respiratory infections, or have chronic rhinitis. However, asymmetric loss (loss of smell in one nostril) is abnormal. Taste may be altered because the sense of smell is diminished or because patients take drugs that decrease salivation. Visual and hearing deficits may result from abnormalities in the eyes and ears rather than in nerve pathways.

Motor Function

Patients can be evaluated for tremor during handshaking and other simple activities. If tremor is detected,

amplitude, rhythm, distribution, frequency, and time of occurrence (at rest, with action, or with intention) are noted.

Muscle Strength

Elderly people, particularly those who do not do resistance training regularly, may appear weak during routine testing. For example, during the physical examination, the clinician may easily straighten a patient's elbow despite the patient's effort to sustain a contraction. If weakness is symmetric, does not bother the patient, and has not changed the patient's function or activity level, it is likely to be due to disuse rather than neurologic disease. Such weakness is treatable with resistance training; for the legs especially, it can improve mobility and reduce fall risk. Strengthening the upper extremities is also beneficial for overall function. Increased muscle tone, measured by flexing and extending the elbow or knee, is a normal finding in elderly people; however, jerky movements during examination and cogwheel rigidity are abnormal.

Sarcopenia (a decrease in muscle mass) is a common age-related finding. It is insignificant unless accompanied by a decline or change in function (e.g. patients can no longer rise from a chair without using chair arms). Sarcopenia affects the hand muscles (e.g. interosseous and thenar muscles) in particular. Weak extensor muscles of the wrist, fingers, and thumb are common among patients who use wheelchairs because compression of the upper arm against the armrest injures the radial nerve. Arm function can be tested by having patients pick up an eating utensil or touch the back of their head with both hands.

Coordination

Motor coordination is tested. Coordination decreases because of changes in central mechanisms and can be measured in the neuro exam; this decrease is usually subtle and does not impair function.

Gait and Posture

All components of gait should be assessed; they include initiation of walking; step length, height, symmetry, continuity, and cadence (rhythm); velocity (speed of walking); stride width; and walking posture. Sensation, musculoskeletal and motor control, and attention, which are necessary for independent, coordinated walking, must also be considered.

Normal age-related findings may include the following; shorter steps, possibly because calf muscles are weak or because balance is poor, reduced gait velocity in patients >70 because steps are shorter, increased time in double stance (when both feet are on the ground), which may be due to impaired balance or fear of falling, reduced motion in some joints (e.g. ankle plantar flexion just before the back foot lifts off, pelvic motion in the frontal and transverse planes), slight changes in walking posture (e.g. greater downward pelvic rotation, possibly due to a combination of increased abdominal fat, abdominal muscle weakness, and tight hip flexor muscles; a slightly greater turn-out of the toes, possibly due to loss of hip internal rotation or to an attempt to increase lateral stability). In people with a gait velocity of <1 m/sec, mortality risk is significantly increased. Aging has little effect on walking cadence or posture; typically, the elderly walk upright unless a disorder is present (Table 25.5).

Overall postural control is evaluated using the Romberg test (patients stand with feet together and eyes closed). Safety is paramount, and a clinician doing the Romberg test must be in position to prevent the patient from falling. With aging, postural control is often impaired, and postural sway (movement in the antero-posterior plane when patients remain stationary and upright) may increase.

REFLEXES

The deep tendon reflexes are checked. Aging usually has little effect on them. However, eliciting the Achilles tendon reflex may require special techniques (e.g. testing while patients kneel with their feet over the edge of a bed and with their hands clasped). A diminished or absent reflex, present in nearly half of elderly patients, may not indicate pathology, especially if symmetric. It occurs because tendon elasticity decreases and nerve conduction in the tendon's long reflex arc slows. Asymmetric Achilles tendon reflexes usually indicate a disorder (e.g. sciatica).

Cortical release reflexes (known as pathologic reflexes), which include snout, sucking, and palmomental reflexes, commonly occur in elderly patients without detectable brain disorders (e.g. dementia). A Babinski reflex (extensor plantar response) in elderly patients is abnormal; it indicates an upper motor neuron lesion, often cervical spondylosis with partial cord compression.

Sensation

Evaluation of sensation includes touch (using a skin prick test), cortical sensory function, temperature sense, proprioception (joint position sense), and vibration sense testing. Aging has limited effects on sensation. Many elderly patients report numbness, especially in the feet. It may result from a decrease in size of fibers in the peripheral nerves, particularly the large fibers. Nonetheless, patients with numbness should be checked for peripheral neuropathies. In many patients, no cause of numbness can be identified.

Many elderly people lose vibratory sensation below the knees. It is lost because small vessels in the posterior column of the spinal cord sclerose. However, proprioception, which is thought to use a similar pathway, is unaffected.

Table 25.5	Some causes of gait dysfunction
Problem	**Possible causes**
Neurogenic claudication (pain, weakness, and numbness that occurs during walking and lessens during sitting)	Lumbar spinal stenosis
Difficulty initiating walking	Frontal or subcortical disorders
	Isolated gait initiation failure
	Parkinson disease
Truncal instability (e.g. sway)	Arthritis in the hips or knees
	Cerebellar, subcortical, or basal ganglia dysfunction
Leaning forward during walking	Osteoporosis with kyphosis
Step asymmetry	Focal neurologic deficit
	Pain or weakness in one leg
	Unilateral musculoskeletal deficit
Step discontinuity	Fear of falling
	Frontal lobe disorder
Step length or height abnormalities	Arthritis
	Foot problem
	Stroke
Stride width abnormalities	Cerebellar disorders
	Hip disorders
	Normal-pressure hydrocephalus

Mental Status

A mental status examination is important. Patients who are disturbed by such a test should be reassured that it is routine. The examiner must make sure that patients can hear; hearing deficits that prevent patients from hearing and understanding questions may be mistaken for cognitive dysfunction. Evaluating the mental status of patients who have a speech or language disorder (e.g. mutism, dysarthria, speech apraxia, aphasia) can be difficult.

Orientation may be normal in many patients with dementia or other cognitive disorders. Thus, evaluation may require questions that identify abnormalities in consciousness, judgment, calculations, speech, language, praxis, executive function, or memory, as well as orientation. Abnormalities in these areas cannot be attributed solely to age, and if abnormalities are noted, further evaluation, including a formal test of mental status, is needed.

With aging, information processing and memory retrieval slow but are essentially unimpaired. With extra time and encouragement, patients do such tasks satisfactorily (unless a neurologic abnormality is present).

Nutritional Status

Aging changes the interpretation of many measurements that reflect nutritional status in younger people. For example, aging can alter height. Weight changes can reflect alterations in nutrition, fluid balance, or both. The proportion of lean body mass and body fat content changes. Despite these age-related changes, body mass index (BMI) is still useful in elderly patients, although it underestimates obesity. Waist circumference and waist-to-hip ratio have been used instead. Risks due to obesity are increased if the waist circumference is >102 cm (>40 in) in men and >88 cm (>35 inches) in women or if the waist-to-hip ratio is >0.9 in men and >0.85 in women.

If abnormalities in the nutrition history (e.g. weight loss, suspected deficiencies in essential nutrients) or BMI are identified, thorough nutritional evaluation, including laboratory measurements, is indicated.

COMPREHENSIVE GERIATRIC ASSESSMENT

Comprehensive geriatric assessment is a multidimensional process designed to assess the functional ability, health (physical, cognitive, and mental), and socio-environmental situation of elderly people.

The comprehensive geriatric assessment specifically and thoroughly evaluates functional and cognitive abilities, social support, financial status, and environmental factors, as well as physical and mental health. Ideally, a regular examination of elderly patients incorporates many aspects of the comprehensive geriatric assessment, making the 2 approaches very similar. Assessment results are coupled with sustained individually tailored interventions (e.g. rehabilitation, education, counseling, supportive services). The cost of geriatric assessment limits its use. Comprehensive geriatric assessment is most successful when done by a geriatric interdisciplinary team (typically, a geriatrician, nurse, social worker, and pharmacist). Usually, assessments are done in an outpatient setting. However, patients with physical or mental impairments and chronically ill patients may require inpatient assessment.

Effects of Age on Laboratory Testing

Basic biochemical and physiological changes accompany the aging process, and these changes can impact an individual's clinical laboratory test results. It is important that laboratorians understand how these changes can impact specific tests. It has been suggested that the presence of age-specific changes may warrant separate reference intervals for the elderly, but these are not readily available. In addition, consideration of preanalytical variables must be factored into the interpretation of laboratory results. How does the aging process affect interpretations of drug levels in the elderly? What are the effects of exercise and nutrition on chemistry results? Table 25.6 describes some of the factors that laboratorians should consider when interpreting test results for the elderly and defines some of the laboratory values that are impacted by these changes.

Muscle

As muscles age, they begin to decrease in number and size. Creatinine levels correlate with both muscle mass and renal function. In the geriatric population, a decrease in muscle mass coupled with the decrease in renal function keeps the creatinine level nearly the same or slightly increased.

Bone

Adequate calcium intake and sufficient vitamin D are important in maintaining bone mass and density.

Osteoporosis incidence is high in the elderly population, and this leads to increased risk of fracture. In addition, osteoporosis incidence coincides with increased risk of vitamin D deficiency. Vitamin D helps with absorption of dietary calcium from the intestine, thus decreased vitamin D levels can impact the amount of dietary calcium that is absorbed. Additionally, vitamin D deficiency leads to inadequate absorption of calcium, which leads to low serum levels and increased PTH levels. This increased PTH then causes increased calcium loss from the bone which increases alkaline phosphatase levels.

Table 25.6	Effects of age on laboratory testing	
	Normal physiological changes with age	**Laboratory values that correlate**
Muscle	↓ Muscle mass	↓ Creatinine
Bone	↓ Mineral content of bone, ↓ cartilage	↑ PTH (females), ↓ calcium, and calcitonin
GI	↓ Gastric motility, vitamin absorption, and drug absorption	↓ Vitamin B12, calcium, and Fe absorption
Kidney	↓ Renal function	↑ Serum ANP, BNP, EPO, and GFR, creatinine
		↓ Renin
Immune	↑ Hematopoietic stem cells, bone marrow activity, thymosin, and T-cell function	↑ ANAs
	↓ Autoimmune antibodies	
Endocrine	↑ Cancer incidence	↓ Aldosterone
		↑ Norepinephrine
Reproductive	↓ Sex hormones	↓ Testosterone, estrogen, progesterone, DHEA-S, and pregnenolone
		↑ GnRH

PTH, parathyroid hormone; GI, gastrointestinal; ANP, atrial natriuretic peptide; BNP, brain natriuretic peptide; EPO, erythropoietin; GFR, glomerular filtration rate; ANA, antinuclear antibody; DHEA-S, sulfated dehydroepiandrosterone; GnRH, gonadotropin-releasing hormone.

Gastrointestinal System

The gastrointestinal (GI) system includes the digestive tract and accessory organs including the pancreas and the liver. There are a number of age-related changes with respect to the liver analytes. C-reactive protein, an acute phase reactant, has been shown to be elevated in the elderly. This elevation is thought to be a nonspecific indicator of inflammation, and typically is a poor prognostic indicator. Gamma-glutamyl transferase (GGT) levels tend to increase with age in a gender-specific manner. Men do not show this age-related increase, but men tend to have higher levels of GGT than women. Fibrinogen, an acute phase reactant, is frequently elevated in geriatric patients, and this increase coincides with inflammatory disease, stroke, coronary dysfunction, and cancer.

Ferritin levels can be low in the elderly population, and when this is seen, it is usually due to iron deficiency anemia, similar to younger people. Transferrin levels can be reduced due to iron-deficient anemia or as a result of acute or chronic stress. Albumin levels are frequently decreased in the elderly population as a result of inflammation, malnutrition, and liver disease. Levels can be high in dehydration, but elevations above the upper limits of normal rarely occur in the elderly due to the prevalence of other health conditions that mask alterations. Total protein levels are also frequently decreased in the elderly for the same reasons that albumin levels are low.

Urinary System

Serum creatinine levels tend to be lower in the elderly. Again, this decreased serum level is associated with decreased muscle mass.

Immune System

As age increases, infection-induced morbidity and mortality rise. This is in part due to a weakened immune system. The innate immune system, commonly referred to as the 'first line of defense,' is the nonspecific antigen activation that confers short-term protection from a pathogen. Adaptive immune system, on the other hand, is activated by the innate system and refers to the protection from antigen that an individual develops throughout the life. Both the innate and adaptive immune systems become damaged and dysfunctional as individuals age, leading to increased prevalence of infection, and potentially also autoimmune disease and cancer.

Gastroenteritis is more frequently observed as individuals' age, but the increased frequency is thought to be a result of a weakened immune system. Pathogenic bacteria can enter and infect the digestive tract and contribute to presentation. Additionally, there is an increase in antinuclear antibody production, which correlates with incidence of arthritis.

Endocrine System

There are a variety of age-related changes to endocrine hormone regulation. These can be subclassified according to whether the hormone level increases or decreases.

INCREASED HORMONE LEVEL

Elevated levels of cortisol, though rarely present, have been reported to be associated with decreased cognitive function and memory loss. A slight increase in thyroid-stimulating hormone (TSH) has been observed, but again, this is not profound. Follicle-stimulating hormone (FSH) levels increase with aging, but with this increase, there is a down regulation of FSH receptors, such that in menopause, there are no longer circulating cells with FSH receptors and thus no responsiveness to the high level of hormone. Atrial natriuretic peptide (ANP) levels increase with age and the levels have been shown to be nearly fourfold higher in healthy elderly individuals than in younger people. Anemia is common in the elderly population, and EPO, a marker for anemia, rises in elderly patients. PTH levels are slightly higher in older individuals than gender-matched pairs.

DECREASED HORMONE LEVEL

In contrast to the finding with cortisol, dehydroepiandrosterone (DHEA) levels have been shown to decrease by 40–60%. Estrogen and progesterone levels decrease with age, and the reduction in estrogen further upregulates FSH levels. Insulin-like growth factor 1 (IGF-1) and growth hormone (GH) levels decrease with age. Secretion rates and serum concentrations of aldosterone decrease with age, and this decrease is a consequence of a decreased level of renin. Pituitary function declines with age and hypothalamic antidiuretic hormone (ADH) levels are increased.

Sex Hormones

Levels of expression of all sex hormone diminish with age. Testosterone levels decrease with age, as do estrogen and progesterone levels.

Glucose Metabolism

Insulin sensitivity decreases with age. As a result of this decreased sensitivity, there is an increase in the prevalence of type 2 diabetes, with the incidence reaching a peak between the ages of 60 and 74.

ESTABLISHING REFERENCE INTERVALS FOR THE ELDERLY

Most laboratory tests have 'gender-specific' reference ranges and/or 'age-specific' reference ranges. The broad categories for the age ranges are very wide, and the adult reference range includes individuals between 18 and about 50 years. As people live longer, age-related criteria for the analysis and interpretation of test results become increasingly important. Because of the need to establish reference ranges in a healthy population, and the increased prevalence of at least one health condition in the aged, there are little data on more appropriate age-specific reference ranges for older adults. Based on this lack of data, there has been an increased interest in determining age-related reference ranges in order to more effectively identify individuals with early stage disease. While the idea has a lot of merit, there are currently no publications establishing age-appropriate reference ranges for the elderly.

Certain analyte fluctuations that are seen as individual's age are clearly the result of aging organs, but other analytes do not lend themselves to such apparent delineation. In addition, coincident medical conditions can further complicate the issue. The requirement that reference values be obtained from healthy, normal individuals unfortunately limits a large number of geriatric patients from contributing to establishing these references. As a result of exclusion criteria, the geriatric population is also vastly under represented in most randomized clinical trials, which further precludes contribution to reference range generation. In addition, there is a wide intraindividual variability among the various analytes, which has been seen as a major obstacle for determining age appropriate reference ranges among the elderly. Instead, the current clinical approach that has been increasingly implemented is careful documentation of laboratory values and paying closer attention to changes over time instead of where the values fit in with the remainder of the population. This is not feasible among all elderly, as there is a small subset that resists treatment and thus does not see a medical professional on a regular basis. A lack of baseline measurements coupled with the lack of age-specific reference ranges continues to make diagnosis challenging. Currently, most physicians that care for the geriatric patient population rely on established patient care, frequent routine examinations, and following changes in laboratory values over time as an early indicator of a problem.

Preanalytical Variables Unique to Geriatric Patients

There are a number of factors that contribute to the accuracy and validity of test results in any population, but several of these factors have a greater impact in the geriatric patient. These include sample collection, sample handing, and physiological variables. Geriatric patients can present a challenge to phlebotomists due to disease, malnutrition, or dehydration. With increased age, there is a reduction in healing rate and an increased risk of acquiring infection due in part to a gradual loss in the capacity of the immune system to fight off infections. Further, the skin and veins are less elastic and can be injured more easily during venipuncture. The decrease in muscle mass and collagen leads to a decrease in vascular stability of veins and a subsequent decrease in blood flow. Physiological changes in the patient may impact laboratory results due to unavoidable issues that arise at the time of collection. Increased hemolysis or insufficient volume can ultimately impact the validity of the result. Other factors that may influence normal laboratory values in geriatric patients include diet, medications, exercise, smoking, alcohol consumption, physical activity, and body composition. While these factors influence results independent of age, geriatric patients are more likely to have one or several of these causing variations in test results. Caution should always be exercised when reporting results in a geriatric patient, but clearly an absurd result (one not compatible with life) should be investigated to identify potential causes of the discrepancy.

Drug Therapy in the Elderly

Among people ≥65, 90% use at least 1 drug per week, >40% use at least 5 different drugs per week, and 12% use ≥10 different drugs per week. Women take more drugs, particularly psychoactive and arthritis drugs. Drug use is greatest among the frail elderly, hospitalized patients, and nursing home residents; typically, a nursing home resident is given 7–8 different drugs on a regular basis.

Providing safe, effective drug therapy for the elderly is challenging for many reasons. They use more drugs than any other age group, increasing risk of adverse effects and drug interactions, and making adherence more difficult, they are more likely to have chronic disorders that may be worsened by the drug or affect drug response, their physiologic reserves are generally reduced and can be further reduced by acute and chronic disorders, aging can alter pharmacodynamics and pharmacokinetics, and they may be less able to obtain or afford drugs.

There are two main approaches to optimizing drug therapy in the elderly; using appropriate drugs as indicated to maximize cost-effectiveness, and avoiding adverse drug effects. Because the risk of adverse drug effects is higher, overprescribing (polypharmacy) has been targeted as a major problem for the elderly. However, underprescribing appropriate drugs must also be avoided.

Pharmacokinetics in the Elderly

Pharmacokinetics is best defined as what the body does to the drug. With aging, there are changes in all these areas; some changes are more clinically relevant. The metabolism and excretion of many drugs decrease, requiring that doses of some drugs be adjusted. Toxicity may develop slowly because levels of chronically used drugs increase for 5–6 half-lives, until a steady state is achieved. For example, certain benzodiazepines (diazepam, flurazepam, and chlordiazepoxide) have half-lives of up to 96 hours in elderly patients; signs of toxicity may not appear until days or weeks after therapy is started.

Absorption

Despite an age-related decrease in small-bowel surface area, slowed gastric emptying, and an increase in gastric pH, changes in drug absorption tend to be clinically inconsequential for most drugs. One exception is Ca

carbonate, which requires an acidic environment for optimal absorption. Age-related increases in gastric pH decrease Ca absorption and increase the risk of constipation. Thus, elderly patients should use a Ca salt (e.g. Ca citrate) that dissolves more easily in a less acidic environment. Another example of altered absorption is early release of enteric-coated dosage forms with increased gastric pH.

Distribution

With age, body fat generally increases and total body water decreases. Increased fat increases the volume of distribution for highly lipophilic drugs (e.g. diazepam, chlordiazepoxide) and may increase their elimination half-lives.

Serum albumin decreases and α1-acid glycoprotein increases with age, but the clinical effect of these changes on serum drug binding is unclear. In patients with an acute disorder or malnutrition, rapid reductions in serum albumin may enhance drug effects because serum levels of unbound (free) drug may increase (only unbound drug has a pharmacologic effect). Phenytoin and warfarin are drugs with a high risk of toxic effects when serum albumin level decreases.

HEPATIC METABOLISM

Overall hepatic metabolism of many drugs through the cytochrome P-450 enzyme system decreases with age. For drugs with decreased hepatic metabolism, clearance typically decreases 30–40%. Theoretically, maintenance drug doses should be decreased by this percentage; however, rate of drug metabolism varies greatly from person to person, and individual dose adjustment is required.

Hepatic clearance of drugs metabolized by phase I reactions (oxidation, reduction, and hydrolysis) is more likely to be prolonged in the elderly. Usually, age does not greatly affect clearance of drugs that are metabolized by conjugation (phase II reactions).

First-pass metabolism (metabolism, typically hepatic, that occurs before a drug reaches systemic circulation) is also affected by aging, decreasing by about 1% per year after age 40. Thus, for a given oral dose, the elderly may have higher circulating drug levels. Important examples of drugs with a high risk of toxic effects include nitrates, propranolol, phenobarbital, and nifedipine.

Renal Elimination

One of the most important pharmacokinetic changes associated with aging is decreased renal elimination of drugs (Table 25.7). After age 30, creatinine clearance decreases an average of 8 mL/min/1.73 m^2/decade; however, the age-related decrease varies substantially from person to person. Serum creatinine levels often

Table 25.7	Effect of aging on metabolism* and elimination of some drugs	
Class or category	**Decreased hepatic metabolism**	**Decreased renal elimination**
Analgesics and anti-inflammatory drugs	Ibuprofen	Meperidine
	Meperidine	Morphine
	Morphine	Oxycodone
	Naproxen	
Antibiotics	—	Amikacin
		Ciprofloxacin
		Gentamicin
		Levofloxacin
		Nitrofurantoin
		Streptomycin
		Tobramycin
Cardiovascular drugs	Amlodipine	N-acetylprocainamide
	Diltiazem	Apixaban
	Lidocaine[†]	Captopril
	Nifedipine	Dabigatran
	Propranolol	Digoxin
	Quinidine	Enalapril
	Theophylline	Enoxaparin
	Verapamil	Heparin
	Warfarin	Lisinopril
		Procainamide
		Quinapril
		Rivaroxaban
Diuretics	—	Amiloride
		Furosemide
		Hydrochlorothiazide
		Triamterene
Psychoactive drugs	Alprazolam[†]	Risperidone
	Chlordiazepoxide	
	Desipramine[†]	
	Diazepam	
	Imipramine	
	Nortriptyline	
	Trazodone	
	Triazolam[†]	
Others	Levodopa	Amantadine
		Chlorpropamide
		Cimetidine
		Exenatide
		Gabapentin
		Glyburide
		Lithium
		Metoclopramide
		Ranitidine
		Sitagliptin

*When aging's effect on hepatic metabolism of a drug is controversial, effects reported in the majority of studies are listed.
[†]The effect occurs in men but not in women.

remain within normal limits despite a decrease in glomerular filtration rate (GFR) because the elderly generally have less muscle mass and are generally less physically active than younger adults and thus produce less creatinine. Maintenance of normal serum creatinine levels can mislead clinicians who assume those levels reflect normal kidney function. Decreases in tubular function with age parallel those in glomerular function.

These changes decrease renal elimination of many drugs; clinical implications depend on the extent that renal elimination contributes to total systemic elimination and on the drug's therapeutic index (ratio of maximum tolerated dose to minimum effective dose). Creatinine clearance is used to guide drug dosing. The daily dose of drugs that rely heavily on renal elimination should be lower and/or the frequency of dosing should be decreased. Because renal function is dynamic, maintenance doses of drugs may need adjustment when patients become ill or dehydrated or have recently recovered from dehydration.

PHARMACODYNAMICS IN THE ELDERLY

Pharmacodynamics is defined as what the drug does to the body or the response of the body to the drug; it is affected by receptor binding, postreceptor effects, and chemical interactions. In the elderly, the effects of similar drug concentrations at the site of action (sensitivity) may be greater or smaller than those in younger people (Table 25.8). Differences may be due to changes in drug-receptor interaction, in postreceptor events, or in adaptive homeostatic responses and, among frail patients, are often due to pathologic changes in organs.

Table 25.8 Effect of aging on drug response

Class	Drug	Action	Effect of aging
Analgesics	Morphine	Acute analgesic effect	↑
	Pentazocine	Analgesic effect	↑
Anticoagulants	Heparin	PTT	↔
	Warfarin	PT/INR	↑
Bronchodilators	Albuterol	Bronchodilation	↓
	Ipratropium	Bronchodilation	↔
Cardiovascular drugs	Angiotensin II receptor blockers	Decreased BP	↑
	Diltiazem	Acute antihypertensive effect	↑
	Dopamine	Increased creatinine clearance	↓
	Enalapril	Acute antihypertensive effect	↑
	Felodipine	Antihypertensive effect	↑
	Isoproterenol	Increased heart rate	↓
		Increased ejection fraction	↓
		Venodilation	↓
	Nitroglycerin	Venodilation	↔
	Norepinephrine	Acute vasoconstriction	↔
	Phenylephrine	Acute venoconstriction	↔
		Acute hypertensive effect	↔
	Prazosin	Acute antihypertensive effect	↔
	Propranolol (and other β-blockers)	Decreased heart rate	↓
	Verapamil	Acute antihypertensive effect, cardiac conduction effects	↑
Diuretics	Bumetanide	Increased urine flow and Na excretion	↓
	Furosemide	Latency and size of peak diuretic response	↓
Oral hypoglycemics	Glyburide	Chronic hypoglycemic effect	↔
	Tolbutamide	Acute hypoglycemic effect	↓
Psychoactive drugs	Diazepam	Sedation	↑
	Diphenhydramine	Psychomotor dysfunction	↑
	Haloperidol	Acute sedation	↑
	Midazolam	EEG activity	↑
		Sedation	↑
	Temazepam	Postural sway	↑
		Psychomotor effect	↑
		Sedation	↑
	Thiopental	Anesthesia	↔
	Triazolam	Sedation	↑
Others	Atropine	Impaired gastric emptying	↔
	Levodopa	Adverse effects	↑
	Metoclopramide	Sedation	↔

↔ = unchanged; ↑ = increased; ↓ = decreased.

DRUG-RELATED PROBLEMS IN THE ELDERLY

Elderly patients are particularly sensitive to anticholinergic drug effects. Many drugs (e.g. tricyclic antidepressants, sedating antihistamines, urinary antimuscarinic agents, some antipsychotic drugs, anti-Parkinsonian drugs with atropine-like activity, many OTC hypnotics and cold preparations) have anticholinergic effects. The elderly, most notably those with cognitive impairment, are particularly prone to CNS adverse effects of such drugs and may become more confused and drowsy. Anticholinergic drugs also commonly cause constipation, urinary retention (especially in elderly men with benign prostatic hyperplasia), blurred vision, orthostatic hypotension, and dry mouth. Even in low doses, these drugs can increase risk of heatstroke by inhibiting diaphoresis. In general, older adults should avoid drugs with anticholinergic effects when possible.

Drug-related problems are common in the elderly and include drug ineffectiveness, adverse drug effects, overdosage, under dosage, and drug interactions. Drugs may be ineffective in the elderly because clinicians under prescribe (e.g. because of increased concern about adverse effects) or because adherence is poor (e.g. because of financial or cognitive limitations).

Adverse drug effects are effects that are unwanted, uncomfortable, or dangerous. Common examples are oversedation, confusion, hallucinations, falls, and bleeding. Among ambulatory people ≥65, adverse drug effects occur at a rate of about 50 events per 1000 person-years. Hospitalization rates due to adverse drug effects are 4 times higher in elderly patients (about 17%) than in younger patients (4%).

REASONS FOR DRUG-RELATED PROBLEMS

Adverse drug effects can occur in any patient, but certain characteristics of the elderly make them more susceptible. For example, the elderly often take many drugs (polypharmacy) and have age-related changes in pharmacodynamics and pharmacokinetics; both increase the risk of adverse effects. At any age, adverse drug effects may occur when drugs are prescribed and taken appropriately, e.g. new-onset allergic reactions are not predictable or preventable. However, adverse effects are thought to be preventable in almost 90% of cases in the elderly (compared with only 24% in younger patients). Certain drug classes are commonly involved antipsychotics, warfarin, antiplatelet agents, hypoglycemic drugs, antidepressants, and sedative-hypnotics.

In the elderly, a number of common reasons for adverse drug effects, ineffectiveness, or both are preventable (Table 25.9). Several of these reasons involve inadequate communication with patients or between health care practitioners (particularly during health care transitions).

DRUG-DISEASE INTERACTIONS

A drug given to treat one disease can exacerbate another disease regardless of patient age, but such interactions are of special concern in the elderly. Distinguishing often subtle adverse drug effects from the effects of disease is difficult (Table 25.10) and may lead to a prescribing cascade.

A **prescribing cascade** occurs when the adverse effect of a drug is misinterpreted as a symptom or sign of a new disorder and a new drug is prescribed to treat it. The new, unnecessary drug may cause additional adverse effects, which may then be misinterpreted as yet another disorder and treated unnecessarily, and so on. Many drugs have adverse effects that resemble symptoms of disorders common among the elderly or changes due to aging. Anti-**psychotics** may cause symptoms that resemble Parkinson disease. In elderly patients, these symptoms may be diagnosed as Parkinson disease and treated, possibly leading to adverse effects from the anti-Parkinson drugs (e.g. orthostatic hypotension, delirium, and nausea). Cholinesterase **inhibitors** (e.g. donepezil) may be

Table 25.9	Preventable causes of drug-related problems
Category	**Definition**
Drug interactions	Use of a drug results in a drug-drug, drug-food, drug-supplement, or drug-disease interaction, leading to adverse effects or decreased efficacy.
Inadequate monitoring	A medical problem is being treated with the correct drug, but the patient is not adequately monitored for complications, effectiveness, or both.
Inappropriate drug selection	A medical problem that requires drug therapy is being treated with a less-than-optimal drug.
Inappropriate treatment	A patient is taking a drug for no medically valid reason.
Lack of patient adherence	The correct drug for a medical problem is prescribed, but the patient is not taking it.
Overdosage	A medical problem is being treated with too much of the correct drug.
Poor communication	Drugs are inappropriately continued or stopped when care is transitioned between providers and/or facilities.
Underprescribing	A medical problem is being treated with too little of the correct drug.
Untreated medical problem	A medical problem requires drug therapy, but no drug is being used to treat that problem.

Table 25.10	Drug-disease interactions in the elderly (based on the American Geriatrics Society 2012 beers criteria update)	
Disease	**Drugs**	**Possible adverse effects**
Cardiovascular		
Heart failure	Cilostazol, COX-2 inhibitors, dronedarone, nondihydropyridine Ca channel blockers* (diltiazem, verapamil), NSAIDs, pioglitazone, rosiglitazone	May promote fluid retention and exacerbate heart failure
Syncope	Acetylcholinesterase inhibitors, chlorpromazine, peripheral α-blockers (doxazosin, prazosin, and terazosin), tertiary TCAs, thioridazine, olanzapine	Increased risk of orthostatic hypotension or bradycardia
CNS		
Chronic seizures or epilepsy	Bupropion, chlorpromazine, clozapine, maprotiline, olanzapine, thioridazine, thiothixene, tramadol	Lowered seizure threshold. Possibly acceptable in patients with well-controlled seizures in whom alternative agents have not been effective
Delirium	All TCAs, benzodiazepines, drugs that have anticholinergic effects, chlorpromazine, corticosteroids, H_2 receptor blockers, meperidine, sedative hypnotics, thioridazine	Worsened delirium in older adults with or at high risk of delirium. If discontinuing drugs used chronically, taper to avoid withdrawal symptoms
Dementia and cognitive impairment	Anti-psychotics (chronic and as-needed use), benzodiazepines, drugs that have anticholinergic effects, H_2 receptor blockers, zolpidem	Adverse CNS effects. For antipsychotics, increased risk of stroke and mortality in patients with dementia
History of falls or fractures	Anticonvulsants, antipsychotics, benzodiazepines, nonbenzodiazepine hypnotics (eszopiclone, zaleplon, zolpidem). TCAs, SSRIs	Ataxia, impaired psychomotor function, syncope, and additional falls; shorter-acting benzodiazepines are not safer than long-acting ones. Can be used if safer alternatives are not available. Avoid anticonvulsants except for seizure disorders
Insomnia	Oral decongestants (pseudoephedrine, phenylephrine), stimulants (amphetamine, methylphenidate, pemoline), theobromines (theophylline, caffeine)	CNS stimulant effects
Parkinson disease	Antiemetics (metoclopramide, prochlorperazine, promethazine), antipsychotics (except for quetiapine and clozapine)	Dopamine receptor antagonists with potential to worsen Parkinsonian symptoms (less likely with quetiapine and clozapine)
GI		
Chronic constipation	Drugs that have antispasmodic and anti-cholinergic effects [antipsychotics, belladonna alkaloids, clidinium-chlordiazepoxide, dicyclomine, hyoscyamine, propantheline, scopolamine, tertiary TCAs (amitriptyline, clomipramine, doxepin, imipramine, and trimipramine)], first-generation antihistamines (brompheniramine carbinoxamine, chlorpheniramine, clemastine, cyproheptadine, dexbrompheniramine, dexchlorpheniramine, diphenhydramine, doxylamine, hydroxyzine, promethazine, triprolidine), nondihydropyridine Ca channel blockers (diltiazem, verapamil), oral antimuscarinics for urinary incontinence (darifenacin, fesoterodine, oxybutynin, solifenacin, tolterodine, and trospium)	Can worsen constipation; agents for urinary incontinence: antimuscarinics overall differ in incidence of constipation; response variable; consider alternative agent if constipation develops
History of gastric or duodenal ulcers	Aspirin (>325 mg/day), non-COX-2 selective NSAIDs	Exacerbate existing ulcers or cause new ulcers. Avoid unless other alternatives are not effective and patients can take a gastroprotective drug (e.g. a proton pump inhibitor or misoprostol)
Kidney and Urinary Tract		
Chronic kidney disease (stages IV and V)	NSAIDs, triamterene	Increased risk of kidney injury

Contd.

Table 25.10	Drug-disease interactions in the elderly (based on the American geriatrics society 2012 beers criteria update)	
Disease	**Drugs**	**Possible adverse effects**
Urinary incontinence (all types) in women	Estrogen, oral and transdermal (excludes intravaginal estrogen)	Worsened incontinence
Lower urinary tract symptoms, benign prostatic hyperplasia	Drugs that have strong anticholinergic effects (except antimuscarinics for urinary incontinence), inhaled agents that have anticholinergic effects	May decrease urinary flow and cause urinary retention in men
Stress or mixed urinary incontinence	α-blockers (doxazosin, prazosin, and terazosin)	Worsened incontinence in women

*Avoid only in patients who have systolic heart failure; COX-2, cyclooxygenase-2; TCAs, tricyclic antidepressants.

prescribed for patients with dementia. These drugs may cause diarrhea or urinary incontinence. Patients may then be prescribed an anticholinergic drug (e.g. oxybutynin) to treat the new symptoms. Thus, an unnecessary drug is added, increasing the risk of adverse drug effects and drug-drug interactions. A better strategy is to reduce the dose of the cholinesterase inhibitor or consider a different treatment for dementia (e.g. memantine) with a different mechanism of action. In elderly patients, prescribers should always consider the possibility that a new symptom or sign is due to drug therapy.

DRUG CATEGORIES OF CONCERN IN THE ELDERLY

Some drug categories (e.g. analgesics, anticoagulants, antihypertensives, Anti-Parkinsonian drugs, diuretics, hypoglycemic drugs, psychoactive drugs) pose special risks for elderly patients. Some drugs, although reasonable for use in younger adults, are so risky they should be considered inappropriate for the elderly. The Beers Criteria are most commonly used to identify such inappropriate drugs (Table 25.11). The 2012 American Geriatrics Society updates to the Beers criteria further categorize potentially inappropriate drugs into 3 groups; (1) inappropriate—always to be avoided, (2) potentially inappropriate—to be avoided in certain diseases or syndromes, (3) to be used with caution—benefit may offset risk in some patients (Table 25.12).

Analgesics

Nonsteroidal anti-inflammatory drugs (NSAIDs) are used by >30% of people aged 65–89, and half of all NSAID prescriptions are for people >60. Several NSAIDs are available without prescription.

Table 25.11	Potentially inappropriate drugs in the elderly (based on the American Geriatrics Society 2012 beers criteria update)
Drug	**Prescribing concern/recommendations**
Anticholinergics*	
First-generation antihistamines, as single agents or in combination products [brompheniramine, carbinoxamine, chlorpheniramine, clemastine, cyproheptadine, dexbrompheniramine,dexchlorpheniramine, diphenhydramine (oral), doxylamine, hydroxyzine, promethazine, and triprolidine]	Highly anticholinergic; greater risk of confusion, dry mouth, constipation, and other anticholinergic effects and toxicity Clearance reduced with advanced age; tolerance develops when used as hypnotics Avoid, except use of diphenhydramine in special situations (e.g. severe allergic reaction) may be appropriate
Antiparkinson drugs [benztropine (oral), trihexyphenidyl]	Not recommended for prevention of extrapyramidal symptoms with antipsychotics; more effective agents available for treatment of Parkinson disease
Antispasmodics (belladonna alkaloids, clidinium-chlordiazepoxide, dicyclomine, hyoscyamine, propantheline, and scopolamine)	Highly anticholinergic, uncertain effectiveness Avoid except short-term use in palliative care to decrease oral secretions
Antiinfectives	
Nitrofurantoin	May cause pulmonary toxicity; safer alternatives available; lack of efficacy in patients with creatinine clearance <60 mL/min due to inadequate drug concentration in the urine; do not use for long-term suppression or in patients with creatinine clearance <60 mL/min
Antithrombotics	
Dipyridamole, oral short-acting† (does not apply to extended-release combination with aspirin)	Possible orthostatic hypotension; more effective alternatives available; avoid, except IV form acceptable for cardiac stress testing
Ticlopidine†	Safer effective alternatives available; avoid

Contd.

Table 25.11 Potentially inappropriate drugs in the elderly (based on the American Geriatrics Society 2012 beers criteria update)

Drug	Prescribing concern/recommendations
Cardiovascular drugs	
Alpha-1 blockers (doxazosin, prazosin, and terazosin)	High risk of orthostatic hypotension; alternative drugs have better risk/benefit ratio; avoid use as an antihypertensive
Alpha agonists, central [clonidine, guanabenz[†], guanfacine[†], methyldopa[†], reserpine (>0.1 mg/day)[†]]	High risk of adverse CNS effects; may cause bradycardia and orthostatic hypotension; avoid clonidine as first-line hypertensive; others not recommended
Antiarrhythmic drugs, classes Ia, Ic, and III (amiodarone, dofetilide, dronedarone, flecainide, ibutilide, procainamide, propafenone, quinidine, and sotalol)	Rate control preferred over rhythm control; avoid as first-line treatment for atrial fibrillation For amiodarone, increased risk of thyroid disease, pulmonary disorders, and QT interval prolongation
Disopyramide[†]	Potent negative inotrope (may induce heart failure); strongly anticholinergic; avoid, other antiarrhythmic drugs preferred
Dronedarone	Worse outcomes in patients who have permanent atrial fibrillation or heart failure; avoid Rate control preferred over rhythm control for atrial fibrillation
Digoxin (> 0.125 mg/day)	In patients with heart failure and/or low creatinine clearance, higher dosages associated with no additional benefit and increased risk of toxicity; avoid
Nifedipine, immediate release[†]	Risk of hypotension and myocardial ischemia; avoid
Spironolactone (> 25 mg/day)	In patients with heart failure, risk of hyperkalemia especially if also taking an NSAID, ACE inhibitor, angiotensin receptor blocker, or K supplement; avoid in heart failure or if creatinine clearance < 30 mL/min
CNS	
Tertiary TCAs, alone or in combination [amitriptyline, chlordiazepoxide-amitriptyline, clomipramine, doxepin (>6 mg/day), imipramine, perphenazine-amitriptyline, trimipramine]	Highly anticholinergic and sedating and cause orthostatic hypotension; avoid
Antipsychotics, first (conventional) and second (atypical) generations	Increased risk of stroke and mortality in patients with dementia Avoid in patients with dementia-related behavior problems unless nonpharmacologic options have failed and patients are a threat to themselves or others
Thioridazine	Highly anticholinergic; risk of QT interval prolongation; avoid
Mesoridazine	
Barbiturates (amobarbital[†], butabarbital[†], butalbital, mephobarbital[†], pentobarbital[†], phenobarbital, secobarbital[†])	High rate of physical dependence and tolerance; risk of overdose at low dosages; avoid
Benzodiazepines, short- and intermediate-acting (alprazolam, estazolam, lorazepam, oxazepam, temazepam, triazolam)	Increased risk of cognitive impairment, delirium, falls, fractures, and motor vehicle crashes
Benzodiazepines, long-acting (clorazepate, chlordiazepoxide, chlordiazepoxide-amitriptyline, clidinium-chlordiazepoxide, clonazepam, diazepam, flurazepam, and quazepam)	May be appropriate for seizure disorders, rapid eye movement sleep disorders, benzodiazepine withdrawal, ethanol withdrawal, severe generalized anxiety disorder, periprocedural anesthesia, end-of-life care Avoid use for insomnia, agitation, or delirium
Chloral hydrate[†]	Can overdose at only 3 times recommended dose; tolerance occurs within 10 days; risks outweigh benefits; avoid
Meprobamate	High rate of physical dependence; very sedating; avoid
Nonbenzodiazepine hypnotics (eszopiclone, zolpidem, and zaleplon)	Similar to benzodiazepines (e.g. delirium, falls, and fractures); minimal improvement in sleep latency and duration Not to be used for >90 days
Ergot mesylates[†] Isoxsuprine[†]	Lack of efficacy; avoid
Endocrine therapy	
Androgens (methyltestosterone[†], testosterone)	Potential for cardiac problems; exacerbation of prostate cancer Avoid except for moderate to severe hypogonadism
Desiccated thyroid	Possible cardiac effects; safer alternatives available; avoid

Contd.

Table 25.11	Potentially inappropriate drugs in the elderly (based on the American Geriatrics Society 2012 beers criteria update)
Drug	**Prescribing concern/recommendations**
Estrogens with or without progestins	Possible carcinogenic potential (breast and endometrium); lack of cardioprotective effect and cognitive protection in older women
	Topical vaginal cream low dose can be used for dyspareunia, lower UTIs, and other vaginal symptoms; evidence that low doses (estradiol <25 mcg twice/week) may be safe in women with breast cancer
	Avoid topical patch and oral
Growth hormone	Little effect on body composition; associated with edema, arthralgia, carpal tunnel syndrome, gynecomastia, impaired fasting glucose
	Avoid except for hormone replacement after pituitary gland removal
Insulin, sliding scale	Higher risk of hypoglycemia without improvement in glucose control regardless of care setting; avoid
Megestrol	Minimal effect on weight; increases risk of thrombotic events and possibly death; avoid
Sulfonylureas, long duration (chlorpropamide, glyburide)	Chlorpropamide: Prolonged half-life; can cause prolonged hypoglycemia, syndrome of inappropriate antidiuretic hormone secretion; avoid
	Glyburide: Greater risk of severe prolonged hypoglycemia; avoid
GI therapy	
Metoclopramide	Can cause extrapyramidal effects including tardive dyskinesia; risk may be greater in frail older adults; avoid except for gastroparesis
Mineral oil, oral	Potential for aspiration; safer alternatives available; avoid
Trimethobenzamide	One of the least effective antiemetics; can cause extrapyramidal effects; avoid
Pain management	
Meperidine	Not an effective oral analgesic in common dosages; may cause neurotoxicity; safer alternatives available; avoid
Non-COX-selective NSAIDs, oral [aspirin (>325 mg/day), diclofenac, diflunisal, etodolac, fenoprofen, ibuprofen, ketoprofen, meclofenamate, mefenamic acid, meloxicam, nabumetone, naproxen, oxaprozin, piroxicam, sulindac, and tolmetin]	Increased risk of GI bleeding and peptic ulcer disease in high-risk groups, including those aged >75 or taking oral or parenteral corticosteroids, anticoagulants, or antiplatelet agents
	Upper GI ulcers, gross bleeding, or perforation occur in about 1% of patients treated for 3–6 months and in about 2–4% of patients treated for 1 years; these trends continue with longer duration of use
	Avoid chronic use unless other alternatives are ineffective and patients are able to take a proton pump inhibitor or misoprostol (which reduce but do not eliminate risk)
Indomethacin	Increases risk of GI bleeding and peptic ulcer disease in high-risk groups (see above non-COX selective NSAIDs)
Ketorolac, includes parenteral	Of all the NSAIDs, indomethacin has most adverse effects; avoid
Pentazocine[†]	CNS adverse effects, including confusion and hallucinations, more common than with other opioids; is also a mixed agonist and antagonist; safer alternatives available; avoid
Skeletal muscle relaxants (carisoprodol, chlorzoxazone, cyclobenzaprine, metaxalone, methocarbamol, and orphenadrine)	Poorly tolerated because of anticholinergic effects; sedation; risk of fracture; effectiveness at dosages tolerated by older adults is questionable; avoid

*TCAs are excluded.

[†]These drugs are used infrequently.

TCAs, tricyclic antidepressants.

Adapted from The American Geriatrics Society 2012 Beers Criteria Update Expert Panel: American Geriatrics Society updated Beers criteria for potentially inappropriate medication use in older adults. Journal of the American Geriatrics Society. 2012; 60: 616–31.

Table 25.12	Drugs to be used with caution in the elderly (based on the American geriatrics society 2012 beers criteria update)
Drug	**Reason for caution**
Aspirin for primary prevention of cardiac events	Use with caution in patients ≥80 years.
	Lack of evidence regarding benefit vs risk in patients >80 years
Dabigatran	Use with caution in patients ≥75 years or with creatinine clearance <30 mL/min. Greater risk of bleeding than warfarin in patients ≥75 years.
	Lack of evidence regarding efficacy and safety in patients with creatinine clearance <30 mL/min
Prasugrel	Use with caution in patients ≥75 years. Increased risk of bleeding; benefit may offset risk in highest-risk elderly (e.g. those with previous MI or diabetes mellitus)
Antipsychotics	May worsen or cause syndrome of inappropriate antidiuretic hormone secretion or hyponatremia
Carbamazepine	Monitor Na level closely when starting or changing dosages
Carboplatin	
Cisplatin	
Mirtazapine	
Serotonin–norepinephrine reuptake inhibitors	
SSRIs	
Tricyclic antidepressants	
Vincristine	
Vasodilators	May increase episodes of syncope in patients with history of syncope

Adapted from the American Geriatrics Society 2012 Beers Criteria Update Expert Panel: American Geriatrics Society updated Beers criteria for potentially inappropriate medication use in older adults. Journal of the American Geriatrics Society. 2012; 60: 616–31.

The elderly may be prone to adverse effects of these drugs, and adverse effects may be more severe because of (1) NSAIDs are highly lipid-soluble, and because adipose tissue increases with age, distribution of the drugs is extensive, (2) plasma protein is often decreased, resulting in higher levels of unbound drug and exaggerated pharmacologic effects, and (3) renal function is reduced in many of the elderly, resulting in decreased renal clearance and higher drug levels.

Serious adverse effects include peptic ulceration and upper GI bleeding; risk is increased when an NSAID is begun and when dose is increased. Risk of upper GI bleeding increases when NSAIDs are given with warfarin, aspirin, or other antiplatelet drugs (e.g. clopidogrel). NSAIDs may increase risk of cardiovascular events and can cause fluid retention and, rarely, nephropathy.

NSAIDs can also increase BP; this effect may be unrecognized and lead to intensification of anti-hypertensive treatment (a prescribing cascade; see drug-disease interactions). Thus, clinicians should keep this effect in mind when BP increases in elderly patients and ask them about their use of NSAIDs, particularly OTC NSAIDs.

Selective COX-2 (cyclooxygenase-2) inhibitors (coxibs) cause less GI irritation and platelet inhibition than other NSAIDs. Nonetheless, coxibs still have a risk of GI bleeding, especially for patients taking warfarin or aspirin (even at a low dose) and for those who have had GI events. Coxibs, as a class, appear to increase risk of cardiovascular events, but risk may vary by drug; they should be used cautiously. Coxibs have renal effects comparable to those of other NSAIDs.

Lower-risk alternatives (e.g. acetaminophen) should be used when possible. If NSAIDs are used in the elderly, the lowest effective dose should be used, and continued need should be reviewed frequently. If NSAIDs are used long-term, serum creatinine and BP should be monitored closely, especially in patients with other risk factors (e.g. heart failure, renal impairment, cirrhosis with ascites, volume depletion, and diuretic use).

ANTICOAGULANTS

Age may increase sensitivity to the anticoagulant effect of warfarin. Careful dosing and routine monitoring can largely overcome the increased risk of bleeding in elderly patients taking warfarin. Also, because drug interactions with warfarin are common, closer monitoring is necessary when new drugs are added or old ones are stopped; computerized drug interaction programs should be consulted if patients take multiple drugs. Patients should also be monitored for warfarin interactions with food, alcohol, and OTC drugs and supplements. The newer anticoagulants (dabigatran, rivaroxaban, apixaban) may be easier to dose and have fewer drug-drug interactions and food-drug interactions than warfarin, but still increase the risk of bleeding in elderly patients, particularly those with impaired renal function.

Antidepressants

Tricyclic antidepressants are effective, but should rarely be used in the elderly. Selective serotonin reuptake inhibitors (SSRIs) and mixed reuptake inhibitors, such as serotonin-norepinephrine reuptake inhibitors (SNRIs), are as effective as tricyclic antidepressants and cause less toxicity; however, there are some concerns about some of these drugs; (1) paroxetine—this drug is more sedating than other SSRIs, has anticholinergic effects, and, like some other SSRIs, can inhibit hepatic cytochrome P-450 2D6 enzyme activity, possibly impairing the metabolism of several drugs, including tamoxifen, some antipsychotics, antiarrhythmics, and tricyclic antidepressants, (2) citalopram—doses in the elderly should be limited to a maximum of 20 mg/day because QT prolongation is a concern, (3) venlafaxine—this drug may increase BP, and (4) mirtazapine—this drug can be sedating and may stimulate appetite/weight gain.

Antihyperglycemics

Doses of antihyperglycemics should be titrated carefully in patients with diabetes mellitus. Risk of hypoglycemia due to sulfonylureas may increase with age (Table 25.11), chlorpropamide is not recommended in elderly patients because of the increased risk of hypoglycemia and of hyponatremia due to the syndrome of inappropriate antidiuretic hormone secretion (SIADH). Risk of hypoglycemia is also greater with glyburide than with other oral antihyperglycemics because its renal clearance is reduced in the elderly.

Metformin, a biguanide excreted by the kidneys, increases peripheral tissue sensitivity to insulin and can be effective given alone or with sulfonylureas. Risk of lactic acidosis, a rare but serious complication, increases with degree of renal impairment and with patient age. Heart failure is a contraindication.

Antihypertensives

In many elderly patients, lower starting doses of antihypertensives may be necessary to reduce risk of adverse effects; however, for most elderly patients with hypertension, achieving BP goals requires standard doses and multidrug therapy. Initial treatment of hypertension in the elderly typically involves a thiazide-type diuretic, ACE inhibitor, angiotensin II receptor blocker, or dihydropyridine Ca channel blocker, depending on comorbidities. β-blockers should be reserved for second-line therapy. Short-acting dihydropyridines (e.g.

nifedipine) may increase mortality risk and should not be used. Sitting and standing BP can be monitored, particularly when multiple antihypertensives are used, to check for orthostatic hypotension, which may increase risk of falls and fractures.

Anti-Parkinsonian Drugs

Levodopa clearance is reduced in elderly patients, who are also more susceptible to the drug's adverse effects, particularly orthostatic hypotension and confusion. Therefore, elderly patients should be given a lower starting dose of levodopa and carefully monitored for adverse effects (Parkinson disease—levodopa). Patients who become confused while taking levodopa may also not tolerate dopamine agonists (e.g. pramipexole, ropinirole). Because elderly patients with Parkinsonism may be cognitively impaired, drugs with anticholinergic effects should be avoided.

Antipsychotics

Antipsychotics should be used only for psychosis. In nonpsychotic, agitated patients, antipsychotics control symptoms only marginally better than placebo and can have severe adverse effects. In people with dementia, studies showed antipsychotics increased mortality and risk of stroke, leading the food and drug association (FDA) to issue a black box warning on their use in such patients. Generally, dementia-related behavior problems (e.g. wandering, yelling, uncooperativeness) do not respond to antipsychotics.

When an antipsychotic is used, the starting dose should be about one quarter the usual starting adult dose and should be increased gradually with frequent monitoring for response and adverse effects. Once the patient responds, the dose should be titrated down, if possible, to the lowest effective dose. The drug needs to be stopped if it is ineffective. Clinical trial data relating to dosing, efficacy, and safety of these drugs in the elderly are limited.

Antipsychotics can reduce paranoia, but may worsen confusion (schizophrenia—conventional antipsychotics). Elderly patients, especially women, are at increased risk of tardive dyskinesia, which is often irreversible. Sedation, orthostatic hypotension, anticholinergic effects, and akathisia (subjective motor restlessness) can occur in up to 20% of elderly patients taking an antipsychotic, and drug-induced Parkinsonism can persist for up to 6–9 month after the drug is stopped.

Extrapyramidal dysfunction can develop even when second-generation antipsychotics (e.g. olanzapine, quetiapine, and risperidone) are used, especially at higher doses. Risks and benefits of using an antipsychotic should be discussed with the patient or the person responsible for the patient's care. Antipsychotics should be considered for behavior problems only when nonpharmacologic options have failed and patients are a threat to themselves or others.

ANXIOLYTICS AND HYPNOTICS

Treatable causes of insomnia should be sought and managed before using hypnotics. Nonpharmacologic measures, such as cognitive-behavioral therapy, and sleep hygiene (e.g. avoiding caffeinated beverages, limiting daytime napping, modifying bedtime) should be tried first. If they are ineffective, nonbenzodiazepine hypnotics (e.g. zolpidem, eszopiclone, and zaleplon) are options for short-term use. These drugs bind mainly to a benzodiazepine receptor subtype and disturb the sleep pattern less than benzodiazepines. They have a more rapid onset, fewer rebound effects, fewer next-day effects, and less potential for dependence. As described in Table 25.11, short-, intermediate, and long-acting benzodiazepines are associated with increased risk of cognitive impairment, delirium, falls, fractures, and motor vehicle crashes in the elderly and should be avoided for the treatment of insomnia. Benzodiazepines may be appropriate for treatment of anxiety or panic attacks in the elderly. Duration of anxiolytic or hypnotic therapy should be limited if possible because tolerance and dependence may develop; withdrawal may lead to rebound anxiety or insomnia.

Antihistamines (e.g. diphenhydramine, hydroxyzine) are not recommended as anxiolytics or hypnotics because they have anticholinergic effects, and tolerance to the sedative effects develops quickly. Buspirone, a partial serotonin agonist, can be effective for general anxiety disorder; elderly patients tolerate doses up to 30 mg/day well. The slow onset of anxiolytic action (up to 2–3 weeks) can be a disadvantage in urgent cases.

Digoxin

Digoxin, a cardiac glycoside, is used to increase the force of myocardial contractions and to treat supraventricular arrhythmias. However, it must be used with caution in elderly patients. In men with heart failure and a left ventricular ejection fraction of ≤45%, serum digoxin levels >0.8 ng/mL are associated with increased mortality risk. Adverse effects are typically related to its narrow therapeutic index. One study found digoxin to be beneficial in women when serum levels were 0.5–0.9 ng/mL but possibly harmful when levels were ≥1.2 ng/mL. A number of factors increase the likelihood of digoxin toxicity in the elderly. Renal impairment, temporary dehydration, and NSAID use (all common among the

elderly) can reduce renal clearance of digoxin. Furthermore, digoxin clearance decreases an average of 50% in elderly patients with normal serum creatinine levels. Also, if lean body mass is reduced, as may occur with aging, volume of distribution for digoxin is reduced. Therefore, starting doses should be low (0.125 mg/day) and adjusted according to response and serum digoxin levels (normal range 0.8–2.0 ng/mL). However, serum digoxin level does not always correlate with likelihood of toxicity.

Diuretics

Lower doses of thiazide diuretics (e.g. hydrochlorothiazide or chlorthalidone 12.5–25 mg) can effectively control hypertension in many elderly patients and have less risk of hypokalemia and hyperglycemia than other diuretics (see also drugs for hypertension—diuretics). Thus, K supplements may be required less often. K-sparing diuretics should be used with caution in the elderly; the K level must be carefully monitored, particularly when these diuretics are given with ACE inhibitors or angiotensin II receptor blockers or when the patient has impaired kidney function.

The Impact of Exercise and Nutrition on Chemistry Results in the Elderly

Research indicates that regular exercise can increase the lifespan and improve the quality of life among geriatric patients. Maintaining physical activity improves physical strength and fitness, as well as balance. Exercise helps prevent depression, and manage and defend against diseases such as diabetes, heart disease, breast and colon cancer, and osteoporosis. Physical activity also improves endurance, flexibility sleep, mood, and self-esteem. Increased physical activity may prevent more rapid deterioration. Fitness-related activities can reduce the risk of falling, and incorporation of exercise into lifestyle has been shown to be one of the best ways to improve bone mass throughout the life. There have also been data linking the positive effects of exercise and long-term maintenance of cognitive function. More importantly, lack of physical activity was shown to be a better predictor of all-cause mortality than being overweight or obese.

The successful management of aging requires proper nutrition in addition to regular exercise. It is reported that 10–40% of hospitalized older adults suffer from malnutrition, which can be defined as any disorder of nutrition status resulting from a deficiency of nutrient intake, impaired metabolism, or over nutrition. The difficulty recognizing the problem makes treatment a challenge. Some of the laboratory values that can indicate undernutrition are low albumin and low pre-albumin.

There are a number of issues with the identification of malnutrition in the elderly. Based on this, there is increasing interest in establishing nutritional assessment tools for identification of undernourished individuals.

Clearly, geriatric dietary intake is a concern in the area of undernourishment, but excessive calorie intake, resulting in obesity and increased prevalence of type 2 diabetes, is also a worry. Based on increasing incidence of diabetes with aging, and the previously discussed benefits of physical activity, increasing numbers of elderly people are being encouraged to become active. Clinicians and laboratorians will need a better understanding of how exercise is likely to impact test results of older individuals. This will require closer attention to baseline measurements and observations of changes over time.

BIBLIOGRAPHY

1. American College of Sports Medicine Position Stand. Exercise and physical activity for older adults. Med Sci Sports Exerc.1998; 30:992-1008.

2. Barron AM, Pike CJ. Sex hormones, aging, and Alzheimer's disease. Front Biosci (Elite Ed). 2012; 4:976-997.

3. Bauer JH. Age-related changes in the renin-aldosterone system. Physiological effects and clinical implications. Drugs Aging.1993; 3:238-245.

4. Baylis C, Schmidt R. The aging glomerulus. Semin Nephrol. 1996; 16: 265–276.

5. Bhutto A, Morley JE. The clinical significance of gastrointestinal changes with aging. Curr Opin Clin Nutr Metab Care. 2008; 11:651-660.

6. Bo-Linn GW, Davis GR, Buddrus DJ, et al. An evaluation of the importance of gastric acid secretion in the absorption of dietary calcium. J Clin Invest. 1984; 73: 640–647.

7. Breitling LP, Claessen H, Drath C, Arndt V, Brenner H. Gamma glutamyl transferase, general and cause-specific mortality in 19,000 construction workers followed over 20 years. J Hepatol. 2011; 55: 594–601.

8. Buell JS, Dawson-Hughes B, Scott TM, et al. 25-Hydroxyvitamin D, dementia, and cerebrovascular pathology in elders receiving home services. Neurology. 2010; 74: 18–26.

9. Burks TN, Cohn RD. One size may not fit all: anti-aging therapies and sarcopenia. Aging (Albany, NY). 2011; 3: 1142–1153.

10. Carlsson L, Lind L, Larsson A. Reference values for 27 clinical chemistry tests in 70-year-old males and females. Gerontology. 2010; 56: 259–265.

11. Castle SC. Clinical relevance of age-related immune dysfunction. Clin Infect Dis. 2000; 31: 578–585.

12. Cockcroft DW, Gault MH. Prediction of creatinine clearance from serum creatinine. Nephron. 1976; 16: 31–41.

13. Cole LA, Khanlian SA, Muller CY. Normal production of human chorionic gonadotropin in perimenopausal and menopausal women and after oophorectomy. Int J Gynecol Cancer. 2009; 19: 1556–1559.

14. Cole LA. HCG variants, the growth factors which drive human malignancies. Am J Cancer Res. 2012; 2: 22–35.

15. Cowie CC, Rust KF, Ford ES, et al. Full accounting of diabetes and pre-diabetes in the U.S. population in 1988-1994 and 2005–2006. Diabetes Care. 2008; 32: 287–294.

16. Dasgupta A. Clinical utility of free drug monitoring. ClinChem Lab Med. 2002; 40: 986–993.

17. Davis KM, Fish LC, Minaker KL, Elahi D. Atrial natriuretic peptide levels in the elderly: differentiating normal aging changes from disease. J Gerontol A BiolSci Med Sci 1996; 51: M95-101.

18. del Val JH. Old-age inflammatory bowel disease onset: a different problem? World J Gastro enterol. 2011; 17: 2734–2739.

19. Drachman DA. Occam's razor, geriatric syndromes, and the dizzy patient. Ann Intern Med. 2000; 132: 403–404.

20. Drion I, Joosten H, van Hateren KJ, et al. Employing age-related cut-off values results in fewer patients with renal impairment in secondary care. Ned TijdschrGeneeskd. 2011; 155:A3091.

21. Engelborghs S, De Vreese K, Van de Casteele T, et al. Diagnostic performance of a CSF-biomarker panel in autopsy-confirmed dementia. Neurobiol Aging. 2008; 29: 1143–1159.

22. Euans DW. Renal function in the elderly. Am Fam Physician.1988; 38: 147–150.

23. Evrin PE, Nilsson SE, Oberg T, Malmberg B. Serum C-reactive protein in elderly men and women: association with mortality, morbidity and various biochemical values. Scand J Clin Lab Invest.2005; 65:23-31.

24. Faulkner WR. Geriatric Clinical Chemistry Reference Values. Washington, DC: American Association for Clinical Chemistry; 1993.

25. Flood C, Gherondache C, Pincus G, et al. The metabolism and secretion of aldosterone in elderly subjects. J Clin Invest.1967; 46: 960–966.

26. Foster AD, Sivarapatna A, Gress RE. The aging immune system and its relationship with cancer. Aging Health. 2011; 7: 707–718.

27. Garcia A, Zanibbi K. Homocysteine and cognitive function in elderly people. CMAJ. 2004; 171: 897–904.

28. Garry PJ. Laboratory Medicine and the Aging Process. Joseph A.Knight. Chicago, IL: ASCP Press; 1996:420 pp., $45.00, ISBN0–89189-397–0. Clin Chem. 1997; 43: 2444–2444.

29. Gerber A. Navigating in evidence-poor waters—how much hydration is needed at the end of life? The recommendations of a Swiss expert group (Bigorio Group). TherUmsch. 2012; 69: 91–92.

30. Gill J, Malyuk R, Djurdjev O, Levin A. Use of GFR equations to adjust drug doses in an elderly multi-ethnic group—a cautionary tale. Nephrol Dial Transplant. 2007; 22: 2894–2899.

31. Glassock RJ, Winearls C. Ageing and the glomerular filtration rate: truths and consequences. Trans Am ClinClimatol Assoc.2009; 120: 419–428.

32. Glassock RJ. The GFR decline with aging: a sign of normal senescence, not disease. Nephrol Times. 2009; 2: 6–8.

33. Gourlay M, Franceschini N, Sheyn Y. Prevention and treatment strategies for glucocorticoid-induced osteoporotic fractures. ClinRheumatol. 2007; 26: 144–153.

34. Gray-Vickrey P. Gathering "pearls" of knowledge for assessing older adults. Nursing. 2010; 40: 34–42.

35. Hausman DB, Johnson MA, Davey A, et al. The oldest old: red blood cell and plasma folate in African American and white octogenarians and centenarians in Georgia. J Nutr Health Aging.2011; 15: 744–750.

36. Hermes GL, McClintock MK. Isolation and the timing of mammary gland development, gonadarche, and ovarian senescence: implications for mammary tumor burden. Dev Psychobiol. 2008; 50: 353–360.

37. Huber KR, Mostafaie N, Stangl G, et al. Clinical chemistry reference values for 75-year-old apparently healthy persons. ClinChem Lab Med. 2006; 44: 1355–1360.

38. Hughes SG. Prescribing for the elderly patient: why do we need to exercise caution? Br J ClinPharmacol. 1998; 46: 531–533.

39. Inouye SK, Studenski S, Tinetti ME, Kuchel GA. Geriatric syndromes: clinical, research, and policy implications of a core geriatric concept. J Am Geriatr Soc. 2007; 55: 730–791.

40. Isaac RM. Nutrition support makes more than sense/cents. J Can Diet Assoc. 1988; 49: 89–91.

41. Koda-Kimble MA, Young LY, Alldredge BK. Applied Therapeutics: The Clinical Use of Drugs. Philadelphia, PA: Lippincott Williams &Wilkins; 2004.

42. Kokotas H, Grigoriadou M, Petersen MB. Age-related macular degeneration: genetic and clinical findings. ClinChem Lab Med. 2011; 49: 601–616.

43. Kraemer G. Epilepsy in the Elderly: Clinical Aspects and Pharmacotherapy. Stuttgart, Germany: Thieme; 1999.

44. Kraft E. Cognitive function, physical activity, and aging: possible biological links and implications for multimodal interventions. Neuropsychol Dev Cogn B Aging Neuropsychol Cogn. 2012; 19: 248–263.

45. Kushner I. C-reactive protein elevation can be caused by conditions other than inflammation and may reflect biologic aging. Cleve Clin J Med. 2001; 68: 535–537.

46. Lapin A, Böhmer F. Laboratory findings in elderly patients: a forgotten aspect of laboratory medicine? Z Gerontol Geriatr. 1999; 32: 41–46.

47. Laughlin GA, Barrett-Connor E. Sexual dimorphism in the influenceof advanced aging on adrenal hormone levels: The RanchoBernardo Study. JCEM. 2000; 85: 3561–3568.

48. Lee J, Vasikaran S. Current recommendations for laboratory testing and use of bone turnover markers in management of osteoporosis. Ann Lab Med. 2012; 32: 105–112.

49. Levey AS, Bosch JP, Lewis JB, et al. A more accurate method to estimate glomerular filtration rate from serum creatinine: a new prediction equation. Modification of Diet in Renal Disease Study Group. Ann Intern Med. 1999; 130: 461–470.

50. Levey AS, Stevens LA, Schmid CH, et al. A new equation to estimate glomerular filtration rate. Ann Intern Med. 2009; 150: 604–612.

51. Llewellyn DJ, Langa KM, Friedland RP, Lang IA. Serum albumin concentration and cognitive impairment. Curr Alzheimer Res. 2010; 7: 91–96.

52. Lombardi G, Di Somma C, Vuolo L, et al. Role of IGF-I on PTH effects on bone. J Endocrinol Invest. 2010; 33: 22–26.

53. Lupien SJ, de Leon M, de Santi S, et al. Cortisol levels during human aging predicthippocampal atrophy and memory deficits. Nat Neurosci. 1998; 1: 69–73.

54. Makarewicz-Wujec M, Kozlowska-Wojciechowska M. Nutrient intake and serum level of gamma-glutamyl transferase, MCP-1and homocysteine in early stages of heart failure. Clin Nutr. 2011; 30: 73–78.

55. Marks BL, Katz LM, Smith JK. Exercise and the aging mind: buffing the baby boomer's body and brain. Phys Sportsmed. 2009; 37: 119–125.

56. Martin P, Midgley E. Immigration: shaping and reshaping America. Popul Bull. 2006; 61: 3–27.

57. Matthews SJ, Lancaster JW. Urinary tract infections in the elderly population. Am J GeriatrPharmacother. 2011; 9: 286–309.

58. Michael L. Bishop. Clinical Chemistry: Principles, Techniques, and Correlations, 7th edition. Philadelphia, Wolters Kluwer/Lippincott Williams & Wilkins, 2013.

59. Morley JE. Diabetes and aging: epidemiologic overview. ClinGeriatr Med. 2008; 24: 395–405.

60. Mulkerrin E, Epstein FH, Clark BA. Aldosterone responses to hyperkalemia in healthy elderly humans. J Am Soc Nephrol. 1995; 6: 1459–1462.

61. Nacif MS, Arai AA, Lima JA, Bluemke DA. Gadolinium enhanced cardiovascular magnetic resonance: administered dose in relationship to United States Food and Drug Administration(FDA) guidelines. J CardiovascMagnReson. 2012; 14:18.

62. Naughton C, Bennett K, Feely J. Prevalence of chronic disease in the elderly based on a national pharmacy claims database. Age Ageing. 2006; 35: 633–636.

63. Pamuk ON, Dönmez S, Cakir N. Increased frequencies of hysterectomy and early menopause in fibromyalgia patients: a comparative study. Clin Rheumatol. 2009; 28: 561–564.

64. Patricia M, Barnes MA, Barbara Bloom MPA, Nahin RL. National Health Statistics Reports. 2008.

65. Phillips K, Aliprantis A, Coblyn J. Strategies for the prevention and treatment of osteoporosis in patients with rheumatoid arthritis .Drugs Aging. 2006; 23: 773–779.

66. Racho D, Teede H. Ovarian function and obesity—interrelationship, impact on women's reproductive lifespan and treatment options. Mol Cell Endocrinol. 2010; 316: 172–179.

67. Reuben DB, Yoshikawa TT, Besdine RW, eds. Geriatric Review Syllabus. 3rd ed. Washington DC: American Geriatrics Society; 1996: 296–297.

68. Rose DJ, Hernandez D. The role of exercise in fall prevention forolder adults. ClinGeriatr Med. 2010; 26: 607–631.

69. Ruiz JG, Array S, Lowenthal DT. Therapeutic drug monitoring in the elderly. Am J Ther. 1996; 3: 839–860.

70. RutgerPersson G. Rheumatoid arthritis and periodontitis—inflammatory and infectious connections. Review of the literature. J Oral Microbiol. 2012; 4: 2066–2074.

71. Shaw ND, Srouji SS, Histed SN, Hall JE. Differential effects of aging on estrogen negative and positive feedback. Am J Physiol Endocrinol Metab. 2011; 301: E351–355.

72. Sherman SS, Hollis BW, Tobin JD. Vitamin D status and related parameters in a healthy population: the effects of age, sex, and season. J Clin Endocrinol Metab. 1990; 71: 405–413.

73. Sim V, Hampton D, Phillips C, et al. The use of brain natriuretic peptide as a screening test for left ventricular systolic dysfunction—cost-effectiveness in relation to open access echocardiography. Fam Pract. 2003; 20: 570–574.

74. Smolina K, Wright FL, Rayner M, Goldacre MJ. Determinants of the decline in mortality from acute myocardial infarction in England between 2002 and 2010: linked national database study. BMJ. 2012; 344:d8059.

75. Tan JC, Workeneh B, Busque S, et al. Glomerular function, structure, and number in renal allografts from older deceased donors. J Am SocNephrol. 2009; 20: 181–188.

76. Tanner GA. Kidney function. In: Rhoades RA, Bell DR, eds. Medical Physiology: Principles for Clinical Medicine. 4th ed. Philadelphia, PA: Lippincott Williams and Wilkins; 2012: 399–426.

77. Tietz NW, Shuey DF, Wekstein DR. Laboratory values in fit aging individuals—sex agenarians through centenarians. Clin Chem. 1992; 38: 1167–1185.

78. Tjia J, Field TS, Fischer SH, et al. Quality measurement of medication monitoring in the "meaningful use" era. Am J Manage Care. 2011; 17: 633–637.

79. Tsutsumi R, Tsutsumi YM, Horikawa YT, et al. Decline in anthropometric evaluation predicts a poor prognosis in geriatric patients. Asia Pac J ClinNutr. 2012; 21: 44–51.

80. Tuljapurkar SR, McGuire TR, Brusnahan SK, et al. Changes in human bone marrow fat content associated with changes in hematopoietic stem cell numbers and cytokine levels with aging. J Anat. 2011; 219: 574–581.

81. Ueda M, Araki T, Shiota T, Taketa K. Age and sex-dependent alterations of serum amylase and isoamylase levels in normal human adults. J Gastroenterol. 1994; 29: 189–191.

82. Uusi-Rasi K, Sievänen H, Pasanen M, Kannus P. Age-related decline in trabecular and cortical density: a 5-year peripheral quantitative computed tomography follow-up study of pre- and postmenopausal women. Calcif Tissue Int. 2007; 81: 249–253.

83. Van Dam RM, Li T, Spiegelman D, Franco OH, Hu FB. Combined impact of lifestyle factors on mortality: prospective cohort study in US women. BMJ. 2008; 337:a1440.

84. Vanasse GJ, Berliner N. Anemia in elderly patients: an emerging problem for the 21st century. Hematology Am SocHematolEduc Program. 2010; 2010: 271–275.

85. Villesen HH, Banning AM, Petersen RH, et al. Pharmacokinetics of morphine and oxycodone following intravenous administration in elderly patients. TherClin Risk Manage. 2007; 3: 961–967.

86. Vukmanovic-Stejic M, Rustin MHA, Nikolich-Zugich J, Akbar AN. Immune responses in the skin in old age. Curr Opin Immunol. 2011; 23: 525-531.

87. Weksler ME, Goodhardt M. Do age-associated changes in "physiologic" autoantibodies contribute to infection, atherosclerosis, and Alzheimer's disease? ExpGerontol. 2002; 37: 971–979.

88. Winzenberg T, van der Mei I, Mason RS, Nowson C, Jones G. Vitamin D and the musculoskeletal health of older adults. Aust Fam Physician. 2012; 41: 92–99.

89. Woon VC, Lim KH. Acute myocardial infarction in the elderly—the differences compared with the young. Singapore Med J. 2003; 44: 414–418.

90. World Health Organization. Assessment of fracture risk and its application to screening for postmenopausal osteoporosis. Report of a WHO Study Group. World Health Organ Tech Rep Ser. 1994; 843: 1–129.

91. Zussman J, Young L. Zoster vaccine live for the prevention of shingles in the elderly patient. ClinInterv Aging. 2008; 3: 241–250.

26

Lean Six Sigma Methodology for Quality Improvement in the Clinical Chemistry Laboratory

INTRODUCTION

Lean six sigma is a combination of two powerful methods: Lean and Six Sigma (Fig. 26.1). Six Sigma at many organizations simply means a measure of quality that strives for near perfection. Six Sigma is a disciplined, data-driven approach and methodology for eliminating defects (driving toward six standard deviations between the mean and the nearest specification limit) in any process, from manufacturing to transactional and from product to service. The Six Sigma methodology is based on the concept that 'process variation' (e.g. customer waiting times at a call center waiting varying between 10 seconds and 3 minutes) can be reduced using statistical tools.

LEAN SIX SIGMA

Lean (also referred to as lean methods or lean speed) is a set of tools developed to reduce the waste associated with the flow of materials and information in a process from beginning to end. The goal of Lean is to identify and eliminate non-essential and non-value added steps in the business process in order to streamline production, improve quality and gain customer loyalty. Methodology is the combination of Six Sigma quality management, developed by Motorola, with Lean manufacturing strategy, pioneered by Toyota, to provide tangible metrics for quality improvement. In its simplest form, Six Sigma asks the question, how can this process be improved? While Lean manufacturing asks the question, does this process (or step) need to exist? Together as Lean Six Sigma, they are being increasingly used to reduce error (Six Sigma) and waste (Lean) within the health-care system.

ADOPTION AND IMPLEMENTATION OF LEAN SIX SIGMA

Using more problem-solving techniques can help solve a larger number and variety of business problems. Starting in the 1980's, consultants trained in both techniques realized the synergy between Lean and Six Sigma and began to push for the combination of the different tools of Six Sigma (focused on improving quality) and Lean (focused on removing waste). Thus, Lean Six Sigma (LSS) was born. Effecting change will not occur without support from senior members within the organization. These leaders select and assign quality improvement projects to teams within the organization.

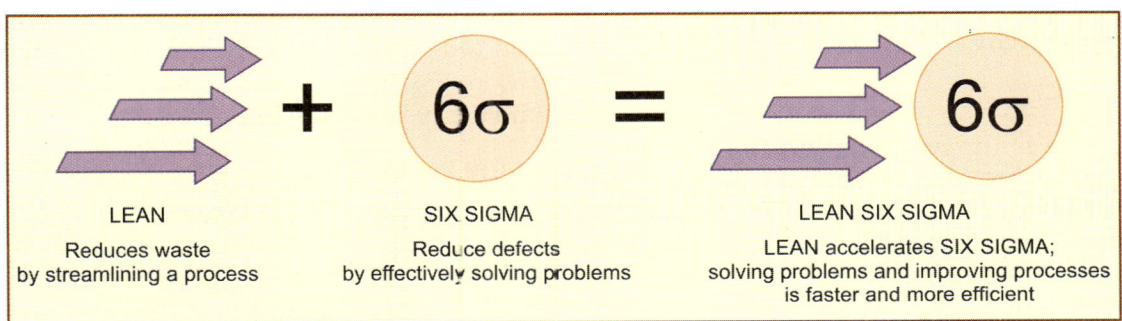

Fig. 26.1: Lean six sigma is a combination of two powerful methods—Lean and Six Sigma

In the laboratory, a team may consist of expert or specialist technologists, supervisors, directors, and an expert consultant who will lead the process. Typically, a full Six Sigma improvement project takes 6–8 months to complete.

The Different Lean Six Sigma Belts

A 'Belt' signifies experience. Practitioners are given a 'belt' title (black belt, green belt, and yellow belt) that corresponds to their level of experience. This roughly corresponds to their hierarchy in martial arts, with darker colored belts indicating more experience (more training, more knowledge and skills).

White Belt

A white belt signifies someone at the **beginning** of their Six Sigma journey and couldn't be easier to attain, taking just a single morning training session to become accredited. Once attained, White belts can **assist problem-solving teams** that sit within larger projects, but which may not necessarily be dedicated Six Sigma projects. White belts possess a **foundation of Six Sigma knowledge** and an awareness of the philosophy that underpins its methodology.

Yellow Belt

Yellow belts are generally employees who have undertaken the basic training in Six Sigma methodologies and who report back to their project leader, typically a green or black belt. At yellow belt, holders focus directly on the process area being reviewed and implement changes at ground level. Their participation in a project is crucial, as they are a core member of the team with specific expertise in the business area being developed. At the start of a project a yellow belt would help to develop 'process maps' using their practical experience, and may be responsible for smaller projects related to their work, within the main objective. Employees with such practical experience are invaluable to any company and by undertaking formalized training in Six Sigma methods, they can gain a professional qualification and have access to a clearly laid-out path to promotion within the Six Sigma hierarchy.

Green Belt

Green belt level is the next step up the Six Sigma hierarchy. At green belt level, an employee would lead a process improvement team alongside their other responsibilities. Being a green belt is not a full time role, but would generally take up around 25–50% of their time. Projects tend to focus on their own work area or department, allowing their expert knowledge and practical business experience within the company to come into play.

Once qualified, a green belt may be selected to lead a project by the management team. A green belt would need to know how to motivate a team, not all members of staff happily embrace the Six Sigma approach, and it would be crucial to the success of a project to have full team engagement. As leader of the process team, a green belt would be expected to gather all relevant data to be used in the project and also validate the measurement system. Leadership qualities are vital to this role in order to make the project a success.

Black Belt

Black belt level is a natural progression from green belt and holders will spend 100% of their time dealing with Six Sigma projects. They are team leaders, guiding green, yellow and white belts in a variety of on-going projects rather than focusing on just one. Black belt level requires strong leadership skills and the ability to clearly explain the philosophy and principles behind Six Sigma. They are key figures in training lower ranked belts, whilst receiving coaching from master black belts. In addition to possessing passion and business acumen, black belts need to have a degree of technical aptitude to collect suitable data and analyze it consistently. They are expected to quickly produce tangible results for the business and explain each step of the process to the corresponding audience, whether that is management executives or workers on the shop floor.

Master Black Belt

Promotion from black belt level to master black belt involves leading the company's Six Sigma program, performing statistical tasks and coaching black belts and green belts. An ability to provide a broad, high-level strategic view of improvements within a company and convey relevant facts to senior executives and departmental managers is paramount for a master black belt. In addition to possessing technical knowledge, an effective master black belt should be able to dispense that knowledge to all levels, from senior executives to workers on the shop floor. Ensuring that six sigma procedures are followed on every project and being able to explain the reason why to workers who may not be fully engaged with the system, is an important part of this role.

SENIOR ROLES

Everyone is accountable to someone and the same is true of six sigma practitioners. Once you attain master black belt level you are directly responsible for the strategic leadership of process improvement projects, but who ensures that you stay on track?

Champions

Champions are responsible for implementing Six Sigma methodology within an organization and work in senior management positions. They appoint and mentor master black belts, select projects and remove barriers that might prevent a project from being successful. These barriers could be financial, or problems associated with clashes of personality, the champion is there to ensure that master black belts and black belts are free to focus on the project without being caught up in office politics.

Executives

Executives include the CEO and other top management personnel. The executive role is to prepare the company 'vision' for Six Sigma, ensure that funds are available to support its introduction and allow role holders in the levels beneath to embrace new ideas to make it successful. Executives focus on Six Sigma as a strategic approach and are there to balance the adoption of Six Sigma with overall company goals.

PROCESS IMPROVEMENT

All work is a dynamic process, and every process has variation, overlap, and waste. Variation results in unpredictable and undesirable outcomes. Waste results in increased cost and delays and thereby limiting efficiency.

Lean Six Sigma uses a problem cause solution methodology to improve any process through waste elimination and variation reduction. The DMAIC (define, measure, analyze, improve, and control) methodology is the quality improvement team's project management road map (Fig. 26.2). The five phases allow for the identification of the root cause for error and waste through establishment of the following: (1) universally accepted framework for quality improvement, (2) common language throughout the organization, (3) a checklist to guide the process, and (4) control measures for long-term monitoring.

The define phase explicitly describes the quality improvement issues. In the measure phase, the team collects data to measure the process. That is, they determine the difference between the current process and the desired one. The analyze phase searches for the root causes of inefficiencies in the process. In the improve phase, the team pilots process changes that seek to remove the identified root problems. The control phase continues to measure the process and ensures changes are maintained.

Let's apply the DMAIC methodology to a real life example in the laboratory. Assume that a high rate of mislabeled aliquot tubes continues to be a chronic problem in the hospital laboratory. Aliquots are currently poured off manually when each specimen arrives in the laboratory either through the tube system or specimen drop-off window. The project would begin in the define phase by setting a goal to reduce by 60%. For example, the number of mislabeled aliquot tubes when the specimens arrive within 2 months. By the end of the define phase, both the project team and the management team have validated the 'project charter.' The project charter states the overall purpose and potential impact, the scope of the project (what is included and what is not), its resources (e.g. who is on the team and what resources are available to implement changes), and expectations, what will be delivered and when. This is a modifiable document intended to keep everyone involved focused on the problem and improving the outcomes.

The measure phase maps, measures, and assesses the current process. For this example, the number of aliquot tubes made on each shift and the number of mislabeled aliquot tubes would be monitored. The data collected would allow the team to calculate the current percentage of mislabeled aliquot tubes that occurs on each shift. In

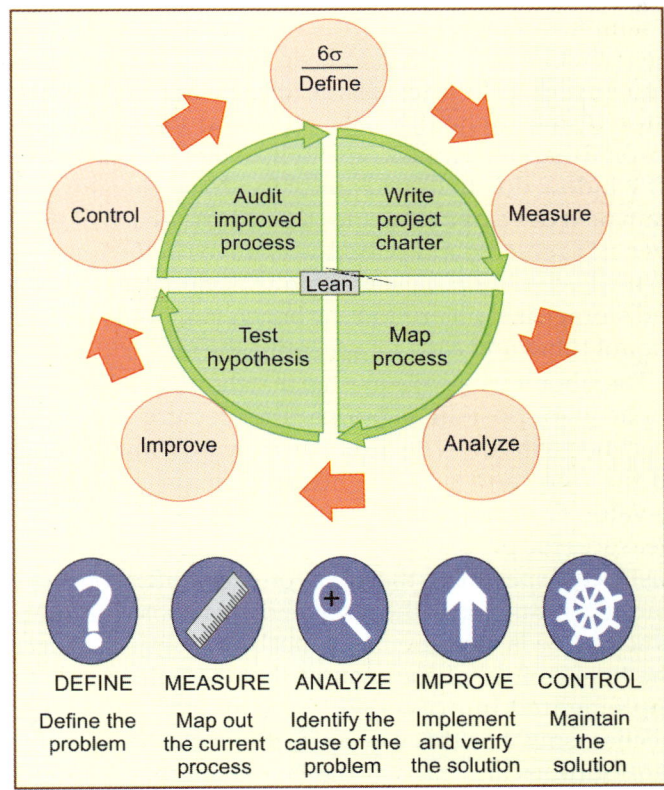

Fig. 26.2: Integration of Six Sigma and Lean principles. The methodologies of Six Sigma manufacturing and Lean process optimization are combined to an iterative cycle of quality improvement. Applications of Lean Six Sigma are now being applied to all aspects of the laboratory and the health-care system as a whole

doing so, the team will also map how the aliquots are made, including the number of specimens received, where labels are printed, where the aliquot tubes are stored, and how many technologists are involved in the process. In this laboratory, it is found that three technologists are responsible for making aliquots and they all share one common label printer. Bags of empty aliquot tubes and caps are stored in the laboratory's surplus room at the back of the laboratory. It is also found that 20 out of every 100 aliquot tubes are mislabeled.

Therefore, the goal of the project is to reduce the number of mislabeled specimens from 20–8 samples for every shift. In the analyze phase, the team identifies the root causes of the problem through cause, effect data analysis. Looking at the data collected, the group identifies several issues that most likely contribute toward the mislabeled aliquots. First, the shared label printer between the three technologists making aliquots creates confusion about which printed label belongs to which technologist. Second, during high-volume times, the technologist frequently runs out of aliquot tubes and caps and must retrieve bags of empty tubes from the surplus room at the back of the laboratory. This results in samples accumulating at the aliquot station and causes the technologists to rush to keep up with demand. It is also found that the technologists are frequently interrupted by health-care staff and visitors in the hospital that stop and ask directions at the specimen drop-off window due to its proximity to a busy elevator. The team next develops strategies that address each of these specific problems and pilots the changes in the Improve phase. Each technologist is given an aliquot label printer and storage is built around the bench that holds enough aliquot tubes and caps for an entire shift.

The laboratory also requested that the hospital facilities department post-signs both at the elevator and at the specimen window with directions toward common units on the floor and provide hospital maps outside the elevator. Once the changes are implemented, the team measures the process again and finds that the number of mislabeled specimens that occur on each shift is four. This is an 80% reduction in the number of mislabeled aliquots, which exceeds the goals of 60% set by the project charter. The final control phase ensures that the gains made by implemented improvements are maintained by QC mechanisms. For this example, this includes stocking aliquot tubes and caps at the beginning of each shift, maintaining three working label printers for the aliquot station, and ensuring that maps are readily available at the elevator. The way the aliquots are made (poured off and labeled by hand) did not change. Instead, modifying the steps around the process was enough to improve the outcome to the level set by the project charter.

Furthermore, these modifications included factors both inside and outside the laboratory. The DMAIC method (Fig. 26.2) was applied to a problem in the laboratory and allowed the team to quantitatively measure the error of the process, identify the root cause(s) of the problem, develop improvement strategies, and monitor the changes in a defined manner.

MEASUREMENTS OF SUCCESS USING LEAN AND SIX SIGMA

Originally, Lean and Six Sigma were separate ideas designed to improve two related metrics—time and error. Lean was designed to eliminate non-value-adding steps and Six Sigma aimed to reduce variation. The metrics for measuring quality improvement with Lean Six Sigma till reflect those original principles. Combination of these two ideas provides a positive synergistic impact on process and quality improvement. The Lean approach seeks to streamline the process by eliminating duplication, excess, and barriers for a more optimized flow. The major measurement for Lean is generally time, but it can also include things such as cost, inventory, and distribution. A common method of Lean improvement is the concept of a Kaizen event.

This is analogous to the DMAIC method used in Six Sigma but can be implemented on a smaller scale. The Kaizen event is 3–5 days of quality improvement by a cross-functional team that analyzes the current steps associated with a particular process and makes changes to improve its efficiency. With detailed study, most teams find unnecessary complexity in their process. This complexity often contributes to errors as well as delays.

Teams typically find that only 5% of the activities in any process add value; this means that a vast majority of activities do not contribute to the process. Graphically, this might look like the redundant and nonlinear process (Fig. 26.3). Lean Six Sigma measures the amount of non-value-adding steps in a process as part of its core metrics. The implemented solutions (based on charter goals) represented by the final process (Fig. 26.3), where inefficiency has been removed illustrate a more stream-lined, efficient process.

Six Sigma metrics seek to quantitatively measure the amount of error or variation that occurs within a system. A **process sigma** represents the capability of a process to meet (or exceed) its defined criteria for acceptability. In the laboratory, this could refer to assay performance, turnaround times, and number of rejected samples, specimen transport, or relay of critical values. The process sigma is usually represented as the number of defects (errors) per million opportunities (DPMO). The sigma(σ) value refers to the number of standard deviations (SDs) away from the mean a process can move before it is outside the acceptable limits (Fig. 26.4). For example, if a

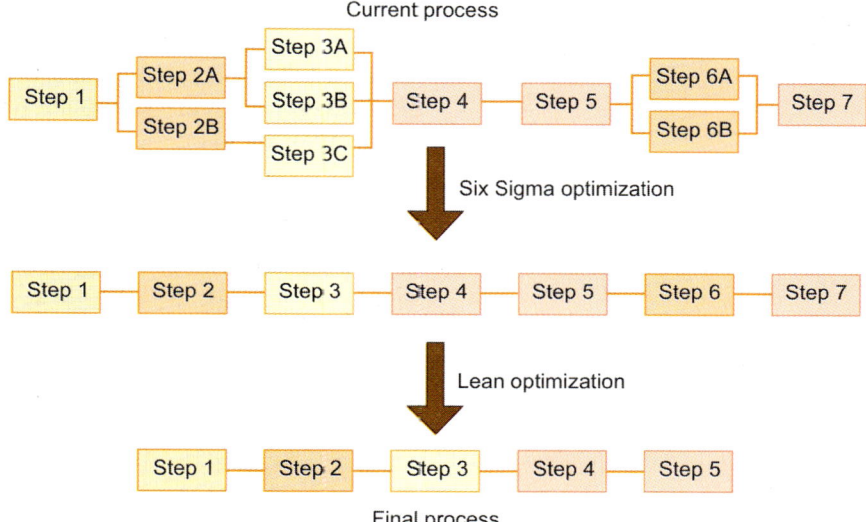

Fig. 26.3: Application of Six Sigma and Lean methodologies toward process improvement. Steps in a process can have duplication, failure, and waste, all of which contribute to delay, increased cost, inefficiency, and longer turnaround times

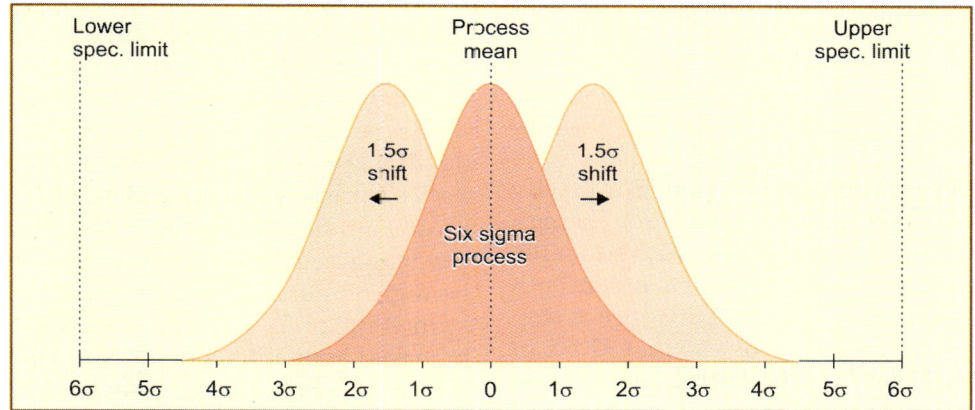

Fig. 26.4: Comparison of Sigma performance for results distributed between the lower satisfactory limit (LSL) and the upper satisfactory limit (USL)

sodium test has Six Sigma performance, then the mean could shift by 6 SDs (6σ) and still meet the laboratory requirements for precision and accuracy for sodium measurement. If a test achieves Six Sigma (6σ), it has an arrow process SD (i.e. it is very precise) and produces only three errors for every million tests performed. A test that performs at a three sigma (3σ) has a much wider process SD and produces about 26,674 errors per million tests (Fig. 26.4).

To calculate the sigma, defects must be clearly defined. In the laboratory, any test that does not meet its requirements (i.e. correctly quantified or delivered on time) is considered a defect. The most straightforward method uses the process yield—the percentage of times that a process is defect free. Another method to calculate the process sigma is to calculate the DPMO.

For example, in the laboratory, this might be measured by the number of errors that occurs for every 1 million tests. The process sigma can be estimated from a process sigma table (Table 26.1) using either the process yield or the DPMO. As stated earlier, eliminating non-value-adding steps and reducing variation have a synergistic positive impact on process performance (Table 26.2). Several examples illustrate this concept. Assume that there are four steps involved in testing a specimen and each step is performed at a 3σ level (each step 93.3% accurate and timely). With this performance, approximately three out of four test results will be accurate and delivered on time (75.8%). Now imagine that a team improves the quality of the process, so that each step is performed correctly and timely at a 4σ level (99.38% accurate and timely). The new level of performance produces 97.5% of the results accurately and delivered on time. Alternatively, if a test has 10 steps, each of which operates at a 3σ level (93.3% accurate and timely) the increase in the number of slightly inaccurate steps, 50%

Table 26.1	Process Sigma table	
Yield	Errors/million results	Process sigma
99.9999%	1	6.27
99.9997%	3	6.04
99.999%	10	5.77
99.99%	100	5.22
99.9%	1,000	4.59

Definition of 'sigma' for a process with a given error rate.

Table 26.2	Example of yield at given performance (σ): % of data reported correctly			
Number of steps	±3 σ	±4 σ	±5 σ	±6 σ
1	93.3%	99.38%	99.977%	99.9999%
3	82.7%	98.16%	99.931%	99.9953%
4	77.4%	97.56%	99.908%	99.9930%
7	61.6%	95.73%	99.839%	99.9976%
10	50.1%	93.96%	99.768%	99.9966%
20	25.1%	88.29%	99.536%	99.9932%
40	6.3%	77.94%	99.074%	99.9864%
80	1.6%	68.81%	98.614%	99.9796%
100	0.4%	60.75%	98.156%	99.9728%

of the tests will be inaccurate and late. Simply by eliminating unnecessary steps and maintaining a high level of performance, the team can drastically reduce the number of total errors. If the improvement team can both eliminate six steps and increase the quality of each step to a 4σ level, the process will improve so that 97.5% of the tests are accurate and on time (Table 26.2). These improvement strategies are designed to be continuous. Once changes have been realized, the improvement process should start again to make the system even better with each cycle.

Lean Six Sigma Applications in the Laboratory and the Greater Health-care System

The popularity of the combination of Lean and Six Sigma principles as an approach to quality management in health care has grown in the last 10 years. In 2004, there were two articles published describing specifically the application of lean six sigma, according to a PubMed search utilizing the phrase 'Lean Six Sigma.' This number has risen to 29 articles published in 2010/2011. Since 1997, there have been 255 publications on Six Sigma quality improvement strategies alone in the health-care field. Application of Lean and Six Sigma methodology at the Virginia Mason Medical Center showed numerous improvements to patient care. Highlights the major improvements achieved in Lean Six Sigma Quality

Management (Table 26.3). Prior to the adoption of Lean Six Sigma strategies, no laboratory result was reported (the time the result was available until mailing) within less than 3 days and every physician had an average of 1,800 results waiting to be reported. After application of Lean methodology, 89% of the test results were reported in less than 3 days. Patient waiting time was significantly reduced for chemotherapy infusion time, clinic waiting time decreased by 50%, and discharge time decreased from 2.5–1.5 hours. All of these aspects for improvement represent tangible metrics that can be measured and quantified by Lean Six Sigma tools. The results of the improvement process provide superior patient care, improve customer service, and positively impact patient satisfaction, which all contribute toward enhanced customer retention by the individual health-care organization.

A similar application of Lean Six Sigma Methodology was used to develop a new phlebotomy staffing model that better matched demand at Brigham and Women's Hospital in Boston. The project was initiated in response to excessive safety reports filed for missed inpatient collections, thereby delaying laboratory results. Discrepancies between estimated and actual collection demand identified periods of under staffing for the phlebotomy service during peak demand times.

After application of the Lean Six Sigma Methodology, new, staggered shifts were implemented to better handle the high-volume times between 5 and 9 am and 7 and 9 pm (Fig. 26.5). Four new shifts were created that increased available personnel during peak hours and decreased available personnel during periods of low collections. The number of full-time equivalents remained the same between the old and new staffing model. The new staffing model improved collection by 17 minutes, accelerated results for basic chemistry such as potassium by 15 minutes, and reduced by 80% the number of filed safety reports from delayed or missed collections.

Table 26.3	Major improvements achieved from Lean Six Sigma quality management	
	Before lean six sigma	After lean six sigma
Results report mailed	100% > 3 d	89% < 3 d
Patient waiting time	[Data not published]	Decreased by 50%
Discharge time	2.5 h	1.5 h
Chemotherapy time	[Data not published]	Decreased by 50%

Source: Bush RW. Reducing waste in US health care systems. JAMA. 2007; 297(8): 871–4.

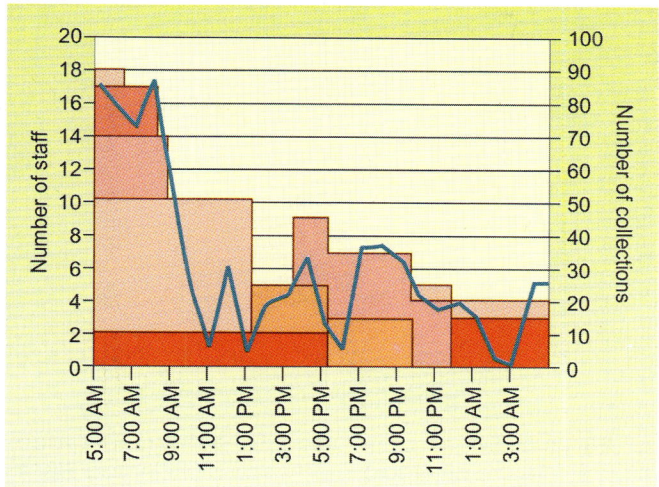

Fig. 26.5: The revised staffing model that better matches the collection pattern (*black line*) modified through Six Sigma quality improvement strategies. Blocked colors represent different staff shifts. A strategy for optimizing staffing to improve the timeliness of inpatient phlebotomy collections.

PRACTICAL APPLICATION OF SIX SIGMA METRICS

Detecting Laboratory Errors

Recent studies have highlighted that medical errors occur with greater frequency than previously thought. As part of the health-care system, the laboratory is a potential source of error. Error rates in laboratory tests have been estimated to occur between 1:164 and 1:8,300 results (Table 26.4). Converting these error rates to the standard Six Sigma metric DPMO, laboratory error rates would be expected to occur at a rate of between 120 and 6,098 DPMO; this corresponds to a 4σ–5σ rating. A 6σ quality level would require less than 3.4 DPMO (Table 26.1).

While an estimated 12.5% of laboratory errors impact patient health, only 37.5 of every 100,000 (0.0375%) errors place patients at risk due to analytical testing mistakes. Previously, laboratory quality improvement focused on errors that occur in the analytic phase of testing. But currently, analytical testing errors comprise only 4–32%

Table 26.4	Rate of laboratory error detection	
Estimated laboratory error rate	**Errors/million (DPMO)**
1:164	6,098
1:214	4,672
1:283	3,534
1:8,300	20
Risk of dying in a plane crash	
1:7,000,000 passengers	0.14

of all errors in the laboratory. Most laboratory errors are now attributed to processes occurring either before (preanalytic) or immediately after (postanalytic) the test. Preanalytic errors are estimated at between 32% and 75%, and postanalytic errors account for 9–55%.

As outlined in (Fig. 26.6), the preanalytic phase involves steps, such as the actual ordering of the tests by physicians, as well as sample collection. Because many of the preanalytic errors are outside the physical laboratory (i.e. phlebotomy), it is imperative that the process as a whole be considered when reorganizing laboratory processes to improve quality. This often requires collaboration between other departments within the system. With the current emphasis on quality improvement in the health-care setting, clinical laboratories have been early adopters of Lean Six Sigma methodology to improve the quality of laboratory testing by identifying and reducing pre- and postanalytical sources of error.

Defining the Sigma performance of an assay from a quality management perspective, Six Sigma metrics can determine how well an analytic process performs and assist in choosing appropriate QC rules based on test performance. For example, if a given test has excellent performance (very precise and accurate over time), then fewer errors will occur. It would take a large shift in the mean for the test to fail the quality requirements.

Accordingly, fewer QC rules would be needed to identify errors. These rules are designed to maximize the chance of detecting a problem, while simultaneously minimizing the risk of rejecting a result when it is actually

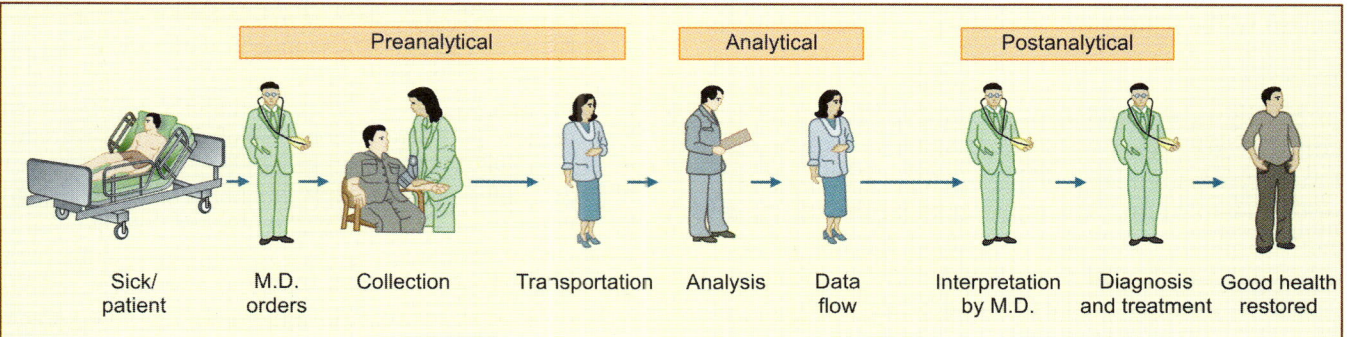

Fig. 26.6: Schematic representation of the process components involved in clinical laboratory testing

correct (false rejection). Six Sigma metrics can be plotted graphically using an operational process specification 'OPSpecs' chart. This chart incorporates many of the measures described in the Method Evaluation chapter into one graph, including (1) total allowable error, (2) systematic error (inaccuracy), and (3) random error (imprecision) (Fig. 26.7).

Plotting the random error of 20% on the x-axis and the systemic error of 70% on the y-axis using the OPSpecs chart (Fig. 26.7) reveals that the assay has a 2σ performance; this is considered poor performance and would require extensive QC measurements to detect the high number of errors. Many rules are needed because only a small shift in the mean would result in a failure (this principle is evident in Fig. 26.4). If the systemic error (bias) could be eliminated (as demonstrated with point 2, Fig. 26.7), the performance would fall into the 5σ range, which is considered to be very good; only a few QC measurements would be necessary with a minimal use of control rules to detect the low number of errors. Choosing the appropriate Westgard Rules.

Recently, a straightforward methodology has been published detailing how Six Sigma metrics can be used to choose appropriate Westgard QC rules for any assay.

A sigma value for every Westgard rule or set of rules can be deduced from the slope of the line it generates in an OPSpecs chart (Fig. 26.7). In short, the slope of the line is equal to the – (negative) sigma value. Furthermore, the sigma value for an assay can be calculated by the following equation:

$$Sigma = \frac{(Total\ allowable\ error - bias)}{Coefficient\ of\ variation}$$

Total allowable error represents the error budget based on the biological variation of the specific analyte. Bias refers to the systematic error of the assay and the coefficient of variation is the analytical SD of the assay. If the calculated sigma for an assay is greater than the sigma of the Westgard rule, that rule is suitable for monitoring the error of the test.

Conclusions

Lean Six Sigma methodology has emerged as a powerful technique to effectively improve the quality and efficiency of the clinical laboratory. It provides a framework to define, measure, and reduce waste and variation associated with the total testing process. Furthermore, it supplies mathematically sound metrics to assess laboratory processes and assay performance, define QC rules, and develop quality improvement strategies.

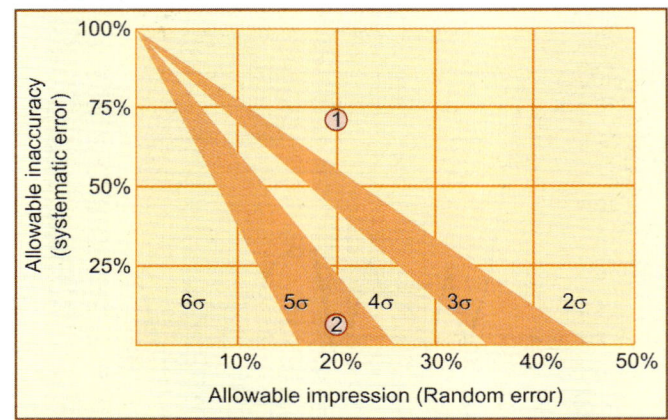

Fig. 26.7: OPSpecs chart used to determine process performance. The allowable imprecision is plotted against the allowable inaccuracy as percentage of the total allowable error. Assay performance changing from point 1 to point 2 by reducing inaccuracy improves the performance from a 2σ process to a 5σ process.

Lean Six Sigma's role in clinical chemistry will continue to grow in importance and scope as the need for improved quality and reduced cost becomes paramount in the health care system. Knowledge of Lean Six Sigma methodology will be critical for laboratorians going forward to achieve the mission of delivering quality health care to patients.

Major hospitals have made institutional-wide commitments to quality improvement using Lean Six Sigma. Yellow belt training is currently offered at certain institutions to all laboratory personnel with the goal of having the entire laboratory staff trained. Supervisors and lead technologists are also trained at the blue, purple, and black belt level to participate in quality improvement projects across departments within the institution. For medical technologists, this training provides an unprecedented opportunity to be an agent for change in the health-care system and allows the laboratorian to take greater ownership in improving patient care and enhancing customer service.

BIBLIOGRAPHY

1. Barnett RN. Medical significance of laboratory results. Am J ClinPathol. 1968; 50:671-676.
2. Bland JM, Altman DG. Statistical methods for assessing agreement between two methods of clinical measurement. Lancet.1986; 1:307-310.
3. Bonini P, Plebani M, Ceriotti F, Rubboli F. Errors in laboratory medicine. Clin Chem. May 2002; 48(5):691-698.
4. Bush RW. Reducing waste in US health care systems. JAMA. February 2007; 297(8):871-874.
5. Centers for Disease Control and Prevention (CDC), Centers for Medicare and Medicaid Services (CMS), Health and Human Services. Medicare, Medicaid, and CLIA programs;

laboratory requirements relating to quality systems and certain personnel qualifications. Final rule. Fed Regist. 2003; 68: 3639–3714.

6. Clinical and Laboratory Standards Institute (CLSI). Statistical Quality Control for Quantitative Measurements: Principles and Definitions. Wayne, PA: CLSI; 2006.

7. Clinical Laboratory Improvement Amendments of 1988; final rule. Fed Regist. 7164 [42 CFR 493.1213]: Department of Health and Human Services, Centers for Medicare and Medicaid Services; 1992.

8. Committee on Identifying Priority Areas for Quality Improvement. Priority Areas for National Action: Transforming Health Care Quality. 1st ed. Washington, DC: National Academies Press; 2003.

9. Committee on Quality of Health Care in America, Institute of Medicine. Crossing the Quality Chasm: A New Health System for the 21st Century. 1st ed. Washington, DC: National Academies Press; 2001.

10. Committee on Quality of Health Care in America. Institute of Medicine. To Err Is Human: Building a Safer Health System. 1st ed. Washington, DC: National Academies Press; 2000.

11. Cornbleet PJ, Gochman N. Incorrect least-squares regression coefficients in method-comparison analysis. Clin Chem. 1979; 25: 432–438.

12. DelliFraine JL, Langabeer JR 2nd, Nembhard IM. Assessing the evidence of Six Sigma and Lean in the health care industry. QualManag Health Care. September 2010; 19(3): 211–225.

13. Ehrmeyer SS, Laessig RH, Leinweber JE, et al. 1990 Medicare/CLIA final rules for proficiency testing: minimum intralaboratory performance characteristics (CV and bias) needed to pass. Clin Chem. 1990; 36: 1736–1740.

14. Feldmann U, Schneider B, Klinkers H, et al. A multivariate approach for the biometric comparison of analytical methods in clinical chemistry. J Clin Chem Clin Biochem. 1981; 19: 121–137.

15. Fraser CG. Biological Variation: From Principles to Practice. Washington, DC: AACC Press; 2001.

16. Fraser CG. Data on biological variation: essential prerequisites for introducing new procedures? Clin Chem. 1994; 40: 1671–1673.

17. Galen RS, Gambino SR. Beyond Normality: The Predictive Value and Efficiency of Medical Diagnoses. New York, NY: Wiley; 1975.

18. Glick MR, Ryder KW, Jackson SA. Graphical comparisons of interferences in clinical chemistry instrumentation. Clin Chem. 1986; 32: 470–475.

19. Glick MR, Ryder KW. Analytical systems ranked by freedom from interferences. Clin Chem. 1987; 33: 1453–1458.

20. Gras JM, Philippe M. Application of the Six Sigma concept in clinical laboratories: a review. ClinChem Lab Med. 2007; 45(6): 789–796.

21. Hollensead SC, Lockwood WB, Elin RJ. Errors in pathology and laboratory medicine: consequences and prevention. J SurgOncol. December 2004; 88(3): 161–181.

22. Institute of Medicine (U.S.). Committee on Crossing the Quality Chasm: Adaptation to Mental Health and Addictive

Disorders. Improving the Quality of Health Care for Mental and Substance-Use Conditions. Washington, DC: National Academies Press; 2006.

23. IOM report: patient safety—achieving a new standard for care. Acad Emerg Med. October 2005; 12(10): 1011–1012.

24. Juran JM. Juran on Leadership for Quality. 1st ed. New York, NY: Free Press; 1989.

25. Kalra J. Medical errors: impact on clinical laboratories and other critical areas. Clin Biochem. December 2004; 37(12): 1052–1062.

26. Krouwer JS, Rabinowitz R. How to improve estimates of imprecision. Clin Chem. 1984; 30: 290–292.

27. Kuo AM-H, Borycki E, Kushniruk A, Lee T-S. A healthcare Lean Six Sigma System for post anesthesia care unit workflow improvement. QualManag Health Care. March 2011; 20(1): 4–14.

28. Lapworth R, Teal TK. Laboratory blunders revisited. Ann Clin Biochem. January 1994; 31(pt 1): 78–84.

29. Levey S, Jennings ER. The use of control charts in the clinical laboratory. Am J Clin Pathol. 1950; 20: 1059–1066.

30. Medicare, Medicaid and CLIA programs; regulations implementing the Clinical Laboratory Improvement Amendments of 1988(CLIA)—HCFA. Final rule with comment period. Fed Regist.1992; 57: 7002–7186.

31. Morrison AP, Tanasijevic MJ, Torrence-Hill JN, Goonan EM, Gustafson ML, Melanson SEF. A strategy for optimizing staffing to improve the timeliness of inpatient phlebotomy collections. Arch Pathol Lab Med. December 2011; 135(12): 1576–1580.

32. National Committee for Clinical Laboratory Standards (NCCLS).Approved Guideline for Precision Performance of Clinical Chemistry Devices. Villanova, PA: NCCLS; 1999 (Document no. EP05-A).

33. National Committee for Clinical Laboratory Standards (NCCLS).Approved Guideline for Method Comparison and Bias Estimation Using Patient Samples. Villanova, PA: NCCLS; 2002 (Document no. EP09-A2).

34. National Committee for Clinical Laboratory Standards (NCCLS).Proposed Guideline for Interference Testing in Clinical Chemistry. Villanova, PA: NCCLS;1986 (Document no. EP07-A).

35. National Committee for Clinical Laboratory Standards (NCCLS).Proposed Guideline for Evaluation of Linearity of Quantitative Analytical Methods. Villanova, PA: NCCLS; 2001 (Document no. EP6-P2).

36. Plebani M. Errors in clinical laboratories or errors in laboratory medicine? Clin Chem Lab Med. 2006; 44(6): 750–759.

37. Plebani M. Exploring the iceberg of errors in laboratory medicine. ClinChimActa. June 2009; 404(1): 16–23.

38. Pocha C. Lean Six Sigma in health care and the challenge of implementation of Six Sigma methodologies at a Veterans Affairs Medical Center. QualManag Health Care. December 2010; 19(4): 312–318.

39. Reibnegger G, Fuchs D, Hausen A, et al. Generalized likelihood ratio concept and logistic regression analysis for multiple diagnostic categories. Clin Chem. 1989; 35: 990–994.

40. Ryder KW, Glick MR. Erroneous laboratory results from hemolyzed, icteric, and lipemic specimens. Clin Chem. 1993; 39: 175–176.

41. Schoenmakers CHH, Naus AJM, Vermeer HJ, van Loon D, Steen G. Practical application of Sigma Metrics QC procedures in clinical chemistry. ClinChem Lab Med. November 2011; 49(11): 1837–1843.

42. Shahzad K, Kim DH, Kang MJ. Analytic evaluation of the beta-human chorionic gonadotropin assay on the Abbott IMx and Elecsys 2010 for its use in doping control. Clin Biochem.2007; 40: 1259–1265.

43. Siebers R. Laboratory blunders revisited. Ann ClinBiochem. July1994; 31(pt 4): 390–391.

44. Siest G, Galteau MM. Drug Effects on Laboratory Tests. Littleton, MA: PSG Publishing; 1988.

45. Signori C, Ceriotti F, Sanna A, et al. Process and risk analysis to reduce errors in clinical laboratories. ClinChem Lab Med. 2007; 45(6): 742–748.

46. Singla P, Parkash AA, Bhattacharjee J. Preanalytical error occurrence rate in clinical chemistry laboratory of a public hospital in India. Clin Lab. 2011; 57(9-10): 749–752.

47. Solberg HE. International Federation of Clinical Chemistry (IFCC), Scientific Committee, Clinical Section, Expert Panel on Theory of Reference Values, and International Committee for Standardization in Haematology (ICSH), Standing Committee on Reference Values. Approved Recommendation (1986) on the theory of reference values. Part 1. The concept of reference values. J Clin Chem Clin Biochem. 1987; 25: 337–342.

48. Solberg HE. International Federation of Clinical Chemistry. Scientific Committee, Clinical Section. Expert Panel on Theory of Reference Values and International Committee for Standardization in Haematology Standing Committee on Reference Values. Approved recommendation (1986) on the theory of reference values. Part 1. The concept of reference values. ClinChimActa. 1987; 165:111-118.

49. Solberg HE. The IFCC recommendation on estimation of reference intervals. The RefVal program. ClinChem Lab Med.2004; 42: 710–714.

50. Standardization of blood specimen collection procedure for reference values. International Committee for Standardization in Haematology (ICSH). Clin Lab Haematol. 1982; 4: 83–86.

51. Stankovic AK. The laboratory is a key partner in assuring patient safety. Clin Lab Med. December 2004; 24(4): 1023–1035.

52. Tonks DB. A study of the accuracy and precision of clinical chemistry determinations in 170 Canadian laboratories. Clin Chem. 1963; 9: 217–233.

53. Van der Helm HJ, Hische EA, Bolhuis PA. Bayes' theorem and the estimation of the likelihood ratio. Clin Chem. 1982; 28: 1250–1251.

54. Van der Meulen EA, Boogaard PJ, van Sittert NJ. Use of small sample-based reference limits on a group basis. Clin Chem. 1994; 40: 1698–1702.

55. Vanker N, van Wyk J, Zemlin AE, Erasmus RT. A Six Sigma approach to the rate and clinical effect of registration errors in a laboratory. J ClinPathol. May 2010; 63(5): 434–437.

56. Wakkers PJ, Hellendoorn HB, Op de Weegh GJ, et al. Applications of statistics in clinical chemistry. A critical evaluation of regression lines. Clin Chim Acta. 1975; 64: 173–184.

57. Westgard JO, Barry PL, Hunt MR, et al. A multi-rule Shewhart chart for quality control in clinical chemistry. Clin Chem.1981; 27: 493–501.

58. Westgard JO, Burnett RW. Precision requirements for cost-effective operation of analytic processes. Clin Chem. 1990; 36: 1629–1632.

59. Westgard JO, Carey RN, Wold S. Criteria for judging precision and accuracy in method development and evaluation. Clin Chem.1974; 20: 825–833.

60. Westgard JO, de Vos DJ, Hunt MR, et al. Concepts and practices in the evaluation of clinical chemistry methods. V. Applications. Am J Med Technol. 1978; 44: 803–813.

61. Westgard JO, de Vos DJ, Hunt MR, et al. Concepts and practices in the evaluation of clinical chemistry methods: IV. Decisions of acceptability. Am J Med Technol. 1978; 44: 727–742.

62. Westgard JO, de Vos DJ, Hunt MR, et al. Concepts and practicesin the evaluation of clinical chemistry methods. I. Background and approach. Am J Med Technol. 1978; 44: 290–300.

63. Westgard JO, de Vos DJ, Hunt MR, et al. Concepts and practicesin the evaluation of clinical chemistry methods. II. Experimental procedures. Am J Med Technol. 1978; 44: 420–430.

64. Westgard JO, Groth T, Aronsson T, et al. Performance characteristics of rules for internal quality control: probabilities for false rejection and error detection. Clin Chem. 1977; 23: 1857–1867.

65. Westgard JO, Groth T. Power functions for statistical control rules. Clin Chem. 1979; 25: 863–869.

66. Westgard JO, Hunt MR. Use and interpretation of common statistical tests in method-comparison studies. Clin Chem. 1973; 19: 49–57.

67. Westgard JO, Seehafer JJ, Barry PL. European specifications for imprecision and inaccuracy compared with operating specifications that assure the quality required by US CLIA proficiency testing criteria. Clin Chem. 1994; 40 (7 pt 1): 1228–1232.

68. Westgard JO. Basic Method Evaluation. 2nd ed. Madison, WI: Westgard Quality Corp; 2003.

69. Westgard JO. Precision and accuracy: concepts and assessment by method evaluation testing. Crit Rev Clin Lab Sci. 1981; 13: 283–330.

70. Young DS. Effects of Drugs on Clinical Laboratory Tests. 4th ed. Washington, DC: American Association of Clinical Chemistry; 2000.

Appendix A

Reference range values are for apparently healthy people and often overlap significantly with values for those who are sick. Actual values may vary significantly due to differences in assay methodologies and standardization. Institutions may also set up their own reference ranges based on the particular populations that they serve, thus regional differences may occur. Consequently, values reported by individual laboratories may differ from those listed in this appendix.

All values are given in conventional and SI units. However, cases where SI units have not been widely accepted, conventional units are used. In case of the heterogenous nature of the materials measured or uncertainty about the exact molecular weight of the compounds, SI measurements cannot be used so that mass per volume remains as the unit of concentration.

Laboratory reference range values		
Tests	Conventional units	SI units
Acetaminophen, serum or plasma (Hep or EDTA)		
Therapeutic	10–30 mcg/mL	66–199 mcmol/L
Toxic	>200 mcg/mL	>1324 mcmol/L
Acetone		
Serum		
Qualitative	Negative	Negative
Quantitative	0.3–2.0 mg/dL	0.05–0.34 mmol/L
Urine		
Qualitative	Negative	Negative
Acid hemolysis test (Ham)	<5% lysis	<0.05 lysed fraction
Adrenocorticotropin (ACTH), plasma		
8 AM	<120 pg/mL	<26 pmol/L
Midnight (supine)	<10 pg/mL	<2.2 pmol/L
*Alanine aminotransferase (ALT, SGPT), serum		
Male	13–40 U/L (37°C)	0.22–0.68 mckat/L (37°C)
Female	10–28 U/L (37°C)	0.17–0.48 mckat/L (37°C)
Albumin		
Serum		
Adult	3.5–5.2 g/dL	35–52 g/L
>60 years	3.2–4.6 g/dL	32–46 g/L
	Avg. of 0.3 g/dL higher in patients in upright position	Avg. of 3 g/L higher in patients in upright position
Urine		
Qualitative	Negative	Negative
Quantitative	50–80 mg/24 h	50–80 mg/24 h
CSF10–30 mg/dL	100–300 mg/L	
*Aldolase, serum	1.0–7.5 U/L (30°C)	0.02–0.13 mckat/L (30°C)
Aldosterone		

Contd.

Laboratory reference range values (Contd.)		
Tests	Conventional units	SI units
Serum		
Supine	3–16 ng/dL	0.08–0.44 nmol/L
Standing	7–30 ng/dL	0.19–0.83 nmol/L
Urine	3–19 mcg/24 h	8–51 nmol/24 h
Amikacin, serum or plasma (EDTA)		
Therapeutic		
Peak	25–35 mcg/mL	43–60 mcmol/L
Trough		
Less severe infection	1–4 mcg/mL	1.7–6.8 mcmol/L
Life-threatening infection	4–8 mcg/mL	6.8–13.7 mcmol/L
Toxic		
Peak	>35–40 mcg/mL	>60–68 mcmol/L
Trough	>10–15 mcg/mL	>17–26 mcmol/L
Aminolevulinic acid, urine	1.3–7.0 mg/24 h	10–53 mcmol/24 h
Amitriptyline, serum or plasma		
(Hep or EDTA);		
trough (≥12 h after dose)		
Therapeutic	80–250 ng/mL	289–903 nmol/L
Toxic	>500 ng/mL	>1805 nmol/L
Ammonia		
Plasma (Hep)	9–33 mcmol/L	9–33 mcmol/L
*Amylase		
Serum	27–131 U/L	0.46–2.23 mckat/L
Urine	1–17 U/h	0.017–0.29 mckat/h
Amylase:creatinine clearance ratio	1–4%	0.01–0.04
Androstenedione, serum		
Male	75–205 ng/dL	2.6–7.2 nmol/L
Female	85–275 ng/dL	3.0–9.6 nmol/L
Anion gap		
$[Na - (Cl + HCO_3)]$	7–16 mEq/L	7–16 mmol/L
$[(Na + K) - (Cl + HCO_3)]$	10–20 mEq/L	10–20 mmol/L
α1-antitrypsin, serum	78–200 mg/dL	0.78–2.00 g/L
Apolipoprotein A-1		
Male	94–178 mg/dL	0.94–1.78 g/L
Female	101–199 mg/dL	1.01–1.99 g/L
Apolipoprotein B		
Male	63–133 mg/dL	0.63–1.33 g/L
Female	60–126 mg/dL	0.60–1.26 g/L
Arsenic		
Whole blood (Hep)	0.2–2.3 mcg/dL	0.03–0.31 mcmol/L
Chronic poisoning	10–50 mcg/dL	1.33–6.65 mcmol/L
Acute poisoning	60–930 mcg/dL	7.98–124 mcmol/L
Urine, 24 h	5–50 mcg/day	0.07–0.67 mcmol/day
Ascorbic acid, plasma (Ox, Hep, EDTA)	0.4–1.5 mg/dL	23–85 mcmol/L
*Aspartate aminotransferase (AST, SGOT), serum	10–59 U/L (37°C)	0.17–1.00 –2 to +3 kat/L (37°C)
Base excess, blood (Hep)	–2 to +3 mEq/L	–2 to +3 mmol/L

*Test values dependent on laboratory methods used.

Contd.

Laboratory reference range values *(Contd.)*		
Tests	**Conventional units**	**SI units**
Bicarbonate, serum (venous)	22–29 mEq/L	22–29 mmol/L
[†]Bilirubin		
Bilirubin, direct		
Birth–death	0.0–0.4 mg/dL	
Bilirubin, total		
Birth–1 day	1.0–6.0 mg/dL	
1–2 days	6.0–7.5 mg/dL	
2–5 days	4.0–13.5 mg/dL	
5 days–death	0.2–1.2 mg/dL	
Total bilirubin, neonatal		
Birth–1 day	1.0–6.0 mg/dL	
1–2 days	6.0–7.5 mg/dL	
2–5 days	4.0–13.5 mg/dL	
5 days–1 month	0.0–1.8 mg/dL	
1 month–death	0.0–1.8 mg/dL	
Bone marrow, differential cell count		
Adult		
Undifferentiated cells	0–1%	0–0.01
Myeloblast	0–2%	0–0.02
Promyelocyte	0–4%	0–0.04
Myelocytes		
Neutrophilic	5–20%	0.05–0.20
Eosinophilic	0–3%	0–0.03
Basophilic	0–1%	0–0.01
Metamyeolocytes and bands		
Neutrophilic	5–35%	0.05–0.35
Eosinophilic	0–5%	0–0.05
Basophilic	0–1%	0–0.01
Segmented neutrophils	5–15%	0.05–0.15
Pronormoblast	0–1.5%	0–0.015
Basophilic normoblast	0–5%	0–0.05
Polychromatophilic normoblast	5–30%	0.05–0.30
Orthochromatic normoblast	5–10%	0.05–0.10
Lymphocytes	10–20%	0.10–0.20
Plasma cells	0–2%	0–0.02
Monocytes	0–5%	0–0.05
CA-125, serum	<35 U/mL	<35 kU/L
CA 15-3, serum	<30 U/mL	<30 kU/L
CA 19-9, serum	<37 U/mL	<37 kU/L
Cadmium, whole blood (Hep)	0.1–0.5 mcg/dL	8.9–44.5 nmol/L
Toxic	10–300 mcg/dL	0.89–26.70 mcmol/L
Cadmium, urine, 24 h	<15 mcg/day	<0.13 mcmol/day
Calcitonin, serum or plasma		
Male	≤100 pg/mL	≤100 ng/L
Female	≤30 pg/mL	≤30 ng/L
Calcium, serum	8.6–10.0 mg/dL (Slightly higher in children)	2.15–2.50 mmol/L (Slightly higher in children)
Calcium, ionized, serum	4.64–5.28 mg/dL	1.16–1.32 mmol/L
Calcium, urine		
Low calcium diet	50–150 mg/24 h	1.25–3.75 mmol/24 h
Usual diet; trough	100–300 mg/24 h	2.50–7.50 mmol/24 h

[†]Bilirubin data – Source: https://labs-sec.uhs-sa.com/clinical_ext/dols/soprefrange.asp

Contd.

Laboratory reference range values *(Contd.)*

Tests	Conventional units		SI units
Carbamazepine, serum or plasma (Hep or EDTA), trough			
Therapeutic	4–12 mcg/mL		17–51 mcmol/L
Toxic	>15 mcg/mL		>63 mcmol/L
Carbon dioxide, total, serum/plasma (Hep)	22–28 mmol/L		22–28 mmol/L
Carbon dioxide (PCO_2), blood, arterial			
Male	35–48 mmHg		4.66–6.38 kPa
Female	32–45 mmHg		4.26–5.99 kPa
Carbon monoxide as carboxyhemoglobin (HbCO), whole blood (EDTA)			
Nonsmokers	0.5–1.5% total Hb		0.005–0.015 HbCO fraction
Smokers			
1–2 packs/day	4–5% total Hb		0.04–0.05 HbCO fraction
>2 packs/day	8–9% total Hb		0.08–0.09 HbCO fraction
Toxic	>20% total Hb		>0.20 HbCO fraction
Lethal	>50% total Hb		>0.5 HbCO fraction
Carotene, serum	10–85 mcg/dL		0.19–1.58 mcmol/L
Catecholamines, plasma (EDTA)			
Dopamine	<30 pg/mL		<196 pmol/L
Epinephrine	<140 pg/mL		<764 pmol/L
Norepinephrine	<1700 pg/mL		<10,047 pmol/L
Catecholamines, urine			
Dopamine	65–400 mcg/24 h		425–2610 nmol/24 h
Epinephrine	0–20 mcg/24 h		0–109 nmol/24 h
Norepinephrine	15–80 mcg/24 h		89–473 nmol/24 h
CEA, serum			
Nonsmokers	<5.0 ng/mL		<5.0 mcg/L
*Cell counts, adult			
Erythrocytes			
Male	$4.7–6.1 \times 10^6$/mcL		$4.7–6.1 \times 10^{12}$/L
Female	$4.2–5.4 \times 10^6$/mcL		$4.2–5.4 \times 10^{12}$/L
Leukocytes			
Total	$4.8–10.8 \times 10^3$/mcL		$4.8–10.8 \times 10^6$/L
Differential	Percentage	Absolute	Absolute (SI)
Myelocytes	0	0/mcL	0/L
Neutrophils			
Band	3–5	150–400/mcL	$150–400 \times 10^6$/L
Segmented	54–62	3000–5800/mcL	$3000–5800 \times 10^6$/L
Lymphocytes	20.5–51.1	$1.2–3.4 \times 10^3$/mcL	$1.2–3.4 \times 10^9$/L
Monocytes	1.7–9.3	$0.11–0.59 \times 10^3$/mcL	$0.11–0.59 \times 10^9$/L
Granulocytes	42.2–75.2	$1.4–6.5 \times 10^3$/mcL	$1.4–6.5 \times 10^9$/L
Eosinophils		$0–0.7 \times 10^3$/mcL	$0–0.7 \times 10^9$/L
Basophils		$0–0.2 \times 10^3$/mcL	$0–0.2 \times 10^9$/L
Platelets	$130–400 \times 10^3$/mcL		$130–400 \times 10^9$/L
Reticulocytes	0.5–1.5% RBCs		0.005–0.015 of RBCs
	24,000–84,000/mcL		$24–84 \times 10^9$/L
Cells, CSF	0–10 lymphocytes/mm³		0–10 lymphocytes/mm³
	0 RBC/mm³		0 RBC/mm³
Ceruloplasmin, serum	20–60 mg/dL		0.2–0.6 g/L
Chloramphenicol, serum or plasma (Hep or EDTA); trough			
Therapeutic	10–25 mcg/mL		31–77 mcmol/L
Toxic	>25 mcg/mL		>77 mcmol/L

*Test values dependent on laboratory methods used.

Contd.

Laboratory reference range values *(Contd.)*		
Tests	**Conventional units**	**SI units**
Chloride		
Serum or plasma (Hep)	98–107 mmol/L	98–107 mmol/L
Sweat		
Normal	5–35 mmol/L	5–35 mmol/L
Cystic fibrosis	60–200 mmol/L	60–200 mmol/L
Urine, 24 h (vary greatly with Cl intake)		
Infant	2–10 mmol/24 h	2–10 mmol/24 h
Child	15–40 mmol/24 h	15–40 mmol/24 h
Adult	110–250 mmol/24 h	110–250 mmol/24 h
CSF118–132 mmol/L (20 mmol/L	118–132 mmol/L (20 mmol/L higher than serum)	higher than serum)
Cholesterol, serum		
Adult desirable	<200 mg/dL	<5.2 mmol/L
borderline	200–239 mg/dL	5.2–6.2 mmol/L
high-risk	≥240 mg/dL	≥6.2 mmol/L
*Cholinesterase, serum	4.9–11.9 U/mL	4.9–11.9 kU/L
Dibucaine inhibition	79–84%	0.79–0.84
Fluoride inhibition	58–64%	0.58–0.64
*Chorionic gonadotropin, intact serum or plasma (EDTA)		
Male and nonpregnant female	<5.0 mIU/mL	<5.0 IU/L
Pregnant female	Varies with gestational age	
Urine, qualitative		
Male and nonpregnant female	Negative	Negative
Pregnant female	Positive	Positive
Clonazepam, serum or plasma (Hep or EDTA); trough		
Therapeutic	15–60 ng/mL	48–190 nmol/L
Toxic	>80 ng/mL	>254 nmol/L
Coagulation tests		
Antithrombin III (synthetic substrate)	80–120% of normal	0.8–1.2 of normal
Bleeding time (Duke)	0–6 min	0–6 min
Bleeding time (Ivy)	1–6 min	1–6 min
Bleeding time (template)	2.3–9.5 min	2.3–9.5 min
Clot retraction, qualitative	50–100% in 2 h	0.5–1.0/2 h
Coagulation time (Lee-White)	5–15 min (glass tubes)	5–15 min (glass tubes)
	19–60 min (siliconized tubes)	19–60 min (siliconized tubes)
Cold hemolysin test (Donath-Landsteiner)	No hemolysis	No hemolysis
Complement components		
Total hemolytic complement activity, plasma (EDTA)	75–160 U/mL	75–160 kU/L
Total complement decay rate (functional), plasma (EDTA)		10–20% Fraction decay rate: 0.10–0.20
	Deficiency: >50%	>0.50
C1q, serum	14.9–22.1 mg/dL	149–221 mg/L
C1r, serum	2.5–10.0 mg/dL	25–100 mg/L
C1s(C1 esterase), serum	5.0–10.0 mg/dL	50–100 mg/L
C2, serum	1.6–3.6 mg/dL	16–36 mg/L
C3, serum	90–180 mg/dL	0.9–1.8 g/L
C4, serum	10–40 mg/dL	0.1–0.4 g/L
C5, serum	5.5–11.3 mg/dL	55–113 mg/L
C6, serum	17.9–23.9 mg/dL	179–239 mg/L
C7, serum	2.7–7.4 mg/dL	27–74 mg/L
C8, serum	4.9–10.6 mg/dL	49–106 mg/L
C9, serum	3.3–9.5 mg/dL	33–95 mg/L

*Test values dependent on laboratory methods used.

Contd.

Laboratory reference range values *(Contd.)*

Tests	Conventional units	SI units
Coombs test		
Direct	Negative	Negative
Indirect	Negative	Negative
Copper		
Serum		
Male	70–140 mcg/dL	11–22 mcmol/L
Female	80–155 mcg/dL	13–24 mcmol/L
Urine	3–35 mcg/24 h	0.05–0.55 mcmol/24 h
Corpuscular values of erythrocytes (values are for adults; in children, values vary with age)		
Mean corpuscular hemoglobin (MCH)	27–31 pg	0.42–0.48 fmol
Mean corpuscular hemoglobin concentration (MCHC)	33–37 g/dL	330–370 g/L
Mean corpuscular volume (MCV)		
Male	80–94 mcm^3	80–94 fL
Female	81–99 mcm^3	81–99 fL
Cortisol, serum		
Plasma (Hep, EDTA, Ox)		
8 AM	5–23 mcg/dL	138–635 nmol/L
4 PM	3–16 mcg/dL	83–441 nmol/L
10 PM	<50% of 8 AM value	<0.5 of 8 AM value
Free, urine	<50 mcg/24 h	<138 mmol/24 h
**+Creatine kinase (CK), serum		
Male	15–105 U/L (30°C)	0.26–1.79 mckat/L (30°C)
Female	10–80 U/L (30°C)	0.17–1.36 mckat/L (30°C)
Note: Strenuous exercise or intramuscular injections may elevate transient CK levels.		
*Creatine kinase MB isoenzyme, serum	0–7 ng/mL	0–7 mcg/L
*Creatinine		
Serum or plasma, adult		
Male	0.7–1.3 mg/dL	62–115 mcmol/L
Female	0.6–1.1 mg/dL	53–97 mcmol/L
Urine		
Male	14–26 mg/kg body weight/24 h	124–230 mcmol/kg body weight/24 h
Female	11–20 mg/kg body weight/24 h	97–177 mcmol/kg body weight/24 h
*Creatinine clearance, serum or plasma and urine		
Male	94–140 mL/min/1.73 m^2	0.91–1.35 mL/s/m^2
Female	72–110 mL/min/1.73 m^2	0.69–1.06 mL/s/m^2
Cryoglobulins, serum	0	0
Cyanide		
Serum		
Nonsmokers	0.004 mg/L	0.15 mcmol/L
Smokers	0.006 mg/L	0.23 mcmol/L
Nitroprusside therapy	0.01–0.06 mg/L	0.38–2.30 mcmol/L
Toxic	>0.1 mg/L	>3.84 mcmol/L
Whole blood (Ox)		
Nonsmokers	0.016 mg/L	0.61 mcmol/L
Smokers	0.041 mg/L	1.57 mcmol/L
Nitroprusside therapy	0.05–0.5 mg/L	1.92–19.20 mcmol/L
Toxic	>1 mg/L	>38.40 mcmol/L

**Test values dependent on laboratory methods used.
+Test values dependent on patient's race.

Contd.

Tests	Conventional units	SI units
Laboratory reference range values *(Contd.)*		
Cyclic AMP		
Plasma (EDTA)		
Male	4.6–8.6 ng/mL	14–26 nmol/L
Female	4.3–7.6 ng/mL	13–23 nmol/L
Urine, 24 h	0.3–3.6 mg/day	1.0–10.9 mcmol/day or
	or 0.29–2.1 mg/g creatinine	100–723 mcmol/mol creatinine
Cystine or cysteine, urine, qualitative	Negative	Negative
*C-peptide, serum	0.78–1.89 ng/mL	0.26–0.62 nmol/L
C-reactive protein, serum	<0.5 mg/dL	<5 mg/L
*≠Cyclosporine, whole blood		
Therapeutic, trough	100–200 ng/mL	83–166 nmol/L
Dehydroepiandrostereone (DHEA), serum		
Male	180–1250 ng/dL	6.2–43.3 nmol/L
Female	130–980 ng/dL	4.5–34.0 nmol/L
Dehydroepiandrosterone sulfate (DHEAS)		
serum or plasma (Hep, EDTA)		
Male	59–452 mcg/mL	1.6–12.2 mcmol/L
Female		
Premenopausal	12–379 mcg/mL	0.8–10.2 mcmol/L
Postmenopausal	30–260 mcg/mL	0.8–7.1 mcmol/L
Desipramine, serum or plasma (Hep or EDTA);		
trough (12 h after dose)		
Therapeutic	75–300 ng/mL	281–1125 nmol/L
Toxic	>400 ng/mL	>1500 nmol/L
Diazepam, serum or plasma (Hep or EDTA); trough		
Therapeutic	100–1000 ng/mL	0.35–3.51 mcmol/L
Toxic	>5000 ng/mL	>17.55 mcmol/L
Digitoxin, serum or plasma (Hep or EDTA); 7.8 h after dose		
Therapeutic	20–35 ng/mL	26–46 nmol/L
Toxic	>45 ng/mL	>59 nmol/L
Digoxin, serum or plasma (Hep or EDTA); ≥12 h after dose		
Therapeutic		
CHF	0.8–1.5 ng/mL	1.0–1.9 nmol/L
Arrhythmias	1.5–2.0 ng/mL	1.9–2.6 nmol/L
Toxic		
Adult	>2.5 ng/mL	>3.2 nmol/L
Child	>3.0 ng/mL	>3.8 nmol/L
Disopyramide, serum or plasma (Hep or EDTA); trough		
Therapeutic arrhythmias		
Atrial	2.8–3.2 mcg/mL	8.3–9.4 mcmol/L
Ventricular	3.3–7.5 mcg/mL	9.7–22 mcmol/L
Toxic	>7 mcg/mL	>20.7 mcmol/L
Doxepin, serum or plasma (Hep or EDTA);		
trough (≥12 h after dose)		
Therapeutic	150–250 ng/mL	537–895 nmol/L
Toxic	>500 ng/mL	>1790 nmol/L
*Estradiol, serum		
Adult		
Male	10–50 pg/mL	37–184 pmol/L
Female	Varies with menstrual cycle	

*Test values dependent on laboratory methods used.
≠Actual therapeutic range should be adjusted for individual patient.

Contd.

Laboratory reference range values *(Contd.)*

Tests	Conventional units	SI units
Ethanol (alcohol), whole blood (Ox) or serum		
Depression of CNS	>100 mg/dL	>21.7 mmol/L
Fatalities reported	>400 mg/dL	>86.8 mmol/L
Ethosuximide, serum or plasma (Hep or EDTA); trough		
Therapeutic	40–100 mcg/mL	283–708 mcmol/L
Toxic	>150 mcg/mL	>1062 mcmol/L
Euglobin lysis	No lysis in 2 h	No lysis in 2 h
α-fetoprotein (AFP), serum	<15 ng/mL	<15 mcg/L
††Fat, fecal, F, 72 h		
Infant, breast-fed	<1 g/day	
Pediatrics (0–6 years)	<2 g/day	
Adult	<7 g/day	
Adult (fat-free diet)	<4 g/day	
§Fatty acids, total, serum	190–240 mg/dL	7–15 mmol/L
Nonesterified, serum	8–25 mg/dL	0.28–0.89 mmol/L
Ferritin, serum		
Male	20–150 ng/mL	20–250 mcg/L
Female	10–120 ng/mL	10–120 mcg/L
Ferritin values of <20 ng/mL (20 mcg/L) have been reported to be generally associated with depleted iron stores.		
Fibrin degradation products	<10 mcg/mL	<10 mg/L
*Fibrinogen, plasma (NaCit)	200–400 mg/dL	2–4 g/L
Fluoride		
Plasma (Hep)	0.01–0.2 mcg/mL	0.5–10.5 mcmol/L
Urine	0.2–3.2 mcg/mL	10.5–168 mcmol/L
Urine, occupational exposure	<8 mcg/mL	<421 mcmol/L
*Folate, Serum RBCs	3–20 ng/mL	7–45 nmol/L
Erythrocytes	140–628 ng/mL RBC	317–1422 nmol/L RBC
*Follicle-stimulating hormone (FSH), serum and plasma (Hep)		
Male	1.4–15.4 mIU/mL	1.4–15.4 IU/L
Female		
Follicular phase	1–10 mIU/mL	1–10 IU/L
Mid-cycle	6–17 mIU/mL	6–17 IU/L
Luteal phase	1–9 mIU/mL	1–9 IU/L
Postmenopausal	19–100 mIU/mL	19–100 IU/L
*Free thyroxine index (FTI), serum	4.2–13	4.2–13
Gastrin, serum	<100 pg/mL	<100 ng/L
Gentamicin, serum or plasma (EDTA)		
Therapeutic		
Peak		
Less severe infection	5–8 mcg/mL	10.4–16.7 mcmol
Severe infection	8–10 mcg/mL	16.7–20.9 mcmol/L
Trough		
Less severe infection	<1 mcg/mL	<2.1 mcmol/L
Moderate infection	<2 mcg/mL	<4.2 mcmol/L
Severe infection	<2–4 mcg/mL	<4.2–8.4 mcmol/L

*Test values dependent on laboratory methods used.

††Reference values vary from laboratory to laboratory, but are generally found within the range of 5–7 g/day. It should be noted that children, especially infants, cannot ingest the 100 g/day of fat that is suggested for the test. Therefore, a fat retention coefficient is determined by measuring the difference between ingested fat and fecal fat, and expressing that difference as a percentage. The figure, called the fat retention coefficient, is 95% or greater in healthy children and adults. A low value indicates steatorrhea.
http://www.labcorp.com/datasets/labcorp/html/chapter/mono/sc008000.htm

§'Fatty acids' include a mixture of different aliphatic acids of varying molecular weight; a mean molecular weight of 284 daltons has been assumed.

Contd.

Laboratory reference range values *(Contd.)*		
Tests	**Conventional units**	**SI units**
Toxic		
Peak	>10–12 mcg/mL	>21–25 mcmol/L
Trough	>2–4 mcg/mL	>4.2–8.4 mcmol/L
Glucose (fasting)		
Blood	65–95 mg/dL	3.5–5.3 mmol/L
Plasma or serum	74–106 mg/dL	4.1–5.9 mmol/L
Glucose, 2 h postprandial, serum	<120 mg/dL	<6.7 mmol/L
Glucose, urine		
Quantitative	<500 mg/24 h	<2.8 mmol/24 h
Qualitative	Negative	Negative
Glucose, CSF	40–70 mg/dL	2.2–3.9 mmol/L
*Glucose-6-phosphate	12.1 ± 2.1 U/g Hb (SD)	0.78 ± 0.13 mU/mol Hb
dehydrogenase	351 ± 60.6 U/10^{12} RBC	0.35 ± 0.06 nU/RBC
in erythrocytes, whole blood (ACD, EDTA, or Hᴇp)	4.11 ± 0.71 U/mL RBC	4.11 ± 0.71 kU/L RBC
γ-glutamyltransfersae serum		
Males	2–30 U/L (37°C)	0.03–0.51 mckat/L (37°C)
Females	1–24 U/L (37°C)	0.02–0.41 mckat/L (37°C)
Glutethimide, serum		
Therapeutic	2–6 mcg/mL	9–28 mcmol/L
Toxic	>5 mcg/mL	>23 mcmol/L
Glycated hemoglobin (hemoglobin A1c), whole blood (EDTA)	4.2–5.9%	0.042–0.059
Growth hormone, serum		
Male	<5 ng/mL	<5 mcg/L
Female	<10 ng/mL	<10 mcg/L
Haptoglobin, serum	30–200 mg/dL	0.3–2.0 g/L
†HDL-lipid panel		
Cholesterol, HDL	>40 mg/dL	
Cholesterol, LDL (calculated)		
optimal	<100 mg/dL	
near optimal	100–129 mg/dL	
borderline high	130–159 mg/dL	
high	>160 mg/dL	
Cholesterol, total		
0–1 year	50–120 mg/dL	
1–2 years	70–190 mg/dL	
2–16 years	120–220 mg/dL	
>16 years	0–199 mg/dL	
desirable	<200 mg/dL	
borderline	200–239 mg/dL	
high	>240 mg/dL	
¶Tryglycerides		
desirable	<150 mg/dL	
borderline high	150–199 mg/dL	
high	>200 mg/dL	
Hematocrit		
Males	42–52%	0.42–0.52
Females	37–47%	0.37–0.47
Newborn	53–65%	0.53–0.65
Children (varies with age)	30–43%	0.30–0.43

*Test values dependent on laboratory methods used.
¶If the triglyceride value is >400 mg/dL, the LDL calculation is invalid.
http://webserver 01.bjc.org/slch/pro/Professional.htm?http://webserver01.bjc.org/labtestguide/Lab%20Test%20Guide
book/slchlabsiteoneline.htm

Contd.

Laboratory reference range values (Contd.)

Tests	Conventional units	SI units
Hemoglobin (Hb)		
Males	14.0–18.0 g/dL	2.17–2.79 mmol/L
Females	12.0–16.0 g/dL	1.86–2.48 mmol/L
Newborn	17.0–23.0 g/dL	2.64–3.57 mmol/L
Children (varies with age)	11.2–16.5 g/dL	1.74–2.56 mmol/L
Hemoglobin, fetal	≥1 year old: <2% of total Hb	≥1 year old: <0.02% of total Hb
Hemoglobin, plasma	<3 mg/dL	<0.47 mcmol/L
Hemoglobin and myoglobin, urine, qualitative	Negative	Negative
Hemoglobin electrophoresis, whole blood (EDTA, Cit, or Hep)		
HbA	>95%	>0.95 Hb fraction
HbA$_2$	1.5–3.7%	0.015–0.037 Hb fraction
HbF	<2%	<0.02 Hb fraction
Homogentisic acid, urine, qualitative	Negative	Negative
β-hydroxybutyric acid, serum, plasma	0.21–2.81 mg/dL	20–270 mcmol/L
17-hydroxycorticosteroids		
Urine		
Males	3–10 mg/24 h	8.3–27.6 mcmol/24 h (as cortisol)
Females	2–8 mg/24 h	5.5–22 mcmol/24 h (as cortisol)
5-hydroxyindoleacetic acid, urine		
Qualitative	Negative	Negative
Quantitative	2–7 mg/24 h	10.4–36.6 mcmol/24 h
Imipramine, serum or plasma (Hep or EDTA); trough (≥12 h after dose)		
Therapeutic	150–250 ng/mL	536–893 nmol/L
Toxic	>500 ng/mL	>1785 nmol/L
Immunoglobulins, serum		
IgG	700–1600 mg/dL	7–16 g/L
IgA	70–400 mg/dL	0.7–4.0 g/L
IgM	40–230 mg/dL	0.4–2.3 g/L
IgD	0–8 mg/dL	0–80 mg/L
IgE	3–423 IU/mL	3–423 kIU/L
Immunoglobulin G (IgC), CSF	0.5–6.1 mg/dL	0.5–6.1 g/L
Insulin, plasma (fasting)	2–25 mcU/mL	13–174 pmol/L
*Iron, serum		
Males	65–175 mcg/dL	11.6–31.3 mcmol/L
Females	50–170 mcg/dL	9.0–30.4 mcmol/L
Iron binding capacity, serum, total (TIBC)	250–425 mcg/dL	44.8–71.6 mcmol/L
Iron saturation, serum		
Male	20–50%	0.2–0.5
Female	15–50%	0.15–0.5
17-ketosteroids, urine		
Males	10–25 mg/24 h	38–87 mcmol/24 h
Females	6–14 mg/24 h (decreases with age)	21–52 mcmol/24 h (decreases with age)
L-lactate		
Plasma (NaF)		
Venous	4.5–19.8 mg/dL	0.5–2.2 mmol/L
Arterial	4.5–14.4 mg/dL	0.5–1.6 mmol/L
Whole blood (Hep), at bed rest		
Venous	8.1–15.3 mg/dL	0.9–1.7 mmol/L
Arterial	<11.3 mg/dL	<1.3 mmol/L
Urine, 24 h	496–1982 mg/day	5.5–22 mmol/day
CSF	10–22 mg/dL	1.1–2.4 mmol/L

*Test values dependent on laboratory methods used.

Contd.

Laboratory reference range values *(Contd.)*

Tests	Conventional units	SI units
*Lactate dehydrogenase		
Total (L → P), 37°C, serum		
Newborn	290–775 U/L	4.9–13.2 mckat/L
Neonate	545–2000 U/L	9.3–34 mckat/L
Infant	180–430 U/L	3.1–7.3 mckat/L
Child	110–295 U/L	1.9–5 mckat/L
Adult	100–190 U/L	1.7–3.2 mckat/L
>60 year	110–210 U/L	1.9–3.6 mckat/L
*Isoenzymes, serum by agarose gel electrophoresis		
Fraction 1	14–26% of total	0.14–0.26 fraction of total
Fraction 2	29–39% of total	0.29–0.39 fraction of total
Fraction 3	20–26% of total	0.20–0.26 fraction of total
Fraction 4	8–16% of total	0.08–0.16 fraction of total
Fraction 5	6–16% of total	0.06–0.16 fraction of total
*Lactate dehydrogenase, CSF	10% of serum value	0.10 fraction of serum value
LDL-cholesterol (LDL-C), serum or plasma (EDTA)		
Adult desirable	<130 mg/dL	<0.2 mmol/L
borderline	130–159 mg/dL	3.37–4.12 mmol/L
high risk	≥160 mg/dL	≥4.13 mmol/L
Lead,		
Whole blood (Hep)	<25 mcg/dL	<0.48 mcmol/L
Urine, 24 h	<80 mcg/day	<0.39 mcmol/day
Lecithin-sphingomyelin (L:S) ratio, amniotic fluid	2.0–5.0 indicates probable fetal lung maturity; >3.5 in diabetic patients	2.0–5.0 indicates probable fetal lung maturity; >3.5 in diabetic patients
Lidocaine, serum or plasma (Hep or EDTA); 45 min after bolus dose		
Therapeutic	1.5–6.0 mcg/mL	6.4–26 mcmol/L
Toxic		
CNS, cardiovascular depression	6–8 mcg/mL	26–34.2 mcmol/L
Seizures, obtundation, decreased cardiac output	>8 mcg/mL	>34.2 mcmol/L
*Lipase, serum	23–300 U/L (37°C)	0.39–5.1 mckat/L (37°C)
Lithium, serum or plasma (Hep or EDTA); 12 h after last dose		
Therapeutic	0.6–1.2 mEq/L	0.6–1.2 mmol/L
Toxic	>2 mEq/L	>2 mmol/L
Lorazepam, serum or plasma (Hep or EDTA), therapeutic	50–240 ng/mL	156–746 nmol/L
*Luteinizing hormone (LH), serum or plasma (Hep)		
Male	1.24–7.8 mIU/mL	1.24–7.8 IU/L
Female		
Follicular phase	1.68–15.0 mIU/mL	1.68–15.0 IU/L
Mid-cycle peak	21.9–56.6 mIU/mL	21.9–56.6 IU/L
Luteal phase	0.61–16.3 mIU/mL	0.61–16.3 IU/L
Postmenopausal	14.2–52.5 mIU/mL	14.2–52.3 IU/L
Magnesium		
Serum	1.3–2.1 mEq/L	0.65–1.07 mmol/L
	1.6–2.6 mg/dL	16–26 mg/L
Urine	6.0–10.0 mEq/24 h	3.0–5.0 mmol/24 h
Mercury		
Whole blood (EDTA)	0.6–59 mcg/L	<0.29 mcmol/L
Urine, 24 h	<20 mcg/day	<0.1 mcmol/day
Toxic	>150 mcg/day	>0.75 mcmol/day

*Test values dependent on laboratory methods used.

Contd.

Laboratory reference range values *(Contd.)*		
Tests	**Conventional units**	**SI units**
Metanephrines, total, urine	0.1–1.6 mg/24 h	0.5–8.1 mcmol/24 h
Methemoglobin	0.06–0.24 g/dL or	9.3–37.2 mcmol/L or
(hemoglobin), whole	0.78 ± 0.37% of total Hb (SD)	mass fraction of total Hb:
blood (EDTA, Hep or ACD)		0.008 ± 0.0037 (SD)
Methotrexate, serum or plasma (Hep or EDTA)		
Therapeutic	Variable	Variable
Toxic		
1–2 week after low dose therapy	≥0.02 mcmol/L	≥0.02 mcmol/L
post IV infusion 24 h	≥5 mcmol/L	≥5 mcmol/L
48 h	≥0.5 mcmol/L	≥0.5 mcmol/L
72 h	≥0.05 mcmol/L	≥0.05 mcmol/L
Myelin basic protein, CSF	<2.5 ng/mL	<2.5 mcg/L
Myoglobin, serum	<85 ng/mL	<85 mcg/L
Nortriptyline, serum or plasma (Hep or EDTA); trough (≥12 h after dose)		
Therapeutic	50–150 ng/mL	190–570 nmol/L
Toxic	>500 ng/mL	>1900 nmol/L
*5'-nucleotidase, serum	2–17 U/L	0.034–0.29 mckat/L
N-acetylprocainamide, serum or plasma (Hep or EDTA); trough		
Therapeutic	5–30 mcg/mL	18–108 mcmol/L
Toxic	>40 mcg/mL	>144 mcmol/L
Occult blood, feces, random	Negative (<2 mL blood/150 g stool/day)	Negative (<13.3 mL blood/kg stool/day)
Qualitative, urine, random	Negative	Negative
Osmolality		
Serum	275–295 mOsm/kg serum water	275–295 mmol/kg serum water
Urine	50–1200 mOsm/kg water	50–1200 mmol/kg water
Ratio, urine:serum	1.0–3.0	1.0–3.0
	3.0–4.7 after 12 h fluid restriction	3.0–4.7 after 12 h fluid restriction
Osmotic fragility of erythrocytes	Begins in 0.45–0.39% NaCl	Begins in 77–67 mmol/L NaCl
	Complete in 0.33–0.30% NaCl	Complete in 56–51 mmol/L NaCl
Oxazepam, serum or plasma (Hep or EDTA), therapeutic	0.2–1.4 mcg/mL	0.70–4.9 mcmol/L
Oxygen, blood		
Capacity	16–24 vol% (varies with hemoglobin)	7.14–10.7 mmol/L (varies with hemoglobin)
Content		
Arterial	15–23 vol%	6.69–10.3 mmol/L
Venous	10–16 vol%	4.46–7.14 mmol/L
Saturation		
Arterial and capillary	95–98% of capacity	0.95–0.98 of capacity
Venous	60–85% of capacity	0.60–0.85 of capacity
Tension		
pO_2 arterial and capillary	83–108 mmHg	11.1–14.4 kPa
Venous	35–45 mmHg	4.6–6.0 kPa
P50, blood	25–29 mmHg (adjusted to pH 7.4)	3.33–3.86 kPa
Partial thromboplastin time activated (APTT)	<35 sec	<35 sec
Pentobarbital, serum or plasma (Hep or EDTA); trough		
Therapeutic		
Hypnotic	1–5 mcg/mL	4–22 mcmol/L
Therapeutic coma	20–50 mcg/mL	88–221 mcmol/L

*Test values dependent on laboratory methods used.

Contd.

Laboratory reference range values *(Contd.)*		
Tests	**Conventional units**	**SI units**
Toxic	>10 mcg/mL	>44 mcmol/L
pH		
Blood, arterial	7.35–7.45	7.35–7.45
Urine	4.6–8.0 (depends on diet)	Same
Phenacetin, plasma (EDTA)		
Therapeutic	1–30 mcg/mL	6–167 mcmol/L
Toxic	50–250 mcg/mL	279–1395 mcmol/L
Phenobarbital, serum or plasma (Hep or EDTA); trough		
Therapeutic	15–40 mcg/mL	65–172 mcmol/L
Toxic		
Slowness, ataxia, nystagmus	35–80 mcg/mL	151–345 mcmol/L
Coma with reflexes	65–117 mcg/mL	280–504 mcmol/L
Coma without reflexes	>100 mcg/mL	>430 mcmol/L
Phenolsulfonphthalein (PSP) excretion, urine	28–51% in 15 min	0.28–0.51 in 15 min
	13–24% in 30 min	0.13–0.24 in 30 min
	9–17% in 60 min	0.09–0.17 in 60 min
	3–10% in 2 h	0.03–0.10 in 2 h
	(After injection of 1 mL PSP intravenously)	(After injection of 1 mL PSP intravenously)
Phenylalanine, serum	0.8–1.8 mg/dL	48–109 mcmol/L
Phenytoin, serum or plasma (Hep or EDTA); trough		
Therapeutic	10–20 mcg/mL	40–79 mcmol/L
Toxic	>20 mcg/mL	>79 mcmol/L
*Phosphatase, acid, prostatic, serum radioimmunoassay	<3.0 ng/mL	<3.0 mcg/L
*Phosphatase, alkaline, total, serum	38–126 U/L (37°C)	0.65–2.14 mckat/L
Phosphate, inorganic, serum		
Adults	2.7–4.5 mg/dL	0.87–1.45 mmol/L
Children	4.5–5.5 mg/dL	1.45–1.78 mmol/L
Phosphatidylglycerol, amniotic fluid		
Fetal lung immaturity	absent	absent
Fetal lung maturity	present	present
Phospholipids, serum	125–275 mg/dL	1.25–2.75 g/L
Phosphorus, urine	0.4–1.3 g/24 h	12.9–42 mmol/24 h
Porphobilinogen, urine		
Qualitative	Negative	Negative
Quantitative	<2.0 mg/24 h	<9 mcmol/24 h
Porphyrins, urine		
Coproporphyrin	34–230 mcg/24 h	52–351 nmol/24 h
Uroporphyrin	27–52 mcg/24 h	32–63 nmol/24 h
Potassium, plasma (Hep)		
Males	3.5–4.5 mEq/L	3.5–4.5 mmol/L
Females	3.4–4.4 mEq/L	3.4–4.4 mmol/L
Potassium		
Serum		
Premature		
Cord	5.0–10.2 mEq/L	5.0–10.2 mmol/L
48 h	3.0–6.0 mEq/L	3.0–6.0 mmol/L
Newborn, cord	5.6–12.0 mEq/L	5.6–12.0 mmol/L
Newborn	3.7–5.9 mEq/L	3.7–5.9 mmol/L
Infant	4.1–5.3 mEq/L	4.1–5.3 mmol/L
Child	3.4–4.7 mEq/L	3.4–4.7 mmol/L

*Test values dependent on laboratory methods used.

Contd.

Laboratory reference range values *(Contd.)*		
Tests	Conventional units	SI units
Adult	3.5–5.1 mEq/L	3.5–5.1 mmol/L
Urine, 24 h	25–125 mEq/d, varies with diet	25–125 mmol/d; varies with diet
CSF70% of plasma level or 2.5–3.2	0.70 of plasma level or 2.5–3.2 mEq/L; rises with plasma hyperosmolality	mmol/L; rises with plasma hyperosmolality
Prealbumin (transthyretin), serum	10–40 mg/dL	100–400 mg/L
Primidone, serum or plasma (Hep or EDTA); trough		
Therapeutic	5–12 mcg/mL	23–55 mcmol/L
Toxic	>15 mcg/mL	>69 mcmol/L
Procainamide, serum or plasma (Hep or EDTA); trough		
Therapeutic	4–10 mcg/mL	17–42 mcmol/L
Toxic (also consider effect of metabolite, i.e. NAPA)	>10–12 mcg/mL	>42–51 mcmol/L
*Progesterone, serum		
Adult		
Male	13–97 ng/dL	0.4–3.1 nmol/L
Female		
Follicular phase	15–70 ng/dL	0.5–2.2 nmol/L
Luteal phase	200–2500 ng/dL	6.4–79.5 nmol/L
Pregnancy	Varies with gestational week	
*Prolactin, serum		
Males	2.5–15.0 ng/mL	2.5–15.0 mcg/L
Females	2.5–19.0 ng/mL	2.5–19.0 mcg/L
Propoxyphene, plasma (EDTA)		
Therapeutic	0.1–0.4 mcg/mL	0.3–1.2 mcmol/L
Toxic	>0.5 mcg/mL	>1.5 mcmol/L
Propranolol, serum or plasma (Hep or EDTA); trough		
Therapeutic	50–100 ng/mL	193–386 nmol/L
*Prostate-specific antigen (PSA), serum		
Male	<4.0 ng/mL	<4.0 mcg/L
*Protein, serum		
Total	6.4–8.3 g/dL	64–83 g/L
Albumin	3.9–5.1 g/dL	39–51 g/L
Globulin		
α_1	0.2–0.4 g/dL	2–4 g/L
α_2	0.4–0.8 g/dL	4–8 g/L
β	0.5–1.0 g/dL	5–10 g/L
γ	0.6–1.3 g/dL	6–13 g/L
Urine		
Qualitative	Negative	Negative
Quantitative	50–80 mg/24 h (at rest)	Same
CSF, total	8–32 mg/dL	80–320 mg/dL
Prothrombin consumption	>20 sec	>20 sec
Prothrombin time-international normalized ratio (see NOTES below)		
INR: birth–6 months	1.0–1.6	
INR: 6 months–adult	0.9–1.2	
Protoporphyrin, total, WB	<60 mcg/dL	<600 mcg/L
Pyruvate, blood	0.3–0.9 mg/dL	34–103 mcmol/L
Quinidine, serum or plasma (Hep or EDTA); trough		
Therapeutic	2–5 mcg/mL	6–15 mcmol/L
Toxic	>6 mcg/mL	>18 mcmol/L

*Test values dependent on laboratory methods used.

Contd.

Tests	Conventional units	SI units
Laboratory reference range values *(Contd.)*		
Salicylates, serum or plasma (Hep or EDTA); trough		
Therapeutic	150–300 mcg/mL	1.09–2.17 mmol/L
Toxic	>500 mcg/mL	>3.62 mmol/L
#Sedimentation rate, erythrocyte		
Westergren		
Male: 0–50 years	0–15 mm/h	
Male: >50 years	0–20 mm/h	
Female: 0–50 years	0–20 mm/h	
Female: >50 years	0–30 mm/h	
Wintrobe		
Males	<10 mm/h	
Females	<20 mm/h	
Critical value	>75 mm/h	
Sodium		
Serum or plasma (Hep)		
Premature		
Cord	116–140 mEq/L	116–140 mmol/L
48 h	128–148 mEq/L	128–148 mmol/L
Newborn, cord	126–166 mEq/L	126–166 mmol/L
Newborn	133–146 mEq/L	133–146 mmol/L
Infant	139–146 mEq/L	139–146 mmol/L
Child	138–145 mEq/L	138–145 mmol/L
Adult	136–145 mEq/L	136–145 mmol/L
Urine, 24 h	40–220 mEq/day (diet dependent)	40–220 mmol/day (diet dependent)
Sweat		
Normal	10–40 mEq/L	10–40 mmol/L
Cystic fibrosis	70–190 mEq/L	70–190 mmol/L
Specific gravity, urine	1.002–1.030	1.002–1.030
*Testosterone, serum		
Male	280–1100 ng/dL	0.52–38.17 nmol/L
Female	15–70 ng/dL	0.52–2.43 nmol/L
Pregnancy	3–4 × Normal	3–4 × Normal
Postmenopausal	8–35 ng/dL	0.28–1.22 nmol/L

NOTE: INR=[(Patient PT)/(Normal PT)] *ISI, where ISI, is the international sensitivity index, a value provided by the reagent manufacturer.

NOTE: Target therapeutic range (international normalized ratio) of 2.0–3.0. http://pediatrics.aappublications.org/cgi/content/full/112/5/e386

NOTE: The American College of Chest Physicians has recommended a therapeutic INR range for adults of 2.0–3.0, except in patients with mechanical cardiac valves who should have an INR of 2.5–3.5. 1.

Target INR range of 2.6–3.8 for children with heart disease and a slightly lower range of 2.1–3.3 for treating children with established venous thrombosis. Clinicians at Toronto's Hospital for Sick Children used an INR range of 2.0–3.0 initially but later found that a lower target of 1.3–1.8 was as effective and resulted in no bleeding complications. http://www.healthsystem.virginia.edu/internet/pediatrics/pharma-news/jan95.pdf

NOTE: The recommended therapeutic target for the treatment and prevention of venous thromboembolisms and pulmonary embolisms in an INR of 2.5 with a range between 2.0–3.0, and children with mechanical prosthetic heart valves have a recommended therapeutic INR range of 3.0 INR range between 2.5–3.5. Evaluate at that time. http://www.warfarinfo.com/pediatrics.htm

*Test values dependent on laboratory methods used.

#http://www.labcorp.com/datasets/labcorp/html/chapter/mono/he005000.htm;

http://www.utmb.edu/lsg/Lab Survival Guide/hem/Sedimentation_Rate.htm

Contd.

Laboratory reference range values *(Contd.)*		
Tests	**Conventional units**	**SI units**
Theophylline, serum or plasma (Hep or EDTA)		
Therapeutic		
Bronchodilator	8–20 mcg/mL	44–111 mcmol/L
Prem. apnea	6–13 mcg/mL	33–72 mcmol/L
Toxic	>20 mcg/mL	>110 mcmol/L
Thiocyanate		
Serum or plasma (EDTA)		
Nonsmoker	1–4 mcg/mL	17–69 mcmol/L
Smoker	3–12 mcg/mL	52–206 mcmol/L
Therapeutic after nitroprusside infusion	6–29 mcg/mL	103–499 mcmol/L
Urine		
Nonsmoker	1–4 mg/day	17–69 mcmol/day
Smoker	7–17 mg/day	120–292 mcmol/day
Thiopental, serum or plasma (Hep or EDTA); trough		
Hypnotic	1.0–5.0 mcg/mL	4.1–20.7 mcmol/L
Coma	30–100 mcg/mL	124–413 mcmol/L
Anesthesia	7–130 mcg/mL	29–536 mcmol/L
Toxic concentration	>10 mcg/mL	>41 mcmol/L
*Thyroid-stimulating hormone (TSH), serum	0.4–4.2 mcU/mL	0.4–4.2 mU/L
Thyroxine serum	5–12 mcg/dL (varies with age, higher in children and pregnant women)	65–155 nmol/L (vaires with age, higher in children and pregnant women)
*Thyroxine, free, serum	0.8–2.7 ng/dL	10.3–35 pmol/L
Thyroxine binding globulin (TBG), serum	1.2–3.0 mg/dL	12–30 mg/L
Tobramycin, serum or plasma (Hep or EDTA)		
Therapeutic		
Peak		
Less severe infection	5–8 mcg/mL	11–17 mcmol/L
Severe infection	8–10 mcg/mL	17–21 mcmol/L
Trough		
Less severe infection	<1 mcg/mL	<2 mcmol/L
Moderate infection	<2 mcg/mL	<4 mcmol/L
Severe infection	<2–4 mcg/mL	<4–9 mcmol/L
Toxic		
Peak	>10–12 mcg/mL	>21–26 mcmol/L
Trough	>2–4 mcg/mL	>4–9 mcmol/L
Transferrin, serum		
Newborn	130–275 mg/dL	1.30–2.75 g/L
Adult	212–360 mg/dL	2.12–3.60 g/L
>60 years	190–375 mg/dL	1.9–3.75 g/L
Triglycerides, serum, fasting		
Desirable	<250 mg/dL	<2.83 mmol/L
Borderline high	250–500 mg/dL	2.83–5.67 mmol/L
Hypertriglyceridemia	>500 mg/dL	>5.65 mmol/L
*Triiodothyronine, total (T_3) serum	100–200 ng/dL	1.54–3.8 nmol/L
*Troponin-I, cardiac, serum	Undetectable	Undetectable
Troponin-T, cardiac, serum	Undetectable	Undetectable
Urea nitrogen, serum	6–20 mg/dL	2.1–7.1 mmol urea/L
Urea nitrogen:creatinine ratio, serum	12:1 to 20:1	48–80 urea:creatinine mole ratio
*Uric acid		
Serum, enzymatic		
Male	4.5–8.0 mg/dL	0.27–0.47 mmol/L
Female	2.5–6.2 mg/dL	0.15–0.37 mmol/L

*Test values dependent on laboratory methods used.

Contd.

Tests	Conventional units	SI units
Child	2.0–5.5 mg/dL	0.12–0.32 mmol/L
Urine	250–750 mg/24 h (with normal diet)	1.48–4.43 mmol/24 h (with normal diet)
Urobilinogen, urine	0.1–0.8 Ehrlich unit/2 h	0.1–0.8 Eu/2h
	0.5–4.0 Eu/day	0.5–4.0 Eu/day
Valproic acid, serum or plasma (Hep or EDTA); trough		
Therapeutic	50–100 mcg/mL	347–693 mcmol/L
Toxic	>100 mcg/mL	>693 mcmol/L
Vancomycin, serum or plasma (Hep or EDTA);		
Therapeutic		
Peak	20–40 mcg/mL	14–28 mcmol/L
Trough	5–10 mcg/mL	3–7 mcmol/L
Toxic	>80–100 mcg/mL	>55–69 mcmol/L
Vanillylmandelic acid (VMA), urine (4-hydroxy-3-methoxymandelic acid)	1.4–6.5 mg/24 h	7–33 mcmol/day
Viscosity, serum	1.00–1 24 cP	1.00–1.24 cP
Vitamin A, serum	30–80 mcg/dL	1.05–2.8 mcmol/L
Vitamin B12, serum	110–800 pg/mL	81–590 pmol/L
Vitamin E, serum		
Normal	5–18 mcg/mL	12–42 mcmol/L
Therapeutic	30–50 mcg/mL	69.6–116 mcmol/L
Zinc, serum	70–120 mcg/dL	10.7–18.4 mcmol/L

*Test values dependent on laboratory methods used.

ABBREVIATIONS

ACD—acid-citrate-dextrose

AMP—adenosine monophosphate

CEA—carcinoembryonic antigen

CHF—congestive heart failure

Cit—citrate

Cl—chlorine

CNS—central nervous system

CSF—cerebrospinal fluid

Cyclic AMP—adenosine 3´,5´-cyclic phosphate

EDTA—ethylenediaminetetraacetic acid

Hb—hemoglobin

HDL—high-density lipoprotein

Hep—heparin

LDL-C—low-density lipoprotein-cholesterol

MB—myoglobin

NaCit—sodium citrate

NAPA—*N*-acetylprocainomide

Ox—oxalate

RBC—red blood cell(s)

RIA—radioimmunoassay

SD—standard deviation

WBC—white blood cell(s)

BIBLIOGRAPHY

1. Burtis CA, Ashwood ER. eds. Tietz textbook of clinical chemistry, 3rd ed. Philadelphia; WB Saunders, 1998.

2. Children's Hospital, St. Louis, The Department of Clinical Laboratories, High Density Lipoprotein Lipid Panel: Cholesterol, HDL, Cholesterol, LDL (calculated), Cholesterol, Total, Triglycerides, Parathyroid Hormone (PTH). Available at
http://webserver01.bjc.org/slch/pro/Professional. htm? http://webserver01.bjc.org/labtestguide/Lab% 20 Test %20 Guidebook/slchlabsiteoutline.htm. Accessed April 20, 2004.

3. Clinical chemistry laboratory: Reference range values in clinical chemistry. Professional services manual. Baltimore, Department of Pathology, University of Maryland Medical System, 1999.

4. Harmening DM, ed. Hematologic values in chemical hematology and fundamentals of hemostasis, 2nd ed. Philadelphia: FA Davis, 1992.

5. Laboratory Corporation of America, Erythrocyte Sedimentation Rate, Westergren. Available at
http://www.labcorp.com/datasets/labcorp/html/ chapter/mono/he005000.htm. Accessed April 20, 2004.

6. Laboratory Corporation of America. Fecal Fat. Quantitative. Available at
http://www.labcorp.com/datasets/labcorp/html/ chapter/mono/sc008000.htm. Accessed April 20, 2004.

7. National cholesterol education program: Report of the expert panel on detection, evaluation, and treatment of high blood cholesterol in adults. Arch Intern Med 1988; 148: 36–69.

8. Triglyceride, high density lipoprotein and coronary heart disease. National Institute of Health Consensus Statement, NIH Consensus Development Conference, 1992;10(2).

9. University of Texas Health Center at San Antonio. Neonatal Bilirubin. Available at http://labs-sec.uhs-sa.com/clinical_ext/dols/soprefrange.aps. Accessed April 20, 2004.

10. University of Texas Medical Branch. Erythrocyte Sedimentation Rate, Wintrobe. Available at http://www.utmb.edu/lsg/LabSurvivalGuide/hem/Sedimentation_Rate.htm. Accessed April 20, 2004.

11. University of Virginia Children's Medical Center. Therapy Review: Warfarin (Coumadin®). *Pediatric Pharmacotherapy*. January 1995;1(5):386.

    Available at http://www.people.virginia.edu/~smb4v/cmchome.html. Accessed April 20, 2004.

12. Wafarin Therapy in Children Who Require Long-Term Total Parenteral Nutrition. *Pediatrics* [electronic article]. November 2003; 112(5):386.

    Available at http://pediatrics.aappublications.org/cgi/content/full/112/5/e386. Accessed April 20, 2004.

Appendix B

CORAL CLINICAL SYSTEMS

(A Division of Tulip Diagnostics (P) Ltd.)

Tulip Diagnostics (P) Ltd., is the leading Indian group of diagnostic companies, which is involved in the manufacture and marketing of *in-vitro* diagnostic reagents and kits both nationally and internationally. It believes in 'Better testing systems for better diagnostics and preventive health'. Most of the group's products are chartered engineer (CE) certified and are exported to over 87 countries worldwide.

Coral Clinical Systems, a division of Tulip Diagnostics (P) Ltd., offers the medical laboratory professionals a comprehensive range of clinical biochemistry products and instrumentation systems that are designed to perform as per internationally accepted standards.

A market leader within *in-vitro* diagnostics industry, Coral Clinical Systems develops innovative diagnostic solutions for hospital, clinical research and molecular labs thus offering customers improved efficiency, quality, cost effectiveness, and flexibility.

Product range	
Clinical chemistry range	Chemical kits
	Enzymatic kits
	Metals and ions
	Calkine kits
	Controls and calibrators
	System packs for coralyzer series of instruments
	System packs for BT1500
Immunoturbidimetry range	Quantia (multistandard)
	Turbilyte (single standard)
	Quantia system packs
Hematology reagents	
Laboratory reagents	
Instruments	Semi-automated clinical chemistry/ Turbidimetry analyzers
	Fully-automated clinical chemistry/turbidimetry analyzers
	Electrolyte analyzers
	Hematology
	Laboratory water purifier

SEMI-AUTOMATED CLINICAL CHEMISTRY/TURBIDIMETRY ANALYZERS

1. Evolution 3000

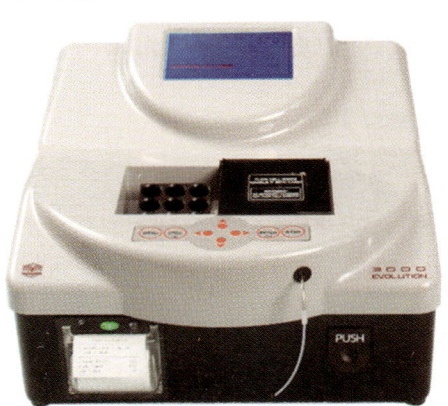

Unique Features

- Accurately executes chemistry and turbidimetry tests
- 120 programming locations
- Wide graphic display
- Filter wavelengths—340, 405, 492, 505, 546, 578, 630 nm; + 1 empty position
- 18 µL flow cell, low reagent consumption
- Online real time graphs for fixed time and kinetic tests
- Menu selection by keyboard arrow keys
- Display real time temperature
- Dual measuring mode-flow cell and cuvette
- Two level QC programmes can be programmed for each test

2. Gr8 Lab

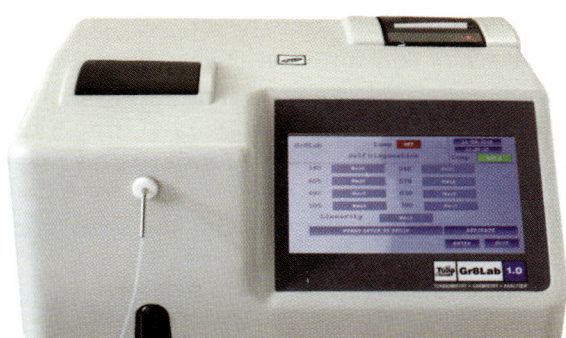

Unique Features

- Accurately executes chemistry and turbidimetry tests
- 200 programming locations
- 7 inches multicolour TFT display with touch screen
- 700 nm filter present
- Sample retrieval option available
- Online real time graphs for fixed time and kinetic tests
- Autodiagnostic features on start
- Dual measuring mode—flow cell and cuvette
- Two level QC programmes can be programmed for each test

FULLY-AUTOMATED CLINICAL CHEMISTRY/TURBIDIMETRY ANALYZERS

1. Coralyzer Mini 100

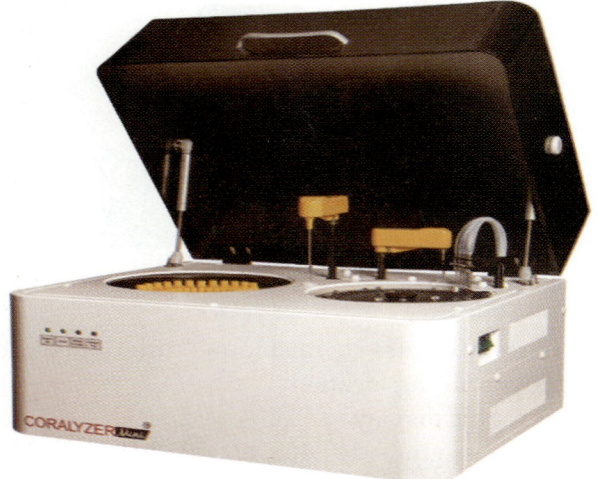

Unique Features

- Fully automatic, random access clinical chemistry analyzer with a throughput of 100 tests/hour
- Excellent on-board cooling for reagents
- Reusable cuvettes with efficient on board laundry
- Dedicated system pack reagents available
- Three level quality control program with L-J graph
- Independent washing station for each sample/reagent probe and mixer
- Automatic sample dilution/retest
- Efficient water consumption
- Accurately executes chemistry and turbidimetry tests running on end-point, kinetic, fixed time methods using 1–2 reagents in multi-standard and reagent/serum blank.
- Fifty sample positions, including standard, controls and samples.
- Sample tray can accommodate both serum cup as well as primary tubes

- STAT facility available on all sample locations, i.e 1–50.
- 36 reagent positions available
- The coralyzer mini is programmed to automatically dilute and retest samples beyond linearity/pathological range
- Results of the diluted sample displayed directly

2. Coralyzer Mini 200

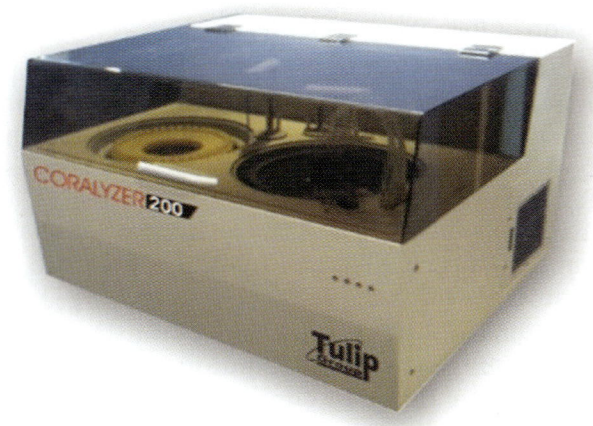

Unique Features

- Fully automatic, random access clinical chemistry analyzer with a throughput of 200 tests/hour
- Excellent on-board cooling for reagents
- Dedicated system pack reagents available
- Three to six level quality control program with L-J graph
- Continuous monitoring of blank Abs to increase accuracy
- Independent washing station for each sample/reagent probe and mixer
- Reagent/sample probe with liquid level sensor
- Automatic sample dilution/retest
- Efficient water consumption (maximum 10 litres for 200 tests)
- Barcode reader for sample and reagents (hand held)
- Accurately executes chemistry tests running on end-point, kinetic, fixed time, differential, sample blanking, mono and bichromatic measurement methods using 1–2 reagents
- 60 sample positions, including standard, controls and samples
- Sample tray can accommodate both serum cup as well as primary tubes
- STAT facility available on all sample locations, i.e 1–60
- 90 reaction cuvettes
- 40 reagent positions available

3. BT1500

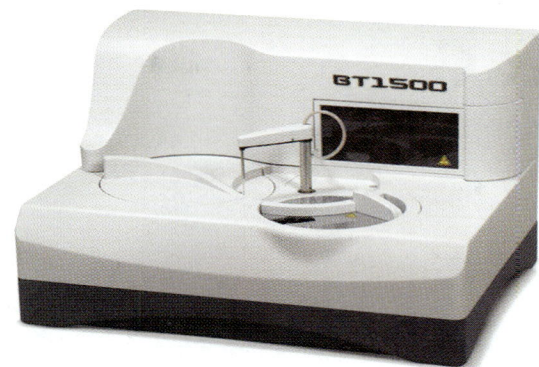

Unique Features

- The BT1500 is small in size and big in performance fully autochemistry and turbidimetry analyzer
- Throughput—up to 250 tests per hour
- Efficient on-board cooling and washing system
- Barcode identification for both reagents as well as samples
- Test mode—random access, batch and STAT
- Reagent tray—48 total; 24 using 50 mL vessels and 24 using 10 mL or 20 mL vessels
- Sample tray—78 total; 62 for samples, 16 standards and 16 controls
- Cuvettes: 32 optical glass cuvettes
- One sampling arm for both samples as well as reagents
- Cycle time of 14.5 seconds
- Reaction time/incubation time and read time to be programmed in seconds
- Addition of sample and reagents can be programmed at any cycle
- Use of three different solutions for daily and weekly maintenance of cuvettes

Appendix C

CORAL CLINICAL SYSTEMS

(A Division of Tulip Diagnostics (P) Ltd.)

Tulip Diagnostics (P) Ltd., is the leading Indian group of diagnostic companies, which is involved in the manufacture and marketing of *in-vitro* diagnostic reagents and kits both nationally and internationally. It believes in 'Better testing systems for better diagnostics and preventive health'. Most of the group's products are chartered engineer (CE) certified and are exported to over 87 countries worldwide.

Coral Clinical Systems, a division of Tulip Diagnostics (P) Ltd., offers the medical laboratory professionals a comprehensive range of clinical biochemistry products and instrumentation systems that are designed to perform as per internationally accepted standards.

A market leader within *in-vitro* diagnostics industry, Coral Clinical Systems develops innovative diagnostic solutions for hospital, clinical research and molecular labs thus offering customers improved efficiency, quality, cost effectiveness, and flexibility.

Product range	
Clinical chemistry range	Chemical kits
	Enzymatic kits
	Metals and ions
	Calkine kits
	Controls and calibrators
	System packs for coralyzer series of instruments
	System packs for BT1500
Immunoturbidimetry range	Quantia (multistandard)
	Turbilyte (single standard)
	Quantia system packs
Hematology reagents	
Laboratory reagents	
Instruments	Semi-automated clinical chemistry/Turbidimetry analyzers
	Fully-automated clinical chemistry/turbidimetry analyzers
	Electrolyte analyzers
	Hematology analyzers (3-part and 5 part)
	Laboratory water purifier

CHEMICAL KITS

Acid Phosphatase KIT

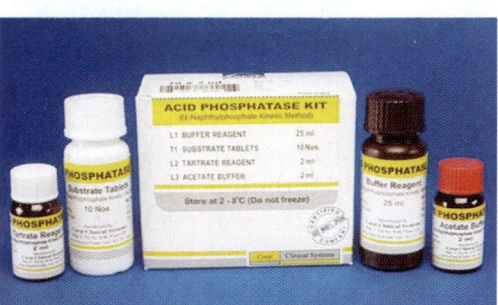

Application	For the determination of acid phosphatase in serum
Method	α-naphthyl phosphate (kinetic)
Principle	Acid phosphatase (ACP) at an acidic pH hydrolyses α-naphthylphosphate to form α-naphthol and inorganic phosphate. The α-naphthol formed is coupled with fast red TR salt to form a diazo dye complex. The rate of formation of this complex is measured as an increase in absorbance which is proportional to the ACP activity in the sample. Tartrate inhibits prostatic ACP and the testing in its presence is done to find the nonprostatic ACP. The difference between the activities of the total and non-prostatic ACP gives the activity of the prostatic ACP.
Benefits and features	• 5 minutes procedure only • Reconstitute ACP tablet with 2.2 mL buffer, useful for both total as well as prostaticfraction • Complete utilization of kit with no wastage of reagent • Provided with serum preservatives • Convenient packs 10 × 2 mL, 30 × 2 mL

ALBUMIN KIT

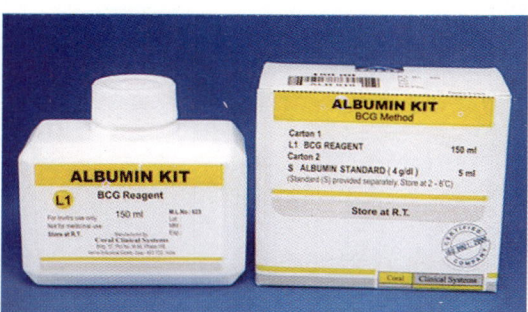

Application	For the determination of albumin in serum or plasma
Method	Bromocresol green (BCG) method
Principle	Albumin binds with the dye bromocresol green in a buffered medium to form a green colored complex. The intensity of the color formed is directly proportional to the amount of albumin present in the sample.
Benefits and features	• Simple procedure • Convenient small pack sizes • Economical and easily available

ALKALINE PHOSPHTASE KIT

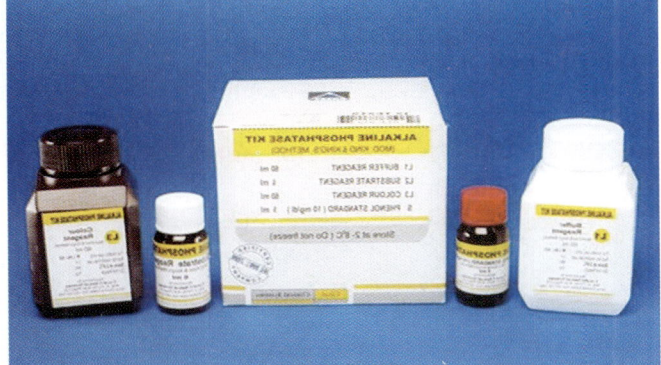

Application	For the determination of alkaline phosphatase (ALP) in serum
Method	Mod. kind and King's method
Principle	ALP at an alkaline pH hydrolyzes disodium phenylphosphate to form phenol. The phenol formed reacts with 4-aminoantipyrine in the presence of potassium ferricyanide, as an oxidizing agent, to form a red colored complex. The intensity of the color formed is directly proportional to the activity of ALP present in the sample.
Benefits and Features	• Simple procedure • Convenient small pack sizes • Economical and easily available

BILIRUBIN KIT

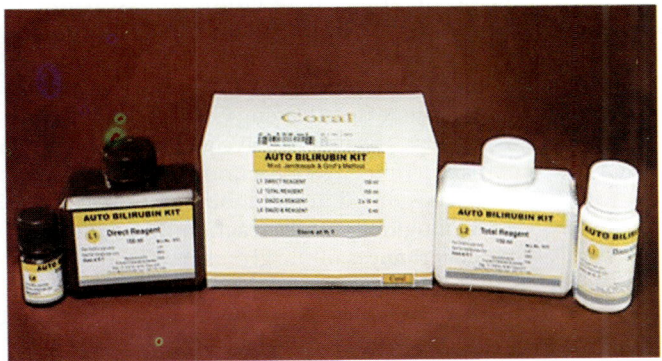

Application	For the determination of direct and total bilirubin in serum
Method	Mod. Jendrassik and Grof's method
Principle	Bilirubin reacts with diazotised sulphanilic acid to form a colored azobilirubin compound. The unconjugated bilirubin couples with the sulphanilic acid in the presence of a caffeinebenzoate accelerator. The intensity of the color formed is directly proportional to the amount of bilirubin present in the sample.
Benefits and Features	• Combi-pack for total and direct bilirubin • Proven caffeine benzoate activator—ensures complete value for total bilirubin • Factor base calculations for 546 filter • Enhanced, proven linearity

CALCIUM (OCPC) KIT

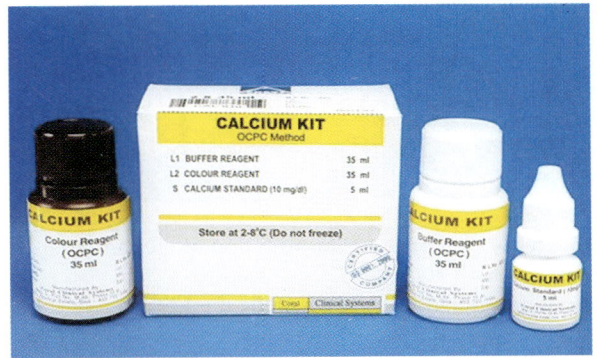

Application	For the determination of calcium in serum or plasma
Method	O-cresolphthalein complex one (OCPC) method
Principle	Calcium in an alkaline medium with OCPC to form a purple colored complex. Intensity of the color formed is directly proportional to the amount of calcium present in the sample.
Benefits and Features	• Very low blanks compared to competition • High linearity • Avoids use of plastic tubes

CREATININE KIT

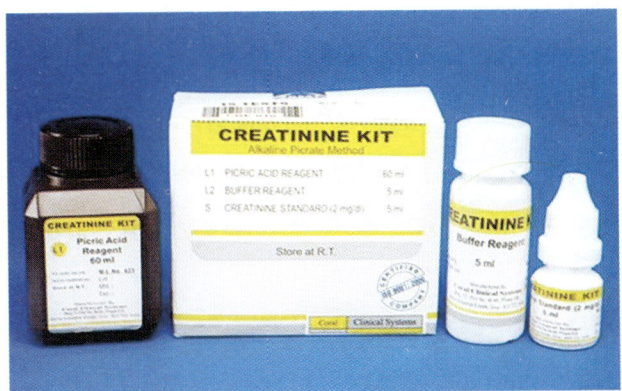

Application	For the determination of creatinine in serum and urine
Method	Alkaline picrate method
Principle	Picric acid in an alkaline medium reacts with creatinine to form an orange colored complex with the alkaline picrate. Intensity of the color formed is directly proportional to the amount of creatinine present in the sample.
Benefits and features	• Classical end-point procedure simplified for low serum samples • Urinary creatinine procedure provided • Convenient pack sizes 15 tests, 35 tests

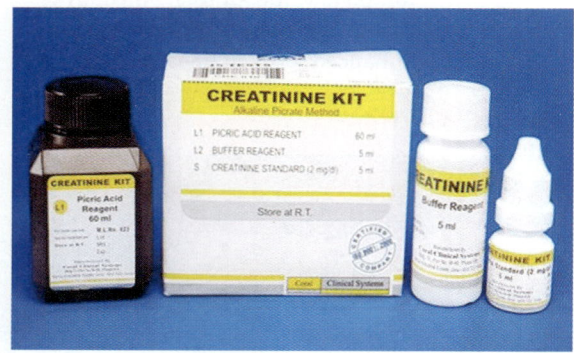

Application	For the determination of creatinine in serum and urine
Method	Mod. Jaffe's Kinetic method
Principle	Picric acid in an alkaline medium reacts with creatinine to form an orange colored complex with the alkaline picrate. Intensity of the color formed during the fixed time is directly proportional to the amount of creatinine present in the sample.
Benefits and Features	• Jaffe's kinetic method—long term used method employed in the kit • Two point fixed time reading • Modified procedure for analysers, 90 seconds only. • Urinary creatinine procedure provided • Convenient pack sizes 2 × 35 mL, 2 × 75 mL

MICROPROTEIN KIT

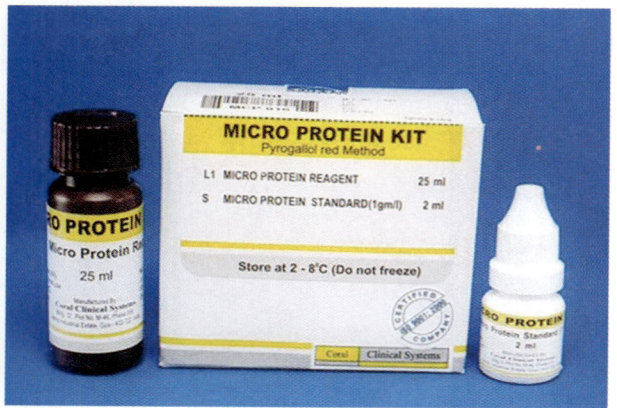

Application	For the determination of proteins in urine and CSF
Method	Pyrogallol red (colorimetric)
Principle	Proteins, in an acidic medium, combines with pyrogallol red and molybdate to form a blue purple colored complex. Intensity of the color formed is directly proportional to the amount of proteins present in the sample
Benefits and features	• Widely accepted pyrogallol red method • Simple one step procedure • Only 5 minutes' incubation at room temperature. • High sensitivity procedure ensures better accuracy over clinically significant range of values • High linearity procedure avoids repetition of test for high value samples • Convenient kit pack of 35 mL with standard

GLYCOSYLATED HEMOGLOBIN KIT (ION EXCHANGE RESIN METHOD)

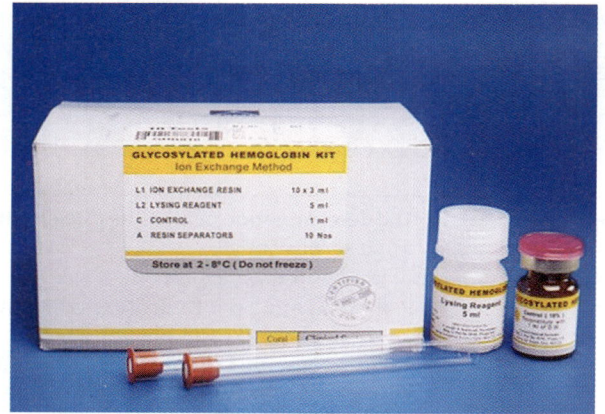

Application	Glycosylated hemoglobin (GHb) test is an important test for the diagnosis of diabetes mellitus and is a reliable indicator of efficacy of therapy.
Method	Ion exchange resin method
Principle	A hemolysed preparation of whole blood is mixed continuously for 5 minutes with a weakly binding cation-exchange resin. The labile fraction is eliminated during the Hemolysate preparation and during the binding. During the mixing, the nonglycosylated hemoglobin (HbAo) binds to the ion exchange resin leaving GHb free in the supernatant. The percent glycosylated hemoglobin is determined by measuring absorbances of the glycosylated hemoglobin fraction and total hemoglobin (THb) fraction. The ratio of the absorbances of the glycosylated hemoglobin and the total hemoglobin fraction of the control and the sample is used to calculate the percent glycosylated hemoglobin in the sample.

Benefits and Features	• Well characterized GHb calibrator included in the kit
	• Lot to lot consistency of results
	• Borate enhanced lysing reagent and resin
	• Two stage removal of schiffs base aldimine forms
	• Minimizes over-estimation errors
	• Predisposed resin tubes
	• Assurance of constant resin volume
	• Resin in zwitter ionic buffered medium
	• Relative temperature independence of assay
	• 4–20% of GHb
	• Consistent performance
	• Low intra and inter assay coefficients of variation (CVs)
	• Convenient reporting
	• Conversion charts provided for
	• converting GHb to HbA1C and mean blood glucose (MBG) values
	• Rapid-less than 10 minutes
	• Very convenient addition sequence
	• High linearity and reproducibility
	• Excellent linearity

CHLORIDE KIT/ ELYTE 2 KIT / ELYTE 3 KIT

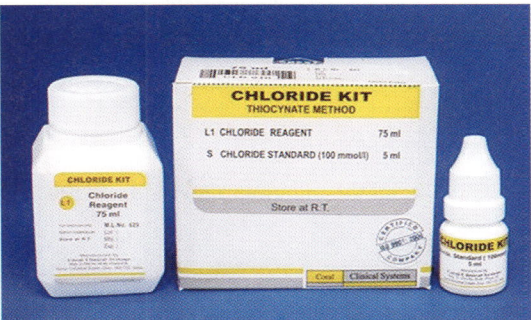

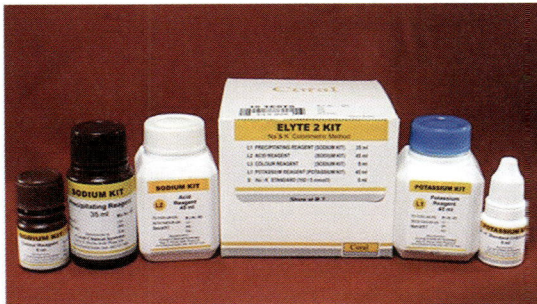

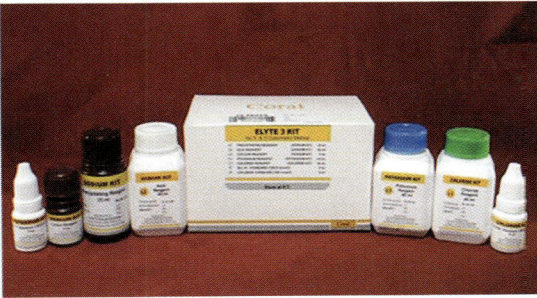

Application	Colorimetric method for the determination of sodium, potassium, and chloride in serum
Method Principle	Thiocyanate method/Na$^+$/K$^+$ colorimetric
	Chloride ions combine with free mercuric ions and release thiocyanate from mercuric thiocyanate. The thiocyanate released combines with the ferric ions to form a red brown ferric thiocyanate complex. Intensity of the color formed is directly proportional to the amount of chloride present in the sample.
	Sodium is precipitated as a triple salt with magnesium and uranyl acetate. The excess of uranyl ions reacts with ferrocyanide in an acidic medium to develop a brownish color. The intensity of the color produced is inversely proportional to the concentration of sodium in the sample.
	Potassium reacts with sodium tetraphenyl boron in a specifically prepared buffer to form a colloidal suspension. The amount of the turbidity produced is directly proportional to the concentration of potassium in the sample.

PHOSPHORUS KIT

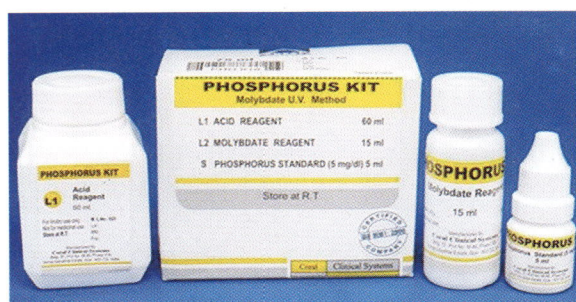

Application	For the determination of inorganic phosphorus in serum, plasma and urine
Method	Molybdate ultraviolet (UV) method
Principle	Phosphate ions in an acidic medium react with ammonium molybdate to form a phosphomolybdate complex. This complex has an absorbance in the ultraviolet range and is measured at 340 nm. Intensity of the complex formed is directly proportional to the amount of inorganic phosphorus present in the sample.
Benefits and features	• Choice of two methods
	• Rapid—less than 10 minutes
	• Convenient addition sequence
	• High linearity and reproducibility

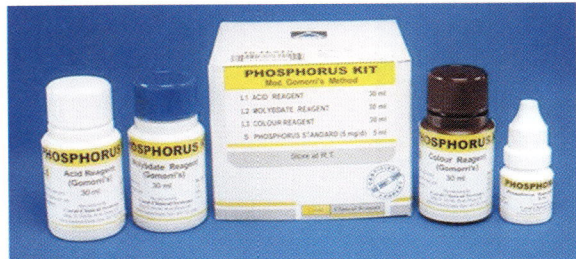

Application	For the determination of inorganic phosphorus in serum, plasma and urine
Method	Modified Gomori (colorimetric) method
Principle	Phosphate ions in an acidic medium react with ammonium molybdate to form a phosphomolybdate complex. This complex reacts with metal and is reduced to a molybdenum blue complex. Intensity of the molybdinum blue complex formed is directly proportional to the amount of inorganic phosphorus present in the sample.
Benefits and features	• Choice of two methods • Rapid—less than 10 minutes • Convenient addition sequence • High linearity and reproducibility

TOTAL PROTEIN KIT

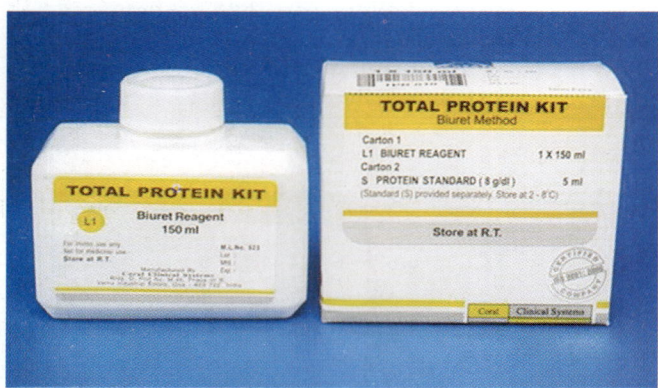

Application	For the determination of total proteins in serum and plasma
Method	Biuret method
Principle	Proteins, is an alkaline medium, bind with the cupric ions present in the biuret to form a blue-violet coloured complex. The intensity of the color formed is directly proportional to the amount of proteins present in the sample.
Benefits and features	• Single reagent—ready to use • Rapid procedure • Kit stored at room temperature

UREA KIT

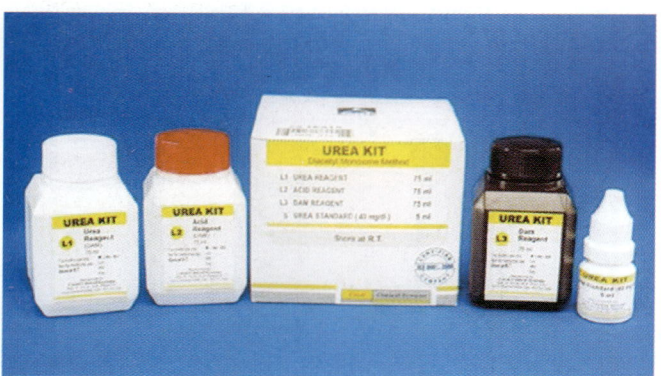

Application	For the determination of urea in serum, plasma.
Method	Diacetyl monoxime (DAM) method
Principle	Urea in an acidic medium condenses with diacetyl monoxime at 100°C to form a red colored complex. Intensity of the color formed is directly proportional to the amount of urea present in the sample.
Benefits and features	• Different methods available • Versatile • Convenient pack size

HEMOCOR-C AND HEMOCOR-D KIT

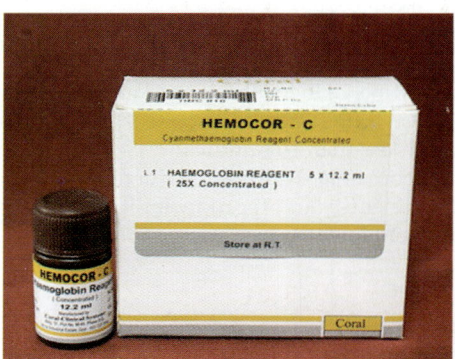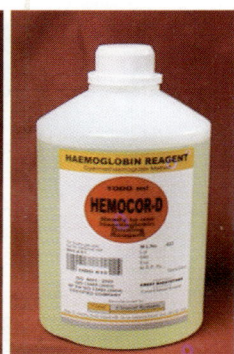

Application	Reagent for quantitative estimation of haemoglobin in blood
Method	Cyanmethaemoglobin method
Principle	Haemoglobin $\xrightarrow{K_3Fe(CN)_6}$ Methaemoglobin Methaemoglobin $\xrightarrow{KCN}$ Cyanmethaemoglobin
Benefits and features	• Both concentrated and dilute forms available • Easy to use

GLUCOSE 6 PHOSPHATE DEHYDROGENASE KIT

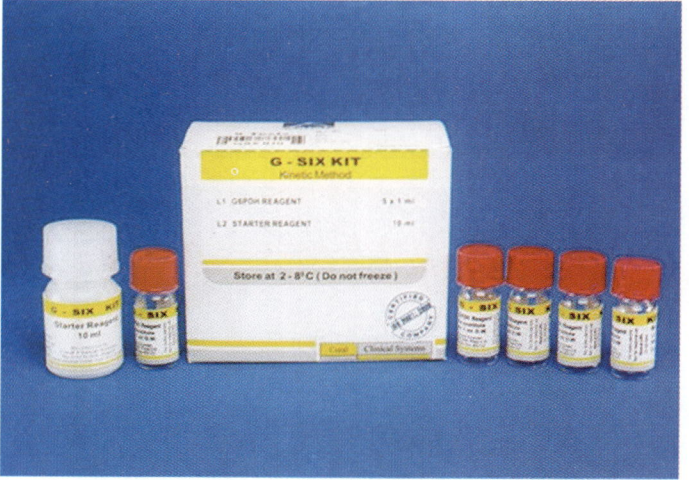

Application Method	For the determination of G6PDH activity in RBC's Cyanmethaemoglobin method
Principle	$G\text{-}6\text{-}P + NADH \xrightarrow{G\text{-}6\text{-}PDH} Gluconate\text{-}6\text{-}P + NADPH + H$
Benefits and features	• Whole blood sample (10 µL) • No loss of enzymes activity due to lysate preparation • Ensures accuracy of estimation • Ideal for neonates and pediatric cases • Two reagent system, simplicity of handling • Excellent reconstituted stability convenient packs • 15-minute assay, start to completion

ENZYMATIC KITS, ACID PHOSPHATASE KIT

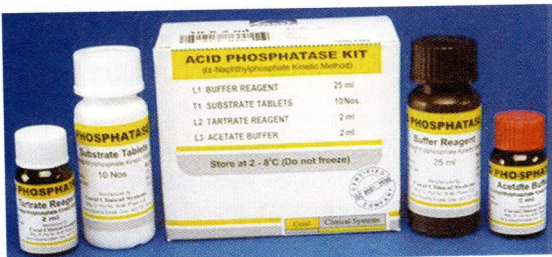

Application	For the determination of acid phosphatase in serum
Method	α-naphthyl phosphate (kinetic)
Principle	ACP at an acidic pH hydrolyses α-naphthyl-phosphate to form α-naphthol and inorganic phosphate. The α-naphthol formed is coupled with fast red TR salt to form a diazo dye complex. The rate of formation of this complex is measured as an increase in absorbance which is proportional to the ACP activity in the sample. Tartrate inhibits prostatic ACP and the testing in its presence is done to find the nonprostatic ACP. The difference between the activities of the total and non-prostatic ACP gives the activity of the prostatic ACP.
Benefits and features	• 5 minutes' procedure only • Reconstitute the tablet with 2.2 mL buffer, useful for both total as well as prostatic fraction • Complete utilization of kit with no wastage of reagent • Convenient packs 10 × 2 mL, 30 × 2 mL

ALKALINE PHOSPHATASE KIT

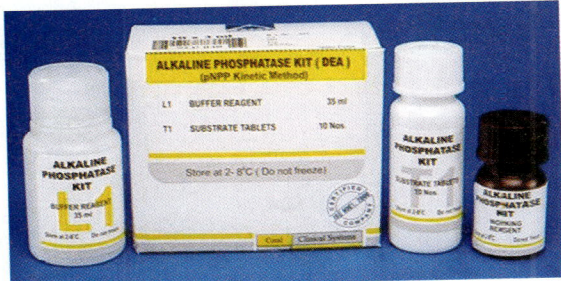

Application	For the determination of alkaline phosphatase in serum
Method	p-nitrophenylphosphate (pNPP) kinetic method
Principle	ALP at an acidic pH hydrolyses p-nitrophenyl-phosphate to form p-nitrophenol and phosphate. The rate of formation of p-nitrophenol as an increase in absorbance which is proportional to the ALP activity in the sample.
Benefits and features	• 3-minute procedure only • Reconstitute ALP tablet with 3.2 mL buffer • Complete utilization of kit with no wastage of reagent • Convenient packs 10 × 3 mL, 5 × 15 mL • Liquid stable (LS) reagent available

α- AMYLASE KIT

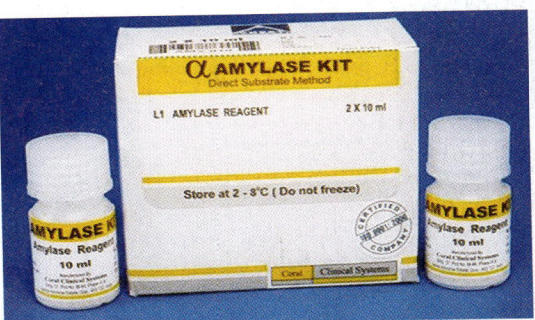

Application	For the determination of α-amylase activity in serum, plasma or urine
Method	Direct substrate
Principle	Amylase catalyze the hydrolysis of a 2-chloro-4 nitrophenol salt to chloronitrophenol (CNP). The rate of hydrolysis is measured as an increase in absorbance due to the formation of chloronitro-phenol which is proportional to the α-amylase activity in the sample. $CNP - Gal - G2 + H_2O \rightarrow CNP + Gal - G2$
Benefits and features	• Substrate is gal g2 CNP—sensitive to both salivary and pancreatic amylase thus avoiding underestimation of total amylase • Reagent contains optimum Ca^{++} ions—maintains functional integrity of amylase in sample • Reagent is buffered to an optimum pH—ensures controlled and consistent hydrolysis conditions • Unaffected by high triglycerides or bilirubin can be used even with lipemic and/or icteric samples

CALCIUM (A III) KIT

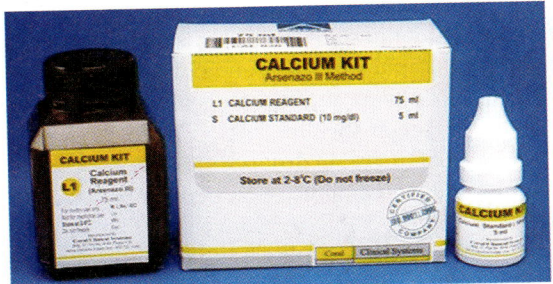

Application	For the determination of calcium in serum or plasma
Method	Arsenazo III method
Principle	Calcium combines specifically with Arsenazo III at a neutral pH to form a blue purple colored complex. Intensity of the color formed is directly proportional to the amount of calcium present in the sample.
Benefits and features	• Choice of two methods • Very low blanks compared to competition • High linearity • Avoids use of plastic tubes

CHOLESTEROL KIT

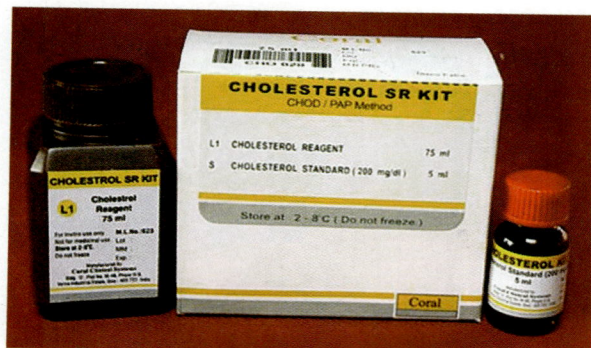

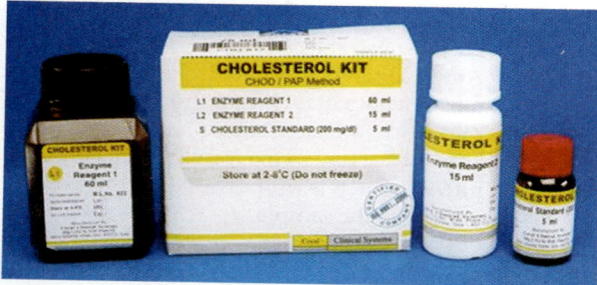

Application	For the determination of cholesterol in serum or plasma
Method	CHOD/PAP method
Principle	Cholesterol esterase hydrolyses esterified cholesterol. The free cholesterol is oxidized to form hydrogen peroxide which further reacts with phenol and 4-aminoantipyrine by the catalytic action to form a red coloured quinoneimine dye complex. Intensity of the color is directly proportional to the amount of cholesterol present in the sample.
Benefits and Features	• Liquid stable ready to use kit • Rapid and stable end points • Enzyme and chromogen provided separately • Larger shelf life • Standard in dropper vials • User flexibility—convenient pack sizes • More stable and convenient than powders • Available in single and double reagent form

CREATINE KINASE (NAC ACT.) KIT

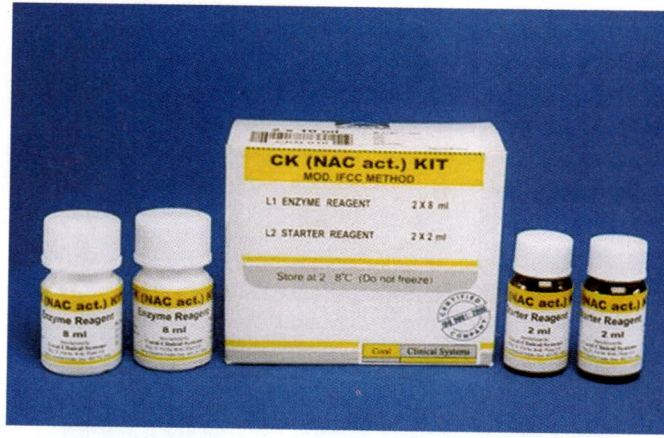

Application	For the determination of creatine kinase (CK) activity in serum
Method	Modified IFCC
Principle:	Creatine kinase catalyse the reaction between creatinine phosphate and adenosine diphosphate (ADP) to form creatine and ATP. The ATP formed along with glucose is catalyzed by hexokinase to form glucose 6 phosphate. The glucose 6 phosphate reduces nicotinamide adenine dinucleotide phosphate (NADP) to NADPH in the presence of glucose 6 phosphate dehydrogenase. The rate of reduction of NADP to NADPH is measured as an increase in absorbance which is proportional to the CK activity in the sample.
Benefits and features	• Thiol activator to reactivate CK in specimen (contains n-acetylcysteine for the maintenance and reactivation of CK activity in serum). • Optimized ethylenediaminetetraacetic acid (EDTA) (protects the thiol activator and prevents CK activity inhibition). • Optimized blend of adenylate kinase inhibitors [adenosine monophosphate (AMP) and DAPP] • Optically clean liquid reagent assay system

CREATINE KINASE (CK-MB) KIT

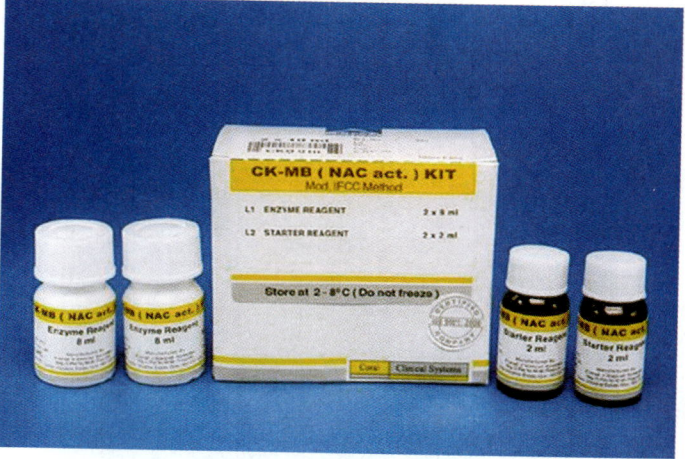

Application	For the determination of creatine kinase muscle-brain (CK-MB) activity in serum
Method	Immunoinhibition/Modified IFCC
Principle	Creatine kinase-muscle (CK-M) fractions of the CK-MM and the CK-MB in the sample are completely inhibited by an anti-CK-M antibody present in the reagent. Then the activity of the creatine kinase-brain (CK-B) fraction is measured by the CK (NAC act.) method. The creatinine (CK-MB) activity is obtained by multiplying the CK-B activity by two.
Benefits and features	• Thiol activator to reactivate CK in specimen (contains n- acetylcysteine for the maintenance and reactivation of CK activity in serum). • Optimized EDTA (protects the thiol activator and prevents CK activity inhibition). • Optimized blend of adenylate kinase inhibitors (AMP and DAPP) • Optically clean liquid reagent assay system do not cause interference from suspended micro-particles • Purified fab fragment-based anti CK-M antibody

CREATININE KIT

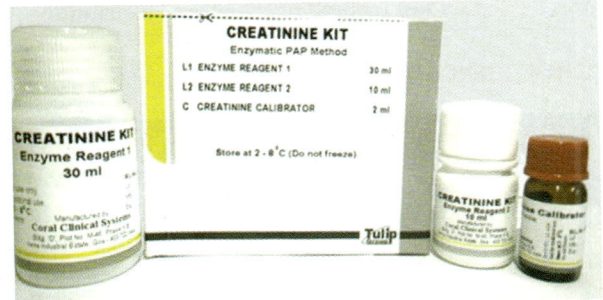

Application	For the determination of creatinine in serum and urine
Method	Enzymatic, fixed time kinetic
Principle	Creatine is converted to sarcosine by creatinase followed by oxidation of sarcosine by sarcosine oxidase (SOD) producing hydrogenperoxide. The hydrogen peroxide formed further reacts with a phenolic cromogen and a 4-aminoantipyrine by catalytic action of peroxidase to form a coloured quinoneimine dye complex. Intensity of colour formed is directly propotional to the amount of creatinine present in the sample. In the presence of peroxidase (POD) the hydrogen peroxide is quantified at 550 nm by the formation of a coloured dye. The endogenous creatine present in the sample is removed by the sarcosine oxidase during pre-incubation.
Benefits and features	• Liquid stable reagent • Ready to use • High linearity and high specificity • Rules out borderline cases • No interference from bilirubin and proteins • Better calibration stability

γ - GLUTAMYL TRANSFERASE KIT

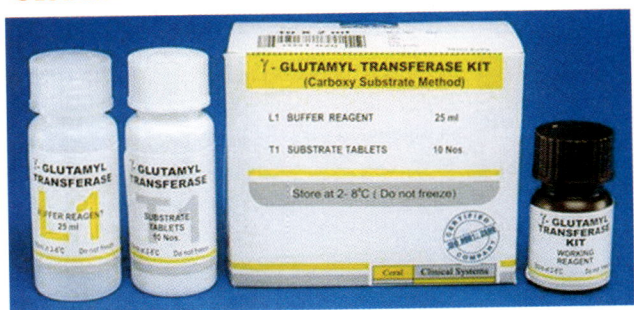

Application	For the determination of γ- glutamyl transferase in serum
Method	Carboxy substrate method
Principle	γ-glutamyl transpeptidase (GGT) catalyzes the transfer of amino group between L-γ-glutamyl-3-carboxy-4 nitroanilide and Glycylglycine to form L-α-glutamylglycylglycine and 5-amino-2-nitrobenzoate. The rate of formation of 5-amino-2-nitrobenzoate is measured as an increase in absorbance which is proportional to the GGT activity in the sample.
Benefits and features	• 3-minute procedure only • Reconstitute 1 tablet with 2.2 mL buffer • Complete utilization of kit with no wastage of reagent • Convenient packs 10 × 2 mL, 35 × 2 mL • Also available in liquid stable (LS) form

GLUCOSE KIT

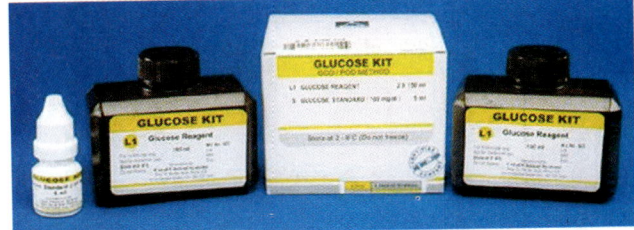

Application	For the determination of glucose in serum, plasma and CSF
Method	Glucose oxidase-peroxidase (GOD/POD) method
Principle	Glucose is oxidized to gluconic acid and hydrogen peroxide in the presence of glucose oxidase. Hydrogen peroxide further reacts with phenol and 4-aminoantipyrine by the catalytic action of peroxidase to form a red colored quinoneimine dye complex. Intensity of the color formed is directly proportional to the amount present in the sample.
Benefits and features	• Purity, grade, and quality of oxidases and peroxidases used ensure that the end • Point is reached fast (approx. 5 minutes) • End points are stable (more than 1 hour) • Liquid stable reagent enables aseptic filtration minimizing biodeterioration • Standard in dropper vials eliminates risk of contamination

SGOT (ASAT) KIT

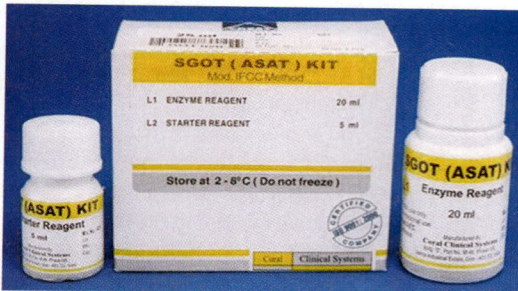

Application	For the determination of serum glutamic-oxalo-acetic transaminase (aspartate aminotransaminase) [SGOT (ASAT)] activity in serum
Method	Mod. IFCC method
Principle	SGOT (ASAT) catalyzes the transfer of amino group between L-aspartate and α-ketoglutarate to form oxaloacetate and glutamate. The oxaloacetate formed reacts with NADH in the presence of malate dehydrogenase to form NAD. The rate of oxidation of NADH to NAD is measured as a decrease in absorbance which is proportional to the SGOT (ASAT) activity in the sample.
Benefits and features	• Sturdy two reagent system. • Flexibility in number of tests • Linearity 500 u/l • Highest initial O.D giving you a large working range and longer shelf life.

SGPT (ASAT)KIT

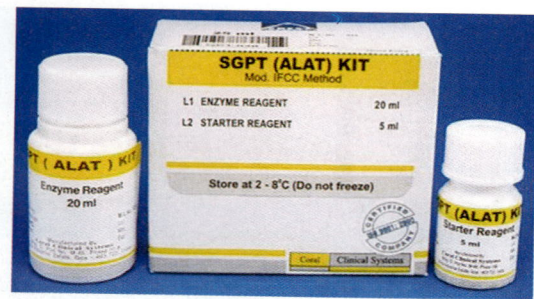

Application	For the determination of serum glutamic pyruvic transaminase (aspartate amino transaminase) SGPT (ALAT) activity in serum
Method	Mod. IFCC method
Principle	SGPT (ALAT) catalyzes the transfer of amino group between L-alanine and α- ketoglurate to form pyruvate and glutamate. The pyruvate formed reacts with NADH in the presence of lactate dehydrogenase to form NAD. The rate of oxidation of NADH to NAD is measured as a decrease in absorbance which is proportional to the SGPT (ALAT) activity in the sample.
Benefits and features	• Sturdy two reagent system • Flexibility in number of tests • Linearity 500 u/l • Highest initial O.D giving you a large working range and longer shelf life

HDL CHOLESTEROL (PPT) KIT

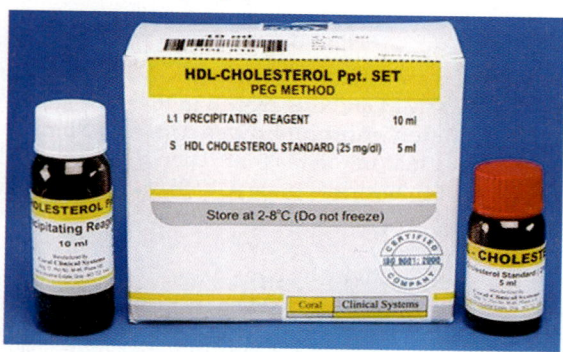

Application	For the determination of high-density lipoprotein (HDL) cholesterol in serum or plasma
Method	Polyethylene glycol (PEG) precipitation method
Principle	When the serum is reacted with the polyethylene glycol contained in the precipitating reagent, all the very-low-density lipoprotein (VLDL) and low-density lipoprotein (LDL) are precipitated. The HDL remains in the supernatant and is then assayed as a sample for cholesterol using the cholesterol (CHOD/PAP) reagent.
Benefits and features	• Easy to use • Oldest method of cholesterol estimation

HDL CHOLESTEROL KIT

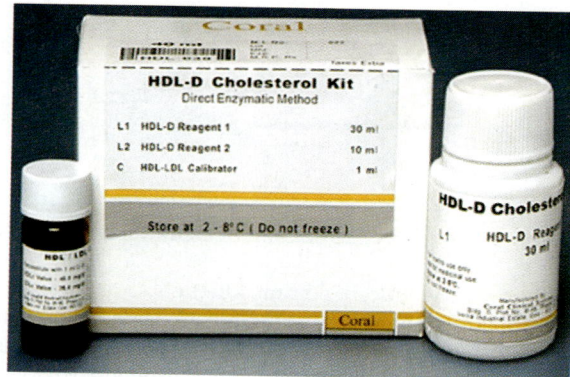

Application	For the determination of high-density lipo-proteins (HDL) cholesterol in serum
Method	Direct enzymatic colorimetric
Principle	Direct determination of serum high-density lipoprotein cholesterol (HDLc) levels without the need for any pretreatment or centrifugation of the sample. The method depends on the properties of a detergent which solubilizes only the HDL so that the HDLc is released to react with the cholesterol esterase, cholesterol oxidase and chromogens to give color. The non-HDL lipo-proteins LDL, VLDL and chylomicrons are inhibited from reacting with the enzymes due to absorption of the detergents on their surfaces. The intensity of the color formed is proportional to the HDLc concentration in the sample.

Benefits and features	• A new generation homogenous method based on an innovative detergent technology
	• Specificity clearance of non-HDL particles in the first reactionstep, offering high specificity for HDL particles
	• Reduced interference from triglycerides, cholesteroland bilirubin for an accurate measurement of HDL cholesterol
	• Fully automated applicable to clinical chemistry analyzers
	• Liquid stable reagents
	• Rapid procedure results obtained within 10 minutes
	• High linearity up to 150 mg/dL
	• Convenient packs economic and minimal wastage of reagents

LACTATE DEHYDROGENASE KIT

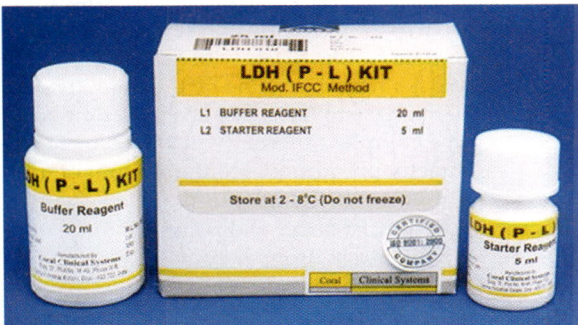

Application	For the determination of lactate dehydrogenase activity in serum
Method	Modified IFCC method
Principle	Lactate dehydrogenase catalyzes the reduction of pyruvate with NADH to form NAD. The rate of oxidation of NADH to NAD is measured as a decrease in absorbance which is proportional to the LDH activity in the sample.
Benefits and features	• Liquid stable reagent system
	• Flexibility in preparing working reagent
	• Complete utilization of kits
	• Easy and convenient procedures
	• Economical

LDL-D CHOLESTEROL KIT

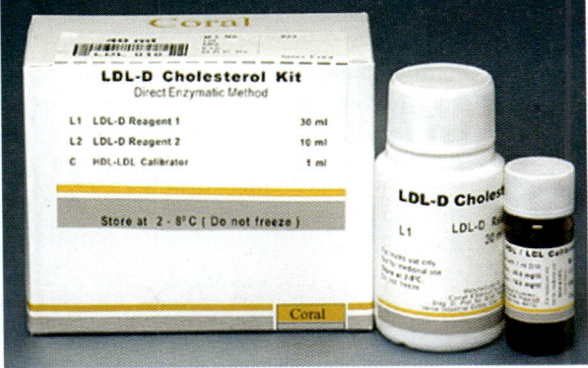

Application	For the determination of LDL cholesterol in serum
Method	Direct enzymatic method
Principle	Direct determination of serum LDLc (low density lipoprotein cholesterol) levels without the need for any pre-treatment or centrifugation steps. The assay takes place in two-steps—first by the elimination of lipoprotein non-LDL cholesterol and then the measurement of LDLc. The intensity of the color formed is proportional to the LDLc concentration in the sample.
Benefits and features	• A new generation method based on an innovative detergent technology
	• Specificity clearance of non-LDL particles in the first reaction step, offering exceptional specificity for LDL particles
	• Applicable to clinical chemistry analyzers
	• Liquid stable reagents
	• Rapid procedure results obtained within 10 minutes
	• No patient fasting required
	• High linearity up to 1000 mg/dL
	• Small and cost effective pack sizes

LIPASE KIT

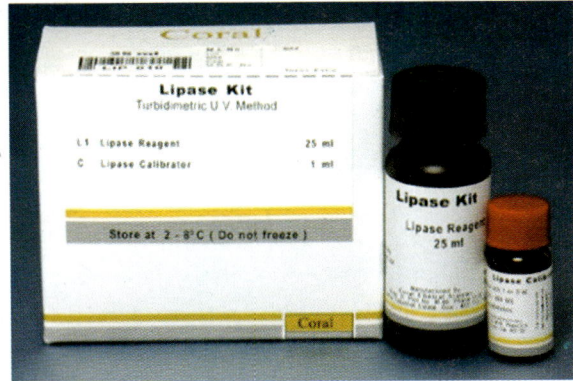

Application	For the determination of lipase activity in serum
Method	Turbidimetric UV method
Principle	Pancreatic lipase catalyzes the hydrolysis of triolein, in the presence of colipase to form mono-glycerides and fatty acids. The rate of decrease in turbidity measured at 340 nm, is proportional to the lipase activity. The activities of other lipases in the serum are inhibited by the cholic acid salts in the reagent.
	Triolein + 2HO → Monoglycerides + 2 Oleic acid
Benefits and features	• Parameter related specifically to the pancreas
	• Sample volume of 40 µL ensures accuracy of estimation
	• Reliable, time tested method—turbidimetric
	• Method measurement using more 'natural' substrate triolein
	• Rapid procedure 9 minutes assay
	• Linearity high linearity up to 700 u/l.
	• Single reagent system simplicity of handling
	• Convenient small packs of 25 mL and 75 mL ensure the economy of the tests

TRIGLYCERIDES KIT/TRIGLYCERIDES SR KIT

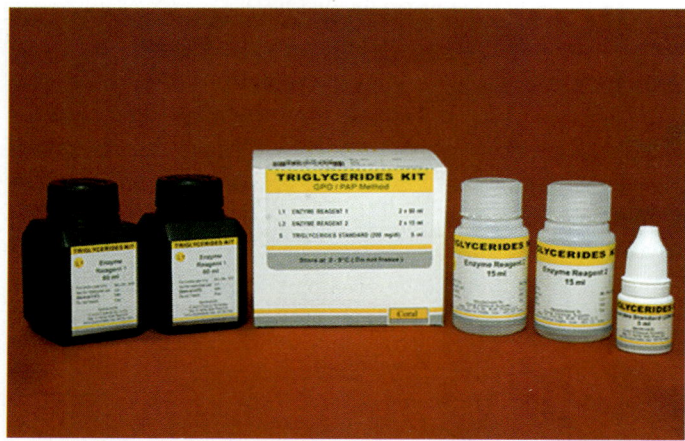

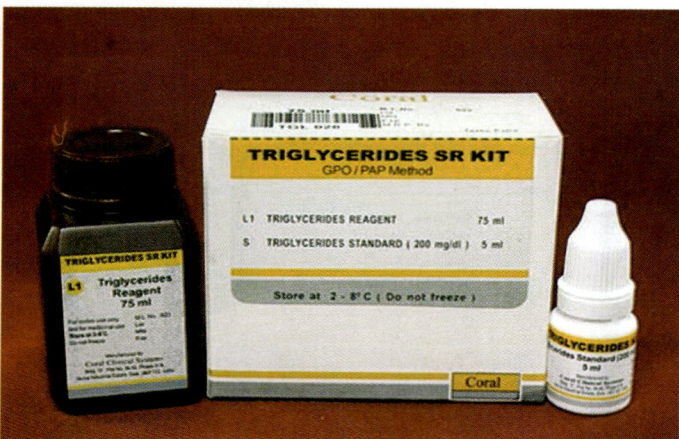

Application	For the determination of triglycerides in serum and plasma
Method	GPO/PAP method
Principle	Lipoproteins lipase hydrolyzes triglycerides to glycerol and free fatty acids. The glycerol formed with ATP in the presence of glycerol kinase forms glycerol 3 phosphate which is oxidized by the enzyme glycerol phosphate oxidase to form hydrogen peroxide. The hydrogen peroxide further reacts with phenolic compound and 4-aminoantipyrine by the catalytic action of peroxidase to form a red colored quinoneimine dye complex. Intensity of the color formed is directly proportional to the amount of triglycerides present in the sample.
Benefits and features	• Liquid stable ready to use kit • Rapid and stable end points; high linearity • Both double and single reagent kits available • Larger shelf life and lower blanks • User flexibility—convenient pack sizes • More convenient than powders

URIC ACID KIT

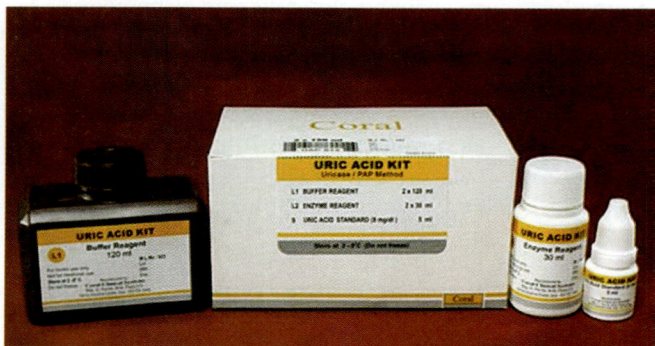

Application	For the determination of uric acid in serum or plasma
Method	Uricase/PAP method
Principle	Uricase converts uric acid to allantoin and hydrogen peroxide. The hydrogen peroxide formed further reacts with a phenolic compound and 4 aminoantipyrine by the catalytic action of peroxidase to form a red colored quinoneimine dye complex. Intensity of the color formed is directly proportional to the amount of uric acid present in the sample.
Benefits and features	• Rapid and stable end point • Standard in dropper bottles • High linearity • Liquid stable and ready to use

UREA KIT

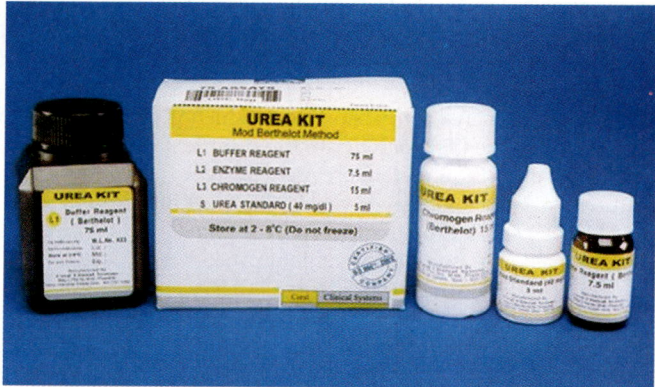

Application	For the determination of urea in serum, plasma.
Method	Modified berthelot method
Principle	Urea hydrolyzes urea to ammonia and CO_2. The ammonia formed further reacts with a phenolic chromogen and hypochlorite to form a green colored complex. Intensity of the color formed is directly proportional to the amount of urea present in the sample.
Benefits and features	• Different methods available • Versatile • Convenient pack size

UREA KIT

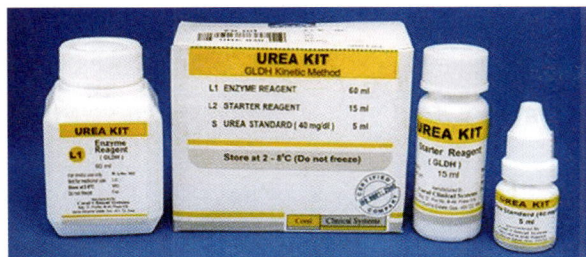

Application	For the determination of urea in serum plasma
Method	Glutamate dehydrogenase (GLDH) (UV kinetic) method
Principle	Urease hydrolyzes urea to ammonia and CO_2. The amount formed further combines with α-ketoglutarate and NADH to form glutamate and NAD. The rate of oxidation of NADH to NAD is measured as a decrease in absorbance in a fixed time which is proportional to the urea concentration in the sample.
	In the GLDH kinetic method, after production of ammonia it is reacted with 2-alphaketoglutarate in the presence of GLDH. The reaction utilizes NADH to produce NAD+ with a decrease in absorbance at 340 nm.
Benefits and features	• Different methods available • Versatile • Convenient pack size

METALS AND IONS, IRON AND TIBC KIT

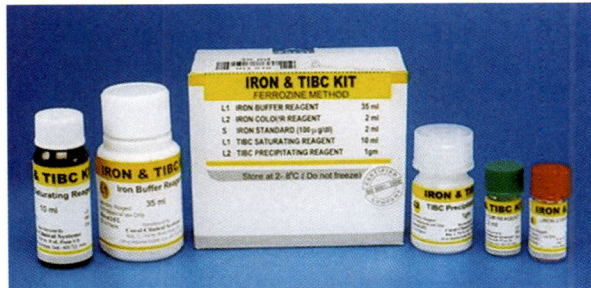

Application	For the determination of iron and total iron binding capacity (TIBC) in serum
Method	Ferrozine method
Principle	Iron, bound to transferrin, is released in an acidic medium and the ferric ions are reduced to ferrous ions. The Fe(II) ions react with ferrozine to form a violet colored complex. Intensity of the complex formed is directly proportional to the amount of iron present in the sample. For TIBC, the serum is treated with excess of Fe(II) to saturate the iron binding sites on transferrin. The excess Fe(II) is adsorbed and precipitated and the iron content in the supernatant is measured to give the TIBC.
Benefits and Features	• Iron assay by accepted ferrozine method • Facility to estimate iron as well as TIBC • Simple procedures

MAGNESIUM KIT

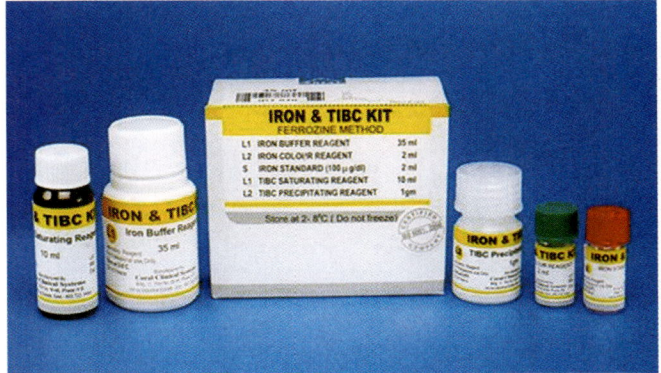

Application	For the determination of magnesium in serum, urine and CSF
Method	Calmagite Method
Principle	Magnesium combines with calmagite in an alkaline medium to form a red colored complex. Interference of calcium and proteins is eliminated by the addition of specific chelating agents and detergents. Intensity of the color formed is directly proportional to the amount of magnesium present in the sample.
Benefits and features	• First indigenous magnesium kit • Simple colorimetric procedures • Highest linearity—10 meq/L • Convenient small pack size

COPPER KIT

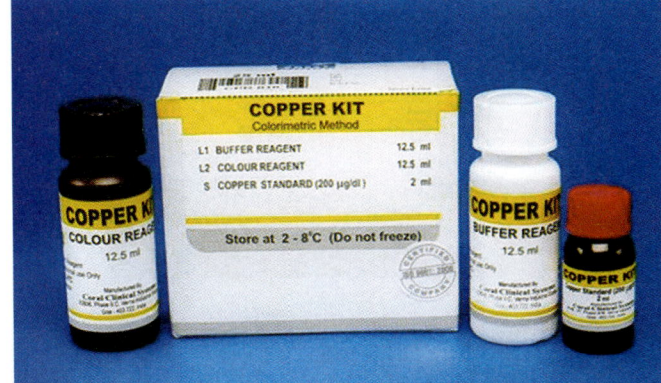

Application	For the determination of copper in serum
Method	Colorimetric method
Principle	Copper, released from cerulcplasmin, in an acidic medium reacts with Di-Br-PAESA to form a colored complex. Intensity of the complex formed is directly proportional to the amount of copper present in the sample.
Benefits and Features	• Convenient pack sizes • Simple colorimetric procedure • Economical and easily available

ZINC KIT

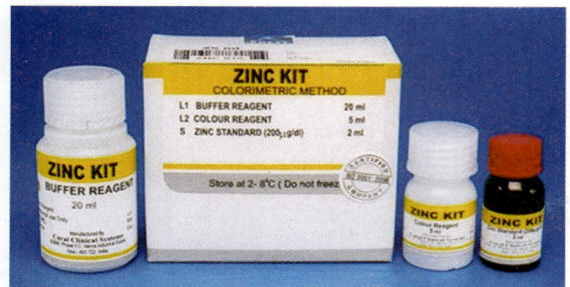

Application	For the determination of zinc in serum
Method	Colometric (nitro-PAPS)
Principle	Zinc in an alkaline medium reacts with nitro-APS to form a purple colored complex. Intensity of the complex formed is directly proportional to the amount of zinc present in the sample.
Benefits and features	• Simple colorimetric procedure • Useful for semen analysis • Convenient small pack sizes • Economical and easily available

SEMI-AUTOMATED CLINICAL CHEMISTRY/TURBIDIMETRY ANALYZERS

1. EVOLUTION 3000

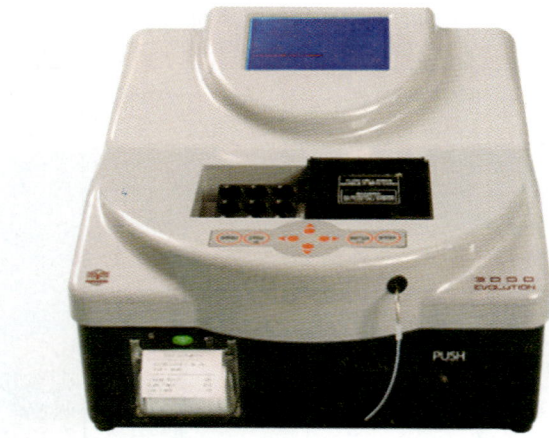

Unique Features

- Accurately executes chemistry and turbidimetry tests
- 120 programming locations
- Wide graphic display
- Filter wavelengths—340, 405, 492, 505, 546, 578, 630 nm; + 1 empty position
- 18 µL flow cell, low reagent consumption
- Online real time graphs for fixed time and kinetic tests
- Menu selection by keyboard arrow keys
- Display real time temperature
- Dual measuring mode—flow cell and cuvette
- Two level QC programmes can be programmed for each test

2. Gr8 Lab

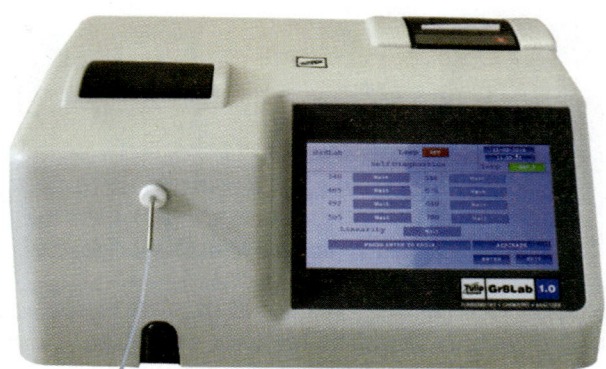

Unique Features

- Accurately executes chemistry and turbidimetry tests
- 200 programming locations
- 7 inches multicolour TFT display with touch screen
- 700 nm filter present
- Sample retrieval option available
- Online real time graphs for fixed time and kinetic tests
- Autodiagnostic features on start
- Dual measuring mode—flow cell and cuvette
- Two level QC programmes can be programmed for each test

FULLY-AUTOMATED CLINICAL CHEMISTRY/TURBIDIMETRY ANALYZERS

1. Coralyzer Mini

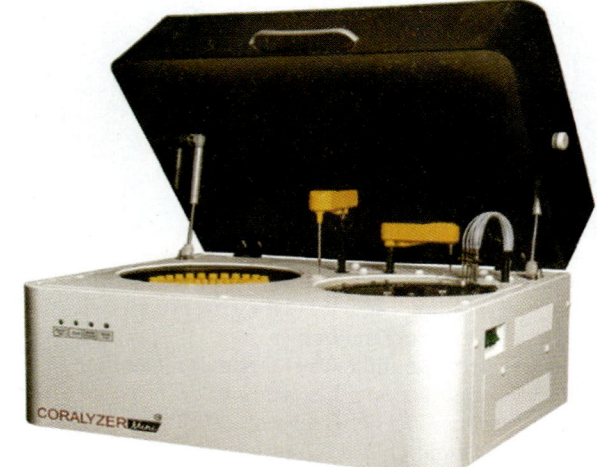

Unique Features

- Fully automatic, random access clinical chemistry analyzer with a throughput of 100 tests/hour
- Excellent on-board cooling for reagents
- Reusable cuvettes with efficient on-board laundry
- Dedicated system pack reagents available

- Three level quality control program with L-J graph
- Independent washing station for each sample/reagent probe and mixer
- Automatic sample dilution/retest
- Efficient water consumption
- Accurately executes chemistry and turbidimetry tests running on end-point, kinetic, fixed time methods using 1–2 reagents in multi-standard and reagent/serum blank.
- Fifty sample positions, including standard, controls and samples.
- Sample tray can accommodate both serum cup as well as primary tubes.
- STAT facility available on all sample locations, i.e 1–50.
- 36 reagent positions available
- The coralyzer mini is programmed to automatically dilute and retest samples beyond linearity/pathological range.
- Results of the diluted sample displayed directly.

2. Coralyzer Mini

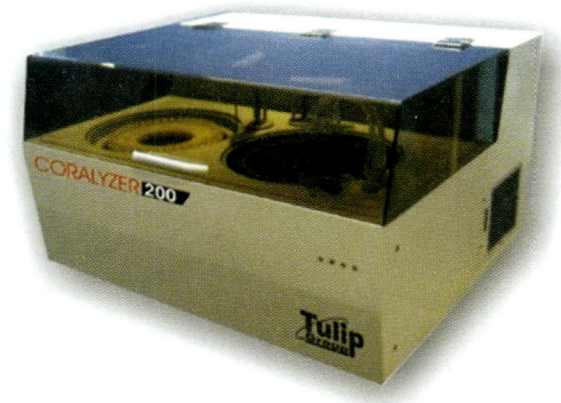

Unique Features

- Fully automatic, random access clinical chemistry analyzer with a throughput of 200 tests/hour.
- Excellent on-board cooling for reagents.
- Dedicated system pack reagents available.
- Three to six level quality control program with L-J graph.
- Continuous monitoring of blank Abs to increase accuracy.
- Independent washing station for each sample/reagent probe and mixer.
- Reagent/sample probe with liquid level sensor.
- Automatic sample dilution/retest.
- Efficient water consumption (maximum 10 litres for 200 tests).

- Barcode reader for sample and reagents (hand held).
- Accurately executes chemistry tests running on end-point, kinetic, fixed time, differential, sample blanking, mono and bichromatic measurement methods using 1–2 reagents.
- 60 sample positions, including standard, controls and samples.
- Sample tray can accommodate both serum cup as well as primary tubes.
- STAT facility available on all sample locations, i.e. 1–60.
- 90 reaction cuvettes.
- 40 reagent positions available.

3. BT1500

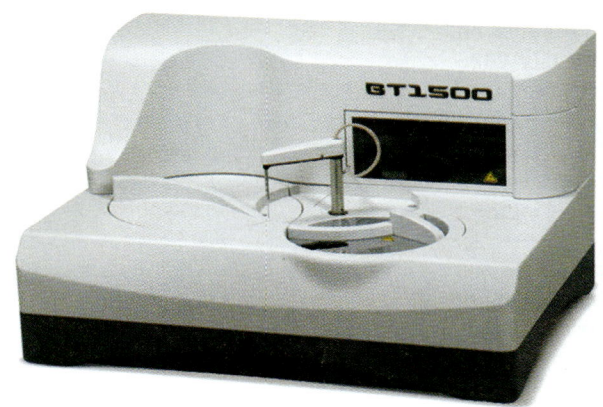

Unique Features

- The BT1500 is small in size and big in performance fully autochemistry and turbidimetry analyzer
- Throughput––up to 250 tests per hour.
- Efficient on-board cooling and washing system.
- Barcode identification for both reagents as well as samples.
- Test mode—random access, batch and STAT.
- Reagent tray—48 total; 24 using 50 mL vessels and 24 using 10 mL or 20 mL vessels.
- Sample tray—78 total; 62 for samples, 16 standards and 16 controls.
- Cuvettes—32 optical glass cuvettes.
- One sampling arm for both samples as well as reagents.
- Cycle time of 14.5 seconds.
- Reaction time/incubation time and read time to be programmed in seconds.
- Addition of sample and reagents can be programmed at any cycle.
- Use of three different solutions for daily and weekly maintenance of cuvette.

Index